Neo-Adjuvant Chemotherapy

Chimiothérapie Néo-Adjuvante

Neo-Adjuvant Chemotherapy

Chimiothérapie Néo-Adjuvante

Proceedings of the Second International Congress on Neo-Adjuvant Chemotherapy held in Paris (France), 19-21 February 1988

Sponsored by the Institut National de la Santé et de la Recherche Médicale (INSERM)

Edited by
Claude Jacquillat
Marise Weil
David Khayat

LES EDITIONS INSERM

John Libbey EUROTEXT LONDON · PARIS

British Library Cataloguing in Publication Data
Neo-adjuvant chemotherapy II.
1. Man. Cancer. Adjuvant therapy
I. Jacquillat, Claude, 1988 II. Series
616.99'4061

ISBN 0 86196 150 1
ISSN 0768-3154

First published in 1988 by

John Libbey & Company Ltd
80/84 Bondway, London SW8 1SF, England. (01) 582 5266
John Libbey Eurotext Ltd
6 rue Blanche, 92120 Montrouge, France. (1) 47 35 85 52
ISBN 0 86196 150 1

Institut National de la Santé et de la Recherche Médicale
101 rue de Tolbiac, 75654 Paris Cedex 13, France.
(1) 45 84 14 41
ISBN 2 85598 349 5

ISSN 0768-3154

Preface

This book presents the Proceedings of the **Second International Congress on Neo-adjuvant Chemotherapy** which took place on February 19th, 20th, 21st, 1988 in Paris under the chairmanship of Professor Claude Jacquillat.

This congress was placed under the patronage of the « Ministère de l'Éducation Nationale », the « Ministère de la Recherche et de l'Enseignement Supérieur », the « Ministère des Affaires Sociales et de l'Emploi », the « Ministère de l'Equipement, du Logement, de l'Aménagement du Territoire et des Transports » and under the scientific patronage of the « Institut National de la Santé et de la Recherche Médicale », of the International Union against Cancer, of the American Cancer Society.

Its aims were to show the present results of neo-adjuvant chemotherapy in cancers where its activity is already well known (breast cancers, head and neck cancers) to promote new indications (infiltrative bladder cancers, œsophageal cancer etc...) and to review the approaches that might improve its activity.

That more than 2 000 congressists did attend this meeting confirms that the scientific community recognizes the impact of this new strategy and indicates that such meetings meet a real need.

The organization of the Congress was made possible solely due to the generous financial support of many sponsors : organizations such as « la Ligue Française Contre le Cancer », « l'Association de Recherches sur le Cancer » (ARC), many pharmaceutical firms which participation was especially active and private funds. The welcome party, given by Monsieur Philippe Clément, Président de la Chambre de Commerce et de l'Industrie de Paris, was again for the participants the best illustration of the « prestige » and of the charm of Paris.

We would like to express our utmost gratitude to all the sponsors and to extend our deep thanks to all those who undertook the scientific and material organization of the Congress : the members of the Scientific Committee, the Administrative staff, particularly Amiral Louis Delorme and our secretaries.

Finally, the success of the Congress should be ascribed to its participants who came from all continents. This book reflects the high standard of their contributions.

Claude Jacquillat, Marise Weil, David Khayat,
Claude Soubrane, Gérard Auclerc

Préface

Ce livre rassemble la plupart des communications du **2e Congrès International sur la Chimiothérapie Néo-adjuvante** que nous avons organisé à Paris entre le 19 et le 21 février 1988, sous la Présidence de Claude Jacquillat.

Le Congrès placé sous le Haut Patronage des Ministères de l'Education Nationale, de la Recherche et de l'Enseignement Supérieur, des Affaires Sociales et de l'Emploi, de l'Equipement et du Logement et de l'Aménagement du Territoire et des Transports, et sous le Patronage Scientifique de l'INSERM, de l'Union Internationale contre le Cancer et de l'American Cancer Society, avait pour but d'actualiser les résultats de la chimiothérapie néo-adjuvante dans des indications déjà connues, de développer ses indications nouvelles, d'étudier enfin les méthodes propres à améliorer son efficacité.

La présence de près de 2 000 participants appartenant à près de 40 nationalités différentes témoigne de l'intérêt de la communauté cancérologique internationale pour cette stratégie d'actualité et confirme que de telles réunions désormais régulières répondent à une attente. A cette attente nous avons pu faire face une fois de plus grâce aux aides financières généreuses qui nous ont été accordées par des organisations comme la ligue Française contre le Cancer, l'Association de Recherche sur le Cancer, des entreprises privées et des particuliers, enfin, par l'industrie pharmaceutique qui a joué un rôle particulièrement important au cours de ce congrès en apportant son soutien actif à différentes sessions.

La réception officielle offerte une fois encore par Monsieur Philippe Clément, Président de la Chambre de Commerce et de l'Industrie de Paris, a été pour les congressistes une nouvelle illustration de l'élégance et du charme de Paris. L'édition de ce livre a été prise en charge par l'INSERM et les Editions John Libbey Eurotext.

Nous adressons des remerciements chaleureux à tous ceux qui ont assuré le succès scientifique et matériel du congrès, les membres du conseil scientifique, le responsable administratif du congrès, l'Amiral Louis Delorme, et à l'ensemble de notre secrétariat. Enfin et surtout, le succès de ce congrès est dû à tous ceux qui, de tous les continents, sont venus y participer. Ce livre reflète la qualité de leurs interventions.

Claude Jacquillat, Marise Weil, David Khayat,
Claude Soubrane, Gérard Auclerc

List and address of contributors

Liste et adresse des auteurs

Abbès M., Centre Antoine Lacassagne, Nice Cedex 06054, France.

Achterrath W., Clin. Research Anticancer, Bristol Myers, New York, États-Unis.

Allouche M., INSERM, U. 268, Hôpital Paul Brousse, BP 200, 94800 Villejuif, France.

Al-Sarraf M., Division of Hematology/Oncology School of Medicine, PO Box 02188, 48201 Detroit, Michigan, États-Unis.

Ambrosini G., Centro Oncologico, Ospedale S. Chiara, Largo Mesaglio d'Oro, 38100 Trento, Italie.

Amichetti M., Ospedale S. Chiara, 38100 Trento, Italie.

Amouroux J., Hôpital Avicenne, 125 rue de Stalingrad, Bobigny Cedex 93009, France.

Armand J.P., Institut Gustave Roussy, 94805 Villejuif Cedex, France.

Arriagada R., Institut Gustave Roussy, 94805 Villejuif Cedex, France.

Asselain B., Unité de Biostatistiques, Institut Curie, 26 rue d'Ulm, 75231 Paris Cedex 05, France.

Auclerc G., SOMPS, 47 boulevard de l'Hôpital, 75651 Paris Cedex 13, France

Azab M.B., Institut Gustave Roussy, 94805 Villejuif Cedex, France.

Baillet F., Radiothérapie, Hôpital Necker, 149 rue de Sèvres, 75730 Paris Cedex, France.

Baiocchi G., Dept of Gynecology and Obstetric, Catholic University, 8 Largo A. Gemelli, Rome 00168, Italie.

Baldeyrou P., Institut Gustave Roussy, 94805, Villejuif Cedex, France.

Banzet P., Service de Chirurgie Plastique, Hôpital Saint-Louis, 2 Place du Dr. A. Fournier, 75475 Paris Cedex 10, France.

Barrelet L., Ctre Pluridiscipl. d'Oncologie, Service de Radiothérapie, Service ORL, CHU Vaudois, Lausanne 1011, Suisse.

Bassot V., Service ORL, Hôpital Laennec, 49 rue de Sèvres, 75007 Paris, France.

Belli L., Institut Curie, 75231 Paris Cedex 05, France.

Benedetti-Panici P., Dept of Gynecology and Obstetric, Catholic University, 8 Largo A. Gemelli, Rome 00168, Italie.

Bernasconi S., Ctre Pluridiscipl. d'Oncologie, Service de Radiothérapie, Service ORL, CHU Vaudois, Lausanne 1011, Suisse.

Bertin F., Institut Gustave Roussy, 94805, Villejuif Cedex, France.

Bertino J. R., Section of Medical Oncology, Yale University, 333 Cedar Street, P.O. Box 3333, 06510-8032 New Haven, CO, États-Unis.

Bertrand-Desvages G., Hôpital Avicenne, 125, rue de Stalingrad, Bobigny Cedex 93009, France.

Biermann W.A., Dept of Medicine and Surgery, Jefferson Medical College, Philadelphia, Pennsylvania 19107, États-Unis.

Blum M., University Hospitals Munster, Hanover, RFA.

Boccon-Gibod L., Hôpital Cochin, 75014 Paris, France.

Bognel C., Institut Gustave Roussy, 94805 Villejuif Cedex, France.

Boissieu (de) F., Ecoute Cancer, Comité de Paris LNFCC, 13 avenue de la Grande Armée, 75017 Paris, France.

Bökkerink J.P.M., Sint Radboudziekenhuis, Universiteit Nijmegen, Pays-Bas.

Bollack C., Département d'Urologie, Hospices Civils de Strasbourg, Strasbourg, France.

Bolner A., Ospedale S. Chiara, 38100, Trento, Italie.

Bonadonna G., Istituto Nazionale per lo Studio e la Cura dei Tumori, Via Venezian, 1, 20133 Milan, Italie.

Boucheix C., INSERM U.268, 16 av. Paul-Vaillant-Couturier, 94800 Villejuif, France.

Bourdin S., Centre René Bauducheau, 44000 Nantes, France.

Brasnu D., Service du Pr. Laccourreyre, Hôpital Laennec, 49, rue de Sèvres, 75007 Paris, France.

Breau J.L., Service du Pr. L. Israël, Hôpital Avicenne, 125, route de Stalingrad, 93000 Bobigny, France.

Brechot J.M., Hôtel Dieu, Service de Pneumologie, 1 pl. du Parvis Notre Dame, 75181, Paris Cedex 04, France.

Brugières L., Institut Gustave Roussy, 94805, Villejuif Cedex, France.

Brunet M., Centre René Huguenin, 35 rue Dailly, 92211 Saint-Cloud, France.

Bünte H., University Hospitals Munster, Hanover, RFA.

Bussel J. B., Dept. of Pediatric Hemat/Onc., Cornell Medical Center, 525 East 58th Street, 10021 New York, N.Y. États-Unis.

Caillaud J.M., Institut Gustave Roussy, 94805 Villejuif Cedex, France.

Calaminus G., Department of Pediatr/Oncol., University of Dusseldorf, Uniklinik, Moorenstr., 5, 04000 Dusseldorf, RFA.

Caldarelli D.D., 1725 West Harrison Street, 60612 Chicago, IL, États-Unis.

Canal M., Laboratoires Delagrange, 1 av. Pierre Brossolette, 91380 Chilly-Mazarin Cedex, France.

Canal P., Centre Claudius Regaud, 20-24 rue du Pont St-Pierre, 31052 Toulouse Cedex, France.

Cantor R.I., Dept of surgery and medicine, Jefferson Medical College, Philadelphia, Pennsylvania 19107, États-Unis.

Capasso P., Ctre Pluridiscipl. d'Oncologie, Service de radiothérapie, Service ORL, CHU Vaudois, Lausanne 1011, Suisse.

Cappelaere P., Centre Oscar Lambret, 1, rue Frederic Combemale, BP 307, 59020 Lille Cedex, France.

Caubel M., Service d'immunochimiothérapie, Centre Val d'Aurelle, rue de la Croix Verte, 34094 Montpellier Cedex, France.

Cerrina M.L., Hôpital Antoine Béclère, 92140 Clamart, France.

Chauveau P., Service d'Urologie, CHU, 1, Avenue de l'Hôtel Dieu, 49033, Angers Cedex, France.

Chauvergne J., Service de Médecine, Fondation Bergonie, 180 rue St-Genès, 33076 Bordeaux Cedex, France.

Chazard M., Bristol Myers, Paris, France.

Chevallier B., Service de Cancérologie, Centre Henri Becquerel, rue d'Amiens, 76038 Rouen Cedex, France.

Choksi A.J., 1515 Holcombe Boulevard, Box 80, Houston, Texas, États-Unis.

Clavier J., Service de Pneumologie, CHU de Brest, 5 avenue Foch, 29279 Brest Cedex, France.

Coldman A.J., Biometry Section CCA, BC 600 West 10th Avenue, V5Z 2E6, Vancouver, B.C., Canada.

Collet J.F., Ctre Cytopathologie Clinique, 49 rue du Ranelagh, 75016, Paris, France.

Conte P.F., Istituto Nazionale per la Ricerca sul Cancro e Clinica Urologica dell'Universita, Viale Benedetto XV, 10, Genova, 16132 Italie.

Contesso G., Service d'Histopathologie C, Institut Gustave Roussy, 94805 Villejuif Cedex, France.

Court B.H. Institut Gustave Roussy, 94805 Villejuif Cedex, France.

Cremoux (de) H., Centre Hospitalier Intercommunal, 94000 Créteil, France.

Cupissol D., Service d'Immunochimiothérapie, Centre Val d'Aureille, rue de la Croix Verte, 34094, Montpellier, France.

Curotto A., Istituto Nazionale per la Ricerca sul Cancro e Clinica Urologica dell'Universita, Viale Benedetto XV, 10 Genova 16132, Italie.

Dalton W.S., Arizona Cancer Center, University of Arizona, Tucson, Arizona 85724, Etats-Unis.

Dautzenberg B., Clinique de Physio-Pathologie Respiratoire, Hôpital de la Salpétrière, Paris, France.

Davi-Armengol E., Hospital Clinic c/o, Casanova, 143, 08036 Barcelone, Espagne.

Debruyne F.M.J., Department of Urology, University Hospital Nijmegen, Pays-Bas.

Delattre C., Lab. de Biochimie et Toxicologie, Hôtel Dieu, 1 place du Parvis Notre Dame, 75181, Paris Cedex 04, France.

Delepine G., Hôpital Paul Brousse, 12-14 av. Paul-Vaillant-Couturier, 94800, Villejuif, France.

Delepine N., Unité d'Oncologie Pédiatrique, Hôpital Hérold-Robert Debré, 7 place Rhin et Danube, 75019 Paris, France.

Delfour C., Lab. de Biochimie et Toxicologie, Hôtel Dieu, 1, place du Parvis Notre Dame, 75181, Paris Cedex 04, France.

Demard F., Directeur Centre Antoine Lacassagne, 36 Voie Romaine, 06054 Nice Cedex, France.

Denck H., I. Surgical Dept. Hosp. Lainz L. Boltzmann, Inst. for clinical Oncology, Vienna A1130, Autriche.

Deneufbourg J.M., Service de Radiothérapie, 66 Boulevard de la Constitution, Bâtiment J 2, 04020 Liège, Belgique.

Desai P.B., Tata Memorial Hospital, Dr. Ernest Borges Marg., Parel, 4000 12 Bombay, Inde.

Desanti C., Laboratoires Delagrange, 1, av. Pierre Brossolette, 91380, Chilly-Mazarin Cedex, France.

Desbois J.C., Service d'Oncologie Pédiatrique, Hôpital Hérold-Robert Debré, 7 place Rhin et Danube, 75019 Paris, France.

Diéras V., Institut Curie, 75231 Paris Cedex 05, France.

Dimery I.W., Dept. Head and Neck Med. Oncology MD, Anderson Hospital, 6723 Bertner Dr., Box No. 8, 77030 Houston, TX, États-Unis.

Dorval T., Service d'Oncologie, Institut Curie, 26, rue d'Ulm, 75005 Paris, France.

Douillard J.Y., Centre René Gauducheau, 44 000 Nantes, France.

Droz J.P., Institut Gustave Roussy, 94805, Villejuif Cedex, France.

Dubousset J., Institut Gustave Roussy, 94805, Villejuif Cedex, France.

Duchatelle V., Hôpital Avicenne, 125 rue de Stalingrad, 93009, Bobigny Cedex, France.

Dufour A., Laboratoires Delagrange, 1 av. Pierre Brossolette, 91380, Chilly-Mazarin Cedex, France.

Dufour B., Service d'Urologie B, Hôpital Necker, 149, rue de Sèvres, 75743 Paris Cedex 15, France.

Dupeyron J.P., Lab. de Biochimie et Toxicologie, Hôtel Dieu, 1 pl. du Parvis Notre Dame, 75181, Paris, Cedex 04, France.

Durand J.-C., Service de Chirurgie Générale, Institut Curie, 26 rue d'Ulm, 75231 Paris Cedex 05, France.

Ehninger G., Medizinische Klinik, University of Tübingen, RFA.

Engert J., Kinderchirurgische Klinik Der Universitat, Bochum, RFA.

Ensley J., Detroit, Michigan 48201, États-Unis.

Eschwege F., Institut Gustave Roussy, 94805, Villejuif Cedex, France.

Extra J.M., Dépt. d'Oncologie Médicale, Hôpital Saint-Louis, 75010 Paris, France.

Fellin G., Ospedale S. Chiara, 38100 Trento, Italie.

Fiorentini G., Department of Oncologia Medica, Ospedale Civile Ravenna, 48100 Ravenna, Italie.

Fisher B., Department of Surgery, University of Pittsburg, 3550 Terrase Street, Room 914, 15216 Pittsburg, PA, États-Unis.

Francini M., Div. Urology, Aviano, Trieste, Italie.

Frei III E., Harvard Medical School, Dana Farber Cancer Institute, 44, Bidney Street, 02115 Boston, MA, États-Unis.

Freireich E. J., Department of Hematology, MD Anderson and Tumor Institute, 1515 Holcome Blvd., Box 5 77030, Houston, Texas, États-Unis.

Frenay M., Centre Antoine Lacassagne, 06054 Nice Cedex, France.

Fumoleau P., Centre René Gauducheau, 44035 Nantes, France.

Gadner H., St Anna Kinderspital, Vienne, Autriche.

Gallo A., Dept. of Gynecology and Obstetric, Catholic University, 8 Largo A. Gemelli, Rome 00168, Italie.

Gehan E. A., Department of Biometrics, MD. Anderson and Tumor Institute, 6723 Bertner Avenue, 77030 Houston, Texas, Etats-Unis.

Gehanno P., Groupe Hospitalier Bichat/Claude Bernard, Service ORL, 46 Rue H. Huchard, 75018 Paris, France.

Génin J., Institut Gustave Roussy, 94805, Villejuif Cedex, France.

George M., Service de Gynécologie, Institut Gustave Roussy, 94805 Villejuif Cedex, France.

Georgoulias V., INSERM U. 268, Hôpital Paul Brousse, BP 200, 94804 Villejuif, France.

Gherlinzoni F., Bone Tumor Center, Istituto Ortopedico Rizzoli, Via Pupilli, 1, 40136 Bologna, Italie.

Ghosn M., Institut Gustave Roussy, 94805, Villejuif Cedex, France.

Giraud C., Laboratoire Cerba, BP 451, 95005 Cergy Pontoise Cedex, France.

Gisselbrecht C., Dept. Hémato-Oncologie, Hôpital Saint-Louis, Place du Dr Fournier, 75010 Paris, France.

Giuliani L., Istituto Nazionale per la Ricerca sul Cancro e Clinica Urologica dell'Universita, Viale Benedetto XV, 10 Genova 16132, Italie.

Göbel U., Abt. Padiatrische Hamatologie und Onkologie der Universitat, Dusseldorf, RFA.

Goldie J.H., Biometry Section, CCA, BC 600 West 10th Avenue V5Z 2E6, Vancouver, BC, Canada.

Gouva S., CHU, 29285 Brest, France.

Graham-Pole J., Dept. Pediatrics and Orthopedics University of Florida, Box J.296, 32610 Gainesville, FL, États-Unis.

Gralla R.J., Memorial Sloan Ketterin, Cancer Center, New York, Etats-Unis.

Gramont (de) A., Service du Professeur Debray, Hôpital Saint-Antoine, 184 rue du Fg St-Antoine, 75571 Paris Cedex 12, France.

Greggi S., Dept of Gynecology and Obstetric, Catholic University, 8 Largo A. Gemelli, Rome 00168, Italie.

Grogan T., Arizona Cancer Center. University of Arizona, Tucson, Arizona 85724, Etats-Unis.

Guillevin L., Hôpital Avicenne, 125 rue de Stalingrad, 93009 Bobigny Cedex, France.

Guittard T., Hôpital Avicenne, 125 rue de Stalingrad, 93009 Bobigny Cedex, France.

Guyon F., Lab. de Biochimie et Toxicologie, Hôtel Dieu, 1 place du Parvis Notre Dame, 75181, Paris Cedex 04, France.

Haas R.J., Abt Padiatrische Hamatologie, und Onkologie der Universitat, München, RFA.

Harms D., Institute fur Paidopathologie der Universitat, Kiel, RFA.

Héry M., Centre Antoine Lacassagne, 06054 Nice Cedex, France.

Hill B. T., Laboratory of Cellular Chemoth. Lincoln's Inn fields, PO. Box 123, WC2A3PX London, Royaume-Uni.

Hiller E., Medizinische Klinik III, University of Munich, Munich, RFA.

Holland J. F., Dep. of Neoplastic Disease Mount Sinai School of Medicine, 100th Street 5th Avenue, 10029 New-York, NY, États-Unis.

Hollinger P.C., 1725 West Harrison Street, 60612 Chicago, IL, États-Unis.

Honegger H. P., Department of Oncology, Triemli Hospital, Birmensdrofers-trasse, 497, 08063 Zurich, Suisse.

Hong W. K., Head and Neck and Thoracic Oncol., MD. Anderson and Tumor Institute, 6723 Bertner Avenue, 77030 Houston, Texas, États-Unis.

Hopkins H.A., Div. of Radiology and Biophysics, Charlottesville, Virginia, États-Unis.

Hortobagyi G. N., Division of Medicine, MD. Anderson and Tumor Institute, 6723 Bertner Avenue, 77030 Houston, Texas, États-Unis.

Housset M., Ctre de Traitement des Tumeurs, Hôpital Necker, 149 rue de Sèvres, 75730 Paris Cedex 15, France.

Hutchingson J.C., 1725 West Harrison Street, 60612 Chicago, IL, États-Unis.

Iglesias J., Dept. of Gynaecology, University of Barcelona, Barcelona, Espagne.

Ihde D. C., Head, Clinical Investigations, SNCI Navy Medical Oncology Branc Naval Hospital, 20814 Bethesda, Maryland, États-Unis.

Israël L., Clinique de Cancérologie, Hôpital Avicenne, 125 route de Stalingrad, 93000 Bobigny, France.

Izar F., Service de Radiothérapie, Centre Claudius Regaud, 20-24 rue du Pont St. Pierre, 31052 Toulouse Cedex, France.

Jacquillat Cl., SOMPS, 47 Boulevard de l'hôpital, 75651 Paris Cedex 13, France.

Jasmin C., Service d'Hématologie, Hôpital Paul Brousse, 14 av. Paul-Vaillant-Couturier, 94804 Villejuif Cedex, France.

Jürgens H., Abt. Padiatrische Hamatologie und Onkologie der Universitat, Düsseldorf, RFA.

Kac J., Institut Gustave Roussy, 94805 Villejuif Cedex, France.

Kalifa C., Institut Gustave Roussy, 94805 Villejuif Cedex, France.

Karrer K., Inst. for Epidemiology of Neoplasms of the University, Vienna A 1090, Autriche.

Kemeny J.L., Hôpital Avicenne 125 rue de Stalingrad, 93009 Bobigny Cedex, France

Khayat D., SOMPS, 47 Boulevard de l'hôpital, 75651 Paris Cedex 13, France.

Kies M., 1725 West Harrison Street, 60612 Chicago, IL, États-Unis.

Kish J., Detroit, Michigan 48201, États-Unis.

Laccourreye H., Service d'ORL, Hôpital Laennec, 42 rue de Sèvres, 75007 Paris, France.

Lailla J.M., Department of Gynecology, Hospital Clinico University, Villarroel n° 170, 08036 Barcelona, Espagne.

Lampidis Th.J., Hôpital Paul Brousse, 94805 Villejuif Cedex, France.

Lasser Ph., Institut Gustave Roussy, 94805 Villejuif Cedex, France.

Lattuneddu A., Ospedale Morgani, Forli I 47100, Italie.

Lavelle F., Dept. de Cancérologie, Centre de Recherches de Vitry, Rhône Poulenc Santé, BP 14, 94403 Vitry sur Seine Cedex, France.

Léandri P., Dept. d'Urologie, Clinique Saint-Jean-Languedoc, 31077 Toulouse Cedex, France.

Lebeau B., Hôtel Dieu, Service de Pneumologie, 1 place du Parvis Notre Dame, 75181 Paris Cedex 04, France.

Leborgne J., Centre René Gauducheau, 44000 Nantes, France.

Le Chevalier Th., Service de Médecine B, Institut Gustave Roussy, 94805 Villejuif Cedex, France.

Lemerle J., Service de Pédiatrie, Institut Gustave Roussy, 94805 Villejuif Cedex, France.

Lenaz L., Clin. Research Anticancer Bristol Myers, New York, États-Unis.

Lepinard V., Service d'Urologie, CHU, 1 Avenue de l'Hôtel Dieu, 49033 Angers Cedex France.

Lesnick G., Cancer and leukemia Group B, Bookline, MA, États-Unis.

Lévi F., Hôpital Paul Brousse, 94804 Villejuif, France.

Leyvraz S., Ctre Pluridiscipl. d'Oncologie, Service de Radiothérapie, Service ORL, CHU Vaudois, Lausanne 1011, Suisse.

Liao M.L., Shanghai Chest Hosp, Shanghai P.R., République de Chine.

Ling V., Bioresearch Division, The Otario Cancer Institute, 500 Sherbourne Street, M4X 1K9, Toronto, Canada.

Lippman M. E., Medicine Branch, National Cancer Institute, Blg n° 10, Ro. 12N226, 20892 Bethesda, MD États-Unis.

Lokiec F., Service Pharmacologie, Centre René Huguenin, 35, rue Dailly, 92210 Saint-Cloud, France.

Looney W. B., Div. Radiobiology and Biophysics; University of Virginia Hospital, University Statio, 22908 Charlottesville, VIR États-Unis.

Luboinski B., Dept. Chirurgie Cervico-Faciale, Institut Gustave Roussy, 94805 Villejuif Cedex, France.

Maeyer (de) E., Institut Marie Curie, Bat. 110, Centre Universitaire, 91405 Orsay, France.

Malhaire J.-P., Service d'Oncologie et de Radiothérapie, CHU de Brest, avenue Foch, 29279 Brest, France.

Malviya V.K., Department Gynecologic-Oncology, Hutzel Hospital, 4707 Street Antoine, 48225 Detroit, MI États-Unis.

Mancuso S., Dept. of Gynecology and Obstetric, Catholic University, 8 Largo A Gemelli, Rome 00168, Italie.

Manfait M., Spectroscopie Biomoléculaire, Faculté de Pharmacie, 51, rue Cognacq-Jay, 51096 Reims Cedex, France.

Manner M., Department of Surgery, Im Neuenheimer Feld 110, 06900 Heidelberg, RFA

Maral J., Service d'Oncologie Médicale Pitié-Salpétrière, Hôpital de la Salpétrière, 47 bd de l'Hôpital, 75013 Paris, France.

Marin J.L., Institut Gustave Roussy, 94805 Villejuif Cedex, France

Martin D., Clinique Sainte-Catherine, Avignon, France.

Martin M., Centre Hospitalier Intercommunal, 94000 Créteil, France.

Martin Ph., Clinique Sainte-Catherine, Avignon, France.

Martorana G., Istituto Nazionale per la Ricerca sul Cancro e Clinica Urologica del l'Universita, Viale Benedetto XV, 10, Genova 16132, Italie.

Marty M., Service d'Hématologie, Hôpital Saint-Louis, 2 place du Dr. Fournier, 75010 Paris Cedex, France.

Mathé G., ICIG, Hôpital Paul Brousse, 16 av. Paul-Vaillant-Couturier, 94800 Villejuif Cedex, France.

Maublanc (de) M. A., Centre Cytopathologie Clinique, 49 rue du Ranelagh, 75016, Paris, France.

Mellat M., Hôpital St-Joseph, 75014 Paris, France.

Merlano M., Istituto Nazionale per la Ricerca sul Cancro e Clinica Urologica dell'Universita, Viale Benedetto XV, 10, Genova 16132, Italie.

Meltzer P.S., Arizona Cancer Center, University of Arizona, Tucson, Arizona 85724, États-Unis.

Meyer J., University Hospitals Munster, Hanover, RFA.

Michel P., Serv. Chir. Maxillo-Faciale, Hôpital Civil de Charleroi, Boulevard Paul Janson, 06190 Charleroi, Belgique.

Michelotti A., Istituto Nazionale per la Ricerca sul Cancro e Clinica Urologica Dell'Universita, Viale Benedetto XV, 10, Genova 16132, Italie.

Milano G., Lab. de Pharmacocinétique, Centre Antoine-Lacassagne, 36 Voie Romaine, 06054 Nice Cedex, France.

Mishina T., Mishina Urological Office, Higashino Toin Sanjo Sagaru, Nakagyo Ku, Kyoto 604, Japon

Missenard G., Institut Gustave Roussy, 94805 Villejuif Cedex, France.

Mittel B., 1725 West Harrison Street, 60612 Chicago, IL, États-Unis.

Montruccoli G.C., Department of Gynecology, Toniolo Hospital, Via Toscana, 34, 40141 Bologna, Italie.

Munck J.N., Institut Gustave Roussy, 94805 Villejuif Cedex, France.

Murthy A., 1725 West Harrison Street, 60612 Chicago, IL, États-Unis.

Nakagawa S., Department of Urology, Kyoto Prefectural University of Medicine, Kyoto 602 Japon.

Nakajima T., Division of Surgery, Cancer Institute Hospital, Toshima-Ku, Tokyo, 170, Japon.

Nakao M., Department of Urology, Kyoto Prefectural University of Medicine, Kyoto 602, Japon.

Namer M., Centre Antoine Lacassagne, 06054 Nice Cedex, France.

Nissen-Meyer R., Tyribakken 10, 00280 Oslo 2, Norvège.

Paineau J., Centre René Gauducheau, 44000 Nantes, France.

Pani G., Ospedale S. Chiara, 38100 Trento, Italie.

Papillon J., 12, Quai Général-Sarrail, 69006 Lyon, France.

Parisot P., Groupe IBM-France, 36 avenue Raymond Poincaré, 75116 Paris, France.

Pasche Ph., Ctre Pluridiscipl. d'Oncologie. Service de Radiothérapie, Service ORL, CHU Vaudois, Lausanne 1011 Suisse.

Perrin J.L., Institut Gustave Roussy, 94805 Villejuif Cedex, France.

Picci P., Bone Tumor Center, Instituto Ortopedico Rizzoli, Via Pupilli, 1 40136, Bologna, Italie.

Piedbois P., SOMPS, 47 boulevard de l'Hôpital, 75651 Paris Cedex 13, France.

Pircher W., University Hospitals Munster, Hanover, RFA.

Ponzio A., Hôpital St-Joseph, 75014 Paris, France.

Possinger K., Medizinische Klinik III, University of Munich, Munich, RFA.

Pouillard P., Institut Curie, 26, rue d'Ulm, 75231 Paris Cedex 05, France.

Preusser P., University Hospital Munster, Hanover, RFA.

Pronzato P., Istituto Nazionale per la Ricerca sul Cancro e Clinical Urologica Dell'Universita, Viale Benedetto XV, 10, Genova 16132, Italie.

Quintens H., Hôpital Pasteur, 06000 Nice, France.

Ragaz J., Department of Medical Oncology, CCA BC 600 West 10th Avenue, Vancouver, BC V5Z4E6, Canada.

Ramaioli A., Centre Antoine Lacassagne, 06054 Nice Cedex, France.

Rebischung J.L., Ser. Pneumologie et Allergologie, Hôpital Saint-Joseph 185, rue Raymond Losserand, 75674 Paris Cedex 14, France.

Reboul F., Clinique Sainte-Catherine, Avignon, France.

Resbeut M., Institut J. Paoli-Calmettes, BP 156, 13273 Marseille Cedex 9, France.

Richard J.M., Dept. Chirurgie Cervico-Faciale, Institut Gustave Roussy, 94805 Villejuif Cedex, France.

Robert J., Service de Biochimie, Fondation Bergonie, 180 rue Saint-Genès, 33076 Bordeaux Cedex, France.

Roche H., Centre Claudius Regaud, 20-24 rue du Pont St-Pierre, 31052 Toulouse Cedex, France.

Rochemaure J., Hôtel Dieu, Service de Pneumologie, 1 Place du Parvis Notre Dame, 75181 Paris Cedex 04, France.

Rosen G., Medical Director, The Cedars-Sinai-Schuman, Big 8700 Beverly Boulevard, 6th Fl., 90048 Los Angeles, CA États-Unis.

Rosso R., Istituto Nazionale per la Ricerca sul Cancro e Clinica Urologica dell'Univ. Viale Benedetto XV, 10 Genova 16132, Italie.

Rouëssé J., Directeur, Centre René Huguenin, 35 rue Dailly, 92211 St-Cloud, France.

Rougier Ph., Service de Gastro-Entérologie, Institut Gustave Roussy, 94805 Villejuif Cedex, France.

Rudelle C., Clinique St-Jean Languedoc, 20 route de Revel, 31077, Toulouse, France.

Ruffié P., Institut Gustave Roussy, 94805 Villejuif Cedex, France.

Saeland S., Unicet, Laboratory for Immunological Research, 69570 Dardilly, France.

Salmon S.E., Dept. of International Medecine, The Arizona Cancer Center, 6th floor Facility, 85724 Tucson, Arizona, États-Unis.

Salzer G.M., II. Surgical Depart, of the University, Innsbruck A 6020, Autriche.

Sancho-Garnier H., Institut Gustave Roussy, 94805 Villejuif Cedex, France.

Sarmini H., Laboratoire Cerba, BP 451, 95005 Cergy Pontoise Cedex, France.

Sauvaget J., Hôpital St-Joseph, 75014 Paris, France.

Savary M., Ctre Pluridiscipl. d'Oncologie, Service de Radiothérapie, Service ORL, CHU Vaudois, Lausanne 1011, Suisse.

Scambia G., Dept of Gynecology and Obstetric, Catholic University, 8 Largo A. Gemelli, Rome 00168, Italie.

Scarpati D., Istituto Nazionale per la Ricerca sul Cancro e Clinica Urologica dell'Universita, Viale Benedetto XV, 10 Genova 16132, Italie.

Scheper R., Dept. of Pathology, Free University of the Netherlands, Amsterdam, Pays-Bas.

Scher H., Solid Tumor Service, Div. Med. Onc Memorial Sloan-Ketterin, 1275 York Avenue, 10021 New-York, États-Unis.

Schlick W., II Surgical Univ. Clinic, Vienna A 1090, Autriche.

Schneider M., Centre Antoine Lacassagne, 36 voie Romaine, 06504 Nice Cedex, France.

Schwartz G.F., Dept of Surgery and Medicine Jefferson Medical College, Philadelphia, Pennsylvania 19107, États-Unis.

Serin D., Clinique Sainte-Catherine, Avignon, France.

Sertoli M.R., Department Oncology, Istituto di Oncologia, Viale Benedetto XV, 1, 16132 Genova, Italie.

Sheen M.-C., Department of Oncology, Kaohsiung Medical College, 100 Shih-Chuan, 1 Rd Kaohsiung, Taiwan, ROC-Kaohsiung, Chine.

Showel J.L., 1725 West Harrison Street, 60612 Chicago, IL, États-Unis.

Simondon F., ORSTOM, UR. G6, 34000 Montpellier, France.

Skipper H. E., Southern Research Institute, 2000 Ninth Avenue South P.O. Box 55305, 35255 5305, Birmingham, AL États-Unis.

Snow G.B., Dept. ORL/Head and Neck Surgery de Boelelaan 1117, 01081 HV Amsterdam, Pays-Bas.

Soloway M. S., Department of Urology UPF, 956 Court Avenue, 2nd Floor, 38163, Memphis, Tennessee, États-Unis.

Soret J.Y., Service d'Urologie, CHU, 1 Avenue de l'Hôtel Dieu, 49033 Angers Cedex, France.

Soubrane C., SOMPS 47 boulevard de l'Hôpital, 75651 Paris Cedex 13, France.

Spielmann M., Institut Gustave Roussy, 94805 Villejuif Cedex, France

Spits H., Unicet, Laboratory for Immunological Research, 69570 Dardilly, France.

Splinter T.A.W., University Hospital Dijkzigt, Dr Molewaterplein 40, 3015 GD Rotterdam, Pays-Bas.

Stephens F.O., Department of Surgery, University of Sidney, 16 Inkerman Street, 02088, Mosman, N.S.W., Australie.

Stettler E.R., Institut Gustave Roussy, 94805 Villejuif Cedex, France.

Stumpf J., Weil Emil Hospital, Budapest, Hongrie.

Subirana R.A., Institut Gustave Roussy, 94805 Villejuif Cedex, France.

Talpaz M., Anderson Hospital, Houston 77030, Texas, États-Unis.

Tapazoglou E., Detroit, Michigan 48201, États-Unis.

Tapiero H., Departement de Pharmacologie Cellulaire et Moléculaire CNRS UA 14, ICIG, 14 av. Paul Vaillant-Couturier, 94804 Villejuif Cedex, France.

Tarrats A., Department of Gynecology, Hospital Clinic Villaroel, 170, 08036, Barcelona, Espagne.

Taylor S. G., Sheridan Road Pavillon, Rush Medical College, 1725 West Harrison Street, 60612 Chicago, IL, États-Unis.

Terrier-Lacombe M.J., Institut Gustave Roussy, 94805 Villejuif Cedex, France.

Théodore C., Institut Gustave Roussy, 94805 Villejuif Cedex, France.

Tran T.M., Hôpital Avicenne, 125 rue de Stalingrad, 93009 Bobigny Cedex France.

Travagli J.P., Institut Gustave Roussy, 94805 Villejuif Cedex, France.

Trifard F., Service du Professeur Dufour, Hôpital Necker, 149 rue de Sèvres, 75015 Paris, France.

Trillet V., Hôpital Louis Pradel, BP Lyon Montchat, 69394 Lyon Cedex 03, France.

Tubiana-Hulin N., Centre René Huguenin, 5 rue Gaston Latouche 92210 St-Cloud, France.

Tursz T., Immuno-Biologie Cellulaire, Institut Gustave Roussy, 94805 Villejuif Cedex, France.

Ulsperger E., Inst. for Epidemiology of Neoplasms of the University, Vienna A 1090, Autriche.

Unkeless J. C., Department of Biochemistry, Mount Sinai Hospital, 19th Floor Ro. 40, 98th St. and Mad, 10029 New York, NY, États-Unis.

Valagussa P., Istituto Nationale Tumori, Milano, Italie.

Valdagni R., Ospedale S. Chiara, 38100 Trento, Italie.

Valleron A.-J., URBB, 263, Université Paris 7, Tour 53, 2 place Jussieu, 75251 Paris Cedex 05, France.

Van der Meijden A.P.M., Department of Urology, University Nijmegen, Pays-Bas.

Vannetzel J.-M., Radiothérapie et Oncologie, Hôpital des Peupliers, 22, rue des Peupliers, 75013 Paris, France.

Venturini M., Istituto Nazionale per la Ricerca sul Cancro e Clinica Urologica dell Universita, Viale Benedetto XV, 10 Genova 16132, Italie.

Verine J.L., Service d'Urologie, CHU, 1 Avenue de l'Hôtel Dieu, 49033 Angers Cedex, France.

Vernant J.P., Hôpital Henri Mondor, 94000 Créteil, France.

Veronesi A., Istituto Nazionale per lo Studio de la Cura dei Tumori, Via Venezian, 1, 20133 Milan, Italie.

Vignoud J., Centre René Gauducheau, 44000 Nantes, France.

Vita (de) V.T., Jr., Director — NCI 9000 Rockville Tyke Bldg 31, Room 11A48, 20892 Bethesda, MD, États-Unis.

Vokes E.E., Div. Hematology/Oncology, Michael Reese Hospital, Ro. L 231 Blood Center, 60616 Chicago, IL, États-Unis.

Voûte P.A., SIOP Nephroblastoma Trial and Study Office, Spinozastraat, 51, 01018 HJ Amsterdam, Pays-Bas.

Vries (de) J.E., Unicet, Laboratory for Immunological Research, 69570 Dardilly, France.

Walther H., Department of Surgery, KKH Trostberg, Siegerthoehe, 1, 08223 Trostberg, RFA

Warrington P.S., Western General Hospital, Edinburgh, Scotland, UK.

Weil M., SOMPS, 47 boulevard de l'Hôpital, 75651 Paris Cedex 13. France.

Wibault P., Institut Gustave Roussy, 94805 Villejuif Cedex, France.

Wiley A.L. Jr., Section of Radiation Oncology, University of Wisconsin, Madison, Wisconsin, États-Unis.

Wilke H., University Hospitals Munster, Hanover, RFA.

Witt T.R., 1725 West Harrison Street, 60612 Chicago, IL, États-Unis.

Zucker J.M., Pédiatrie Oncologique, Institut Curie, 26, rue d'Ulm, 75231 Paris Cedex 05, France.

Contents

Sommaire

RADIO-CHEMOTHERAPY COMBINATIONS/*ASSOCIATIONS RADIOTHÉRAPIE-CHIMIOTHÉRAPIE*

Presidents : W.B. Looney, J. Papillon

BREAST CANCER II/*CANCER DU SEIN II*
(Sponsored by ICI Laboratory/Sponsorisé par les Laboratoires ICI)

Presidents : B. Fisher, Cl. Jacquillat

BREAST CANCER III/*CANCER DU SEIN III*
(Sponsored by ICI Laboratory/Sponsorisé par les Laboratores ICI)

Presidents : M.E. Lippman, M. Weil

GYNECOLOGY/*GYNÉCOLOGIE*

Presidents : J.F. Holland, M. George

PHARMACOKINETICS/*PHARMACOCINÉTIQUE*

Presidents : R.S. Benjamin, J.P. Cano

SYMPOSIUM CARBOPLATINUM (PARAPLATIN)/*CARBOPLATINE (PARAPLATINE)*

(Sponsored by Bristol Laboratory/Sponsorisé par le Laboratoire Bristol)

Presidents : S.K. Carter, M. Marty

WORKSHOP ON LYMPHOKINES AND OTHER IMMUNOLOGICAL TOOLS IN MEDICINE/*LYMPHOKINES ET AUTRES OUTILS IMMUNOLOGIQUES EN MÉDECINE*

(Sponsored by Unicet Laboratory/Sponsorisé par le Laboratoire Unicet)

Presidents : J.F. Bach, J.C. Unkeless

Inaugural Lecture

Conférence inaugurale

Neo-Adjuvant Chemotherapy. Ed. Cl. Jacquillat, M. Weil, D. Khayat. Colloque INSERM/John Libbey Eurotext Ltd. © 1988. Vol. 169, pp. 3-14.

On the value of response criteria in therapeutic research

Vincent T. de Vita, Jr.

National Cancer Institute, Bethesda, Maryland, USA

ABSTRACT

Primary chemotherapy is the use of anticancer drugs as the first treatment in patients with localized tumor presentations for which there is an alternative but less than satisfactory treatment. Its most important feature is the preservation of the primary tumor mass as a biologic marker of response and in this sense it shares the same response criteria as induction chemotherapy for advanced cancer for which there is no alternative treatment. The use of chemotherapy as the primary treatment for patients with localized tumor presentations is experimental except in localized forms of tumors such as diffuse large-cell lymphomas, small-cell lung cancers, and some pediatric malignancies. Complete remission rates and the relapse-free survival are the best current way of quantifying the cytoreductive effect of primary chemotherapy. The use of full dose chemotherapy used with a flexible number of induction cycles is recommended. Protocol design should not obscure these endpoints by adding alternative therapies before a best response to primary chemotherapy is attained.

KEYWORDS

Adjuvant, primary therapy, biologic marker, lymphomas, lung cancer, pediatric malignancies, endpoints, cytoreduction, protocol design, primary chemotherapy, response criteria, therapeutic research

The steady movement of the use of chemotherapy towards early stages of cancer relates to four factors (Skipper, 1986). 1.) In rodents there is an invariable inverse relationship between cell number and curability by chemotherapy, an observation now confirmed in human tumors such as childhood leukemia, Wilms' tumor, choriocarcinoma, diffuse large-cell lymphoma, Hodgkin's disease, osteogenic sarcoma, small-cell lung cancer, ovarian cancer, breast cancer, and probably now, colo-rectal cancers. 2.) A given dose of chemotherapy kills a constant fraction of cells not a fixed number; the two choices facing clinicians to enhance cure rates are to increase the dose or reduce the cell burden. The factor most easily manipulated in clinical studies is the reduction of cell number by the selection of patients with early stage disease for treatment with chemotherapy. 3.) Most common cancers are systemic illnesses even when they present as localized disease as evidenced by the high recurrence rate in common cancers that present as localized tumors. Recurrence rates are strongly influenced by the size of the primary tumor, the depth of tumor invasion, and the extent of local spread to draining lymph nodes. These prognostic factors, have allowed the selection of high-risk subgroups for additional treatment after local excision or radiotherapy (DeVita, 1983). 4.) By 1970 chemotherapy had been demonstrated to cure a fraction of patients with some types of far advanced cancers with tumor cell masses estimated to be in the range of 10^{11} cells, far in excess of the tumor volume present in most patients with localized presentations (DeVita, 1987).

Concomitant with these advances, the specialty of medical oncology was founded to deliver these complicated drug treatments in medical practice. Because curative chemotherapy has not yet been developed for most common cancers, the need for palliative approaches in medical practice has led to undue emphasis on protocol design that stresses treatments that prolong survival with minimal toxicity. Yet, neither toxicity nor survival are adequate guideposts to direct therapeutic research in humans (DeVita, 1987). At a time when the use of chemotherapy as the primary treatment for localized cancer is under test, it may be useful to reflect on the value of endpoints in research protocols. Fig. 1 illustrates the current uses of chemotherapy. There are three circumstances where

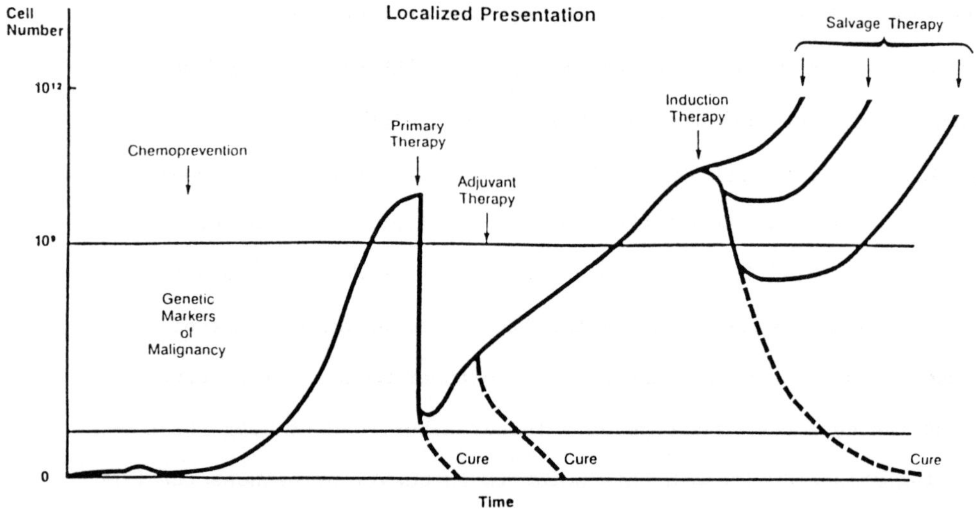

Fig. 1 Localized Presentation

chemotherapy is used. 1.) The term "induction chemotherapy" has generally been used to describe drug or other systemic therapy as the primary treatment for patients who present with advanced cancer for which no alternative treatment exists (Holland, 1986). Selection of treatment is based on the effectiveness of the agents in rodent models. Combinations of drugs are fashioned based on the effectiveness, level of cross-resistance, and limiting toxicity of the available drugs used alone in similar patient populations. Patients who fail after one drug treatment, and require further chemotherapy, represent a particularly difficult circumstance because of drug resistance. This form of induction therapy is referred to as "salvage treatment." 2.) Adjuvant chemotherapy refers to the use of systemic treatment after the primary tumor has been removed by an alternative method. The selection of treatment is based on response rates in separate groups of patients with advanced cancers of the same histologic type, and selection of suitable populations of patients for adjuvant treatment is based on disease variables known to adversely influence prognosis. 3.) The use of chemotherapy as initial treatment, the subject of this conference, may be defined as the use of induction chemotherapy as the primary treatment for patients who present with localized cancer for which there is an alternative but less than satisfactory treatment. This has variously been described as neoadjuvant chemotherapy (Frei, 1987), or as primary chemotherapy (Muggia, 1985), although the latter is a more accurate representation of its case. Since the likelihood of development of spontaneous resistant cell lines relates to tumor mass, earlier drug treatment may have the advantage of a lesser likelihood of drug resistant lines being present, although this point is in question, because the time interval between chemotherapy used as an adjuvant treatment and as primary treatment is now only a matter of a few weeks in most cases (Goldie, 1987). Primary chemotherapy has the potential to down-stage tumors by decreasing the size and extent of the tumor mass. This can influence both the need for and radical nature of subsequent alternative treatments by influencing operability, and/or decreasing tumor hypoxia and increasing the effectiveness of a given dose of radiotherapy. The theoretical disadvantages of primary chemotherapy are that by leaving the primary tumor mass in place, even temporarily, the tumor volume is actually larger than if surgery and/or radiotherapy are used first and chemotherapy is used as an adjunct. Also, the favorable influence of resection of the primary tumor on the kinetics of proliferation of the residual micrometastases may be lost (Simpson-Herren, 1976) although this has not been a universal observation in rodent systems and no comparable cell kinetic data are available in human tumors. In addition, toxicity of chemotherapy may impair the effectiveness and increase the side effects of subsequent alternative treatments, and may delay the use of an alternative treatment sufficiently to adversely impact on the outcome, if no provisions are made for rapid progression to an alternative treatment in the presence of a poor response to primary chemotherapy. Also, as in the use of adjuvant chemotherapy, patients who would otherwise be cured by local treatment alone are exposed to the acute and chronic side effects of chemotherapy in combined modality programs.

RESPONSE CRITERIA IN CLINICAL TRIALS

Endpoints in clinical trials differ depending on whether or not investigators are evaluating and refining a new treatment for introduction into medical practice or aiming at testing a hypothesis that may define a new curative approach to a previously incurable tumor. The clinical investigator uses different endpoints in each of the three major uses of chemotherapy shown in Fig. 1. These are listed in Table 1.

Table 1. Signal Endpoints for Clinical Investigators Using Chemotherapy for:

Induction therapy of Advanced Disease	Adjuvant therapy	Primary therapy
1. Response rate	1. Effect against advanced disease	1. Complete response rate
2. Complete response rate	2. Relapse-free survival	2. PR rate with pathologic confirmation
3. RFS of complete responders	3. Treatment mortality	3. RFS of complete responders
4. Treatment and tumor mortality	4. Chronic toxicity	4. RFS of PR's after resection or RRX
		5. Treatment mortality
		6. Chronic toxicity

In induction chemotherapy for advanced cancer it is possible to determine the individual response to chemotherapy on a case-by-case basis. The overall response rate, usually defined as a reduction of measurable tumor masses by greater than 50%, a small reduction in actual cell number, is usually not of clinical value and is only useful in testing new drug programs for activity to determine whether the particular experimental approach is worth pursuing further. The most important indicator of effectiveness, however, is the complete response rate. It is a prerequisite for cure. The qualitative and quantitative difference in value between a complete and partial response is such that they should never be reported as combined complete/partial response rates (or overall response rates) as they often are. When new programs consistently produce more than an occasional complete remission, they have invariably later proven of practical value in medical practice. The dramatic total disappearance of tumor in a patient with advanced cancer raises the question of whether that tumor has been permanently eradicated and the most important indicator of the quality of the remission is relapse-free survival of complete responders. This is the only clinical counter-part of the quantifiable cytoreductive effect of drugs in rodent systems. The current trend in many clinical protocols testing new approaches in patients with advanced cancer to use freedom from progression, of complete and partial responders combined, as an indicator of the practical potential of a new treatment, obscures the value of relapse-free survival of complete responders as the major determinant of the quality of remission. Other endpoints such as median response duration or median survival are of little practical value until treatment results have been refined to the point that the complete response rate is over 50%. Toxicity only serves as a limiting endpoint in seminal therapeutic research protocols.

There was great excitement concomitant with the move to the use of chemotherapy as an adjuvant to local treatments. The promise was great because tumor volume is at a minimum when adjuvant chemotherapy is initiated after all visible tumor has been removed, and it was assumed that either a much higher cure rate could be achieved, or treatment intensity could be reduced, with the same therapeutic effect, and thereby diminish side effects. The failure to appreciate the circumstances surrounding the assessment of response to adjuvant chemotherapy is the source of some of the current disillusionment with the positive, but less than dramatic, results in the adjuvant chemotherapy of common tumors such as breast and colo-rectal cancer (DeVita, 1983). First, the practice of arbitrarily reducing doses and prolonging intervals between cycles of treatment because of the smaller tumor volume in the adjuvant situation has been detrimental, was never justified by experimental data (Skipper, 1986) and should be condemned (DeVita, 1987). Second, and most important, the major indicator of effectiveness, the complete remission rate, is lost since the primary tumor has been removed. Treatment is selected for individual patients based on response rates in an entirely different population of patients with advanced disease of the same histologic type. While relapse-free survival remains the major endpoint, the treated patients represent those whose tumor could have been either sensitive or resistant to chemotherapy. Thus relapse-free survival, in the adjuvant setting, measures the duration of remission of complete and partial responders, as well as those who would have been classified as non-responders, and is equivalent to the use of freedom from progression in patients with advanced disease. Attempts to overcome the shortcomings of the absence of an indicator of individual response by the use of *in vitro* assays of drug sensitivity, from biopsy material from the primary tumor, will be reviewed elsewhere in this symposium, but have not proven practical. Since some patients would have been cured with the use of localized treatment only, another factor is introduced: the effect of acute and chronic toxicity, most especially the latter, in patients who need not have received chemotherapy to achieve their cure.

The unique feature of primary chemotherapy in patients with localized tumor presentations is the preservation of the presenting tumor mass as a biologic marker of responsiveness to anticancer drugs. Thus, as with induction chemotherapy, it is possible to determine, on a case-by-case basis, the potential effectiveness of a new treatment program. By definition the presenting tumor mass is the largest aggregate of tumor in the body, and historically the oldest, and thus the aggregate of tumor cells most likely to contain one or more resistant cell lines (Goldie, 1979). It is also the mass with the least favorable cell kinetics. It is reasonable to assume, then, that whatever the effect of the chemotherapy on the primary tumor, a similar or greater effect is occurring fairly uniformly in micrometastatic deposits unless the phenotype of metastasizing cells coincides with those which spontaneously develop drug resistance. Such a circumstance would explain the clinical observation of the control of the primary with chemotherapy with death resulting from metastases at a distant site. Nonetheless, a poor response of the primary tumor to chemotherapy clearly defines a group of patients for which alternative methods of treatment should be used, and used quickly.

Another unique feature of primary chemotherapy is the ability to delineate partial responders, with varying degrees of prognosis, as determined by the presence of residual tumor masses after an initial good response. Examination of residual masses histologically enables the determination of viability of the remaining tissue. Obviously, response duration of these categories of responders needs to be determined separately. Treatment mortality, and the potential for serious chronic toxicities, should be viewed only as limiting endpoints in these protocols as well. Survival, it should be noted, is not now a major endpoint to evaluate whether or not, and how, this unique approach to the treatment of localized cancer should be pursued, but improvements in survival will follow improvements in complete response rates as it did with induction chemotherapy in advanced cancer.

The major issues facing investigators at this conference are listed in Table 2.

Table 2. Important Issues in the Design of Protocols to Assess the Value of Chemotherapy as the Primary Treatment of Localized Disease

1. Does the degree of sensitivity to drugs (complete versus partial response) predict the ultimate outcome?
2. The need for other therapy in complete responders.
3. Can pathologic examination of tissue in residual masses identify subsets of partial responders who are sensitive to chemotherapy?
4. The value of continued adjuvant drug treatment of partial or nonresponders.

The most important issue is whether or not an effective primary chemotherapy treatment, pursued flexibly and intensively to the point of complete remission, plus two or more cycles of treatment, will define a significant fraction of cured patients with or without the addition of alternative treatments. In carefully selected patients, with some stages of most of the common tumors that currently have less than satisfactory end results with available standard treatments, such a protocol design is ethically and theoretically sound. Such an approach may also result in shorter duration, less morbid, and more effective treatment programs. In some tumor types, such as localized diffuse large-cell lymphomas, limited-stage small-cell cancers, some pediatric malignancies, and now even in some categories of head and neck cancers, such approaches already are becoming the standard of treatment.

RESUME

A major problem in clinical therapeutic research is the failure to draw a distinction between the requirements for the development of curative and palliative treatments. The distinction occurs at the level of endpoints used to evaluate the treatment programs. The main indicator of the curative potential of new systemic treatments is the ability to produce complete remissions and the durability of these remissions. Many investigators persist in using overall survival as an endpoint in therapeutic research, but this is a misleading assessment of the value of a new approach to treatment in early clinical trials if the complete remission rate is too low to affect survival but high enough to warrant further work with the new approach on an investigational basis. Survival is of value once some level of assurance has been reached to indicate that a treatment is ready to become a standard of care. Toxicity, while important, should only serve as a limiting endpoint in early clinical studies.

The distinction of the importance of endpoints is particularly useful as new fields of treatment research emerge. The use of chemotherapy as the primary treatment of patients who present with localized cancers is such a new field. It defines the use of chemotherapy in a population of patients for which there is an alternative, but not entirely effective, treatment already available. The selection of key endpoints for evaluation of its effectiveness is therefore an important feature of early studies. The unique feature of primary chemotherapy is the preservation of the primary tumor mass as a biologic marker of the effectiveness of a systemic treatment program. The value of a primary chemotherapy program, therefore, can be determined by noting the capacity to eradicate the presenting tumor mass on a case-by-case basis. The question of quality of these remissions can be isolated and examined by their duration without further treatment. Adjuvant drug treatment is more complex because when the presenting tumor has been removed, the endpoints are blurred. Relapse-free survival in adjuvant studies measures the effect of adjuvant drugs on tumor cells, which may have been sensitive, insensitive, or unresponsive to chemotherapy. The sequence of steps that proved so useful in developing curative therapy in some types of very advanced cancers should be as useful in determining the proper role of primary chemotherapy as a standard treatment in properly designed primary chemotherapy protocols.

REFERENCES

Skipper, H.E. (1986) Critical variables in the design of combination chemotherapy regimens to be used alone or in adjuvant setting. Neo-adjuvant Chemotherapy. Colloque Inserm 137, 11-22.

DeVita, V.T., Hubbard, S.M., Longo, D.L. (1987): The chemotherapy of lymphomas: looking back, moving forward - The Richard and Hinda Rosenthal Foundation Award Lecture. Cancer Res. 47, 5810-5824.

DeVita, V.T. (1983): The relationship between tumor mass and resistance to chemotherapy: implications for surgical adjuvant treatment of cancer. *Cancer 51,* 1209-1220.

Holland, JF. (1986): Induction chemotherapy: an old term for an old concept. *Neo-adjuvant chemotherapy. Colloque INSERM 137,* 45-47.

Frei, A. III, Clark, J.R., and Miller, D. (1987) The concept of neo-adjuvant chemotherapy. *Adjuvant Therapy of Cancer V* , p. 67. San Francisco, Grune and Stratton.

Muggia, F.M. (1985) Primary chemotherapy: concepts and issues. *Primary Chemotherapy in Cancer Medicine,* 377-383. New York, NY, Alan R. Liss.

Goldie J.H. (1987): Scientific basis for adjuvant and primary (neo-adjuvant) chemotherapy. *Sem. Oncol. 14,* 1-7.

Simpson-Herren, L., Sanford, A.H. and Holmquist, J.P. (1976) Effects of surgery on the cell kinetics of residual tumor. *Cancer Treatment Reports 60,* 1749-1760.

Résumé

Le problème principal de la recherche thérapeutique en clinique est le fait qu'on n'a pu faire une distinction entre les exigences de la mise au point des traitements curatifs et palliatifs. La distinction se fait au niveau des points finals employés dan l'évaluation des programmes de traitement. L'indicateur principal du potentiel curatif de nouveaux traitements généraux est la capacité de produire des rémissions complètes et la durée de ces rémissions. Un grand nombre de chercheurs continuent à employer la survie globale comme point final dans la recherche thérapeutique, mais cela est une appréciation trompeuse de la valeur d'une nouvelle approche au traitement dans les premières études cliniques si la fréquence de rémission complète est trop diminuée pour influencer la survie mais assez élevée pour justifier de plus amples recherches employant cette nouvelle approche. Une fois qu'un niveau de confiance est établi, la survie a une valeur indice que le traitement est prêt à devenir un standard des soins. La toxicité, quoiqu'importante, ne devrait servir que comme point final limitant dans les premières études cliniques.

La distinction de l'importance du point final est spécialement utile au fur et à mesure que de nouveaux champs de recherches thérapeutiques apparaissent. L'emploi de la chimiothérapie comme traitement principal des malades affectés par un cancer localisé est un très nouveau champ. Il détermine l'emploi de la chimiothérapie dans une population des malades pour lesquels il y a un traitement alternatif, mais pas complètement efficace, déjà disponible. La sélection des points finals clefs pour l'évaluation de son efficacité est donc une particularité importante des premiers travaux. La caractéristique tout à fait particulière de la chimiothérapie principale est la conservation de la masse tumorale primitive comme marqueur biologique de l'efficacité du programme de traitement général. La valeur d'un programme de chimiothérapie principale donc peut être déterminée par la constation de la capacité d'élimination de la masse tumorale présentée, basée sur l'étude de chaque cas. La question de la qualité de ces rémissions peut être étudiée en la dégageant et en examinant leur durée sans traitement additionel. Le traitement médicamenteux avec adjuvant est plus complexe car quand le tumeur présenté a été extirpé, les points finals sont brouillés. La survie san récidive dans les études employant les adjuvants mesure l'effet des médicaments adjuvants sur les cellules tumorales qui peuvent être sensibles, insensibles, ou sans réponse à la chimiothérapie. Les étapes successives qui se sont affirmées si utiles dans la mise au point du traitement curatif pour quelques types de cancers très avancés devraient être utiles dans la détermination du propre rôle de la chimiothérapie principale comme traitement standard dans les protocoles de chimiothérapie principale proprement établis.

Scientific Basis

Bases scientifiques

Neo-Adjuvant Chemotherapy. Ed. Cl. Jacquillat, M. Weil, D. Khayat. Colloque INSERM/John Libbey Eurotext Ltd. © 1988. Vol. 169, pp. 17-23.

Relevance of multidrug resistance to neo-adjuvant therapy of cancer

S.E. Salmon*, T. Grogan*, R. Scheper**, P.S. Meltzer* and W.S. Dalton*

** Arizona Cancer Center, University of Arizona, Tucson, Arizona 85724, USA and ** the Department of Pathology, Free University of the Netherlands, Amsterdam, The Netherlands*

ABSTRACT

Neoadjuvant therapy is administered when the risk of multidrug resistance is considered low. In this paper we review evidence that MDR1 can be present prior to all therapy and potentially be reversed using therapeutic approaches focused on inhibiting the function of a cell membrane drug efflux pump.

KEY WORDS

gene amplification, multidrug resistance (MDR1), P-glycoprotein, calcium antagonists, verapamil, amiodarone, monoclonal antibody

INTRODUCTION

Neoadjuvant therapy of cancer is given at a time when there has been no prior exposure to cancer therapy including surgery, radiation, cytotoxic drugs, hormonal or biologic agents and when tumor burden is relatively small. Conventional wisdom would suggest that the likelihood of mutation and selection of a drug resistant neoplasm is potentially reduced in that setting. Nonetheless, recent information on multidrug resistance suggests that the drug resistant phenotype may be intrinsic in certain tumor types and in fact a property of the normal tissues from which some tumors arise (Fojo et al., 1987b). Advances in molecular and cellular biology and pharmacology are currently changing our concepts on resistance to cytotoxic anticancer drugs. In this paper we will review some of this evidence, and report some of our preliminary observations in both detecting the multidrug resistant phenotype in human cancer specimens, and on early efforts to develop strategies to attack multidrug resistant tumor cells.

A MOLECULAR VIEW OF DRUG RESISTANCE

Acquired forms of drug resistance are those which occur at the cellular level and usually result from molecular abnormalities in the genome of malignant cells which result in a quantitative or qualitative change in a gene product that is a critical cellular determinant for anticancer drug action, inactivation, or elimination. Such altered gene products can be specific enzymes, cell surface or intracellular receptors or critical intermediaries. Potential alterations in the genomic apparatus which can result in a drug resistant phenotype are summarized in Table 1.

Table 1. Possible Molecular Mechanisms of Drug Resistance in Cancer

Molecular Abnormality in Genome	Effect on Gene Product
1. Gene Amplification	Increased amount
2. Altered Gene Regulation	Changed amount
3. Point Mutation in Gene	Altered activity
4. Translocation of Gene	Changed amount/ Altered activity

While some forms of drug resistance are specific for a single chemotherapeutic agent, in other instances the molecular abnormality results in multidrug resistance to a number of apparently unrelated agents. Even in the instance of multidrug resistance, one or more of the molecular mechanisms summarized in Table 1 may still be operative. Gene amplification is an important means by which a cancer cell can increase the number of gene copies coding for a specific enzyme or transport pump (Schimke, 1984). Similarly, altered gene regulation resulting in increased transcription of the message for a given gene product; this may be the result of a change in the function of a regulatory gene or mutations in a regulatory region of the drug resistance gene itself.

MOLECULAR MECHANISMS OF MULTI-DRUG RESISTANCE

A general form of multidrug resistance (MDR1) was first described by Ling and his colleagues, who applied the term "pleiotropic drug resistance" (Ling, 1975; Riordan, 1979; Gerlach, 1986). The pleotropic drug resistant phenotype has been studied using both molecular probes for the MDR1 gene, its RNA product, or its ultimate protein product on the cell membrane. The recent development of monoclonal antibodies to the P-glycoprotein has greatly increased the facility with which the expression of MDR1 can be identified (Scheper, 1987; Hamada and Tsuruo, 1986). Multidrug resistance is mediated by expression on the tumor cell membrane of increased quantities of the 170 kilodalton glycoprotein that conveys resistance to a wide variety of drugs such as actinomycins, anthracyclines, chytochalasins, podophyllotoxins, and vinca alkaloids (Ling, 1975; Riordan, 1979; Gerlach, 1986; Beck, 1979, 1984). Cancer cells derived from normal progenitors may retain or enhance the expression of gene products that eliminate environmental toxins including anticancer drugs (Cowan, 1986). There is evidence for structural homology between the P-glycoprotein and the bacterial transport proteins (Chen, 1986).

Characteristics of MDR1 are summarized in Table 2. Other forms of MDR will likely be identified in the future.

Table 2. Characteristics of Multidrug Resistance (MDR1)

1) Selected normal tissues (colon, renal tubules, bile canaliculi, breast ductules, and adrenal medulla) as well as tumor cells express increased amounts of the cell-surface P-glycoprotein.

2) The P-glycoprotein functions as an energy-dependent transport pump which increases the extrusion of a wide variety of potentially toxic compounds. (The normal substrate, however, is unknown).

3) Intracellular accumulation of anticancer drugs is diminished in MDR1 cells in comparison to cells not expressing the P-glycoprotein.

4) The P-glycoprotein appears to be a structural homolog of bacterial transport proteins (i.e., hemolysin β for transport of α hemolysin).

5) Tumor cells lines that do not normally express the P-glycoprotein can be selected to do so after prolonged passage in the presence of vinblastine, doxorubicin or etoposide.

6) Tumor cells lines selected to express the P-glycoprotein after exposure to one of these agents exhibit cross resistance to a wide variety of anticancer drugs.

MDR1 AND NEOADJUVANT CHEMOTHERAPY

Pleotropic multidrug resistance associated with P-glycoprotein may be relevant to neoadjuvant chemotherapy from several perspectives. Firstly, some normal tissues (e.g., colon, kidney) express relative increases in the amount of RNA specific for production of the P-glycoprotein (Fojo, 1987a). Untreated neoplasms derived from these tissue types are notoriously drug resistant and also can express the P-glycoprotein (Fojo, 1987b). The assumption which may be drawn is that tumors derived from tissues that normally express MDR1 will frequently show resistance to cancer chemotherapy, even in the neoadjuvant setting. High baseline P-glycoprotein expression in untreated cancer cells may thus reflect either a normal differentiated phenotype of the tissue of origin or a genetic variation resulting from cellular damage or mutation resulting from carcinogen exposure (Cowan, 1986). Of interest, forms of cancer that are known to result from exposure to chemical carcinogens (e.g., lung, bladder cancer) frequently express high levels of resistance to chemotherapy or acquire it relatively quickly after the initiation of systemic chemotherapy. The finding of P-glycoprotein expression in untreated human tumors provides a scientific basis for considering that there may be biochemical features in common between tumor cells expressing inherent drug resistance and those exhibiting acquired drug resistance after exposure to chemotherapy (Fojo, 1987b). The presence of a limited number of MDR1 cells in an untreated tumor could therefore lead to their selective advantage after exposure to neoadjuvant chemotherapy.

In preliminary studies using a monoclonal antibody to the P-glycoprotein (JSB-1), we have observed that biopsies from some patients with breast cancer are positive for the expression of the P-glycoprotein. When these initial immunohistochemical studies were correlated with the results of doxorubicin testing with the human tumor clonogenic assay (HTCA), we found that breast cancers that were strongly positive for the P-glycoprotein were also quite resistant to doxorubicin, whereas those that were weakly positive or negative exhibited greater degrees of chemosensitivity. Positive staining was observed in some untreated breast cancer but only occasional tumor cells within such tumors stained positively. In contrast, tumor cells from patients in relapse with high degrees of clinical and in vitro resistance stained uniformly positively. We have only recently initiated these studies and it will be necessary to study a large number of tumor specimens and correlate the results with in vitro chemosensitivity and clinical cancer chemotherapy. However, our initial observations support the contention that MDR1 is an important clinical phenomenon that likely will need to be addressed.

STRATEGIES TO OVERCOME PLEOTROPIC DRUG RESISTANCE

The finding that multidrug resistance (MDR1) has a specific molecular mechanism provides a basis for developing therapeutic strategies to either overcome multidrug resistance via a directed pharmacologic or immunologic attack on cells expressing this phenotype. Potential strategies for therapeutic attack on tumor cells expressing the P-glycoprotein are summarized in Table 3.

Table 3. Strategies for Neoadjuvant Therapy for Tumor Types Exhibiting Inherent P-glycoprotein Expression

1) Add antiarrhythmic drugs or calmodulin inhibitors to combination chemotherapy.

2) Exploit collateral sensitivity of MDR1 cells to hormones, selected cytotoxic drugs and cytokines.

3) Utilize monoclonal antibodies to cell surface epitopes of P-glycoprotein together with vinca alkaloids or as monoclonal antibody conjugates.

Tsuruo and his colleagues (1982) first demonstrated that in a murine leukemia-lymphoma model, acquired resistance to vinca alkaloids and anthracyclines could be reversed both in vitro and in vivo with the calcium channel blocker, verapamil or with quinidine (Tsuruo, 1984). It is now recognized that verapamil can also at least partially reverse doxorubicin resistance, and that this form of reversal appears to be specific for tumors which express increased quantities of the P-glycoprotein. Dalton et al. (1986) have recently reported on their development of a doxorubicin-resistant human multiple myeloma cell line which expresses increased amounts of P-glycoprotein and the characteristic MDR1 phenotype. Of interest, this cell line also exhibits enhanced sensitivity to glucocorticoids (Dalton, 1986). This doxorubicin-resistant myeloma line also exhibits reversal of resistance with the addition of verapamil. The antiarrhythmic agents appear to inhibit drug efflux in drug resistant cells by inhibiting binding of drugs to the P-glycoprotein (Cornwell, 1986, 1987). We have recently analyzed P-glycoprotein expression in patients with B-cell neoplasms (multiple myeloma and non-Hodgkin's lymphoma) and found that it is expressed in some patients who have developed resistance to the combination of vincristine, doxorubicin and dexamethasone (VAD) administered as reported by Barlogie et al. (1984). In studies using HTCA, we have observed that in fresh lymphoma and myeloma specimens tested in vitro, pharmacologically achievable doses of verapamil can reverse doxorubicin resistance, and that this agent on some occasions exhibits single agent activity as well. Accordingly, we have initiated clinical trials of VAD plus verapamil in patients with known VAD or doxorubicin resistance. These studies have been most encouraging, as we have found that some patients with these neoplasms can enter complete remissions when treated with VAD plus verapamil (Dalton, 1988). Such strategies can be most quickly tested initially in the advanced cancer setting, but likely also warrant early neoadjuvant testing in tumor types that frequently exhibit clinical multidrug resistance but would otherwise be amenable to neoadjuvant chemotherapy. Evidence recently published suggests this approach may be worthwhile in both lung (Milroy et al., 1987; Chauffert, 1987) and kidney cancer (Fojo, 1987b). The use of verapamil plus doxorubicin has also been studied in ovarian cancer by Ozols et al. (1987), but in that setting did not appear to induce doxorubicin sensitivity, however in that series, P-glycoprotein expression was not reported.

It has also been observed that other antiarrhythmic drugs such as amiodarone can also reverse the MDR1 phenotype in vitro on various tumor cell lines at pharmacologically achievable concentrations (Chauffert, 1987). In preliminary studies using HTCA on fresh specimens, we have confirmed the ability of amiodarone to reverse doxorubicin or vincristine resistance. Our group has also observed that several tumor cell lines exhibiting the MDR1 phenotype exhibit increased sensitivity to tumor necrosis factor (Salmon, 1987). Finally, Hamada and Tsuruo (1986) have recently reported the development of a monoclonal antibody to the P-glycoprotein which binds to the surface of viable drug resistant tumor cells, and is capable of inhibiting cell proliferation and enhancing vincristine but not doxorubin sensitivity. Conjugating this antibody to toxins, drugs and especially to radioisotopes may also provide an approach to direct therapeutic attack on just those cells exhibiting the MDR1 phenotype. If such approaches are found active in advanced cancer without excessive toxicity, they likely will also be examined in neoadjuvant chemotherapy as well.

REFERENCES

Barlogie, B., Smith, L., Alexanian, R. (1984): Effective treatment of advanced multiple myeloma refractory to alkylating agents. New Engl. J. Med. 310, 1353-1356.

Beck, W.T., Mueller, T.J., Tanzer, L.R. (1979): Altered surface membrane glycoproteins in vinca alkaloid resistant leukemic lymphoblasts. Cancer Res. 39, 2070-2076.

Beck, W.T. (1984): Cellular pharmacology of vinca alkaloid resistance and its circumvention. Advances in Enzyme Regulation 22, 207-227.

Chauffert, B., Rey, D., Coudert, B., Dumas, M., Martin, F. (1987): Amiodarone is more efficient than verapamil in reversing resistance to anthracyclines in tumour cells. Br. J. Cancer 56, 119-122.

Chen, C.J., Chin, J.E., Ueda, K. (1986): Internal duplication and homology with bacterial transport proteins in the MDR1 (P-glycoprotein) gene from multidrug resistant human cells. Cell 47, 381-389.

Cornwell, M.M., Safa, A.R., Felsted, R.L., et al. (1986): Membrane vesicles from multidrug resistant human cancer cells contain a specific 150-170 kDa protein detected by photoaffinity labeling. Proc. Natl. Acad. Sci. USA 83, 3847-3850.

Cornwell, M.M., Pastan, I., Gottesman, M.M. (1987): Certain calcium channel blockers bind specifically to multidrug resistant KB carcinoma membrane vesicles and inhibit binding to P-glycoprotein. J. Biol. Chem. 262, 2166-2170.

Cowan, K.H., Batist, G., Tulpule, A., et al. (1986): Similar biochemical changes associated with multidrug resistance in human breast cancer cells and carcinogen-induced resistance to xenobiotics in rats. Proc. Natl. Acad. Sci. 83, 9328-9332.

Dalton, W.S., Durie, B.G.M., Alberts, D.S., et al. (1986): Characterization of a new drug resistant human myeloma cell line which expresses P-glycoprotein. Cancer Res. 46, 5125-5130.

Dalton, W.S., Grogan, T.M., Durie, B.G.M., Meltzer, P.S., Scheper, R.J., Taylor, C.W., Miller, T.P., Salmon, S.E. (1988): Drug resistance in multiple myeloma and non-Hodgkin's lymphoma: Detection of P-glycoprotein and potential circumvention by addition of verapamil to chemotherapy. Submitted, New Engl. J. Med.

Fojo, A.T., Ueda, K., Slamon, D.J., et al. (1987a): Expression of a multidrug resistance gene in human tumors and tissues. Proc. Natl. Acad. Sci. 84, 265-269.

Fojo, A.T., Shen, D.W., Mickley, L.A., Pastan, I., Gottesman, M.M. (1987b): Intrinsic drug reistance in human kidney cancer is associated with expression of a human multidrug resistance gene. J. Clin. Oncol. 5, 1922-1927.

Gerlach, J.H., Kartner, N., Bell, D.R., et al. (1986): Multidrug resistance. Cancer Surveys 5, 25-46.

Hamada, H., Tsuruo, T. (1986): Functional role for the 170-180-kDa glycoprotein specific to drug resistant tumor cells as revealed by monoclonal antibodies. Proc. Natl. Acad. Sci. 83, 7785-7789.

Ling, V. (1975): Drug resistance and membrane alterations in mutants of mammalian cells. Canad. J. Genetics and Cytol. 17, 503-515.

Milroy, B., Connery, L., Banham, S., et al. (1987): A randomised trial of verapamil in addition to chemotherapy for small cell lung cancer. Thorax 47, 209.

Ozols, R.F., Cunnion, R.E., Klecker, R.W., Hamilton, T.C., Ostchega, Y., Parrillo, J.E., Young, R.C. (1987): Verapamil and adriamycin in the treatment of drug resistant ovarian cancer patients. J. Clin. Oncol. 5, 641-647.

Riordan, J.R., Ling, V. (1979): Genetic and biochemical characterization of multidrug resistance. Pharmacol. and Therapeutics 18, 51-75.

Salmon, S.E. (1987): Drug resistance and adjuvant therapy of cancer. In Adjuvant Therapy of Cancer V, ed S.E. Salmon, pp 3-12. Orlando: Grune and Stratton Press.

Scheper, R.J., Bulte, J.W.M., Wuak, J.J., Brakkee, J.G.P., Broxterman, H., Kuiper, C.M., Lankelma, J. (1987): Production of a monoclonal antibody (JSB-1) with high affinity for multidrug (MDR) resistant tumor cells. Proc. Amer. Assoc. Cancer Res. 28, 360.

Schimke, R.T. (1984): Gene amplification in cultured cells. Cell 37, 705-713.

Tsuruo, T., Iida, H., Tsukagoshi, S., Sakurai, Y. (1982): Increased accumulation of vincristine and adriamycin in drug resistant P388 tumor cells following incubation with calcium antagonists and calmodulin inhibitors. Cancer Res. 42, 4730.

Tsuruo, T., Iida, H., Kitatani, Y., et al. (1984): Effects of quinidine and related compounds on cytotoxicity and cellular accumulation of vincristine and adriamycin in drug resistant tumor cells. Cancer Res. 44, 4303-4307.

Résumé

La chimiothérapie néoadjuvante est administrée quand le risque de résistance pléïotropique est considéré comme faible. Dans cet article nous rappelons les arguments qui montrent que la résistance pléïotropique peut être présente avant tout traitement et qu'elle peut être potentiellement corrigée en utilisant des approches thérapeutiques visant à inhiber la fonction de pompe à efflux de médicaments, de la membrane cellulaire.

Neo-Adjuvant Chemotherapy. Ed. Cl. Jacquillat, M. Weil, D. Khayat. Colloque INSERM/John Libbey Eurotext Ltd. © 1988. Vol. 169, pp. 25-30.

On design of combination chemotherapy regimens to be used alone or in an adjuvant setting

Howard E. Skipper

President Emeritus, Southern Research Institute, PO Box 55305, Birmingham, Alabama, USA

ABSTRACT

In this presentation I will try to use a question and response format in pointing to some tumor variables and treatment variables that are important in combination chemotherapy design.

KEY WORDS

Tumor variables; Treatment variables; Combination design.

INTRODUCTION

It is always a pleasure to return to this beautiful city on the Seine. The older I get, the more beautiful Paris seems to become--perhaps because I now take more time to enjoy the city and the delightful people who live here.

It is a double pleasure to follow Dr. DeVita and to speak in this first session in the company of other friends, Drs. Tubiana, Jasmin, Salmon, and Goldie.

Today I will talk briefly about the importance of the design of combination chemotherapy regimens to be used alone or in an adjuvant setting when treating disseminated cancers.

Much of what I will have to say is based on detailed analyses of hundreds of multiarmed trials carried out in animals bearing different cancers at different stages of advancement--and treated with all sorts of single drugs and combinations of drugs delivered in different ways.

In order to make the points I want to make, I will have to oversimplify. If I had time, I would stop after each conclusion offered and amplify or qualify its implications.

This morning I plan to pose some broad questions and respond to them briefly, but as carefully as I can.

QUESTION 1. What are the major phenomena underlying the responsiveness of different cancers to different drugs and combinations of drugs when used alone or in an adjuvant setting?

RESPONSE

1. The total tumor stem cell burden at the initiation of treatment.
2. The fraction of tumor stem cells committed to DNA replication and division per unit time (the "Growth Fraction").
3. The proportions and absolute numbers of diverse and limiting T/R cells (local and disseminated) at a given stage of disease advancement.
4. What I mean by T/0 and limiting T/R cells is indicated in Fig. 1.

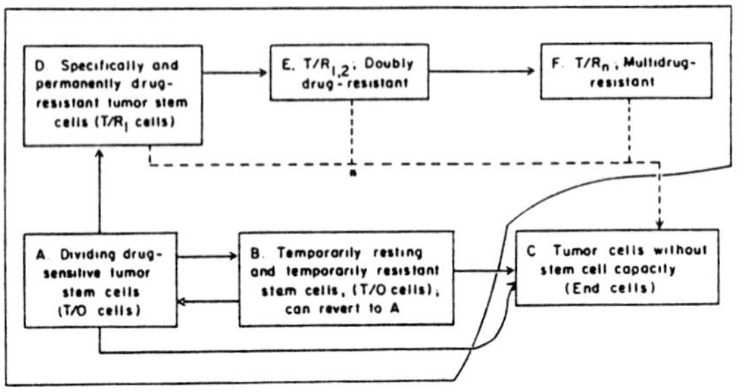

Tumor Stem Cell Compartments

*Resistant phenotypes may go into and out of resting phase but they remain T/R_1 or $T/R_{1,2}$ or T/R_n cells.

Fig. 1. Tumor stem cell heterogeneity and response to chemotherapy

1. There is strong evidence that the origin of diverse T/R cells is as follows: $T/0 \rightarrow T/R_1 \rightarrow T/R_{1,2} \rightarrow T/R_n$.

2. Prior to treatment, one may expect the following relative proportions of tumor stem cells in almost any type of cancer: $T/0 > T/R_1 > T/R_{1,2} > T/R_n$ (if any).

3. Local treatment (when feasible) reduces the burden of T/0 and T/R cells.

4. Cure with Drug A only will be impossible if T/A cells are present. Cure with Drug B only will be impossible if T/B cells are present. Cure with any combination of Drug A and Drug B only will be impossible if T/A/B cells are present at the initiation of chemotherapy or emerge during treatment. The more rapid the reduction of T/0 cells, the lower the probability of continuing emergence of limiting T/R cells.

5. There is an invariable inverse relation between the tumor stem cell burden and curability with chemotherapy, albeit with wide differences in the total burden curable by a given drug or combination in different cancers. There is a direct relation between the total tumor stem cell burden and the probability of the presence of limiting T/R cells, but with significant differences in this probability in different types of cancer at a given stage of advancement.

QUESTION 2. Why is adjuvant chemotherapy (when feasible) often superior to chemotherapy alone, or local treatment alone, when treating disseminated cancers?

RESPONSE

1. Because local treatment reduces the burden of both T/0 and T/R cells, sometimes to levels curable by near optimally selected and delivered combination chemotherapy.

2. When adjuvant chemotherapy fails, I presume that the residual tumor stem cell burden <u>after local treatment</u> was too high to be eradicated by the combination chemotherapy design employed.
3. Curves <u>ac</u> and <u>e</u> in Fig. 2 provide idealized illustrations.

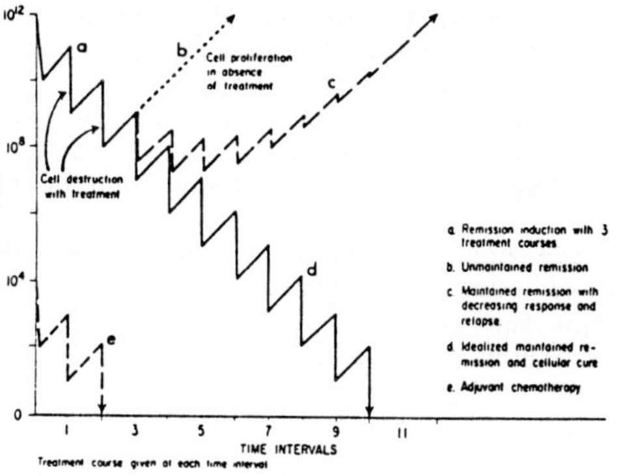

Fig. 2. Idealized time-action response curves for the total tumor stem cells (T/O + T/R)

<u>Curve ab</u>: Cessation of treatment after three courses. A second response with the same drug or drugs might or might not be possible, depending on the T/R to T/O stem cell ratio at the cessation of treatment and at relapse (see Fig. 3).

<u>Curve ac</u>: A classical illustration of tumor response followed by tumor progression during continuing undiminished treatment with the same drug or combination of drugs. A nadir will be reached when the surviving tumor stem cell burden is comprised of about 50% limiting T/R cells (T/R to T/O ratio = 1.0). Tumor progression will be observed when the T/R to T/O ratio exceeds 1.0 (see Fig. 3).

<u>Curve ad</u>: This type of curve would almost never be expected on treating individuals bearing, say, 10^9 or > tumor stem cells with a single drug because of the high probability of the presence of T/R cells with specific resistance. Burkitt's lymphoma and choriocarcinoma may or may not be exceptions to this generalization.

<u>Curve e</u>: Cure of relatively small numbers of metastatic stem cells after local surgery or radiation that left no T/R cells that were resistant to the drug or drugs employed.

<u>QUESTION 3</u>. What are the reasons for the superiority of near optimally delivered combination chemotherapy over single drug treatment?

<u>RESPONSE</u>

1. Well designed combination chemotherapy regimens offer the chance of eradicating the T/R cells that would overgrow during continuing maximum tolerated treatment with a single drug.
2. In addition, some drug combinations are less than strictly additive in toxicity. This is a bonus.

QUESTION 4. What are the major problems faced in designing curative combinations to be used alone or in an adjuvant setting?

RESPONSE

1. Toxicity.
2. Matching the dose intensity of each drug in a combination in a manner that will eradicate the T/0 and T/R cells or, failing that, provide the longest possible relapse-free survival.
3. The models of Goldie and Coldman (1979, 1982, and 1983) and the retrospective analyses of clinical combination chemotherapy trials by Hryniuk and associates (1984, and In Press) have been helpful to me.

QUESTION 5. What are the dose and schedule variables which affect both toxicity and therapeutic response? Or, in other words, what variables do we have to work with in trying to design the best possible combinations from the drugs available today--and new agents as they come to hand in the years ahead?

RESPONSE

1. The dose and schedule variables that influence both toxicity and therapeutic response are these:

Treatment Variables	Type
1. Individual dose level	Dose
2. Interval between doses	Schedule
3. No. of doses	Schedule
4. Duration of Rx (2 X 3)	Schedule
5. Total dose (1 X 3)	Dose
6. Dose intensity (1 X 3) / (2 X 3)	Dose per unit time

2. When designing any combination chemotherapy regimen, one is forced to make decisions regarding each of the six dose and schedule variables for each drug in the combination. Needless to say, choosing a near optimum combination chemotherapy design becomes increasingly complicated as we add more drugs to the combination.
3. In large numbers of internally controlled combination chemotherapy trials carried out in uniformly staged animals bearing a given cancer, we have consistently observed the following:

   (a) Poorly designed multidrug combinations are not nearly as effective as well designed 2-drug combinations.

   (b) Poorly designed 2-drug combinations are not nearly as effective as the optimum delivery of the best single drug in the 2-drug combination.

   In other words, it is common, all too common, to discover (after much effort) that combination chemotherapy design can be more important than the number of drugs in a combination. Furthermore, a combination design that is near optimum for one cancer may be a poor one for another cancer--for fairly obvious reasons.

QUESTION 6. Has 25+ years of intuitive and trial-and-error manipulation of combination chemotherapy designs--at both the experimental and clinical levels--taught us anything that might be useful in prospective design of more effective combination regimens for treating disseminated human cancers?

RESPONSE

1. I think so, but some of the newer concepts based on (a) theory or (b) computer simulations or (c) retrospective analyses of available experimental and clinical combination trial results have yet to be tested in many human cancers.
2. It seems to me that the clinical analyses of Hryniuk and Bush were an important step in developing better guidelines for designing combinations to be used alone or in an adjuvant setting. They noted a direct relation between the average relative dose intensity of the drugs in combinations and observed therapeutic response.
3. In retrospective analyses of many combination trials carried out in experimental cancers, we have seen good correlations between the avg. RDI and the degree and duration of therapeutic response--but with some notable exceptions. I think that the circumstances and the reasons for such exceptions may have important implications.

   The exceptions were seen in 2-drug combinations comprised of one very effective and one moderately effective drug. The exceptions were traceable to regimens in which the dose intensity of the most effective drug was reduced below a critical level. Then poor results were achieved, regardless of the RDI of the less effective drug or the avg. RDI (Skipper, 1986 and 1987).

   The matching of the dose intensities of both drugs was not so critical in 2-drug combinations comprised of two very effective drugs. It appears to me that the "most of the best" rule holds in combination chemotherapy design with one fairly obvious qualification. The dose intensity of the less effective drug (or drugs) must be high enough to eradicate the phenotypes that are resistant to the most effective drug (or drugs) if cure is to be achieved.

   A little study of the idealized nomogram in Fig. 3 might help to indicate both the tumor and treatment variables that I think are important in combination chemotherapy design.

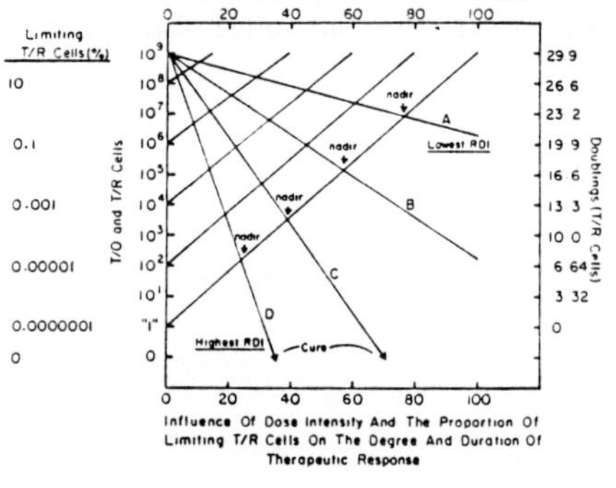

Fig. 3. An idealized nomogram illustrating the influence of the dose intensity of single drugs or combinations of drugs and the proportion of limiting T/R cells on the degree and duration of therapeutic response

1. Follow lines A, B, C, or D (for T/O cells) down to where they cross lines for various assumed burdens of limiting T/R cells. The nadir will be reached when the surviving burden is about 50% T/R and 50% T/O cells. Continuing the same treatment past the nadir will result in tumor progression.

2. Increasing the dose intensity of a single drug or the average relative dose intensity of a combination will increase the net rate of reduction of T/0 cells and result in (a) a shorter duration of treatment required to reach the nadir, (b) a lower total surviving burden at the nadir, and (c) a longer duration of remission after the nadir is reached.

3. If two non-cross-resistant drugs are used in combination (Drug A and Drug B) the net rate of T/0 cell reduction is influenced by the dose intensity of both drugs (avg. RDI). On the other hand, the net rate of decrease or increase of T/A cells will be related to the dose intensity of Drug B and the net rate of reduction or increase of T/B cells will be related to the dose intensity of Drug A. It is important to match the dose intensities of all drugs in a combination in a manner that offers the possibility of eradicating the T/0 cells and the T/R cells that are resistant to each drug in the combination. (When feasible, adjuvant chemotherapy improves the chances for cure, because local treatment reduces the absolute numbers of T/0 and T/R stem cells.)

4. Different cancers of a given size containing, say, 0.1% or > T/R cells that are resistant to the chemotherapy employed might be classified as very refractory, while those containing 0.00001% or < might be classified as very responsive.

REFERENCES

Goldie, J.H. and Coldman, A.J. (1979). A mathematic model for relating the drug sensitivity of tumors to their spontaneous mutation rate. Cancer Treat. Rep. 63, 1727-1731.

Goldie, J.H., Coldman, A.J. and Gudauskas, G.A. (1982). Rationale for the use of alternating non-cross-resistant chemotherapy. Cancer Treat. Rep. 66, 439-449.

Goldie, J.H. and Coldman, A.J. (1983). Quantitative model for multiple levels of resistance in clinical tumors. Cancer Treat. Rep. 67, 923-931.

Hryniuk, W. and Bush, H. (1984). The importance of dose intensity in chemotherapy of metastatic breast cancer. J. Clin. Oncol. 2, 1281-1288.

Hryniuk, W. (In press). Importance of dose intensity on the outcome of chemotherapy. In Advances in Oncology, ed V.T. DeVita, Jr., S. Hellman, and S.A. Rosenberg, Philadelphia: J.B. Lippincott Co.

Skipper, H.E. (1986, 1987). Informal reports from Southern Research Institute to Division of Cancer Treatment of the National Cancer Institute.

Neo-Adjuvant Chemotherapy. Ed. Cl. Jacquillat, M. Weil, D. Khayat. Colloque INSERM/John Libbey Eurotext Ltd. © 1988. Vol. 169, pp. 31-35.

Leukemic stem cells and the chemocurability of human leukemia and lymphoma

C. Jasmin, V. Georgoulias and C. Boucheix

Unité d'Oncogenèse Appliquée, INSERM U.268, Hôpital Paul Brousse, 14-16 Avenue Paul Vaillant-Couturier, 94800 Villejuif, France

RESUME

We postulate the existence of two levels of chemoincurability of human leukemia and lymphomas : a) when the malignant transformation has occurred on the compartement of pluripotent stem cells, the disease is chemoincurable and chemoresistant leukemic cells will invariably develop during the prolonged course of the disease. Bone marrow transplantation is the only curative approach which is presently available. b) When the disease involves only the transformation of committed precursors, it is chemocurable unless chemoresistant clones are present or/will develop during treatment. Bone marrow transplantation can be used as a salvage treatment after relapse.

MOTS CLEFS

Chimiocurabilité, leucémies et lymphomes, cellules souches pluripotentes, précurseurs commis, greffe de moelle osseuse.

KEY WORDS

Chemocurability, leukemias and lymphomas, pluripotent stem cells, committed precursors, bone marrow transplantation.

The advent of chemotherapy constitutes a turning point in the treatment of human malignancy. Chemotherapy permits the treatment and cure of various malignancies including acute leukemias, lymphomas (Table 1) and a number of solid tumors even when disease is disseminated and involves a large tumor mass. According to the current prevailing ideology, the present limitations of the chemocurability of human cancer result from the insufficiency of available active antimitotic drugs and from their infra-optimal utilisation.

Table 1. The chemocurability of human leukemias and lymphomas

Chemocurable	Chemo-incurable
Hodgkin's disease	Low grade malignancy non-Hodgkin lymphomas.
Burkitt's lymphomas	Myeloma
A fraction of diffuse lymphomas belonging to the high or intermediate grade of malignancy	A fraction of acute leukemias (mainly adults and non-lymphocytic leukemias)
Some acute lymphocyte and non lymphocytic leukemias (mostly in children and young adults).	All chronic leukemias.

Modern cancer chemotherapy is based on the remarkable work of Skipper, Schabel and coworkers (1984), the Goldie and Coldman hypothesis (1979) and the more recent concepts of late intensification (Norton and Simon, 1977 et 1986). In all these theories, chemoincurability of malignant diseases depends only of a genetic (preexisting or induced) chemoresistance similar to the antibioresistance of bacteria. However, it is important to note that the most recent model of Goldie and Coldman (1984) has taken into account the role of stem cell differentiation in the development of chemoresistance.

Thus the aims and hopes of modern cancer chemotherapy have focused on : a) the development of new families of antimitotic drugs, b) the use of massive or even lethal doses agents combined with bone-marrow auto-grafts, c) the development of combinations of drugs administered in alternating cycles in order to minimise the chemoresistance of tumor stem cells.

Although we lack sufficient hindsight to fully evaluate the efficacy of these new strategies, it seems that such strategies has increased the cure rate of some chemocurable leukemias and lymphomas but has not allowed the cure of cancers considered to be chemoincurable despite the uses of new drugs and therapeutic trials designed according to the above mentioned new concepts.

This body of clinical results raise the question of whether the chemocurability of certain tumors and not others is due to quantitative differences in the chemosensitivity of various malignant human tumors or rather to qualitative differences between chemocurable and chemoincurable tumors reflecting fundamental biological differences between the cells of these two categories of tumors. Several characteristics suggest that chemocurable tumors do indeed differ in their basic biological properties : chemocurable cancers are rare, occur essentially in children or young adults, are often poorly differentiated and/or of embryonic origin, and grow rapidly. Relapses usually occur within the first years of follow-up, and most, if not all, patients can be considered as cured with or without chemotherapy after three years without relapse. These features are found in chemocurable acute leukemias and lymphomas, with the exception of Hodgkin's lymphoma which represents a rather particular pathologic entity. The low frequency of late relapses in these tumors suggests that the vast majority of them do not contain tumor stem cells capable of unlimited proliferation.

In contrast, chemoincurable tumors include the majority of the most frequent human cancers and usually occur after fifty years of age. Chronic leukemias and lymphomas show varying degrees of differentiation. Many of them have a slow doubling time and a prolonged course lasting up to 10 years, as for example, chronic lymphoïd leukemia or polycythemia vera even in the absence of treatment. Nodular lymphomas are also good examples of indolent chemocurable diseases.

The fact that chemotherapy can eradicate the malignant cells of certain cancers without causing irreversible destruction of the normal stem cells of essential tissues such as the bone marrow or digestive mucosa suggests that differences exist between the phenotype of normal stem cells and precursor cells of those human tumors which are cured by chemotherapy. Therefore, the study of the biological properties of precursor cells of chemocurable tumors compared with those of chemoincurable tumors and their normal counterparts, may provide valuable insight into the reasons why chemotherapy succeds in some cancers and fails in others. We postulate that malignant leukemias and lymphomas conserve the same organisation as the normal tissues with unlimited proliferative capacity from which they are derived (Jasmin and al., 1984, 1986, 1988). Normal tissues such as the bone marrow which undergo continuous renewal contain both primitive pluripotent stem cells and committed precursor cells. Thus our model would predict that for the most part chemocurable leukemias and lymphomas derive from the malignant transformation of committed precursor cells. These cells are actively dividing with a short doubling time and are thus sensitive to cycle dependant antimitotic agents. Such tumors do not give rise to late relapses or metastases due to the absence of malignant primitive stem cells. Furthermore in these types of cancers the possibility exists that committed malignant precursor cells may be eliminated by a process of terminal differentiation.

In differentiated leukemias such as chronic myeloid leukemias, known to involve transformation of the pluripotent hematopoietic stem cells, although the disease is not chemocurable the tumor cells are in fact chemosensitive. This is also the case of erythroïd, lymphoid, myelomonocytic and hairy cell leukemia. It should be emphasized that only histocompatible allogeneic bone marrow grafts are capable of curing chronic myeloid leukemia.

But the involvement of a primitive hematopoietic stem cells may also determine the chemocurability of acute leukemias. Indeed, the recent results of Fialkow et al (1987), based on the study of the X-chromosome linked-enzyme glucose-6-phosphate dehydrogenase, provide strong evidence for the existence of two clonal forms of acute non-lymphocytic leukemia. In one form of the disease prevalent in children and young adults, clonal leukemic committed myeloid progenitor cells are detected and nonclonal remission are frequent with repopulation of the bone marrow by normal stem cells. In contrast, the study shows that the other form of acute non-lymphocytic leukemia which occurs mainly in the elderly, arises from multipotent stem cells and that in these patients, marrow stem cells remain clonal even during remission. According to our model, cases of acute non-lymphocytic leukemia cured by chemotherapy would all belong to the form of the disease characterized by the absence of primitive leukemic stem cells.

Indeed, the presence of pluripotent leukemic stem cells would make selective eradication of the tumor extremely difficult in the absence of a specific antitumor action of the drugs currently employed. The recent results of Tachibana et al. (1987) also provide strong support for our hypothesis. Their results show that pluripotent stem cells are involved in the pathogenesis of some types of Philadelphia-chromosome-positive acute lymphoblastic leukemia and may indeed contribute to the poor prognosis of this form of the disease which contrasts with the great chemocurability of acute lymphocytic leukemia in children. It is clear that it would be difficult to eradicate completely pluripotential leukemic stem cells by the use of myelotoxic drugs unless such drugs are used in conjunction with bone marrow grafts as is the current trend.

In conclusion, we postulate the existence of two levels of chemoincurability of human leukemia and lymphomas : a) when the malignant transformation has occurred on the compartement of pluripotent stem cells, the disease is chemoincurable and chemoresistant leukemic cells will invariably develop during the prolonged course of the disease. Bone marrow transplantation is the only curative approach which is presently available. b) When the disease involves only the transformation of committed precursors, it is chemocurable unless chemoresistant clones are present or/will develop during treatment. Bone marrow transplantation can be used as a salvage treatment after relapse.

The discovery of substances such as growth factors, which control the division and proliferation of normal and malignant cells, holds promise for the development of new approaches to cancer therapy in the near future. It can be hoped that new biologic approaches such as immunotherapy, the use of differentiating agents, growth factors, or growth factors agonists, could help to alter the primitive tumor stem cell compartment for therapeutic purposes (Jasmin, 1987). Although there are currently no means of identifying primitive stem cells in normal and malignant tissues of solid tumors, it is to be hoped that, as in the case of hematopoietic precursors, specific and early genetic markers of commitment of tumor stem cells will be found.

REFERENCES

Fialkow F.J., Singer G.W., Raskind W.H., Adamson J.W. and al. (1987) : Clonal development, stem cell differentiation and clinical remission in acute non-lymphocytic leukemia. New Eng. J. of Med. 317, 468-473.

Goldie J.H., Coldman A.J. (1979) : A mathematical model for relating the drug sensitivity of tumors in their spontaneous mutation rate. Cancer Treat. Rep. 63, 1727-1733.

Goldie J.H., Coldman A.J. (1984) : The genetic origin of drug resistance in neoplasms. Implications for systemic therapy. Cancer Res. 44, 3643-3653.

Jasmin C. (1988) : The chemocurability of human cancer. Cancer Therapy Update, In press.

Jasmin C. (1987) : Le traitement biologique des cancers. La recherche 18, N°189, 754-764.

Jasmin C., Judde J.G., Georgoulias V. (1984) : Models for adjuvant therapy. Adjuvant Therapy of Cancer IV (Edited by Salmon S.) 35-45, Grune and Stratton, Tucson, N.Y.

Jasmin C., Poupon M.F., Smadja-Joffe F. and al. (1986) : Tumor stem cells and their ecosystem : Therapeutic implications of a new concept. R and B Symposium, Local immunity in cancer. Edition E. Macher and C. Sorg, Regensberg and Biermann Publ., Munchen, 114-123.

Norton L. and Simon R. (1977) : Tumor size, sensitivity to therapy, and design of treatment schedules. Cancer Treat. Rep. 61, 1307-1317.

Norton L. and Simon R. (1986) : The Norton-Simon hypothesis revisited. Cancer Treat. Rep. 70, 163-170.

Skipper H.E., Schabel F.M. Jr (1984) : Tumor stem cell heterogeneity : implications with respect to classification of cancers by chemotherapeutic effect. Cancer Treat. 60, 43-61.

Tachibana N., Raimondi S.C., Lauer S.J., Sartain P. and Dow L.W. (1987) : Evidence for a multipotential stem cell disease in some childhood Philadelphia chromosome positive acute lymphoblastic leukemia. Blood 70, N°5:1458-1461.

Résumé

Nous postulons l'existence de deux niveaux de chimio-incurabilité des leucémies et lymphomes humains : a) quand la transformation maligne est survenue au niveau du compartiment des cellules souches pluripotentes, la maladie est chimio-incurable et des cellules leucémiques chimio-résistantes se développeront toujours sous chimiothérapie. La greffe de moelle osseuse est le seul traitement potentiellement curatif quand elle est possible ; b) quand la leucémisation porte uniquement sur les compartiments des précurseurs hématopoïétiques commis, la maladie est chimiocurable sauf s'il se développe des clones chimio-résistants. Dans ce cas, la greffe de moelle osseuse pourrait servir de traitement de rattrapage en cas de rechute de la maladie.

Neo-Adjuvant Chemotherapy. Ed. Cl. Jacquillat, M. Weil, D. Khayat. Colloque INSERM/John Libbey Eurotext Ltd. © 1988. Vol. 169, pp. 37-41.

Drug resistance, heterogeneity and neo-adjuvant chemotherapy

Andrew J. Coldman and James H. Goldie

Cancer Control Agency of British Columbia, 600 West 10th Avenue, Vancouver, British Columbia, V5Z 4E6 Canada

ABSTRACT

Neo-adjuvant chemotherapy has been proposed as a therapeutic manoeuvre which may be utilised to reduce the likelihood that a tumor will develop drug resistance. The effect of tumor heterogeneity and in particular, the effect of variation in post-surgical tumor burdens and tumor growth rates is shown to diminish the benefits (which may otherwise be expected) of neo-adjuvant chemotherapy. The conclusions from this analysis are discussed with respect to the neo-adjuvant chemotherapy of breast cancer. Although the exact increase in the probability of no resistance cannot be calculated without error, it is found that the range for the reduction in this probability is 1% to 4%. For neo-adjuvant chemotherapy to be demonstrably better in breast cancer clinical trials it will also have to influence other (than drug resistance) clinical parameters which control prognosis.

Key words: neo-adjuvant chemotherapy, drug resistance, tumor heterogeneity

INTRODUCTION

Neo-adjuvant chemotherapy was originally proposed for the treatment of disease whose extent indicated that definitive surgery (and/or radiotherapy) was not initially possible (Frei, 1982). It has also been recomended for use in situations where definitive treatment is possible and it is then used for the control of micrometastases. The rationale for the use of neo-adjuvant chemotherapy need not be the same in each of these situations and a variety of reasons for making this change in the timing of treatment have been suggested. Prominent among the justifications suggested for its' likely superiority in the treatment of micrometastatic disease has been the idea that neoadjuvant chemotherapy will reduce the likelihood that drug resistant cells will emerge and cause treatment failure (Fisher, 1986; Ragaz, 1986). We will examine whether this assertion is supported by consideration of a mutational model for drug resistance.

MODELLING NEO-ADJUVANT CHEMOTHERAPY

Clinical drug resistance, that is the insensitivity of tumors to chemotherapy, can arise from a number of specific causes. Such causes include problems involved with drug metabolism, drug access, location of the tumor etc (Hall, 1986). We will only be concerned with one of the possible causes; the development of permanently drug resistant cells. These cells may emerge at either the genesis of the tumor or spontaneously develop as it grows (Skipper, 1978). Available evidence from in-vivo and in-vitro experimentation would lead one to expect that the development of resistance followed laws of somatic mutation theory

(Ling, 1983). Under this hypothesis the development of resistance is a random event occurring in a cell and this resistance is subsequently inherited by all the progeny of the original cell. Somatic mutation theory may be simply analyzed in mathematical terms so that the implications of this theory may be quantitatively expressed (Goldie and Coldman, 1979). Using this mathematical theory it is a simple matter to show that the likelihood that a tumor will have no resistant cells, P, at first treatment is given by (Goldie and Coldman, 1979)

$$P=e^{-\alpha(T-1)}. \tag{1}$$

where α is the probability that a cell resistant to the drug will arise upon division of one which was sensitive and T is the number of tumor cells at first treatment. More precisely T should be interpreted as the number of tumor cells with clonogenic capacity, although for simplicity we will continue to refer to it as the number of tumor cells.

Equation (1) only applies prior to the commencement of therapy and must be modified to accomodate the effects of treatment (Coldman and Goldie, 1983). However we may use equation (1) to see why early treatment may be beneficial. Using chemotherapy earlier has the effect of bringing about a reduction in T since the earlier a tumor is treated the smaller it will be. If we assume, for the purposes of this discussion, that the change in the probability of no resistant cells is directly related to the likelihood of cure then one may use equation (1) to estimate the effect of earlier application of therapy as follows.

For simplicity we will use equation (1) to give an approximate expression for the increase in the probability of no resistant cells achieve by the use of neo-adjuvant chemotherapy although the calculated magnitude of the effect will only be approximate. We will not specify the drug or drugs used in the chemotherapy regimen, but will assume in all cases that the drugs used in the neo-adjuvant cycle or cycles are the same as those used in the adjuvant programme. Let T_N be the size of the tumor at the time of neo-adjuvant therapy and T_A the size when adjuvant therapy would normally be applied and let P_N and P_A be the respective probabilities of no resistant cells, then

$$P_N-P_A = P_A[e^{\alpha(T_A-T_N)}-1]. \tag{2}$$

The expression P_N-P_A measures the gain in the likelihood of no resistant cells and shows that this is a function of the probability of no resistant cells for the standard adjuvant programme, P_A, the mutation rate, α, and the difference in tumor sizes, T_N-T_A. Examination of equation (2) reveals that the expected improvement in the probability of no resistant cells associated with neo-adjuvant chemotherapy depends upon:

- the magnitude of the probability of no resistant cells when treated with usual adjuvant therapy;
- the change in tumor size which would occur in the absence of neo-adjuvant therapy and
- the mutation for the drug or combination.

It is not possible to view these as three independent factors which influence the effect of neoadjuvant chemotherapy since P_A depends upon α and T_A (as expressed in equation (1). In neo-adjuvant therapy we attempt to increase the magnitude of T_A-T_N by administering therapy earlier. Clearly the earlier it is applied the better, however in situations where P_A is effectively zero (i.e. adjuvant chemotherapy cures few if any patients), then giving the same therapy earlier is unlikely to have a great effect on the probability of no resistant cells.

In a previous discussion of the effect of neo-adjuvant chemotherapy on the prevention of drug resistance it was assumed that the size, mutation rate and growth rate of each tumor is the same (Ragaz, 1986). Comparitively little is known about mutation rates in spontaneous human neoplasms, indeed it has not been directly demonstrated that clinical resistance arises via a somatic mutation process. Examination of results from different murine leukemias would suggest that there is some variation in the mutation rates for each drug although this may not be great so that the assumption of a common α for each tumor may be reasonable (Skipper, 1965). Variation in tumor burden, even in similarly staged patients, is clearly considerable; more importantly variation in post surgical tumor burden can be large so that it is not reasonable to assume that the predicted values of T_A (and thus P_A) are the same for each of the tumors. Similarly variation in tumor doubling times, in situations in which it can be reliable measured, are known to be considerable so that T_A-T_N will also be variable.

In attempting to use equation (2) to predict the likely benefit of neo-adjuvant chemotherapy we are thus faced with a situation where not only is there considerable uncertainty in the average values of many of the important clinical parameters but it is certain that they vary within any group of patients. Since the results of neo-adjuvant therapy can only be assesed within a group, and not on an individual, this presents a number of problems in attempting to predict the likely increase (in the probability of no resistant cells) which will occur when using neo-adjuvant chemotherapy. One possibility is to use the group averages for each of these parameters and calculate the likely net benefit. Unfortunately in most situations this will not yield a reasonable estimate of the therapeutic gain since the effect of inhomogeneity in parameter values do not 'balance out'. To see this, consider the following extreme situation. A group of patients is to be treated using neo-adjuvant therapy is composed (unknown to the investigator) of two subgroups; subgroup I which consists of patients with very high mutation rates to resistance and subgroup II which have very low mutation rates to resistance to the drug to be used. Patients from the first subgroup respond poorly to therapy whether given in the adjuvant or neo-adjuvant setting since their disease is very likely to be insensitive even when therapy is given early. Similarly patients in subgroup II are likely to be sensitive at both the neo-adjuvant and adjuvant times of therapy application so that neo-adjuvant chemotherapy is again unlikely to be of great benefit. In fact it is possible to show (theoretically using reasonable assumptions) that the effect of variability in the mutation rates to resistance, or variability in tumor burden at first treatment is always to diminish the amount of benefit which might otherwise be expected from the application of neo-adjuvant therapy.

In general we have little idea of the heterogeneity of tumor parameters prior to treatment. Tumor burden variation is reduced by staging however it is unlikely that this also significently reduces any (natural) variation in growth or mutation rates. However given that we do see a substantial relationship between stage of disease and survival after adjuvant treatment, does suggest (again) that the variation in mutation rates is not too great. It is important to note that it is the post-surgical tumor burden which is important and not just the pre-surgical burden. The distribution of recurrence times of those treated with surgery alone displays considerable variability indicating (after allowing for differences in growth rates) that substantial variation exists in post-surgical burdens. The exact magnitude of this variation is difficult to estimate due to ignorance of the doubling time of each tumor. Despite considerable uncertainty as to the value of these unknown parameters it is possible to carry out some calculations of the effect of neo-adjuvant chemotherapy. We will now illustrate such a calculation for breast cancer.

Example: Breast Cancer

Typically neo-adjuvant programmes for operable breast cancer consist of advancing the first course of a 'standard' adjuvant programme to immediate pre- or post-surgery. To simplify presentation we will treat the chemotherapy regimen as if it were a single drug and use the theory previously outlined. We will also assume that the neo-adjuvant cycle is given one day pre-operatively. Assuming that drug resistance is the only reason for therapeutic failure then the increase in curability is a function of the following factors (i) the log-kill of the regimens on sensitive calls, (ii) the value of the mutation rate, (iii) the variation (between individuals) in post-operative tumor burden and (iv) the variation in growth rates. Using data from the recurrence times on women with breast cancer receiving no chemotherapy (Valagussa et al, 1978). it is possible to estimate the distribution of post-operative tumor burden assuming some pre-defined distribution of tumor doubling times (Skipper, 1979). Clearly there is considerable uncertainty in the actual values of many of the parameters used, however, they are constrained. For example, although we do not accurately know the individual doubling times and post-operative tumor burdens, we know that they must combine together to yield a distribution of recurrence times on which we have quite good information. Similarly we may not know the parameter values for the chemotherapy (i.e. mutation rates, log-kill) but we do have good information about the increase in survival associated with adjuvant chemotherapy (Fisher, 1986) which again constrains the values these parameters can take. Using this knowledge we can carry out sensitivity analysis whereby these parameters are systematically altered, yet required to satisfy the basic constraints, and the outcome calculated. Ideally one would hope for a situation in which the calculated impact of the neo-adjuvant cycle varied little with the particular parameter values chosen. Calculation shows that this is reasonably true with predicted increases in curability in the range of 1% to 4% for an extra neo-adjuvant cycle given as described. Smaller increases being found for post-menopausal women especially those with 4+positive modes. Further details of the mathematics of this calculation are given elsewhere (Coldman and Goldie, 1986; Coldman, 1987). This range of rather low estimates suggest that for neo-adjuvant chemotherapy of breast cancer to be reliably demonstrated to be superior in clinical trials either (i) this model or data used are not applicable, (ii) the major benefit of neo-adjuvant therapy cases from some other (unspecified) mechanism or (iii) other factors important to the development of drug resistance have not been included (e.g. growth spurts produced by surgery).

In this presentation we have calculated the effect of neo-adjuvant chemotherapy on the development of drug resistance. However the mathematics used is not specific to this concept and may be used to calculate the effect on preventing the establishment of metastases since these have also been hypothesized to arise by mechanisms which have a mathematical representation analogous to that for drug resistance. Thus similar considerations should apply and the magnitude of the benefit should be comparable. However, one may not simply add the predicted benefits of neo-adjuvant therapy upon each effect as they assume different reasons for the failure of adjuvant chemotherapy.

CONCLUSION

We have examined the effect of neo-adjuvant chemotherapy on the development of permanent drug resistance in cells not removed by 'definitive' therapy. We find that neo-adjuvant chemotherapy is likely to have an effect upon the prevention of drug resistance. The effect of tumor heterogeneity is found to decrease the likely benefit of neo-adjuvant chemotherapy, which indicates the need for accurate staging of patients (and any other techniques which place patients into more homogenous groups). For breast cancer we do not anticipate that the use of an extra neo-adjuvant cycle will have a large effect upon the likelihood of permanent drug resistance. However, growth stimulation of micrometastases caused by the removal of the primary tumor could lead to greater estimated benefits.

REFERENCES

Coldman, A J.(1987): The development of resistance to anti-cancer agents. Ph.D. Thesis, University of British Columbia.

Coldman, A.J. and Goldie, J.H.(1983): A model for the resistance of tumor cells to cancer chemotherapeutic agents. Mathematical Biosciences 65: 291-307.

Coldman, A.J. and Goldie, J.H.(1986): Factors affecting the development of permanent drug resistance and its impact upon neo-adjuvant chemotherapy. In: Pre-operative (Neo-adjuvant) Chemotherapy pp 69-78. Eds: J. Ragaz, P.R. Band and J.H. Goldie, Springer-Verlag. New York.

Fisher, B.(1986): Adjuvants therapy for breast cancer: a brief overview of the NSABP experience and some thoughts on neo-adjuvant chemotherapy. In: Pre-operative (Neo-Adjuvant) Chemotherapy pp 54-68. Eds: J. Ragaz, P.R. Band and J.H. Goldie, Springer-Verlag. New York.

Frei, E.III.(1982): Clinical cancer research: an embattled species. Cancer 50: 1979-1992.

Goldie, J.H. and Coldman, A.J.(1979): A mathematic model for relating the drug sensitivity of tumors to their spontaneous mutation rates. Cancer Treatment Reports 63: 1727-1733.

Hall, T.C.(1986): Conference summary. In: Cancer Drug Resistance, pp 219-228. Ed. T.C. Hall. and Alan R. Liss, New York.

Ling, V.(1983): Genetic basis of drug resistance in mammalian cells. In: Drug and Hormone Resistance in Neoplasia, vol 1. pp 1-19. Eds. N. Bruchovsky and J.H. Goldie. C.R.C. Press, Boca Raton.

Ragaz, J.(1986): Pre-operative (neo-adjuvant) chemotherapy for breast cancer: outline of the British Columbia In: Pre-operative (Neo-Adjuvant) Chemotherapy pp 85-94. Eds: J. Ragaz, P.R. Band and J.H. Goldie, Springer-Verlag, New York.

Skipper, H.(1979): Repopulation rates of breast cancer cells after mastectomy (judged from break-points in remission-duration curves) Booklet 12, Southern Research Institute, Birmingham, Al.

Skipper, H.E., Schabel, F.M.Jr. and Lloyd, H.(1978): Selection and overgrowth of specifically and permanently drug resistant tumor cells. Experimental Therapeutics and Kinetics 15: 207-19.

Skipper, H.E., Schabel, F.M.Jr. and Wilcox, W.S.(1965): Experimental evaluation of potential anti-cancer drugs XIV, further study of certain basic concepts underlying the chemotherapy of leukemia. Cancer Chemotherapy Reports 45: 5-113.1965.

Valagussa, P., Bonadonna, G. and Veronesi, U. Patterns of relapse and survival in operable breast carcinoma with positive and negative axillary nodes. Tumori 64: 241-258.

Résumé

La chimiothérapie néo-adjuvante a été proposée comme une manoeuvre thérapeutique qui peut être utilisée pour réduire la probabilité qu'une tumeur a de développer une résistance aux drogues. En utilisant un modèle de mutation somatique pour la chimiorésistance, nous analysons la situation et montrons que la chimiothérapie néo-adjuvante va rèduire l'éventuelle résistance permanente aux drogues. L'effect d'hétérogénéité de la tumeur et en particulier l'effet de variation dans le masse tumorale post-opératoire et dans les taux de croissance tumoral, a tendance à diminuer les bénéfices (que l'on pouvait attendre) de la chimiothérapie néo-adjuvante du cancer du sein. Bien que l'augmentation exacte de la probabilité de non-résistance ne puisse être calculée sans erreur, on trouve que la diminution de cette probabilité se situe entre 1% et 4%. Si l'on veut que la chimiothérapie néo-adjuvante démontre son effect dans les essais cliniques sur le cancer du sein, elle se doit d'avoir également une influence sur les autres paramètres cliniques pronostiques (autres que la chimiorésistance).

Radio-chemotherapy combinations

Associations radiothérapie-chimiothérapie

Neo-Adjuvant Chemotherapy. Ed. Cl. Jacquillat, M. Weil, D. Khayat. Colloque INSERM/John Libbey Eurotext Ltd. © 1988. Vol. 169, pp. 45-49.

Further experimental studies on alternating chemotherapy and radiotherapy

H.A. Hopkins and W.B. Looney

Division of Radiobiology and Biophysics, University of Virginia Medical Center, Charlottesville, VA 22908, USA

ABSTRACT

The effect of giving cyclophosphamide or radiotherapy as the first agent in alternating treatment schedules was examined in ACI rats with 3924A tumors. The radiation was given as daily fractions or as multiple fractions per day (MFD). Growth delays were not different for daily radiation fractions and MFD alone (27.1 and 29.8 days), or for cyclophosphamide given 7 days before or after MFD radiation (52.1 and 48.5 days). Growth delays differed ($P<.005$) when the drug was given 7 days before daily radiation versus 7 days after daily radiation (50.2 and 42.4 days, respectively). In terms of growth delay, MFD was more effective than daily fractions when the radiation was given first ($P<.025$) but not when cyclophosphamide was given first. Only for cyclophosphamide prior to MFD did the tumor volume regress below initial volume. These results indicate that intensive treatment with effective chemotherapeutic agents or with MFD radiation is preferable to daily radiation fractions as the first agent in schedules which alternate the two modalities for treatment of tumors which are responsive to both modalities.

KEY WORDS

Combined radiotherapy and chemotherapy, multiple fractions per day (MFD) radiotherapy, radiotherapy alternated with cyclophosphamide

INTRODUCTION

Previous studies with the experimental tumor 3924A have demonstrated the effectiveness of treatment schedules in which short intensive courses of radiotherapy are alternated with chemotherapy (Looney et al., 1983, 1984, 1985). Cure rates >50% were obtained with these schedules with acceptable damage to normal tissues, compared with no cures with either therapy alone at similar doses or even at doses exceeding normal tissue limits. Sequential treatment with all of one modality before initiating the other modality was ineffective in obtaining cure of these tumors.

Radiation was the modality given first in these earlier alternating schedules, on the premise that the modality believed to be most generally effective in a particular type of cancer should be first, to reliably reduce the number of tumor cells and minimize the risk of build-up of resistant cells, in accordance with the hypothesis set forth by Goldie and Coldman (1979). However, in the alternating regimens the second modality is initiated very soon after the first, which minimizes the opportunity for resistant cells to arise between modalities. Therefore, mechanisms of interaction which can be achieved when the drug is given first might conceivably have a greater impact on tumor control. The studies reported here were done to determine whether the order in which the treatments are given and the intensity of the radiotherapy, that is, daily fractions and multiple daily fractions (MFD) affect the response obtained.

MATERIALS AND METHODS

The tumors were obtained by injecting 3924A tumor cells into the flank of ACI inbred rats so that the primary tumor could be irradiated with minimal radiation to the host, accomplished by shielding. Viable tumor tissue was minced with scissors, loaded into 1-ml syringes, and 0.1 ml containing ~2 x 10^7 cells was delivered s.c. into the animals through a 14-gauge needle.

Tumors were irradiated with a 250-kV 15 ma GE Maximar 250-III with a half-value layer of 1.39 mm Cu at a rate of 270 rad/min. Filtering was through 0.5 mm Cu and 1.0 mm Al. Before irradiation animals were anesthetized with ether and placed in a lead shield through which the tumor protruded. Cyclophosphamide (CP), supplied by Mead Johnson Research Center, Evansville, Ind., was dissolved in 0.9% NaCl solution and given by i.p. injection. Treatments were initiated when the tumor volumes were approximately 330 mm^3. The time required for individual tumors to reach 40 times the initial volume ($40V_0$) was determined by interpolation between measurements. Median times to $40V_0$ were determined from Kaplan-Meier plots. Statistical comparisons utilized log rank analysis (Peto et al., 1977).

RESULTS AND DISCUSSION

The effects of radiation alone on volume of 3924A are shown in Fig. 1. The radiation dose used was 2500 rad. Two schedules were compared. The more intensive MFD treatment given as ten 250-rad fractions in 2 days halted growth of the tumor earlier than did the daily fractions for 10 days, but regrowth began earlier, so that growth delays (taken at $40V_0$ when constant growth rates had been reestablished) were not significantly different (Table 1). The similarity between these two regrowth curves suggests that sublethal damage repair has been completed within the 2 hr period between fractions in the MFD schedule.

Cyclophosphamide was given at the LD10 dose, 150 mg/kg (0.9 g/m^2). When CP was given alone, tumor volume continued to increase for 2 days, then regressed to the original volume by day 8 (Fig. 2). Growth delay was 19.6 days for CP at this dose (Table 1), considerably less than for the radiation alone even though regression did not occur with the radiation treatments. Apparently tumor cells die and are cleared faster after CP than after the radiation treatments employed here.

Daily irradiations were completed on day 9. Cyclophosphamide administered 7 days after the daily radiation gave only a slight regression of tumor volume but markedly prolonged the time required to reestablish growth rates (Fig. 3). Daily radiation given after the CP also delayed regrowth of the tumor, but in this case a constant growth rate was achieved earlier and at a lower volume than when CP was given after the radiation (Fig. 3). Growth delays (Table 1) were significantly less when daily radiation was given first than when the order was reversed ($p<.005$). This significant difference may result from a change in proliferative rate of the tumor cells. If proliferative activity is decreased for a time

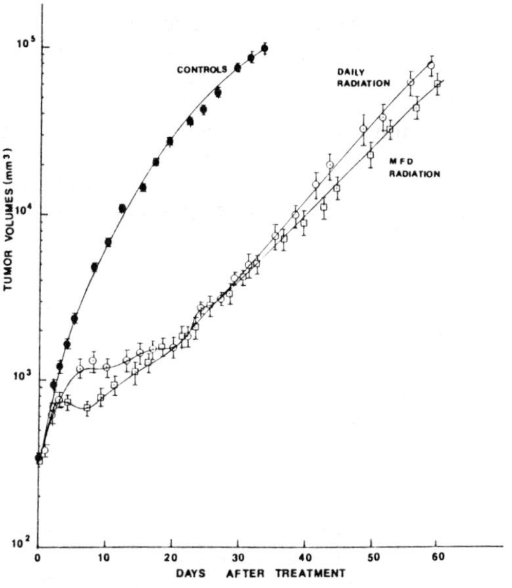

Fig. 1. Changes in volume of 3924A after 2500 rads radiation given as 10 fractions in 10 days (daily radiation) or in 2 days (MFD radiation).

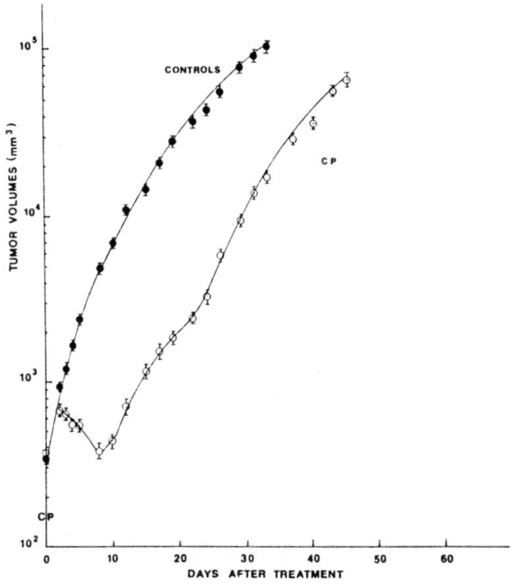

Fig. 2. Changes in volume of 3924A after 150 mg/kg cyclophosphamide (CP).

following daily radiation, cells might be less responsive to the drug. However, it can not be stated with certainty that the stable tumor volume reflects the proliferative status at that time. Removal of dead cells and short-term proliferation of cells eventually destined to die would also contribute to the shape of the tumor volume curve. Another possibility is that the cells which survive the

Table 1. Minimum volumes and growth delays for 3924A after daily or MFD radiation and cyclophosphamide

Group	Treatment[1]	Number of Rats	V_0	V_{min}[2] Day	Volume	Growth Delay
B:	CP+DF[3]	10	334	22	444	50.2[4]
C:	DF+CP	9	321	21	1323	42.4[4]
D:	CP+MFD	9	327	16	181	52.1
E:	MFD+CP	9	328	16	528	48.5[4]
F:	CP	10	371	8	380	19.6
G:	DF	10	330	10	1207	27.1
H:	MFD	9	322	7	681	29.8

[1]Treatments shown in the order given, from left to right. An interval of 7 days separated the modalities in the combined treatments.
[2]The minimum tumor volume observed after completion of treatment.
[3]CP=cyclophosphamide; DF=daily fractions; MFD=multiple fractions per day.
[4]Group C was significantly different from Group B ($p < .005$) and from Group E ($p < .025$) by log rank test.

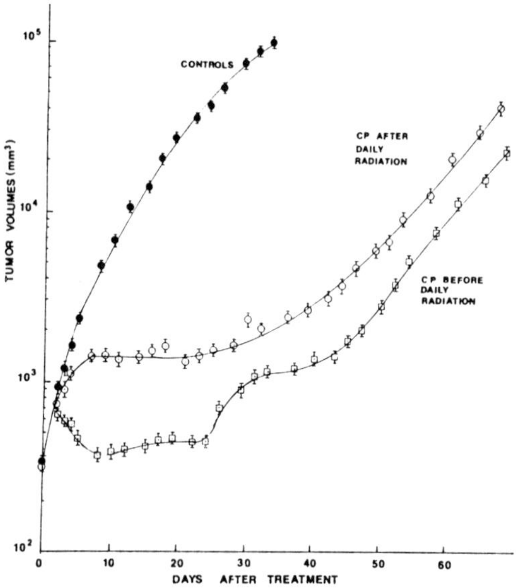

Fig. 3. Changes in volume of 3924A for CP given 7 days before or after daily radiation.

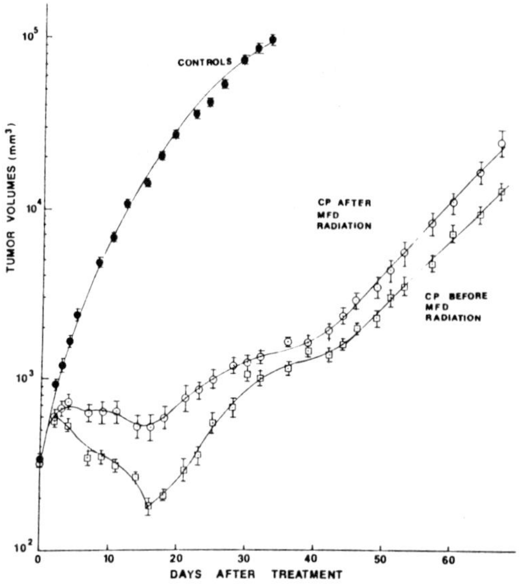

Fig. 4. Changes in volume of 3924A for CP given 7 days before or after MFD radiation.

daily radiation also tend to be somewhat more resistant to CP. The increased size of the tumor at the time the CP was given in this treatment group is not likely to be a factor, since the size of tumor at CP treatment can be varied from 250 to 10,000 mm^3 with no change in the time to reach $8V_0$ or $40V_0$ (Hopkins and Looney, 1988). CP given after MFD radiation also stabilized tumor volume for a time (Fig. 4), as happened after daily fractions (Fig. 3). However, in the group given MFD radiation after CP the regression begun with CP alone continued, so that on day 16 the mean volume was approximately half the initial volume (Table 1: V min for group D). Since recovery of bone marrow and gut is completed within 11 days after this dose of CP (Hopkins and Looney, 1988), this result allows subsequent courses of combined therapy to be given to continue the regression and eventually to cure the tumor. Although the other treatment in this comparison (Fig. 4), CP after MFD radiation, did not achieved comparable tumor regression, nevertheless, regression does continue with further treatments and cures are possible with 3 courses of the combined therapy as has been shown elsewhere (Looney et al., 1985). Growth rates were reestablished at similar times for these 2 groups given MFD radiation and CP, and growth delays, although favoring the group given CP first, were not significantly different (Table 1).

Curative therapy depends upon the killing of all clonogenic tumor cells by the end of the treatment period, including those cells added by repopulation between the individual courses in the treatment. The cell kill for each course of treatment must be greater than the repopulation between courses, and the total number of courses required must not exceed the limits of toxicity to the animal, otherwise cure will not be possible. The data presented here illustrate the principle that interruptions in radiation treatment, such as occur in schedules which alternate chemotherapy and radiotherapy, do not necessarily compromise the outcome , providing that each course of treatment is sufficiently intensive. In the experimental tumor 3924A, intensive treatment with CP or with MFD radiation is preferable to daily radiation fractions as the first agent in schedules which alternate the two modalities.

ACKNOWLEDGMENTS
We thank D. Reto for technical assistance. This work was supported in part by Public Health Service grant CA-35372, "Cross Resistance or Sensitivity in Multimodal Therapy," from the National Cancer Institute, National Institutes of Health, Department of Health and Human Services.

REFERENCES

Goldie, J.H., Coldman, A.J. (1979): A mathematic model for relating the drug sensitivity of tumors to their spontaneous mutation rate. Cancer Treat.Rep. 63, 1727-1733.

Hopkins, H.A., Looney, W.B. (1988): Interactions between cyclophosphamide and radiation. In Interactions between Antitumour Drugs and Radiation, ed B.T. Hill and A. Bellamy, in press. Boca Raton: CRC Press.

Looney, W.B., Longerbeam, M.B., Hopkins, H.A., Carter, Jr., W.C. (1983): Solid tumor models for the assessment of different treatment modalities. XXI. Comparison of different radiation dose schedules alone or in combination with cyclophosphamide. Cancer 51, 1012-1020.

Looney, W.B., Hopkins, H.A., Carter, Jr., W.C. (1984): Solid tumor models for the assessment of different treatment modalities. XXII. The alternate utilization of radiotherapy and chemotherapy. Cancer 54, 416-425.

Looney, W.B., Hopkins, H.A., Carter, Jr., W.C. (1985): Solid tumor models for the assessment of different treatment modalities. XXIII. A new approach to the more effective utilization of radiotherapy alternated with chemotherapy. Int.J.Radiat. Oncol.Biol.Phys. 11, 2105-2117.

Peto, R., Pike, M.C., Armitage, P., Breslow, N.E., Cox, D.R., Howard, S.V., Mantel, N., McPherson, K., Peto, J., Smith, P.G. (1977): Design and analysis of randomized clinical trials requiring prolonged observation of each patient. II. Analysis and examples. Br.J.Cancer 35, 1-39.

Résumé

Chez des rats ACI porteurs de tumeur 3924 A, nous avons examiné les conséquences du premier traitement Cyclophosphamide ou radiothérapie dans des traitements alternant ces deux possibilités. L'irradiation a été donnée en fraction quotidienne ou en multiple fractions par jour (MFD). Les retards de croissance n'ont pas été différents selon que l'irradiation ait été donnée de façon quotidienne ou en MFD, ou selon que le Cyclophosphamide ait été donné 7 jours avant ou après l'irradiation MFD. Par contre, il y a une différence ($p < 0{,}005$) quand le Cyclophosphamide a été donné 7 jours avant ou 7 jours après l'irradiation quotidienne. En terme de retard de croissance la MFD a été plus efficace que le fractionnement quotidien lorsque l'irradiation a été donnée en premier et non lorsque le Cyclophosphamide est donné en premier. Ce n'est que pour les traitements où le Cyclophosphamide a été donné avant le MFD que le volume de la tumeur a régressé au-dessous du volume initial. Ces résultats indiquent que un traitement intensif avec une chimiothérapie efficace et une irradiation en MFD est préférable à une irradiation quotidienne comme premier agent dans des traitements qui alternent ces deux modalités pour le traitement de tumeur qui sont sensibles à ces deux modalités.

Neo-Adjuvant Chemotherapy. Ed. Cl. Jacquillat, M. Weil, D. Khayat. Colloque INSERM/John Libbey Eurotext Ltd. © 1988. Vol. 169, pp. 51-56.

Concomitant radiochemotherapy in the management of epidermoid carcinoma of the anal canal

J. Papillon

12 quai Général-Sarrail, 69006 Lyon, France

Optimal treatment of anal canal carcinoma aims to achieve a high cure rate with sphincter preservation. The management of this tumor has long been a subject of controversy between surgeons and radiation therapists. Surgery alone, i.e., abdomino-perineal resection (APR) with permanent colostomy results in a 5-year survival of about 50% on the average. Morbidity and mortality with APR are not negligible, especially in elderly patients. Radical radiation therapy has been used by many investigators. If the results of radiotherapy are good in early lesions, the rates of cure in case of large infiltrating tumors differ markedly according to the radiation technique. In 1974, NIGRO[1] et al considering that the results of APR were disappointing initiated a preoperative radio-chemotherapy combined treatment. The radiotherapy was given at a low dose (30 Gy over 3 weeks). Chemotherapy using 5 fluorouracil (5FU) on day 1 to 5 and mitomycin C (MTC) on day one was associated with the first days of irradiation. Among the three patients reported by NIGRO two were operated upon and had tumor-free operative specimens. The third patient refused to be operated and was clinically disease-free.

Since 1974 many investigators have utilized simultaneous radio-chemotherapy in attempts to minimize or avoid surgery and confirmed the data published by NIGRO[2] et al. MICHAELSON[3] et al at the Memorial Hospital N.Y. used chemotherapy prior to radiotherapy. The results obtained demonstrate that induction chemotherapy followed by irradiation is less effective than concomitant radio-chemotherapy as suggested by NIGRO[2] et al. The efficacy of this protocol is due to an additive effect of both modalities or to a potentiation of radiotherapy by chemotherapy. These studies led to substantial changes in the treatment strategy applied to patients with anal canal carcinoma in many institutions. Radical surgery as initial treatment has been abandoned at the Memorial Hospital (N.Y.) and questioned at St Mark's Hospital (London) (1981) and at the Mayo Clinic (1984) in favor of a systematic radio-chemotherapy approach.

The current problem is to identify the most effective combined treatment modalities by refining 1/ radiotherapy technique, 2/ chemotherapy methods.

1/ Protocol of radiotherapy

Radiotherapy by itself must be capable to control large proportion of tumors. In most radiotherapy centers the irradiation aims to deliver an homogeneous dose (40 to 50 Gy) to the whole pelvis by box technique, plus a boost to the anal area. The anatomical and clinical behavior of anal canal carcinoma demonstrated that it is not rational to irradiate the whole pelvis in the absence of clinically involved inguinal lymph nodes. It is the reason why the protocol used at the Centre Léon Bérard since 1974 consists in concentrating irradiation to anal and posterior pelvic areas (35 Gy in 19 days). After a two-month rest the second stage is an iridium-192 implant aiming to give a booster dose to the bed of the tumor. The split-course protocol has proven a real superiority on external beam irradiation alone especially for large infiltrating lesions. (4,5)

2/ Chemotherapy

Chemotherapy associated with low dose irradiation is well tolerated. Combined with radical radiotherapy (50 Gy in 4 to 7 weeks) chemotherapy may result in severe acute and late toxicity. CUMMINGS[6] (1984) reported a series of 55 patients with 15 cases (27%) of severe toxicity requiring colostomy. These complications jeopardized the beneficial effect of the combined treatment. Chemotherapy is used to enhance the effectiveness of radiotherapy without giving rise to complications, which would compromise the beneficial effect of the combined treatment.

At the Centre Léon Bérard the dosage of chemotherapy was intentionally reduced to allow a good tolerance. Between 1977 and 1984, 5FU was used at a dose of 600 mgr/m² per day from day 1 to4 and MTC was used at a dose of 12 mgr/m² on day 1. This combined treatment was applied to 89 robust, middle aged patients with T_3 tumor larger than 4 cm. Retrospectively the results of radiochemotherapy were compared with a group of 78 patients with matched tumors treated with the same protocol of irradiation without chemotherapy (Table 1) because of their age or general condition.

TABLE 1

Epidermoid Carcinoma T_3 of the anal canal

Radiotherapy alone vs Radiotherapy + concomitant chemotherapy
Series of the Centre L. Bérard

	No. of cases	Rate of local failures
RT Alone (Co^{60} + Ir^{192})	78	30%
RT (Co^{60} + Ir^{192}) + 5FU, MTC	89	10% p=0.02

The study of the rates of local failures shows a difference statistically significant. These results prompted us to use systematically concomitant radio-chemotherapy since 1985 in all patients with anal canal carcinoma, regardless of stage of the disease and age of the patients. In case of elderly, frail patients in poor condition, the dosage of 5FU is reduced to 500 mgr/m² for four days and MTC is excluded. In robust patients 5FU is applied at a dose of 750 mgr/m² and MTC at 12 mgr/m².

This experience which demonstrates that concomitant radiotherapy and chemotherapy improves the chance of control of epidermoid carcinoma of the anal canal, without altering the radiotherapy protocol, may be extended to others epidermoid carcinomas such as those of uterine cervix or those of the pharynx and larynx. In this latter field a study has been conducted at the Centre Léon Bérard, using a concomitant chemotherapy protocol similar to that applied to anal canal carcinomas[7]. The preliminary results are reported in Table 2.

TABLE 2

Concomitant radio-chemotherapy (5FU, MTC)
in the treatment of carcinomas of the pharynx ans larynx

Series of the Centre L. Bérard
Preliminary results

	Nb. of cases	Rate of death at 3 years	Rate of death at 5 years
RT alone	22	59%	77%
RT + 5FU, MTC	25	36%	38%

The difference of death rates is not statistically significant but these data are encouraging and prompt us to carry on this study, which tends to confirm that concomitant radio-chemotherapy is more efficient than induction chemotherapy followed by irradiation in the management of epidermoid carcinomas.

REFERENCES

1. NIGRO ND, VAITKEVICIUS VK, CONSIDINE B Jr. Combined therapy for cancer of the anal canal : a preliminary report. Dis. Colon Rectum 1974 ; 17 : 354-356.

2. NIGRO ND. An evaluation of combined therapy for squamous cell cancer of the anal canal. Dis. Colon Rectum 1984 ; 27 : 763-766.

3. MICHAELSON RA, MAGILL GB, QUAN SH, LEAMING RH, NIKRUI M, STEARNS MW. Preoperative chemotherapy and radiation therapy in the management of anal epidermoid carcinoma. Cancer 1983 ; 51 : 390-395.

4. PAPILLON J. Rectal and anal cancers. Conservative treatment by irradiation : an alternative to radical surgery. New York, Springer Verlag, 1982.

5. PAPILLON J, MONTBARBON JF. Epidermoid carcinoma of the anal canal. A series of 276 cases. Dis. Colon Rectum 1987 ; 30 : 324-333.

6. CUMMINGS B, KEANE T, THOMAS G, HARWOOD A, RIDER W. Results and toxicity of the treatment of anal canal carcinoma by radiation therapy or radiation therapy and chemotherapy. Cancer 1984 ; 54 : 2062-2068.

7. MONTBARBON JF, ARDIET JM, CHAUVIN F, GIGNOUX B, CHASSARD JL, PAPILLON J. Concomitant radiation and chemotherapy (mitomycin C and 5-fluorouracil) in the treatment of head and neck carcinomas. In New trends in cancer chemotherapy with mitomycin C. Taguchi T, Andrysek O, Excepta Medica 1987 ; 38-43.

Résumé

En 1974 NIGRO, chirurgien à Détroit, expérimenta une association de radiothérapie à doses faibles (30 Gy en 3 semaines) et d'une courte chimiothérapie concomitante (5FU, MTC) à titre préopératoire pour chercher à améliorer les résultats jugés par lui décevants de l'amputation abdomino-périnéale. Chez les 3 patients concernés la tumeur fut contrôlée. Depuis lors, cette méthode, avec des modifications multiples, a été utilisée par de nombreux auteurs qui ont confirmé les bons résultats obtenus par NIGRO. An Centre Léon Bérard (LYON) où plus de 300 cas de cancer du canal anal ont été traités depuis 1971, l'association d'une chimiothérapie (5FU, MTC) à une irradiation intensive en split-course combinant irradiation externe (19 jours) et curiethérapie à l'Iridium 192 deux mois plus tard, a été expérimentée depuis 1977 pour un certain nombre de patients (89) porteurs de gros cancers T3 de plus de 4 cm. Une étude rétrospective de cas similaires traités par irradiation seule (78) a permis une comparaison des deux groupes. L'analyse des échecs locaux montre une différence statistiquement significative en faveur de la radio-chimiothérapie. Dans cette association l'accent est mis sur l'intérêt de l'utilisation concomitante de la chimiothérapie et de la radiothérapie alors qu'une série de cas traités au Memorial Hospital (N.Y.) où la chimiothérapie a précédé l'irradiation, a eu une efficacité nettement moins marquée.

Ce type de protocole peut être employé pour traiter d'autres cancers épidermoïdes tels que ceux du pharyngo-larynx. Dans la série lyonnaise randomisée comportant 47 cas, les résultats sont encourageants, mais la différence de survie n'est pas encore significative.

Neo-Adjuvant Chemotherapy. Ed. Cl. Jacquillat, M. Weil, D. Khayat. Colloque INSERM/John Libbey Eurotext Ltd. © 1988. Vol. 169, pp. 57-62.

Chimiothérapie néo-adjuvante dans les carcinomes épidermoïdes évolués du canal anal : étude pilote

Ph. Rougier*, J.L. Marin**, Ph. Lasser+, P. Wibault**, C. Bognel°, J. Kac*, C. Théodore§, J.P. Droz§ et F. Eschwege**

Institut Gustave-Roussy, 94805 Villejuif Cedex, France

INTRODUCTION

La radiothérapie est le traitement électif des petites tumeurs épidermoïdes du canal anal T1 et T2 car elle permet d'obtenir d'excellents résultats sans perte de la fonction sphinctérienne (2). En revanche la radiothérapie seule donne des résultats décevants lorsque les tumeurs sont volumineuses et envahissantes localement : T4 N0, N1, ou N2, M0 selon la classification UICC 1987) (7). Dans ces cas la survie est médiocre et inférieure à 25 % à 5 ans (2, 5) et la conservation sphinctérienne rare puisque la plupart des patients doivent avoir une amputation abdomino-périnéale en raison de la persistance de reliquats tumoraux après radiothérapie externe ou de la destruction fréquente du sphincter anal par la tumeur.

----

* Sce de Gastro-Entérologie; ** Service de Radiothérapie B;

+ Sce de Chirurgie Digestive; ° Sce d'Anatomopathologie B;

§ Sce de Médecine B.

Des protocoles de chimiothérapie associée à la radiothérapie ont été utilisés en pré opératoire avec l'association 5FU + Mitomycine C (3, 6) avec des résultats encourageants en terme de stérilisation tumorale mais dont le bénéfice sur la survie n'est pas démontrée.

Dans le cadre d'une étude pilote nous avons testé la faisabilité d'une polychimiothérapie, associant des produits potentiellement efficaces sur les carcinomes épidermoïdes, administrés avant la radiothérapie.

Patients et Méthodes : Entre 1985 et 1987, 9 patients ont été inclus dans ce protocole. Il y avait 8 femmes et 1 homme, leur âge moyen était de 59 ans (35 à 72 ans). La tumeur était étendue à la marge anale 6 fois/9, et elle remontait au niveau du rectum 4 fois/9. Sa taille moyenne était de 5,25 cm (3,2 à 7,7 cm). Une extension vaginale ou à la cloison recto-vaginale était notée 7 fois/8.

Selon la classification de l'UICC, 5 avaient une tumeur T4 N2 M0, 3 une tumeur T4 N0 M0 et 1 une tumeur T3 N3 M0. Deux de ces patients avaient une fistule recto-vaginale.

La chimiothérapie consistait en deux cycles séparés de 4 semaines et associant : Velbé 5 mg: J1, en bolus IV ; Bléomycine 10 mg/24h en perfusion continue de j1 à J4 ; 5FU: 300 mg/m² en bolus IV J2, 3 et 4 ; Endoxan 200 mg/m² en perfusion courte IV en J2, 3 et 4 et Cisplatinum: 100 mg/m² avec hyperhydratation en J5.

La radiothérapie externe était ensuite délivrée 3 semaines après le 2ème cycle de chimiothérapie, après réévaluation tumorale, à la dose de 40 Gy (3 cas) ou 45 Gy (6 cas) avec un fractionnement classique

(16 à 22 fractions) et un étalement de 4 à 5 semaines (29 à 34 jours). Le volume irradié incluait le volume tumoral (9/9) et les aires ganglionnaires inguinales (8/9).

Une intervention chirurgicale a été pratiquée chez 7 patients (amputation abdomino-périnéale : AAP) de principe en raison de l'importance de l'envahissement initial. Deux patients n'ont pas été opérés (l'un par refus, l'autre en raison d'une extension ganglionnaire inguinale très importante : N3).

RESULTATS

La tolérance à la chimiothérapie a été acceptable avec, selon les critères de l'OMS, des vomissements grade 3 chez 8/9 patients et grade 4 : 1/9 ; une leucopénie grade 2 : 2/9 et grade 3 : 1/9 ; une alopécie grade 3 : 9/9.

La tolérance à la radiothérapie a été bonne : avec une toxicité cutanée grade 2 : 3/9 et grade 3 : 4/9 ; une mucite anale grade 2 : 4/9 et grade 3 : 2/9 ; une diarrhée grade 2 : 1/9 et grade 3 : 2/9 ; une proctite grade 2 : 1/9 et grade 3 : 3/9.

La réponse à la chimiothérapie selon les critères de l'OMS, évalué 3 semaines après le 2ème cycle a été : réponse complète 0/9, réponse partielle : 7/9 (77 %) et stabilisation : 2/9. Tous les patients ayant eu une réponse à la chimiothérapie ont amélioré cette réponse avec la radiothérapie et 4/9 avaient une réponse complète 4 semaines après la fin de la radiothérapie, qui a été confirmée pour 3/7 lors de l'AAP, par l'examen histologique de la pièce opératoire qui n'a retrouvé que des lésions cicatricielles.

Sur le plan de la survie, aucun décès n'a été observé avec un recul moyen de 17 mois (3 à 31 mois), cependant seuls 5/9 patients restent en rémission complète alors que 2 des patients sont en poursuite évolutive locale malgré les traitements associés et que 2 autres ont une récidive locale à 4 et 12 mois après le début du traitement.

DISCUSSION

Cet essai de phase II d'une chimiothérapie néoadjuvante dans les volumineuses tumeurs du canal anal montre que celle-ci est réalisable avec une tolérance acceptable et nous a permis d'observer des régressions tumorales objectives 7 fois sur 9. Par ailleurs nous n'avons pas observé de progressions tumorale sous chimiothérapie et la toxicité de la radiothérapie n'est pas augmentée. Il faut remarquer que les deux patients n'ayant pas eu de réponse à la chimiothérapie, n'ont pas eu de réponse importante à la radiothérapie (à la dose de 45 Gy).

Enfin, malgré une stratégie lourde et agressive dans ce groupe de patients ayant des facteurs de mauvais pronostic, nous avons observé pour 4 des 9 patients une poursuite évolutive (2 cas) ou une récidive locale précoce (2 cas) qui soulignent l'agressivité de certaines formes de carcinome épidermoïde du canal anal.

Cela pose la question de l'efficacité de cette chimiothérapie choisie sur le contrôle tumoral et la survie et, si des arguments existent, pour utiliser l'association cisplatinum et 5FU en perfusion continu (4), les autres produits n'augmentent probablement que peu l'efficacité du traitement au prix d'une toxicité accrue. Une évaluation de l'efficacité de l'association 5fu continu + CDDP semble donc licite avant d'entreprendre une étude randomisée. Cela pose également la question de la reprise de la chimiothérapie après la fin de la radiothérapie ou en post-opératoire lorsqu'elle a été efficace en pré opératoire, car il est possible que l'effet de deux cycles soit marginal,en terme de survie, sur ces volumineuses tumeurs.

Quoiqu'il en soit la constatation que 4 patients sur 9 ont eu une RC avec l'association chimiothérapie + radiothérapie fait espérer diminuer le taux de récidives locales.

CONCLUSION

Cet essai de chimiothérapie néoadjuvante dans les cancers épidermoïdes montre que celle-ci est faisable et partiellement efficace. Mais que d'autres études, en particulier l'association 5FU perfusion continue + CDDP sont necessaires avant que ne soit menés des essais randomisés pour évaluer l'efficacité sur la survie de ces nouvelles stratégies associant la chimiothérapie à la radiothérapie et à l'exérèse chirurgicale qui restent actuellement les deux traitements de référence de ces tumeurs évoluées.

BIBLIOGRAPHIE

1. CUMMINGS B., KEANE T., THOMAS G., HARWOOD A., RIDER W.: Results and toxicity of the treatment of anal canal carcinoma by radiation therapy or radiation therapy and chemotherapy. Cancer 1984, 54: 2062-2068.

2. ESCHWEGE F., LASSER P., CHAVY A., WIBAULT P., KAC J., ROUGIER Ph., BOGNEL C. Squamous cell Carcinoma of the anal canal: treatment by external irradiation. Radiotherapy and Oncology 1985, 3: 145-150.

3. NIGRO N.D.: Multidisciplinary management of cancer of the anus. World J Surg 1987, 11: 446-451.

4. SALEM P.A., HABBOUBI N. et col. Cisdichlorodiamine platinum (II) is effective in the treatment of anal squamous cell carcinoma. Proc Am Soc Clin Oncol 1985, 4, C 303.

5. SALMON R.J., FENTON J., ASSELAIN B., MATHIEU G., GIRODET J., DURAND J.C., DECROIX Y., PILLERON J.P., ROUSSEAU J. Treatment of epidermoid anal canal cancer. Am J Surg 1984, 147: 43-48.

6. SISCHY B. The use of radiation therapy combined with chemotherapy in the management of squamous cell carcinoma of the anus and marginally resectable adenocarcinoma of the rectum. Int J Radiat Oncol Biol Phys 1985, 11: 1587-1595.

7. TNM Classification of malignant tumours. UICC International Union Against Cancer. Hermanek P. and Sobin L.H. Ed.; Springer-Verlag Berlin-Heidelberg. New York - Paris - Tokyo 1987, p 57.

Résumé

NEOADJUVANT CHEMOTHERAPY(CT)IN ADVANCED ANAL EPIDERMOID CARCINOMA (AAEC) : A PILOTE STUDY

PH.ROUGIER, J.L.MARIN, PH.LASSER, P. WIBAULT, A.LUSINCHI,C.BOGNEL, C.THEODORE, J.P.DROZ, F.ESCHWEGE : Institut Gustave-ROUSSY - 94800 VILLEJUIF

Locally advanced anal epidermoid carcinoma (AAEC) have a very poor prognosis 35% at 5 years. To try to improve the survival rate and to decrease the risk of local reccurence we have conducted a pilote study on neoadjuvant chemotherapy. Nine patients with AAEC have been included : 5 pts T4 N2 M0; 3 pts T4 N0 M0 and 1 pt T3N3M0 according to the UICC classification. Two patients had recto-vaginal fistulaes. Two cyles of CT was given d1 and d28 with : Velban 5 mg/sqm IV bolus d1, Bleomycin 10mg (CI) d1-d4 and d29-d31, 5FU IV bolus 300mg/sqm d2,3,4 and d29,30,31 ; Cyclophosphamide 300mg/sqm IV perfusion d2,3 and d30, 31 and CDDP : 100 mg/sqm with hydration d5 and d32. At the end of CT external radiation therapy (RT) has been delivered at the total dose of 40 to 45 Gy with a standard fractionnation in the tumor field(9/9) and the inguinal area (8/9). Surgery has been performed in 6 cases (AAP) is planed in 1 pt, was conterindicated in 1 pt and refused by 1 pt. Results : The CT tolerance (WHO grade)has been acceptable : vomiting grade (g) 3 :8/9 and g4 :1/9 ; leucopenia g2 : 2/9 and g3 : 1/9. The response rate (WHO criteria) to CT has been : CR: 0/9 ; PR : 7/9 (77%) ; no change : 2/9. All the pts with PR after chemotherapy improved their response on RT and two achieved a CR confirmed at pathological examination in one pts. The 2 pts who were not responding to chemotherapy have been resistant to radiation therapy as well as to surgical treatment. The survival rate is 100% with a median follow up of 17 mths, however only 5/9 pts are free of disease. Two pts have recurred at 4 and 12 mths and two other have never been controlled by the treatment. Conclusion : Neoadjuvant chemotherapy is feasible however and less toxic protocol have to be developped to improve the quality of tumoral response.

Neo-Adjuvant Chemotherapy. Ed. Cl. Jacquillat, M. Weil, D. Khayat. Colloque INSERM/John Libbey Eurotext Ltd. © 1988. Vol. 169, pp. 63-65.

Conservative treatment of 115 breast cancers greater than 3 cm by initial chemotherapy followed by a special radiotherapy technique

F. Baillet*, Cl. Jacquillat**, C. Alapetite, B. Dessard-Diana, P. Gomez, M. Housset, C. Journel, P. Michel-Langlet and G. Boisserie

* *Centre de Traitement des Tumeurs, Hôpital Necker, 149 rue de Sèvres, 75015 Paris, France*
** *Service d'Oncologie Médicale, Hôpital de la Salpêtrière, 47 Bd de l'hôpital, 75013 Paris, France*

SUMMARY

In France there is a consensus for the conservative treatment of tumours of the breast ≤3 cm. It was interesting to show that excellent results could be obtained by conservative treatment of larger tumours. We have treated 115 cancers > 3 cm by a combination of initial chemotherapy and external and implantation radiation treatment. There were 33 T2 > 3 cm, 82 T3-T4, 43% of forms with clinical adenopathy and 36% with clinical aggressive disease (PEV). After a 3 to 7 years follow-up, the 5 year survival for T2 > 3 cm was 85%, breast conservation in 97% and an excellent aesthetic result in 79,5% of cases.

KEY WORDS

Breast cancer. Conservative treatment. Radiotherapy. Chemotherapy.

INTRODUCTION

In France there is a consensus for the conservative treatment of breast tumours ≤3 cm (3). Elsewhere, others place the limit at 4 cm (2), or even 5 cm. It was interesting to show that excellent results can be obtained by conservative treatment of tumours beyond these limits.

MATERIAL AND METHODS

We have conservatively treated 115 breast cancers greater than 3 cm by a combination of initial chemotherapy and radiotherapy. The lesions were carefully demarcated and the extent of any metastases assessed before starting treatment. Chemotherapy was given with the dual aims of possibly reducing the risk of metastasis and facilitating the radiotherapy by reducing the tumour size prior to irradiation. The therapy consisted of 3 to 6 injections in 2 months of vinblastin 6mg/m2, thiotepa 6mg/m2, methotrexate 25mg/m2, fluoro-uracil 350mg/m2 with adriamycin 30mg/m2 for the most advanced tumours (T > 7 cm, N2 or N3, clinical aggressive disease (PEV)). The frequency of the injections was adapted to the tolerance of the patients and the number of agents used was reduced in elderly patients. Tamoxifen was systematically administered to post-menopausal women. In non-menopausal patients, this medication was initially given in a randomized manner but later it was systematically administered. The breast and axillary nodes were treated by external radiation using standard fractionation (5 Gy x 1,8 Gy per week) or by hypofractionation using a dose that we consider to be equivalent (5 Gy on D1 and D3 and 6,5 Gy on D15 and D17). The booster dose of 20-30 Gy was then given by implantation to the primary tumour and 20 Gy (or 2 x 5 Gy on D29 and D31) at the site of possible clinical adenopathy. Following this, the chemotherapy was recommenced for 3 to 18 months depending on the aggressiveness. The study included 33 T2 > 3 cm, 62 T3 and 20 T4. The mean tumour diameter was 7 cm (range 3,5 to 17 cm) with 43% with clinical adenopathy and 36% with PEV. The mean age was 54 years (range 30 to 83 years).

RESULTS

Following chemotherapy, the mean tumour diameter decreased from 7 to 3,5 cm and after external irradiation it decreased from 3,5 to 1,2 cm. There was no early failure after local regional treatment. After an interval of 3 to 7 years, the 5 year actuarial survival was 85% for the T2 > 3 cm, 67% for the T3, 79% for the T4 and 70% for the combined T3-T4. There was a 9% local regional recurrence rate for the T2 > 3 cm, 16% for the T3 and 10% for the T4. Five of the 15 local regional recurrences underwent local conservative treatment. Two isolated lymph node recurrences were treated by axillary dissection and 3 distal tumour recurrences were treated by lumpectomy with per operative implantation therapy at doses of 30 Gy. Until now, none of these treatments has been followed by further local regional recurrence. Three other recurrences were treated by mastectomy. Seven recurrences were treated by palliative chemotherapy because of the simultaneous appearance of metastases. Another recurrence became inoperable as the patient refused mastectomy.

For the 32 T2 > 3 cm, there was breast conservation in 97% and an excellent aesthetic result in 91% (no, or only minimal traces). In the 82 T3-T4 there was 97,5% mammary conservation and 82% had excellent aesthetic results.

This protocol improved survival. In a study of 6719 cases of T3-T4, the Enquête Permanente Cancer (1) reported a 5 year survival of 52% compared to 70% in our study. The incidence of breast conservation was also very high. In the T3 > 7 cm + T4 + N2 + N3 group without PEV, the only study with which comparison is possible reported 40% of secondary mastectomies compared to 4% in our study (4). The aesthetic results were usually excellent.

REFERENCES

1 - Fédération Nationale des Cancers de Lutte contre le Cancer. Enquête Permanente Cancer. Paris, Dion, 1982.

2 - Fisher B., Bauer M., Margolese R. et al. Five year results of a randomized clinical trial comparing total mastectomy and segmental mastectomy with or without radiation in the treatment of breast cancer. New Eng. J. Med., 1985, 312, 11, 665-72.

3 - Pujol H. Conclusions In : les traitements conservateurs du cancer du sein, Montpellier : Sauramps Medical, 1984, 157-9.

4 - Vilcoq J.R, Fourquet A., Julien D., Gautier C., Calle R., Ghossein N.A. Pronostic significance of clinical nodal involvement in patients treated by radical radiotherapy for a locally advanced breast cancer. Am. J. Oncol., 7 : 1984, 625-8.

Résumé

En France il y a un consensus pour un traitement conservateur des tumeurs du sein de moins de 3 cm. Il est intéressant de montrer que d'excellents résultats peuvent être obtenus par le traitement conservateur de tumeurs plus volumineuses. Nous avons traité 115 malades avec des tumeurs de plus de 3 cm par une association de chimiothérapie initiale et une irradiation externe et interstitielle. Il y avait 33 T2 supérieurs à 3 cm, 82 T3,T4, 3 % de formes avec des adénopathies cliniques et 36 % de maladie évolutive (PeV). Après un suivi de 3 à 7 ans, la survie à 5 ans, pour les T2 de plus de 3 cm est de 85 %, la conservation mammaire de 97 % et un résultat esthétique excellent est observé dans 79,5 % des cas.

Neo-Adjuvant Chemotherapy. Ed. Cl. Jacquillat, M. Weil, D. Khayat. Colloque INSERM/John Libbey Eurotext Ltd. © 1988. Vol. 169, pp. 67-70.

Combined modality therapy in patients with locally advanced squamous cell carcinoma of the head and neck : Wayne State University (WSU) experience

M. Al-Sarraf, J. Kish, J. Ensley and E. Tapazoglou

Division of Hematology and Oncology, Wayne State University and Harper-Grace Hospitals, Detroit, Michigan 48201, USA

ABSTRACT

Since 1977 nine sequential prospective induction chemotherapy pilots of platinol based combination in patients with locally advanced head and neck cancer were carried out. Results based on the three largest studies with minimal follow-up of five years, that clinical (54%) and histological (50%) complete responses and over-all survival of three courses of cisplatin and 120 hour 5-FU infusion are superior than other combination. Four other pilots to investigate the timing of chemotherapy as part of combined modality therapy were also carried out. These studies were activated on the cooperative group level. Efforts to continue to improve on the effectiveness and the safety of induction chemotherapy are under way in WSU.

KEYWORDS

Head and neck cancer, chemotherapy, combined modality therapy, cisplatin, 5-FU

INTRODUCTION

The results of standard treatment of surgery and/or radiotherapy in patients with locally advanced cancer are poor and unacceptable. Extensive efforts are under way to improve the results in this group of patients. Part of these efforts is the utilization of adjuvant chemotherapy as part of multi-modality therapy in patients with locally advanced cançer. Since 1977 efforts at WSU, Detroit, Michigan, have been to study the effectiveness and the feasibility of induction (proto) chemotherapy as part of combined modality treatment (Al-Sarraf 1984a, 1987, 1988).

RESULTS AND DISCUSSION

Induction Chemotherapy

Since the introduction of cisplatin as an active agent for SCC H&N, it became clear to us that high response rate could be achieved when cisplatin combinations were used in previously untreated patients. So far nine of such induction chemotherapy regimens have been investigated at WSU (Table 1). Our three largest and mature trials are the two courses of COB (Al-Sarraf 1979), two courses of cisplatin and 96 hour 5-FU infusion (Al-Sarraf 1981, Kish 1982), and three courses of cisplatin and 120 hour 5-FU infusion (Al-Sarraf 1984, Jacobs 1987). Table 2 shows the response rate to each of these pilots. All patients entered on study were evaluated for response and survival with minimum follow-up of 5 years. The type of induction chemotherapy did influence the overall survival of these patients regardless of the subsequent definitive therapy. Significantly better survival was in favor of the cisplatin and 5-FU groups. Also, patients achieving clinical CR to the initial chemotherapy have significantly superior survival than those patients with less than CR to chemotherapy (Table 3). More important, those CR patients after chemotherapy who were found to have no microscopic cancer after surgical resection had

Table 1. Prospective Induction (Proto) Chemotherapy Trials at WSU - 1977-1988

	Type of Combination	No. of Courses	No. of Patients	References
1.	Cisplatin, Oncovin, Bleomycin (COB)	2	77	Al-Sarraf 1979
2.	COB - Methotrexate	2	6	--
3.	Cisplatin, 5-FU 96 hr. infusion	2	26	Al-Sarraf 1981, Kish 1982
4.	Cisplatin, 5-FU 120 hr. infusion	3	88	Al-Sarraf 1984, Jacobs 1987
5.	Cisplatin, 5-FU 120 hr. infusion	6	6	--
6.	Cisplatin 40 mg/M^2 d 1-5 and 5-FU 120 hr. infusion	3	12	Kish 1984, 1988
7.	Sequential Cisplatin, 5-FU 120 hr. infusion and Methotrexate and 5-FU (L)	5	46	Ensley 1988
8.	Sequential Cisplatin, 5-FU 120 hr. infusion and Methotrexate, 5-FU (L)	6	18	--
9.	Carboplatin, 5-FU 120 hr. infusion	3-6		

Table 2. Response to Induction (Proto) Chemotherapy. WSU - 1977-1982

	COB 2 courses	Cisplatin, 5-FU 2 courses	Cisplatin, 5-FU 3 courses	
CR	22 (28.6%)	5 (19.3%)	48 (54.5%)	p=0.04
PR	39 (50.6%)	18 (69.2%)	35 (39.8%)	
NP	16 (23.8%)	3 (11.5%)	5 (5.7%)	
CR+PR	61/77 (79.2%)	23/26 (88.5%)	83/88 (94.3%)	N.S.

statistically superior survival when compared to those clinical CR who had residual disease at surgery (Al-Kourainy 1987). The patient's nodal status (T4NO vs T4N3) did influence the clinical CR to chemotherapy and the overall survival rate.The results of three courses of cisplatin and 5-FU infusion led to the activation of the same trial in the cooperative group (Al-Sarraf 1985).

One important finding during these trials was that response to initial cisplatin combination usually mean a response to subsequent radiotherapy (Ensley 1984). This led to offering chemotherapy for those patients with locally advanced cancer refusing surgery, and for the responders to go for radiotherapy and for no response surgery have to be considered. This observation led to the protocol for organ preservation and the activation of the V.A. Laryngeal Cancer study in the United States.

Our most recent completed study is five courses of alternate chemotherapy with cisplatin and 120 hour 5-FU infusion given courses one, three and five and high dose methotrexate (MTX) and 5-FU bolus and leucovorin given weekly for three weeks course two and four (Ensley 1988). Forty-six patients, all with stage IV cancer, with 85% had T4 and 58% had N3 disease were entered. Thirty-one patients completed the planned chemotherapy. The CR rate was 46% (21/46) of all patients entered, and CR rate of 40% (10/25) of patients with N3 disease; 8 did not complete the study. The CR rate in patients who completed this trial was 65% (20/31). The overall toxicities were acceptable and reversible. This led to more intensification of this alternate chemotherapy by giving initially two courses of cisplatin and 5-FU infusion followed by alternated two courses of MTX and 5-FU and two courses of cisplatin and 5-FU infusion with shortening the time between courses. This pilot will also be activated on the cooperative group level.

Chemotherapy after Surgery

To study the efficacy of active chemotherapy in these patients the timing of this treatment as part of definitive therapy was investigated at WSU. One of these studies was to give effective chemotherapy after surgery and before radiotherapy (Al-Sarraf 1982). This led in 1981 to the activation of the same pilot on the cooperative group level (Al-Sarraf 1985). In 1983 a randomized phase III study of surgery, chemotherapy and radiotherapy vs surgery and post-op radiotherapy was activated at the cooperative group level. This trial was adopted by the Head and Neck Cancer Intergroup in the United States in 1985.

Table 3. Prognostic Factors, Median Survival and Significance to Induction Chemotherapy - WSU - 1977-1987

Group	Weeks	p Value
Response		
CR	138	0.0000
PR	45	
NR	29	
Stage		
III	110	0.0072
IV	50	
Stage IV		
CR	108	0.0000
PR	43	
NR	28	
T&N		
T4N0	139	0.0029
T4N3	36	

Concurrent Chemo-radiotherapy

Another possible sequence of giving chemotherapy is combining chemotherapy with concurrent radiotherapy. Since the late 1960's efforts to combine individual or combinations of chemotherapy drugs (MTX, 5-FU, Bleomycin, Hydrea, etc.) simultaneously with radiotherapy have been investigated. These trials ended with increase of oral mucosa side effects, problems in continuation of treatments, and without improvement of survival in randomized trials.
The combination of cisplatin with radiotherapy seemed very attractive from the clinical and basic aspects. A small pilot of cisplatin 100 mg/m2 I.V. with hydration and mannitol diuresis day 1 and every 3 weeks for 3 courses with total radiotherapy in patients with unresectable and/or inoperable cancer was conducted at WSU. When the feasibility of this combined modality treatment was established, the same trial was activated at the cooperative group level in late 1981 (Al-Sarraf 1987a). The combination of chemo-radiotherapy post surgery or induction chemotherapy are being investigated in our Institution.

REFERENCES

Al-Sarraf, M., Binns, P., Vaishampayan, G., et al. (1979): The adjuvant use of cis-platinum, Oncovin and bleomycin (COB) prior to surgery and/or radiotherapy in untreated epidermoid cancer of the head and neck. Adjuvant Therapy of Cancer II. Ed. SE Jones, SE Salmon, Grune & Stratton, Inc. New York, p. 421-428.

Al-Sarraf, M., Drelichman, A., Peppard, S., et al (1981): Adjuvant cis-platinum and 5-fluorouracil 96 hour infusion in previously untreated epidermoid cancers of the head and neck. Proc. ASCO-AACR 22, 428.

Kish, J .A., Drelichman, A., Jacobs, J., et al. (1982): Clinical trials of cis-platinum and 5-FU infusion as initial treatment for advanced squamous carcinoma of the head and neck. Cancer Treat. Rep. 66, 471-474.

Al-Sarraf, M., Kish, J.A., Ensley, J.F., et al. (1984): Induction cis-platinum and 5-fluorouracil infusion before surgery and/or radiotherapy in patients with locally advanced head and neck cancer. Progress report. Proc. AACR 25, 1986.

Jacobs, J.R., Weaver, A., Ahmed, K., et al. (1987): Proto-chemotherapy in

advanced head and neck cancer. Head and Neck Surg. 10, 93-98.
Al-Sarraf, M. (1984a): Chemotherapy strategies in squamous cell carcinoma of the head and neck. CRC Crit. Rev. Oncol. Hematol. 1, 323-355.
Al-Sarraf, M. (1987): Chemotherapeutic management of head and neck cancer. Cancer Metas. Rev. 6, 181-198.
Al-Kourainy, K., Kish, J.A., Ensley, J.F., et al. (1987): Achievement of superior survival for histologically negative vs histologically positive clinically complete responders to cis-platinum combination in patients with locally advanced head and neck cancer. Cancer 59, 233-238.
Al-Sarraf, M., Pajak, T.F., Marcial, V.A., et al. (1987a): Concurrent radiotherapy and chemotherapy with cisplatin in in-operable squamous cell carcinoma of the head and neck. RTOG study. Cancer 59, 259-265.
Al-Sarraf, M., Kinzie, J., Jacobs, J., et al. (1982): New way of giving chemotherapy as part of multi-disciplinary treatment for patients with head and neck cancers. Preliminary report. Proc. AACR 23, 134.
Ensley, J.F., Jacobs, J.R., Weaver, A., et al. (1984): The correlation between response to cis-platinum combination chemotherapy and subsequent radiotherapy in previously untreated patients with advanced squamous cell cancers of the head and neck. Cancer 54, 811-814,
Al-Sarraf, M. (1988): Head and neck cancer: chemotherapy concepts. Sem. Oncology (in press).
Ensley, J.F., Kish, J.A., Tapazoglou, E., et al. (1988): An intensive five course alternating combination chemotherapy induction regimen employed in patients with advanced unresectable head and neck cancer. J. Clin. Oncol. (in press).
Kish, J.A., Ensley, J.F., Jacobs, J., et al. (1984): Investigation of optimal initial chemotherapy in patients with advanced head and neck cancer (HNC) utilizing "high dose" cis-platinum (CACP)-phase I-II. Proc. AACR 25, 173.
Kish, J.A., Ensley, J.F., Jacobs, J.R., et al. (1988): Evaluation of high dose cisplatin and 5-FU infusion as initial therapy in advanced head and neck cancer. Amer. J. Clin. Oncol. (in press).
Al-Sarraf, M., Pajak, T., Laramore, G., et al. (1985): Timing of chemotherapy as part of definitive treatment for patients with advanced head and neck cancer. An RTOG study. Proc. ASCO 4, 141.

Résumé

Combinaisons de différentes modalités thérapeutiques dans les patients atteints d'un epithélioma épidermoide localement avancé tête et cou: Wayne State University

Depuis 1977, huit études pilotes consécutives et prospectives de chimiothérapie d'induction sur base de Cisplatine étaient conduites a la W.S.U. dans le cas de cancer tête et cou, localement avancé. Les résultats des trois études, les plus larges, avec une durée de follow-up de plus que cinq ans, ont démontrés des réponses complètes cliniques (56%) et histologigues (50%), et la survie des traitements par Cisplatine et 5-FU, infusée pendant 120 hours, est supérieure aux autres combinaisons. Deux autres études pilotes ont été effectuées pour investiger le "timing" de la chimiothérapie dans un traitement consistant de différentes modalités thérapeutiques. Dans une, trois cycles de Cisplatine et 5-FU en infusion étaient données après chirurgie et avant radiothérapie, et dans l'autre, un traitement de Cisplatine et radiothérapie simultane était investigé. Ces deux études pilotes étaient faisables et d'une toxicitée tolérable.

Neo-Adjuvant Chemotherapy. Ed. Cl. Jacquillat, M. Weil, D. Khayat. Colloque INSERM/John Libbey Eurotext Ltd. © 1988. Vol. 169, pp. 71-77.

Accelerated treatment with alternating hyperfractionated radiotherapy and chemotherapy of advanced, inoperable squamous cell carcinoma of the head and neck

S. Leyvraz, S. Bernasconi, P. Capasso, Ph. Pasche, M. Savary and L. Barrelet

Centre Pluridisciplinaire d'Oncologie, Service de Radiothérapie, Service d'ORL, Centre Hospitalier Universitaire Vaudois, 1011 Lausanne, Switzerland

ABSTRACT

We explored the possibility of using accelerated hyperfractionated radiotherapy, alternating with chemotherapy in 33 patients with advanced or inoperable squamous cell carcinoma of the head and neck. Two different treatment schedules were tested. In the first, ten patients were treated with radiotherapy; 2.0 Gy three time per day on days 1, 2, 8, 9 and 22, 23, 29, 30. The chemotherapy consisted of a continuous infusion 5 Fluorouracil, 1250 mg/m2/day, on days 4 - 7 and 25 - 28, Vindesine 3 mg/m2 on days 4, 11, 25, 32 and Cis-Platinum 80 mg/m2 on days 4 and 25. Because of the acute toxicity, the schedule was modified with the radiotherapy given on days 1, 2, 3, 11, 12 and 29, 30, 39, 40. The doses and timing of chemotherapy were also reduced, with 5 Fluorouracil (in a continuous infusion of 1000 mg/m2) on days 8 to 10 and 36 to 38, Vindesine 3 mg/m2 and Cis-Platinum 100 mg/m2 on days 8 and 36. From the 33 patients entered in the trial four were ineligible, two because of other tumors and two because of performance status 3. 20 patients had stage IV disease (69%), 4 stage III (14%),one stage II, one multicentric, and 3 recurrent disease. Of the 29 eligible patients 24 were male and 5 female. The median age was 63 (43-76) and the median P.S. was 1 (0-2). At the end of the treatment 28 patients had responded (96%), with 7 in PR (24%) and 21 in CR (72%). 5 patients underwent an adenectomy; two of which had no residual histological tumor while the remaining 3 became surgical complete responders. The total CR rate was 83%. With a median follow-up of 12 months (3-24) 19 patients are alive NED. 4 patients died in CR of unrelated causes, 2 of treatment toxicity and 4 with PD. The acute toxicity was severe. According to the WHO scale: mucositis 3 (0-3), skin 2 (0-3), nausea and vomiting 2 (0-3), weight loss 6 kg (1,3-17,4) were not different in the two treatment schedule. The median leucocyte nadir was 0.9 G/l (0.3-6.5) and 1.3 G/l (0.1-4.7) in the two schedules respectively. Temperature developed in 7 of 10 patients in the first schedule and 7 of 19 patients in the second. A documented case of sepsis and one of pneumonia were found in both regimens. In the second schedule however, the patient with sepsis expired of septic shock while the one with pneumonia expired of bronchial aspiration. In conclusion, this combined treatment was effective, with a higher CR rate than either modality alone, but the toxicity was severe and further modifications of the treatment schedule have been planned.

KEY WORDS: Advanced squamous cell carcinoma of head and neck, accelerated hyperfractionated radiotherapy, alternating radiotherapy and chemotherapy.

INTRODUCTION

Two thirds of the patients with head and neck carcinoma present with stage III or IV disease. In spite of advances in the surgical and radiotherapeutic techniques, the prognosis of these patients remains poor and local recurrence occurs in 50-80%. Furthermore, the required surgery is often mutilating, resulting in major sequellae and disfigurement. Conventional radiotherapy controls 29-50% of locally advanced tumors (Marcial, 1985). No improvement of local control or survival could be shown by hyperfractionated radiotherapy in large randomized trials (Marcial, 1987; Van der Bogaert, 1986) even though some studies (Wang, 1985) have shown potential benefits. Chemotherapy produces a response rate between 50-80% with 10-53% complete local control, but resistance and recurrence appear rapidly, without any consistent improvement in survival (Tannock, 1986). In order to improve these results, concomittant administration of chemotherapy and radiotherapy have been tried (Taylor, 1985; Adelstein, 1986), with increased effectiveness on local control, but with a prohibitive toxicity during the 3 months needed to complete these regimens.

Based on Looney's (1985) experimental data and following the Goldie-Coldman hypothesis on tumor resistance, we devised a treatment protocol using quickly alternating radiotherapy and chemotherapy. Our main objectives were to explore different treatment schedules in order to obtain a lower overall toxicity, an increased complete response rate, and a shorter treatment time.

MATERIALS AND METHODS

Radiotherapy

Radiation therapy was delivered by super-voltage equipment with 60 Co or a 6 meV linear accelerator at a source-to-axis distance of 60-100 cm with a boost on spinal areas with electrons of 3-6 meV. The areas treated included all those of known gross disease. The dose was calculated mid-plane for bilateral and central tumors and loaded two third-one third for unilateral tumors. Because of the exploratory nature of the study, we designed two treatment schemes. In the first, radiotherapy was given as three 2.00 Gy on days 1, 2, 8, 9 and 22, 23, 29, 30; for a total of 4.80 Gy and a tissue dose fraction (TDF) of 120 rets. In the second treatment scheme it was given on days 1, 2, 3, 11, 12 and 29, 30, 39, 40 for a total of 5.40 Gy and a TDF of 131 rets. The interval between fractions was 4 hours.

Chemotherapy

A three drug combination of Cis-Platinum (80 mg/m2) on days 4 and 25, Vindesine (3 mg/m2) on days 4, 11, 25, 32 and Fluorouracil (1250 mg/m2/day) in continuous infusion, from days 4 to 7 and 25-28 was given in the first treatment schedule. It was modified in the second scheme with Cis-Platinum (100 mg/m2) and Vindesine (3 mg/m2) on days 8, 36 and 5 Fluorouracil (1000 mg/m2) from days 8 to 10 and 36 to 38. The regimen was chosen for the following reasons: 1) Cis-Platinum - 5 Fluorouracil is one of the most active combinations for ENT carcinoma (Weaver, 1984). 2) A Synergistic antitumor effect has been described between Cis-Platinum and Vindesine (Gralla, 1981). 3) Vindesine has a 17-25% overall response rate as a single agent and synchronizes cells in their mitotic cycle as other vinca alkaloïds. 4) These three agents have also been shown to be radiosensitizers.

The treatment schemes are summarized in Figue 1.

FIGURE 1: TREATMENT SCHEMES

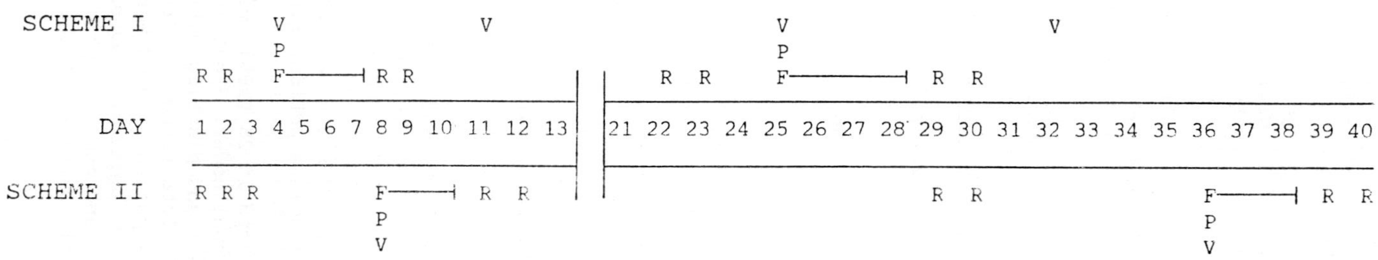

R: 3 x 2.0 Gy/DAY

SCHEME I:	5 FLUOROURACIL	1250	$mg/m^2/day$ x 4
	CIS PLATINUM	80	mg/m^2
	VINDESINE	3	mg/m^2
SCHEME II:	5 FLUOROURACIL	1000	$mg/m^2/day$ x 3
	CIS PLATINUM	100	mg/m^2
	VINDESINE	3	mg/m^2

PATIENTS

All patients with proven squamous cell carcinoma, with a performance status 0 - 2, normal marrow, hepatic and renal functions, with no other malignancy, who were declared inoperable by a multidisciplinary team, or who refused a mutilating operation were eligible for this study. A total of 33 patients were entered in the study. Four were ineligible, either because of a performance status 3 or of the presence of a second malignancy. From the remaining 29 eligible patients, 10 were treated with the first regimen and 19 with the second. There were 24 males and 5 females. The median age was 63 years old (range: 43-76). The median performance status was 1 (range: 0-2). The distribution of patients according to localisation of the primary and the TNM classification is shown in the table I. Seven patients were truly inoperable and 22 were due for mutilating surgery.
The definition of complete response (CR), partial response (PR), no change (NC) and progression (PD) were done according to the ECOG scale.

Table I Head and neck status (No. of patients)

Stage		TNM		Localisation	
II	(3,5%)	T2 NO MO	1	Oral cavity	5
III	(14%)	T3 NO MO	3	Oropharynx	15
		T3 N1 MO	1	Hypopharynx	3
IV	(69%)	T4 NO MO	3	Larynx	3
		T4 N1 MO	4	Maxillary sinus	1
		T2 N3 MO	3	Middle ear	1
		T3 N3 MO	7	Unknown primary	1
		T4 N3 MO	2		
		TX N3 MO	1		
Recurrence	(10%)		3		
Multicentric	(3,5%)		1		

RESULTS

Patients were evaluated for clinical response 6 weeks after the end of therapy. Two major protocol violations occured in the first treatment scheme, where the second part of the hyperfractionated radiotherapy was modified to conventional radiotherapy. At time of protocol violation one patient was in PR and the other already in CR. Two early deaths were noted, one because of bronchial aspiration and the other because of septic shock, the latter occuring in a patient with recorded PR.
Of the 29 eligible patients a clinical response was noticed in 28 (96%), with 7 in PR (24%) and 21 in CR (72%). Because of persistent residual nodes, 5 patients had adenectomies. In 2 patients, no residual tumor could be found histologically. After adenectomy 24 of the 29 patients (83%) were in complete response. With a median follow-up of 12 months (range 3-24), 18 of the 24 patients in CR were alive without evidence of disease. Six patients expired : four of unrelated causes in CR and 2 in PD. Of the 4 partial responders, 3 expired (2 of PD and one of septic shock) while one was still alive with disease. The median overall survival of the patients was 18 months.

Toxicity

As seen in table 2, the acute toxicity was severe and not significantly different in the two treatment schemes. Temperature developed in 7 of the 10 patients in scheme I and 7 of 19 patients in scheme II. One documented sepsis, one pneumonia, 3 oral candidiasis, and one oral herpes occured in treatment I. One sepsis with shock and one bronchial aspiration, both followed by death occured with treatment II, as well as one case of urinary tract infection, 3 of oral candidiasis and one of oral herpes. The follow-up was too short to define the chronic toxicities, and no difference could be noted in the two treatments. Chronic edema developed in 6 patients, moderate xerostomia in 7, skin induration in 2 and slow wound healing in 3 patients.

The treatment was easier to manage in the second scheme, with no delay, protocol violation and only 6 minor chemotherapy modifications. All patients successfully completed the protocol. On the other hand, the first scheme was associated with 4 treatment delays, two protocol violations, 8 chemotherapy modifications, while two patients were unable to complete the regimen.

Table 2

Acute toxicity (WHO scale)	Scheme I (No: 10 p.)		Scheme II (No: 19 p.)	
	median	(range)	median	(range)
Mucositis	3	(0 - 3)	3	(0 - 3)
Skin	2	(0 - 3)	2	(0 - 3)
Nausea Vomiting	2	(0 - 3)	2	(0 - 3)
Leucocyte nadir	0.9 G/l	(0.3 - 6.5)	1.3 G/l	(0.1 - 4.7)
Platelets nadir	100 G/l	(55 - 256)	92 G/l	(13 - 180)
Hemoglobin nadir	89 g/l	(76-114)	107 g/l	(86 - 132)
Weight loss	6 kg	(1.3 - 17.4)	6 kg	(1.5 - 11)

CONCLUSIONS

This combined treatment was effective, producing a response rate of 96% with 83% complete responders. It produced a higher overall response rate and CR rate than each modality alone. The treatment time (40 days) was shorter than in conventional radiotherapy or in any other combined treatment. This had a major impact on the quality of life of these patients. The acute toxicity was severe. Mucositis and skin toxicity could not be avoided. Myelosuppression and toxic deaths were a major concern and have lead to a modification of the chemotherapeutic schedule. The chronic toxicity was minimal, although one must consider the inadequate follow-up time at present. A longer follow-up is also needed to better define a possible impact on overall survival.

In the future a trial should explore the possibility that such a treatment could decrease the need of mutilating surgery. We cannot exclude that our results could have been obtained by accelerated hyperfractionation radiotherapy alone and only a randomized trial could clarify the role of each treatment modality.

REFERENCES

Adelstein D.J., Sharan V.M., Scott E. et al (1986). Chemoradiotherapy as initial management in patients with squamous cell carcinoma of the head and neck. Cancer Treat. Rep. 70: 761-767.

Gralla R.J., Casper E.S., Kelsen D.P. et al (1981). Cisplatin and Vindesine combination chemotherapy for advanced carcinoma of the lung: a randomized trial investigating two dosage schedules. Ann. Intern. Med. 95: 414-420.

Looney W.B., Goldie J.H., Little J.B. et al (1985). Alternation of chemotherapy and radiotherapy in cancer management. 1. Summary of the division of Cancer Treatment Workshop. Cancer Treat. Rep. 69: 769-775.

Marcial V.A., Pajak T.F. (1985). Radiation therapy alone or in combination with surgery in head and neck cancer. Cancer 55: 2259-2265.

Marcial V.A., Pajak T.F., Chang C. et al (1987). Hyperfractionated photon radiation therapy in the treatment of advanced squamous cell carcinoma of the oral cavity, pharynx, larynx and sinuses, using radiation therapy as the only planned modality (Preliminary Report) by the Radiation Therapy Oncology Group (RTOG). Int. J. Radiat. Oncol. Biol. Phys. 13: 41-47.

Tannock I.F., Browman G. (1986). Lack of evidence for a role of chemotherapy in the routine management of locally advanced head and neck cancer. J. Clin. Oncol. 4: 1121-1126.

Taylor S.G., Murthy A.K., Showel J.L. et al (1985). Improved control in advanced head and neck cancer with simultaneous radiation and Cisplatin/5 FU chemotherapy. Cancer Treat. Rep. 69: 933-939.

Van den Bogaert W., Van der Schueren E., Horiot J.C. et al (1986). Early results of the EORTC randomized clinical trial on multiple fractions per day (MFD) and misonidazole in advanced head and neck cancer. Int. J. Radiat. Oncol. Biol. Phys. 12: 587-591.

Wang C.C., Blitzer P.H., Suit H. (1985). Twice-a-day radiation therapy for cancer radiation therapy for cancer of the head and neck. Cancer 55: 2100-2104.

Wearer A., Fleming S., Ensley J. et al (1984). Superior complete response and survival rates with initial bolus Cis-Platinum and 120 hour 5 FU infusion before definitive therapy in patients with locally advanced head and neck cancer. Am. J. Surg. 148: 525-530.

Résumé

Nous avons exploré la possibilité d'utiliser la radiothérapie hyperfractionnée alternée avec de la chimiothérapie chez 33 malades atteints de cancers épidermoïdes avancés et inopérables de la tête et du cou. Deux différents modes de traitement ont été testés. D'une part 10 malades ont été traités par de la radiothérapie 2 Gy trois fois/jour, aux jours 1, 2, 8, 9, 22, 23, 29, 30. La chimiothérapie a consisté en une perfusion continue de 5.Fluorouracile 1250 mg/m2/jour aux jours 4, 7, 25, 28, plus Vindésine 3 mg/m2 aux jours 4, 11, 25, 32, du Cis.Platyl, 80 mg/m2 aux jours 4 et 25. En raison de la toxicité aigue, la séquence a été modifiée, la radiothérapie a été donnée aux jours 1, 2, 3, 11, 12, 29, 30, 39,40. Les doses et la chronologie de la chimiothérapie ont été également réduites : le 5.Fluorouracile donné en perfusions continue de 1000 mg/m2 du jour 8 au jour 10, du jour 36 au jour 38 ; la Vindésine 3 mg/m2 et le Cis.Platyl 100 mg/m2 aux jours 8 et 36. Sur 33 malades entrés dans l'étude, 4 ne sont pas exploitables, 2 en raison de l'apparition d'autres tumeurs, et 2 en raison de l'altération de l'état général (performance III). 20 malades avaient un stade IV (69 %), 4 malades stades III (14 %), un malade au stade II, un malade avec une maladie multicentrique et 3 une rechute. 29 malades exploitables, 4 étaient des hommes, 5 des femmes. L'âge médian était de 63 ans (43-76) et le PS médian était 1 (0-2). A la fin du traitement, 28 malades avaient répondus (96 %) : 17 rémissions partielles (24 %), 21 rémissions complètes (72 %). 5 malades ont subi une adénectomie chez deux d'entre eux il n'y avait pas de tumeur résiduelle histologique alors que les trois autres sont devenus des répondeurs complets chirurgicaux. Le pourcentage de rémission complète est de 83 % avec un suivi médian de 12 mois (3 - 24), 19 malades sont en vie sans rechute. 4 malades sont morts en rémission complètes pour d'autres causes, 2 de toxicité, 4 de maladie progressive. La toxicité aigue a été sévère selon l'échelle de l'OMS. Les complications : muqueuses (3), cutanées (2), nausées et vomissements (2), perte de poids (6 kilos) n'ont pas été différentes dans les deux schémas thérapeutiques. La leucopénie maximum était de 0,9 G/l et de 1,3 G/l dans les deux schémas. Une élévation de la température a été notée chez 7 des 10 malades du 1er schéma et chez 7 des 19 malades du second. Dans les deux régimes on a observé 1 cas de septicémie et 1 cas de pneumonie. Cependant, avec le second schéma, le malade avec la septicémie est mort d'un choc septique tandis que celui atteint de pneumonie est mort d'une aspiration bronchique. En conclusion ce traitement combiné a été efficace avec un taux de rémission complète plus élevé qu'avec chacune des modalités seules. La toxicité a été sévère et d'autres modifications de ce traitement sont prévues.

Neo-Adjuvant Chemotherapy. Ed. Cl. Jacquillat, M. Weil, D. Khayat. Colloque INSERM/John Libbey Eurotext Ltd. © 1988. Vol. 169, pp. 79-84.

Use of concurrent chemotherapy and radiation in head and neck cancer

S.G. Taylor, A. Murthy, D.D. Caldarelli, J.L. Showel, J.C. Hutchingson, P.C. Hollinger, T.R. Witt, M. Kies and B. Mittel

Sheridan Road Pavillon, Rush Medical College, 1725 West Harrison Street, 60612 Chicago, Ill, USA

ABSTRACT

Whereas induction chemotherapy with current regimens has failed to produce any survival advantage, concurrent radiation and 5-FU has shown improved survival over radiation alone in 2 randomized studies. Using a combination of cisplatin, 5-FU infusion and radiation in 52 patients we showed a 55% 3 year survival for predominantly stage IV inoperable patients (8 stage III, 35 IV, 9 recurrent) with a median follow-up of 45 months. There is strong evidence to indicate that optimal results with cisplatin, 5-FU infusion and radiation may be expected from giving these modalities together as much as possible. Such coordination requires split course fractionation of the radiation and, when given in this way, can produce high local control rates.

INTRODUCTION

Concomitant chemotherapy and radiation in head and neck cancer is a treatment approach that had initially been pursued during the 1960's and early 1970's. Use of induction chemotherapy largely replaced this approach when dramatic responses were described; however, no survival benefit has been shown from several randomized trials. With awareness of the radiation sensitizing properties of many active antineoplastic drugs, there is renewed interest in integrating chemotherapy with regional treatment.

Review of past experience with combined radiation and various antineoplastics indicates that only bleomycin and 5-FU have caused a survival advantage. Positive results with combined bleomycin and radiation, however, have been predominantly in tumors characterized by a high degree of histologic differentiation. Such tumors are uncommon in Western countries so that most such trials in Europe and the U. S. have shown limited results (1).

5-FU, on the other hand, has caused a significant survival advantage when given with radiation in the only 2 randomized trials with this agent, of which I am aware (1). While one used intra-arterial infusion and the other intravenous bolus, both had remarkably similar conclusions: 1) A survival advantage was seen, 2) this survival advantage occurred despite more radiation therapy interruptions and with less total dose of radiation delivered than for the control group, and 3) future trials with combined radiation and 5-FU should use planned treatment interruptions (1,2).

Byfield has exploited the integration of 5-FU with radiation therapy, giving maximal exposure during and after radiation by giving 5-FU as a high dose infusion and using a planned split course fractionation. This enables each radiation treatment to be combined with 5-FU (4). We have extended this concept by combining the radiation with cisplatin and 5-FU infusion together (5), based on reports of high activity of this drug combination (6), and on the radiation sensitizing properties of cisplatin.

SUBJECTS AND METHODS

Subjects

Patients had inoperable stage IV disease of any site or stage III nasopharynx, hypopharynx and tongue carcinomas or regional recurrence following prior surgery. This report includes only those patients treated with curative intent (not M1 and no prior radiation therapy that would prevent delivery of at least 60 Gy to the tumor bed). All patients had normal hematologic parameters, a serum creatinine less than 1.5 mg% and bilirubin less than 1.9 mg%. Creatinine clearance was not performed. Characterics of the patients is shown in Tables 1 and 2.

Treatment

Each cycle consisted of cisplatin 60 mg/m^2, 15 minutes infusion, day 1, 5-FU 800 mg/m^2, 24 hour infusion, days 1-5 (120 hours), and radiation with 2 Gy once daily, days 1-5. The treatment cycles were repeated after a 9 day rest period (every other week treatments) to a total of 7 cycles (70 Gy). The schedule for dose modification based on toxicity and the methods of analysis of response has been reported (5).

Radiation was delivered by supervoltage equipment using conventional techniques with multiple fields. The spinal cord was shielded after 44 Gy and only gross disease treated after 50 Gy. In the event of a week with a holiday, 2.5 Gy daily fractions were used for 4 days, but the chemotherapy schedule was not altered.

RESULTS

Fifty-two patients have entered this study and all are included in the analysis. Nine had recurred following prior surgery and one had received 3 cycles of induction cisplatin-5-FU therapy at another institution with stable disease prior to starting the combined treatment.

Table 1 Patient Characteristics

Characteristic	Values	Sites:	
% Female	23%	Oral Cavity	19%
		Oropharynx	10%
Median Age (range)	63 (36-83)	Nasopharynx	6%
		Hypopharynx	19%
Performance Status:		Larynx	12%
		Tongue	27%
0/1/2/3	38%/40%/19%/6%	Sinus	4%
		Unknown	4%
Histologic Differentiation			
Well/Mod. Well/ Poor	12%/58%/30%		

TABLE 2: T and N Staging (AJC 1978)

Nodes	Tumor 0	1	2	3	4	Total
0				5R	7R	12
1				5R	8R	13
2		1	3	3R	4R	11
3	4R	2	1R	2	7	16
Total	4	3	4	15	26	52

RESPONSE

Clinical response to this regimen was 56% complete and 42% partial. One patient who suffered a stroke after 2 cycles was never reevaluated. Destructive lesions involving bone rarely normalized even with prolonged follow-up. Twelve patients underwent subsequent neck dissections (3 with resections of the primary as well) and 3 others had biopsies. Five of 6 patients who had a complete response clinically were pathologically free of disease as were 4 of 9 partial responders.

TOXICITY

The major dose limiting toxicities have been mucositis and myelotoxicity, while weight loss was the most frequent side effect. Five patients had leukocyte counts less than 1,000/mm^3 and none had platelet counts less than 20,000/mm^3. Grade 3 mucositis occurred in 26 (50%) of patients. Fifteen had an one week delay and 2 had 2 weeks delay in treatment. Two patients refused to complete therapy and two were removed from the treatment with the development of severe cerebral vascular occlusion in one and a vertebral fracture from a fall in another. Four patients have died during treatment: One aspiration pneumonia and renal failure with aminoglycoside antibiotics, two sudden deaths during one of the rest weeks off therapy, and one bowel perforation. A serum creatinine over 2.5 from the cisplatin has occurred in only one patient. All other patients completed the planned 6 (9 patients) or 7 (34 patients) cycles of treatment.

SURGERY

Only 12 of these patients underwent subsequent surgery. All had a radical neck dissection. Two patients also had a planned resection of the primary (one base of tongue and one hypopharynx). An additional patient with a T4 supraglottic cancer required laryngectomy for repeated aspiration. Five had had a complete response to the combined chemotherapy and radiation treatment and 7 a partial response.

While difficult to quantitate, surgery was felt to be more difficult than following radiation alone. Fibrosis and loss of tissue planes were worse. Neck dissections were accomplished without long-term toxicity but initial wound healing was often problematic with partial breakdown of incisions requiring healing by secondary intent. One patient had a persistant seroma requiring reexploration of the neck and treatment with a sclerosing agent. All 3 patients who underwent surgery on the primary site had major post-operative morbidity consisting of osteomyelitis in the patient having a partial glossectomy and prolonged pharyngocutaneous fistulas in the laryngectomy patients. Edema of the pharynx and larynx was common following combined chemotherapy and radiation making wound healing even from local biopsies compromised. One patient, not included in this series because of having had prior radiation, had severe laryngeal edema following repeated biopsies that ultimately required a laryngectomy for relief of airway obstruction. With that experience we have discouraged biopsying treated areas unless progression is suspected clinically.

RECURRENCE AND SURVIVAL

Follow-up ranges from 6 to 80 months (median 45 months). However, 43 (83%) have had at least 2 years follow-up. Eleven (21%) have recurred regionally in the radiation fields including the two patients who refused further treatment after 4 and 5 cycles respectively. While all of these involved recurrence at the primary site, only 2 of these have thus far failed in the neck. Eight (15%) have had only distant failure. Time to progression of those who failed varied from 3.8 to 50.5 months (median 8.5 months), but all 3 failures after 27 months have been due to distant disease.

Survival has been affected by both disease recurrence and other causes as is usual for this disease. Twenty-five patients (48%) have died, 14 (27%) from cancer and 11 (21%) due to other causes, including the 4 deaths during treatment. The 1,2, and 3 year survivals are 73%, 66%, and 55% respectively for all 52 patients.

DISCUSSION

These results of combining radiation with cisplatin and 5-FU infusion chemotherapy in inoperable, predominantly stage IV, head and neck cancer are better than those reported with surgery and radiation used for less advanced stage II-IV, operable disease. The relatively high proportion of patients failing at distant sites reflects both the excellent regional control as well as the advanced nature of the disease in our patients, as 5 of the 8 distant failures were in patients with N3 neck disease, and the other 3 all had T4 primaries. Despite the advanced disease status only 21% have had local failure and only 2 of these have shown failure in the irradiated neck.

It is difficult to accept these results outside of a randomized trial. We are currently randomizing inoperable head and neck cancer patients to either induction chemotherapy with 3 cycles of cisplatin and 5-FU infusion followed by radiation or to concurrent cisplatin, 5-FU infusion and radiation. Others are also beginning to publish phase II trials of combined cisplatin, 5-FU and radiation. Those trials emphasize the need to give the radiation and chemotherapy together for optimal results. Two studies have sandwiched the radiation in between chemotherapy treatments and both have median survivals less than 1 year (although both have entered very advanced patients with predominantly recurrent disease) (6). The Cleveland Clinic study using cisplatin and high dose infusion 5-FU only gave chemotherapy for the first week of each 3 week cycle of radiation (6). Although 53% of their patients were less than stage IV, their one year survival was almost identical to ours (74%).

Wendt et al have treated patients with cisplatin, 5-FU infusion and leucovorin and twice daily fractionation of radiation (7). The chemotherapy was given for the 1st of every 2 weeks of radiation. This schedule would allow only very low dose 5-FU (350 mg/m^2) because the mucosal toxicity from 5-FU would be expected to peak during the second week of radiation. Nevertheless, this schedule did give more chemotherapy during radiation than the other studies, and has produced a 58% 2 year survival in predominantly stage IV disease patients. Both twice daily fractionation and the use of leucovorin are interesting concepts to explore.

In conclusion, our results do appear promising but derive principally from a single institution. They certainly require confirmation by others. Nevertheless, they are, we believe, based on sound principles and are provocative enough to warrant testing in a randomized trial.

RÉSUMÉ

Tandis que la chimiothérapie antérieure n'a pas montre une amélioration de la survie dans les éssais randomises des carcinomes de la tête et du cou, les résultats de deux éssais randomisés avec 5 FU pendant la radiothérapie sont concordants en donnant la survie mieux. Nous avons montre une 3 an survie de 55% pour 52 patients (8 stade III, 35 IV, 9 recidive) avec une association de cisplatinum, 5 FU et radiothérapie. Nous croyons que les mieux résultats avec cette association sont quand on donne la radiothérapie autant que possible avec 5 FU.

REFERENCES

1) Taylor SG IV, Murthy AK. Concurrent chemotherapy and radiation in head and neck cancer: A review. Submitted to Cancer Communication, 1988.
2) Wiley AL Jr, Ramirez G, Johnson RO, Brandenburg JH, Lieberman LM, Lo TCM, Vermund H: Treatment of carcinoma of base of tongue with radiation therapy and 5-fluorouracil. Acta Radiologic Oncology, 18:235-243. 1979
3) Byfield JE, Sharp TR, Frankel SS, Tang SG, Callipari FB: Phase I and II trial for five-day infused 5-fluorouracil and radiation in advanced cancer of the head and neck. J Clin Oncol. 2:406-413, 1984.
4) Murthy AK, Taylor SG IV, Showel J, Caldarelli DD, Hutchinson J Jr, Holinger LD, Witt TR, Hoover S. Treatment of advanced head and neck cnacer with concomitant radiation and chemotherapy. Int. J. Radiation Oncology Biol Phys. Vol. 13, 1807-1813, 1987.
5) Weaver A, Fleming S, Kish J, et al. Cis-platinum and 5-fluorouracil as induction therapy for advanced head and neck cancer. Am J Surg 144:445-448, 1982.
6) Taylor SG IV, Head and Neck Cancer in Cancer Chemotherapy and Biological Response Modifiers. Annual 9. HM Pinedo, DL Longo, BA Chabner, ed. Elsevier Science Publ., Amsterdam. 226-238, 1987.
7) Wendt TG, Wustrow TPU, Hartensten RC, Rohloff R, Trott KR: Accelerated split-course radiotherapy and simultaneous cis-dichlorodiammine-platinum and 5-fluorouracil chemotherapy with folinic acid enhancement for unresectable carcinoma of the head and neck. Radiotherapy and Oncology, 10 277-284, 1987.

Résumé

Alors que la chimiothérapie d'induction avec les protocoles actuels n'a pas montré d'avantage de survie, une association de 5.Fu et d'irradiation a montré une survie supérieure à celle d'une irradiation seule dans deux études randomisées utilisant une association de Cis.Platyl-5.Fu et d'irradiation chez 52 malades, nous avons obtenu une survie à 3 ans de 55 % pour des malades ayant le plus souvent un stade IV inopérable (8 stade III, 35 stades IV, 9 rechutes), avec un recul médian de 45 mois. Il y a des arguments très forts pour indiquer que les résultats les meilleurs sont obtenus lorsque les modalités Cis.Platyl-5.Fu et irradiation sont données aussi rapprochés que possible. Une telle coordination nécessite un fractionnement intermittent de l'irradiation et donné de cette façon ce traitement produit un taux élevé de contrôle local.

Neo-Adjuvant Chemotherapy. Ed. Cl. Jacquillat, M. Weil, D. Khayat. Colloque INSERM/John Libbey Eurotext Ltd. © 1988. Vol. 169, pp. 85-88.

Combination of cisplatin and radiotherapy in advanced head and neck cancer: an update

G. Ambrosini, M. Amichetti, A. Bolner, G. Fellin, G. Pani and R. Valdagni

Centro Oncologico, Ospedale S. Chiara, 38100 Trento, Italy

ABSTRACT

Between April 1984 and August 1986, 53 patients with advanced squamous cell carcinoma of the head and neck were entered into this study.
A combination of Cisplatin 20 mg/sq.m. i.v. once a week and standard Radiation Therapy (65-70 Gy total dose) was administered.
Responses to therapy were the following: 36 C.R. (76,6%), 8 P.R. (17%), 2 S.D. (4,3%), 1 P.D. (2,1%).
Actuarial overall survival at 36 months was 45%, disease-free survival 34,1%.
Toxicity was mild.

KEYWORDS

Cisplatin, Radiation Therapy, head and neck cancer.

INTRODUCTION

Radiation therapy is the treatment of choice in the management of advanced inoperable head and neck squamous cell carcinoma. Despite this, local control and survival rates are very meager.
In an attempt to improve these discouraging results, chemotherapy has been added to Radiation Therapy in neoadjuvant, sequential or simultaneous setting.
Many drugs (MTX, BLM, 5 FU, HU etc...) have been tested in contemporary combination to irradiation with conflicting results and enhanced toxicity.
In recent years, Cisplatin has shown particular radiopotentiating properties in experimental models and in clinical studies.
This report is an update of our experience in the treatment of advanced head and neck cancer with the association of Radiation Therapy and weekly administration of Cisplatin as radioenhancer.

MATERIALS AND METHODS

From August 1984 to April 1986, 53 untreated patients affected by squamous cell carcinoma of the head and neck were entered into the study.
Criteria for eligibility were the following: age 70 years, no prior treatments, no distant metastases, Performance Status $\geq$2 (ECOG scale), serum creatinine $\leq$ 1,2 mg/100 ml, creatinine clearance $>$70 ml/minute, leukocite count $\geq$4000/mm^3, platelet count $\geq$100.000/mm^3, and haemoglobin $\geq$11 g/100 ml. Patient characteristics are shown in Table 1.
Physical examination, laringoscopy, bilateral audiogram, chest x-ray, head and neck CT, and routine haematologic tests were performed before therapy.
Radiation therapy was delivered by megavoltage equipments (60 CO or 6-12 MV L.A., photon and electron beam) with a total dose ranging from 65 to 70 Gy, 2-2,5 Gy per fraction with usual treatment techniques.
Cisplatin was administered i.v., once a week, at a dose of 20 mg/sq.m. during the whole course of radiation therapy, and was injected within two hours after irradiation. No special hidration was used.
Responses and toxicity were evaluated according to W.H.O. criteria (Miller, 1981) survival and disease-free data were calculated by Kaplan and Meier method.

RESULTS

Up to April 1986 fifty three patients entered the study: 47 were evaluable. One month after the end of combined therapy responses were the following: 36 C.R. (76,6%), 8 P.R. (17%), 2 S.D. (4,3%), 1 P.D. (2,1%). At time of analysis, 38 months after the start of the study, median follow-up is of 17 months (5-37 months), actuarial overall survival is 45%,disease free-survival is 34,1%. The probability of local regional control at 36 months is 42,5%.
Toxicity is summarized in Table 2. Four patients developed distant metastases, four patients had a metachronous cancer, two patients died of cancer unrelated to disease or to therapy.

DISCUSSION

Cisplatin has been used as radioenhancer mainly in lung and head and neck cancer (Tobias, 1987) with interesting results. Complete response rates in head and neck tumors range between 31% (Snyderman, 1986) and 90% (Coughlin, 1986) and the superiority of combined treatment over Radiation Therapy alone has been suggested by many Authors.
The best timing schedule and the optinum dose of Cisplatin in combination with irradiation is still debated. We chose our schedule (20 mg/sq. m. once a week after RT) on the basis of Haselow at al's (1983) suggestions and also for logistic reasons.
The ongoing results of our study (76,6% C.R. with 93,6% overall responses) are within the range of the reports published in the literature and they confirm our preliminary results (Ambrosini, 1986). Toxicity seems to be mild: the most frequent side effects noted were haematological but always of grade 1 or 2. Radiation therapy side effects did not appear to be increased by the addition of Cisplatin. No severe late effects were seen. If the combination of Radiation Therapy and Cisplatin is superior to Radiation Therapy alone, it will only be

demostrated through carefully controlled prospective randomized studies.
The use of different fractionation (multiple fractions per day), the use of less toxic but equal radiopotentiating analogues such as Carboplatin, and the use of different schedules could furtherly improve these preliminary encouraging results.

Table 1. Patients characteristics

No. of patients	53
median age in years (range)	52 (17-69)
SEX: Male/Female	51/2
Hystology	squamous cell ca.
Sites of disease:	
oral cavity	13
oropharynx	21
hypopharynx	10
larynx	6
nasopharynx	1
maxillary sinus	2
Stage: III / IV	17/36

Table 2. Toxic effects

	GRADE 1	GRADE 2	GRADE 3	GRADE 4
Haematological	30%	17%	-	-
Gastrointestinal	5,5%	5,5%	11%	-
Infection	5,5%	-	-	-
Renal	2%	-	-	-
Allergic	-	-	2%	-
Oral-Cutaneous	80%	8%	10%	2%

REFERENCES

Haselow R.E., Adams G.S., Oken M.M., Goudsmit A., Lerner H.J., Marsh J.H. (1983): Cis-platinum (DDP) with Radiation therapy (RT) for locally advanced unresectable head and neck cancer. Proc. Am. Soc. Clin. Oncol. 1, 160.

Miller A.B., Hoogstraten B., Staquet M., Winkler A. (1981): Reporting results of cancer treatment. Cancer 47, 207-214.

Snyderman N.L., Wetmore S.J., Suen J.Y. (1986): Cisplatin sensitization to radio therapy in stage IV squamous cell carcinoma of the head and neck. Arch. Otolaryngol head neck surg. 112, 1147-1150.

Coughlin C.T., Richmond R.C. (1985): Platinum based combined modality approach for locally advanced head and neck carcinoma. Int. J. Radiat. Oncol. Biol. Phys. 11, 915-919.

Ambrosini G., Amichetti M., Piffer S., Valdagni C. (1986): Combination of cisplatin and radiotherapy in advanced head and neck cancer: preliminary report. In: Neo-adjuvant chemotherapy. Jacquillat C., Weil M., Khayat D., eds. pp 383-386. London - Paris: J. Libbey Eurotext.

Tobias J.S., Smith B.J., Blackman G., Finn G. (1987): Concurrent daily cisplatin and radiotherapy in locally advanced squamous carcinoma of the head and neck bronchus. Radiother. Oncol. 9, 263-268.

Résumé

De août à mai 1986. Cinquante quatre patients porteurs d'un carcinome épidermoïde de la tête et du cou au stade III et IV, ont été traités par une association chimiothérapie-radiothérapie, consistant en irradiation classique à visée radicale plus cisplatinum deliverée une fois par semaine. Quarant sept patients sont évaluables. Les pourcentages de réponses sont les suivantes: 36 régressions complètes (76,6%) 8 régressions partielles (17%), 2 stabilisation (4,3%) et 1 progression tumoral (2,1%). La médiane de durée de surveillance est de 17 mois (5-37), la survie calculée par le méthode actuarielle de Kaplan-Meyer est du 45%, la survie libre de maladie est du 34,1%. La toxicité hématologique concerne presque esclusivement la numération leucocitaire et plaquettaire. Le vomissement liés au cisplatinum a été frequente mais pas importante. Aucun aggravation des complications cutanéo-muqueses n'a été observée.
Les notres resultats ont confirmé l'efficacité objettive immediate de la combination chimiothérapie-radiothérapie dans les carcinones épidermoides de vads.

Neo-Adjuvant Chemotherapy. Ed. Cl. Jacquillat, M. Weil, D. Khayat. Colloque INSERM/John Libbey Eurotext Ltd. © 1988. Vol. 169, pp. 89-93.

Carcinomes bronchiques à petites cellules limités. Résultats d'un protocole d'alternance de chimiothérapie et de radiothérapie chez 165 malades

Thierry Le Chevalier [1], Rodrigo Arriagada [1], Pierre Baldeyrou [1], Pierre Ruffié [1], Hubert de Cremoux [2], Marie-Lise Cerrina [3], Michel Martin [2], Hélène Sancho-Garnier [1] et le GROP

[1] *Institut Gustave-Roussy, 94805 Villejuif Cedex, France*
[2] *Centre Hospitalier Intercommunal, 94000 Créteil, France*
[3] *Hôpital Antoine Béclère, 92140 Clamart, France*

RESUME

De 1980 à 1986, 165 malades porteurs de cancers bronchiques à petites cellules limités ont été inclus dans trois études consécutives de faisablité selon un protocole d'alternance de 6 cycles de chimiothérapie et de 3 séries d'irradiation. Les cures de chimiothérapie étaient administrées toutes les 4 semaines et un intervalle libre d'une semaine était prévu entre les cures de chimiothérapie et les séries d'irradiation. La chimiothérapie comportait : doxorubicine 40 mg/m2 jour 1 ; VP 16213 75 à 100 mg/m2 jours 1 à 3 ; cyclophosphamide 300 mg/m2 jours 3 à 6 et méthotrexate 400 mg/m2 ou cis-platinum 100 à 120 mg/m2 jour 2. La dose totale de radiothérapie thoracique était de 45 à 65 Gy.

Notre population, 140 hommes et 25 femmes, avait un âge moyen de 54 ans et un index de Karnofsky moyen de 83 % ; 91 % des malades étaient stade III.

Le taux de réponses complètes est de 77 % et le taux de récidives locales de 14 %. Le taux de survie sans récidive ni métastase est de 33 % à 18 mois et de 21 % à 48 mois (19 malades sont vivants à plus de 4 ans). La tolérance a été dans l'ensemble acceptable mais la toxicité hématologique constante (létale dans 3 % des cas).

La dose de la première cure de chimiothérapie s'est révélée d'importance pronostique majeure et nous a conduits à renforcer la première cure de chimiothérapie et à délivrer une première série d'irradiation précoce hyperfractionnée dans notre protocole actuel.

MOTS-CLEFS

Cancer bronchique à petites cellules limité. Combinaison chimiothérapie-radiothérapie.

La chimiothérapie (CT) constitue depuis 15 ans le traitement de base des cancers bronchiques à petites cellules (CPC). Les résultats en règle spectaculaires, sont, on le sait, souvent éphémères du fait de l'apparition précoce de clônes résistants. Goldie et Coldman (1) ont développé un modèle mathématique basé sur l'alternance de combinaisons de drogues sans résistance croisée et cette approche est particulièrement intéressante en cas de tumeurs instables génétiquement et à temps de doublement rapide (2).

Le rôle de la radiothérapie thoracique (RT) dans les CPC a été l'objet de nombreuses discussions (3) mais il semble que, associée à la chimiothérapie, elle augmente significativement le taux de rémissions complètes et probablement la durée de survie malgré une toxicité accrue (4, 5). Le problème de telles associations thérapeutiques est en effet celui de leur mode d'administration, ces deux traitements sans résistance croisée évidente (6) devant être délivrés précocément mais leur administration simultanée diminuant indéniablement leur tolérance respective.

L'alternance de CT et de RT permet a) de débuter la CT d'emblée, b) de l'administrer chaque mois sans interruption, c) de réaliser une RT précoce à doses suffisantes (3) et d) grâce à un intervalle d'une semaine entre les cures de CT et les séries de RT, d'améliorer la tolérance des tissus sains.

C'est ainsi que le schéma proposé par Tubiana et col. (7) à partir de ces concepts nous a conduits à traiter les CPC par un protocole d'alternance de CT et de RT dont nous rapportons ici les résultats.

MALADES ET METHODES

De 1980 à 1987, 165 malades ont été inclus dans trois protocoles prospectifs consécutifs. Un bilan d'extension initial complet (8) permettait de définir la notion de maladie limitée (explorations cérébrale, hépatique, surrénalienne, osseuse et médullaire négatives). Tous les malades étaient âgés de moins de 70 ans et devaient avoir un index de Karnofsky supérieur à 40 %. Le schéma du protocole d'induction était le suivant :

CT---CT-RT-CT-RT-CT-RT-CT-CT,

(-) représentant un intervalle d'une semaine.

Dans le premier protocole (002, 28 malades inclus de Mai 1980 à Octobre 1981), la CT associait : doxorubicine 40 mg/m^2 jour 1 ; VP16213 75 mg/m^2 jours 1-3 ; cyclophosphamide 300 mg/m^2 jours 3-6 et méthotrexate 400 mg/m^2 jour 2 (+ acide folinique). La dose de chacune des 3 séries de RT était de 15 Gy en 6 séances sur 10 jours par des champs antéro-postérieurs (dose totale 45 Gy).

Dans le second protocole (004, 81 malades inclus de Novembre 1981 à Décembre 1984), le méthotrexate a été remplacé par du cisplatinum à la dose de 100 mg/m^2 jour 2 et la dose des deux premières séries d'irradiation a été portée à 20 Gy en 8 séances sur 12 jours par des champs antéro-postérieurs, la troisième série délivrant 15 Gy en 6 séances sur 10 jours par des champs latéraux évitant la moelle épinière (dose totale 55 Gy).

Les malades de ces deux premiers protocoles recevaient au terme du traitement d'induction six à huit cures de chimiothérapie d'entretien (8).

Dans le troisième protocole (006, 56 malades inclus de Janvier 1985 à Mai 1987), les doses de VP16213 et de cisplatinum ont été augmentées (respectivement 100 mg/m^2 jours 1 - 3 et 120 mg/m^2 jour 2) lors des deux premiers cycles de CT. La dose de la troisième série de RT a été portée à 25 Gy en 10 séances sur 17 jours par des champs latéraux et obliques (dose totale 65 Gy). Ces malades n'ont pas reçu de chimiothérapie d'entretien.

Une irradiation de principe de l'encéphale (IPC) à la dose de 30 Gy en 10 séances sur 12 jours a été administrée chez tous les malades des protocoles 002 et 004 après la seconde cure de chimiothérapie, tandis qu'elle a fait l'objet d'une randomisation dans le protocole 006 pour les seuls malades en rémission complète au terme de leur traitement d'induction, un malade sur deux recevant une IPC à la dose de 24 Gy en 8 séances sur 12 jours.

Notre population était composée de 140 hommes et 25 femmes et l'âge moyen était de 54 ans. L'index de Karnofsky moyen était de 83 % (allant de 50 à 100 %) et 91 % des malades étaient stade III (16 présentaient des adénopathies sus-claviculaires). Il n'y a pas de différence entre les caractéristiques des malades des trois protocoles.

RESULTATS

Tous les malades ont été réévalués après 6 mois, au terme du traitement d'induction, et le taux de rémissions complètes était alors de 79 % dans les protocoles 002 et 004 et 73 % dans le protocole 006. Le taux de récidives locales a été de 15 % dans les protocoles 002 et 004 et de 11,5 % dans le protocole 006. Le taux de métastases cérébrales (comme premier site de rechute) a été de 17 % dans les protocoles 002 et 004 et de 25 % dans le protocole 006.

La survie médiane sans récidive ni métastase de l'ensemble de la population est de 13,7 mois.

Les taux de survie sans récidive ni métastase sont présentés dans le tableau ci-dessous.

Taux de survie sans récidive ni métastase

	002 + 004		006	
mois	n (109)	%	n (56)	%
6	101	93	48	91
12	69	64	28	58
18	35	33	15	35
24	28	27		
36	20	21		
48	19	21		

Tous les malades ont présenté une toxicité hématologique. Elle a été de grade IV OMS dans 29 % des cas. Cinq malades sont décédés en aplasie lors du traitement d'induction. La tolérance a été par ailleurs acceptable. Les 18 premiers malades en vie à 30 mois ont fait l'objet d'une évaluation de leur fonction respiratoire (9) et une dyspnée d'effort a été retrouvée chez 8 d'entre eux. Des séquelles endoscopiques ont été notées dans 65 % des cas. Les gaz du sang étaient dans les limites de la normale chez tous les malades. Par contre, un épanchement péricardique a été retrouvé dans la majorité des cas à l'échographie ; il n'était symptomatique que chez une malade. Enfin l'index de Karnofsky moyen de ces malades était de 90 %.

Une étude rétrospective des facteurs pronostiques réalisée chez les malades des protocoles 002 et 004 a mis en évidence l'importance de la première cure de chimiothérapie et en particulier l'effet dose constaté avec la cyclophosphamide et le cisplatinum qui se révèlent d'importance pronostique majeure sur la survie sans récidive ni métastase de même que le volume tumoral, en analyse multivariate (10).

DISCUSSION

Les trois protocoles consécutifs rapportés ici ont permis d'obtenir des résultats comparables et reproductibles en termes de résultats.

Sur l'ensemble de la population, le taux de rémission complète, de 77 %, et le faible pourcentage de récidives locales (inférieur à 15 %) confirment l'intérêt d'associer la RT à la CT (3, 4, 5).

La faisabilité des protocoles d'alternance de CT et RT est démontrée dans notre étude, tant en ce qui concerne les résultats à court terme que les survivants à plus de trente mois.

Le rôle de la première cure de chimiothérapie paraît majeur sur le plan pronostique et nous a conduits à augmenter les doses de chimiothérapie initiales et à débuter dès la seconde semaine de traitement une irradiation hyperfractionnée. Ce nouveau protocole thérapeutique est en cours d'évaluation.

REFERENCES BIBLIOGRAPHIQUES

1.- Goldie, J.H., Coldman, A.J. (1979) : A mathematical model for relating the drug sensitivity of tumors to their spontaneous mutation rate. Cancer Treat. Rep. 63, 1727-1733.

2.- Evans, W.K., Feld, R., Murray, N. (1987) : Superiority of alternating non cross resistant chemotherapy in extensive small cell lung cancer. Multicenter randomized clinical trial by the National Cancer Institute of Canada. Ann. Int. Med. 107, 451-458.

3.- Morstyn, G., Ihde, D.C., Lichter, A.S. et al. (1984) : Small cell lung cancer 1973-1983 : early progress and recent obstacles. Int. J. Rad. Oncol. Biol. Phys. 10, 515-539.

4.- Bunn, P.A., Lichter, A.S., Makuch, R.W. et al. (1987) : Chemotherapy alone and chemotherapy with chest radiation therapy in limited stage small cell lung cancer. Ann. Int. Med. 106, 655-662.

5.- Perry, M.C., Eaton, W.L., Propert; K.H. et al. (1987) : Chemotherapy with or without radiation therapy in limited small cell carcinoma of the lung. N. Engl. J. Med. 316, 912-918.

6.- Looney, W.B., Ritenour, E.R., Hopkins, H.A. (1981) : Solid tumor models for the assessment of different treatment modalities : XVI. Sequential combined modality (cyclophosphamide, radiation) therapy. Cancer 47, 860-869.

7.- Tubiana, M., Arriagada, R., Cosset, J.M. (1982) : New types of fractionation for optimization of combinations of radiotherapy and chemotherapy. In : Progress in Radiation Oncology II, Karcher ed., New-York, Raven Press, pp. 387-391.

8.- Arriagada, R., Le Chevalier, T., Baldeyrou, P. et al. (1985) : Alternating radiotherapy and chemotherapy schedules in small cell lung cancer, limited disease. Int. J. Radiat. Oncol. Biol. Phys. 11, 1461-1467.

9.- De Cremoux, H., Baldeyrou, P., Martin, M. et al. (1987) : Séquelles respiratoires après chimiothérapie et radiothérapie alternées pour cancer anaplasique à petites cellules. Bull. Cancer 74, 575-580.

10.- Le Chevalier, T., De The, H., Arriagada, R. et al. (1986) : Prognostic value of initial chemotherapy drug doses in patients with small cell lung cancer. Cancer Chemoth. Pharmacol. 18, suppl. 1, A43.

LIMITED SMALL CELL LUNG CARCINOMA. RESULTS OF AN ALTERNATING RADIOTHERAPY AND CHEMOTHERAPY SCHEDULE IN 165 PATIENTS

Thierry LE CHEVALIER[1], Rodrigo ARRIAGADA[1], Pierre BALDEYROU[1], Pierre RUFFIE[1], Hubert DE CREMOUX[2], Marie-Lise CERRINA[3], Michel MARTIN[2], Hélène SANCHO-GARNIER[1], and The G.R.O.P.

1. Institut Gustave-Roussy, 94805 VILLEJUIF Cédex - France.
2. Centre Hospitalier Intercommunal, 94000 Créteil - France.
3. Hôpital Antoine Béclère, 92140 Clamart - France.

Résumé

Combination chemotherapy is the basic treatment of small cell lung carcinoma (SCLC) and thoracic radiotherapy (RT) improves local control in patients with limited disease. In order to avoid the toxicity of concurrent CT and RT, we alternated these therapeutic modalities and we report here the results obtained with the following schedule :

CT---CT-RT-CT-RT-CT-RT-CT---CT

were (-) represents one week interval.

From 1980 to 1986, 165 patients were entered in three consecutive phase II studies (002, 004, 006) based on this alternating combination. The CT regimen included : doxorubicin 40 mg/m2 day 1, Etoposide 75 to 100 mg/m2 day 1-3, cyclophosphamide 300 mg/m2 day 2-5 and methotrexate 400 mg/m2 or cis-platinum 100 to 120 mg/m2 day 2. The total RT dose was 45 to 65 Gy and most patients received prophylactic cranial irradiation (PCI). Twenty eight patients with limited disease were included in protocol 002 (1980-1981), 81 in protocol 004 (1981-1984) and 56 in protocol 006 (1985-1987). There were 140 males and 25 females and median age was 54 y.o. Mean performance status was 83 % (range 50-100 %) and 91 % of patients presented with stage III (16 with supraclavicular lymph nodes). Complete response rate was 79 % in protocols 002 and 004 ; it was 73 % in protocol 006. Local recurrence was observed in 15 % of patients in protocols 002 and 004, 11.5 % in protocol 006. Brain metastases rate (as first site of relapse) was 17 % in protocols 002 and 004 where all patients had received PCI and 25 % in protocol 006 where patients had been randomized to receive or not PCI. Median disease free survival of our population is 13.7 months. Eighteen month disease free survival rate is 33 % in protocols 002 and 004, 35 % in protocol 006. Nineteen patients are alive disease free at 4 years (survival rate 21 %). Tolerance was acceptable but bone marrow toxicity was observed in all patients (lethal in 3 %). The dose of the first CT cycle was the major prognostic factor in a retrospective multivariate analysis. From these conclusions, we have currently increased doses in the first CT cycle and we deliver earlier a first multifractionated RT course in our ongoing trial.

Neo-Adjuvant Chemotherapy. Ed. Cl. Jacquillat, M. Weil, D. Khayat. Colloque INSERM/John Libbey Eurotext Ltd. © 1988. Vol. 169, pp. 95-98.

Combination chemotherapy and hyperfractionated large fields radiotherapy for limited small cell lung cancer

Véronique Trillet*

from the Groupe Lyonnais d'oncologie Thoracique, Lyon, France
**Lung Department, Pr. Brune, Pr. Cordier, Hôpital Louis Pradel, 28, avenue Doyen Lépine, 69394 Lyon Cedex 03, France; Lung Department, Pr. Emonot, Hôpital Nord Saint-Etienne; Lung Department, Pr. Kalb, Pr. Guérin, Hôpital de la Croix-Rousse; Lung Department, Pr. Bernard, Hôpital Jules Courmont, Pierre-Bénite; Medical Oncology Department, Dr Clavel, Centre Léon Bérard, Lyon; Lung Department, Pr. Perrin-Fayolle, Hôpital Ste Eugénie, Pierre-Bénite; Lung Department, Dr Van Straaten, Hôpital St Joseph, Lyon; Radiotherapy Department, Pr. Chassard, Centre Léon Bérard, Lyon; Radiotherapy Department, Dr Schmidt, Hôpital Nord, Saint- Etienne; Radiotherapy Department, Pr. Gérard, Hôpital Jules Courmont; Biostatistics Department, Dr Chauvin, Centre Léon Bérard, Lyon, France*

SUMMARY

From January 1 st 1986 to February 15 th 1988, 160 patients (pts) were included in a multicentric pilot study for small cell lung cancer (SCLC). All pts received 4 courses of the "AVI" CT : Doxorubicin 50 mg/m2, Etoposide 150 mg/m2 x 2 and Ifosfamide 2 g/m2 x 2 every 3 weeks. 53 (33%) pts were shown to have LD (disease limited to the chest) including pts with contro-lateral hilar involvement and ipsilateral pleural effusion. The overall response rate after 3 courses of CT is 84% (48% CR). Hematologic toxicity was constant and the Nadir was 0,6 x 10^9 /l for PN. The RT programm consisted in a split course hyperfractionated (twice-a-day) treatment with a large initial field including all an hemithorax, combined with te "VI" CT ("AVI" without Doxorubicin) as follows :

```
/__/_____/_____/__/_____/_____/            /___/ : 1 semaine
 RT        CT   RT        CT    RT
(15 Gy)   (VI) (18 Gy)   (VI)  (18 Gy)
```

28 pts fully completed the RT programm on February 15th 1988. 5 out of 11 pts who were in PR after CT achieved CR after RT and 6 remained in PR. 15 out of these 28 patients have already relapsed, 10 (35%) in the central nervous system and 6 (21%) in irradiated areas, but 3 out of these 6 initially had pleural effusion and relapsed in the same area where the radiation dose had been decreased from 18 to 9 Gys since the first 2 pts presented severe pneumonitis.
We conclude that "VI" is an effective regimen, and that sequential RT + CT increases the CR rate to first line CT. Hyperfractionation resulted in decreased gastro-intestinal toxicity. Although too preliminary, our results on survival (actuarial median survival time 14 months, 2 years disease free survival rate 35%) are very promising.

KEY WORDS : Small cell lung cancer, combination radio-chemotharapy.

Small cell lung cancer (SCLC) is one of the best tumor models to test sequential chemo-radiotherapy combinations.
We present here the results of a large multicentric pilot study using a combination chemotherapy (CT) and hyperfractionated large fields radiotherapy (RT) for limited SCLC. The rationale for first line chemotherapy in SCLC is obviously the need for micrometastases control and also the usefulness of tumor debulking before starting RT. We choosed a

combination of Doxorubicin, Etoposide and Ifosfamide because of the good response rates obtained in the EORTC protocols with the combination Doxorubicin, Etoposide, Cyclophosphamide (1) and because of the very high response rate to Ifosfamide alone in phase II trials for SCLC where Ifosfamide appeared to be a more effective agent than Cyclophosphamide (2).
The use of alternating chemo-radiotherapy schedules in SCLC is based on the mathematic model describ by Goldie and Coldmann (3) and it allows decreased toxicity and decreased delay for CT (4). Furthermore, the long-term results of the first clinical trials using these schedules are very encouraging (5).
Hyperfractionated radiotherapy is an interesting approach in SCLC since it has been shown that there is no or minimal shoulder on radiation curves in SCLC cell lines (6).
Since local recurrences observed in our previous protocols (7) appeared to be often located on the margin of irradiated areas, we tried to improve local control by the use of larger radiation fields.

MATERIAL AND METHODS

Inclusion criteria in the protocol (GLOT PC 86/01) included age under 70 years, Karnofsky index over 50%, biopsy proven SCLC, no prior therapy, no feasible surgical resection, no cardiac, renal or hepatic failure and possible follow-up during and after treatment. 171 patients were included from January 1st 1986 to February 15th 1988.

"Limited disease" was defined based on the use of large radiation fields : a patient was considered to have limited disease when the entire tumor burden could be included in one radiation field and treated with a "curative intent". Therefore, limited disease patients included patients with contro-lateral hilar involvement and/or homolateral pleural effusion but not patients with supra clavicular nodes. Out of the 160 now fully staged patients (staging procedures including blood routine tests, chest X rays, fiberoptic bronchoscopy with multiple biopsies, CT scan of the thorax, brain and abdomen, liver ultrasonography, radionucleide bone scan and bone marrow cytology and biopsy), 53% (33%) were considered as limited with this definition.

The treatment protocol started for all patients with 4 courses of the "AVI" regimen, consisting in Doxorubicin 50 mg/m2 day 1, Etoposide 150 mg/m2 day 1 and day 2, and Ifosfamide 2 g/m2 day 1 and day 2 using I.V. Mesna 2 g half an hour before and 1 g 4 and 8 hours after infusion.
Responding patients with "extensive disease" received a total of 10 courses of the same chemotherapy.
Patients with "limited disease" then started radiotherapy alternating every 2 weeks with the so-called "VI" regimen (same protocol as "AVI" without Doxorubicin) for initial responders, and with Cisplatinum 100 mg/m2 day 1 and Etoposide 120 mg/m2 per os day 4, 6 and 8 for non responders to "AVI".

Hyperfractionated RT consisted in a "split course" twice-a-day RT with 3 consecutive courses : RT "A" was given through a large radiation field including one hemithorax and the controlateral hilum. In our first 2 patients, the dose delivered was 15 Grays to the tumor and to the mediastinum and 18 Grays to the homolateral lung, but it resulted in 2 severe radiation pneumonitis and the dose to the homolateral hemithorax was then decreased from 18 to 9 Grays, without changing our definition of "limited disease"patients. RT "B" (18 Grays) was reduced to the mediastinum and both hilums. RT "C" consisted in 18 additional Grays on the tumor only.

After completing the RT schedule, patients received 2 more courses of "AVI".

RESULTS

Out of the 53 "limited disease" patients included, 49 were males, 4 were females, and the mean age was 56 years.
Response evaluation to the different modalities of treatment was assessed using the following criterias : complete response (CR) was defined as complete regression of the tumor both on the chest X rays and CT scan, with complete endoscopic normalization and negative cytologiesand biopsies. Partial response (PR) was defined as a regression of the tumor superior to 50%, or complete regression on chest X rays and CT scan with

persistance of positive cytologies and/or biopsies by fiberoptic bronchoscopy. Response inferior to 50% or no response was considered as stabilisation.
Out of the 44 patients now evaluable for response to induction CT alone, 21 (48%) were complete responders, 16 (36%) partial responders and 7 (16%) non responders for an overall response rate of 84%. 28 patients have now completed the CT-RT schedule and 5 out of 11 patients who were in PR before starting RT, achieved CR after RT-CT combination and 6 remained PR. 2 CR patients progressed in the central nervous system (CNS) during RT. 21 patients have now fully completed the protocol and 15/28 are in CR.

The "AVI" CT induced constant hematologic toxicity (medium neutrophils Nadir of 0,6 10^9/l), no neurologic toxicity as previously described with Ifosfamide + Mesna, and mild gastro-intestinal toxicity. There were no treatment-related deaths in this group of patients.
The combination of RT and "VI" was thought responsible for 3 cardiac complications(one moderate pericarditis and 2 congestive heart failures) and induced 2 severe pneumonitis as mentionned before. All patients had mild oesophagitis and other gastro intestinal toxicities.

15/28 patients evaluable for response to CT + RT have already relapsed : CNS was the most frequent site of relapse since 10 (35%) presented cerebral metastases, and CNS was the first metastatic site in 7 (25%). Local relapse was seen in 6 (21%) patients and in 3/28 (10,5%) was the first site of relapse. But it is to be noted that 3 out of these 6 relapsing patients initially had pleural effusion and relapsed in the pleura.

The actuarial median survival time is 14 months with a 35% 2 years actuarial survival rate and a 35% 2 years actuarial disease free survival rate.

CONCLUSIONS

The "AVI" combination (Doxorubicin, Etoposide, Ifosfamide) is a very tolerable and effective regimen with an overall response rate of 84%.

Sequential CT-RT allows an increased CR rate since 5 patients were restaged from PR to CR after this combination. Compared to standard RT previously used in our group, hyperfractionation resulted in a significant decrease of gastro intestinal toxicity. Large radiation fields did not improve local control because the dosage warranted to control on hemithorax was constantly too toxic on lung tissue.

CNS relapse was a major problem and there is a need for prophylactic cranial irradiation or chemoprevention.

Although the time of follow up is not long enough yet to publish long term survivalship, our preliminary results on survival are prom sing.

REFERENCES

(1) Klastersky J., Sculier J.P., Dumont J.P. et al
Combination chemotherapy with Adriamycine, Etoposide and Cyclophosphamide for small cell carcinoma of the lung. A study by the EORTC lung cancer Working Party (Belgium)
Cancer, 56 : 71-75, 1985

(2) Kokron O., Sheiner W., Flicker M. et al
High dose Ifosfamide as continuous infusion in small cell lung cancer. 13th International congress of chemotherapy, Vienna, Symposium Sy 83

(3) Goldie J.M., Coldman A.J.
Quantitative model for multiple levels of drug resistance in clinical tumors
Cancer Treat Rep, 67 : 923-931, 1983

(4) Tubiana M.
Les associations radiothérapie-chimiothérapie
J. Eur. Radiother, 3 : 107-114, 1980

(5) Arriagada R., LeChevalier T., Baldeyrou P. et al
Alternating radiotherapy and chemotherapy schedules in small cell lung cancer, limited disease
Int. J. Radiation Oncol. Biol. Phys, 11 : 1461-1467, 1985

(6) Carney D.N., Mitchell J.B., Kinsella T.J.
In vitro radiation and chemotherapy sensitivity of established cell lines of human small cell lung cancer and its large cell morphological variants
Cancer Res., 43 : 2806-2811, 1983

(7) Trillet V., Guerin J.C., Chauvin F.
Cancers anaplasiques à petites cellules dupoumon : résultats à 2 ans du protocole "CHEP" du Groupe Lyonnais d'Oncologie Thoracique.
Société Européenne de Pneumologie, réunion de la commission de cancérologie, Paris, 4 septembre 1987.

Résumé

Du 1er janvier 1986 au 15 février 1988, 160 patients (pts) ont été inclus dans un protocole de traitement multicentrique du cancer du poumon à petites cellules (CPC). Tous les patients reçoivent d'abord 4 cures de chimiothérapie (CT) ("AVI" : Doxorubicine 50 mg/m2 J1, Etoposide 150 mg/m2 J1 et J2, Ifosfamide 2 g/m2 J1 et J2), toutes les 3 semaines. A l'issue du bilan d'extension, 53 (33%) pts ont été considérés comme porteurs d'une maladie limitée au thorax (atteintes du hile controlatéral et de la plèvre homolatérale inclues). Le taux de réponse après 3 cures de CT est de 84% (dont 48% de réponses complètes) (RC)). La toxicité hématologique est constante et le Nadir moyen est de 0,6 x 10^9/l pour les polynucléaires neutrophiles. L'irradiation (RT) consiste en une formule "split-course" bi-fractionnée avec 3 champs consécutifs alternant tous les 15 jours avec une CT "VI" sans Adriamycine. Le premi er champ englobe tout un hémithorax, le 2e est reduit aux 2 hiles et le 3ème est un surdosage sur la tumeur.

28 pts ont maintenant reçu l'ensemble du programme de radiothérapie. 5 des 11 pts qui étaient en réponse partielle (RP) après la CT d'incudction passent en RC après la RT et 6 restent en RP. 15 de ces 28 patients ont déjà rechuté, 10 (35%) au niveau du système nerveux central et 6 (21%) au niveau de zones irradiées. 3 de ces 6 pts avaient initialement un épanchement pleural et ont récidivé au niveau de la plèvre ou la dose totale d'irradiation n'est que de 9 Gy (la dose initiale de 18 Gy a du être réduite du fait de 2 pneumopathies radiques sévères).

L'irradiation bi-fractionnée a permis uner éduction intéressante de la toxicité digestive. Nos résultats en terme de survie (médiane actuarialle : 14 mois, taux de survie sans récidive à 2 ans : 35%) sont préliminaires mais prometteurs.

Neo-Adjuvant Chemotherapy. Ed. Cl. Jacquillat, M. Weil, D. Khayat. Colloque INSERM/John Libbey Eurotext Ltd. © 1988. Vol. 169, pp. 99-104.

Phase II study of concomitant radiotherapy and chemotherapy in inoperable non small cell lung cancer

J.L. Rebischung [(1)], J.M. Vannetzel [(2)], M. Mellat [(1)], A. Ponzio [(1)] and J. Sauvaget [(1)]

[1] *Unité d'oncologie médicale (Pr. Sauvaget). Hôpital St Joseph 7, rue Pierre Larousse, 75014 Paris, France*
[2] *Centre de radiothérapie et d'oncologie médicale. Hôpital des Peupliers 22, rue des Peupliers 75013 Paris, France*

RESUME

Fourty-five patients with inoperable non small cell lung cancer stage II, III, Mo have been treated with a cyclic concomitant association of Vindesin, 5 Fluoro-Uracile, Cis-Platinum and radiotherapy.
After three and six cycles (36 and 72 Gy), the objective response rates are respectively of 77 and 86 %, with a median survival of one year.
Such results suggest the utilisation of this therapeutic modality as first line treatment before surgery in selected stage III patients.

MOTS CLEFS - KEY WORDS

Inoperable non metastatic non small cell lung cancer ; cyclic concomitant chemo-radiotherapy.

INTRODUCTION

Inoperable non small cell lung cancer keeps very poor prognosis

At the last world Conference in Toronto, in August 1985 it was clearly established that :

- radiotherapy alone can induce a local control of the disease, with a dose tumor response but that the survival remains poor because the rapid development of metastasis specially cerebral metastasis in adeno-carcinomas and undifferenciated carcinomas.

The efficacy of chemotherapy is limited with response rate of 25 to 35 % specially with combination of Vindesine and Cis Platin but without significant improvement of survival in most of the randomized trials.

Recently, some experimental and clinical datas, pointed out the inter-actions of radiation therapy and chemotherapy, and specially of 5 FU Cis Platinum and radiotherapy.

So we start in March 1986 a phase II trial of cyclic concomitant radiotherapy and chemotherapy with Vindesine, 5 Fluoro-Uracile and Cis platinum in inoperable non small cell lung cancer (NSLC), which first results are here reported.

MATERIAL AND METHODS

- Pre-inclusion explorations included :
  - clinical examination
  - X Ray
  - CT scan
  - Fibroscopy with biopsies
  - Functionnal explorations
  - ECG
  - Metastatic evaluation by brain scan, liver echography and bone scintigraphy.

- Conditions of eligibility were :
  - histological proof of NSCLC
  - stage II orIII Mo disease
  - age less than 75 years
  - performance status more than 60 (Karnofsky index)
  - adequate renal and hematological status
  - no prior chemo or radiotherapy

- 45 patients have been included

It was 4 females, 41 men of median age 61 y. (range 39-74). The repartition by histology and stage are reported in table I.

TABLE I : REPARTITION BY STAGE AND HISTOLOGY

	Sq CLC	Adenoc.	Undif.	Total
Stage II	4	-	-	4
Stage III	32	8	1	41
Total	36	8	1	45

- Criterias of inoperability have been
  - Respiratory insufficency for seven patients :
    2 T2 No ; 2 T2 N1 ; 2 T2 N2 ; 1 T3 Nx
    with post-operative MEF 1 < 1L.
  - Mediastinal or pleural involvement determined by initial CT scan and/or histological analysis for 38 cases.

- Patients have been treated with six cycles of combined therapy including :

  - Vindesin 0,6 mg/m2 by continuous infusion d. 1-4
  - 5 FU 600 mg/m2 by continuous infusion d. 1-4
  - Cis Platin 20 mg/m2 daily after radiation 3 Gy/day, days 1 to 4.

  each four weeks.

Radiation therapy was delivered on tumor mass, mediastinum and supra clavicular aeras by antero-posterior fields for the four first cycles. The two last cycles necessit lateral fields; the spinal cord receives 48 Gy in 16 fractions and four months.

RESULTS

The results have been evaluated after 3 and 6 cycles by the repetition of initial explorations, with the usual criterias of complete and partial responses.

- Among the 45 patients, it was two early deaths and three patients are under treatment,and 40 are evaluable for response.

After 3 cycles, 36 Gy, for 40 patients it was noted 1 complete remission 30 partial responses, 3 stable diseases, and 6 progressions so 77,25 % of objective responses (Table II).

TABLE II

	Sq. CLC	Adeno.	Undif.	Total
CR	1	-	-	1
PR	24	5	1	30
SD	3	-	-	3
PD	3	3	-	6

CR + PR = 31/40 77,25 %

PD = 6/40 15 %

After 6 cycles, 72 Gy, for twenty- nine evaluable patients, the response rate is 86 % for 24 % of progressive disease TABLE III .

TABLE III :

	Sq CLC	Adeno.	Undif.	Total
CR	11	3	1	15
PR	8	-		8
PD	5	1		6

- Actually, twenty-two patients died :

  - four with metastasis
  - nine by local relaps with metastasis
  - three by local recurrence only
  - and six by intercurrent pathology ;
    . acute respiratory insufficency
    . acute migration
    . sepsis.

  with 5 patients NED at autopsy.

  The median survival is 385 days.

- Toxicities have been noted monthly for 210 cycles and are reported in table IV.

TABLE IV

Hemato.	4 grades III	with dose reduction
	7 grades II	
	18 grade I	
Neuro.	17 grades I	
	10 grades II	
G.I.	20 grades I	
	18 grades II	
	2 grades III	
Nephro.	6 grades I	
	4 grades II	
Alopecia.	constant	

We notedalso four cardiac events with :

- One regressive pericarditis after 36 Gy
- two cases of spastic coronaropathy, suggesting 5 FU cardiotoxicity.
- one rythmic disorder treated by Amiodarone.

In term of pulmonary toxicity, it must be distinguished between :

- the risk of acute complication with three cases of lung necrosis.
  . one completely regressive after 36 Gy
  . one after 60 Gy, associated with chronic sepsis
  . one after 72 Gy complicated by fatal hemoptysis in a patient in a complete remission at autopsy.

and

- The modifications of functionnal parameters after radio and chemotherapy which analysis for 20 patients is showned in Table V and demonstrate a progressive restrictive syndrom better evaluated by VC and TPC than by DCO without modification of blood gaz levels.

TABLE V

	Pre-TT value	At 36 Gy	At 72 Gy	At 72 Gy + 6 months
VC	2.85	2.86	2.57	2.28 - 30 %
MEF1	1.66	1.68	1.44	1.45
RV	2.59	2.57	2.76	2.15
TPC	5.59	5.5	5.47	4.6 - 18 %
DCO	20	18.9	17.5	15.8 - 21 %

CONCLUSION

- These combined modality of treatment for inoperable NSCLC seems to be able to induce a high response rate, and confirm the results obtained by Taylor and Trybula.

- Because the difficulties of response appreciation, specially in mediastinal involvement, and the possible role of residual lesions in term of local recurrence of the disease and metastatic progression , we propose the utilisation of these cyclic concomitantchemo-radiotherapy as neo-adjuvant treatment delivering non more than 40 Gy before surgery for responders and start in January 1988 such a prospective study in stage III NSCLC.

REFERENCES

- Fourth World Conference on Lung Cancer
  Abstracts ; Toronto , August 25-30, 1985

- The interaction of radiation therapy and chemotherapy
  Abstracts ; Williambsurgh ; Sept. 28, Oct. 1 ; 1986

- Taylor S.G. W. and Al.
  The Interaction of Radiation therapy and Chemotherapy. September 28 October
- 1, 1986. Williamsburg, Virginia.

- Preoperative simultaneous 5 FU - Cis DDP and radiotherapy in clinical
  stage III - NSCLC
  Trybula M. and Al. Asco March 1984.

Résumé

Quarante-cing patients porteurs de carcinomes bronchiques primitifs inopérables non anaplasiques, stade II, III, Mo, ont été traités par une association concomitante cyclique de Vindésine, 5 Fluoro-Uracile, Cis Platýl et radiothérapie.

Après trois et six cycles (36 et 72 Gy), les taux de réponses objectives respectifs sont de 77 et 86 % avec une survie médiane d'un an.

Ces résultats suggèrent l'utilisation d'une telle association en première intention dans le traitement des cancers bronchiques stade III.

Neo-Adjuvant Chemotherapy. Ed. Cl. Jacquillat, M. Weil, D. Khayat. Colloque INSERM/John Libbey Eurotext Ltd. © 1988. Vol. 169, pp. 105-108.

Diffuse interstitial pneumonitis following bone marrow transplantation : possible role of the combination cyclophosphamide and single fraction total body irradiation

P. Piedbois*, C. Cordonnier**, C. Lévy*, G. Ganem*, M. Kuentz**, G. Karianakis**, J.F. Bernaudin***, J.P. Vernant**, J.M. Boigné**** and J.P. Le Bourgeois*

** Department of Oncology, ** BMT unit; *** LHPD; **** Department of MBG Henri Mondor Hospital, Créteil 94000, France*

ABSTRACT

The role of the conditioning regimen before BMT in the incidence of diffuse nonbacterial nonfungal interstitial pneumonitis (nBnF IPn) has been analysed in a serie of 170 patients with hematological malignancies. The conditioning regimen included chemotherapy (Cyclophosphamide alone at d-5 and d-4 for 148 patiens) and single fraction TBI at d-1 with respect to BMT (10 Gy abdomen, 8 Gy lung, low dose rate). Among 162 evaluable patients 39 (24%) experienced nBnF IPn. GVHD ≥ II strongly increased the incidence of nBnF IPn. Among other parameters, only mediastinal and pulmonary shielding ≤ 70% of thoracic area was found to increase this incidence. The role of the combination Cyclophosphamide (cy) plus TBI could be investigated. Experiments with mice or rats and some clinical data have shown that there could be a potentiation between Cy and irradiation with respect to lung toxicity. These data are discussed and compared with our protocol.

KEYWORDS

Bone marrow transplantation, total body irradiation, cyclophosphamide, diffuse interstitial pneumonitis.

INTRODUCTION

Diffuse interstitial pneumonitis (IPn) is one of the most frequent and serious complications of bone marrow transplantation (BMT). Among IPn, nonbacterial and nonfungal IPn (nBnF IPn) have been a subject of special attention because their high incidence and mortality rates. This retrospective study was performed to assess the role of conditioning regimen in the incidence of nBnF IPn following BMT.

METHODS AND MATERIALS

Between 1980 and 1986, 170 patients with hematological malignancies underwent BMT (tab. I).

Table I : Population

Hematological malignancies :	
AML	59 (58)
ALL	59 (55)
CML	37 (34)
NHL	9 (9)
Other	6 (6)
BMT :	
Allogeneic	155 (149)
Syngeneic	2 (2)
Autologous	13 (11)

( ) evaluable patients for nBnF IPn

The conditioning regimen included chemotherapy and single fraction total body irradiation (TBI). Most of the chemotherapy regimens (n=148) consisted of Cyclophosphamide (cy) alone (Fig.1).

Figure 1 : Conditioning regimen

day	-5	-4	-3	-2	-1	0	+1	+2	+3	+4
	cy	cy			TBI	BMT				

cy : 60 mg/kg/day

TBI was performed with a cobalt unit at a low dose rate : 4.10 +/- 0.62 cGy/min for instantaneous and 2.85 +/- 0.75 cGy/min for average pulmonary dose rate, patient lying in lateral position. The required doses were 10 Gy at the abdominal mid-plane and 8 Gy at lungs. In patients receiving allogeneic BMT, prophylaxis with methotrexate according to the Seattle protocol was used. Eighteen patients only were grafted with T-cell depleted marrow.
All patients with radiological IPn except 8 (excluded from analysis) were investigated by at least a bronchoalveolar lavage (Cordonnier and coll., 1986).

RESULTS

Among 162 evaluable patients, 39 (24%) experienced nBnF IPn (tab.II).

Table II : 39 patients with nBnF IPn

CMV alone	22
CMV + P.carinii	1
Other virus**	3
Idiopatic	13

* excluded from nBnF IPn analysis
** 2 respiratory syncitial virus and 1 zooster virus

The mortality rate with nBnF IPn was 17/39 (44%).
GVHD ⩾ II strongly increased the incidence of nBnF IPn.
The following parameters did not influence this incidence : age (mean = 26 y.), sex (100 males and 62 females), malignancy (8/58 AML, 15/55 ALL, 12/34 CML, 2/9 NHL, 2/6 Others), drug conditioning regimen, recorded doses at abdomen (9.92 +/- 0.51 Gy) or at lung (7.57 +/- 0.41 Gy), pulmonary dose rate. Only pulmonary and mediastinal shielding < 70% of thoracic area was found to increase significantly the incidence of nBnF IPn (46% when ⩽ 70% vs 20% when > 70% of thoracic area ; $p < 0.01$).

DISCUSSION

Lung dose and pulmonary dose rate have not be found to be predictive factors of nBnF IPn, probably because of the narrow values ranges, but pulmonary shielding needs special attention.
The role of the combination cyclophosphamide plus TBI could be investigated. Experiments with mice or rats and some clinical data have shown that cyclophosphamide at high doses induces lung toxicity (Rodin and coll., 1970 ; Stentoft J., 1987). Cyclophosphamide increases the pulmonary level of hydroxyproline and causes acute alveolar type I cells death, which is followed by alveolar type II cells proliferation. This proliferation can be measured by (C^{14}) thymidine incorporation into pulmonary DNA. The peak of thymidine incorporation occurs 7 days after injection (Hakkinen P.J. and Coll., 1982).
The pulmonary toxicity of irradiation is well recognized, especially with high dose rate or if delivered 1 to 2 days before the proliferation of alveolar type II cells proliferation (Hakkinen P.J. and coll., 1982). In mouse, the ratio LD_{50} at low dose rate / LD_{50} at high dose rate after thoracic irradiation was found about 1.8 (Hill, 1983).
Experiments (Varekamp and coll., 1986 ; Phillips and coll., 1975 ; Collis and coll., 1980 ; Steel and coll. 1979) and some clinical data (Trask C.W.L. and coll., 1985 ; Sostman and coll., 1981) have shown that there could be a potentiation between cyclophosphamide and irradiation with respect to lung toxicity, especially with low dose rate. For Varekamp and coll. (1986), a possible explanation of this observation is that cyclophosphamide decreases the repair capacity of lung. Hakkinen and coll. (1982) did not found this potentiation, but they used a high dose rate (233 cGy/min). Thus, the actuarial advantage of low dose rate is reduced by cyclophosphamide (Hill, 1983). In mice, if cyclophosphamide were given at -5 and -4 days with respect to BMT, the peak of the proliferation of alveolar type II cells would occur 7 days later, that is at +2 day. Therefore, the theorical moment at which the irradiation would be most dangerous for the lung is the day 0. This is close to when TBI is given in our protocol (-1 day).

CONCLUSION

These data led us 1) to consider with special attention the area of pulmonary shielding;
2) to perform further experimental studies about pulmonary effects of various combinations and timing of cyclophosphamide - TBI;
3) by this way to determine the conditioning regimen which in man could result in the lowering of lung toxicity.

REFERENCES

Collis C.H., Wilson C.M., Jones J.M. (1980) : Cyclophosphamide-induced lung damage in mice : protection by a small preliminary dose. Br. J. Cancer 41, 901-907.

Cordonnier C., Bernaudin J.F., Bierling P., Huet Y., Vernant J.P. (1986) : Pulmonary complications occurring after allogeneic bone marrow transplantation (a study of 130 consecutive transplanted patients). Cancer 58, 1047-1054.

Hakkinen P.J., Whiteley J.W., Witschi H.R. (1982) : Hyperoxia, but not thoracic X-irradiation, potentiates Bleomycin- and Cyclophosphamide-induced lung damage in mice. Am. Rev. Respir. Dis. 126, 281-285.

Hill R.P. (1983) : Response of mouse lung to irradiation at different dose-rate. Int. J. Radiation Oncology Biol. Phys. 9, 1043-1047.

Phillips T.L., Wharam M.D., Margolis L.W. (1975) : Modification of radiation injury to normal tissues by chemotherapeutic agents. Cancer 35, 1678-1684.

Rodin A.E., Haggard M.E., Travis L.B. (1970) : Lung changes and chemotherapeutic agents in childhood (Report of a case associated with cyclophosphamide therapy). Amer. J. Dis. Child. 120, 337-340.

Sostman H.D., Putman C.E., Gamsu G. (1981) : Diagnosis of chemotherapy lung. AJR 136, 33-40.

Steel G.G., Adams K., Peckham M.J. (1979) : Lung damage in C57BI mice following thoracic irradiation : enhancement by chemotherapy. Br.J. Radiol. 52, 741-7.

Stentoft J. (1987): Progressive pulmonary fibrosis complicating cyclophosphamide therapy. Acta Med. Scand. 221, 403-407.

Trask C.W.L., Joannides T., Harper P.G., Tobias J.S., Spiro S.G., Geddes D.M., Souhani R.L., Beverly P.C.L. (1985) : Radiation-induced lung fibrosis after treatment of small cell carcinoma of the lung with very high-dose cyclophosphamide. Cancer 55, 57-60.

Varekamp A.E., Vries A.J., Hagenbeek A. (1986) : Lung damage in the rat after irradiation and treatment with cytotoxic drugs. Br. J. Cancer 53,suppl. VII, 347-350.

Résumé

Entre 1980 et 1986, 170 patients porteurs d'une hémopathie maligne ont reçu une greffe de moelle osseuse à l'Hôpital Henri Mondor. La responsabilité du conditionnement à la greffe dans la survenue des pneumopathies interstitielles diffuses non bactériennes et non fungiques (IPn nBnF) a été analysée. Le conditionnement comportait une chimiothérapie (cyclophosphamide seule à J-5 et J-4 par rapport à la greffe pour 148 patients) et une irradiation corporelle totale (ICT) en une seule fraction à J-1 (10 Gy abdomen ; 8 Gy poumon ; faible débit de dose). Sur 162 patients évaluables, 39 (24%) ont présenté une IPn nBnF. Une réaction du greffon contre l'hôte d'un degré $\geqslant$ II augmente fortement le risque d'IPn nBnF. Parmi les autres paramètres étudiés, seul un cache médiastino-pulmonaire $\leqslant$ 70% de la surface thoracique a augmenté le risque d'IPn nBnF de façon statistiquement significative. Le rôle de l'association cyclophosphamide - ICT doit être évoqué. Plusieurs expériences chez l'animal et quelques observations cliniques ont montré qu'il pouvait y avoir une potentialisation entre la cyclophosphamide et l'irradiadion pour la toxicité pulmonaire. Ces données sont discutées et comparées à notre propre protocole.

Breast cancer I

Cancer du sein I

Neo-Adjuvant Chemotherapy. Ed. Cl. Jacquillat, M. Weil, D. Khayat. Colloque INSERM/John Libbey Eurotext Ltd. © 1988. Vol. 169, pp. 111-116.

One single, short perioperative cyclophosphamide course in breast cancer. Results from the scandinavian adjuvant chemotherapy study 1 (SACS — 1) and the cancer research campaign II trial (CRC — II)

R. Nissen-Meyer[a], M. Baum[b], J. Houghton[b], D. Riley[b] and R. A'Hern[b]

[a] *SACS group, Tyribakken 10, 0280 Oslo 2, Norway*
[b] *CRC Clinical Trials Centre, 123 Coldharbour Lane, London SE5 9NU, England, UK*

ABSTRACT

The 1026 patients in SACS-1 were randomised Jan.1965 - Sept. 1975. Median followup time of living patients is 17.1 years. The treatment group received a single i.v. cyclophosphamide course, 5 mg/kg/day for 6 days, first dose immediately after mastectomy. The effect on RFS was significant, increasing during the first 4 years, then kept at a level of 10% up to 20 years after mastectomy. If started 2-4 weeks after mastectomy, the same course had no effect.
The 2230 patients in the CRC-II trial were randomised Sept. 1981 - Dec. 1985 to 4 groups: control, one short perioperative course as given in the SACS-1 study, Tamoxifen for 2 years, and combination of the two treatments. By comparing the two groups with the short cyclophosphamide course with the two without, a significant effect on RFS was found, mirroring the effect observed in the SACS-1 study during the first 5 followup years.
The effect in the two studiescombined was most pronounced in the node negative group and in the patients less than 50 years old.

KEY WORDS

Breast cancer, adjuvant chemotherapy, perioperative cyclophosphamide.

MATERIAL AND METHODS

This paper is based on the results from two independent studies: The first was the Scandinavian Adjuvant Chemotherapy Study 1 (SACS-1) with 27 clinicians in 11 clinics in Finland, Norway and Sweden, as listed in Table 1. The 1026 patients were randomised between one control group and one treatment group with one single i.v. cyclophosphamide course, 5 mg/kg/d for 6 days perioperatively.
The Scandinavian study was then repeated in the Cancer Research Campaign Adjuvant Breast Trial II (CRC-II). The 2230 patients in this trial were randomised according to a factorial 2x2 design, with the same short cyclophosphamide course, Tamoxifen for 2 years, and combination of the two treatments as the experimental arms (Table 2). The two arms with the perioperative cyclophosphamide course may be

Table 1. Participants in the Scandinavian Adjuvant Chemotherapy Study 1 (SACS-1)

IN FINLAND:

IV.Surg.Univ.Clin.HELSINKI: AA.Järvinen*
Univ.Radiother.Clin.HELSINKI: L.Holsti, K.Malmio*
Univ.Hosp. OULU: G.Blanco, T.Larmi
Centr.Hosp.VASA: P.-O.Grönblom

IN NORWAY:

Univ.Hosp.BERGEN: O.Dahl, T.Kolsaker, B.Rosengren, M.Tangen, J.E.Varhaug
Centr.Hosp.LILLEHAMMER: I.Hareide, S.K.Hjort
Aker Hosp.OSLO:R.Nissen-Meyer (coordinator)

IN SWEDEN:

Centr.Hosp.BORÅS: S.Ahlström, C.-A.Ekman, B.Månsson*
Centr.Hosp.GÄVLE: G.Hellström, T.Norin,G.Odén
Centr.Hosp.JÖNKÖPING: I.Iacobaeus, B.Mårtensson
RegionalHosp.LINKÖPING: J.Sääf, D.Turesson
Centr.Hosp.NORRKÖPING: H.O.Ahnlund, K.Kjellgren, R.Peterhoff

*deceased

Table 2. Cancer Research Campaign Adjuvant Breast Trial II (CRC-II)

79 SURGEONS FROM 61 CENTRES IN
UK, AUSTRALIA AND GREECE

ADMINISTERED BY
CRC CLINICAL TRIALS CENTRE, LONDON

RANDOMISATION

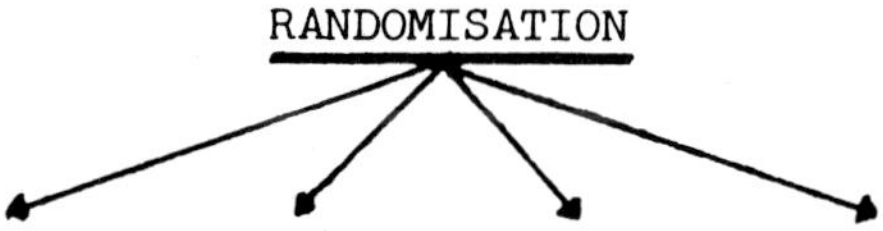

TAMOXIFEN 20 mg/day 2 years	CONTROL	CYCLOPHOSPHAMIDE iv. 6 days peri-operatively	COMBINATION

compared with the two arms without, but when we want to pool the results from SACS-1 and CRC-II together, we use only the cyclophosphamide arm and the control arm, since the delaying effect of Tamoxifen in the other two arms may tend to reduce the number of events during the first 5 years, and obscure the cyclophosphamide effect.
The two studies are further described and compared in Table 3.

Table 3. Comparison of SACS-1 and CRC-II

Cyclophosphamide i.v. 5 mg/kg/d for 6 days in both studies

	SACS - 1 A	CRC - II
Number of cases	1026	2230
Mean age	55.5 years	55.0 years
Intake period	Jan. -65 - Sept. -75	Sept. -81 - Dec. -85
Median follow-up	17.1 years	4.3 years
First injection	day 0	day 1

RESULTS

The results in SACS-1 are shown in Figs. 1 and 2. In terms of relapsefree % the difference between the groups increased with increasing time after mastectomy, and was 13.5% after 20 years. The results in terms of survival were influenced by the high age of the patients, with many deaths due to causes other than breast cancer. The difference in RFS is nethertheless significant (P=0.0009).
When the same short cyclophosphamide course was given 2-4 weeks after mastectomy, no effect was found (Nissen-Meyer et al. 1986).

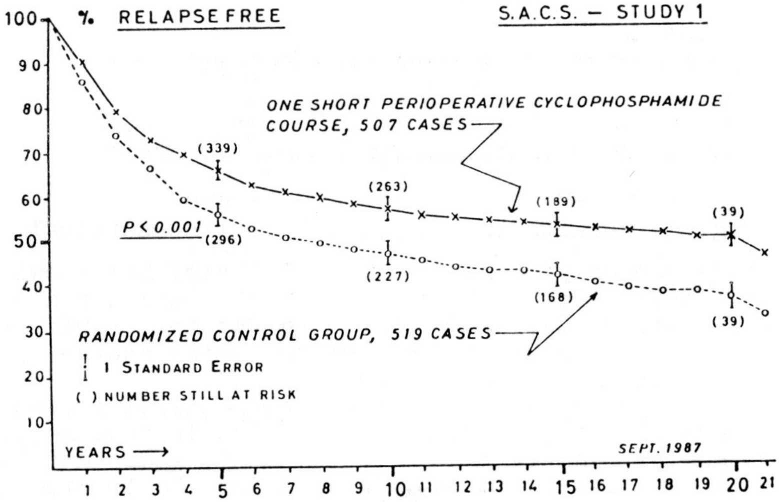

Fig. 1. Results in SACS-1, relapsefree percent.

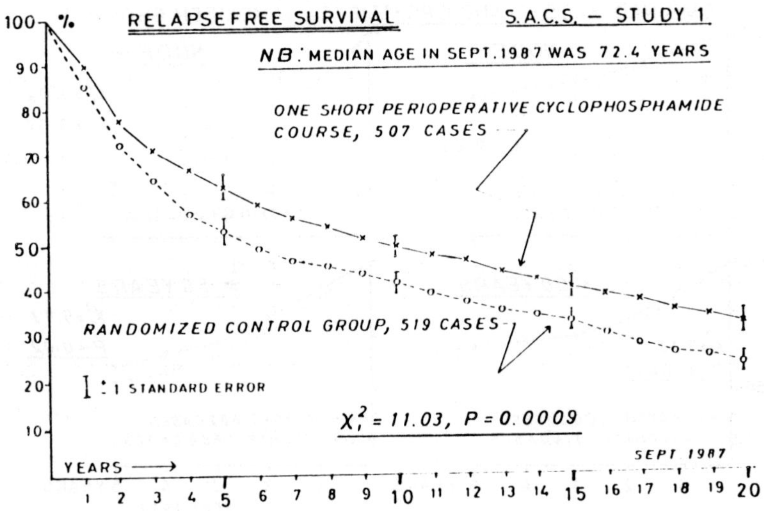

Fig. 2. Results in SACS-1, relapsefree survival.

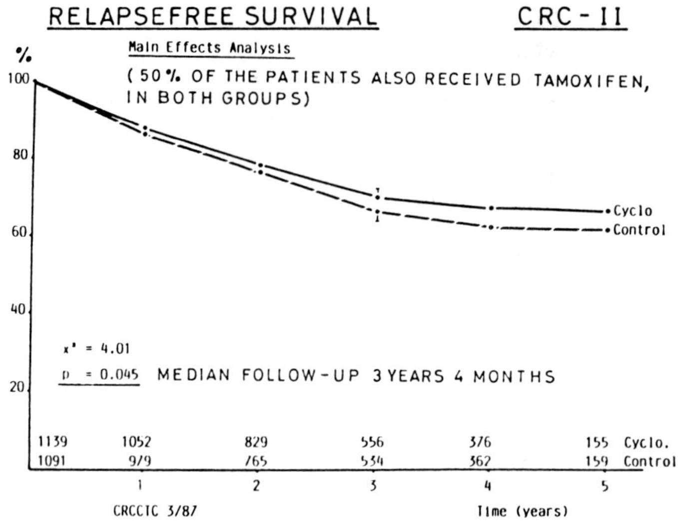

Fig. 3. Results in CRC-II, relapsefree survival.

The CRC-II study can only be followed for 5 years, but shows already a significant benefit (Fig.3). Since 50% of the patients also had Tamoxifen treatment, we may assume that some of the events are delayed, and the difference due to the cyclophosphamide course may accordingly be higher than shown here at 5 years.
In Fig. 4 the cyclophosphamide groups and the control groups from the two studies are pooled together, and stratified in node negative and node positive groups, and in groups less than 50 years and 50 years or more. in all 4 strata there is a benefit for the treated group, not significant for the node positive, significant for the others. Best is the effect for the node negative and the younger categories.

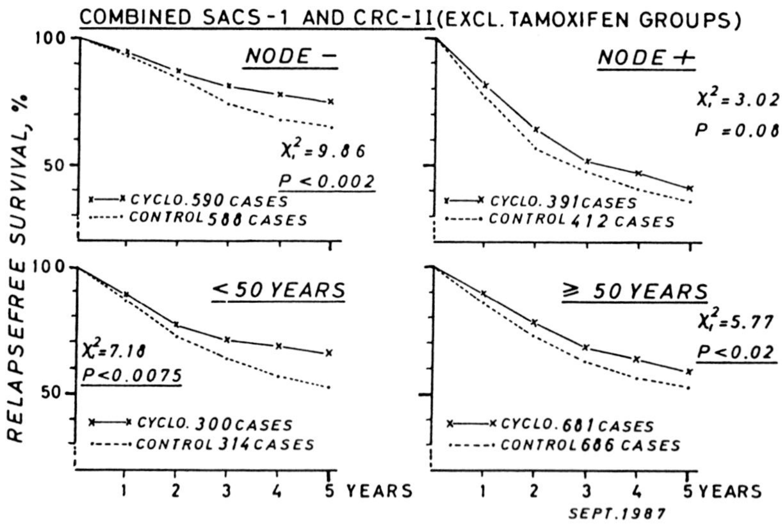

Fig. 4. Results after stratification, relapsefree survival.

The immediate side effects were moderate and of short duration. The usual nausea was easy to palliate, since the patient was still in hospital after the mastectomy. The treatment did not interfere with a normal healing of the surgical wound, and the short, but deep bone marrow suppression caused no problem. Secondary malignant diseases were found as frequently in the control group as in the cyclophosphamide group, and occurred earlier in the control group (Table 4).

Table 4. Secondary malignant diseases observed in SACS-1 (excl. ca. mammae and ca. basocellulare)

	Cyclo:	Control:
Leucaemia & lymphoma	1	4
Gynecological cancer	4	6
Gastro-intest. cancer	11	8
Other neoplasms	9	6
Total	25	24
Mean time to diagnosis	125.7 months	74.4 months

CONCLUSION

The conventional procedure in most centres has been to wait after mastectomy until all prognostic factors are evaluated, and then decide if adjuvant treatment shall be given - usually only to those with the worst prognosis. Taking into consideration the significant effect, most pronounced in the node negative cases, and the clinically insignificant side effects of the short perioperative chemotherapy course, it seems reasonable to give such a course to all cases. After evaluation of the individual prognosis of the patients we may then continue with longterm adjuvant treatment (chemo- or hormonal) in selected cases, within a clinical trial or as routine treatment.

REFERENCES

Nissen-Meyer, R., Høst, H., Kjellgren, K., Månsson, B., Norin, T. (1986): One short chemotherapy course given immediately after mastectomy: experience of the Scandinavian Adjuvant Chemotherapy Study Group. Neoadjuvant chemotherapy. Colloque INSERM/ John Libbey Eurotext Ltd. Vol. 137, pp 157-164.

Résumé

1026 patients du protocole SACS.1 ont été randomisées entre janvier 1965 et septembre 1975, le recul médian des malades vivantes est de 17,1 an.
Le groupe traité a reçu une seule cure de Cyclophosphamide par voie intraveineuse 5 mg/kg/jour, pendant 6 jours, la première dose ayant été commencée tout de suite après la mastectomie. L'effet sur la survie sans rechute a été significatif, augmentant durant les 4 premières années puis se maintenant à un niveau de 10 %, durant 20 ans après la mastectomie. Si la chimiothérapie était commencée 2 à 4 semaines après la mastectomie, la même cure n'a plus aucun effet sur la survie.

2230 patientes du protocole SRC.2 ont été randomisées entre septembre 1981 et décembre 1985 en 4 groupes : groupe contrôle, groupe avec une cure brève de chimiothérapie pré-opératoire comme dans l'étude SACS.1, Tamoxifène pendant 2 ans, association des deux traitements.
En comparant les deux groupes traités par une cure de Cyclophosphamide aux autres groupes, un bénéfice significatif sur la survie sans rechute est retrouvé, reproduisant l'effet observé dans l'étude SACS.1. avec un recul de 5 ans. L'effet a été plus prononcé dans le groupe des ganglions négatifs chez des malades de moins de 50 ans.

Neo-Adjuvant Chemotherapy. Ed. Cl. Jacquillat, M. Weil, D. Khayat. Colloque INSERM/John Libbey Eurotext Ltd. © 1988. Vol. 169, pp. 117-122.

The rationale for an NSABP trial to evaluate preoperative systemic therapy in primary operable breast cancer

Bernard Fisher

Chairman of the NSABP and Professor of Surgery, University of Pittsburgh, School of Medicine, Pittsburgh, PA 15261, USA

INTRODUCTION

The National Surgical Adjuvant Breast and Bowel Project (NSABP) has designed and will shortly implement a major trial (Protocol B-18) in the United States and Canada to (1) determine whether pre-operative chemotherpay will more effectively prolong disease-free survival and survival than does the same chemotherapy given post-operatively, (2) evaluate the response of the primary tumor to pre-operative chemotherapy and correlate the response with disease-free survival and survival, (3) determine whether pre-operative chemotherapy by reducing the size of the primary tumor will permit more conservative surgery and decrease the incidence of ipsilateral breast tumor reoccurrence, and (4) determine whether patterns of DNA histograms (ploidy and S phase) and changes in them resulting from chemotherapy can be correlated with disease-free survival and survival. The following stresses the rationale for conducting the study.

BIOLOGICAL RATIONALE FOR PREOPERATIVE CHEMOTHERAPY

Several biological premises formed justification for evaluating the use of such therapy.

Effect of primary tumor removal on the growth kinetics of metastases: Experimental systems indicate that noncurative reduction of tumor cell burden results in an increase in the proliferation of residual tumor cells.[1-3] Investigations by us from six different tumor-host systems demonstrate that 24 hours following removal of a primary tumor there is an increase in the labeling index (LI) of the metastases which persists for a variable period of time (e.g. 5-7 days) and results in a decrease in tumor doubling time with a measurable increase in tumor size.[4] Primary tumor radiation also results in kinetic changes in distant tumors similar to those obtained following tumor removal. Studies elucidating the mechanism whereby removal of a primary tumor exerts its effect on metastases indicate that the stimulation of cell growth following tumor removal or radiation is due to a serum growth factor. Serum from mice following tumor removal or radiation when transferred to isologous recipient bearing tumors of the same type as in the donor result in kinetic alterations identical to those observed when a primary tumor was removed. Investigations by us indicate that chemotherapy (cyclophosphamide), tamoxifen, or radiation therapy given prior to operation prevent the kinetic events, suppress tumor growth, and prolong survival.[5] Serum from mice so treated (pre-operative) fail to stimulate DNA synthesis in contrast to what occurs when serum is obtained from untreated mice following tumor removal.

Goldie-Coldman hypothesis: The Goldie-Coldman hypothesis contends that as a tumor cell population increases there is an ever-expanding number of drug-resistant phenotypic variants arising due to spontaneous somatic mutations which become more difficult to eradicate.[6] Their thesis is that the risk of resistant cells being present can be minimized by initiating combinations of non-cross resistant drugs as soon as possible, i.e., when a tumor population contains the fewest number of cells. The Goldie somatic mutation theory does not provide an alternative and independent rationale to the previous one involving cell kinetic principles. The two are not mutually exclusive. With the growth of a tumor, not only are the absolute numbers of resistant cells increased but so is the percentage of resistant cells in the total cell population. The latter is presumed to occur because resistant phenotypes not only multiply as a result of their own intrinsic growth rates but as a consequence of the addition of new mutations from the pool of non-resistant (sensitive) cells (Goldie 1982).[7] As a consequence of the enhanced proliferation of cells following tumor removal, it becomes more likely that the number of resistant phenotypes will increase in the metastic population. Thus, appropriate pre-operative therapy should not only destroy cells made more sensitive by their kinetic alteration but also prevent cell proliferation and so prevent an increase in resistant cells.

Skipper and Schabel principles: In the 1960's Skipper and his associates promulgated a series of concepts which resulted in the justification for the use of adjuvant chemotherapy such as has been employed for the past 15 years. In brief, they proposed that, (1) growth fractions and doubling times of primary tumors may differ from those in micrometastases. Consequently, responsiveness to chemotherapy may differ, (2) the magnitude of response of a primary tumor in the plateau of gomperzian growth need not reflect the response of micrometastases in exponential growth, (3) first order kinetics relative to cell kill by cytocidal agents apply to those cells with constant growth fractions in exponential growth, i.e. micrometastases of $\leq 10^6$ cells, (4) the degree of sychronization of cell cycle times of a primary tumor and its micrometastases may differ and may respond to cyclical chemotherapy differently, (5) ablation of a primary tumor with a resultant decrease in total tumor cell burden may alter the growth characteristics of residual micrometastases so that there is a decrease in tumor doubling time, an increase in growth fraction and an improved sychronization of cell cycle times enhancing the sensitivity of micrometastases to chemotherapy.

Despite the innumerable clinical trials which have been conducted no evidence exists which correlates primary tumor response to therapy with patient outcome, i.e. response of metastases. In our protocol information will be obtained with the intent of carrying out such a correlation. Concomitantly the principles of Skipper and Schabel will be tested.

In summary, while there is no assurance that similar kinetic changes observed in animal models occur following removal of tumors in the human and that the temporal pattern of the kinetic changes (should they occur) are similar, nor is there certainty that the Goldie-Coldman hypothesis has relevance in patients who already have tumors of long standing, and there may be question whether the Skipper-Schabel concepts are testable in this setting, there is ample justification to evaluate the worth of pre-operative therapy in patients. Aside from the potential clinical benefits, a trial to evaluate the efficacy of such therapy will provide more definitive biological information relative to human neoplasms than will additional *in vivo* animal models and *in vitro* preparations as they relate to this particular problem.

CLINICAL RATIONALE FOR PREOPERATIVE CHEMOTHERAPY.

Limited clinical information exists to support the importance of the timing of chemotherapy in the treatment of Stage I and II breast cancer.

Timing of Post-operative chemotherapy: Two trials are frequently referred to as indicating the importance of early post-operative therapy. In NSABP B-01, Thiotepa was administered for three successive days starting on the day of surgery.[8] The results of that study demonstrated an improvement in both disease-free survival and survival in some patients - the first evidence indicating the worth of adjuvant chemotherapy. A Scandinavian trial in which cyclophosphamide was administered for six consecutive days starting on the day of operation also indicated an advantage.[9] Unfortunately, the NSABP trials did not have a proper control group of patients who were treated precisely the same way but at a longer interval following operation so as to be able to address the issue of the timing of therapy. Similarly, by today's standards regarding clinical trial design, the evidence from the Scandinavian trial to indicate that the use of early post-operative chemotherapy is better than delaying it two to four weeks after operation is tenuous. In that study findings were obtained from 1,026 patients at 10 hospitals (surgical subseries) randomized between early post-operative chemotherapy and no-chemotherapy (post-operative radiation in all). The findings were compared with those obtained from 110 patients who entered a radiotherapy institute 2 to 4 weeks after operation for radiation therapy (radiation subseries) and who in a separate randomization process were allocated to the same two groups as those in the surgical subseries. Their chemotherapy was begun on average 21 days after mastectomy instead of at time of operation. They failed to demonstrate a benefit from the therapy.

In a more recent study, Jones, et al., employing AC therapy for Stage II patients reported a greater disease-free survival at 48 months for 1-3 positive node patients (48) who received their adjuvant therapy ≤4 weeks than for those (37) getting it >4 weeks (85% vs 59%, P=0.02).[10] In the same report they paradoxically noted that in those with >3 positive nodes (46 and 38 patients) the results were better (15%, P=0.06) if drugs were given >4 weeks after operation. Buzdar et al. observed no adverse effect from a delay in administering therapy.[11] They evaluated the outcome from patients receiving therapy <10 weeks, 10-13, 14-17 and ≥18 weeks. Precisely when the therapy was given in the <10 weeks group is not stated. This study would hardly be considered a test of "early" versus "late" therapy. Whereas Senn et al., observed that a delay between the diagnosis and first day of chemotherapy was higher in relapsing than in nonrelapsing patients (32 vs 23 days; P=0.5),[12] data from the SWOG could not confirm an adverse effect from delay in starting CMF, vincristine and prednisone.[13] A critical review of the studies noted indicates that they are really "no contest" of the importance of the timing of administration of systemic adjuvant therapy.

One prospectively randomized trial evaluating early post-operative therapy is in progress. The Ludwig Breast Cancer Study Group is comparing patients receiving conventionally timed post-operative CMFp X6 courses with those administered one course of perioperative therapy (within 36 hours after operation) or one course of perioperative therapy followed by conventionally timed chemotherapy[14,15]. Data from that trial has recently been reported and, in general, fails to discern a benefit for the early administered therapy as employed in the study.

In summary, when considered overall, there is currently insufficient information to indicate the significance of the timing of the onset of post-operative chemotherapy.

Pre-operative chemotherapy: Almost all information regarding the clinical worth of pre-operative chemotherapy has come from its use for the treatment of osteosarcoma[16], head and neck tumors[17] and esophageal cancers.[18] Its worth for locally-advanced (stage III) breast cancers has been dramatically demonstrated.[19,20] Lippman et al. have shown that with the use of primary chemotherapy in stage III disease there was an objective response of 90%.[21] Complete response was observed in 50% and 40% were partially responsive. Although this information was not derived from a randomized trial, the importance of the findings for earlier stage disease is worthy of serious consideration. Others have also reported a similar experience with locally advanced breast cancer.[22] From all of these studies has come evidence to indicate the safety of such therapy relative to overall systemic toxicity and local (regional) wound-healing. Moreover, as a result of the marked decrease in tumor size resulting from such therapy it has been possible to utilize less extensive surgery, e.g., lumpectomy, to achieve local regional control. Not only does such therapy ensure the earlier treatment of micrometastases, but it also permits assessment of response of a tumor to a particular drug regimen. Such responsiveness can then be correlated with the effectiveness of the therapy on micrometastases as evidenced by freedom from distant disease and prolongation of survival. Unfortunately, none of the studies were able to answer the question: Does the use of pre-operative therapy more effectively control disseminated disease than does the same therapy administered after operation.

To our knowledge only two groups of investigators are currently evaluating the worth of pre-operative chemotherapy in patients with earlier stage (less than stage III) breast cancer. Jacquillat et al., (Paris) using a non-randomized treatment protocol has administered combination chemotherapy after diagnosis by drill biopsy to patients with any tumor stage (T_1-T_4).[23] Ragaz from Vancouver initiated a randomized study of pre-operative versus post-operative chemotherapy in 1983.[24] In that study the diagnosis of cancer is made using needle aspiration cytology or "open" biopsy. One group of patients received a single cycle of CMF prior to definitive operation and those at high risk received 8 cycles of CMF after operation. In the second group all patients received 9 cycles of therapy after operation.

In summary, it may be concluded that practically no information is available from a randomized study to evaluate the worth of pre-operative chemotherapy in the management of primary breast cancer.

SUMMARY OF THE NSABP STUDY.

Patients with palpable operable (T_1, T_2, T_3) breast cancer in whom the diagnosis has been established by needle aspiration cytology or core needle biopsy will be stratified by age, clinical tumor size, clinical nodal status and randomly assigned to one of two groups. Group I will receive a total or segmental (lumpectomy) mastectomy plus axillary dissection followed by four cycles (courses) of Adriamycin and cyclophosphamide given every 21 days. Group II will receive four cycles of Adriamycin and cyclophosphamide followed by a total or segmental mastectomy plus axillary dissections within 4 weeks of the fourth course of chemotherapy, i.e. when counts allow.

All patients in either Group I or Group II who are ≥50 years will begin tamoxifen 10mg b.i.d. at the completion of chemotherapy. For patients undergoing segmental mastectomy, breast radiation will be given after the completion of all chemotherapy. Patients in Group II who, after four cycles of chemotherapy, have a complete response (no evidence of residual disease clinically or mammographically) may undergo (a) total mastectomy and axillary node dissection, or (b) segmental mastectomy, axillary node dissection and ipsilateral breast irradiation.

Group II patients who progress (>50% in size) despite either two or three courses of AC will have mastectomy or segmental mastectomy at that time followed by the remainder of their chemotherapy post-operatively.

BIBLIOGRAPHY

Gunduz N, Fisher B, and Saffer EA: "Effect of surgical removal on the growth and kinetics of residual tumor," Cancer Res., 39:3861-3865, 1979.

Fisher B, Gunduz N, and Saffer EA: "Influence of the interval between primary tumor removal and chemotherapy on kinetics and growth of metastases," Cancer Res., 43:1488-1492, 1983.

Fisher B, Saffer EA, and Deutsch M: "Influence of irradiation of a primary tumor on the labeling index and estrogen receptor index in a distant tumor focus," Int. J. Radiat. Oncol. Biol. Phsy., 12:879-885, 1986.

Fisher B, Gunduz N, and Saffer EA: "Evidence for a growth factor in serum following primary tumor removal," IN PRESS

Fisher B, Gunduz N, and Saffer EA: "Effect of local or systemic treatment prior to primary tumor removal on inhibitions of a growth factor in serum following operation," IN PRESS

Goldie JH, Coldman AJ: "A mathematical model for relating the drug sensitivity of tumors to their spontaneous mutation rate," Cancer Treat. Rep., 63:1727-1733, 1979.

Goldie JH: "Drug resistance and chemotherapeutic strategy," IN: TUMOR CELL HETEROGENEITY: ORIGINS AND IMPLICATIONS, Eds.: Owens AH Jr., Coffey DS and Baylin SB, Academic Press, New York, 1982, pp. 115-125.

Fisher B, Slack NH, Katrych D, and Wolmark N: "Ten years of follow-up results of patients with carcinoma of the breast in a cooperative clinical trial evaluating surgical adjuvant chemotherapy," Surg. Gynecol. Obstet., 140:528-534, 1975.

Nissen-Meyer R, Kjellgren K, Malmio K, Mansson B, and Norin T: "Surgical adjuvant chemotherapy: results with one short course with cyclophosphamide after mastectomy for breast cancer," Cancer 41:2088-2098, 1978.

Jones SE, Brooks RJ, Takasugi BJ, et al.: "Current results of the University of Arizona adjuvant breast cancer trials," In: RECENT RESULTS IN CANCER RESEARCH: ADJUVANT CHEMOTHERAPY OF BREAST CANCER, Ed: Senn SJ, Springer-Verlag, New York, 1984, Vol. 96, pp. 131-141.

Buzdar AU, Smith TL, Powell KC, et al.: "Effect of timing of initiation of adjuvant chemotherapy of disease free survival in breast cancer," Breast Cancer Res. Treat., 2:163-169, 1982.

Senn JH, Jungi WF, Amgwerd R: "Chemo(immuno)therapy with LFMP plus BCG in node negative and node positive breast cancer," In: ADJUVANT THERAPY OF CANCER III, Eds.: Salmon SE and Jones SE, Grune and Stratton, San Francisco, 1981, pp. 385-395.

Glucksberg H, Rivkin SE, Rasmussen S, et al.: "Combination chemotherapy (DMFVP) versus L-phenylalanine mustard (L-PAM) for operable breast cancer with positive axillary nodes," Cancer, 50:423-434, 1982.

Ludwig Breast Cancer Study Group: "Toxic effcts of early adjuvant chemotherapy for breast cancer," Lancet, II:542-544, 1983.

Goldhirsch A and Gelber R: "Perioperative and conventionally timed chemotherapy in operable breast cancer: The Ludwig Breast Cancer Study V," In: RECENT RESULTS IN CANCER RESEARCH, Eds.: Ragaz J, Band PR, and Goldie JH, Springer-Verlag, New York, 1986, Vol. 103, pp 103-112.

Rosen G: "Preoperative chemotherapy for osteogenic sarcoma," Cancer, 49:1221-1230, 1982.

Schuller DE: "Preoperative reductive chemotherapy for locally advanced carcinoma of the oral cavity, oropharynx, and hypopharynx," Cancer, 51:15-19, 1983.

Leichman L, Seydel HG and Steiger Z: "Pre-operative adjuvant therapy for squamous cell cancer (SCC) of the esophagus: SWOG & RTOG clincial trials,"

Perloff M, Lesnick J: "Chemotherapy before and after mastectomy in Stage III breast cancer," Arch. Surg 117:879-881, 1982.

Shick P, Goodstein J, Moor J, et al.: "Preoperative chemotherapy followed by mastectomy for locally advanced breast cancer," J. Surg. Oncol., 22:278-282, 1983.

Sorace RA, Bagley CS, Lichter AS, et al.: "The management of nonmetastatic locally advanced breast cancer using primary induction chemotherapy with hormonal synchronization followed by radiation therapy with or without debulking surgery," World J. Surg., 9:775-785, 1985.

Jacquillat CI, Baillet F, Blondon J, et al.: "Preliminary results of 'neoadjuvant' chemotherapy in initial management of breast cancer (BC)," Proc. Am. Soc. Clin. Oncol., 2:C-437,112, 1983.

Jacquillat CI, Weil M, Auclerc G, et al.: "Neoadjuvant chemotherapy in the conservative management of breast cancers: Study of 143 patients," In: RECENT RESULTS IN CANCER RESEARCH, Eds.: Ragaz J, Band PR and Goldie JH, Springer-Verlag, New York, 1986, Vol. 103, pp. 113-119.

Ragaz J: "Preoperative (neoadjuvant) chemotherapy for breast cancer: Outline of the British Columbia Trial," In: RECENT RESULTS IN CANCER RESEARCH, Eds.: Ragaz J, Band PR and Goldie JH, Springer-Verlag, New York, 1986, Vol. 103, pp. 85-94.

Neo-Adjuvant Chemotherapy. Ed. Cl. Jacquillat, M. Weil, D. Khayat. Colloque INSERM/John Libbey Eurotext Ltd. © 1988. Vol. 169, pp. 123-127.

Locally advanced breast cancer. Ten-year results after combined treatment

P. Valagussa, M. Zambetti, R. Zucali and G. Bonadonna

Istituto Nazionale Tumori, Milano, Italy

ABSTRACT

The paper presents the 10-year results achieved at the Milan Cancer Institute with combined modality therapy in 277 patients with non inflammatory locally advanced breast cancer. Freedom from progression, survival and local control were significantly improved by the addition of drug therapy following primary chemotherapy and local-regional treatment.

KEY WORDS

Breast cancer, combined modality, Adriamycin.

INTRODUCTION

Locally advanced breast cancer can be defined either as disease presenting in patients who are technically inoperable or who show clinical-pathologic signs of inflammatory carcinoma. The 1978 TNM classification describes as T3b a tumor more than 5 cm in greatest dimension with fixation to underlying pectoral fascia and/or muscle, and as T4 a tumor of any size with direct extension to chest wall (to include ribs, intercostal muscles and serratus anterior muscle but not pectoral muscle) or skin. Although many publications on treatment for T3b-T4 breast cancer appeared during the past 15 years (Henderson et al., 1987, Swain et al., 1987, Valagussa et al., 1988), the natural history of locally advanced breast cancer remains today widely misunderstood. From the prognostic point of view, although patients who are inoperable may be considered incurable, not all women who are incurable have a universal short-term prognosis. This paper will briefly condensate the experience achieved with combined modality approach at the Istituto Nazionale Tumori of Milan.

PATIENTS AND METHODS

A total of 277 women with the clinical diagnosis of T3b-T4 breast cancer were enrolled in two prospective clinical trials as previously described (De Lena et al., 1978, De Lena et al., 1981, Valagussa et al., 1983). In the first study, following primary chemotherapy and radiotherapy, patients with no disease progression were randomized to no further therapy (CT+RT) versus additional chemotherapy (CT+RT+CT). In the second study patients were randomly allocated to receive CT+RT+CT versus chemotherapy-surgery-chemotherapy (CT+S+CT). The main patient characteristics are listed in Table 1. Tumor size and lymph node status were evenly distributed among treatments.

TABLE 1
MILAN CASE SERIES WITH T3b - T4
NON-INFLAMMATORY BREAST CANCER

Total patients 277		%
Extent	T3b	7
	T4	93
Tumot size*	≤ 5 cm	20
	5-10 cm	69
	> 10 cm	11
Lymph nodes*	N_0	23
	N_1	52
	N_2	25

* On clinical examination

Treatment modalities are summarized in Table 2.

TABLE 2
TREATMENT MODALITIES

Primary Chemotherapy	Adriamycin 60-70 mg/m² q. 3 wks Vincristine 1.2 mg/m², day 1 + 8 Total cycles: 3 to 4
Radiotherapy	60 Gy to breast + 10 Gy "boost" in 70% 40-60 Gy to regional nodes
Surgery	Radical mastectomy
Subsequent Chemotherapy	Adriamycin (50 mg/m² + vincristine for 6-7 cycles in responders to primary chemotherapy or CMF for 6-7 cycles

Primary chemotherapy consisted of adriamycin plus vincristine (AV). Surgery was planned in 79 women while high-energy radiotherapy was planned in all remaining patients. Chemotherapy post local-regional treatment consisted of the same AV regimen, without exceeding the total dose of 500 mg/m² for adriamycin, in women who had achieved partial remission after primary chemotherapy. Patients who had attained with primary AV only a minor objective response were given CMF following radiotherapy or surgery.

Objective tumor response was assessed by combining physical examination and mammography.

RESULTS

A total of 72 women were treated with CT+RT and 79 with CT+S+CT, respectively. The remaining 126 women receiving CT+RT+CT were derived by grouping together patients from two different study protocols and who received the same treatment program. These patients presented with similar pretreatment characteristics and treatment outcome was superimposable.

For the entire series, complete tumor response as the end of combined modality therapy was 74%, and progressively increased from CT+RT (64%) to CT+RT+CT (75%) to CT+S+CT (82%) (Valagussa et al., 1983).

TABLE 3
10-YEAR RESULTS
ACCORDING TO TREATMENT MODALITY

	FFP %	Survival %	Local-regional control %
CT + RT	1.5	14	44
CT + RT + CT	14	26	56
CT + S + CT	22	28	72
	P=0.0001	P=0.002	

Tables 3 to 5 summarize the 10 year results. Freedom from progression (FFP), total survival and local control were significantly improved by the addition of drug therapy following local-regional treatment. This finding was also clearly evident in patients who were complete responders at the end of therapy. The 10-year results for the entire series of patients were inversely related to tumor size and clinical nodal status with no difference between pre and postmenopausal women. It is important to stress that the addition of chemotherapy post surgery or radiotherapy was able to significantly influence treatment outcome when analyzed both singly as well as in the presence of the two above mentioned prognostic factors (tumor size and nodal status).

TABLE 4
10-YEAR RESULTS IN COMPLETE RESPONDERS
ACCORDING TO TREATMENT MODALITY

	RFS %	Survival %
CT + RT	2	18
CT + RT + CT	19	27
CT + S + CT	26	35
	P=0.0001	P=0.01

TABLE 5
10-YEAR RESULTS
REGARDLESS OF TREATMENT MODALITY

		FFP %	Survival %
Total patients		13	23
Tumor size	≤ 5 cm	27	48
	5-10 cm	9	20
	> 10 cm	4	4
Lymph nodes	N_0	21	27
	N_1	13	28
	N_2	5	12

No difference between pre and post

CONCLUSION

Present findings indicate that T3b-T4 non inflammatory breast cancer is a heterogeneous group of diseases. This group is characterized by a key prognostic factor, the tumor cell burden. Variables affecting the 10-year results are represented by primary tumor size, nodal status, and intensity of treatment.

REFERENCES

De Lena, M., Zucali, R., Viganotti, G., Valagussa, P., Bonadonna, G. (1978): Combined chemotherapy-radiotherapy approach in locally advanced (T3b-T4) breast cancer. Cancer Chemother. Pharmacol. 1, 53-59.

De Lena, M., Varini, M., Zucali, R., Rovini, D., Viganotti, G., Valagussa, P., Veronesi, U., Bonadonna, G. (1981): Multimodal treatment for locally advanced breast cancer. Results of chemotherapy-radiotherapy versus chemotherapy-surgery. Cancer Clin. Trials 4, 229-236

Henderson, I.C., Hayes, D.F., Come, S., Harris, J.R., Canellos, G. (1987): New agents and new medical treatments for advanced breast cancer. Semin. Oncol. 14, 34-64

Swain, S.M., Sorace, R.A., Bagley, C.S., Danforth, D.N. Jr., Bader J., Wesley M.N., Steinberg, S.N., Lippman, M.E. (1987): Neoadiuvant chemotherapy in the combined modality approach of locally advanced non-metastatic breast cancer. Cancer Res. 47, 3889-3894

Union Internationale contre le cancer (UICC) (1978): TNM classification of malignant tumors. 3rd Edition.

Valagussa, P., Zambetti, M., Bignami, P., De Lena, M., Varini, M., Zucali, R., Rovini, D., Bonadonna, G. (1983): T3b-T4 breast cancer: factors affecting results in combined modality treatments. Clin. Expl. Metastasis 1, 191-202

Valagussa, P., Brambilla, C., Bonadonna, G. (1988): Chemotherapy of metastatic breast cancer and the management of stage III disease. In Breast Cancer, Hoogstraten, B. (ed), Springer Verlag (in press).

ACKNOWLEGMENTS

Supported in part by Contract NO1-CM-07338 with DCT, NCI, NIH.

Neo-Adjuvant Chemotherapy. Ed. Cl. Jacquillat, M. Weil, D. Khayat. Colloque INSERM/John Libbey Eurotext Ltd. © 1988. Vol. 169, pp. 129-136.

Results of a conservative treatment combining neo-adjuvant chemotherapy and radiotherapy in 252 patients with breast cancer

Cl. Jacquillat, M. Weil, G. Auclerc, G. Forget, F. Baillet*, Cl. Soubrane, M.F. Auclerc, M.A. de Maublanc**, L. Thill, M. Housset*, J. Maral and D. Khayat

SOMPS Service d'Oncologie Médicale, Hôpital de la Salpétrière, 47 boulevard de l'hôpital, 75013 Paris, France
**Service de Radiothérapie, Hôpital Necker, Paris, France*
***Laboratoire de Cytologie, rue du Ranelagh, Paris, France*

INTRODUCTION

The activity of chemotherapy is now widely recognized in locally advanced breast cancer. Significant tumor regression and increase in DFS are observed by most authors (3)(4)(6)(10).

However, histological sterilisation is observed only in a fraction of responders (20 % to 25 %) by those who advocate surgery as the local control. On the other hand, the rate of CR after radiotherapy is not entirely satisfactory for many who use irradiation as local treatment.

Therefore, we have initiated in 1980 a protocol intensifying initial chemotherapy by shortening the interval between perfusions, using external and interstitial radiotherapy as local treatment ; in addition, in most patients, the schedule was designed to interdigitate hypofractioned radiotherapy with chemotherapy. Moreover, this Neo-Adjuvant Chemotherapy was extended to all stages of infiltrating breast cancers considering that although the 5 year survival of localised breast cancers varies between 65 % and 85 %, 80 % of the patients once diagnosed as having breast cancer will die from this cancer within 20 years (5).

On the other hand, primary or neo-adjuvant chemotherapy represents the most logical way to apply chemotherapy since it allows the assessment of the activity of a given combination in a given patient by measuring the tumor regression, it improves the local control and allows more often conservative treatment, it ensures the early management of micrometastases and might prevent their development.

MATERIAL & METHODS

The 252 consecutive patients with infiltrated breast cancer who were treated at the Department of Medical Oncology of the Salpétrière Hospital and at the Department of Radiotherapy of Necker Hospital between May 1980 and May 1986, were stratified into 4 groups.

Group 1 included 50 patients (pts) with tumors less than 3 cm diameter (19 T1) without clinical axillary involvement

Group 2 included 87 pts whose tumors was over 3 and under 7 cm (79 T2) ; 15 of them were N1b.

Group 3 included 43 pts with tumors over 7 cm or with fixed axillary lymphnodes (42 T3 - 14 N1b - 3 N2)

Group 4 included 72 pts with skin extension and inflammatory symptoms limited to a breast portion (PeV2) or extended to the whole breast in 7 pts (PeV3), realizing the clinical picture of carcinomatous mastitis. 1 pt had supra-clavicular fixed axillary lymph nodes. PeV1 pts (6 weeks clinical doubling time) were not included to group 4 but entered other groups according to their tumor size and to their clinical lymph nodes status.

Table I summarizes the pre-treatment characteristics of the patient population.

TABLE I

		N
Tumor size (cms)	⩽2	14
	⩽3	62
	>3 <7	131
	>7	45
Clinical Lymph nodes Status	N 0	143
	N 1a	33
	N 1b	66
	N 2	9
	N 3	1
Age	20-30	4
	⩾30-40	27
	⩾40-50	63
	⩾50-69	84
	⩾60 <80	74
Groups	G1	50
	G2	87
	G3	43
	G4	72
PeV	0	185
	1	25
	2	30
	3	7

The diagnosis relied on drill biopsy or more often on needle biopsy providing the histological grade (SBR index) or the cytopronostic index.

Oestrogen and progesterone receptors were not available in most patients. All pts had a complete blood count and serum chemistry, urinalysis, chest roentgenogram, bone scan, liver sonogram, bilateral mammogram, and CEA estimations. The initial treatment consisted of an intra-venous infusion combining Vinblastine 6 mg/m2, Thiotepa 6 mg/m2, Methotrexate 25 mg/m2, and Fluoro.5.Uracil 400 mg/m2 which was delivered for one hour. Adriamycin was combined to these drugs in Groups 3 & 4 pts. In addition, Prednisone 30 mg/m2/day was given oraly for 5 days after each infusion.

VTMF was given every 14 days for 3 cycles in Group 1, every 10 days for 4 cycles in Group 2.

VTMFA was planned every 7 days for 4 cycles in Group 3 and every 7 days for 6 cycles in Group 4.

Delays were allowed based upon the neutrophiles and the platelets counts. Before the third course neutropenia of under 1 000 neutrophils/mm3 and less frequent thrombopenia of under 100 000/mm3 led to a delay of the infusion for several days in Groups 3 & 4 in contrast to Groups 1 & 2 pts whose hematological tolerance was good.

Generally, the 4 courses would be given within 5 weeks in Group 3 and 6 courses within 8 weeks in Group 4.

Before any infusion one of us (F.B.) saw the patients in order to determine the appropriate radiotherapy plan according to the tumor size and site. Cobaltotherapy was delivered by tangential fields to the whole breast. Supra-clavicular and internal mammary lymph nodes were treated by direct beam and axillary lymph nodes by anteroposterior ports.

By randomisation, Groups 1 & 2 pts were treated according to the classical schedule (45 Gy within 5 weeks) or according to hypofractioned schedule (5 Gy on days 1 & 3, 6.5 Gy on days 15 & 17).

All Group 3 & 4 pts were treated by the hypofractioned schedule. Prior clinical studies have demonstrated that the 23 Gy delivered by this schedule were equivalent to 45 Gy by classical schedule (1)(2).

In those pts, an infusion devoid of Adriamycin and of Methotrexate was interspaced between day 3 and day 15.

Two weeks after the teletherapy after an additional infusion of chemotherapy without Adriamycin & Methotrexate, a boost at the initial tumor site, by wire implants of Irridium 192, was delivered. The dose was 20 to 30 Gy according to the initial size of the tumor and to its clinical persistance or not at the time of endocurietherapy.

Thereafter, maintenance chemotherapy with the initial combination was given for 5 monthly cycles to Group 1, 6 bimonthly cycles and 12 monthly cycles to Group 2, 6 bimonthly cycles followed by every 12 monthly cycles for Group 3 & 4. In addition, although the protocol planned to give Tamoxifen to all post-menopausal pts and to randomize its administration in other pts, this randomization could not be respected in all pts. Among the 80 pts who did not receive Tamoxifen, 50 were post-menopausal and had an history of thrombosis.

RESULTS

Induction chemotherapy induced a significant tumor regression (>75 % largest tumor diameter) in 71 % pts. 28 % of pts reached complete clinical remission before radiotherapy and in all pts complete clinical tumor regression was achieved after interstitial irradiation.

Table II summarizes the relationship between various parameters and response to chemotherapy.

TABLE II

		Nb of patients	Tumor regression incidence (%) (≥75% and 100 %)	Statistical significance	Relapse incidence (%)	Statistical significance
Groups	1	50	72		10	$p < 0.005$
	2	87	69		14	
	3	43	71		39	
	4	72	73		37	
Histological or Cytological grade	1	41	66		5	$p < 0.05$
	2	109	73		26	
	3	41	80		24	
	not verif.	61	63		32	
Age	<50	94	69		30	
	≥50	158	72		21	
PeV	0	185	71		19	$p < 0.005$
	1	25	84		36	
	2	30	60		40	
	3	7	86		57	
Regression	<75 %	73			36	$p < 0.05$
	≥75 %	179			20	
Tamoxifen Administration	TAM +	194	77	$p < 0.05$	20	$p < 0.02$
	TAM -	58	50		34	

Few parameter seem to influence tumor regression except perhaps Tamoxifen administration. The incidence of relapses depends on groups, on histology (only 2 relapses occured among 41 pts with cytopronostic index 1). It is also significantly influenced by clinical doubling time (PeV1) and inflammatory symptoms (PeV2 and PeV3) and also, by initial regression above 75 %. The combination of Tamoxifen seems to decrease relapses incidence.

The distribution of relapses is shown on Table III.

TABLE III

Groups	Loco regional recurrences	Contro lateral cancer	Distant metastasis	Local recurr. and synchrono. distant metast	Total
1 (50	1		4		5
2 (87)	6		4	2	12
3 (43)	3		12	3	18
4 (72)	5	1	18	2	26
Total	15	1	38	7	61

15 patients had exclusively locoregional recurrences (10 breast lumps, 3 lymph nodes, 2 skin nodules), 7 pts had simultaneously loco-regional recurrences and distant involvements, 1 pt had a controlateral breast cancer. A mastectomy was performed in 5 pts and a tumorectomy in 5 pts.

Actuarial disease free survival according to groups are overall survival are shown on Figure 1 and 2.

Death occured in 46 pts : 43 pts died from breast cancer (3 pts died in complete remission), 2 pts from groups 2 who did not receive Adriamycin died from myocardial infarction (62 y.-69 y.old), another pt died during anesthesia for minor surgery (70 y.old) from cardiac arrest.

Toxicity is indicated in Table IV.

TABLE IV.

Toxicity (252 pts)	Grade 1	Grade 2	Grade 3
Bone marrow	224	25	3
Neurol..	200		
G.I.	252		
Cardiac	*		
Hair loss		10	212
Performance status	226	20	3

(*) = 2 unrelated myocardial infarction in patients not receiving Adriamycin.

Hematological toxicity obliged us to spread the initial treatment and to delay some perfusions. Neutropenia managed by ambulatory antibiotics was observed in 25 pts whereas sepsis and aplasia required hospitalisation in 3 pts.

Mild symptoms of Vinblastine neuropathy were frequent, as well as nausea. Despite application of cold, alopecia was observed in most pts. No clinical or subclinical cardiotoxicity checked by sonography was noted.

Despite the large volume of most tumor, cosmetic results were excellent or good in 85 % pts. No major functional or cosmetic sequelae was observed.

DISCUSSION

With more followed we confirm the encouraging results that we have already published in several papers in all stages of breast cancers (7)(8)(9)(10) or in locally advanced breast cancers using intensive neo-adjuvant chemotherapy, radiotherapy and hormonotherapy, the problem being now to improve these results.

Chemotherapy intensity should be further increased specially in pts with poorly differentiated tumors leading to revise pts stratification. Tumor regression after 3 doses might indicate whether we may pursue the same treatment or try another combination. A synchronisation of tumor cells by Premarin may be attempted in locally advanced patients in a controled way considering Lipman's encouraging results. Anyway we may conclude that neo-adjuvant chemotherapy is now adopted by almost everybody in locally advanced breast cancers and several papers on this topic are presented in this book.
In operable cancers, several preliminary studies are comparing neo-adjuvant chemotherapy and adjuvant chemotherapy. In a retrospective study presented elsewhere in this book, comparing 02SR80 results to results achieved in pts who had mastectomy followed by adjuvant chemotherapy in nodes positive pts no significant difference is observed in survival and in DFS except for large tumors for which 02SR80 results are significantly better. Controlled studies will be valuable only if they use intensive treatment achieving complete clinical remission in most pts.

In our Department our aim is now to achieve complete clinical remission before radiotherapy in most patients.

REFERENCES

1 - Baillet F., Cussac A., Deluen F., Bessard B., Misset N., Marin JL., Maylin C., Rhein-Bachellerie B. (1983) : Comparaison des effets d'une irradiation classique de 45 Gy et d'une forme particulière d'irradiation hypofractionnée considérée comme équivalente. A propos de 417 cas. Bull. Cancer, 3 : 228-335.

2 - Baillet F., Dessard-Diana B., Diana C., Housset M., Maylin C. and Thomas F. (1987) : Therapeutics and Cost-Effectiveness of Special Type of Hypofractionaled Radiotherapy. Health Care. Edt Joint Commission, Chicago : 112.

3 - Bedwinek J., Ratkin G., Philpott G., Wallack M., Perez C. (1983) : Concurrent chemotherapy and radiotherapy for nn metastatic stage IV breast cancer. Am. J. Clin. Oncol, 6: 159-165.

4 - De Lena M., Varini M., Zucali R., Ravino D., Vignotti G., Valagussa P., Veronesi U., Bonadonna G. (1981) : Multinodal treatment for locally advanced breast cancer. Results of chemotheray-radiotherapy versus chemotechrapy-surgery. Cancer Clin. Trials, 4 ; 3 : 229-236

5 - Ferguson D.J., Meier P., Karrison J., Dawson P.J., Straus F.H., Lowenstein F.G. (1982) : Staging of Breast Cancer and Survival Rates. JAMA, 248 : 1337-1341.
6 - Hortobagyi G.N., Blumenschein G.R., Spanos W., Montague E.D., Buzdar A.U., Yap H.Y. and Schell F. (1983) : Multimodality treatment of loco-regionally advanced breast cancer. Cancer, 51 : 763-768.
7 - Jacquillat Cl., Baillet F., Auclerc G. and coll (1982) : Initial Chemotherapy and Conservative Radiotherapy in Stage I, II and III Breast Cancer. Proceedings 13th International Cancer Congress : 52.
8 - Jacquillat Cl., Baillet F., Blondon J. and coll (1983) : Preliminary Results of "Neo-adjuvant" Chemotherapy in Initial Management of Breast Cancer (BC). Proceedings A.S.C.O. : 112.
9 - Jacquillat Cl., Baillet F., Auclerc G., and coll (1984) : Cancer du sein : Chimiothérapie Précédant le Traitement Loco-Régional avec Extensiton des Indications du Traitement COnservateur. Bull. Cancer, 71,4 : 354-360.
10 -Jacquillat Cl., Baillet F., Weil M. and coll (1988) : Results of a conservative treatment combining induction (neoadjuvant) and consolidation chemotherapy, hormonotherapy and interstitial irradiation in 98 pts with locally advanced breast cancer (IIIa-IIIb). Cancer (1988), 61 : 1977-1982

Acknowledgment :
We are grateful to Brigitte Cédreau for her technical help.

Résumé

Entre mai 1980 et mai 1986, 252 patientes consécutives (pts) atteintes d'un cancer du sein ont été incluses dans un protocole thérapeutique prospectif associant chimiothérapie (CT) néoadjuvante et radiothérapie (RT)(03SR80). Quatre groupes thérapeutiques avaient été préalablement définis : gr.I (50 pts) T$\leq$3cm NO N1a ; gr.II (87 pts) T$>$3$\leq$7 cm ou N1b ; gr. III (43 pts) T$>$7 cm ou N2 ; gr IV (73 pts) T4 ou PeV. Chaque cycle de CT associait en mg/m2 : le premier jour (J1) : Velbé 6 ; Thiotépa 6 ; Méthotrexate 25 ; Fluoro-5-uracile 350 ; Adriamycine 30 (gr III et IV) et de J1 à J5 per os : Prednisone 20. L'espacement des cycles, leur nombre et la durée du traitement d'entretien après la RT dépendaient du gr thérapeutique. Les femmes ménopausées et quelques unes non ménopausées recevaient du tamoxifène. La RT externe (45 Gy ou 45 Gy eq) a été délivrée en fractionnement classique pour la plupart des patients des gr I et II ou en hypofractionnement pour les pts des gr III et IV. L'importance du complément par Irridium 192 dépendait du reliquat. Après CT d'induction, une régression tumorale$\geq$75% a été obtenue chez 179 pts (71%), taux de réponse encore meilleur sous tamoxifène (75%). Après RT, une RC a été obtenue dans tous les cas. 15 malades ont présenté une récidive loco-régionale, 38 (8 gr I et II ; 30 gr III et IV) des métastases à distance et 7 une rechute mixte locale et générale. La survie globale a été de 75 % à 5 ans (84% grI+II 63% gr III+IV) et la survie NED de 62% (75% grI+II ; 47% gr III+IV) (méthode actuarielle). Plusieurs facteurs ont influencé la survie NED à 5 ans ($p<0{,}01$) : le cytopronostic (SBR 1/2+3), la PeV (PeV0/1+ 2+3), le T (T1+2/3+4), le groupe thérapeutique (gr I+II/III+IV) et l'importance de la régression tumorale avant le RT$\geq$75%/$<$75%). Les résultats esthétiques ont été excellents ou très bons chez 85% des patientes.

Ainsi, les survies globales et NED à 5 ans (75 et 62%) sont au moins égales à celles rapportées après des traitements comportant une chirurgie mutilante.

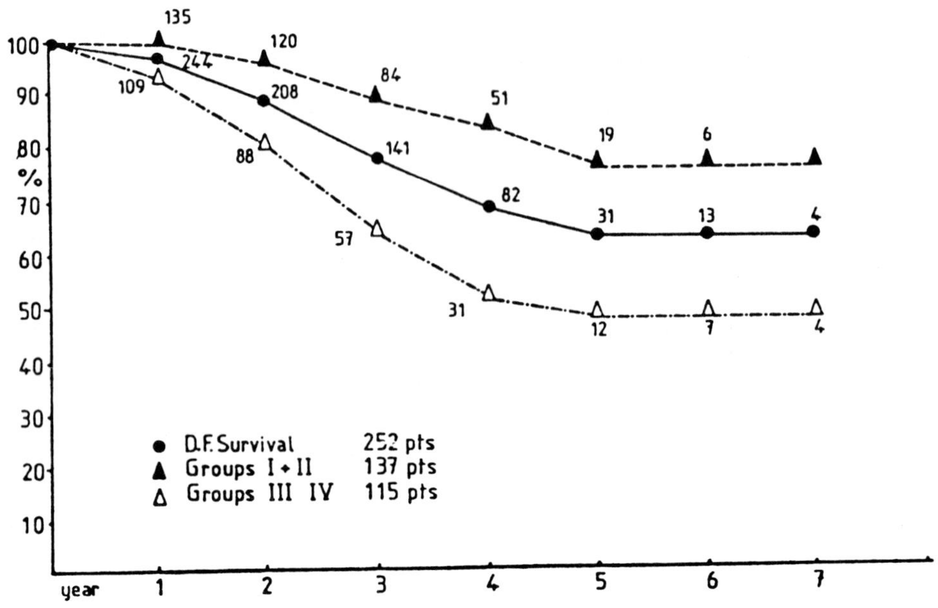
D.F. Survival 252 pts
Groups I + II 137 pts
Groups III IV 115 pts
%
year

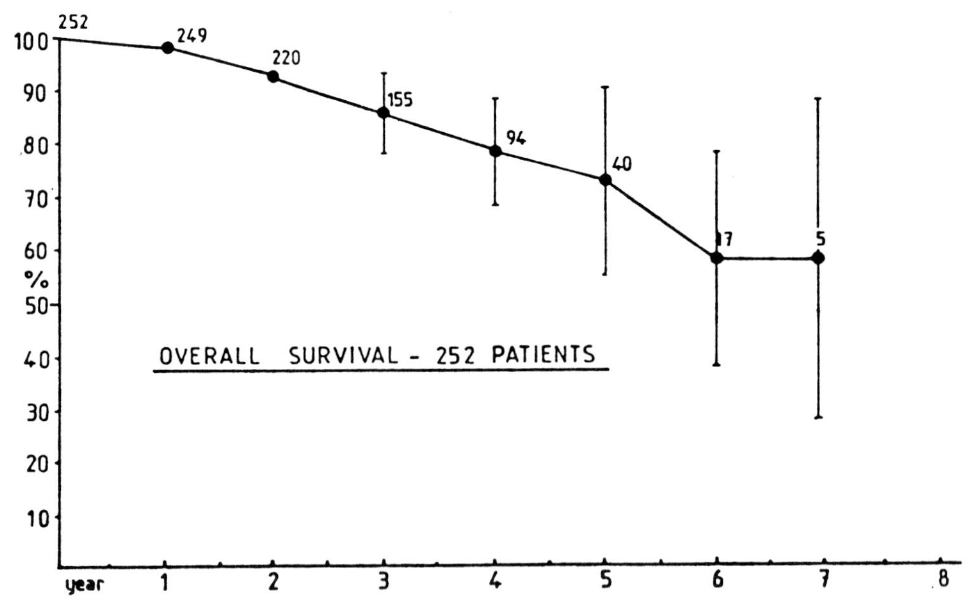
OVERALL SURVIVAL - 252 PATIENTS
%
year

Neo-Adjuvant Chemotherapy. Ed. Cl. Jacquillat, M. Weil, D. Khayat. Colloque INSERM/John Libbey Eurotext Ltd. © 1988. Vol. 169, pp. 137-142.

Neo-adjuvant chemotherapy in the management of advanced primary carcinoma of the breast

G.N. Hortobagyi [1], A.U. Buzdar [1], F.C. Ames [2] and M.D. McNeese [3]

From the Departments of Medical Oncology [1], Surgery [2] and Radiotherapy [3], The University of Texas M.D. Anderson Hospital and Tumor Institute at Houston, Houston, Texas, 77030 USA

In May 1973 we began using combined modality treatment including primary chemotherapy followed by surgery, or radiation, or both, and adjuvant chemotherapy for patients with both inflammatory, and non-inflammatory, locally advanced breast cancers. Although initially designed for patients with inoperable, locally advanced disease, in more recent years all patients with stage III breast cancer were treated with this strategy. We present here our experience with this multimodal treatment over the last 14 years.

PATIENTS AND METHODS

Between May 1973 and June 1987, 360 patients with stage III breast carcinoma were entered on the trial. Patients with large primary (T3, T4) or advanced regional node involvement (N2, N3) were candidates for this protocol if no evidence of distant metastases was detected. Prior invasive malignancies, prior treatment, or major organ failure excluded patients from participation.

Treatment started with induction chemotherapy. On day 1 500 mg/m^2 of fluorouracil (F), 50 mg/m^2 of doxorubicin (Adriamycin), and 500 mg/m^2 of cyclophosphamide (C) (FAC) were given intravenously. The dose of fluorouracil was repeated on day 8 after three initial cycles of induction chemotherapy responding patients were treated with a total mastectomy with level 2 axillary dissection or a radical mastectomy, or primary radiotherapy to the breast and regional lymphatics, or both, and systemic therapy was continued with the same chemotherapy combination (1). After reaching 450 mg/m^2 of doxorubicin, maintenance therapy consisting of C, methotrexate, F (CMF) was administered for two years. However, maintenance therapy was not administered to patients registered after 1980.

Radiation therapy was administered with a cobalt-60 machine to a tumor dose of 5000 rad to the breast (or chest wall), the internal mammary, and supraclavicular areas. The axilla was included only for patients without an axillary dissection. An additional 1500 to 2000 rad were given to a restricted field in areas of residual tumor. When possible, the electron beam was employed to treat the internal mammary nodes to decrease the risk of cardiac toxicity. Patients with inflammatory breast cancer were treated only with FAC chemotherapy and radiotherapy from 1973 to 1981 (first protocol) (2). Since 1982, induction chemotherapy was followed by a total mastectomy and then by additional chemotherapy and radiotherapy (second protocol) (3).

In March 1985 a new protocol was designed for patients with non-inflammatory stage III breast cancer. This consisted of induction chemotherapy with vincristine, doxorubicin (Adriamycin), C, and prednisone (VACP) administered in 21-day cycles, with doses escalated to maximum tolerance. After three cycles of induction chemotherapy, all patients underwent a total mastectomy with level 2 axillary dissection. Patients with minimal, or no residual disease in the mastectomy specimen continued the same chemotherapy regimen until completing 500 mg/m^2 of doxorubicin, and then received radiation therapy to the chest wall and regional lymph node bearing areas. Patients with no response to induction chemotherapy were treated with radiation therapy to the breast and regional lymphatics followed by a total mastectomy and axillary dissection (if possible), and adjuvant chemotherapy with a combination of vinblastine, methotrexate, and 5-fluorouracil (VMF). Patients who responded to induction chemotherapy, but still had substantial residual disease, were randomly allocated to continue postoperatively either the induction regimen (VACP), or a different adjuvant chemotherapy (VMF) for five cycles, and then received radiation therapy to the chest wall and regional lymphatics.

The initial evaluation included a history and physical examination, complete blood count, biochemical survey, and appropriate radiologic and radioisotopic exams to rule out distant metastases. Weekly blood counts were done during chemotherapy, and the biochemical survey was repeated before each cycle of treatment. A complete metastatic evaluation was repeated every 4 to 6 months for the first five years, and yearly thereafter. A written informed consent was obtained from each patient according to institutional and federal guidelines.

Survival curves were calculated according to the Kaplan-Meier method and differences between them were assessed by the Gehan-Wilcoxon technique (5,6).

RESULTS

Non-Inflammatory Breast Cancer:

Between 1973 and March 1985, 1974 patients with stage III non-inflammatory breast cancer were treated under the initial protocol (1). The median age was 51 years and 48% of the patients were premenopausal. Forty-eight patients had stage IIIA (operable) breast cancer and 126 had stage IIIB (inoperable) breast cancer (Table 1). Estrogen receptor status was available in 66% of the patients and, of those, slightly less than half had positive estrogen receptor status (>10 fmoles/mg of protein) (Table 2). The overall response rate to induction chemotherapy, assessed by clinical measurements, was 87%, of which 17% represented complete remissions. One hundred sixty-eight of the 174 patients (96%) were disease-free after induction chemotherapy and local treatment, whereas six patients had residual disease. The minimal follow-up was 30 months and the maximum, 156 months (median follow-up:

Table 1. Distribution of Patients According to Clinical T and N Categories

		Primary Tumor			
		T1-2	T3	T4	Total
Regional	N0	-	4	9	13
Nodal	N1	-	18	35	53
	N2	0	17	37	63
Involvement	N3	8	5	32	45
	Total	17	44	113	174

Table 2. Patient Characteristics

	Non-Inflammatory	Inflammatory First Protocol	Inflammatory Second Protocol
Median age (range)	51 (24-78)	51 (27-78)	52 (30-70)
T1-3	61	-	-
T4	113	63	43
N0-1	66	26	25
N2	63	21	14
N3	45	16	4
Estrogen receptor			
Positive	51	-	10
Negative	64	-	20
Unknown	59	-	13
Median follow-up (months)	59	98	30
No. of patients	174	63	43

59 months). The median disease-free survival (DFS) for patients with stage IIIA disease had not been reached and that for patients with stage IIIB was 30 months. The 5-year DFS were 71% and 33% for stages IIIA and IIIB disease, respectively. The median survival (S) for patients with stage IIIA disease had not been reached, and that for patients with stage IIIB disease was 48 months (Figure 1). It is projected that the 10-year S for patients with stages IIIA and IIIB disease will be

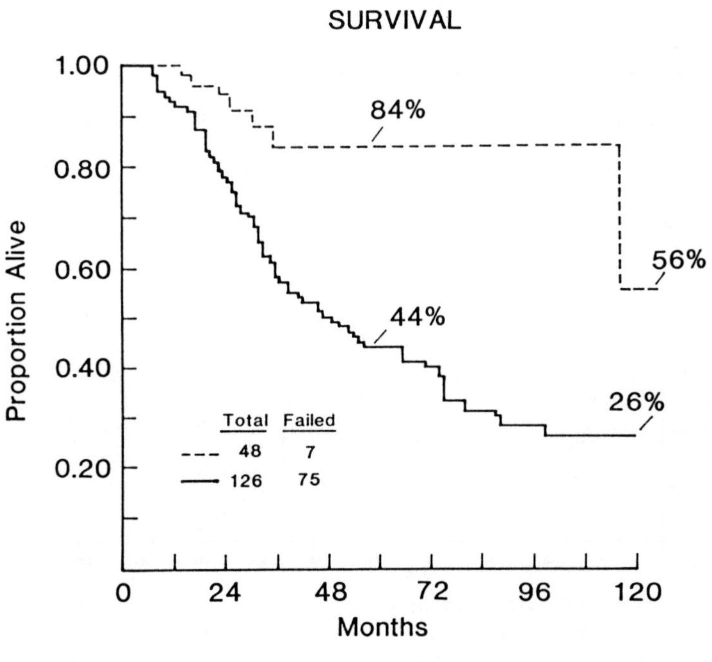

Fig. 1

56% and 26%, respectively. Patients with estrogen receptor-positive tumors, those with a good response to induction chemotherapy, and those with good compliance with treatment had a higher DFS and S rates than patients with estrogen receptor-negative tumors, no response to induction chemotherapy, or poor compliance. The local regional failure rate was 15%.

Since March 1985, 80 additional patients with non-inflammatory stage III breast cancer were treated with the second protocol. It is too early to evaluate fifteen of these patients but for the remaining 65 the overall and complete response rates were similar to our earlier experience. It is too early to state whether the second protocol will result in better DFS or S.

Inflammatory Breast Cancer:

Between May 1973 and December 1986, 106 patients with inflammatory breast carcinoma were treated on two consecutive phase II protocols. The chemotherapy for the first was identical to that described for the first protocol for non-inflammatory breast cancer (FAC-CMF) (2). For the second inflammatory protocol vincristine and prednisone were added to FAC (3). Radiation therapy was administered after all planned systemic therapy had been given. After induction chemotherapy 67% of patients with inflammatory breast cancer achieved a major objective regression; after induction chemotherapy and local treatment 93% of patients on both protocols were rendered disease-free. The rest had persistent disease. Figure 2 shows the DFS of patients with inflammatory breast carcinoma treated on these two protocols.

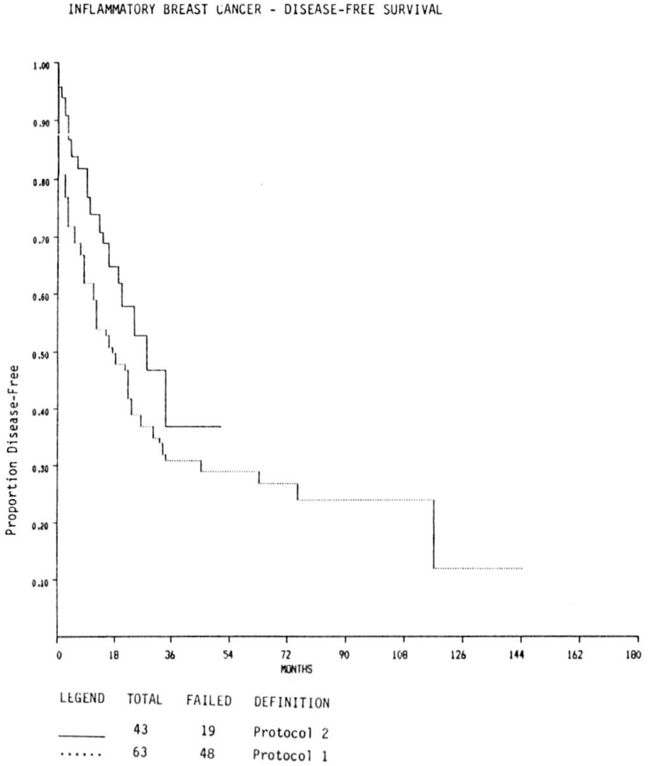

Fig. 2

The median DFS was 24 months; the median S was 43 months for patients treated with the first protocol. The local regional failure rates were 14% and 12% for patients with inflammatory breast cancer treated with the first and second protocol, respectively. A major response to induction chemotherapy correlated very closely with outcome and responding patients had higher DFS and S rates than nonresponders.

These regimens caused nausea, vomiting, alopecia, and myelosuppression. Clinical cardiotoxicity related to doxorubicin was observed in 4% of patients, but only one patient died because of progressive irreversible cardiomyopathy.

COMMENTS

Over the last ten years we have acquired extensive experience with neoadjuvant, or induction chemotherapy for breast cancer. We have demonstrated that the majority of patients with primary breast cancer respond to the chemotherapy programs used in this report. In addition, almost all can be rendered disease-free by combining systemic and local therapies. Compared with extensive historical experience at our institution (7,8), and reported in the literature (9,10), the local control rate of patients treated with these multimodality regimens is far superior to that obtained with local regional treatments alone.

These multimodality regimens have resulted in a major change in survival for inflammatory breast carcinoma (11). Previously a uniformly fatal disease, now 30-50% of patients survive five years or longer. The heterogeneity of non-inflammatory breast carcinoma makes conclusions about survival less solid. However, it is certain that patients with stage IIIB locally advanced breast cancer survive longer with these multimodality programs. The information obtained during primary systemic therapy, the ability to assess in vivo response to systemic treatment, the decreased tumor bulk, and the early introduction of antimetastatic therapy are all substantial, practical advantages for this strategy. The development of better staging and prognostic criteria, and, more important, effective non-cross-resistant systemic regimens for nonresponders should help improve the survival in this group of high risk patients.

REFERENCES

1. Hortobagyi GN, Kau KW, Buzdar AU, et al: Induction chemotherapy for stage III primary breast cancer. IN Adjuvant Therapy of Cancer V, SE Salmon (ed), Grune & Stratton, Orlando, 1987, pp. 419-428.
2. Fastenberg NA, Buzdar AU, Montague ED, et al: Management of inflammatory carcinoma of the breast. A combined modality approach. Am J Clin Oncol (CCT) 8: 134-141, 1985.
3. Buzdar AU, Hortobagyi G, Frye D, et al: Inflammatory carcinoma of the breast: Preliminary result of combined modality approach. Presented at the 15th International Congress of Chemotherapy, Istanbul, Turkey, July 1987.
4. Hayward JL, Carbone PP, Heuson JC, et al: Assessment of response to therapy in advanced breast cancer. A project of the programe of clinical oncology of the International Union Against Cancer, Geneva, Switzerland. Cancer 39:1289-1294, 1977.
5. Kaplan EL, Meier P: Nonparametric estimation from incomplete observations. J Amer Stat Assoc 53:457-481, 1958.
6. Gehan EA: A generalized Wilcoxon test for comparing arbitrarily singly-censored samples. Biometrics 52:203-223, 1965.
7. Barker JL, Nelson AJ, Montague ED: Inflammatory carcinoma of the breast. Radiology 121:173-176, 1976.
8. Hortobagyi GN, Blumenschein GR, Spanos W, et al: Multimodal treatment of locoregionally advanced breast cancer. Cancer 51:763-768, 1983.
9. Treves N: The inoperability of inflammatory carcinoma of the breast. Surg, Gynecol & Obstet 109:240-242, 1959.

10. Sicher K, Waterhouse JAH: Evaluation of TNM classification of carcinoma of the breast. Br J Cancer 28:580-588, 1973.
11. Hortobagyi GN, Buzder AU: Progress in inflammatory breast cancer: Cause for cautious optimism. J Clin Oncol 4:1727-1729, 1986.

Neo-Adjuvant Chemotherapy. Ed. Cl. Jacquillat, M. Weil, D. Khayat. Colloque INSERM/John Libbey Eurotext Ltd. © 1988. Vol. 169, pp. 143-148.

Neo-adjuvant chemotherapy in the combined modality approach of locally advanced non-metastatic breast cancer

M.E. Lippman, S.M. Swain, E.F. Egan, D.N. Danforth Jr., J. Bader and S.M. Steinberg

Medicine Branch, Surgery Branch, Radiation Oncology, and Biostatistics and Data Management Section, National Cancer Institute, Bethesda, Maryland 20892 USA

ABSTRACT

We have treated 100 patients with locally advanced breast cancer, 43 with stage III A, 53 with stage III B, and 4 with stages IV disease, with primary induction chemotherapy including an attempted hormonal synchronization. All were treated to maximum objective clinical response before proceeding to any local therapy. Patients achieving a pathologic complete response generally received radiation therapy while patients with residual disease, partial response (PR) or no change (NC) status received debulking surgery prior to radiation therapy. Regardless of response to induction chemotherapy, patients received at least 6 additional months of chemotherapy following local therapy. Initial doses of combination chemotherapy were escalated to targeted myelosuppression. The objective response rate to induction chemotherapy was 95% with 46% complete response (CR), 49% PR and 5% NC. Of 44 patients achieving a CR to chemotherapy, 42 were assessed by biopsies to determine pathologic evidence of response. Twenty-seven of the 44 patients (61%) were proven to be pathologic complete responders with negative biopsies. Median time to progression is 30 months and median survival is 49 months for all patients. This aggressive primary chemotherapy regimen with hormonal synchronization followed by local therapy appears to provide excellent local control and encouraging early results on systemic disease control.

KEY WORDS

Neoadjuvant, Breast Cancer, Hormonal Synchronization

INTRODUCTION

Locally advanced, non metastatic breast cancer is associated with poor local control and dismal survival (Haagensen, 1971). Combined programs of surgery and radiation have resulted in 5-year survivals of 35 to 55% in some selected series (Balawajder, 1983; Fletcher, 1972; Pearlman, 1976; Zucali, 1976; Bedwinek, 1982). The majority of patients succumb to metastatic disease, suggesting that disseminated micrometastases exist at initial presentation in virtually all patients.

Chemotherapy has been used in conjunction with local therapy to treat locally advanced breast cancer (Bruckman, 1979; Grohn, 1984; DeLena, 1978; Hortobagyi, 1983). Generally speaking, these studies have verified the general efficacy of systemic therapy in improving both local control and survival.

Since 1977 patients with locally advanced breast cancer have been treated with combination chemotherapy given to the point of maximum objective clinical response. Simultaneous tamoxifen and premarin were given sequentially before the administration of cell cycle specific agents in the hopes of synchronizing DNA synthesis and thus making them more susceptible to cytotoxic chemotherapy. The rationale for this approach has its foundation in prior studies from our laboratory (Donehower, 1980; Lippman, 1976; Nawata, 1981) which demonstrated that antiestrogen-induced inhibition of breast cancer cell growth could be reversed by estrogen rescue. In a randomized study from our institution (Lippman, 1984) using CAMF chemotherapy with or without hormonal synchronization in patients with metastatic and inflammatory breast cancer, improvement in overall survival and time to progression was observed in objective responders in the treatment arm including tamoxifen and premarin.

MATERIALS AND METHODS

Patient Selection

From January 1977 through October 1987, we have treated 100 women with locally advanced breast cancer. These patients' stages were defined as stage III A and III B according to the 1983 American Joint Committee staging system. To be eligible for treatment, all patients were required to have a histologically documented diagnosis of mammary cancer with evidence of measurable disease. Details of evaluation and therapy have been published (Swain, 1987).

RESULTS

Distribution of Prognostic Variables

At the time of this evalution, 100 patients have been started on treatment and are evaluable for toxicity, time to progression and survival. Patient characteristics are shown in Table 1. TNM status of patients at presentation is shown in Table 2.

Table 1. Patients Entered on Study

Total Number of Patient on Study:	100
Stage IIIA	43
Stage IIIB	53
Inflammatory	43
Non-Inflammatory	10
Stage IV	4
Median Age	51.7
Menopausal Status	
Premenopausal	40
Postmenopausal	60
Estrogen Receptor	
Positive	27
Negative	38
Unknown	35

Table 2. Clinical T-N-M Stage at Presentation

	N0	N1	N2	N3	Total
T2	1	0	2	1	4
T3	15	15	12	4	46
T4	12	21	11	6	50
	28	36	25	11	100

Chemotherapy Response

Overall objective response rate (CR + PR) was 95%. Forty-four patients (46%) achieved a CR, 47 patients (49%) achieved a PR and 5 patients (5%) showed no change. Median number of chemotherapy cycles to achieve a CR, PR, or NC was 5,3, and 5 respectively with a range of cycles of 2 to 11, 2 to 9, and 4 to 6 respectively. There was no impact on response rate of TNM stage. In addition, there is no indication that estrogen receptor status, histology, nodal status, menopausal status or age were predictive of a patient's best clinical response to induction chemotherapy.

Toxicities

The white blood cell nadir reached 3000-3999 in 17% of patients, 2000 to 2999 in 35%, 1000-1999 in 40% and below 1000 in 7%. There were four infection-related admissions occuring during periods of neutropenia while on chemotherapy and no deaths. Two patients developed cardiomyopathies secondary to doxorubicin. One patient received a total dose of 490 mg/m^2 of doxorubicin and is doing well with compensated congestive heart failure. The second patient received 513 mg/m^2 of doxorubicin and died of progressive congestive heart failure with no evidence of breast cancer. There has been one serious wound infection after local treatment with surgery and radiation, one radiation neuropathy resulting in a non-functioning arm which is improving, and one methotrexate pneumonitis. One patient developed a severe rash with blistering skin from 5-flourouracil and this agent was discontinued in this patient only.

Histologic Evaluation of Response

Patients achieving a clinical CR were evaluated histologically to determine if a pathologic CR had been attained (Table 3). Seven of the 27 biopsy negative patients (or 26%) have relapsed in their irradiated breasts.

Table 3. Results of Biopsy in Clinical Complete Responders

Complete Responders		
Biopsy Negative Treated wtih radiation therapy	27/44	(61%)
Biopsy Positive Treated with mastectomy and radiation therapy	15/44	(34%)
Biopsy Not Done	2/44	(5%)

Local Therapy
All patients achieving a clinical CR received radiation therapy with the exception of a single patient who refused any local therapy after acheiving a complete response with negative repeat biopsy. One hundred percent of the patients were NED following the completion of induction chemotherapy and local therapy.

Outcome of Patients Completing Combined Modality Treatment
There have been 38 patients (38%) who have relapsed to date. Thus far no predictive value for eventual relapse has been found for estrogen receptor status, menopausal status, age, addition of hormonal synchronization, or number of cycles to best chemotherapy response. The most important predictor of relapse was the clinical TNM stage at the start of treatment. Patients with advanced nodal metastasis who relapsed tended to have inflammatory breast cancer. Of the 38 relapsed patients, 12 were stage III A (29% of patients with IIIA disease), 24 were stage IIIB (47% with stage IIIB) and two were stage IV (50% with stage IV). Ten failures were locoregional, 21 distant and 7 locoregional and distant. At 2 years the probability of local control is 83% for all patients. Median time to progression is 30 months for all patients. The median survival is 49 months.

DISCUSSION

We treated locally advanced breast cancer by giving initial chemotherapy for as many cycles as necessary to achieve maximal response. This approach has yielded significant response rates in both stage III A and stage III B breast cancer. The concept of giving a variable initial amount of chemotherapy is unique to our study design. By giving a variable number of chemotherapy cycles until the maximum objective clinical response was attained, our induction chemotherapy regimen produced objective responses, without significant morbidity, in 95% of patients.

In the present study, patients achieving a clinical CR to chemotherapy underwent biopsy evaluation in the area of the breast previously known to be involved with tumor. Using this approach the overall pathologic complete response rate for this induction chemotherapy regimen was 27%. In a recent report from the M.D. Anderson Hospital (Feldman, 1984) only 6 patients (7%) had no evidence of microscopic disease. While great efforts were made to utilize clinical and radiologic information in guiding each biopsy in our series, this method is still subject to sampling errors. Nevertheless, the multiple biopsy procedure has appeared useful in identifying clinical CR patients with no or only microscopic residual tumor burden. These patients appear likely to do well with radiation alone, thereby avoiding the need for disfiguring surgery. At the present time, 27 of our patients have finished combined modality therapy and been rendered disease free with a cosmetically intact breast. While cosmetic issues have not been our primary concern in the treatment of locally advanced breast cancer, the possibility of being able to maintain an intact breast after aggressive treatment may provide an important psychologic incentive in a population of patients, some of whom initially delayed seeking medical attention for fear of losing their breast.

The combined modality approach used in this series has achieved a local and systemic disease free state for all those patients who completed both induction chemotherapy and local therapy, irrespective of their clinical stages at presentation or best local response to induction therapy. This aggressive regimen appears to provide excellent local control. Stage III B patients still have a high rate of relapse and an overall shorter survival. This is most apparent in those patients with inflammatory breast cancer. An effort is being made to improve systemic control in inflammatory patients in this study. After they are rendered disease free by this combined modality regimen, they are randomized to receive either high dose chemotherapy plus autologous bone marrow transplant followed by maintenance chemotherapy, or maintenance chemotherapy alone. It is hoped that this very aggressive chemotherapy can improve survival in these poor prognosis patients. We have also expanded our study to poor prognosis stage II patients with extensive lymph node involvement.

REFERENCES

Balawajder, I., Antich, P.P., Boland, J. (1983): An analysis of the role of radiotherapy alone in combination with chemotherapy and surgery in the management of advanced breast carcinoma. Cancer 51, 574-580.

Bedwinek, J., Rao, D.V., Perez, C., Lee, J., Finberg, B. (1982): Stage III and localized stage IV breast cancer: Irradiation alone versus irradiation plus surgery. Int. J. Radiat. Oncol. Biol. Phys. 8, 31-36.

Bruckman, J.E., Harris, J.R., Levene, M.B., Chaffey, J.T., Hellman, S. (1979): Results of treating stage III carcinoma of the breast by primary radiation therapy. Cancer 43, 985-993.

DeLena, M., Zucali, R., Viganotti, G., Valagussa, P., Bonadonna, G. Combined chemotherapy-radiotherapy approach in locally advanced (T_{3b}-T_4) breast cancer. Cancer Chemother Pharmacol 1:53-59, 1978.

Donehower, R., Allegra, J.C., Lippman, M.E., Chabner, B. (1980): Combined effects of methotrexate and 5-fluoropyrimidine on human breast cancer cells in serum-free culture. Eur. J. Cancer 16, 655-661.

Feldman, L., Hortobagyi, G., Buzdar, A., Blumenschein, G. (1984): Pathologic complete remission in patients with inflammatory breast cancer and locally advanced breast cancer. Proc. Am. Soc. Clin. Oncol. 25, 197 (Abstr).

Fletcher, G.H. (1972): Local results of irradiation in the primary management of localized breast cancer. Cancer 29, 545-551.

Grohn, P., Heinonen, E., Klefstrom, P., Tarkkanen, J. (1984): Adjuvant Post-Operative Radiotherapy, Chemotherapy and Immunotherapy in Stage III Breast Cancer. Cancer 54, 670-674.

Haagensen, C.D. (1971): Diseases of the Breast, 2nd edn, p. 629. Philadelphia: W.B. Saunders.

Hortobagyi, G.N., Blumenschein, G.R., Spanos, W., Montague, E.D., Buzdar, A.U., Yap, H.Y., Schell, F. (1983): Multimodal treatment of locoregionally advanced breast cancer. Cancer 51, 763-768.

Lippman, M.E., Bolan, G., Huff, K. (1976): The effects of estrogens and anti-estrogens on hormone-responsive human breast cancer in long-term tissue culture. Cancer Res. 36, 4595-4601.

Lippman, M.E., Cassidy, J., Wesley, M., Young, R.C. (1984): A randomized attempt to increase the efficacy of cytotoxic chemotherapy in metastatic breast cancer by hormonal synchronization. J. Clin. Oncol. 2, 28-36.

Nawata, H., Chong, M., Bronzert, D., Lippman, M.E. (1981): Estradiol independent growth of a subline of MCF-7 human breast cancer cell line in culture. J. Biol. Chem. 256, 6895-6902.

Pearlman, N.W., Guerra, O., Fracchia, A.A. (1976): Primary inoperable cancer of the breast. Surg. Gynecol. Obstet. 143, 909-913.

Swain, S.M., Sorace, R.A., Bagley, C.S., Bader, J., Wesley, M.N., Steinberg, S.M., Lippman, M.E. (1987): Neoadjuvant Chemotherpay in the Combined Modality Approach of Locally Advanced Nonmetastatic Breast Cancer. Cancer Res. 47, 3889-3894.

Zucali, R., Uslenghi, C., Kenda, R., Bonadonna, G. (1976): Natural history of survival of inoperable breast cancer treated with radiotherapy and radiotherapy followed by radical mastectomy. Cancer 37, 1422-1431.

Résumé

Nous avons traité 100 patients atteintes de cancer du sein localement avancé, 43 stades IIIA, 53 stades IIIB, 4 stades IV par une chimiothérapie d'induction primaire incluant un essai de synchronisation hormonale. Toutes ont été traitées jusqu'à la réponse clinique maximum avant tout traitement local. Les patientes chez lesquelles une réponse histologique complète a été observée ont reçu une radiothérapie, tandis que les malades qui avaient une maladie résiduelle ou une réponse partielle, ou pas d'amélioration ont reçu un traitement chirurgical avant l'irradiation. Quelqu' ait été la réponse à la chimiothérapie d'induction, les malades ont reçu au moins 6 mois supplémentaires de chimiothérapie après le traitement local. Les doses initiales de chimiothérapie ont été augmentées jusqu'à la myélosuppression qui a été recherchée. Le taux de réponse objective à la chimiothérapie d'induction a été de 95 % avec 46 % de réponse complète, 49 % de réponse partielle, 5 % d'échec. Chez les 44 malades chez lesquels la chimiothérapie a induit une réponse clinique complète. 42 ont été étudiés dpar biopsie pour déterminer la réponse histologique, 27 de ces 44 malades soit 61 % ont eu des biopsies négatives. La durée médiane de rémission est de 30 mois, la survie médiane a été de 49 mois pour toutes les malades. Une chimiothérapie primaire aggressive avec synchronisation hormonale suivie de traitement local parait apporter un très bon contrôle local et des résultats préliminaires encourageants sur le contrôle de la maladie systémique.

Breast cancer II

Cancer du sein II

Neo-Adjuvant Chemotherapy. Ed. Cl. Jacquillat, M. Weil, D. Khayat. Colloque INSERM/John Libbey Eurotext Ltd. © 1988. Vol. 169, pp. 151-156.

Récepteurs hormonaux, cyto-ponctions et cancer du sein

M.A. de Maublanc*, Ch. Giraud**, F. Simondon***, J.F. Collet* et H. Sarmini**

** Centre de Cytopathologie Clinique, 49 rue du Ranelagh 75016 Paris, France*
*** Laboratoire Cerba, BP 451, 95005 Cergy Pontoise Cedex, France*
**** ORSTOM, UR.G6, Montpellier, France*

RESUME

De janvier 1986 à septembre 1987, 532 dosages de Récepteurs Hormonaux, Estrogènes: RE, et Progestérone : RP (méthode au charbon dextran), ont été effectués sur Cyto-Ponctions (C-P) à l'aiguille fine (23 gauge). 470 cas (89%) sont des adéno-carcinomes mammaires diagnostiqués par C-P avant tout traitement, 34 cas (6,8%) des récidives mammaires locales et 24 cas (4,5%) des métastases ganglionnaires ou sous-cutanées. Le contrôle de la cellularité de la C-P est assuré par la mesure de l'Acide désoxyribonucléique (ADN>10µg/ml cytosol). 94,9 % des C-P sont significatifs en ADN. 69,3% des C-P sont RE+ et 60,8% RP+ (RE-RP>500 fmol/mg ADN). Un grade Cyto-Pronostique de Malignité (CPM) est possible dans 93,7% des Adéno-carcinomes de Forme Commune : CPM I : 21,7%, CPM II : 54,9%, CPM III : 23,3%. La positivité des RP est corrélée au CPM : 85% RP+ CPM I - 52% RP+ CPM III.

MOTS CLEFS

Cyto-Ponctions. Récepteurs Hormonaux. Cancer du Sein.

KEY WORDS

Fine needle Aspiration. Hormonal Receptors. Breast Cancer.

INTRODUCTION

La Cyto-Ponction (C.P.) à l'aiguille fine (23 gauge = 6/10) utilisée depuis 30 ans (Zajdela et coll., 1975) fait partie du bilan diagnostique préthérapeutique du cancer du sein, et prend toute sa valeur dans les traitements conservateurs, en particulier chimiothérapie et/ou radiothérapie, premières et/ou exclusives. L'objectif de ce travail, effectué de janvier 1986 à septembre 1987, est l'étude de la valeur de la C.P. dans le diagnostic du cancer du sein, et surtout dans l'appréciation des facteurs pronostiques, tels que : variété tumorale, cyto-pronostic de malignité (CPM) et dosages des Récepteurs Hormonaux (RH), Estrogènes (RE) et Progestérone (RP) et leurs corrélations avec la taille (T) de la tumeur selon le système T.N.M.

MATERIEL ET METHODES

Importance de l'étude. Parmi les 5.194 C.P. à l'aiguille fine que nous avons effectuées de janvier 1986 à septembre 1987, 532 ont été transmises au Laboratoire Cerba pour dosage de Récepteurs Hormonaux : R.E. et R.P. Les localisations mammaires : 499/532 représentent 93,8% des C.P., et notre étude porte sur 470/532 (89%) C.P. pour adénocarcinome avant tout traitement. Nous avons éliminé les 34 (6,8%) récidives mammaires locales et les 24 (4,5%) métastases ganglionnaires ou sous-cutanées. L'âge moyen des femmes est de 57,1 ans (extrêmes 27 et 91 ans).
La saisie des données a été effectuée à partir d'un questionnaire pré-encodé à l'aide d'un logiciel de saisie contrôlée. L'analyse a été faite avec le logiciel BMDP, sur un ordinateur Olivetti M 28.
Les effectifs peuvent varier d'un tableau à un autre, certains renseignements n'étant pas disponibles pour la totalité des sujets; en particulier pour les R.P.

Technique de dosage des Récepteurs Hormonaux et mesure de l'Acide Désoxyribonucléique. Tous les dosages des R.E. et R.P. ont été effectués dans le même Laboratoire Cerba par méthodes radio-chimiques utilisant des radio-ligands. Les traceurs radio-actifs sont des stéroïdes de synthèse : R 2858 (Roussel-Uclaf) pour le R.E. et O 2058 (Organon) pour le R.P.
Un prélèvement par C.P. est significatif de la tumeur s'il est suffisamment riche en cellules tumorales. Afin de contrôler cette cellularité, un dosage d'Acide Désoxyribonucléique (ADN) est effectué sur le culot d'ultra-centrifugation : le seuil de positivité de l'ADN a été fixé à 10µg/ml = 10^6 cellules tumorales. Les résultats des R.E. et R.P. sont exprimés en femtomoles de stéroïde lié, ou de récepteur par mg d'ADN. Pour les C.P., les seuils de positivité des R.E. et R.P. sont fixés à 500 fmol/mg ADN.

La Cyto-Ponction à l'aiguille fine (23 gauge : 6/10°), radiée et pluridirectionnelle fournit de 10^3 à 10^7 cellules tumorales, prises à différents endroits de la tumeur, et réprésentatives de son éventuelle hétérogénéité. La technique souvent décrite(A. Zajdela, M.A. de Maublanc, 1975-1981) est la même pour le diagnostic et pour le dosage des R.E.-R.P., et utilise soit l'aiguille seule, soit le pistolet -seringue (10ml) avec un contrôle extemporané microscopique de la cellularité.

La variété tumorale de l'Adénocarcinome est précisée en référence à la classification O.M.S. : Forme Commune ou Particulière.

Un grade Cyto-Pronostique de Malignité CPM, peut être établi sur certaines C-P très cellulaires en se référant aux critères histo-pathologiques de Scarff et Bloom (1957) : différenciation, anisonucléose, structure chromatinienne.
La Taille T. de la Tumeur est évaluée selon le système T.N.M.

RESULTATS

Parmi les 470 adénocarcinomes mammaires primitifs diagnostiqués par C.P., avant tout traitement, la variété tumorale a pu être précisée 449 fois, soit dans 95,5% des cas. Les 397 adénocarcinomes de Forme Commune représentent 88,5% des cas et les 52 Formes Particulières 11,5% des cas : Adénocarcinomes colloïdes 2,8%, Médullaires 0,5%, Comédo-carcinomes 6,2%, Papillaires 1,5%, Apocrines 0,5%.

Le Cyto-Pronostic de Malignité (CPM) ne peut être établi que pour les adéno-carcinomes de Forme Commune. Il est exprimé en 3 grades : I, II, III de malignité croissante. Nous avons volontairement démembré le groupe II, le plus important numériquement, en deux sous groupes II et II+. Les résultats sont les suivants : sur 382 cas, la précision du CPM a été possible 358 fois (93,7%) et impossible 24 fois (6,3%). Les 382 adénocarcinomes de Forme Commune se répartissent ainsi :

C.P.M.		NOMBRE		POURCENTAGE %	
	I		78		21,7
II	II	196	142	54,9	39,9
	II+		54		15
	III		84		23,3
Impossible			24		

TABLEAU I. Cyto-Pronostic de Malignité = C.P.M. Répartition des 382 Cyto-Ponctions d'Adénocarcinomes mammaires selon le grade C.P.M.

Dosage des Récepteurs, R.E-R.P., et contrôle de la cellularité par la mesure de l'A.D.N. Parmi 468 C.P. d'adénocarcinomes mammaires transmises pour dosages des Récepteurs, 444 (94,9%) étaient significatives en A.D.N.> 10µg/ml cytosol. Les R.E. ont été dosés sur 466 C.P. : 444 (69,3%) sont R.E+ et 143 (30,7%) sont R.E-. Les R.P. ont été dosés sur 316 C.P. 192 (60,8%) sont R.P+ et 124 (39,2%)R.P-

R.E.	C.P.n=466	%
Positifs *	323	69,3
Négatifs	143	30,7
R.P.	n=316	
Positifs *	192	60,8
Négatifs	124	39,2

* R.E+ et R.P+ > 500 fmol/mg ADN

TABLEAU II. Fréquence des Récepteurs d'Estrogènes R.E., et de la Progestérone R.P. dans les Cyto-Ponctions C.P. d'Adénocarcinomes mammaires.

L'ensemble R.E. et R.P. étudié sur 246 C.P. est comparé aux résultats histologiques de la littérature. (Mc Guire et coll. 1977, ROUESSE et coll. 1985, YOUNG et coll. 1980).

	EXAMENS HISTOLOGIQUES			CYTO-PONCTIONS
	Young	Mc Guire	I.G.R.	M.A. de Maublanc n=276
R.E+. R.P+	51,4%	52%	51%	55,4%
R.E+. R.P-	22,0%	17%	15%	17,4%
R.E-. R.P+	5,2%	6%	8%	5,8%
R.E-. R.P-	21,2%	25%	26%	21,4%
R.E.+		69%	66%	69,3%
R.P.+		58%	59%	60,8%

I.G.R. = Institut Gustave Roussy.

TABLEAU III. Fréquence des différents types de Récepteurs, Estrogènes R.E., Progestérone R.P. dans les Adénocarcinomes mammaires. Comparaisons histo-cytologiques.

Les corrélations entre R.E., R.P., et C.P.M. ont été étudiées. La positivité en R.P., élevée dans les C.P.M. I : 85 %, décroît progressivement jusqu'à 52,4 % dans les C.P.M. III. Il est intéressant de noter que les R.P+ 59,5% dans les C.P.M. II+ sont bien identifiés, entre II (69,4%) et III (52,4%).

C.P.M.	R.P. Positifs * n	%	Négatifs n	%	Total n
I	34	85	6	15	40
II	68	69,4	30	30,6	98
II+	22	59,5	15	40,5	37
III	33	52,4	30	47,6	63
Impossible	4		4		8
Total = n	161		85		246

* R.P. Positifs : > à 500 fmol/mg ADN.

TABLEAU IV. Variations des Récepteurs de Progestérone R.P., en fonction du grade Cyto-Pronostic de Malignité C.P.M., eétudiées sur 246 Cyto-Ponctions d'Adénocarcinomes mammaires.

Les 470 Adénocarcinomes de l'étude se répartissent en 196 T1, 179 T2, 34 T3, 57 T4 et 4 données manquantes.

Les relations entre la Taille de la Tumeur T. et les Récepteurs Hormonaux sont les suivantes : il n'y a pas d'association entre T. et R.E +, par contre, il existe une association entre T. et R.P. : les T1 sont plus souvent R.P.+ (70,5%) que les autres (T4 : 52,6%).
Pour les T1 et les T2, la positivité en R.P. décroît lorsque le C.P.M. augmente.

	TAILLE	C.P.M.	*R.P.+	%	R.P.-	%
T1*	28	I	25	89,3	3	10,7
	47	II	35	74,5	12	25,5
	12	II+	8	66,7	4	33,3
	20	III	13	65	7	35
T2*	9	I	8	88,9	1	11,1
	35	II	23	65,7	12	34,3
	20	II+	10	50	10	50
	20	III	9	45	11	55

* R.P.+ > 500 fmol/mg ADN. *T1<20mm de diamètre. *T2 = 20 à 50mm.

TABLEAU V. Etude des relations entre Récepteurs de Progestérone R.P. et grade Cyto-Pronostic de Malignité C.P.M. dans 246 Cyto-Ponctions d'Adénocarcinomes mammaires T1 et T2.

En conclusion : à condition d'être très cellulaire, la C.P. à l'aiguille fine assure le diagnostic du cancer du sein avec une fiabilité de 89% (Zajdela et coll. 1975), d'autant plus grande qu'elle est associée dans le Triplet diagnostique, à la mammographie et la clinique (99%. Cornillot, 1981). Elle fournit également les éléments du pronostic : variété tumorale. C.P.M. et dosages des récepteurs : R.E. et R.P. avec la même fiabilité que les forages biopsies (H. Magdelenat et coll., 1983-1987, M.A. de Maublanc et coll. 1987). L'étude des relations Taille de la Tumeur, C.P.M. et RP permet d'isoler des petites tumeurs T1 avec de mauvais facteurs de pronostic : C.P.M. II+ et III, R.P.-, et de les traiter en conséquence.

REFERENCES BIBLIOGRAPHIQUES

BENYAHIA B., MAGDELENAT H., ZAJDELA A., VILCOQ J.R. (1982) : Ponction aspiration à l'aiguille fine et dosage des récepteurs d'estrogènes dans le cancer du sein. Bull. Cancer (Paris) 69, 456-460.

BLOOM H.J.G., RICHARDSON W.W. (1957) : Histological grading and prognosis in breast cancer. Brit. J. Cancer 11, 359-366.

BOLLA M., BONNABEL P., CHEDIN M., VILLEMAIN D., ZINS M., MOUSSEAU M., CHAMBAZ E., (1987) : Etude de la valeur pronostique des récepteurs à l'estradiol et à la Progestérone, dans les cancers du sein stade I-II UICC, soumis à un traitement adjuvant. Bull. Cancer 74. 623-630.

CHUA W'Y PANG, RAUFF, SWEE-ENG, CHAN AW. SOH-HA, (1985) : Correlation of steroïd Receptors with histologic differentiation in mammary carcinoma. A Singapore Experience. Cancer 56. 2228-2234.

CORNILLOT M. (1981) : Le triplet diagnostique du cancer du sein. Evaluation des moyens de diagnostic du cancer du sein. J.M.T. Conseil Editeur, 129-141.

ELLIS F. (1947) : Needle biopsy in the clinical diagnosis of tumors. Brit. J. Surg. 34, 240.

KLINE T.S., KANNAN V., KLINE I. (1985) : Appraisal and Cytomorphologic Analysis of Common Carcinomas of the Breast. Diagn. Cytopath. Vol 1, N°3, 188-193.

Mc GUIRE W.L., HORWITZ K.B., PEARSON Q.H. SEGALOFF A. (1977) : Current status of estrogen ans progesterone receptors in breast cancer. Cancer 39, 2934-2947.

MAGDELENAT H., LAINE-BIDRON C., MERLE S., ZAJDELA A. (1987) : Estrogen and progestin receptor assay in fine needle aspirates of breast cancer : methodological aspects. Eur. J. Cancer Clin. Oncol. Vol. 23, n°4, 425-431.

MASON M.B., HOLDAWAY I.M., LUMMINS P.R. (1983) : Progesterone receptors and oestrogene Receptors as prognostic variables in breast cancer. Cancer Res. 43 - 2985-2990.

de MAUBLANC M.A., ZAJDELA A. (1981) : Actualités de la cytologie mammaire par ponction aspiration. Evaluation des moyens de diagnostic du cancer du sein. J.M.T. Conseil Editeur, 143-151.

de MAUBLANC M.A., DENYS I., VILCOQ J.R., VEITH F., ASSELAIN B., CALLE R., (1987): Valeur du forage-biopsie dans le cancer mammaire. Bull. Cancer Vol. 74, n°1, 23-30.

de MAUBLANC M.A., (1986) : Cyto-ponctions et cancer du sein : diagnostic - pronostic - dosage des récepteurs hormonaux. Neo-adjuvant chemotherapy. Colloque INSERM/John Libbey Eurotext Ltd. Vol. 137, 181-188.

ROUESSE J., CONTESSO G. (1985) : Le cancer du sein. Hermann p.33.

SAEZ S., PICHON M.F. (1984) : Recepteurs hormonaux et pronostic du cancer du Sein. Sem. Hop. Paris. 60, 852-859.

SILFVERSWARD C., HUMLA S. (1980) : Estrogen receptor analysis on needle aspirates from human mammary carcinoma. Acta Cytol. 24, 54-57.

YOUNG PEM., EHRLICH CE., EINHORN LH. (1980) : Relationship between steroïd receptors and response to endocrine therapy and cytotoxic chemotherapy in metastatic breast cancer. Cancer 1980. 46. 2916-2963.

ZAJDELA A., GHOSSEIN N.A., PILLERON J.P., ENNUYER A. (1975) : The value of aspiration cytology in the diagnosis of breast cancer : experience at the Fondation Curie. Cancer 35, 499-506.

Résumé

From january 1986 to september 1987, 532 Hormonal Receptors, for Estrogens : E.R., and Progesterone : P.R. (dextran coal method), were performed on Fine Needle Aspiration (FNA) (23 gauge).
470 cases (89%) are breast carcinomas diagnosed by F.N.A. before any treatment, 34 cases (6,8%) are local breast recurrences, and 24 cases (4,5%) are lymphnodes or sub-cutaneous metastasis from breast carcinoma. The control of the F.N.A. cellularity is performed by the measurement of Desoxyribo Nucleic Acid (DNA>10µg/ml cytosol).
94,9 % F.N.A. show significant DNA.
69,3 % F.N.A. are E.R. + and 60% F.N.A. are P.R. + (Positivity threshold for E.R. and P.R. was set at 500 fmol/mg DNA).
A Cytological Prognosis grade of Malignancy (C.P.M.) comparable to Scarff-Bloom histo-pathological grade, is possible on 93,7% of Common type Carcinomas (not otherwise specified N.O.S.) : C.P.M. grade I = 21,7%, grade II = 54,9%, grade III = 23,3%.
P.R. positivity is related to C.P.M. grade : 85 % in C.P.M. I, 52 % in C.P.M. III.
There is an association between Tumor size (T) and P.R. positivity : 70,5% T1 are P.R.+ and only 52,6% T4 are P.R.+
In T1 , P.R. positivity decreases as C.P.M. increases : 89,3% P.R.+ in C.P.M. I, 65% P.R.+ in C.P.M. III.

Neo-Adjuvant Chemotherapy. Ed. Cl. Jacquillat, M. Weil, D. Khayat. Colloque INSERM/John Libbey Eurotext Ltd. © 1988. Vol. 169, pp. 157-167.

Role of preoperative (neo-adjuvant) therapy for breast cancer in stage I and II disease

J. Ragaz, R. Baird, J.H. Goldie, A.J. Coldman and P. Rebbeck

Cancer Control Agency of B.C., Vancouver, Canada

RESUME

In 1983 a randomized study of preoperative vs postoperative adjuvant CMF chemotherapy for stages I and II breast cancer patients started at CCABC. Overall, 124 patients were randomized until July 1987, with 66 and 58 patients in the two arms respectively. The 3 year overall and disease free survival for both groups (all 124 patients) was 91 and 78% respectively. The interval between the diagnosis and mastectomy was not changed from the conventional postoperative treatment, and was 13.2 vs 14.0 days in both randomized groups. The interval between the diagnosis and the first day of chemotherapy was reduced in both groups compared to conventional postoperative timing, being 8.2 vs 14.3 days in the preoperative and the postoperative groups respectively (p=0.02). 21 out of 124 patients had fine needle aspiration (FNA) as the only diagnostic procedure, and 26 had open biopsy in addition to FNA. Fifty two out of all randomized patients had negative axillary lymph nodes. Node negative, low risk patients (absence of lymphangitic and vascular invasion) received only 1 course of preoperative CMF, if allocated to the preoperative group. The high risk patients (+ve axillary nodes or +ve lymphangitic vascular invasion) received 6 months of CMF chemotherapy. The main emphasis of this study is on the organizational aspects of the conduct of randomized neoadjuvant trials. These include frequent communications with peripheral surgeons - practitioners, and family physicians. Presently, there is no sufficient evidence for a clear superiority of neoadjuvant chemotherapy in stages I and II breast cancer over the postoperative adjuvant treatments. Therefore, the role of preoperative treatment of this population of patients should be determined from randomized studies.

INTRODUCTION

The purpose of this report is to update our work on preoperative (neoadjuvant) chemotherapy for breast cancer and discuss its impact in the management of breast cancer.

Despite encouraging results from randomized trials of postoperative adjuvant chemotherapy (NCI Monographs, 1986) the overall mortality of breast cancer in North America has not decreased significantly. The likely explanation is that during the years of the mortality analysis, only a minority of the overall population of breast cancer patients has been receiving adjuvant chemotherapy consistently. Hence, whatever survival advantage from a given treatment is documented in an individual trial, it cannot emerge as significant if such a treatment is not given to the whole population. In addition, however, the modesty of therapeutic gains from presently available postoperative adjuvant therapies remains a consistent problem.

Preoperative timing of adjuvant chemotherapy is an example of a new approach, and along with questions on the dose intensity, it remains one of the few exciting and potentially fruitful areas of clinical breast cancer research. Its theoretical appeal confirmed in several animal systems is enhanced by the fact that virtually no new drugs for breast cancer are available. Also, clinical data on effective downstaging of initially inoperable breast tumors (Morris, 1978; Ragaz, 1987) confirm not only the safety, but also indicate a possible therapeutic benefit of the preoperatively timed chemotherapy (Morris, 1978; Hortobagyi, 1987).

The rationale justifying the testing of preoperative chemotherapy has been outlined by our group in the past (Ragaz, 1985). All arguments, mostly theoretical, have been partially confirmed in animal experiments (Simpson-Herren, 1976; Gunduz, 1979) and clearly justify its testing in clinical trials.

In recent years, our group has introduced the preoperative chemotherapy of stage I and II breast cancer in our region and popularized its implementation in North America (Ragaz, 1985; Ragaz, 1986; Ragaz, 1986). This report is an update of our preoperative chemotherapy trial of stages I and II breast disease.

THE NEOADJUVANT TRIAL - STAGES I AND II BREAST CANCER

In the first phase, 43 patients with clinical stages I and II disease were tested in a pilot study (Ragaz, 1985). In this, we have confirmed the safety of one cycle of preoperative CMF chemotherapy. Preoperative CMF did not delay healing of the chest wall mastectomy scar, nor were other toxicities noted.
Also, an important part of the study was the introduction of fine needle biopsy (FNA) as the only diagnostic procedure for breast cancer in our region.

In 1983, a randomization between the preoperative and postoperative CMF chemotherapy was begun, and presently, an interim report on the first 124 randomized patients is provided.

MATERIALS AND METHODS

Details of materials and methods have been described in the past (Ragaz, 1985; Ragaz, 1986). Briefly, premenopausal patients with tissue diagnosis of breast cancer were eligible for the randomization. Altogether, 150 patients were randomized, of whom the first 124 are presently analyzed. Of those, 66 were randomized to the preoperative, and 58 into the postoperative arms. The tissue diagnosis was obtained either by the help of FNA, or via open biopsy. After the staging procedures, premenopausal patients without metastatic spread were eligible for the randomization.

PREOPERATIVE ARM: Patients randomized to the preoperative arm received one cycle of chemotherapy with Cyclophosphamide 600 mg/m2 i.v., Methotrexate 40 mg/m/2 i.v. and 5-FU 600 mg/m/2 i.v. Afterwards, patients were scheduled for their definitive surgery. Postoperatively, patients with high risk tumors (positive axillary lymph nodes; or negative axillary nodes with tumor signs of lymphangitic, vascular or neurovascular bundle invasion) continued 8 more cycles of post operative adjuvant chemotherapy with CMF given i.v. every 3 weeks. Patients with low risk tumors received no further chemotherapy after the mastectomy.

POSTOPERATIVE ARM: Patients randomized to the postoperative arm were scheduled for their definitive surgery after the biopsy. High risk patients subsequently received postoperative chemotherapy with 9 cycles of CMF.

Table I shows the patients' main characteristics. Both randomized groups were comparable in the mean age, tumor size, nodal stage, and in the interval between the diagnosis and the mastectomy. They differed in the interval between the diagnosis and the first cycle of chemotherapy (p=0.02), and in the number of low risk node negative patients receiving one cycle of CMF preoperative chemotherapy (p=<0.0001).

Sixty five percent of patients randomized to preoperative chemotherapy had modified radical mastectomy as their definitive surgical procedure, while 35% had partial mastectomy. In the group randomized to the post operative treatment, the corresponding figures were 59 and 41%.

To exclude any adverse effects of the preoperative chemotherapy on the whole population of the neoadjuvant study, the 3 and 4 year survival figures of patients who participated in the previous British Columbia postoperative adjuvant breast cancer study, are available. In that study, premenopausal axillary node positive patients receiving postoperative adjuvant chemotherapy with CMF, were randomized for locoregional radiotherapy given between the fourth and the fifth CMF cycles.

RESULTS

In this report, the first 124 patients were analyzed, 66 randomized to the preoperative and 58 to the postoperative arms.

Emphasis for the initial diagnosis was on fine needle aspiration (FNA), without open biopsy. Altogether, 21 patients had FNA as the only diagnostic procedure and 26 additional patients had open biopsy together with FNA.

Fifty two percent of all 124 randomized patients had negative axillary lymph nodes. Within each nodal category, patients with negative nodes, 1-3 nodes, and the 4+ nodal subgroup, were evenly distributed between our randomized groups (Tables I and II). In the preoperative arm, 27/33 node negative patients (the low risk subgroup) received one cycle of preoperative chemotherapy cycle, while 6/33 (the high risk subgroup) had postoperative CMF. As seen in Table III, the corresponding figures for the node negative patients from the post operative arm were 0/32 and 9/32, p=<0.0001).

Analysis of the time intervals has shown that the mean duration between the diagnosis and the mastectomy in patients from the preoperative arm was 13.2

compared to 14.0 days in the post-operative group (Table IV).

The mean interval between the diagnosis and the first day of chemotherapy was 8.2 in the preoperative arm, and 14.3 days in the post operative group (p=0.02).

The survival analysis for all 124 patients randomized to the neoadjuvant study shows the 3 and 4 year overall survival of 91 and 85% respectively (Table V). The disease free survival for the corresponding population of patients was 78 and 68% respectively (Table VI).

The survival analysis comparing the two randomized groups has not been performed, as the study continues.

Table VI shows the 3 and 4 year overall and disease free survivals of the neoadjuvant study (combined preoperative and the postoperative arms), compared to the postoperative adjuvant CMF chemotherapy study.

DISCUSSION:

The survival gains after therapy with conventional postoperative chemotherapy are modest, and trials of new treatment scheduling constitute an exciting aspect of clinical breast cancer research. Theoretical and animal data indicate a potential for improvement with the preoperative timing of the systemic treatment, and testing of this approach in human malignancies has started in the last few years. Our ongoing neoadjuvant study is presently the only preoperative randomized trial of this design for breast cancer. The main emphasis of the study is on the organizational aspects of the conduct of the study, where the randomization, and the initial explanation of the rationale for the trial are all done by surgeons practicing from private practice throughout the province of British Columbia. A consistent upgrading of the practitioners, with formal slide-talk presentations is the mainstay for the coordination between the institute and the unfunded practitioners.

Taking the frequency of the incisional open biopsy for breast cancer, and the potentially adverse effects of a noncurative surgery as seen in animal studies, the introduction of FNA as the only diagnostic procedure is considered of importance. Despite frequent interactions of the principal investigators with the surgeons, only a minority of patients had FNA as the main diagnostic procedure. This is likely due to problems with the technical aspects of aspiration, as well as due to the lack of experience and confidence with the cytological interpretation by locoregional pathologists. Increasing popularization, and experience will be needed for a more uniform adoption of FNA as the main initial diagnostic procedure for breast cancer.

It is possible that one cycle of CMF chemotherapy before the surgery may not detect the survival difference of the preoperative timing. Utilization of more dose intensive regimens, the importance of which has recently been emphasized (Frei, 1980; Hryniuk, 1984) as well as inclusion of several Anthara - cycline - contai for a fair trial of preoperative chemotherapy.

Long term results of the subset of node negative patients may be of some interest, particularly when the survival and recurrence analysis of the impact of one cycle of preoperatively administered CMF chemotherapy become available.

Other aspects of the neoadjuvant approach are emerging as important. A more refined risk assessment at the time of diagnosis (the neoadjuvant staging) will clearly be needed. Such information will have to be available in the preoperative time period, as the pathological assessment of axillary lymph nodes will not be available. The risk assessment will likely include, in addition to the clinical T and N stage, also combined information of several individual prognostic factors, such as tumor grade (Fisher, 1980; Andersen, 1981; Fisher, 1988), receptor status (McGuire, 1974; Godolphin, 1981; Shek, 1987), data from DNA assessment as seen from flow cytometry (Hedley, 1985; Kute, 1985; Meyer, 1983), labelling index (Meyer 1983; Silvestrini, 1986) and oncogenic survey (Bishop 1983; Varmus, 1984; Lundy, 1986; Slamon, 1987). Only high risk patients would be considered for preoperative chemotherapy. Low risk patients, on the other hand, would require no adjuvant treatment as the chance for cure by surgery will be high.

A comparison of the overall and disease free survivals of the present neoadjuvant study with the historical British Columbia postoperative CMF study shows no adverse survival effect of preoperative administration of CMF chemotherapy. Such information is important as previous reports from the Ludwig's perioperative chemotherapy showed, in the initial phase of their study, increased mortality in patients given CMF chemotherapy close to their surgery.

In this study, the timing of the definitive surgery was not altered when compared to our historical post operative adjuvant chemotherapy controls, so as not to introduce several major changes in the management of breast cancer in our region at the same time. With the data on prolonged and more dose-intense preoperative therapy of locally advanced breast cancer (Morris, 1978; Hortobagyi, 1987; Lippmann 1986; Ragaz, 1987), it looks as though the postponement of surgery by several months may be a safe approach. The possibility of a dissemination of resistant cells from the unresected primary, however, will have to be considered potentially as the main adverse outcome of surgical delay. Hence, until the benefit of such an approach is more clearly confirmed from prospective trials, delays of mastectomy should be considered only within the context of clinical studies. Plans for such studies on a larger scale are presently underway in North America, as anounced at the most recent NSABP convention (NSABP, Tampa, Florida, 1988).

CONCLUSION:

In summary, our group provided the rationale and theoretical data in the past justifying the initiation of preoperative (neoadjuvant) chemotherapy studies for breast cancer. In this report the methodology and some observations of the British Columbia Randomized Preoperative Chemotherapy Trial for Stages I and II is described. We conclude that preoperative chemotherapy for stages I and II should continue within the context of randomized trials. Despite its theoretical appeal as seen from experimental data, insufficient evidence is available for its superiority in stage I and II breast cancer over the post-operative treatment. All efforts should be exerted towards the completion of randomized trials testing the preoperative concept.

TABLE I

COMPARISON OF THE MAIN CHARACTERISTICS BETWEEN THE RANDOMIZED GROUPS

	PRE	POST	p
Diagnosis-mastectomy Interval (days)	13.2	14.0	N.S.
% With Negative Axillary Nodes	50.0	55.2%	N.S.
% With 4+ Nodes	18.2%	17.2%	N.S.
Mean Size of Tumor (cm)	2.8	2.6	N.S.
Diagnosis-Chemotherapy Interval (days)	8.2	14.3	0.02
1 Cycle of CMF Given To Low Risk Node Negative Pts No of Pts (%)	27/33 (82%)	0/32(0%)	< 0.0001

TABLE II

DISTRIBUTION OF AXILLARY NODES

NUMBER OF NODES	PRE* (66)	POST** (58)	p
0	33 (50%)	32 (55.2%)	N.S.+
1-3	21 (31.8%)	16 (27.6%)	N.S.
4+	12 (18.2%)	9 (17.2%)	N.S.

*Preoperative

**Postoperative

+ Not Significant

NUMBER OF CHEMOTHERAPY COURSES FOR NODE NEGATIVE PATIENTS

	PRE (33)	POST (32)	p
0 Cycles	0	23	<0.0001
1 Cycle of Preop CMF	27	0	
Postoperative CMF*	6	9	

*Postoperative chemotherapy given to high risk node negative patients (positive vascular, lymphangitic, neurovascular bundle involvement).

TABLE IV

INTERVAL BETWEEN DIAGNOSIS AND MASTECTOMY

DAYS	PRE (66)	POST (58)	p
0-6	24 (36.3%)	23 (39.7%)	
7-13	18 (27.3%)	17 (29.3%)	
14-20	14 (21.2%)	8 (13.8%)	0.9
>21	10 (15.2%)	10 (17.2%)	
Mean (days)	13.2	14.0	

TABLE V

NEOADJUVANT STUDY - DISEASE FREE SURVIVAL (DFS)
(ALL 124 PATIENTS)

YEARS		DFS%
0		100.0%
1		95.4%
2		83.5%
3		78.2%
4		68.7%
Events (Recurrences)	19/124	

TABLE VI

COMPARISON OF BRITISH COLUMBIA PREOPERATIVE (NEOADJUVANT) AND POSTOPERATIVE* (ADJUVANT) STUDIES

YEARS	NEOADJUVANT	ADJUVANT
	OVERALL SURVIVAL	
1	97%	99.3%
2	96%	92.6%
3	91%	84.8%
4	85%	80.6%
	DISEASE FREE SURVIVAL	
1	95.4%	95.5%
2	83.5%	82.0%
3	78.2%	71.0%
4	68.7%	64.7%

*Premenopausal patients with pathologically positive axillary lymph nodes, randomized between CMF vs CMF + Locoregional Radiotherapy.

REFERENCES

Andersen, J.A. (1981): Selection of high risk groups among prognostically favourable patients with breast cancer: in analysis of the value of prospective grading of tumor anaplasia in 1048 patients. Ann. Surg 194, 1-3.

Bishop, J.M. (1983): Cellular oncogenes and retroviruses. Annu. Rev. Biochem 52, 301-54.

Fisher, E. (1988): Identification of risk factors by conventional pathological ancillary techniques in women with breast cancer. In High Risk Breast Cancer - Diagnosis, ed J. Ragaz, I. Ariel. Heidelberg: Springer-Verlag, in press.

Fisher, E.R. (1980): Histologic grading of breast cancer. Pathol. Annu.15, 239-251.

Frei, E, (1980): Dose: A critical factor in cancer chemotherapy. Am. J. Med 69, 4, 585-594.

Godolphin, W. (1981): Estrogen receptor quantitation and staging as complimentary prognostic indicators in breast cancer: A study of 583 patients. Int. J. Cancer 28, 677-683.

Gunduz, N. (1979): Effects of surgical removal on the growth and kinetics of residual tumor. Cancer Res. 39, 3861-3865.

Hedley, W. (1985): Application of DNA Flow Cytometry to Paraffin Embedded Archival Material for the Study of Aneuploidy and its Clinical Significance. Cytometry 6, 327-333.

Hortobagyi, G. (1987): Effective multidisciplinary therapy of inoperable stage III breast cancer. Proc. Amer. Soc. Clin. Oncol. 6, 64.

Hryniuk, W. (1984): The importance of dose intensity in chemotherapy of metastatic breast cancer. J. Clin. Oncol.2, 1281-1288.

Kute, T.E. (1985): Relationship of flow cytometry results to clinical and steroid receptors in human breast cancer. Breast Cancer Res. Treat 6, 113-121.

Lippmann, M.E. (1986): Treatment of locally advanced breast cancer using primary induction chemotherapy with hormone synchronization followed by radiation therapy with or without debulking surgery. NCI Monogr. 1, 153-159.

Lundy, J. (1986): Elevated RAS oncogene expression correlate with lymph node metastases in breast cancer patients. J. Clin. Oncol. 4, 1321-1325.

McGuire, W.L. (1975): Estrogen receptors in human breast cancer: an overview. In Estrogen Receptors in Human Breast Cancer, ed W.L. McGuire, P.P. Carbone, E.P. Vollmer, pp 1-7. New York: Raven Press.

Meyer, J.S. (1983): Prediction of early course of breast cancer by Thymidine labelling. Cancer 51, 1879-1886.

Morris, D.M. (1978): Mastectomy as an adjunct to combination chemotherapy. Arch. Surg. 113, 282-284.

National Surgical Adjuvant Project for Breast and Bowel Cancers (NSABP) Convention, Tampa, Florida, U.S.A. 1988.

Proceedings of the NIH Consensus Development Conference on Adjuvant Chemotherapy and Endocrine Therapy for Breast Cancer. NCI Monogr. 1, 1986.

Ragaz, J. (1986): Emerging Modalities for Adjuvant Therapy of Breast Cancer: Neoadjuvant Chemotherapy. NCI Monogr 1, 145-153.

Ragaz, J. (1986): Preoperative (neoadjuvant) chemotherapy for breast cancer: Outline of the British Columbia Trial In Preoperative (Neoadjuvant) Chemotherapy ed J. Ragaz, P. R. Band, J.H. Goldie, pp 85-94. Heidelberg: Springer-Verlag.

Ragaz, J. (1985): Neoadjuvant (Preoperative) Chemotherapy for breast cancer. Cancer 56, 719-724.

Ragaz, J. (1987): Preoperative combined modality (neoadjuvant) therapy for locally advanced inoperable breast cancer. In Fundamental Problems in Breast cancer, ed A.H.G. Paterson, A.W. Lees, pp 383-391. Norwell, MA.: Kluwer Academic Publ.

Ragaz, J. (1987): Role of mastectomy in preoperative (neoadjuvant) combined modality therapy of locally advanced breast cancer. Proc Amer Soc Clin Oncol 6, 55.

Shek, L.L.M. Estrogen receptors, nodes and stage as predictors of post recurrence survival in 457 breast cancer patients. Br J Cancer 57, 825-829.

Silvestrini, R. (1986): Prognostic implication of labelling index versus estrogen receptors and tumor size in node negative breast cancer. Breast Cancer Res Treat 7, 161-169.

Simpson-Herren, L. (1976): Effects of surgery on the cell kinetics of residual tumor. Cancer Treat Rep 60, 1749-1760.

Slamon, D.J. (1987): Human breast cancer: correlation of relapse and survival with amplification of the HER-2 NEU oncogene. Science 235, 177-182.

Varmus, H.E. (1984): The Molecular kinetics of cellular oncogenes Annu Rev Genet 18, 553-612.

Neo-Adjuvant Chemotherapy. Ed. Cl. Jacquillat, M. Weil, D. Khayat. Colloque INSERM/John Libbey Eurotext Ltd. © 1988. Vol. 169, pp. 169-176.

Chimiothérapie adjuvante dans les cancers du sein opérables. Résultats préliminaires d'un essai contrôlé

V. Diéras, P. Pouillard, S. Scholl, T. Dorval, R. Vilcoq, M. Jouve, J.C. Durand, G. Mathieu, V. Mosseri, B. Asselain, T. Palangie, E. Garcia-Giralt, P. Beuzeboc, L. Belli, R.J. Salmon et A. Livartowski

Institut Curie, 75231 Paris Cedex 05, France

RESUME

Chez 296 patientes porteuses d'un cancer du sein histologiquement prouvé, du stade I au stade III, un programme de chimiothérapie première comportant Adriamycine, Cyclophosphamide et 5 Fluoro-uracile a été appliqué. L'analyse des taux de réponse, de la durée de survie sans récidive et de survie globale à 4 ans fait apparaitre :
- que le taux de réponses initiales à la chimiothérapie est d'autant plus élevé que la tumeur est de petite taille,
- que la signification statistique des paramètres usuels du pronostic n'est pas modifiée (SBR, RO RP, stade clinique),
- que le risque de rechute locale est indépendant de tous les paramètres pronostiques.
Dans une étude complémentaire contrôlée incluant 161 patientes, 86 ont été traitées par chimiothérapie première. Avec un recul de 3 ans, une réduction significative du taux de récidive métastatique est observée (p = 0,04) alors que le taux de récidive locale est significativement plus élevé (p = 0,03).

MOTS CLEFS

Cancer du sein, chimiothérapie adjuvante, paramètres pronostiques.

INTRODUCTION

L'application d'une chimiothérapie chez les patients porteurs d'une tumeur solide a pour objet :

1. de traiter au plus tôt la dissémination métastatique,
2. de réduire le volume de la tumeur initiale et de son éventuelle extension ganglionnaire,
3. de simplifier le traitement loco-régional nécessaire et le rendre plus conservateur.

De plus, elle permet d'évaluer objectivement l'efficacité réelle du programme de chimiothérapie appliqué.
Afin d'analyser au mieux les caractéristiques de la réponse au traitement, deux études contrôlées ont été effectuées chez des patientes porteuses de cancer mammaire.

MATERIEL ET METHODES

Etude S5 : 161 patientes âgées de 25 à 65 ans (médiane 48 ans) sont entrées dans une étude contrôlée. Les caractéristiques anatomo-cliniques des 86 patientes traitées par chimiothérapie première et des 75 patientes traitées par chimiothérapie adjuvante conventionnelle, sont présentées sur le tableau I. Aucune différence dans la répartition entre les deux groupes n'est observée.

Tableau I : Présentation des patientes.

Nombre	159 patientes	
Age 25-30 ans	(médiane 48 ans)	
	Chimio 1ère (n = 86)	Tt loco-rég. (n = 75)
T2	37	27
T3	49	48
N0, 1a	22	21
N1b	64	52
SBR I	6	7
II faible	20	28
II fort	24	11
III	19	23
R.O. +	14	16
R.O. -	29	25
R.P. +	22	27
R.P. -	42	40
ACTIVITE GENITALE		
. Pré-ménop.	41	46
. Post-ménop.	45	29

Etude S'5 : 296 patientes présentant au moins un paramètre de mauvais pronostic (âge, siège de la tumeur, évolutivité clinique) ont été traitées systématiquement par 3 à 4 cycles de chimiothérapie avant tout traitement loco-régional. Les caractéristiques de cette population sont présentées sur le tableau II.

TABLEAU II : Présentation des patientes.

Nbr de patientes 296
. Recul actuel : 12 à 78 mois (méd. = 36 mois)
. AGE MEDIAN (extrêmes) 48,3 (26-80)
ETAT HORMONAL
. ménopause 76
. castration 17
. non ménopausées 167
. péri-ménopause 36
Age médian ménopause (ou castration)(extrêmes) 50 ans (34-58)

TAILLE TUM.		N		T & N		GRADE HISTO.	
. T1	12	N0, N1a	71	T1, T2 N0 N1a	20	Non gradable	30
. T2	98	N1b	190	T1, T2 N1b	82	SBR I	24
. T3	129	N2	19	T3 N0, N1a	40	SBR II faible	67
. T4	57	N3	16	T3 N1b	80	SBR II fort	87
				T4 N2, N3	74	SBR III	72

TEMPS DE DOUBLEMENT CLINIQUEMENT RAPIDE PEV 1 : . non 186
. oui 37

RECEPTEURS HORMONAUX : R.O. - 69 R.P. - 128
R.O. + 49 R.P. + 85

TRAITEMENT

Le protocole comprend l'administration mensuelle d'un cycle de chimiothérapie (protocole CFA) associant :
. Adriamycine : 25mg/m2, J1 et J8
. Cyclophosphamide : 500mg/m2, J1 et J8
. 5 Fluoro-uracile : 600mg/m2 J1, J3, J5, J8
. Prednisone : 30mg, J1 à J10.
En cas de bonne tolérance hématologiqueet générale, la dose d'Adriamycine était portée à 30mg/m2 lors du 2ème cycle.
Dans l'étude S5, les patientes recevaient 3 cycles de chimiothérapie avant et après le traitement loco-régional dans le groupe I. Les patientes du groupe II ont reçu 6 cycles après la fin du traitement loco-régional.
Dans la 2ème étude S'5, les patientes ont reçu 2 à 5 cycles de chimiothérapie avant le traitement loco-régional et 3 cycles après la fin de celui-ci.
Après le traitement, une surveillance régulière a été instituée. Le recul médian de surveillance est de 36 mois dans la 2ème étude (12 à 78 mois).

EVALUATION DES REPONSES

La réponse de la tumeur mammaire et ganglionnaire a été évaluée cliniquement dans les deux études.
La réponse complète (R.C.) a été définie par la disparition de toute anomalie clinique mammaire et ganglionnaire.
La réponse partielle supérieure à 50% (RP ≥ 50%) a été définie par la régression de plus de 50% de chacun des 2 diamètres perpendiculaires et mesurables de la tumeur.
La réponse partielle minime a été définie selon les mêmes critères.
La stabilité a été définie par la régression inférieure à 20% du produit des 2 diamètres.
La progression a été définie par la croissance de la tumeur ou par l'apparition d'une nouvelle localisation intra-mammaire ou ganglionnaire.

RESULTATS

Etude S5 : Le taux de réponse objective dans le groupe I du protocole S5 a été de 45% (R.C. + RP ≥ 50%). 7 patientes sur 83 actuellement évaluables dans le 1er groupe ont présenté une localisation métastatique et 11 sur 71 dans le 2ème groupe. La différence est actuellement significative (p = 0,04) en faveur du groupe de traitement par chimiothérapie de 1ère intention.
Parallèlement, 9 patientes sur 83 ont présenté une rechute locale dans le 1er groupe contre 1 patiente sur 71 dans le 2ème groupe ; cette différence est significative (p = 0,03). Il n'apparait pas de différence actuellement en terme de survie. (tableau IV).

Tableau IV : Résultats à 3 ans de l'essai S5.

	RECUL 3 ans	
SURVIE		
. GROUPE I (chimiothérapie)	4/83	p = 0,23
. GROUPE II (Tr local)	7/71	N.S.
METASTASE		
. GROUPE I	7/83	p = 0,04
. GROUPE II	11/71	S.
RECHUTE LOCALE		
. GROUPE I	9/83	p = 0,03
. GROUPE II	1/71	S.

Etude S'5 : sur les 296 patientes de ce protocole d'étude, 294 étaient clairement évaluables pour la réponse clinique à 2 mois et 209 à 4 mois. Entre 2 et 4 mois, le taux de réponse majeure passe de 33,6% à 54,5%.

Tableau V : Réponse à la chimiothérapie.

	APRES 2 CYCLES Nbr	%	APRES 4 CYCLES Nbr	%
RC	16	5,4	35	16,7
RP $\geq$ 50 %	83	28,2	79	37,8
RP $\leq$ 50 %	151	51,4	76	38,4
STAB.	42	14,3	18	8,6
PROGRESSION	2	0,7	1	0,5
	Nbr = 294		Nbr = 209	

Dans cette population diversifiée et hétérogène dans sa répartition, l'analyse de la réponse clinique à la chimiothérapie selon les paramètres cliniques est présentée sur le tableau VI.

Tableau VI : Réponse clinique selon les paramètres cliniques.

PARAMETRES CLINIQUES		RC + RP (%) 2 cycles		RC + RP (%) 4 cycles	
T	T1 T2	45		69	
	T3	31	p = 0,01	51	p = 0,006
	T4	18		40	
N	N1b	33,9		54	
	N2	38,9	p = 0,85	53,3	p = 0,99
	N3	25		54,5	
STADE	T1 T2 N0 N1a	55		90	
	T3 N1a	27,5		52	
	T1-2 N1b	41	p = 0,04	62	p = 0,06
	T3 N1b	34		53	
	T4 N2 N3	23		44	
TOTAL		294		209	

A 4 mois, le taux de réponse majeure passe de 69% pour les T1 T2 à 40% pour les T4 (p = 0,006). En revanche, la régression des adénopathies parait indépendante de leur siège et de leur nombre. Le taux de réponse majeure passe de 54% pour les adénopathies N1b à 54,5 % pour les N3 (p = 0,99).
La stratification selon le stade clinique de la tumeur fait également apparaitre une différence puisque le taux de réponses majeures passe de 90% pour les T1 T2 N0 N1 à 44% pour les T4 N2 N3 (p = 0,06).
L'analyse du taux de réponse majeure selon les critères histologiques (SBR) et biologiques (RO et RP) est présentée sur le tableau VII.

Tableau VII : Réponse majeure selon SBR, RO/RP.

	RC + RP ≥ 50%(%) 2 mois		RC + RP ≤ 50%(%) 4 mois	
SBR I	12		41	
SBR II faible	14	$p = 0{,}001$	39	$p = 0{,}12$
SBR II fort	36		57	
SBR III	45		60	
R.O. +	17		41	
R.O. -	35	$p = 0{,}02$	59	$p = 0{,}1$
R.P. +	20		49	
R.P. -	35	$p = 0{,}01$	49	$p = 0{,}9$

Le taux de réponse majeure est significativement différent à 2 mois entre les grades histologiques faibles (SBR I et SBR II faible) et les tumeurs de grades histologiquesélevés (II fort et III). Cette différence s'estompe à 4 mois. De même, les taux de réponse significativement différents à 2 mois entre les RO + et RO -, RP + et RP - deviennent identiques à 4 mois.

En tenant compte des réponses observées à la chimiothérapie, le traitement loco-régional s'est ramené 82 fois à une amputation mammaire, 211 fois un essai de conservation mammaire a pu être fait (72%), une irradiation à visée exclusive a été réalisée dans 147 cas, une irradiation suivie d'une chirurgie de complément (évidement axillaire) a été réalisée 23 fois, une tumorectomie suivie d'une irradiation 39 fois.

L'évaluation actuarielle à 4 ans fait apparaitre dans les taux de survie une différence entre les stades cliniques ($p = 0{,}03$). Le grade histologique SBR, l'expression des récepteurs et la réponse objective à la chimiothérapie conservent leur signification pronostique.

Actuellement, 42 patientes ont présenté une rechute locale et/ou ganglionnaire soit 14% ; 76 patientes ont présenté une évolution métastatique (26%) soit un échec chez 93 patientes (31%) (tableau VIII).

Tableau VIII : Situation évolutive - Essai S'5

	METASTASE non	METASTASE oui	
0	203	51	
Rec. locale	16	14	30
Rec. ganglionnaire	0	8	8
Rec. loc. + ganglionnaire	1	3	4
	Echecs locaux (14 %)		42

Les rechutes locales sont apparues dans tous les types de tumeur (T2 N1b, T3 N0, T3 N1b, T4 N2 N3) de façon homogène. Le risque est de 11% chez les patientes qui avaient présenté une réponse initiale majeure et de 12% chez celles qui n'avaient pas présenté de réponse. Il est indépendant de l'état des récepteurs (RO et RP) et du grade histologique (SBR).

La survenue de métastases varie de 13% dans le groupe T1 T2 N0 N1a à 59% dans le groupe T4 N2 N3. Le risque de survenue de métastases est de 20% chez les patientes ayant présenté une réponse majeure à la chimiothérapie première contre 31% chez celles n'ayant pas présenté de réponse : différence modérément significative. Cette différence est très marquée pour l'expression des récepteurs hormonaux RO et RP (p respectivement de 0,006 et 0,007). (tableau IX).

Tableau IX : Résultats à 4 ans.

	RECHUTE LOCALE à 4 ans			SURVIE S/METASTASE			SURVIE A 4 ANS		
	DC	% s/rechute	p	DC	%	p	DC	%	p
PRESENTATION CLINIQUE									
. T1 T2 N0 N1a	0/19			2/19	81		1/19	88	
. T3 N0 N1a	4/39	85		6/39	77		2/39	81	
. T1 T2 N1b	10/81	81	0,56	15/81	73	0,02	8/81	83	0,03
. T3 N1b	9/79	82		25/79	58		13/79	70	
. T4 N2 N3	11/73	73		28/73	47		23/73	65	
SBR I	1/24	95		4/24	83		1/24	96	
II faible	3/67	95	0,2	11/67	83		4/67	94	0,03
II fort	13/87	85		24/87	72		14/87	84	
III	11/72	85		25/72	65		19/72	74	
R.H. R.O. -	20/69	71	0,14	38/69	45	0,006	17/69	75	0,16
R.O. +	7/49	86	NS	12/49	76		6/49	88	
R.P. -	26/128	80	0,12	58/128	55	0,007	32/128	75	0,01
R.P. +	12/85	86		24/85	72		9/85	89	
REPONSE CLINIQUE CHIMIO.									
RC	5/41	88		3/41	93		1/41	97	
RP ≥ 50%	11/101	89	0,88	25/101	75	0,03	13/101	88	0,02
RP ≤ 50% + NR	18/153	88		47/153	69		32/153	79	
REP. MAJEURES	16/142	89	0,94	28/142	80	0,05	14/142	90	0,02
NON REPONDEURS	18/153	88		47/153	69		32/153	79	

L'analyse de l'évolution de la maladie selon l'état hormonal ne fait apparaitre une différence que pour le risque métastatique qui parait significativement moins important pour les patientes avant la ménopause que pour les patientes ménopausées (tableau X).

Tableau X : Evolution selon l'état hormonal des patientes.

	PRE-MENOPAUSE	POST-MENOPAUSE	
DECES	27/201	19/95	p = 0,11
RECHUTE LOCALE	28/201	7/95	p = 0,16
REC. METASTATIQUE	44/201	32/95	p = 0,01

DISCUSSION

L'extension des indications de la chimiothérapie cytotoxique dans le cadre de stratégies multidisciplinaires à visée curatrice pose un problème d'évaluation de son efficacité et de la détermination précise de ses indications.
L'avantage de la chimiothérapie néoadjuvante peut se ramener à 3 points :
1. traitement précoce de la dissémination métastatique potentielle,
2. réduction posssible de la tumeur initiale,
3. évaluation immédiate de l'efficacité potentielle du protocole thérapeutique appliqué (Skipper, 1986).
Sur le plan technique et théorique (Goldie et Goldman, 1979) se posent outre le problème du choix de l'association cytotoxique, le problème de la durée du traitement. Le risque d'un traitement trop bref est de sous-estimer l'efficacité potentielle du schéma thérapeutique retenu. Parallèlement, le risque d'un traitement trop prolongé est de sélectionner de façon apparente une population cellulaire résistante à la chimiothérapie et susceptible d'un comportement local, régional et général très différent de celui de la population cellulaire moyenne initialement présente.
Avec une durée d'application de la chimiothérapie de 3 à 4 mois en moyenne, il apparait certain qu'au terme de 4 ans, la prévention des rechutes métastatiques est certaine. Même s'il est possible d'extrapoler de cet effet relativement précoce, une conclusion à plus long terme, il parait probable que la chimiothérapie proposée soit capable de réduire (ou de détruire) complètement les clones micrométastatiques.
En revanche, deux points essentiels émergent de l'étude ouverte.
D'une part, la signification statistique des paramètres essentiels du pronostic n'est pas altérée par la chimiothérapie première. Leur importance reste fondamentale sur le risque de survenue de métastases et la survie, qu'il s'agisse du grade histologique, des taux de R.O. et de R.P., de la classification T.N.M. Ce résultat laisse suspecter que la chimiothérapie n'est pas active de façon prédominante sur les formes de cancer qui rassemblent divers paramètres de mauvais pronostic. D'autre part, l'absence de toute relation entre le risque de rechute locale et les habituels paramètres du pronostic, y compris le T et le N., ceci laisse supposer qu'il existe peut être dans la séquence thérapeutique retenue une défaillance responsable de l'expression de ce risque.

REFERENCES BIBLIOGRAPHIQUES

Goldie J.H., Goldman A.J. (1979) : A mathematical model for relating the drug sensitivity of tumors to their spontaneous mutation rate.
Cancer Treat. Rep. 63, 1727-1733.
Skipper H.E. (1986) : Critical variables in the design of combination chemotherapy regimens to be used alone or in an adjuvant setting. In "Neoadjuvant chemotherapy". Colloque Inserm. John Libbey Eurotext Ltd., vol. 137, pp 11-22

Résumé

296 patients with an histologically proven stage 1 to 3 breast cancer were given a neoadjuvant program of cytotoxic chemotherapy including Adriamycin, Cyclophosphamide and 5 Fluoro-uracile. A preliminary analysis of results after 4 years of follow-up shows :

- that initial response rate to chemotherapy is depending upon size of local tumor (the smaller the tumor, the higher the response rate).
- that statistical signification of common parameters of prognosis as histological grading, E.R., PgR, clinical sstaging, is entirely preserved.
- that the risk of local relapse is independant of these parameters.

In a complementary controlled study including 161 patients, 86 of them were given a neoadjuvant program of chemotherapy : with a mean follow up of 3 years, a significant reduction of metastatic relapse is observed (p = 0,04) but the rate of local relapse is increased (p = 0,03).

Neo-Adjuvant Chemotherapy. Ed. Cl. Jacquillat, M. Weil, D. Khayat. Colloque INSERM/John Libbey Eurotext Ltd. © 1988. Vol. 169, pp. 177-181.

Influence of the response rate obtained by neo-adjuvant chemotherapy on the survival of patients with locally advanced breast cancer

M. Namer, M. Héry, M. Abbes, M. Frenay and A. Ramaioli

Centre Antoine-Lacassagne, 06054 Nice Cedex, France

ABSTRACT

Since 1977, 170 locally advanced nonmetastatic breast cancers have been treated with 3 courses of neoadjuvant chemotherapy before starting locoregional treatment: 1977-81 protocol A; 1982-84 protocol B; 1985-87 protocol C. Response was assessed by clinical (UICC) and radiologic criteria. A gradual improvement was seen in the objective response rate between these 3 protocols. Disease-free survival and overall survival were improved between A and B, and an improvement is expected in the survival of protocol C patients. This treatment modality may thus be of real benefit and not due merely to patient selection.

KEYWORDS
Breast cancer, chemotherapy, survival

INTRODUCTION

Locally advanced breast cancer (LABC) has a very poor prognosis. These patients cannot be cured by locoregional treatment alone. Starting treatment by neoadjuvant chemotherapy has certain advantages:

- administration of systemic treatment as early as possible to a population that experimental and clinical studies have shown has a 70% risk of having subclinical micrometastases
- obtainment of an in vivo sensitivity assay that will permet the selection of a responder population and thereby improve the cost benefit ratio
- in the case of significant remission, allow proposal of a conservative treatment that is totally impossible to envisage at the time of initial diagnosis
- reduce the number of circulating cells observed by certain workers in the days after surgery.

Since 1977, we have treated 170 consecutive cases of LABC with the following chronology: (1) neoadjuvant chemotherapy (2) locoregional treatment (3) adjuvant chemotherapy associated with hormonotherapy (tamoxifen) for patients with positive receptor levels. Three different chemotherapy protocols were used for the induction step.

This study was designed:
- to evaluate the effect of each protocol on breast tumors
- to determine any correlations between the effect on the breast tumor and survival
- to search for parameters that would predict sensitivity to treatment

MATERIAL AND METHODS

From 1977-1980, 70 patients were given protocol.A, from 1981-1984 protocol B was used for 47 patients, and from 1985-87 a total of 53 patients were treated with protocol C (Table 1). A total of 56 patients (33%) were less than 50 years old; 97 (57%) were aged 50-70 years, and 17 (10%) were over 70 years old. Distribution by TNM stage was : 42 (25%) T2, 79 (47%) T3, and 47 (28%) T4. Two patients had a multifocal tumor. 35 patients (21%) had no clinically palpable axillary lymph node; 16 (68%) were N1, and 19 (11%) were N2 or N3. Receptors were assayed before treatment in those patients for whom a Trucut biopsy was performed for diagnosis, and after treatment on surgically excised tumors . The cut-off value for positivity was calculated per mg of protein: 10 fm for estrogen receptors (ER) and 15 fm for progesterone receptors (PR). The Scarff, Bloom and Richardson (SBR) grade was calculated only for those Trucut biopsies obtained prior to treatment. Analysis of the distribution of these different parameters did not reveal any difference between the 3 populations (Table 2).

TABLE 1: Consecutive protocols from 1977 to 1987
(protocols repeated every 28 days)

1977 to 1980 : 70 patients received Protocol A:	ADM	40 mg/m2/iv Day 1
	VCR	1 mg/m2/iv Day 2
	5-FU	500 mg/m2/iv Days 3,4,5
	CPA	300 mg/m2/iv Days 3,4,5
1981 to 1984: 47 patients received Protocol B:	ADM	40 mg/m2/iv Day 1
	VDS	3 mg/m2/iv Day 2
	5-FU	500 mg/m2/iv Days 3,4,5
	CPA	300 mg/m2/iv Days 3,4,5
1985 to 1987: 53 patients received Protocol C:	ADM	30 mg/m2/iv Days 1 + 8
	5-FU	500 mg/m2/iv Days 1 + 8
	CPA	100 mg/m2/po Days 1-14
	Prednisone	40 mg/m2/po Days 1-14

The neoadjuvant chemotherapy protocol consisted in 3 courses: 7 patients received less than 3 courses because of intolerance and 20 others received 4 courses as part of a trial aimed at obtaining greater locoregional efficacy. Locoregional treatment consisted in surgical resection in 145 cases (138 radical and 7 partial mastectomies) followed by postoperative radiotherapy. Axillary node sampling revealed no metastatic nodes in 38 patients; 107 patients were node-positive. In 28 cases, tumor reduction was such that only radiotherapy was given, without surgery. Adjuvant chemotherapy was always included in the locoregional treatment. Groups A and B received the same treatment regimen as that used for induction purposes. Group C received courses of FAC (5-FU 500 mg/m2/D1; ADM 50 mg/m2/D1; CPA 500 mg/m2/D1 repeated every 21 days). The number of postoperative courses varied from 3 to 6 depending on the degree of regression observed after the induction treatment. Hormonotherapy (tamoxifen for 24 months) was prescribed after the locoregional therapy for 88 patients who had positive receptor levels (ER or PR).

Statistical analysis consisted in the chi-square test for all percentage comparisons and the Wilcoxon test for curve comparisons. The software used was BMDP.

TABLE 2: PATIENT CHARACTERISTICS

		Total	A	B	C	p (chi-2)
Age:	< 50 yr	56	23	12	21	)
	51-70	97	40	28	29	) NS
	> 70 yr	17	7	7	3	)
Menopausal status:						
- premenopausal		61	27	15	19	)
- post menopausal		109	43	32	34	) NS
TNM stage:						
- T2		42	14	11	17	)
- T3		79	30	33	27	) NS
- T4		47	26	14	7	
- N0		35	9	10	16	)
- N1		116	50	33	33	) NS
- N2-3		19	11	4	4	)
Hormone receptors after induction chemotherapy:						
- ER-		48	16	16	16	)
- ER+		63	23	24	16	) NS
- PR+		51	23	15	13	)
- PR-		60	17	25	18	) NS
Scarff, Bloom & Richardson grade:						
- SBR 1		17	6	5	6	)
- SBR 2		60	14	16	30	) NS
- SBR 3		9	3	2	4	)

RESULTS

Induction chemotherapy

The efficacy of neoadjuvant chemotherapy was assessed both clinically and radiologically using the breast tumor and lymph nodes as targets. Results obtained using these two methods correlated well in 65% of cases. Radiologic findings were worse than the clinical data in 29% and were better for 6% of patients. Using clinical parameters, an objective response (CR + PR) was obtained in 23/70 (33%) protocol A patients, in 22/47 (47%) protocol B patients, and in 36/53 (68%) protocol C patients: A vs B = $p < 0.05$; B vs C = $p < 0.05$; A vs C = $p < 0.01$. For the entire study population, an objective response was obtained in 81/170 (48%) of the patients. This response did not vary with age (≤ 50 yr, > 50 yr), tumor size or receptor status.

Disease-free survival and overall survival

The median disease-free survival (DFS) and the overall survival (OS) for the entire population were 65 and 80 months: these figures are much higher than the results of classical treatments that do not begin with chemotherapy (1). The DFS and OS were better for responders than for nonresponders ($p < 0.002$, $p< 0.001$). This positive difference persisted and even increased with time (Figures 1 and 2).

In order to prove the utility of induction chemotherapy, we compared the outcome of the 3 populations studied. Owing to the fact that the objective remissions were different with the 3 protocols, we feel that if the survival can be improved when the objective remission rate is improved, the induction chemotherapy is beneficial. The DFS and OS improved between protocols A and B ($p = 0.06$, $p < 0.04$) (Figures 3 and 4). It was not possible to compute the DFS and the OS for protocol C patients owing to the insufficient follow-up interval and because few events have yet occurred.

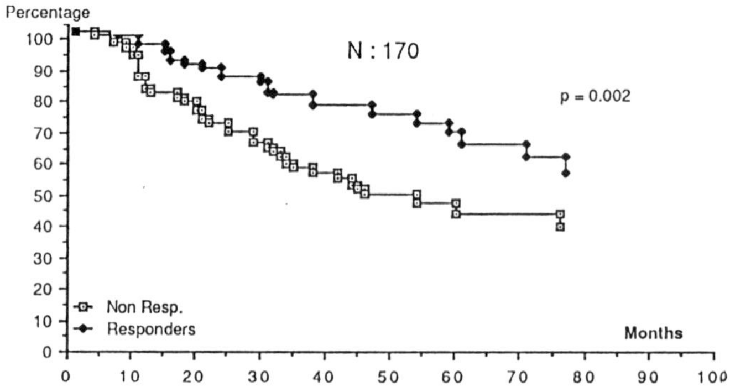

Fig. 1 : Disease-free survival : responders vs nonresponders

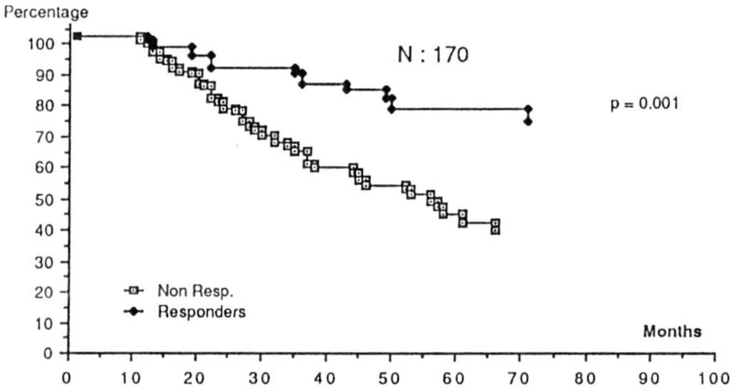

Fig.2 : Overall survival : responders vs nonresponders

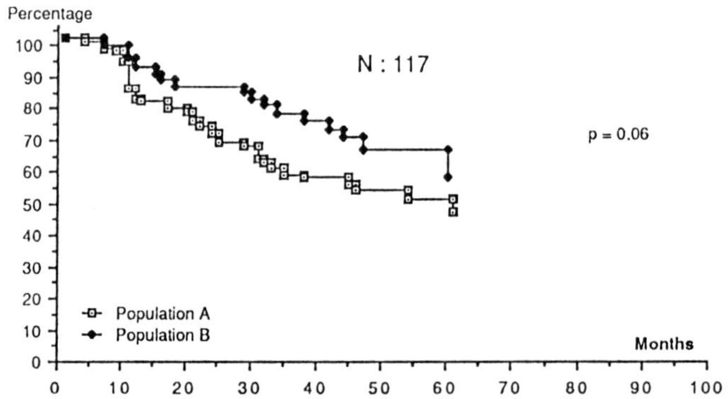

Fig.3 : Disease-free survival: Population A vs B

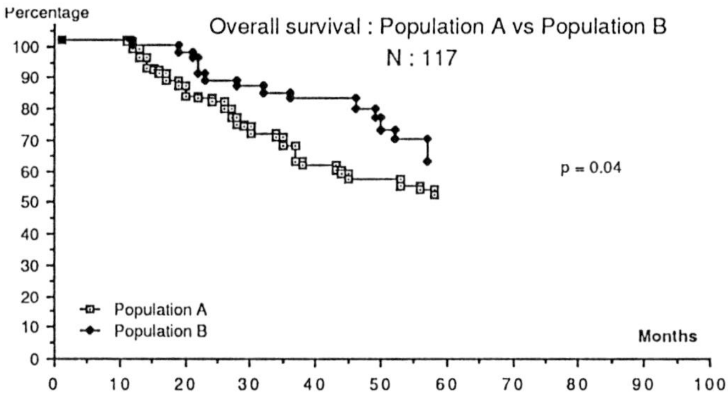

Fig. 4: Overall survival: Population A vs B

However, owing to the gradual improvement in the objective response rate between these 3 protocols, we expect to see an improvement in the survival curves of patients treated with protocol C. In addition, the DFS and OS of responders in protocols A and B were not different ($p = 0.13$, $p = 0.7$). The survival of N- patients was better than that of N+ patients ($p < 0.02$).

CONCLUSION

The objective remission rate obtained for breast tumors and adjacent lymph nodes rose with the search for a more effective chemotherapy regimen. Obtainment of remission, however, was not correlated with patient age, tumor size, or ER or PR status. The most significant number of remissions was obtained after 3 courses; however, 20 patients required a fourth course. In addition, for 7 patients, intolerance necessitated the halt of treatment after the 2nd course.

The DFS and OS are influenced by achievement of objective remission; this is all the more so when the protocol used is more effective on the breast tumor. When a remission is obtained, the DFS and OS are just as good, regardless of the chemotherapy protocol that produces it. Survival is better when axillary node sampling evidences the absence of nodal metastases.

REFERENCES

Ackland S.P., Bitran J.D., and Dowlatshahi K (1985): Management of locally advanced and inflammatory carcinoma of the breast

Résumé

Depuis 1977, nous avons traité 170 cancers du sein inopérables par une chimiothérapie néo-adjuvante. Trois différents protocoles ont été successivement utilisés : protocole A (AVCF) de 1977-81, protocole B (AECF) de 1982-85, protocole C (CAFPred) de 1985-87. Les réponses objectives ont augmenté de manière significative entre A,B et C. L'augmentation du pourcentage de réponses sur la tumeur du sein s'accompagne d'une amélioration de l'intervalle libre et de la survie. Ceci tend à prouver que la chimiothérapie néo-adjuvante est réellement bénéfique pour le malade et n'est pas simplement le reflet d'une sélection.

Breast cancer III

Cancer du sein III

Neo-Adjuvant Chemotherapy. Ed. Cl. Jacquillat, M. Weil, D. Khayat. Colloque INSERM/John Libbey Eurotext Ltd. © 1988. Vol. 169, pp. 185-188.

Neo-adjuvant chemotherapy for stage III breast cancer- 5 year report of CALGB 7784

G. Lesnick, M. Perloff, A. Korzun, F. Chu, J.F. Holland, M. Thirwell, R. Ellison, R. Carey, L. Leone, V. Weinberg, M. Rice and W. Wood

Cancer and leukemia Group B (CALGB), Bookline, MA, USA

ABSTRACT

In 1978 the CALGB initiated a trial of chemotherapy (CHEMO) preceding and following local and regional therapy (LOC RX) with radiotherapy (XRAY) or surgery (SURG) for treatment of locally advanced (stage III) breast cancer. Initial CHEMO consisted of three 28 d. cycles of cyclophosphamid 100mg/m^2 po QD x 14 d., adriamycin 25 mg/m^2 iv d. 1 & 8, vincristine 1.4 mg/m^2 iv d. 1 & 8, and prednisone 40 mg/m^2 po QD x 14d. 113 eligible patients received initial chemotherapy. There were 78 complete or partial responses (69%) including 7 responses among 14 patients with inflammatory cancer. 91 patients (81%) were considered suitable for LOC RX but 4 refused randomization. 43 were randomized to SURG, the majority having a modified radical mastectomy. 44 received XRAY (55 Gy/5 wks. + 15-22 Gy boost to tumor and axilla). Patients randomized to XRAY were comparable to those randomized to SURG in age, ER status, stage, tumor size, and response to initial chemotherapy. By definition all patients treated by SURG had a complete remission. 23 patients (52%) had complete remissions to XRAY + subsequent CHEMO. Following LOC RX, CHEMO was continued for 2 years. There was no significant differences in duration of disease control, survival, incidence or location of recurrences in both groups. Toxicities were generally acceptable. Median survival was 42.9 months for SURG and 40.1 months for XRAY. 5 year survival estimates were 35% for all 113 eligible patients, 39% for those 87 randomized to SURG or XRAY.

KEY WORDS

Breast, cancer, noadjuvant chemotherapy, surgery, radiotherapy

INTRODUCTION

Locally advanced breast cancer is seldom cured by conventional regional therapy be it mastectomy or radiotherapy. There is a high incidence of both local and systemic recurrence. In addition, the local involvement often is of such extent that complete surgical excision cannot be achieved without unacceptable deformity. The advent of chemotherapeutic agents that are effective in advanced breast cancer encouraged the expectation that their use would change this dismal prospect.

In December of 1978, after pilot data from the Mount Sinai Medical School had indicated that preoperative chemotherapy was both safe and effective, the Cancer and Leukemia Group B instituted a trial of combined therapy with initial chemotherapy followed by either mastectomy or radiotherapy for patients with locally advanced breast cancer. Early data from this trial were presented at the First International Conference on Neoadjuvant Chemotherapy. Additional observation now permits this report of the status of these patients after a median follow-up of five years.

METHODS

The trial was limited to patients with a poor prognosis following conventional therapy. Patients with Stage III breast cancer by criteria of the UICC including patients with inflammatory cancers were included. Since patients with large tumors without axillary involvement have a relatively good prognosis, they were excluded. The study population thus consisted of patients with previously untreated breast cancer in the following subgroups: T3 NIB MO; T 1,2,3, N2 MO; T4 NO, 1,2 MO.

Initial treatment consisted of three monthly cycles of chemotherapy. Each 28 day cycle included 14 daily oral doses of cyclophosphamid 100 mgm/m^2 and prednisone 40 mgm/m^2 plus on days 1 & 8, intravenous doses of adriamycin 25 mgm/m^2, 5-fluorouracil 500 mgm/m^2, and vincristine 1, 4 mgm/m^2 (maximum single dose of 2 mg.).

Within six weeks of completion of the chemotherapy the patients were re-evaluated. If their disease was considered operable and there was no evidence of metastases the patient was randomly assigned to receive either radiotherapy or mastectomy. For those assigned to surgery modified mastectomy was the recommended technique but radical mastectomy was acceptable. Radiotherapy patients received treatment five days a week to the entire breast, the axilla, the internal mammary and supraclavicular lymph node areas. The prescribed dose was 50 Grays in 5 weeks. Residual tumor in the breast was boosted with 22 Grays, axillary nodes were boosted by 15 to 20 Grays in two weeks. Chemotherapy identical to the initial treatment was resumed after regional treatment for a total duration of two years. However when a cumulative dose of 550 mgm/m^2 was reached, adriamycin was discontinued and methotrexate 40 mgm/m^2 (30 mgm/m^2 for patients over 60 years old) was substituted on the same schedule. Chemotherapy dose was modified as necessary for evidence of hematologic, hepatic, mucosal and cardiac toxicity. The treatment was generally well tolerated. There was only one death that was possibly treatment related.

RESPONSE TO INITIAL CHEMOTHERAPY

Initial chemotherapy was administered to 113 eligible patients. The median age was 54, 63% were post menopausal. Estrogen receptors were positive in 19 patients, negative in 27 and unknown in 63. T3 tumors were present in 36 patients, T4 tumors in 76. Inflammatory cancer was present present in 14 of the 113 patients who received initial chemotherapy. A complete or partial response was seen in 7 (50%). In the remaining 99 non-inflammatory tumors, the total response rate was 72% and the complete response rate was 18%. After initial chemothrapy 91 of the 113 (81%) were considered operable and suitable for radiotherapy. Four refused randomization. Randomization assigned 43 to receive surgery and 44 to radiotherapy.

RESULTS OF RANDOMIZED TREATMENT

The two groups were comparable in age, stage, tumor size and response to initial chemotherapy. The only major difference was a longer delay from completion of radiotherapy to resumption of chemotherapy than from time of mastectomy to resumption of chemotherapy. All patients treated by mastectomy were, by definition, complete responders. Twenty-three of 44 (52%) of radiotherapy patients attained a complete response. Eleven (25%) maintained or achieved a partial response. Four patients achieved improvement or stable disease. Six patientswere unevaluable. No patient had progressive disease during radiotherapy.

DURATION OF DISEASE CONTROL

Duration of disease control was measured from the date of entry on study to the date off study if the patient relapsed or to the date of death if the patient died without relapse. Those who were alive without relapse were censored on the date last seen.

There was no significant difference in the rate of either local or systemic relapse between the patients treated with surgery and those treated with radiotherapy. Local relapse was the initial recurrence in 21% of the surgery patients and in 27% of those treated with radiotherapy. Median duration of disease control was 29 months for the surgery patients and 28 months after radiotherapy.

SURVIVAL

Survival was measured from the date of entry on study to the date of death from any cause. Patients still alive were consored at the date of last contact. The median follow-up time for the 113 eligible patients was 5 years with a minimum of 4 years. The median survival time estimate was 40.1 months. The estimated 5 year survival was 35%. In this relatively small sample, the only factors with possible prognostic significance were ER status (p=.094) and inflammatory cancer (p=.26) Among the 87 randomized patients, there was no difference in survival between the two regional treatments: median 43 months after surgery and 39 months after radiotherapy (p=.42). Five year survival estimates were 34% for the entire group, 34% for those treated with surgery and 41% for those treated by radiotherapy.

CONCLUSIONS

1. This study demonstrates that prolonged control of locally advanced breast cancer can be achieved by combined therapy with cytotoxic chemotherapy that both precedes and follows local ablation of the primary tumor by either surgery or radiotherapy.

2. There was no indication of any aggravation of the disease from either delay in instituting regional therapy or the employment of surgery in advanced disease.

3. Surgery and radiotherapy proved to be equally effective when used in conjunction with pre and post therapy chemotherapy.

4. Chemotherapy in the doses used did not iterfere with either post surgical wound healing or administration of adequate doses of radiation.

5. The 34% 5-year survival is disappointing and indicates the need for more effective chemotherapeutic agents.

Résumé

Le groupe coopératif CALGB a commence, en 1978, un essai thérapeutique avec chimiothérapie (CHEMO) precedant et suivant le traitement loco-régional (LOC RX) avec radiothérapie (XRAY) ou chirurgie (SURG) pour le traitement des cancers du sein localement avances (stade III). La chimiothérapie d'emblée comprenait 3 cycles de 28 jours de Cyclophosphamide: 100 mg/m2 jx14 jours, Adriamycine: 25 mg/m2 iv, j 1 et 8, 5-Fluorouracile 500 mg/m2 iv, j 1 et 8, Vincristine 1.4 mg/m2 iv, j 1 et 8 et Prednisone 40 mg/m2, po x 14 jours. 113 malades reçurent la chimiothérapie d'emblée. Il y eut 78 rémissions complètes ou partielles (69%) y compris 7/14 malades avec cancer inflammatoire. 91 malades (81%) furent considerées acceptables pour (LOCRX), mais 4 refusèrent randomisation. 43 malades furent randomisées pour (SURG), la majorite desquelles eurent une mastectomie radicale modifiée. 44 malades recurent XRAY (55 Gy/5 semaines + 15-22 Gy surdosage sur la tumeur et axillaire). Les malades randomisée a XRAY ou SURG étaient comparables en âge, recpteurs oestrogèniques, dimensions de la tumeur et en reponse a la chimiotherapie d'emblée. Par définition, touts les malades traitées par SURG étaient en rémission complète. 23 malades (52%) achevèrent une remission complète par XRAY + chimiothérapie par la suite. Apres LOCRX, CHEMO fut continuée pour 2 ans. Il n'y eut pas de difference significative en durée de controle de la maladie, survie, incidence our localisation des récidives dans les deux groupes. Les toxicités furent en general acceptables cependant les malades recevant CHEMO après XRAY subirent une toxicité hématologique plus sévère. La survie mediane a été de 42.9 mois pour SURG et de 40.1 mois pour XRAY. La survie estimée à 5 ans était de 35% pour la totalité des 113 malades admissibles a l'essai et 39% pour les 87 malades randomisées à SURG ou XRAY

Neo-Adjuvant Chemotherapy. Ed. Cl. Jacquillat, M. Weil, D. Khayat. Colloque INSERM/John Libbey Eurotext Ltd. © 1988. Vol. 169, pp. 189-200.

Etude comparative de deux stratégies thérapeutiques du cancer du sein

M. Brunet*, F. Baillet**, M. Weil***, K. Hacene*, G. Auclerc***, P. Guérin[1], D. Khayat***, J.L. Floiras*, J. Rouëssé* et Cl. Jacquillat***

* *Centre René Huguenin, 35 rue Dailly, 92211 Saint Cloud, France*
** *Service de Radiothérapie, Hôpital Necker, 149 rue de Sèvres, 75015 Paris, France*
*** *Service d'Oncologie Médicale, Hôpital de la Salpétrière, 47 boulevard de l'Hôpital 75013, Paris, France*
[1] *Service de Radiothérapie, Hôpital de la Salpétrière, 47 boulevard de l'Hôpital, 75013 Paris, France*

Cette étude compare les résultats du traitement du cancer du sein unilatéral, non métastatique, non traité antérieurement, chez des femmes, sans autre lésion maligne, traitées de 1980 à 1985 et suivies régulièrement d'une part au Centre René Huguenin et d'autre part dans le Service d'Oncologie Médicale de la Pitié-Salpétrière et le Service de Radiothérapie de l'Hopital Necker. Durant cette période, le Centre René Huguenin a traité 2.154 patientes en privilégiant le traitement loco-régional, chirurgie avec ou sans radiothérapie, avec ou sans chimiothérapie adjuvante, pour toutes les formes sauf les cancers inflammatoires. Les équipes de la Pitié et de Necker ont traité 205 patientes par chimiothérapie première, suivie d'irradiation.

Pour l'ensemble des deux groupes, on dispose des informations suivantes : l'âge au moment du diagnostic, la taille clinique de la tumeur, le TNM, la notion de poussée évolutive cotée de 0 à 3.

Les traitements ont été décrits et commentés par les équipes respectives. Le groupe Pitié-Necker a utilisé quatre protocoles différents de chimiothérapie première, en fonction des facteurs de gravité, mais ne sera retenu ici que la stratégie globale : chimiothérapie suivie d'irradiation. Au CRH, 86 % de l'effectif a été traité par chirurgie première : mastectomie radicale modifiée avec curage pour 60 % de ces cas et tumorectomie avec curage pour 40 %. Une irradiation post-opératoire a été réalisée chez plus de la moitié des patientes. Il faut noter qu'une chimiothérapie péri-opératoire a été faite dans tous ces cas : une injection de 10 mg de Thiotépa en cours d'intervention, puis les 4 jours suivants. Une chimiothérapie adjuvante a été réalisée en cas d'envahissement ganglionnaire axillaire.

Lors de la surveillance des évènements carcinologiques, récidive loco-régionale ou métastases à distance sont survenues pour 19 % de l'effectif du CRH et 25 % pour la Pitié-Necker, et respectivement 13 et 15 % des patientes sont décédées.

Les courbes de survie globale et de survie sans évènement ont été établies pour les deux groupes, par la méthode du produit limite et la comparaison assurée par le logrank test. Pour les deux critères, les courbes correspondantes ne présentent aucune différence significative.

Mais la comparaison des deux populations, vis à vis des facteurs de pronostic connus pour l'ensemble, montre qu'elles diffèrent de façon importante. La population de la Pitié-Necker est un peu plus jeune, 53,8 ans contre 56,6, et elle comporte des tumeurs plus volumineuses, 54,3 mm contre 36,3 mm. De la même façon, la comparaison du T du N et de la Pev, avec le test du Khir 2, les montre significativement différente au risque de $p = 10^{-5}$. Ces différences peuvent, bien entendu, jouer un rôle important lors de la comparaison globale des résultats. Ce problème est abordé par trois approches méthodologiques différentes.

Comparaison partielle dans chacune des mortalités des facteurs

En utilisant la même méthode que pour la comparaison globale, les deux groupes sont donc comparés dans chaque modalité de l'âge, du T, du N, de la Pev, et vis à vis de la survie globale et de la survie sans évènement. Au total, 24 comparaisons ont été réalisées, deux se sont révélées significatives du risque de 5 % : pour les T_4 vis à vis de la survie, en faveur du groupe Pitié-Necker ; pour les N_1 vis à vis des évènements en faveur du CRH. Les deux sous-groupes pourraient être le point de départ d'une étude sur des effectifs plus importants, mais cependant la théorie des tests statistiques peut expliquer, à elle seule, un pourcentage de signification lors de la réalisation de tests multiples.

Analyse globale à l'aide du modèle de Cox

Les variables candidates à la sélection sont : le groupe 0 pour CRH et 1 pour Pitié-Necker ; l'âge en année, la taille clinique en millimètre, le N avec $0 = N_0$, $1 = N_1$, $2 = N_2$; la poussé évolutive 0 = Pev 0, 1 = Pev 1. Dans cette analyse, les tumeurs en poussée évolutives 2 et 3 ont été écartées de façon à ne garder que les cas correspondant à une stratégie différente. L'effectif total est alors de 2.234 patientes.

L'analyse pour la survie, avec 261 décès soit 241 + 20, a sélectionné dans l'ordre d'importance de contribution à la prévision, la taille, l'âge, le N et la Pev.

L'analyse pour la survie sans évènement, avec 388 évènements soit 353 + 35, a sélectionné la taille et le N.

Le modèle de Cox, qui isole les variables ayant de l'importance par leur valeur de prévision, compte tenu de leur intervention, n'a pas sélectionner la variable appartenance à l'un ou l'autre groupe.

Stratification, appariement avec tirage aléatoire

Une stratification a été réalisée sur les deux séries, qui consiste à regrouper les patientes ayant le même profil, basé sur les variables suivantes : âge en 4 classes, N en 3 classes, Pev en 2 classes, taille clinique en 6 classes.

Après élimination des profils existant dans une série et non dans l'autre, on obtient une stratification commune qui comporte 54 profils distincts. La taille des séries est ramenée à respectivement 1.751 et 177 patientes. Puis ont été tirés au sort, dans la population CRH, 12 échantillons de 177 patientes, chacun ayant dans chaque strate le même effectif que celui existant dans la strate correspondante de la population de la Pitié-Necker.

L'ensemble des méthodes décrites a été appliqué successivement, pour la survie globale et la survie sans évènement, dans les 12 comparaisons entre chacun des échantillons du CRH et la population de la Pitié-Necker.

Aucun logrank test ne s'est révélé significatif parmi les 24 tests réalisées.

Pour les 24 applications du modèle de Cox, de façon très uniforme, la taille et le N clinique ont été sélectionnés. Seule la comparaison, correspondant à l'échantillon n°10 du CRH, a sélectionné l'appartenance au groupe, avec un avantage pour la Pitié-Necker. Cependant, la fluctuation d'échantillonnage est susceptible d'expliquer cet aspect.

Cette étude est certes criticable, car elle ne comporte pas une attribution des traitements au hasard. Cependant, l'attitude de l'équipe la Pitié-Necker a été uniforme pendant cette période. De même, la population du CRH a été extraite du dossier médical informatisé de cet établissement. Il est le reflet de l'activité d'équipes pluridisciplinaires avec des protocoles thérapeutiques structurés et bien définis. Par ailleurs, la saisie prospective des données initiales, des traitements et de la surveillance élimine tous biais possible de saisie pour une étude précise. Enfin, l'utilisation de plusieurs approches méthodologiques de comparaison, qui convergent dans leurs résultats, fourni une forte probabilité à la réalité des conclusions.

Au total, chacune des équipes peut revendiquer des avantages aux traitements qu'elles appliquent, mais vis à vis de la survie et de la survie sans évènement, on peut considérer que globalement deux stratégies thérapeutiques différentes se révèlent fournir des résultats équivalents.

COMPARAISONS PARTIELLES

- **24 comparaisons** Survie
  Évènement.
- **2 significatives**

T4 survie en faveur du groupe Pitié Neker
N1 évènement en faveur du CRH.

LES DEUX POPULATIONS 1980-85

CRH 2154		**Pitié-Neker 205**
	âge	
	taille clinique	
	T	
	N	
Chirurgie	PeV	**Chimio première**
irradiation		**irradiation**
chimio adjuvante		
Chimio péri opératoire		
chimio première pour :		
PeV 2-3, N, 3	**évènement carcinologique**	
	décès	

MODÈLE DE COX

L'établissement 0 = CRH - 1 = Pitié Neker - Age en années - Taille clinique en mm —N 0 = N0 - 1 = N1 - 2 = N2 - 3 = N3. Poussée évolutive 0 = PeV0 - 1 = PeV 1.

SURVIE		SURVIE SANS ÉVÈNEMENT	
Taille	$p < 0{,}000001$	Taille	$p < 0{,}000001$
Age	$p < 0{,}000001$	N	$p < 0{,}00075$
N	$p < 0{,}000028$		
PeV	$p < 0{,}027$		

LES FACTEURS DE PRONOSTIC

		Médiane	Moyenne	
Age	CRH	55	56,6	$p = 0{,}004$
	Pitié-Neker	53	53,8	
Taille		30	36,3	$p = 10^{-8}$
		54	54,3	
T				
N		répartion significativement différente		
PeV				$p = 10^{-5}$

APPROCHES MÉTHODOLOGIQUES

1 - Comparaison partielle dans chaque modalités des facteurs.

2 - Analyse globale : modèle de Cox.

3 - Stratification - appariement avec tirage aléatoire.

LES CRITÈRES DE PRONOSTIC

Décès		
CRH	279	13 %
Pitié-Neker	31	15 %
Évènement		
	401	19 %
	52	25 %

SURVIE

Échantillon	Variables sélectionnées	Valeur du p
1	Taille PeV	0.0001 0.032
2	Taille N	0.0001 0.028
3	Taille	0.00002
4	Taille N	< 0.00001 0.006
5	Taille N	0.00002 0.014
6	Taille N PeV	< 0.00003 0.012 0.038
7	Taille N	< 0.00001 0.012
8	Taille N	< 0.00001 0.038
9	Taille N	0.00007 0.027
10	N Taille Centre	0.00004 0.0058 0.0375
11	Taille N	< 0.00015 0.014
12	Taille N	< 0.0003 0.046

SURVIE SANS ÉVÈNEMENT

Échantillon	Variables sélectionnées	Valeur du p
1	Taille	< 0.00001
	N	0.046
2	Taille	< 0.00001
	N	0.021
3	Taille	0.00003
	Age	0.009
	N	0.28
4	Taille	< 0.00001
	N	0.003
5	N	< 0.00001
	Taille	0.003
	Centre	0.049
6	Taille	< 0.00001
	N	0.007
	Age	0.020
7	Taille	< 0.00001
	N	0.004
8	Taille	< 0.00001
	N	0.0098
9	Taille	< 0.00001
	N	0.034
10	Taille	< 0.00001
	N	0.001
	Centre	0.015
11	Taille	< 0.00001
	N	0.012
12	Taille	< 0.00001
	N	0.023

Stratification - appariement - tirage aléatoire variables : âge 4 classes - N 3 classes - PeV 4 classes - taille 6 classes

54 profils communs	CRH n = 1751
	Pitié-Neker n = 177

CRH	Pitié-Neker
177 x 12	177
Le logrank test x 12 x 2	N.S.

SURVIE SANS ÉVÈNEMENT

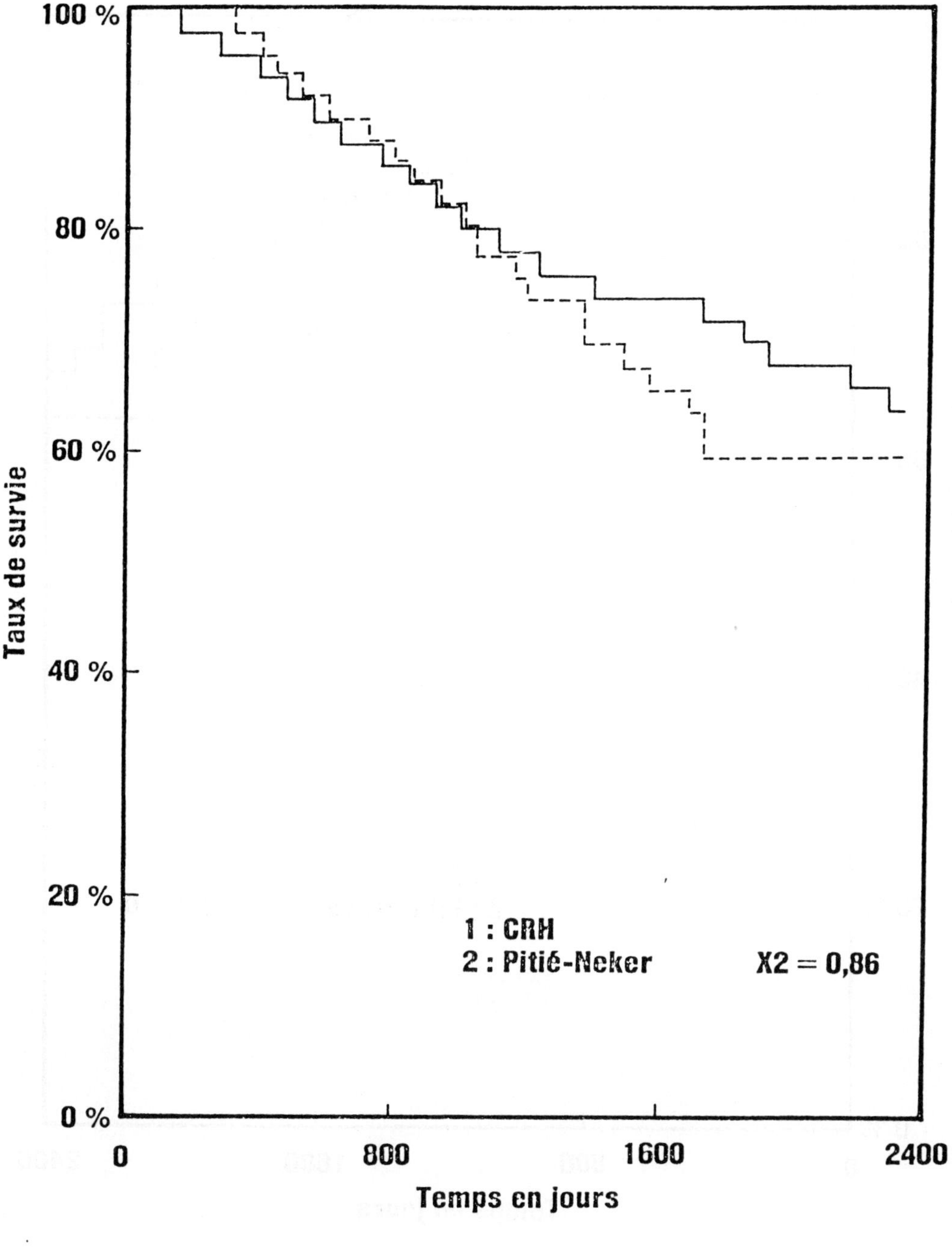

SURVIE

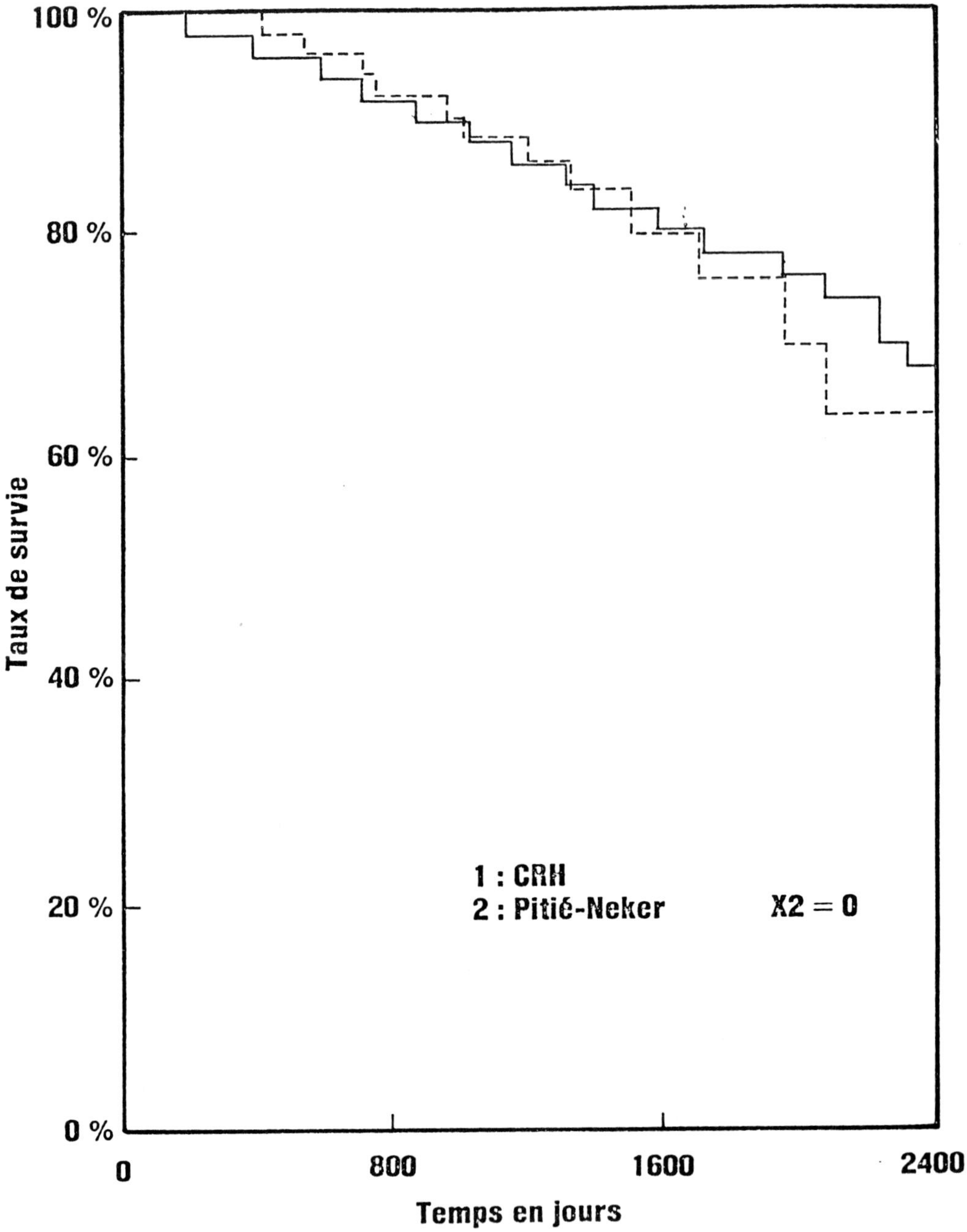

100 %
80 %
60 %
40 %
20 %
0 %
Taux de survie
0
800
1600
2400
Temps en jours
1 : CRH
2 : Pitié-Neker
X2 = 0

Neo-Adjuvant Chemotherapy. Ed. Cl. Jacquillat, M. Weil, D. Khayat. Colloque INSERM/John Libbey Eurotext Ltd. © 1988. Vol. 169, pp. 201-206.

Neo-adjuvant chemotherapy prior to definitive treatment for stage III carcinoma of the breast

Gordon F. Schwartz, Ronald I. Cantor and William A. Biermann

From the departments of surgery and medicine (medical oncology), Jefferson Medical College, Philadelphia, Pennsylvania, 19107, 1015 Chestnut Street, Suite 510, Philadelphia, PA 19107 USA

One hundred women with Stage III breast cancer were treated with neoadjuvant chemotherapy prior to any other treatment of the local disease. Response was assessed after three cycles of treatment and responders treated until the tumor and/or axillary nodes failed to show further regression, and definitive surgery was then performed. Chemotherapy was resumed following surgery to total twelve cycles. Ninety patients are evaluable; 70% responded to chemotherapy. Radical mastectomy without post-operative radiotherapy seems to be the preferable surgical treatment for responders. Median followup of the evaluable patients was 27 months; projected five year disease free-survival of the responders is >65%, and projected overall five year survival of this group is >85%.

In 1979 we began to treat women with locally advanced breast cancer, or AJC Stage III, (not N-3), by "neo-adjuvant" chemotherapy, prior to any surgical treatment other than initial biopsy to confirm the diagnosis and obtain tissue for hormone receptors. All women with clinical Stage III breast cancers were considered candidates for this study, excluding women with suspicious supraclavicular nodes (N-3). Metastatic work-up (chest Xray, bone scan and liver function studies) was performed to rule out the presence of overt systemic disease.

Cyclic chemotherapy was instituted with CMF, plus tamoxifen in post-menopausal women if hormone receptors were positive. Serial measurements of tumor and involved lymph nodes were used to assess the effect of chemotherapy, and response was evaluated after the third cycle. Responders were defined as women whose tumors decreased in diameter by at least 25%. Also considered responders were women whose axillary lymph nodes decreased in diameter by at least 50%. Although CMF was used initially in all patients, if there was no sign of response after the first or second cycle, one cycle of Adriamycin was added to the regimen before a patient was considered a non-responder. If some response was noted with Adriamycin, then this was continued and the patient remained eligible for consideration as a responder according to the above criteria. If there was no response to Adriamycin, then she was considered a non-responder. Early in the study, responders underwent definitive treatment after the initial three cycles of chemotherapy. As we became impressed by the magnitude of the response seen in many patients, responders were treated cyclically until there was no further objective decrease in size of tumor or nodes; operation was performed when this plateau was reached. Radical mastectomy was the operation chosen because so many of the lesions were so large that they involved multiple quadrants, or they could not be easily separated from the underlying pectoralis major muscle. If the original tumor had been located laterally in the breast and was not in proximity to the underlying pectoralis major muscle, modified radical mastectomy was considered. The size and location of the original tumor at the time of diagnosis were the criteria for the operation chosen, not the response of the tumor to chemotherapy. Several patients refused mastectomy, and they were treated by "lumpectomy," axillary dissection, and irradiation, although two of these patients underwent only "lumpectomy" and irradiation because they refused axillary dissection as well. Nonresponders underwent radiation therapy without mastectomy.

Subsequent to definitive treatment, chemotherapy was resumed and continued for a total of twelve cycles or for an additional six months, whichever was longer. The outcomes of responders and non-responders were analyzed according to age, clinical stage of disease, definitive treatment, microscopic findings in axilla and breast, estrogen and progesterone receptor status, recurrence (local vs systemic), and survival.

Between July 1, 1979, and October 31, 1986, 100 women with Stage III breast cancer entered this study. Their ages at diagnosis ranged from 30 to 84. Included within this group are 51 women with Stage III-A carcinoma, 32 women with Stage III-B carcinoma, and 17 women with inflammatory carcinoma. The diagnosis of inflammatory carcinoma was a clinical one. Of the 100 women, 10 are still in the initial chemotherapy phase of treatment, so that there are 90 women evaluable, followed for a median of 27 months since diagnosis, the longest follow-up being 92 months. The clinical stages of patients entered into the study along with their response to chemotherapy is noted in Table 1.

Table 1
PATIENT POPULATION

STAGE	T?,N?	RESPONDERS	NON-RESPONDERS	ON RX.	
III-A	T2,N2	12	3	2	17
	T3,N0	6	2	1	9
	T3,N1	14	1	1	16
	T3,N2	4	4	1	9
TOTAL III-A		36	10	5	51
III-B	T4,N0	2	2	0	4
	T4,N1	3	5	1	9
	T4,N2	10	7	2	19
TOTAL III-B		15	14	3	32
INFLAMMATORY CA.		12	3	2	17
GRAND TOTAL		63	27	10	100

Responders to chemotherapy numbered 63, or 70%, and 27 women, or 30%, were considered non-responders. No patient's cancer progressed systemically during treatment. Patients with Stage III-A cancer were more likely to respond than women with Stage III-B cancers, 78% vs 52%, but, of the 17 women with inflammatory carcinoma, 12 (80%) of the 15 evaluable patients responded; two are still undergoing treatment.

The median time of treatment before definitive surgery in the patients who responded to their chemotherapy was 7 months (cycles), the vast majority falling between 6 and 9 months. Only an initial group of 5 patients underwent surgery after only three cycles of treatment.

Most patients, 44 of the 63 responders (71%), underwent radical mastectomy. Nine women underwent modified radical mastectomy, and ten women were treated by irradiation following "lumpectomy" and levels I and II axillary dissection. Of the women who underwent modified mastectomy, two women also had post-operative irradiation to the chest wall because the tumor extended microscopically to within 0.5 cm. of the posterior margin of the pectoralis major fascia. None of the patients undergoing radical mastectomy also had irradiation, even though penetration of tumor to the underlying muscle fascia could be documented in several. No residual breast cancer could be found in four of the women undergoing mastectomy, and three of these four also had negative axillary lymph nodes. Two more women undergoing mastectomy were found to have only non-invasive ductal carcinoma in their breasts and no positive lymph nodes, so that five of the 53 women, or 9%, who underwent mastectomy after responding to chemotherapy, had no remaining invasive cancer in their breast or axilla.

Node status of 61 responders undergoing axillary dissection as part of subsequent treatment is noted in Tables 2 and 3. Fifty-three of these women (87%) were thought to have involved nodes, based upon the clinical findings when initially seen, including 33 women (54%) with multiple, matted axillary nodes (N-2).

Table 2
CLINICAL ASSESSMENT OF AXILLA
VS. FINAL PATHOLOGY

	INITIAL IMPRESSION	OPERATIVE FINDINGS	
T-N STATUS	NUMBER	NODES NEG	NODES POS
N-0	8	5	3
N-1	20	10	10
N-2	33	10	23
TOTAL	61	25	36

At operation, however, 20 of the 53 women with clinically involved nodes initially had negative microscopic axillary findings, including five women who also had no residual cancer in their breast (Table 3).

Table 3
RESPONDER NODE STATUS AT OPERATION

STAGE	NEGATIVE	POSITIVE		
		ONE ONLY	2-3+	=/>4+
III-A	18	1	4	11
III-B	5	1	4	5
INFLAMMATORY	2	2	3	5
TOTAL		4	11	21

25 PATIENTS WITH NEGATIVE NODES = 41%
36 PATIENTS WITH POSITIVE NODES = 59%

Overall, 25 of the 61 women who underwent axillary dissection, or 41%, had no microscopic evidence of axillary metastasis, including two of the women with inflammatory cancer. Many of the women with positive nodes, as might be expected, had multiple involved nodes at all axillary levels.

With respect to patient survival, patients, both responders and non-responders have been followed for a median of 27 months from diagnosis, the longest followup being 92 months. The differences between the responders and the non-responders is noteworthy, for both freedom from recurrence and for survival. Projected five year status for non-responders is 43% survival and 28% disease-free, whereas for those women responding to chemotherapy, these projections are 87% survival and 67% disease-free. Concerning local or regional recurrence, only one of the responders has subsequently had a local failure, a chest wall recurrence in a young woman with a Stage III-B carcinoma. No patient has had an axillary recurrence.

Neoadjuvant chemotherapy has been used prior to definitive treatment with radiotherapy since at least 1973, as reported by Brambilla, et al. in 1974 (1). Zucali et al. reported a response rate of 73% (2). More recently, Morrow et al. reported 77% success with two preliminary cycles of CAF +\- T in 31 women with Stage III disease (3). Hortobagyi et al., Lesnick et al., and Aisner et al. have also reported similar success with initial response to chemotherapy, allowing radiotherapy and\or surgery to be employed following a fixed period of chemotherapy (4,5,6).

Lippman et al. have been among the first to employ a flexible approach to neo-adjuvant chemotherapy as we have, using the maximal clinical response rather than a fixed number of cycles of therapy to determine timing of local treatment (7). We recognized the surgical advantages of this approach early in our own study. The median number of cycles of chemotherapy to achieve maximal response was seven. Seven months was also the mean and the mode. The likelihood of patient response to chemotherapy was not predicted by age, tumor size, lymph node status or presence of hormone receptors, although 87% of patients with T-3, N-0 or T-3, N-1 cancers responded and only 52% of the Stage III-B (non-inflammatory) cancers did. However, 80% of the inflammatory cancers responded, so that if one includes the inflammatory cancers with the other Stage III-B's, then 61% of the III-B cancers did respond to chemotherapy.

Microscopic examination of breast and axillary nodes was interesting. Although only three patients had histologic proof of axillary node disease (aspiration biopsy) prior to treatment by chemotherapy, the axillary node findings in those patients considered to be node-positive were not equivocal. We have previously reported our own high accuracy in the clinical assessment of axillary nodes (8), and virtually all of these patients left little in doubt. As noted previously, there were 20 patients (38%) with clinical N-1 or N-2 disease who had negative microscopic axillary findings. We do not attribute these negative findings to error in clinical assessment of the axilla, but rather to the effect of chemotherapy. Also, since incisional rather than excisional biopsy was used initially to confirm the diagnosis, chemotherapy must be given credit for eradicating the disease in the four women whose breasts failed to demonstrate evidence of any residual invasive cancer in the mastectomy specimen and the two more with only non-invasive carcinoma.

Only one patient has had local chest wall recurrence, although none of the 44 women undergoing radical mastectomy underwent post-operative irradiation. The only patients who did have radiotherapy, other than the 10 who chose irradiation as primary treatment instead of mastectomy, were two women who underwent modified radical mastectomy whose tumors were found to extend within 0.5 cm. of the posterior margin of the pectoralis fascia. It has been a common practice when dealing with locally advanced breast cancer to employ both mastectomy and post-operative irradiation in those patients who respond to neo-adjuvant chemotherapy. Our results thus far strongly militate against the need for irradiation as a supplement to mastectomy except in specific situations.

We continue to advocate radical mastectomy for these patients, even those who respond remarkably to their chemotherapy. We are uncomfortable about removing only the mass that remains after chemotherapy with a small margin of contiguous normal breast in order to achieve an aesthetically acceptable breast. Most of the cancers we have encountered have been 6-8 cm. in diameter, if not larger, and we have always used the original measurements of the cancer at time of initial biopsy to guide the surgical margins of resection. The patients who underwent modified radical mastectomy rather than radical mastectomy had "small" (5-6 cm.) T-3 cancers, laterally placed in relatively large breasts, so that there was an apparent comfortable distance between the posterior tumor margin and the chest wall; nevertheless, as noted, two of these women had permeation of tumor to within 0.5 cm. of the pectoralis major fascia and did receive post-operative irradiation. If radical mastectomy is the surgical procedure chosen, irradiation should not be necessary except under the most unusual circumstances. This spares the patient from the very high likelihood of arm edema, which almost inevitably accompanies the combination of axillary dissection and post-operative irradiation, as well as the other complications of irradiation added to mastectomy.

Disease-free and overall five year actuarial survival data are considerably better than anticipated for the women who responded to chemotherapy. The projected 5-year survival for this group is over 85% and the disease free survival is more than 65%. Our results thus far are most encouraging. As might be expected, those women who did not respond to chemotherapy failed relatively rapidly.

In summary, we have now employed neo-adjuvant chemotherapy in 100 women with Stage III breast carcinoma. Significant tumor regression has been noted in a majority of patients, 70%, permitting definitive local treatment with greater success than heretofore expected. No patient's disease progressed systemically while she was undergoing neo-adjuvant therapy. Radical mastectomy without supplementary irradiation was used in the majority of these women with excellent local control of disease and much better than anticipated disease-free intervals and absolute survival. Our previously dismal outlook for these unfortunate patients with advanced local disease has been replaced by a more optimistic attitude.

References

1. Brambilla, C., DeLena, M., and Bonadonna, G.: Combination chemotherapy with adriamycin (NSC-123127) in metastatic mammary carcinoma. Cancer Chemother. Rep., 1974; 120: 67-73.
2. Zucali, R., Uslenghi, C., Kenda, R., et al.: Natural history and survival of inoperable breast cancer treated by radiotherapy and radiotherapy followed by radical mastectomy. Cancer, 1976; 37: 1422-31.
3. Morrow, M., Braverman, A., Thelmo, W., et al.: Multimodal therapy for locally advanced breast cancer. Arch. Surg., 1986; 121: 1291-1296.
4. Hortobagyi, G.N., Buzdar, A.U., Montague, E., et al.: Neo-adjuvant chemotherapy for primary breast cancer, in **Neo-Adjuvant Chemotherapy**, edited by Jacquillat, C., Weil, M., and Khayat, D. Paris, Colloque INSERM/John Libbey Eurotext, 1986, pp. 189-196.
5. Lesnick, G., Perloff, M., Korzun, A., et al.: Combination chemotherapy prior to surgery or radiotherapy in locally advanced breast cancer, in **Neo-Adjuvant Chemotherapy**, pp. 207-211.
6. Aisner, J., Morris, D., Elias, E.G., et al.: Mastectomy as an adjuvant to chemotherapy for locally advanced breast cancer. Arch. Surg., 1982; 117: 882-887.
7. Lippman, M.E., Sorace, A., Bagley, C.S., et al: Treatment of locally advanced breast cancer using primary induction chemotherapy with hormonal synchronization followed by radiation therapy with or without debulking surgery. NCI Monographs, Number 1, 1986; 153-159.
8. Schwartz, G.F., Rosenberg, A.L., Danoff, B.F., et al: Lumpectomy and level I axillary dissection prior to irradiation for "operable" breast cancer. Ann. Surg., 1984; 200: 554-5560.560.

Résumé

100 malades atteintes de cancer du sein au stade III ont été traitées par chimiothérapie néoadjuvante avant tout traitement local. La réponse a été jugée après 3 cycles de traitement et chez les répondeurs, le traitement a été continué, jusqu'à ce que la tumeur ou les ganglions axillaires ne montrent plus aucune régression. A ce moment une chirurgie a été pratiquée, puis la chimiothérapie a été reprise après la chirurgie pour un total de 12 cycles. 90 malades sont évaluables. 70 % ont répondu à la chimiothérapie. A notre avis la mastectomie radicale sans radiothérapie post-opératoire semble le meilleur traitement pour les répondeurs. Le suivi médian pour les malades évaluables est de 27 mois. La survie sans rechute des répondeurs est supérieure à 65 % et la survie globale de ce groupe est supérieure à 85 %.

Neo-Adjuvant Chemotherapy. Ed. Cl. Jacquillat, M. Weil, D. Khayat. Colloque INSERM/John Libbey Eurotext Ltd. © 1988. Vol. 169, pp. 207-210.

Neo-adjuvant chemotherapy without radiation therapy in inflammatory breast carcinoma

L. Israël, J.L. Breau and J.F. Morère

Centre Hospitalier Universitaire Avicenne, 125 route de Stalingrad, 93000 Bobigny, France

SUMMARY

Neoadjuvant chemotherapy has already been in use in the field of inflammatory breast ca for several years, before the formulation of the concept, and some of its advantages are clearly seen in this situation. We report here two studies : The first entered 25 patients between november 1978 and September 1983 and has a median follow-up of 68 months. Median age was 48 years, with 13 patients post menopausal. All were submitted to a high dose Cyclophosphamide and a 5 days FU regimen given every 3 weeks with total mastectomy at 3 months, and a two years total chemotherapy without radiation. The median disease free survival has been 48 months and the median survival (including one toxic death and two unrelated deaths) is 52+ months. No complete histologic response was observed. The number of involved lymph nodes retained its prognostic significance. The second current study, with a rotation of CTX-FU-VCR and Cis DDP-BLM includes so far only 10 patients with a median follow-up of 13 months (7+-40+). We have seen 2 complete histologic responses, one relapse and no death. Saving time through immediate chemotherapy, and sparing bone marrow reserves by excluding radiation therapy seem definitely beneficial in the management of this disease.

It is still debatable, in the absence of any long term controlled and randomized study, whether preoperative chemotherapy is of definitive advantage in tumors such as head and neck cancer, and squamous cell ca of the lung, in which the major risk is local, or in slow growing tumors such as conventional breast cancer.

If fast growing tumors, from which the risk is essentially of distant metastases, it seems obvious that the systemic disease be controlled first, by means of the most potent available chemotherapy. This is the case in localized small cell carcinoma of the lung, and in breast cancer of the inflammatory type. The problem of the local control arises some weeks later, when it becomes apparent that the metastatic risk is at least temporarily controlled and that chemotherapy is not effective enough to eradicate the local disease.

Along these lines of evidence we have designed for inflammatory breast carcinoma two consecutive phase II studies in which the local control is of the surgical type and follows 3 courses of intensive chemotherapy, cytostatic drugs being applied afterwards for two years in a less intensive fashion.

THE FIRST STUDY IS NOW COMPLETED

25 patients with inflammatory breast ca involving the entirely of the cutaneous area - and excluding cases which are sometimes counsidered as inflammatory and that involve only a part of this area - were entered from November 1978 to September 1983 with a median follow-up that is presently of 70 months.

Median age was 48 years at the onset of therapy, with 13 patients post menopausal. All were submitted to a chemotherapy regimen described earlier and applied first to metastatic cases (Israël, 1984). It consisted of two drugs applied every 3 weeks, cytoxan at the dose of 1 gram per m2, on day 1, and 5 FU at the dose of 600 mg/m2/day for 5 consecutive days. Total mastectomy was performed 15 to 20 days after the third course and chemotherapy was resumed 3 weeks after surgery and continued for two years (Israël, 1986).

In fact the above doses had to be decreased by 10 to 20 % in a majority of patients due to hematologic toxicity, and cytoxan was further decreased during the course of therapy for 8 additional patient.

Besides, a second line regimen, including Vinblastin, Adriamycin and Mitomycin C was prescribed to 7 patients before the completion of the 2 years, scheme due to recurrent disease. No radiation therapy was given at any time, except lately for control of bone metastasis.

The results were as follows :

Preoperative responses :
24 out of 25 patients were subjected to mastectomy, the 25th patient having died from uncontrolled septicœmia after the second course. 24 objective response were registered, with 2 apparently complete.

Pathologic results at surgery
In 4 cases were only found microscopic remnants scattered throughout the gland. In 20 cases tumor was found, with large areas of necrosis. In 10 cases out of 24 a single tumor mass existed. As for the lymph nodes they were involved in 19 of 24 patients.

Disease free survival
Median DFI was reached at 48 months (8-110). Eight patients are in DFI at 50+, 53+, 54+, 80+, 86+, 94+, 96+ and 110+ months. Among the patients that reached 48 months, 8 out of 12 are surviving and in DFI.

Survival
Median survival is 53+ months, with 12 patients surviving from 50+ to 110+ months, eight of them disease free.

Overall toxicity
Except for one early death, toxicity through moderate to severe has always been manageable.

oOo

The second study was undertaken in an attempt to prolong the median DFI and to increase the cure rate, by means of a more intensive chemotherapy.

Drug regimen

A rotation was designed of a first combination, Cyclophosphamide, FU and Vincristin, given over a 5 day period, every 4 weeks, and a second non myelotoxic combination, Cis-DDP and bleomycin given also over a 5 day period, every 4 weeks in between, so that patients were treated 5 days every 2 weeks. The doses of the initial therapy were reduced, Cyclophosphamide 800 mg/m2 day 1, and 5 FU 500 mg/m2 day 1 through 5, plus Vincristin 1 mg/m2 on day 1. Platine is given at the dose of 20 mg/m2/day for 5 days and bleomycin 5 mg/m2/day for 5 days. Renal and respiratory function are regularly monitored together with blood counts.

Interim results

So far 11 patients have been subjected to total mastectomy with 2 complete responses histologically controlled. The median follow-up is 15 months (9+-42+) with no death but one relapse. 25 patients will be entered.

CONCLUSION

Counsidering only the first study, the registered results compare very favorably with all the results published so far in the litterature.

From the point of view of neoadjuvant chemotherapy, we would like to submit the following remarks :

1. The concept seems to be now universally accepted in the field of inflammatory breast cancer. It is a a matter of topic in a situation where the tumor doubling time is short an the chance of the patient having already metastatic disease virtually 100 %.

2. In such a situation it seems obvious that long term results will be correlated to the rapidity and the intensity of chemotherapy. Hence the necessity to give high doses and to accept severe toxicity.

3. Prolonged chemotherapy seems also in order, since we have registered 16 recurrences out of 24 cases, the majority of them being after cessation of therapy. It follows that surgery for local control is better suited than radiation therapy, due to the importance of sparing bone marrow reserves.

4. Future improvements should rely on more potent chemotherapies, as in our study number II, but also probably on additional procedures designed to control pleiotropic resistance.

REFERENCES

Israël, L., Breau, J.L., Aguilera, J. (1984) : High dose cyclophosphamide and high dose 5 fluoro-uracil : A new first line regimen for advanced breast cancer. Cancer 53, 1655-1659.

Israël, L., Breau, J.L., Morère, J.F. (1986) : Two years of high-dose cyclophosphamide and 5-fluorouracil followed by surgery after 3 months for acute inflammatory breast carcinomas. A phase II study of 25 cases with a median follow-up of 35 months. Cancer, 57, 24-28.

Résumé

Les résultats d'une chimiothérapie première, avant mastectomie puis reprise d'une chimiothérapie prolongée, sans irradiation, sont rapportés dans les cancers inflammatoires du sein. Dans une première étude, 25 patientes ont été traitées par Cyclophosphamide et 5 Fluorouracile, 3 cycles avant mastectomie, suivie de la même chimiothérapie durant 2 ans, avec un suivi médian de 70 mois. Malgré l'absence de réponse complète histologique, les médianes de survie sans récidive et la survie sont de 48 et 52+ mois. La chimiothérapie a été renforcée dans une deuxième étude en cours, par l'association Cisplatine-Bléomycine. 11 patientes ont été opérées, avec un recul médian de 13 mois. Une récidive sans décès a été observée.

Neo-Adjuvant Chemotherapy. Ed. Cl. Jacquillat, M. Weil, D. Khayat. Colloque INSERM/John Libbey Eurotext Ltd. © 1988. Vol. 169, pp. 211-214.

Inflammatory breast cancer : neo-adjuvant chemotherapy with vindesin, adriamycin and cyclophosphamide

J.P. Malhaire [1], B. Chevallier [2], D. Barral [3], J.Y. Genot [4], M.J. Goudier [5], P. Kerbrat [6], D. Gedoin [6] and M.F. Morice [5]

[1] *Centre Hospitalier Régional et Universitaire, Service d'Oncologie et de Radiothérapie, Avenue Foch, 29279 Brest Cedex, France*
[2] *Centre H. Becquerel, 76038 Rouen Cedex, France*
[3] *Laboratoire Lilly France, 203 Bureaux de la Colline, 92213 Saint Cloud, France*
[4] *Centre F. Baclesse, 14021 Caen Cedex, France*
[5] *Centre Hospitalier Régional, 56322 Lorient Cedex, France*
[6] *Centre E. Marquis, 35011 Rennes Cedex, France*

SUMMARY : 44 unilateral nonmetastatic inflammatory breast cancer patients have been included in this prospective multicentric pilot study. The protocol of neo-adjuvant chemotherapy was a combination of IV administration of Vindesin, Adriamycin and Cyclophosphamide. The number of courses repeated every 3 weeks was of 2, 4 or 6 before loco-regional treatment depending on the response to chemotherapy. Complete response rates on tumor and inflammatory signs were respectively of 9 % and 48 % after 2 courses and 15 % and 75 % after 4 courses. But the percentage of total response did not improve after 2 more courses. Radical modified mastectomy with axillary node dissection was performed on 15 patients (CR = 3, PR = 12) : 4 were actually in complete histological response. The main toxicity of the chemotherapy regimen was haematologic, with profound nadir but rapid recovery allowing next course at D21 in 80 % of the cases. One death from a septic shock concomitant of an aplasia grade 4 was to deplore. These results suggest that this chemotherapy regimen has a major antitumor effect on inflammatory breast cancer. Its impact on overall survival is still to be evaluated.

Key-words : Inflammatory breast cancer, neo-adjuvant chemotherapy
Mots-clés : cancer du sein inflammatoire, chimiothérapie néo-adjuvante

Inflammatory Carcinoma of the breast represents 1 % to 7 % of all breast cancers (1, 2, 3, 4, 5) and is defined mainly by clinical features such as skin erythema, skin edema or peau d'orange and increase in local heat (2, 4, 6). Some authors also include the ridging of the skin (7). The invasion of dermal lymphatics by neoplasic cells has been proposed as the characteristic histological criterion (4, 7, 8). Although there has been definite progresses with the introduction of neo-adjuvant chemotherapy within the last decade, the prognosis remains very disappointing as regards survival and it looks as if only a complete histological response might allow a better prognosis.

The aims of this nonrandomized and multicentric trial were first to assess the response rate and particularly the number of complete clinical and histological responses to this protocol which associates Vindesin, Adriamycin (doxorubicin hypochloride) and Cyclophosphamide, and next to try to determine the optimal number of courses to carry out before loco-regional treatment.

Patients and Methods

* Patients characteristics :

Between June 30th 1986 and October 1st 1987, 44 patients aged 32-69 (average 53,6) with a unilateral inflammatory breast cancer were included in the multicentric trial. 21 patients were still actively menstruating and 23 were postmenopausal. All carcinomas had been confirmed by biopsy and inflammatory cancer corresponded to the clinical criteria given above. The extent of inflammatory signs was localized in 32 patients (PEV 2) and diffuse to the whole breast (PEV 3) in 12. None of the cancers was metastatic, according to standard methods of evaluation : clinical examination, standard biology, chest X ray, bone scintigraphy and liver echography.

Patients were all under 70 years old and no previous treatment had been given. TNM classification was as follows : T4b N0 : 5 ; T4b N1a : 1 ; T4b N1b : 29 ; T4b N2 : 4 ; T4b N3 : 4 ; T4c N 3 : 1.

* Treatment schedule :

Chemotherapy consisted of intravenous administration of Vindesin, 1 mg/m² from day 1 to day 4 and of Adriamycin, 15 mg/m² and Cyclophosphamide, 200 mg/m² from day 1 to day 3. Each course was repeated every 3 weeks. In order to respect as much as possible the 3 week interval between courses, an adaptation of the doses had been elaborated if neutrophils were under 2,000/mm³ and/or platelets were under 100,000/mm³, and the course was postponed for one week if neutrophils were < 1,000/mm³ and/or platelets were < 50,000/mm³.
The theoretical number of courses was 6 but chemotherapy was i nterrupted after 2 courses in case of tumor progression within these first two courses and after 4 courses if at least a partial response had not been obtained. As the aim of this trial was only to test neo-adjuvant chemotherapy, loco-regional and adjuvant treatments were performed according to each centre's protocol currently in use.

* Evaluation of response and toxicity :

- Tumor response was defined by clinical examination and mammography according to WHO criteria [complete (CR), partial (PR), no change (NC), progression (PD)] after 2, 4 and 6 courses.

- Response on inflammatory signs was defined as follows : CR (complete disappearance of all inflammatory signs for at least 3 weeks), PR (partial disappearance of all inflammatory signs for at least 3 weeks), NC (no change), PD (progression)

- Toxicity corresponded to WHO grading (0 to 4).

Results :

- Toxicity : 42 courses of chemotherapy had to be postponed for one week for hematological toxicity. None was postponed for more.
The most tragic side-effect to deplore is one death due to a septic shock which occured during aplasia stage 4. Other infectious complications were only grade I and 2.
Alopecia was found grade 3 in 37 patients and grades I or 2 for the others.
Nausea and vomiting were very frequent but mainly grade I and 2.
A peripheral neuropathy stage 3 imposed to stop Vindesin in one patient. Another patient was taken out of the protocol for cardiac toxicity grade I.

- Response rate :

* after 2 courses 21 patients were in CR as regards inflammatory signs (48 %), 13 in PR (CR + PR : 77 %) ; tumor regressed totally in 4 patients (9 %) and partially in 20 (CR + PR : 55 %) ; out of 39 patients with clinical metastatic nodes 11 were in CR (28 %) and 19 in PR (CR + PR : 77 %). 2 patients were taken out of the protocole after 2 courses because of progression of the disease (PD), one for mild cardiac toxicity and are for a psychiatric probleme unrelated to the chemotherapy.

* after 4 courses, out of the remaining patients 27 were in CR (68 %) and 9 in PR (CR + PR : 90 %) for inflammatory signs, 6 in CR (15 %) and 24 in PR (CR + PR : 75 %) for the tumor, and 18 in CR (52 %) and 12 in PR (CR + PR : 88 %) for the nodes.

* but none of the patients in partial remission at 4 courses who received 2 more courses of chemotherapy could reach a complete response.

- It should be added that 15 patients were operated (mastectomy with axillary lymph node dissection), 3 of whom were considered on clinical CR and 12 on clinical PR ; in fact 4/15 were actually on complete histological response.

Discussion

This study avaluated the effectiveness of neo-adjuvant chemotherapy in the induction treatment of inflammatory breast cancer. Most of the inflammatory signs retroceded rapidly after the first 2 to 4 courses of chemotherapy. The results obtained both on inflammation and tumor rejoin those of other studies with, after 4 courses of chemotherapy,15% of complete response and 75 % of partial response compared to 14 % and 81 % for Chauvergne and al (8), 9,8 % and 53 % for Mignot and al (4), 19 % of complete response for De Lena and al (6), 8 % and 88 % for Israël and al (3) and 20 % and 73 % for Ravina and al (6).
In spite of their bad prognosis, it confirms the high response rate of these inflammatory tumors to chemotherapy, which not only facilitates loco-regional treatment but also, as all recent essays confirm improves notably disease - free and overall survivals (1, 3, 5, 6, 8,10, 11, 12, 13) even if the curve does not seem to reach any plateau (2, 4, 7).

The other results of this trial was to point out that maximal response rates were already observed among our patients after 4 chemotherapy courses and that continuing chemotherapy did not seem to improve the quality of the inital local response. Most of the trials mentioned above consisted of 2 to 5 courses of chemotherapy before loco-regional treatment. Nevertherless, two groups (5, 6) notice in their studies that although clinical signs of inflammation totally receded within the very first courses, it might require 4 to 7 courses to reach a thermographic return to normal.

Finally, the toxicity of our induction chemotherapy regimen in spite of one death by infection in aplasia stage 4, remains acceptable when compared to other trials. In this pilot study, the effect of chemotherapy on disease- free survival and overall survival has not been evaluated.

REFERENCES

1 - A.V. Buzdar, E.D. Montague, J.L. Barker, G.N. Hortobagyi, G.R. Blumenschein : Management of Inflammatory Carcinoma of the Breast with Combined Modality Approach. An Update : Cancer, 47 : 2537-2542, 1981.
2 - B. Chevallier, B. Asselain, A. Kunlin, C. Veyret, P. Bastit, Y. Graïc : Inflammatory Breast Cancer - determination of Prognostic Factors by Univariate and Multivariate Analysis : Cancer, 60 : 897-902, 1987.

3 - L. Israël, J.L. Breau, J.F. Morere : Two years of High Dose Cyclophosphamide and 5-Fluorouracil followed by surgery after 3 Months for Acute Inflammatory Breast Carcinomas : Cancer , 57 : 24-28, 1986.
4 - L. Mignot, M. Espie, F. Morvan, A. De Roquancourt, D. Belpomme, A. Gorins, M. Marty : Cancers du sein en poussée évolutive - Expérience du groupe St Louis-Beaujon. A propos de 71 cas : Gynécologie, 35 : 175-180, 1984.
5 - B. Zylberberg, J. Salat-Baroux, J.H. Ravina, D. Dormont, J.P. Amiel, P. Diebold, V. Izraël : Initial Chemoimmunotherapy in Inflammatory Carcinoma of the Breast : Cancer, 49 : 1537-1943, 1982.
6 - J.H. Ravina, J. Salat, A. Letessier, X. Ayral, P. Madelenat, B. Zylberberg : Immuno-polychimiothérapie dans les cancers inflammatoires primitifs du sein. Essai thérapeutique : Chirurgie, 108 : 32-36, 1982.
7 - N.A. Fastenberg, A.U. Buzdar, E.D. Montague, J.M. Jessup, R.G. Martin, G.N. Hortobagyi, G.R. Blumenschein : Management in inflammatory Carcinoma of the Breast : a combined modality approach : Am. J. Clin. Oncol., 8 : 134-141,1985
8 - J. Chauvergne, M. Durand, M.H. Dilhuydy, B. Hoerni, T. Germain, C. Lagarde : Traitement des cancers du sein inflammatoires : Etude contrôlée d'un programme d'association thérapeutique : Rev. Fr. Gynéc. Obstét., 76 : 227-235, 1981.
9 - M. De Lena, R. Zucali, G. Viganotti, P. Valagussa, G. Bonadonna : Combined chemotherapy - radiotherapy approach in locally advanced breast cancer - Cancer Chemother. Pharmacol., 1 : 53-59, 1978.
10 - P. Pouillart, T. Palangie, M. Jouve, E.Garcia-Giralt, J.R. Vilcoq, J.P. Bataini, B. Asselain : Cancer Inflammatoire du sein traité par une association de chimiothérapie et d'irradiation, Bull. Cancer, 68 : 171-186, 1981.
11 - J. Rouëssé, M. Spielmann, T. Le Chevalier, R. Arriagada, H. Mouriesse, J.P. Munck, J.L. Amiel, C. Toussaint, D. Sarrazin, F. May-Levin : Chimiothérapie première dans le traitement des cancers du sein inflammatoires : 230 observations La Presse Médicale, 16 : 475-478, 1987.
12 - C. Wiseman, J.P. Jessup, T.L. Smith, E. Hersh, J. Bowen, G. Blumenshein : Inflammatory Breast Cancer Treated With Surgery, Chemotherapy and Allogeneic Tumor Cell/BCG Immunotherapy : Cancer 49 : 1266-1271, 1982.
13 - N. Mourali, F. Tabbanc, L. Muenz, J.Bahi, S. Belhassen, L. Kamaraju, P. Levi : Preliminary results of primary systemic chemotherapy in association with surgery or radiotherapy in rapidly progressing breast cancer. Br. J. Cancer, 45, 367-374, 1982.

Résumé

44 patientes présentant un cancer du sein inflammatoire, unilatéral,non métastasé ont été incluses dans cet essai pilote prospectif multicentrique. Le protocole de chimiothérapie néo-adjuvante associant la Vindésine, l'Adriamycine et le Cyclophosphamide administrés par voie IV. Le nombre des cures, répétées toutes les 3 semaines, a été de 2,4 ou 6 avant traitement loco-régional en fonction de la réponse à la chimiothérapie. Les taux de réponses complètes sur la tumeur et les signes inflammatoires ont été recpectivement de 9% et 48% après 2 cures et de 15% et 75 % après 4 cures. Mais le pourcentage de réponses complètes n'a pu être amélioré par 2 cures supplémentaires. 15 Patientes ont subi une mammectomie avec curage axillaire (CR = 3, PR = 12) ; en fait 4 ont été retrouvées en RC histologique. La toxicité éssentielle a été hématologique avec un nadir profond mais une récupération rapide autorisant la cure suivante à J 21 dans 80% des cas. Un décès par choc septique contemporain d'une aplasie de grade4 est à déplorer. Ces résultats suggèrent que l'association testée possède une efficacité antitumorale majeure dans le cancer du sein inflammatoire. Son effet sur la survie globale reste à préciser.

Breast cancer IV

Cancer du sein IV

Neo-Adjuvant Chemotherapy. Ed. Cl. Jacquillat, M. Weil, D. Khayat. Colloque INSERM/John Libbey Eurotext Ltd. © 1988. Vol. 169, pp. 217-223.

Experimental comparative study of adjuvant and/or neo-adjuvant chemotherapy, or hormonotherapy or immunotherapy applied to a hormone receptor carrying murine mammary tumor

G. Mathé, C. Bourut, E. Chenu, Y. Kidani, Y. Mauvernay, A.V. Schally and P. Reizenstein

Institut du Cancer et d'Immunogénétique (Université Paris-Sud, CNRS UA 04-1163), Hôpital Paul-Brousse, 94800 Villejuif, France

ABSTRACT

MA 16/C is a spontaneous, hormone-dependent, mouse mammary adenocarcinoma. It was injected s.c. on C3H/He female mice on day 0. Tumors were excised on day 15.
Neoadjuvant treatments were applied from day 1 to day 21 for hormonotherapy and immunotherapy, and on days 1, 5 and 9 for chemotherapy.
Adjuvant treatments were applied from day 21 to day 42 for hormonotherapy and immunotherapy, and on days 21, 25 and 29 for chemotherapy.
Mixed (neoadjuvant and adjuvant) treatments combined the two patterns.
Chemotherapy consisted of an oxalato-platinum complex of trans-l-dach (l-OHP) at the dose of 5 mg/kg i.p. Hormonotherapy consisted of D-Trp6-LH-RH at the dose of 100µg/kg i.p.. Immunotherapy consisted of zinc gluconate, known to regulate CD8 cells at the dose of 6mg/kg per os, and of bestatin, known to regulate CD4 cells at the dose of 6mg/kg per os.
In the condition where surgery alone did not cure any animal, adjuvant or neoadjuvant chemotherapy or the combination of both, induced about 40% cure at the second month, which is a highly significant benefit as compared to surgery alone. Adjuvant hormonotherapy or neoadjuvant or the combination of both and finally the combination of both neoadjuvant and adjuvant immunotherapy give a benefit which is not significantly different from that of chemotherapy.

Key words: adjuvant - neo-adjuvant - chemotherapy - hormonotherapy - immunotherapy

INTRODUCTION

The general failure of so-called adjuvant (A) chemotherapy (CT) is recognized in the case of solid tumors (13), except breast cancer in non menopaused patients on which CMF (cyclophosphamide, methotrexate, 5-fluorouracil) has been calculated by Peto (17), to give a 9% benefit in survival, and AVCF (adriamycin, vincristine, cyclophosphamide, 5-fluorouracil) has been shown by OncoFrance (12) to give 30% more than CMF at the seventh year.

As the effect of both combinations is not found after menopausis and as it correlates with the incidence of amenorrhea induced by CMF (3) and by ours AVCF (12), one cannot eliminate a hormonosuppressive action of chemotherapy.

Facing this post-surgical so-called adjuvant chemotherapy failure in solid tumors, several groups, including ours, have shifted to presurgical so-called "neo-adjuvant (NA) chemotherapy" based on never confirmed experimental preliminary result (16) and a few clinical trial results including ours for head and neck tumors (11) and breast cancer (6).

For both these tumors our objective today attained was to avoid all functional and esthetic mutilations and deteriorating action of intensive chemotherapy (4).

MATERIALS AND METHODS

The murine adenocarcinoma used is MA16/C which is known to bear estrogen and progestative receptors, which we have checked up.

Forteen groups of 16 C3H/He female mice received subcutaneous implants of carcinoma on day 0. Tumors of 10 groups were excised on day 15: three groups (CT), were given neoadjuvant chemotherapy on days 1, 5 and 9 (NACT) or adjuvant CT on days 21, 25 and 29 (ACT) with an oxalato-platinum complex of trans-l-dach (l-OHP, 5mg/kg body weight intraperitoneally, i.p.) or the combination of NACT and ACT. Another three groups, hormonotherapy (HT), were given neo-adjuvant hormonotherapy (NAHT) with the LH-RH agonist D-Trp6-LH-RH (100μg/kg i.p.) on days 1-21, or adjuvant HT (AHT) on days 21-42 or the combination of both NAHT and AHT. The last three groups, immunotherapy (IT), were given neo-adjuvant treatment (NAIT) with zinc gluconate (6mg/kg orally, daily) and with bestatin (6mg/kg p.o. every second day) on days 1 to 21 or adjuvant IT (AIT) on days 21 to 42 or the combination of NAIT and AIT. The tenth group was the surgery control group. Four groups without excision received treatment alone (CT, IT or HT) or no treatment (tumor control). The end-point was mouse survival.

The reasons of the choice of these four agents were that: a) 1-OHP has been shown by us maximally acting without renal toxicity in our screening murine tumors (8), and in man in a phase I trial with intra-patient escalation method (9); b) D-Trp-6-LH-RH has been shown to be efficient in human breast cancer (5) as well as in prostate cancer (14) and in gynecological papilloma virus in situ carcinoma and dysplasias (7); c) finally bestatin has been shown by us, experimentally (2) and clinically (15), to regulate CD4 (helper) lymphocytes, and zinc gluconate has been shown to regulate CD8 (cytotoxic-suppressor) lymphocytes (10).

RESULTS

Surgery: alone does not cure any animal. It has a positive effect in combination with HT. Its effect is weak incombination with CT which is active by itself and IT which is middly efficient even with surgery (Table 1).

TABLE 1

% CURED ANIMALS AT DAY 60 AFTER: CT, HT, IT AND SURGERY ALONE

	TREATMENT ALONE	NEOADJUVANT	ADJUVANT	NEOADJUVANT + ADJUVANT
1-OHP	40	62	66	43
D-Trp-6-LH-RH	10	55	40	50
ZINC GLUCONATE + BESTATINE	0	0	6	21
SURGERY	0			

CHEMOTHERAPY: 1-OHP 5mg/kg i.p., days 1,5,9 Neoadjuvant (NA); days 21,25,29 Adjuvant (A), or days 1,5,9,21,25,29 (NA+A)
IMMUNOTHERAPY: Zinc gluconate: 6mg/kg p.o. + bestatine 6mg/kg p.o. days 1 —— 21 for NA, 21 —— 42 for A, or 1 —— 42 (NA+A)
HORMONOTHERAPY: D-Trp-6-LH-RH 100μg/kg i.p. days 1 —— 21 for NA, 21 —— 42 for A, or 1 —— 42 (NA+A)

CT and HT. There is no significant difference neither between patterns of treatment administration: NA, A or NA+A, nor between CT or HT treatments taken as a whole: percentages of alive mice at day 60, are similar in all groups treated by surgery and CT or HT (Tables 1 and 2).

TABLE 2

COMPARISON BETWEEN CR, HT AND IT TREATMENTS OF MA 16/C: STATISTICS

			CHEMOTHERAPY			HORMONOTHERAPY			IMMUNOTHERAPY		
		SURGERY	NA	A	NA+A	NA	A	NA+A	NA	A	NA+A
	NA	NS	S	S	S	S	S	S		NS	S
IMMUNOTHERAPY	A	NS	S	S	S	S	S	S			S
	NA+A	S	S	S	NS	S	S	NS			
	NA	S	NS	NS	NS		NS	NS			
HORMONOTHERAPY	A	S	NS	NS	NS			NS			
	NA+A	S	NS	NS	NS						
	NA	S		NS	NS						
CHEMOTHERAPY	A	S			NS						
	NA+A	S									

STATISTICS: χ_2 TEST
NS: NOT SIGNIFICANT
S: SIGNIFICANT

IT. It must be long-dated (NA+A) administered so it is efficient. In this case only, result of IT treatment is statistically equivalent to those obtained with CT and HT.

DISCUSSION

In this experimental system, the remaining of residual disease after surgical excision can be either prevented or cured in 20-60% of the animals, ie, in a non significantly different proportion whether it consist of preoperative (neoadjuvant) or/and postoperative (adjuvant) therapy, and whether it is chemotherapy or hormonotherapy. Combined pre and post operative immunotherapy, hormonotherapy and chemotherapy give an identical benefit.

The fact that for chemotherapy and hormonotherapy, the combinations of both presurgical and post-surgical applications do not increase the proportions of cured animals is in favor of our previously published concept according to which 30% only of the patients in a population affected by a certain tumor are sensitive to chemotherapy, and 30% by hormonotherapy, those affected by immunotherapy being other subjects, as we showed by the survival curve analysis (1).

Our object is to develop our experimental model in order it may detect these three populations respectively, sensitive to the different therapies.

In practice, the presently published result autorises clinical trials on neo-adjuvant or neo-adjuvant + adjuvant chemotherapy or hormonotherapy or immunotherapy.

ACKNOWLEDGEMENT

We thank Nicole Vriz for their excellent editorial assistance.

REFERENCES

1. Eriguchi, M., and Mathé, G. (1986): New survival curve model for comparison of adjuvant therapy of malignant diseases. Biomed. & Pharmacother., 40, 143-147.
2. Florentin, I., Mathé, G., and Bruley-Rosset, M. (1984): Do tuftsin and bestatin constitute a biopharmacologic immunoregulatory system? In Progress in cancer chemo-immunotherapy, ed G. Mathé and H. Umezawa, pp. 180-192, Tokyo, Japan Antibiotics Research Association.
3. Howell, A., George, W.D., Crowther, D., Rubens, R.D., Bulbrook, R.D., Bush, H., Howat, J.M.T., Sellwood, R.A., Hayward, J.L., Fentiman, I.S., and Chaudary, M. (1984): Controlled trial of adjuvant chemotherapy with cyclophosphamide, methotrexate, and fluorouracil for breast cancer. Lancet ii, 307-311.
4. Jacquillat C., Baillet F., Auclerc G., Khayat D., Blondon J., Auclerc M.F., Facchin T., Lefranc J.P., and Weil M. Neoadjuvant chemotherapy of breast cancer. In Clinical trials in oncology: Ethics, errors, methods and results. eds P. Reizenstein, G. Mathé & M. Dicato (eds), pp. 147-152, Geneva: Bioscience Ediprint, 1986.
5. Keiling, R., Mathé, G., Misset, J.L., VoVan, M.L., Gastiaburu, J. 1988): D-Trp-6-LH-RH in breast carcinoma. Biomed. & Pharmacother., in press.
6. Mathé, G., Baruch, J., Umezawa, U., Umezawa, K., Misset, J.L., Jasmin, C., Musset, M., Ribaud, P., Despax, R., and Brienza, S. (1988): THP-adriamycin or pirarubicin combined to a vinca alcaloid, an alkylating agent and fluorouracil for the treatment of advanced breast cancer and the primary (neoadjuvant) treatment of breast cancer: toward a breast cancer primary neoadjuvant chemotherapy followed by immediate plastic surgery. In 15th International Congress of Chemotherapy, Istanbul, July 1987 (in press).
7. Mathé, G., Busuttil, M., Reynes, M., Hagipantelli, R., Mauvernay, Y., and Schally, A.V. (1988): D-Trp-6-LH-RH (Decapeptyl) in the treatment cervical and vaginal dysplasias related to 16 or 18 papilloma virus. Submitted to The Lancet.
8. Mathé, G., Kidani, Y., Noji, M., Maral, R., Bourut, C., and Chenu, E.

(1985): Antitumor activity of 1-OHP in mice. Cancer Letters 27, 135-143.

9. Mathé, G., Kidani, Y., Triana, K., Brienza, S., Ribaud, P., Goldschmidt, E., Ecstein, E., Despax, R., Musset, M., and Misset, J.L. (1986): A phase I trial of trans-1-diamino-cyclohexane oxalato-platinum (1-OHP). Biomed. & Pharmacother., 40, 372-376.

10. Mathé, G., Misset, J.L., Gil-Delgado, M., Musset, M., Reizenstein, P., and Canon C. (Stat. Anal.: Itzhaki M., and Gaget H.) (1986): A phase II trial of immunorestoration with zinc gluconate in immunodepressed cancer patients. Biomed. & Pharmacother., 40, 383-385.

11. Mathé, G., Musset, M., Abitbol, J., Misset, J.L., Breteau, N., Favre, A., Deboise, J., Goldschmidt, E., Benkemoun, J.P., and Hagipantelli, R. (1988): Primary (neo-adjuvant) chemotherapy in larynx cancer. A phase II study. In 2nd Internat. Congress on Neo-Adjuvant Chemotherapy, Paris, Februrary 19-21, 1988 (abstract).

12. Mathé, G., Plagne, R., Morice, V. & Misset, J.L. for the OncoFrance Breast Cancer Trial Group (1987): Consistencies and variations of observations during serial analyses of a trial of adjuvant chemotherapy in breast cancer. In Adjuvant therapy of Cancer V, ed S.E. Salmon, pp. 271-280, Orlando: Grune & Stratton.

13. Mathé, G., Reizenstein P., and Eriguchi M. (1986): Clinical trials of the treatment of minimal residual tumours. In Clinical trials in oncology: Ethics, errors, methods and results. eds P. Reizenstein, G. Mathé & M. Dicato (eds), pp. 83-98, Geneva: Bioscience Ediprint, 1986.

14. Mathé, G., Schally, A.V., Comaru-Schally, A.M., Mauvernay, R.Y., VoVan M.L., Machover, D., Misset, J.L., Court, B., Bouchard, P., Duchier, J., Morin, P., Keiling, R., Schwarzenberg, L., Kerbrat, P., Achille, E., Tronc, J.C., Fendler, J.P., Pappo, E., Metz, R., and Prevot, G. (1986): Phase II trial with D-Trp-6-LH-RH in prostatic carcinoma: comparison with other hormonal agents. Prostate, 9, 327-342.

15. Mathé, G., Umezawa, H., Misset, J.L., Brienza, S., Canon, C., Musset, M., and Reizenstein, P. (Stat. Anal.: Itzhaki, M., and Gaget, H.) (1986): Immunomodulating properties of bestatin in cancer patients. A phase II trial. Biomed. & Pharmacother., 40, 379-382.

16. Papaioannou, A. (1981): Preoperative chemotherapy for operable solid tumors. Europ. J. Cancer 17, 263-269.

17. Peto, R. (1985): Private meeting on early breast cancer trial, BCTCS, NCI UICC, WHO, Washington, Sept. 1985.

Résumé

Le MA 16/C est un adénocarcinome mammaire murin, spontané, hormonodépendant. Il a été injecté par voie sous-cutané chez des souris femelles C3H/He au jour 0. Les tumeurs ont été excisées au jour 15. Des traitements neoadjuvants ont été appliqués du jour 1 au jour 21 pour l'hormonothérapie et pour l'immunothérapie, ainsi qu'aux jours 1, 5 et 9 pour la chimiothérapie. Des traitements adjuvants ont été appliqués du jour 21 au jour 42 pour l'hormonothérapie et l'immunothérapie, ainsi qu'aux jours 21, 25 et 29 pour la chimiothérapie. Des traitements mixtes (neoadjuvants et adjuvants) ont combiné les deux systèmes. La chimiothérapie était constituée par un complexe oxalato-platine de "trans-I-dach" (1-OPH) à une dose de 5 mg/kg par voie intrapéritonéale. L'hormonothérapie était constituée par le "D-Trp6-LH-RH" à la dose de 100 μg/kg par voie intrapéritonéale. L'immunothérapie était constituée par du gluconate de zinc, connu pour réguler les cellules CD8, à la dose de 6 mg/kg par voie orale et par de la bestatine, connue pour réguler les cellules CD4 à la dose de 6 mg/kg par voie orale. Dans la situation dans laquelle la chirurgie seule n'assurait la guérison d'aucun animal, la chimiothérapie adjuvante ou neoadjuvante, ou la combinaison des deux systèmes, a provoqué une guérison d'environ 50% des animaux au second mois, ce qui est un avantage hautement important par rapport à la chirurgie seule. L'hormonothérapie adjuvante ou neoadjuvante, ou la combinaison des deux systèmes, ainsi que l'immunothérapie neoadjuvante et adjuvante ont donné des résultats qui ne sont pas notablement différents de ceux obtenus pour la chimiothérapie.

Neo-Adjuvant Chemotherapy. Ed. Cl. Jacquillat, M. Weil, D. Khayat. Colloque INSERM/John Libbey Eurotext Ltd. © 1988. Vol. 169, pp. 225-230.

Traitement combiné de 270 cancers mammaires localement étendus : résultats d'un programme thérapeutique contrôlé

J. Chauvergne, M. Durand, L. Mauriac, M. David, J. Pigneux, M.-H. Dilhuydy, A. Avril, R. Denépoux, D. Marée et F. Bonichon

Fondation Bergonié, 180, rue de Saint Genès, 33076 Bordeaux Cedex, France

RÉSUMÉ

Une chimiothérapie initiale, une radiothérapie et/ou une chirurgie d'exérèse d'un reliquat tumoral, puis une chimiothérapie complémentaire, suivie ou non d'une immunostimulation par lévamisole, ont été successivement appliqués de mai 1981 à juin 1985 à 270 malades non métastatiques, porteuses d'adénocarcinomes mammaires évolués, inopérables d'emblée.

L'induction chimiothérapique, sans différence significative selon l'ordre d'application des schémas d'association (doxorubicine + vincristine + méthotrexate et mitomycine C + thiotepa + vindésine), dans le cadre d'un premier essai randomisé, a permis d'obtenir 222 réponses de plus de 50 % (82,2 % des cas) dont 69 réponses apparemment complètes (25,5 %) ; 180 patientes ont été ensuite radiothérapées (dont 20 après exérèse) et 90 ont été uniquement opérées de façon large. Après confirmation de la rémission complète en fin de traitement adjuvant (appliqué chez 225 patientes) il a été fait une randomisation (2ème essai) en vue d'une immunothérapie complémentaire.

Les résultats se sont maintenus chez 158 malades (58,5 %) avec une médiane de rémission et une médiane de survie globale non atteintes à 70 mois. L'évolution a été influencée par la qualité de la réponse à la chimiothérapie initiale ($p < 0,01$) mais les facteurs pronostiques prédominants ont été les signes inflammatoires, l'atteinte ganglionnaire ($p < 0,01$) et la présence de récepteurs d'estrogènes ($p = 0,01$). Le type de traitement locorégional et la chimiothérapie adjuvante n'ont pas modifié l'évolution d'ensemble. Les différences de survie, selon qu'il y ait eu ou non du lévamisole, ne sont pas significatives. Ces résultats sont sensiblement supérieurs à ceux obtenus dans une étude antérieure similaire (1975-78) en termes de rémissions immédiates et de durée de survie, chez des malades présentant le même pronostic péjoratif. Ils fournissent en outre d'utiles indications pour les orientations thérapeutiques ultérieures (allègement pour les malades en évolution favorable prévisible et renforcement de l'induction pour les cas à très hauts risques).

MOTS CLEFS

Cancers mammaires inopérables, chimiothérapie d'induction, traitement combiné, facteurs pronostiques.

INTRODUCTION

Le mauvais pronostic général des cancers du sein évolués sur le plan locorégional ou rapidement évolutifs est lié à la grande fréquence des métastases à distance déjà présentes à la mise en traitement. La chimiothérapie a pour but d'agir sur cette maladie générale inapparente. Quand elle est faite précocément, elle peut en outre apporter une contribution au contrôle durable des lésions locales inopérables d'emblée (2). La présente étude porte sur les résultats obtenus dans une série de 270 cancers mammaires de ce type traités de mai 1981 à juin 1985 selon un programme thérapeutique homogène (3).

MALADES et MÉTHODES

Les malades traitées étaient des femmes de moins de 75 ans présentant un cancer localement avancé mais sans métastase décelable au terme d'un bilan préthérapeutique complet (clinique, radiographique, scintigraphique et biologique). Elles ont été dans tous les cas déclarées inopérables d'emblée pour des raisons locales ; 270 malades ont été retenues pour l'étude complète, avec une durée d'observation allant de deux à six ans après le début du traitement, qui a été intégralement appliqué ; elles avaient un âge médian de 52 ans, 56 % étaient ménopausées et 88 % avaient des conditions de vie initiales très satisfaisantes (catégorie 0 du code OMS).

Les cancers traités étaient tous des adénocarcinomes infiltrants, diagnostiqués par drill biopsie ou prélèvement ganglionnaire, classés cliniquement en majorité dans la catégorie T4 (74 % des cas) et présentant des adénopathies axillaires mobiles (57 %) ou fixées et sus-claviculaires (27 % des cas).

TRAITEMENTS

a - ***Protocoles de chimiothérapie*** : il a été utilisé deux schémas d'association de médicaments sans résistance croisée, administrés en perfusions uniques, répétées toutes les trois semaines et comportant pour le schéma DVM : de la doxorubicine (50 mg/m^2), de la vincristine (1 mg/m^2), du méthotrexate (20 mg/m^2) et pour le schéma MTV : de la mitomycine C (10 mg/m^2), du thiotépa (20 mg/m^2),de la vindésine (4 mg/m^2). Dans le cas d'une réponse insuffisante à la chimiothérapie initiale il a été appliqué en adjuvant le protocole CMF en perfusions uniques toutes les trois semaines (cyclophosphamide 600 mg/m^2, méthotrexate 40 mg/m^2, fluorouracile 600 mg/m^2). En plus de la chimiothérapie, les malades ayant des récepteurs hormonaux ont reçu du tamoxifène à la dose de 30 mg/jour de façon continue pendant deux ans. Les malades n'ayant pas de récepteurs ont reçu de la prednisone associée aux cycles de chimiothérapie par série de cinq jours débutant le même jour que la chimiothérapie et renouvelée toutes les trois semaines à la dose quotidienne de 40 mg/m^2.

b - ***Traitement locorégional*** : la radiothérapie a été appliquée à la dose de 60 Gy sur le sein et 45 Gy sur les aires ganglionnaires axillo-sus-claviculaires et mammaires internes. L'irradiation a été poussée jusqu'à 80 Gy sur le siège tumoral (électrons) en l'absence d'une chirurgie complémentaire et jusqu'à 60 à 75 Gy sur les territoires lymphatiques. Quand la décision d'exérèse a été prise, il a été réalisé, chaque fois que possible, une tumorectomie avec évidement axillaire et dans les autres cas une mastectomie avec curage selon la technique de Patey.

c - *Le programme thérapeutique général* a comporté quatre phases successives :

1°) Une chimiothérapie d'induction comportant trois cycles de chacune des deux associations ; à ce niveau un premier essai comparatif a été réalisé pour déterminer si l'ordre de succession des deux types de traitement (fixés par randomisation) pourrait influer sur les résultats immédiats ou à plus long terme.

2°) Le traitement locorégional modulé en fonction de la réponse obtenue : chirurgie d'exérèse en présence d'un reliquat tumoral opérable ou irradiation dans les autres cas.

3°) Une chimiothérapie adjuvante de consolidation faisant appel au même schéma que la chimiothérapie initiale dans le cas de réponses supérieures à 50 % ou au CMF si le taux de réponse a été inférieur.

4°) Une immunostimulation éventuelle chez les patientes restant en rémission apparemment complète au terme de la chimiothérapie précédente : deuxième essai randomisé comportant une branche avec lévamisole per os pendant un an ou rien (sauf le tamoxifène dans le cas de récepteurs positifs).

RÉSULTATS

Tolérance : pour la chimiothérapie initiale elle a été dans l'ensemble plus satisfaisante que celle observée dans la phase de consolidation. Les différences constatées entre les deux groupes définis suivant l'ordre d'application des schémas sont à la limite de la signification ($p < 0,05$) avec 4 arrêts pour toxicité et 55 modifications du traitement (21,6 % dans le groupe I : DVM puis MTV) contre 7 arrêts et 73 modifications (29,8 % dans le groupe II : MTV puis DVM). Les réactions sévères ont été essentiellement d'ordre hématologique. Les incidents relatifs à la seconde phase loco-régionale ne se sont manifestés qu'à l'occasion de la chirurgie : ils sont survenus dix fois chez les 109 malades opérées (9,2 %) sous forme de désunion dans six cas avec problèmes de surinfection ou de lymphocèle dans quatre cas.

Efficacité immédiate en fin de chimiothérapie initiale (6 cycles) : 29 malades du groupe I ont présenté une réponse complète (RC) et 81 une réponse partielle (RP) soit 80,3 % et dans le groupe II 40 une RC, 72 une RP (84,2 %). La différence n'est pas statistiquement significative. La réponse immédiate n'a pas été fonction de l'atteinte ganglionnaire, du grade, des récepteurs ou du type histologique mais de la taille tumorale qui s'est révélée le facteur prédictif majeur (plus ou moins de 40 ou 60 mm : $p < 0,01$). Au terme du traitement locorégional 90 % des malades étaient en rémission complète, 140 après radiothérapie, 88 après chirurgie, 17 après association des deux. Au terme de la chimiothérapie adjuvante 210 malades restaient en rémission apparemment complète soit 78 %.

Pour l'ensemble de la série au cours de la période d'observation (72 mois), 57 récidives locorégionales ont été observées (soit 21 %) et 95 évolutions métastatiques (35 %).

Survie : 183 malades étaient vivantes (68 %) à 72 mois après le début du traitement (dont 158, soit 58,5 % en rémission) et la médiane de survie, n'a pas été atteinte à ce délai. Les paramètres étudiés ont eu une influence variable sur cette évolution en analyse monofactorielle. La différence de survie en fonction du taux des récepteurs hormonaux (inférieur ou supérieur à 10 fmol pour les estrogènes et à 15 pour la progestérone) a été très significative ($p = 0,0001$) avec médiane à 48 mois pour les taux les plus bas. L'évolution a été également influencée par l'efficacité de la chimiothérapie d'induction avec une différence ($p < 0,01$) entre les sujets répondants et non répondants. Aucune corrélation significative n'a pu être établie en fonction du type de traitement loco-régional, de la durée de la chimiothérapie adjuvante (quel que soit le protocole utilisé) ou de l'immunostimulation complémentaire (1). La survie est à 60 % à

72 mois quand la rémission complète a été obtenue au terme des trois premières phases du programme thérapeutique alors qu'il n'y a aucune survivante à 48 mois dans le cas contraire. L'analyse multifactorielle utilisant le modèle de Cox a fait apparaître quatre variables prédictives principales (signes inflammatoires, envahissement ganglionnaire, présence de récepteurs et grade histologique) dont l'association a permis de définir trois catégories de malades à évolution différente : un groupe à très bon pronostic (97 % à 4 ans) ne présentant aucun facteur de risque, un groupe à mauvais pronostic avec trois à quatre facteurs de risques (35 % de survie) et un groupe intermédiaire avec deux ou trois facteurs (63% de survie).

DISCUSSION

L'adjonction d'une chimiothérapie systémique au traitement locorégional des cancers mammaires localement étendus et/ou inflammatoires, inopérables d'emblée, modifie à long terme une évolution globalement péjorative (4,9). En induction, la chimiothérapie agit en même temps sur le plan général et local, son efficacité est rapide, elle a peu d'influence défavorable sur les temps locorégionaux et sert de test de chimiosensibilité à l'adaptation du traitement adjuvant (6). En élevant le taux de rémission complète, elle permet de limiter le temps local à une seule radiothérapie et en réduisant le volume tumoral elle peut rendre opérable le plus grand nombre de reliquats tumoraux (7). L'obtention d'une rémission complète paraît la condition préalable essentielle pour une évolution favorable ultérieure : la proportion obtenue en fin d'application du programme (78 %) est supérieure à celle des schémas peu différents qui étaient utilisés antérieurement de 1975 à 1978 (5) et du même ordre que ceux publiés par d'autres auteurs avec des protocoles assez proches (8). La survie est également améliorée : la médiane n'est pas atteinte au cours de la sixième année alors que dans la série précédente elle était située à 43 mois. Cette survie est également supérieure à celle de l'ensemble des cas recensés dans l'Enquête Permanente Cancer et correspondant à une population très voisine.

CONCLUSION

La chimiothérapie première contribue à améliorer en durée et qualité la survie des malades présentant un cancer mammaire évolué non métastatique. En renforçant le traitement locorégional elle permet d'élever le taux de rémission complète et réalise un traitement adjuvant précoce en maintenant un bon équilibre coût-efficacité, compte tenu du risque métastatique élevé de ces cancers. L'analyse des différents paramètres aide enfin à la définition de groupes pronostiques significatifs dont la connaissance doit guider les choix thérapeutiques ultérieurs (allègement pour les évolutions favorables prévisibles et renforcement initial pour les cas à très hauts risques).

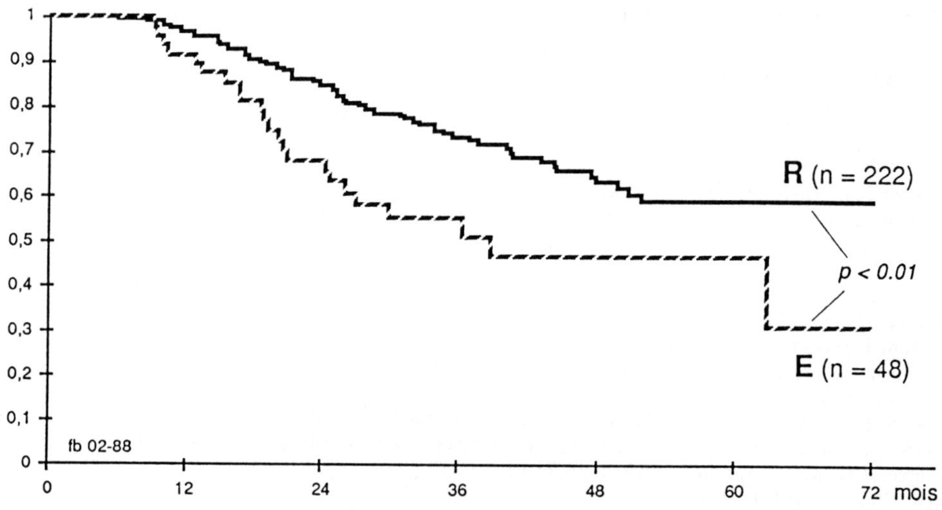

SURVIE ACTUARIELLE GLOBALE
en fonction de la réponse à la chimiothérapie d'induction
(**R** = réponses , **E** = échecs)

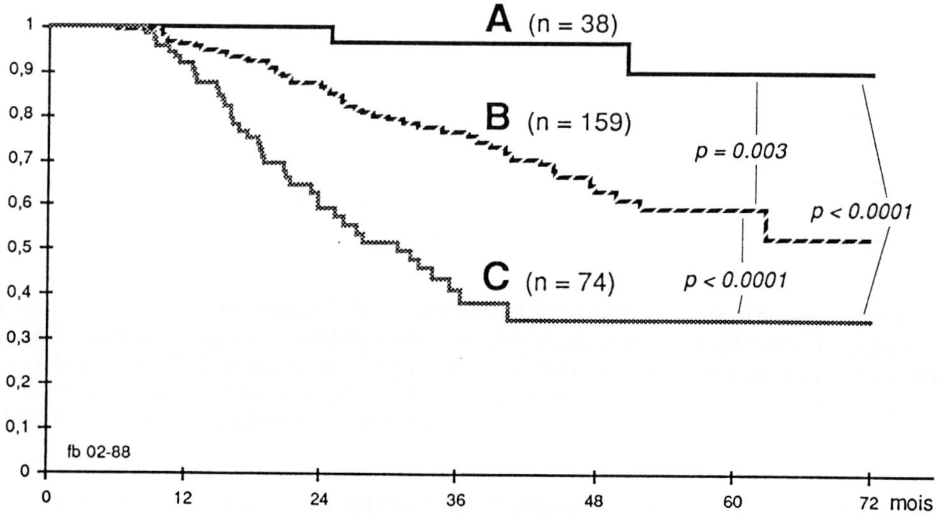

SURVIE ACTUARIELLE
en fonction des principaux groupes pronostiques
(**A** = 0 , **B** = 2 à 3 , **C** = 4 facteurs)

RÉFÉRENCES BIBLIOGRAPHIQUES

1. **Carpenter J.T., Smalley R.V., Raney M., Vogel C.L., Weiner R.S. (1986) :** Ineffectiveness of levamisole in prolonging remission or survival of women treated with cyclophosphamide, doxorubicin, and 5-fluorouracil for good-risk metastatic breast carcinoma : A southeastern cancer study group trial. *Cancer Treat. Rep. 70*, 1073-1079.

2. **Chauvergne J., Hœrni B., Durand M., (1982) :** Traitement des cancers (du sein) localement avancés ou inflammatoires. Intérêt d'une chimiothérapie d'induction. In : Bremond A. Les cancers gynécologiques et mammaires. Progrès en cancérologie 2, ed. Doin, Paris, pp 97-109.

3. **Chauvergne J., Durand M., Mauriac L., Hœrni B., David M. (1986) :** Chimiothérapie des cancers mammaires. Évolution coordonnée des schémas thérapeutiques de 1975 à 1985. *Rev fr. Gynécol. Obstét. 81*, 119-122.

4. **Chauvergne J., Durand M., Dilhuydy M.H., Hœrni B., Germain T., Lagarde C. (1981) :** Traitement des cancers du sein inflammatoires. Étude contrôlée d'un programme d'association thérapeutique. *Sem. Hôp. Paris, 58*, 1813-1819.

5. **Chauvergne J., Durand M., Richaud P., Avril A., Hœrni B., Lagarde C. (1981) :** Traitement combiné des cancers mammaires localisés à haut risque métastatique. Résultats d'une étude prospective contrôlée. J. *Gynécol. Obstet. Biol. Reprod., 10*, 75-85.

6. **Hœrni B., Chauvergne J., (1984) :** Rationalisation de la chimiothérapie adjuvante par une chimiothérapie d'induction. *Bull Cancer Paris, 71*, 297-300.

7. **Jacquillat C., Auclerc G., Baillet F., Auclerc M.F., Khayat D., Facchini T., Weil M. (1986) :** Chimiothérapie initiale avec traitement locorégional conservateur dans les cancers du sein (à propos de 205 malades). *Sem. Hôp. Paris, 62*, 3021-3023.

8. **Jacquillat C., Baillet F., Auclerc G., Blondon J., Auclerc M.F., Facchini T., Lefranc J.P., Weil M. (1984) :** Cancer du sein : chimiothérapie précédant le traitement locorégional avec extension des indications du traitement conservateur. *Bull Cancer, 71*, 354-360.

9. **Rouëssé J., Friedman S., Sarrazin D., Mouriesse H., Le Chevalier T., Arriagada R., Spielmann M., Papacharalam bous A., May-Levin F. (1986) :** Primary chemotherapy in the treatment of inflammatory breast carcinoma : a study of 230 cases from the Institut Gustave-Roussy, J. *Clin. Oncol., 4*, 1765-1771.

Résumé

Primary chemotherapy, radiotherapy and/or residual tumor removal then adjuvant chemotherapy followed or not by immunostimulation have been successively administrated from May 81 to June 85 to 270 patients with inoperable, locally advanced breast adenocarcinomas free of metastases.

Primary chemotherapy lead in a first randomized trial (doxorubicin + vincristine + methotrexate or mitomycine C + thiotepa + vindesine) to 222 objective responses (82.2 %), among which 69 were apparently complete (25.5 %). No significant difference was exhibited according to the sequence of drug administration. 160 patients underwent then radiotherapy, 20 conservative surgery and radiotherapy and 90 mastectomy. At the end of the adjuvant treatment, patients in complete remission were randomized between immunostimulation by levamisole and no further treatment.

These achievements were maintained in 158 patients (58.3 %) with medians of remission and overall survival not yet reached at 70 months. The evolution was affected by the quality of the initial chemotherapeutic response ($p < 0.01$) but the main prognostic factors were : inflammatory signs, lymph node involvement ($p < 0.01$) and presence of estrogen receptors ($p = 0.01$). The type of the local treatment and the adjuvant chemotherapy did not modify the overall evolution. The effect of levamisole on survival was not significant. These results, in terms of immediate response and survival rate, are better than those obtained in a previous study (1975-78).

Neo-Adjuvant Chemotherapy. Ed. Cl. Jacquillat, M. Weil, D. Khayat. Colloque INSERM/John Libbey Eurotext Ltd. © 1988. Vol. 169, pp. 231-235.

La chimiothérapie néo-adjuvante peut-elle augmenter le taux de conservation mammaire ?

J.C. Durand, P. Pouillard, B. Asselain, J.P. Bataini, G. Mathieu, R. Vilcoq, R.J. Salmon et J.P. Pilleron

Institut Curie, 26 rue d'Ulm, 75231 Paris Cedex 05, France

RESUME

Un essai thérapeutique portant sur 187 patientes compare la chimiothérapie adjuvante suivant un traitement locorégional à visée conservatrice et une chimiothérapie néoadjuvante suivie d'un traitement locorégional. Cette étude montre qu'une réponse majeure (>50 %) à la chimiothérapie néo-adjuvante est obtenue dans 44,7 %, une réponse complète dans 12 % des cas, ce qui permet un traitement conservateur dans 78,1 % des cas ce qui est significativement plus important qu'en cas de traitement locorégional 1er (62,6 %). Le taux de conservation est supérieur dans les T2. Bien que les delais de surveillance soient insuffisants les récidives locorégionales apparaissent plus fréquentes en cas de chimiothérapie néo-adjuvante.

MOTS CLEFS

Cancer du sein, Chimiothérapie néo-adjuvante, traitement conservateur.

INTRODUCTION

Si la chimiothérapie première a montré son efficacité dans les formes aigues du cancer du sein, si la chimiothérapie adjuvante parait utile dans les cancers du sein avec envahissement ganglionnaire en préménopause, la place exacte de cette chimiothérapie est mal précisée. Est-il préférable de pratiquer d'abord le traitement locorégional en particulier chirurgical et de réaliser ensuite la chimiothérapie adjuvante ? Le foyer tumoral principal est alors excisé, la chimiothérapie n'agit plus que sur les micrométastases. Est-il préférable de commercer le traitement par une chimiothérapie précoce, tumeur en place, vascularisation sans modification, mais avec un volume tumoral important ? La réponse à cette question n'est pas encore claire. C'est pourquoi à l'INSTITUT CURIE nous avons en 1983 décidé de pratiquer un essai thérapeutique comparant une chimiothérapie première suivie du traitement locorégional à un traitement locorégional suivi de chimiothérapie. L'efficacité de cette chimiothérapie première se juge à deux niveaux : une augmentation du taux de survie sans récidive et une augmentation du pourcentage de conservation mammaire. En raison de l'absence de recul suffisant nous n'étudierons pas la survie mais nous nous intéresserons aux possibilités de traitement conservateur en particulier par association radiochirurgicale après chimiothérapie initiale.

MATERIEL ET METHODES

De novembre 1983 à Novembre 1986, 187 patientes de moins de 65 ans ont été incluses dans cet essai (S5) dont 91 avec un traitement locorégional premier (TLR 1er) et 96 avec une chimiothérapie première (CH 1re)
Les patientes entrant dans l'essai S5 sont classées selon la classification TNM : T2N1bMo, T3NoN1aMo, T3N1bMo. Les tumeurs T3 de plus de 7 cm sont exclues de l'essai. Les tableaux 1 et 2 précisent cette classification en remarquant que les T2 ainsi que les N1b sont plus fréquents dans les cas traités par chimiothérapie première ou néoadjuvante.

Tableau I. Répartition TNM

	T2	T3
TLR 1er	29	62
CH 1re	44	52

Tableau II. Répartition TNM

	NoN1a	N1b
TLR 1er	29	62
CH 1re	23	73

Le tableau III montre qu'il existe un bon équilibre de l'envahissement axillaire entre les 2 branches de l'essai.

Tableau III. Pourcentage d'envahissement ganglionnaire axillaire (si curage)

	N-	N+(1à3)	N+ >3
TLR 1er	21	21	18
CH 1re	18	20	13

Le tableau IV précise la répartition des cas traités par chimiothérapie première

Tableau IV. Chimiothérapie première

	NoN1a	N1b
T2	0	44
T3	23	29

Le tableau V donne un schéma de l'essai thérapeutique.

Tableau V.

Diagnostic T2N1b, T3NoN1a, T3N1b
Randomisation

Chimiothérapie 2 cycles	Traitement locorégional
↓	↓
Traitement locorégional	
↓	
Chimiothérapie 4 Cycles	Chimiothérapie 6 cycles

Le diagnostic histologique initial est toujours obtenu par drill biopsie sur la tumeur. La chimiothérapie comporte de l'Adriblastine (ADM), du Methotrexate (CPM) et du 5 Fluorouracil (5 FU) à raison de 1 cycle toutes les 4 semaines.
Le traitement locorégional a été :
- en cas de TLR 1er une radiothérapie initiale à la dose de 55 grays et un bilan à cette dose. En fonction du reliquat tumoral et ganglionnaire est décidée soit
  . une mammectomie
  . une tumorectomie large + évidement axillaire
  . une tumorectomie large
  . un évidement axillaire et un surdosage local par curiethérapie
- en cas de CH 1re le traitement locorégional comporte soit :
  . une mammectomie
  . une tumorectomie large avec évidement axillaire suivie ou précédée d'une irradiation
  . soit une tumorectomie large suivie ou précédée d'irradiation
  . soit un évidement axillaire suivi ou précédé d'irradiation.

Le tableau VI précise la répartition des différents types de traitement loco régional

Tableau VI.

	Tumorectomie + Evidement + RX	RX	Mammectomie +/- RX	Total
TLR 1er	26	31	34	91
CH 1re	33	42	21 (6 sans RX)	96

Cet essai a été arrêté en novembre 1986 car il nous est apparu nécessaire de faire des modifications : étude des patientes en période préménopausique, intégration des T2 NoN1a, changement du type de chimiothérapie et du nombre de cycle. En 1987 a été commencé un essai S6 avec ces nouvelles données.

RESULTATS

Tableau VII.: réponse au traitement

Réponse complète	12,8 %)	
Réponse > 50 %	31,9 %)	44,7 %
Réponse < 50 %	39,4 %	
Pas de réponse	14,9 %	
Progression	1,1 %	

Le tableau VII expose les réponses obtenues avec une chimiothérapie première ou néoadjuvante : 45 % environ de régression supérieure à 50 %, 40 % de réponse très partielle et 15 % sans aucune efficacité.
Cette réponse varie en fonction du volume tumoral puisque le taux des réponses majeures (>50%) est de 51 % pour les T2 et 39 % pour les T3 (P=0,05). Par contre le statut ganglionnaire axillaire n'a pas d'influence puisque le taux de réponse majeure est de 48 % en cas de NoN1a et de 43 % en cas de N1b (Non significatif).
Le tableau VIII précise les taux de conservation mammaire en fonction des traitements initiaux et du TNM.

Tableau VIII

	T2	T3	Total
TLR 1er	72 %)	58 %	62,6 %)
CH 1re	91 %)P=0,04	67 %	78,1 %)P=0,02
Total	84 %	62 %	

Ce taux est de 78,1 % en cas de chimiothérapie premiere et de 62,6 % en cas de traitement loco régional premier. Lachimiothérapie première augmente donc nettement la conservation mammaire (P=0,02) Ce taux est aussi significativement plus élevé (P=0,04) dans les T2 par chimiothérapie première, par contre la différence dans les T3 67 % contre 58 % n'est pas statistiquement prouvée. Cependant il est intéressant de noter que les taux globaux de conservation ont été de 84 % pour les T2 et de 62 % pour les T3.
Après chimiothérapie première la conservation mammaire a été obtenue 42 fois par radiothérapie exclusive, 33 fois par association radio-chirurgicale (20 tumorectomies larges avec évidement axillaire, 4 tumorectomies larges et 9 évidements axillaires). En cas de traitement locorégional premier la radiothérapie a été exclusive dans 31 cas, suivie de chirurgie conservatrice dans 26 cas (19 tumorectomies avec évidement axillaire, 1 tumorectomie large, 6 évidements axillaires).
Il n'est bien entendu, pas possible, en l'absence de recul suffisant, d'apprécier l'efficacité sur la survie de la chimiothérapie première. De même la valeur du traitement conservateur devra être modulée en fonction de l'évolution, des récidives locorégionales et des métastases.
Le tableau IX montre les récidives, les métastases et les associations récidive/métastase.

Tableau IX

	Rec.	Métastase	Rec+métastases
TLR 1er	3	8	4
CH 1re	7	7	2
TOTAL	10	15	6

Bien que le recul soit encore faible il faut remarquer la plus grande fréquence des récidives locorégionales isolées dans les cas de chimiothérapie première

CONCLUSION

L'étude d'un essai thérapeutique dans les cas de T2N1b, T3NoN1a, T3N1b comparant une chimiothérapie première suivie de traitement locorégional à un traitement locorégional suivie de chimiothérapie, montre un taux de réponse majeure (> 50%) à la chimiothérapie de 44,7 %, de 39,4 % de réponse partielle et de 16 % d'absence d'efficacité.
Ce taux de réponse majeure est meilleur dans les T2 : 51 %, que dans les T3 : 39 % (P=0,05), par contre l'état ganglionnaire entraine peu de modification. Le taux de conservation mammaire a été de 78,1 % en cas de chimiothérapie première pour 62,6 % en cas de traitement locorégional premier (P=0,02).
Par contre les récidives locorégionales semblent plus fréquentes en cas de chimiothérapie première. Les délais de surveillance sont cependant encore insuffisants pour permettre une conclusion définitive.

Résumé

A protocol dealing with 187 pts compares Adjuvant Chemotherapy after conservative surgery and Neo-adjuvant Chemotherapy followed by locoregional treatment. This study shows that a major response (> 50%) to Neo-Adjuvant Chemotherapy is achieved in 44,7 %, a C.R. in 12 % pts allowing a conservative treatment in 78,1 % pts : the breast preservation is thus significantly more frequent than with primary locoregional treatment especially in T2.
Although the follow-up is too short for definitive assessment, locoregional recurrences seem more frequent with Neo-Adjuvant Chemotherapy.

Neo-Adjuvant Chemotherapy. Ed. Cl. Jacquillat, M. Weil, D. Khayat. Colloque INSERM/John Libbey Eurotext Ltd. © 1988. Vol. 169, pp. 237-240.

Pre-operative chemotherapy as a treatment of breast cancer. Analysis of 95 cases

T.M. Tran, T. Guittard, V. Duchatelle, G. Bertrand-Desvages, J.L. Kemeny, J. Amouroux and L. Guillevin

Hôpital Avicenne, 125 rue de Stalingrad, 93009 Bobigny Cedex, France
Correspondance and reprints : T.M. Tran

Long term prognosis of breast cancer remains poor in some cases as a consequence of metastasis and local relapses.
Preoperative chemotherapy has been proved to be effective in preventing such an evolution.
95 patients afflicted of breast cancer with a tumor greater than two cm were included in our study. Twenty nine out of them were classified as T2 (20 NO ; 9 N+), 26 as T3 (20 NO ; 6 N+) and 4O as T4 (28 NO ; 12 N+). Menopause was present in 51 % of cases at time of our study.
After 4 sessions of chemotherapy, before mastectomy and axillary nodes dissection,the tumor disappeared in 18 cases and had a significant reduction in another 81 patients.
27.5% of the T2 patients ,20% of the T3 patients and 12.5% of the T4 had a complete response. 89.5% of the T2 patients,96% of the T3 patients,and 87.7% of the T4 patients had a partial response.The hormonotherapy did not influence patient's reactions to chemotherapy.
Twenty one % of patients showed multiples sites of cancer after a histopathological examination of the mastectomy specimen. The overall survival was 92 % after 36 months of follow-up(no metastasis was noticed)and 80 % after 60 months of follow up.

KEY WORDS

Cancer du sein, chimiothérapie pré-opératoire, métastases.
Breast cancer, pre-operative chemotherapy, metastasis.

INTRODUCTION

The long term prognosis of breast cancer is based not only on the size and local extention of the tumor to nodes but also on the presence of undetectable metastasis by all means of diagnosis available to date. These metastasis persist even after local and regional treatment of the cancer. Therefore we propose chemotherapy as a co-treatment of the breast cancer as well as pre operative and post operative therapy in our study.
The therapeutic strategy used in our service since 1976, consists of initial chemotherapy followed by mastectomy and ganglion curage regardless of the size of the tumor. This strategy is carcinologicaly satisfying; more over our study has allowed us to quantify the tumor reduction, to study the multifocality and finally to indicate the most adapted post operative therapy.

PATIENTS AND METHODS.

Between 1980 and 1985 we have studied 95 patients presenting a breast cancer classified in T2, T3 and T4 stage. Before any treatment the repartition of the patients has been clinically determined as follow :

- 29 patients were classified as T2; 20 were NO, 9 were N+
- 26 patients were classified as T3; 20 were NO, 6 were N+
- 40 patients were classified as T4; 28 were NO. 12 were N+

The malignancy of the tumor has been confirmed by drill biopsy.

The average age was 49 years old (3O-74). At the time of diagnosis, 51 % of the patients were menopaused. Every patient had a mammography and a thermography before any treatment; these exams were renewed after 4 sessions of chemotherapy , and before surgery. Before any chemotherapy initiation a complete check up for the search of an extention has been performed including hepatic and pelvic echography, pulmónary X-ray, skeletal scanning, skeletal X-ray, and CEA test. These tests allowed us to select patients having detectable metastasis.

Patients presenting nephropathy, hepatopathy, or heart failure were excluded of this study.

TREATMENT

Before any surgical resection four cycles of chemotherapy have been performed every four weeks. Each cycle consisted of 45 mg/m2 of DOXORUBICINE on the first day ,1 mg/m2 of VINCRISTINE on the 2nd day ; on the 3 rd, 4th and 5 th days 25O mg/m2 of CYCLOPHOSPHAMIDE and 5OO mg of 5 FU were delivered by bolus.On the 6 th day 12O mg/m2 of CIS PLATINIUM were delivered by bolus. All other treatments, especially hormonotherapy have been excluded from our study.

The doses have been adapted according to the hematologic tolerance, especially for the leucocyte count, which was checked up between 10 th and 15 th days after the beginning of the chemotherapy.

After four sessions of chemotherapy, a modified radical mastectomy has been performed. The whole specimen was sent for histopathological examination. The size of the residual tumor was noted, as well as an eventual multifocality.

Chemotherapy was stopped or pursued according to the pathological results, including the size of tumor, and the number of metastatic nodes.

RESULTS

During these four months of treatment the size of the tumor did not increase in any of our 95 patients. On the opposite the tumor size decreased in 81 out of the 95 patients (85%), and a complete regression was noticed in 18 out of 95 patients (18%). Complete desappearance was present in 27.5% of T2 patients, 20% of T3, and 17.5% of T4. Objective regression (more than 50 %) was present in 89.5% of T2 patients, 96% of T3 patients, and 97.5% of T4 patients.

The hormonal status of the patients had no influence on the treatment. There were no statistically significant differences between menopaused and non-menopaused patients; 27% of the non-menopaused patients and 16% of the menopaused patients had a complete response. 88 % of the non-menopaused and 84 % of the menopaused patients had a total or a partial response .

Thermography has proved a total disappearance of any extensive evolution in all cases, as well as edema around the tumor. Pathological examination showed complete disapearance of the tumor in 22%.

Nevertheless 21 % of the patients had distance metastasis .

An average 12 nodes (6 to 17) was present in the lymph nodes resection.

Table I shows node invasion regardless of initial size of the tumor.

We have found in 9 % of cases, after chemotherapy, depleted nodes without any metastasis.

21 % of the patients had a multifocal tumor. During these four months of treatment, however, none of our patients died or showed any side effect especially aplastic anemia which might have required antibiotherapy. We did not observed renal insufficiency.

Nevertheless few episodes of diarrhea were quickly controled by a symptomatic treatment. The survival after 36 months was 92 % without any relapses.

COMMENTAIRES discussion

At present the pre operative chemotherapy is widely used. Since we are using it , positive results allow us to use this treatment before any surgical act.
The results that are mentionned above, which are limited to T2, T3 and T4 stages, allow us to appreciate the accuracy of the responses and the absence or persistance of tumoral residue in the mastectomy specimen. Pre operative chemotherapy appears to be of great interest for the treatment of local and regional breast cancer. We can expect it to be usefull for the destruction of undetectable metastasis (especially for liver and bones metastasis), which are the main cause of treatment failure. Our study can demonstrate ,in all cases, the regression of *clinically detectable tumors* . The rate of our response is higher than those of other protocols. The adjonction of CIS PLATINIUM has improved our own results of 1O %. However this *drug* is not always efficient ; only 22% of the patients had a complete tumor regression , controled by pathological examination. The others had partial tumor reduction, and even multifocality.
This multifocality demonstrates that polychemotherapy could not be the only radical treatment of breast cancer. Therefore it is necessary to complete the treatment either by radiotherapy, or by a modified radical mastectomy. However, we think that mastectomy is justified by carcinologic security.To minimise the psychologic trauma resulting from mastectomy, especially in young patients, we propose reconstructive surgery. The results are at present satisfying.

		O	N≤3	N>3
T2	29	21	4	4
T3	22	22	2	2
T4	4O	19	13	8
	95	62	19	14

TABLE I : node invasion

REFERENCES

1 - BONNADONA and coll.
The CMF program for operable breast cancer with positive axillary nodes. Update analysis on the disease free interval site of relapse and drug tolerance.
Cancer, 1977, 39, 2904-2915

2 - CANELLOS G.P.
The treatment of local advanced breast cancer.
J.Clin.Onc., 1984, 2, 149-151

3 - CHAUVERGNE J. and coll.
Traitement des cancers du sein inflammatoire. Etude contrôlée d'un programme d'association thérapeutique.
Sem. Hôp. Paris, 1982, Tome 58, 1813-1819

4 - DARGENT D. and coll.
Lambeau cutané abdominal transversal pédiculisé sur le muscle grand droit.
Presse Méd., 1987, 16, 533-536

5 - FISCHER B. and coll.
The evolution of breast cancer surgery : past, present and future.
Semin. Oncol. , 1978, 5, 385-394

6 - GALITCHI E. and coll.
Tentative d'association radio chirurgicale conservatrice dans le traitement des cancers du sein non accessibles à une tumorectomie première.
Congrès de Sénologie Avignon (abstract), 14, 15, 16 octobre 1987

7 - JACQUILLAT C. and coll.
Initial chemotherapy and conservative radiotherapy in stage I and II and III breast cancer.
Proceedings of the 13 th International Cancer Congress, 1982, 52, (abstract 3218)

8 - JACQUILLAT C. and coll.
Preliminary results of "neoadjuvant" chemotherapy in initial management of breast cancer.
Proceedings ASCO, 1983, 112 (abstract C 437)

9 - JACQUILLAT C. and coll.
Cancer du sein. Chimiothérapie précédant le traitement loco-régional avec extension des indications du traitement conservateur.
Bull. Cancer, 1984, 71, 354-360

10 - MAYLIN C.
Traitement conservateur du cancer du sein T1-T2 (UICC). Etude critique multifactorielle des récidives locales sur 466 cas (oct 1979 à déc 1984).
Congrès de Sénologie Avignon (abstract), 14, 15 ,16 octobre 1987

11 - RAGAZ J. and coll.
Neoadjuvant (pre operative) chemotherapy of breast cancer.
Cancer,1985, 56, 719-724

12 - ROUESSE J. and coll.
Initial chemotherapy in the treatment of inflammatory breast cancer. 230 cases.
Presse Med., 1987, 16, 475-478

Résumé

DE 1980 à 1985 nous avons étudié 95 femmes porteuses d'un cancer du sein non métastatique dont la taille tumorale était supérieure à 2 cm. Elles ont été traitées par polychimiothérapie pré-opératoire, mammectomie, curage axillaire.

Une régression objective de la masse tumorale a été observée dans 87,36 % des cas dont 18,9 % de rémission complète.

La survie à trois ans est de 92 % et à cinq ans de 80 %.

Neo-Adjuvant Chemotherapy. Ed. Cl. Jacquillat, M. Weil, D. Khayat. Colloque INSERM/John Libbey Eurotext Ltd. © 1988. Vol. 169, pp. 241-244.

Tumor proliferative activity and prognosis of locally advanced breast cancer patients treated with neo-adjuvant chemotherapy

P.F. Conte, G. Gardin, P. Pronzato, A. Alama, A. Nicolin, G. Bertelli, D. Amoroso and R. Rosso

Istituto Nazionale per la Ricerca sul Cancro, V. le Benedetto XV 10, 16132 Genova, Italy

INTRODUCTION

Tumor proliferative activity is a reliable prognostic parameter and a higher Thymidine Labeling Index (TLI) identifies a subset of patients with a worse prognosis in the case of non Hodgkin lymphomas (4), multiple myeloma (5) and primary breast cancer (6, 7, 9). The experience in locally advanced breast cancer is more limited: R. Silvestrini and coworkers (8) have reported a poorer survival for patients with a highly proliferating non inflammatory locally advanced breast cancer. In the present paper we evaluate the prognostic relevance of tumor proliferative activity in 43 cases of locally advanced breast cancer (including inflammatory carcinoma).

ABSTRACT

Thymidine Labeling Index (TLI) and Primer dependent α DNA polymerase (PDP-LI) have been determined in 43 patients with locally advanced breast cancer (11 stage III A, 32 stage B).
Median TLI and PDP-LI were 1.8 and 5.25 respectively. TLI and PDP-LI were not significantly related to other prognostic variables (age, ER status, stage, presence or not of inflammatory findings). The patients have been treated with 3 cycles of chemotherapy (5-FU + Doxorubicin + Cytoxan) followed by surgery and 6 more cycles of chemotherapy. Four years survival (S) and progression free survival (PFS) are 76% and 72.1% respectively in the case of high TLI; 4 years S and PFS are 67.1% and 37.1% in the case of low TLI. An objective response (CR+PR) was achieved in 80.9% of patients with high TLI and 68.2% in patients with low TLI. These differencies are not significant.

PATIENTS AND METHODS

Tumor proliferative activity was determined in 43 women with locally advanced breast cancer; the relevant patient characteristics are reported in Table 1.

Table 1. Patient characteristics.

Characteristics	N. Pts.	(%)
≤ 50 yrs	15	(34.9)
> 50 yrs	28	(65.1)
ER+	15	(34.9)
ER-	23	(53.5)
ER unknown	5	(11.6)
III a	11	(25.6)
III b	32	(74.4)
I.B.C.	14	(32.6)
non I.B.C.	29	(67.4)

ER= estrogen receptor
I.B.C.= inflammatory breast carcinoma

These patients were entered into two consecutive trials: 29 patients come from a pilot study recently published (2, 3) and have been treated with DES-FAC (Dietilstilbestrol 1 mg/die for 3 days followed by 5-FU 600 mg/mq + Doxorubicin 50 mg/mq + Cytoxan 600 mg/mq on day 4) for 3 cycles, surgery and 6 more cycles of DES chemotherapy; 14 patients come from an ongoing prospective randomized trial comparing presurgical DES-FAC to FAC alone.
Tumor proliferative activity was evaluated by Thymidine Labeling Index (TLI) and the Primer dependent α DNA polymerase assay (PDP-LI) on single cell suspensions obtained with mechanical disaggregation of tumor samples taken at diagnosis.
The TLI represents the percentage of S-phase cells while the PDP-LI is a measure of tumor growth fraction.
The two kinetic techniques have been described in detail elsewhere (1, 2).

RESULTS

Median TLI was 1.8% (range 0.1 - 19.4) while median PDP-LI was 5.25% (range 0.4 - 41.2). TLI and PDP-LI were not significantly related to age, stage, receptor status, presence or not of inflammatory findings. An objective response (OR= CR+PR) after 3 cycles of chemotherapy was achieved in 74.4% of patients: 80.9 % in the case of high TLI and 68.2% in the case of low TLI (p= 0.6).
TLI and PDP-LI do not significantly affect survival or disease free survival (DFS) (Table 2).

Table 2. 4 years survival (S) and DFS according to TLI and PDP-LI

	4 yrs S %		4 yrs DFS %	
High TLI	76	p=0.9	72.1	p=0.6
Low TLI	67.1		37.1	
High PDP-LI	74.6	p=0.5	61.6	p=0.7
Low PDP-LI	64.4		49.4	

The only significant influence of TLI was evident in the subsets of patients older than 50 years: the 4 years DFS was 83.5% in the case of high TLI and 37.4% in the case of low TLI (p=0.03).

DISCUSSION

Our present study does not confirm the report from Silvestrini et al. (8) which demonstrates a negative influence of a high TLI in patients with locally advanced breast cancer. The series from Silvestrini and ours differ from three main characteristics: the kinetic technique employed (TLI performed on tumor fragments in the Silvestrini's report, TLI and PDP-LI on cell suspensions in ours), the selection of patients (inflammatory carcinomas were excluded in the Milan study), the type of chemotherapy (Doxorubicin + Vincristine in the first study and FAC in the present report). Undoubtely the cell disaggregation of tumor samples results in a lower median TLI, however it is unlikely that this could alter the discrimination between slowly and rapidly proliferating tumors.

On the contrary the inclusion of inflammatory carcinomas and the utilization of a more aggressive chemotherapy could explain the disagreament between the two studies. Inflammatory carcinomas are characterized by a rapidly fatal outcome unless treated with very aggressive combination chemotherapy. Despite this rapid clinical course, in our series medium TLI of inflammatory carcinomas was lower than that observed in non inflammatory carcinomas (1.1 vs 2.5, p=0.2).

As a consequence the majority of inflammatory carcinomas are included in the group of slowly proliferating tumors and these cases are responsible for the majority of treatment failures (3/29 non inflammatory carcinomas relapsed in comparison to 10/14 inflammatory carcinomas, p=0.0001).

Even more important seems to be the effect of treatments: patients in the Milan trial have been treated with doxorubicin and vincristine while our patients received a more aggressive three drugs regimen (5-FU + Doxorubicin + Cytoxan); interestingly this results in the same 4 years survival for slowly proliferating tumors (68.1% in Milan and 67.1% in our study) while a large difference is evident in the case of highlyproliferating tumors (36.7% in Silvestrini's study and 76.0% in ours).

In conclusion tumor proliferative activity which has been reported to be an important prognostic parameter, loses its unfavourable effect if patients with locally advanced breast cancer are treated with more aggressive chemotherapy.

Supported in part by a Grant from the Italian National Research Council, Special Project "Oncology", Contract 87.01516.44

Acknowledgment: we thank Miss M. Pratolongo for typing the manuscript.

REFERENCES.

1) Alama A., Conte P.F., Di Marco E. et al. (1986). In vitro proliferative activity of human solid tumors evaluated by Thymidine Labeling Index and Primer dependent α DNA polymerase. Oncology 43, 385-389.

2) Conte P.F., Fraschini G., Alama A. et al. (1985). Chemotherapy following estrogen induced expansion of the growth fraction of human breast cancer. Cancer Res. 45, 5926-5930.

3) Conte P.F., Alama A., Bertelli G. et al. (1987). Chemotherapy with estrogenic recruitment and surgery in locally advanced breast cancer: clinical and cytokinetic results. Int. J. Cancer 40, 490-494.

4) Costa A., Bonadonna G., Villa E. et al. (1981). Labeling Index as a prognostic marker in non Hodgkin lymphomas. J.N.C.I., 66, 1-5.

5) Durie B.G.M., Salmon S.E., Moon T.E. (1980). Pretreatment tumor mass, cell kinetics and prognosis in multiple myeloma. Blood 55, 364-372.

6) Gentili C., Sanfilippo O., Silvestrini R. (1981). Cell proliferation and its relationship to clinical features and relapse in breast cancer. Cancer 48, 974-979.

7) Meyer J.S., Friedman E., Mc Crate M. et al. (1983). Prediction of early course of breast carcinoma by Thymidine Labeling Index. Cancer 51, 1879-1986.

8) Silvestrini R., Daidone M.G., Valagussa P. et al. (1987). Cell kinetics as a prognostic marker in locally advanced breast cancer. Cancer Treat. Rep. 71, 375-375.

9) Tubiana M., Pejovic M.H., Chavaudra G. et al. (1984). The long term prognostic significance of the Thymidine Labeling Index in breast cancer. Int. J. Cancer 33, 441-445.

Neo-Adjuvant Chemotherapy. Ed. Cl. Jacquillat, M. Weil, D. Khayat. Colloque INSERM/John Libbey Eurotext Ltd. © 1988. Vol. 169, pp. 245-247.

Pre-operative chemotherapy and differentiated surgery in the treatment of breast cancer

Gian Carlo Montruccoli, Antonia d'Errico, Daniele Barnabé, Daniele Montruccoli-Salmi and Walter Franco Grigioni

Toniolo Hopital, via Toscana 34, 40141 Bologna, Italy

ABSTRACT

1) There is no single ideal technique for breast cancer surgery. 2) Before surgery it is impossible to know with certainty the true histopathologic-biological condition of the tumor or of the so-called healthy tissue surrounding it. 3) The effectiveness of chemotherapy on this type of neoplasm has been documented. 4) It is considered prudent and absolutely necessary to carry out preliminary therapy which can sterilize the tumor, reduce its size and in short destroy as much as possible of what could be defined as the "local tumor system". The intention was to use preoperative chemotherapy to make surgery adequate, not to correct the inadequacies of surgery. For all these reasons, in 1975, we instituted a therapeutic approach combining chemotherapy and surgery in various ways.

INTRODUCTION

Almost all breast cancer patients wish to minimize esthetic impairment. This means that the surgeon requires a rationalisation of breast surgery whereby the decision whether to undertake radical or "conservative" surgery can be justified on the basis of accurate safety criteria. These considerations led us in 1975 to begin a non-randomized approach involving pre-operative chemotherapy followed by various surgical techniques.

METHODS

Between January 1975 and December 1987 129 cases were treated. A few minor variations were made to our method during this period, but the following principles were always applied: i) to traumatize the tumor as little as possible during the diagnostic stage, drill-biopsy alone was used wherever possible; ii) chemotherapy was always initiated before performing surgery, administering three cycles with Adriblastine 40 mg/m2, Vincristine 1 mg/m2, Endoxan 250 mg/m2 and 5 Fu 500 mg over 4 days, every 21 days. After the operation a further 3-5 cycles were administered every 4 weeks. Tamoxifene was administered to women in menopause for 2 to 3 months before the operation at a dosage of 30 mg daily.

iii) In general we use quadrantectomy for women in menopause and the Patey technique in very large or inflammatory tumors, while a special technique was developed for premenopausal women called "enlarged subcutaneous mastectomy" (ESM). The latter consists of the total and bilateral removal of the mammary gland, followed by immediate subpectoral replacement with a silicone prosthesis.

Table 1. Incidence of locoregional recurrences and overall survival rate for T_0 and T_1 tumors.

Surgery	Patients (No.)	No.Nodes involved		Metastasis (No.)	Locoregional recurrence				Metastasis (No.)				Dead (No.)			
		<3	>3		> 10 years	> 5 years	> 3 years	> 18 months	> 10 years	> 5 years	> 3 years	> 18 months	> 10 years	> 5 years	> 3 years	> 18 months
Quadrantectomy																
premenopausal																
postmenopausal	8	5	1				1			2						
ESM																
premenopausal	65	7	1				2							23		
postmenopausal	7	2	2					2								
Patey																
premenopausal	4	2	1													
postmenopausal	9		1				1									

(Total, no.=93; survival at 10 years, no.=8; at >5 years, no.=31; at >3 years, no.=27; at >18 months, no.=22. Results from January 1975 to December 1987)

Table 2. Incidence of locoregional recurrences and overall survival rate for T_2, T_3, T_4 tumors.

Surgery	Patients (No.)	No.Nodes involved		Metastasis (No.)	Locoregional recurrence				Metastasis (No.)				Dead (No.)			
		<3	>3		>10 years	> 5 years	> 3 years	> 18 months	> 10 years	> 5 years	> 3 years	> 18 months	> 10 years	> 5 years	> 3 years	> 18 months
Quadrantectomy																
premenopausal																
postmenopausal																
ESM																
premenopausal	16	2	1			1	2		1	2					3	
postmenopausal	1	1	3					1								
Patey																
premenopausal	8	2	3													
postmenopausal	10	1	5					1							1	1

(Total, no.=36; survival at >10 years, no.=3; at >5 years, no.=8; at >3 years, no.=12; at >18 months, no.=8. Results from January 1975 to December 1987)

An axilla was performed with an additional incision on the diseased side.

RESULTS (See tables 1 and 2)

DISCUSSION

After a little more than 10 years, we can conclude from our data that pre-operative chemotherapy:

1) makes a large number of tumors operable which would otherwise be non-operable;
2) facilitates surgery by effectively sterilizing any undetected foci;
3) significantly reduces the number of local and regional recurrences especially in cases of large or inflammatory tumors;
4) reveals the sensitivity of the individual tumor to chemotherapy and acts immediately on distant micrometastasis;
5) in no way modifies the post-operative period, either generally or locally, as regards hematomas and infections;
6) significantly improves the prognosis of inflammatory tumors, both as regards local recurrences and the length of disease-free survival; the number of cases with non-inflammatory tumors were too few and the follow-up too brief to determine whether there was in fact a significant improvement in the long-term survival rate.

REFERENCES

Liotta L.A., Rao C.N., Barsky S.H. (1983): Tumor invasion and extracellular matrix. Lab. Invest. 49, 636-649.

Montruccoli G.C. (1979) In Abstracts, 9th World Congress of Gynaecology and Obstetrics, pp 171-175. Tokyo.

Montruccoli G.C. et al (1980): La mastectomia sottocutanea nella prevenzione e nel trattamento dei tumori delle mammella. Riv. Ital. Chir. Plast. 12, 317357.

Montruccoli G.C. (1986) Gynecology and Obstetrics, Ed. H. Ludwig and K. Thompson, pp 592-598. Berlin Heidelberg: Springer-Verlag.

Résumé

1) Il n'y a pas une technique idéale unique pour pouvoir effectuer une intervention chirurgicale concernant le cancer du sein. 2) Avant d'opérer, il est impossible de connaître avec certitude quelle est la condition histopathologique-biologique réelle de la tumeur ou de la partie soi-disant saine qui l'entoure. 3) L'efficacité de la chimiothérapie sur ce genre de néoplasme a été documentée. 4) Il est prudent et absolument nécessaire d'effectuer une thérapie préliminaire qui est à même de stériliser la tumeur, de réduire ses dimensions et en bref de détruire autant que possible ce qui est défini comme "système tumoral local". Le but était celui d'effectuer une chimiothérapie préopératoire afin de permettre une chirurgie adéquate et non afin de corriger des interventions chirurgicales inadéquates.

Neo-Adjuvant Chemotherapy. Ed. Cl. Jacquillat, M. Weil, D. Khayat. Colloque INSERM/John Libbey Eurotext Ltd. © 1988. Vol. 169, pp. 249-256.

Analysis of the British Columbia study of pre-operative (neo-adjuvant) therapy of breast cancer in stage III disease

J. Ragaz, M. Manji, I.H. Plenderleith, M. Knowling, I. Olivotto, V. Basco, J. Hardman, A. Worth and U. Kuusk

Cancer Control Agency of B.C., Vancouver, Canada

RESUME

This study is a follow up of our previous report on the role of preoperative (neoadjuvant) combined modality therapy in patients with inoperable stage III breast cancer (Ragaz, 1987). Using a combined chemotherapy - radiotherapy treatment protocol, 75 of all registered patients were rendered operable and considered for mastectomy. Of those, 47 underwent the surgery, while because of their physician's or their own noncompliance, 28 patients had no mastectomy. As both groups were comparable in their main prognostic characteristics (clinical tumor and nodal stage, age) and in their objective response (CR + PR) to the preoperative treatment, we were able to obtain information on the role of mastectomy in stage III breast cancer. Our analysis showed a significant trend for an improved disease free survival in the patients with mastectomy. Also, importance of the surgery was further reinforced by the documention of residual invasive or in-situ disease in 72.8% of the mastectomy specimens. Our study indicates that patients rendered operable by the preoperative chemotherapy-radiotherapy treatment combination may benefit by a subsequently performed mastectomy. Longterm survival impact of the surgery in those patients will, however, require a longer follow up. Alternatively, a randomized trial controlling for mastectomy will be required. We conclude, that the majority of patients presenting with inoperable stage III breast cancer could be rendered operable by effective neoadjuvant treatment, and considered subsequently for a resection with curative intent.

INTRODUCTION

Risks for both locoregional recurrence and systemic dissemination are the main reasons for inoperability of patients with stage III disease

(Haagensen, 1932). According to internationally set criteria from the U.I.C.C., this category excludes inflammatory breast cancer, and includes stages T3a-4c, any N, MO; or any T, N2-3, MO. Past reviews have shown poor survival with locoregional therapies alone (Harris, 1983; Baclesse, 1949); and a trend for improved outcome with combination chemotherapy (Davila, 1984). Presently, most centres routinely use chemotherapy in the management of stage III disease, while no uniformity exists for the use of surgery and radiotherapy.

Preoperative (neoadjuvant) chemotherapy is being used in a variety of tumors (Frei, 1986; Ragaz, 1986). The preoperative downstaging of primarily inoperable tumors, and subsequent easier conduct of the surgical procedure (Morris, 1978; Schick 1983; Ragaz, 1987) is considered the main clinical application of the neoadjuvant approach. Experimental data indicate a low growth fraction in the bulky primary tumor, with poorly vascularized central core, and admixture of older necrotic and presumably resistant cells. It is believed that these factors cause chemotherapy to induce a pathological complete remission at the primary site in only a minority of patients. However, it is possible, that in a subset of patients, younger and more actively cycling systemic micrometastases could be eliminated by the same chemotherapeutic agents. On theoretical grounds, the subsequently performed surgery in these cases could be a potentially curative procedure. Hence, the addition of locoregional treatments (radiotherapy and surgery) in responding stage III breast cancer patients aiming for treatment with curative intent is an appealing concept. In 1982, our group started a study to test such an approach. Since then, 75 stage III breast cancer patients, seen at the British Columbia Cancer Control Agency, have received combined chemotherapy - radiotherapy preoperative therapy. The treatment started with an Adriamycin-containing chemotherapy regimen for 3 months. Subsequently, locoregional radiotherapy was given, followed by 3 more months of chemotherapy. Patients rendered operable were offered definitive surgery (a modified radical mastectomy). Due to the physicians or patients noncompliance, some registered patients (group 1) did not have surgery. These patients were found to be comparable in main prognostic factors and characteristics with patients who had the mastectomy (group 2), as judged not only from their initial T, and N staging and age, but also from the response to the 7 months of induction combined modality treatment (Table I). Hence, a comparison of the outcome in these two groups allowed us to analyze the impact of mastectomy on patients with stage III breast cancer. To reduce the possibility of a selection bias, only patients in clinical complete remission (CR) or partial remission (PR) are compared and analyzed for the overall and disease free survivals (Table II).

MATERIALS AND METHODS

Up to December 1987, 75 patients diagnosed as stage III breast cancer have been registered under the locally advanced protocol. This analysis includes patients with a pathological diagnosis of breast cancer with clinical stage T3a-b, T4a-c, NO-2, MO; or any T, N2, MO (UICC 1978).

Patients with N3 (supraclavicular) disease or a clinical diagnosis of inflammatory carcinoma, were excluded from this analysis. Out of 75 registered patients, 28 had no mastectomy (group 1) and 47 had mastectomy (group 2). Twenty six out of 28 patients without mastectomy (group 1), and 42 out of 47 cases with mastectomy (group 2) were found to be in clinical CR or PR after 6 cycles of chemotherapy and radiotherapy. Patients in both groups had a similar distribution of prognostic characteristics, particularly age (p=0.33), T stage (p=0.6), N stage (p=0.92), and response to preoperative treatment (Table 1). Treatment started with 3 cycles of chemotherapy before locoregional radiotherapy, followed by 3 additional chemotherapy courses. Each cycle consisted of an A and B portion, given 2 weeks apart, cycles repeated q 4 weeks. (Portion A = Adriamycin 40 mg/m2 i.v., day 1, Cyclophosphamide 200 mg/m2 p.o. days 3-6. Portion B = Methotrexate 350 mg/m2 i.v. day 15; 5-fluorouracil 1000 mg/m2 i.v. day 15; Folinic acid rescue 15 mg p.o. q 6 hrs x 6, day 16. Locoregional radiotherapy was given using 5 field technique. Both internal mammary nodal chains were treated with enface portal employing a given dose of 3750 cGy in 16 daily fractions. Whole breast was treated with tangent pairs to deliver maximum dose of 4000 cGy in 16 daily fractions. Supraclavicular and axillary regions were treated with a semi - parallel opposed portal, delivering a given dose of 3750 cGy in 16 fractions, and a tumor dose of 3500 cGy in 16 fractions respectively. Patients rendered operable were considered for surgery.

RESULTS

Forty two of 47 patients (89.3%) from group 2 (mastectomy) had an objective response (CR + PR) before the surgery. Of those, 30 were in CR and 12 in PR. Of the 28 patients in group 1 (without mastectomy), 26 (92.8%) were in CR (16) or PR (10). Hence, the objective response rate (CR + PR) for all patients was 90.6% (68/75).

The following analysis includes only patients who were in CR or PR after the preoperative treatment. The 2 and 3 year overall survival (Table II) for patients with mastectomy was 93 and 73%, compared to 100 and 72% for patients without the mastectomy (p = 0.9). The 2 and 3 year disease free survival (Table II) in patients with mastectomy was 87 and 71% respectively, compared to 63 and 34% in patients without the surgery (p = 0.0089).

The analysis of the mastectomy specimens in patients with surgery showed pathological complete response (no residual invasive or in-situ disease) in 10/47 patients (21.2%). Three patients (6.3%) had residual in situ disease. The remaining 34 patients (75.5%) had residual invasive disease, either at the primary site axilla or both (table III).

The analysis of the mastectomy specimen in 30 patients who were in clinical complete remission before mastectomy showed 30% pathological complete response. In the remaining 70% of patients, residual in-situ or invasive disease was found (Table III).

Analysis correlating pathological response with outcome showed that in the group of 37 patients with residual disease in the mastectomy specimen, 81% were alive with no recurrence, 8% were alive with disease, and 11% died from metastatic disease. The corresponding figures for the 10 patients with pathological complete remission were 70, 10 and 20% (Table IV). There was no instance of postoperative wound abscess, sepsis or failure of primary healing of the mastectomy wound.

DISCUSSION:

The design of this study offered routine mastectomy in all patients rendered operable by the preoperative therapy. However, because of patient or physician non-compliance, a group of patients without mastectomy was available for comparative analysis. The prognostic factors, including tumor size, nodes, clinical stage, and age, as well the response to the preoperative therapy, were similar in both groups. Hence, a comparison of the two groups enabled some conclusions on the role of mastectomy in patients treated with preoperative therapy. The data show the disease free survival at 2 and 3 year followup to be improved by the surgical procedure. Longer followup, however, will be needed to assess the impact of mastectomy for overall survival. Of importance is the repeatedly documented safety of modified radical mastectomy performed after 6 months Adriamycin - containing chemotherapy regimen combined with locoregional radiotherapy (Ragaz, 1987). Virtually no delays of healing or infection of the mastectomy wound were seen.

Also of interest is the detection of the residual disease in the locoregional site in 78.8% of the mastectomy specimens. Such findings suggest that without the mastectomy, a regrowth and dissemination of the disease from the site of the residual disease could be a possible outcome. On the other hand, at the present time we cannot entirely rule out a loss, or a reduction of the metastatic potential in the surviving cells as a result of pretreatment by chemotherapy and radiotherapy. Such an outcome, as indicated from recent data on differentiation (Sartorelli, 1986) is a plausible mechanism of chemotherapy and radiotherapy treatments, and may explain a lack of correlation between the pathological response, and the recurrence and mortality rates in our patients.

Results of longterm followup, however, and of randomized studies testing the role of mastectomy will be required before conclusions on the impact of surgery and of the combined modality neoadjuvant treatment in the management of locally advanced breast cancer can be reached more definitely.

TABLE I

PREOPERATIVE (NEOADJUVANT) CHEMOTHERAPY AND RADIOTHERAPY - COMPARISON OF PATIENTS CHARACTRISTICS IN GROUPS WITH AND WITHOUT MASTECTOMY

MASTECTOMY	NO (28 pts)	YES (47 pts)	p
AGE < 50	40.7%	59.3%	0.33
CLINICAL STAGE			
T0	11.1%	4.3%	
T1a,b	3.7%	0.0%	
T2a,b	0.0%	6.4%	0.63
T3a,b	25.9%	44.7%	
T4a-c	59.3%	44.7%	
N0	25.9%	36.2%	
N1	40.7%	36.1%	0.92
N2	33.3%	27.7%	
N3	-	-	
CLINICAL RESPONSE TO PREOPERATIVE THERAPY (CT+XRT)			
(CR+PR)	92.8% (26/28)	89.3% (42/47)	
CR	61.5% (16/28)	63.8% (30/47)	>0.5
PR	35.7% (10/28)	25.5% (12/47)	

TABLE II

COMBINED MODALITY (NEOADJUVANT) THERAPY FOR PATIENTS IN CR or PR AFTER PREOPERATIVE THERAPY - SURVIVAL ANALYSIS

	MASTECTOMY		
	NO (26)	YES (42)	p
OVERALL SURVIVAL (Years)			
1	100%	97%	
2	100%	93%	
3	72%	73%	0.91
DISEASE FREE SURVIVAL (Years)			
1	85%	94%	
2	63%	87%	
3	34%	71%	0.0089

TABLE III

ANALYSIS OF PATHOLOGICAL RESPONSE IN 47 STAGE III BREAST CANCER PATIENTS WHO HAD MASTECTOMY AFTER PREOPERATIVE CHEMOTHERAPY AND RADIOTHERAPY

	CLINICAL RESPONSE	
	CR+PR	CR
RESIDUAL DISEASE (PATHOLOGY)		
NO	10/47 (21.2%)	9/30 (30.0%)
IN SITU ONLY	3/47 (6.3%)	3/30 (10.0%)
INVASIVE		
primary only	17/47 (36.0%)	6/30 (20.0%)
axilla only	4/47 (8.5%)	4/30 (13.3%)
primary and axilla	13/47 (28.0%)	8/30 (26.6%)
ANY RESIDUAL	78.8%	70%

TABLE IV

ANALYSIS OF 47 PATIENTS WITH MASTECTOMY - CORRELATION OF THE PATHOLOGICAL COMPLETE RESPONSE (CR) WITH OUTCOME

PATHOLOGICAL CR	ALIVE NED*	ALIVE RECURRENCE	DEAD
YES (10 pts)	7 (70%)	1 (10%)	2 (20%)
NO (37 pts)	30 (81%)	3 (8%)	4 (11%)

*NED = No evidence of disease

REFERENCES

Baclesse, F. (1949): Roentgen therapy as the sole method of treatment of cancer of the breast. Am. J. Roentgenol.Radium. Ther. 62, 311.

Chu, A.M. (1980) Treatment of early stage breast cancer by limited surgery and radical irradiation. J.Rad.Oncol.Biol.Phys. 6, 25-30.

Davila, E. (1984): Management of locally advanced breast cancer (stage III): a review. Int Advan Surg Oncol 7, 297-327.

Frei, E. (1986): Clinical and scientific considerations In Preoperative (Neoadjuvant) Chemotherapy. ed J. Ragaz,In Preoperative Neoadjuvant Chemotherapy P.R. Band, J.H. Goldie, pp 1-5. Heidelberg: Springer-Verlag.

Haagensen, C.D. (1932): Carcinoma of the breast: criteria of operability. Ann.Surg 118, 859-870, 1032-1051.

Harris, J.R. (1985): Cancer of the Breast. In Cancer Principles and Practice of Oncology, ed V.T. De Vita Jr., S. Hellman, S.A. Rosenberg, pp 1148-50. Philadelphia: J.B. Lippincott.

Harris, J.R. (1983): Management of locally advanced carcinoma of the breast by primary radiation therapy. Int. J. Rad. Oncol. Biol.Phys.9, 345-349.

Jacquillat, C. (1986): Neoadjuvant chemotherapy in the conservative management of breast cancer - study on 205 patients. In Neoadjuvant Chemotherapy, ed C. Jacquillat, M. Weil, D. Khayat, 137: pp 197-207, John Libbey.

Morris, D.M. (1978): Mastectomy as an adjunct to combination chemotherapy. Arch. Surg.113, 282-284.

Ragaz, J. (1985): Neoadjuvant (preoperative) chemotherapy for breast cancer. Cancer 56, 719-725.

Ragaz, J. (1986): Preoperative neoadjuvant chemotherapy, Heidelberg: Springer-Verlag.

Ragaz J. (1987): Preoperative combined modality (neoadjuvant) therapy for locally inoperable breast cancer. In Fundamental Problems in Breast Cancer ed H.G.A. Patterson, A.W. Lees, pp 383-391. Boston: Martinus Nijohoff.

Rosen, G. (1979): Primary osteogenic sarcoma. The rationale for preoperative chemotherapy and delayed surgery. Cancer 43, 2163-2177.

Sartorelli, A.C. (1986): Mechanisms Involved in the induction of malignant cell differentiation. Adv Enzyme Regul 25, 507-529.

Schick, P. (1983): Preoperative chemotherapy followed by mastectomy for locally advanced breast cancer. J. Surg. Oncol 22, 278-282.

Head and neck I

Voies aérodigestives I

Neo-Adjuvant Chemotherapy. Ed. Cl. Jacquillat, M. Weil, D. Khayat. Colloque INSERM/John Libbey Eurotext Ltd. © 1988. Vol. 169, pp. 259-273.

Neo-adjuvant chemotherapy for head and neck cancer. Problems and prospects

Emil Frei III, John R. Clark and Daniel Miller

Harvard Medical School, Dana Farber Institute, 44 Bidney Street, 02115 Boston, MA, USA

This is the Second International Congress of Neoadjuvant Chemotherapy. Controversy persists as to the appropriateness of the name neoadjuvant chemotherapy.(1) In Figure 1 various terms often used for neoadjuvant chemotherapy are presented with comments. Anterior chemotherapy and protochemotherapy are too broad and imprecise. All it means is that chemotherapy is used initially which is true, for example, for the leukemias and the lymphomas. Induction chemotherapy is an old term with a precise and restricted meaning for the leukemias. To extend such a term is to dilute its precision. Upfront chemotherapy is too trivial a term and preoperative chemotherapy is too restricted since many patients receiving neoadjuvant chemotherapy have surgery and/or radiotherapy. One should build on the term adjuvant since it is precise. Proto adjuvant chemotherapy is a precise term. However, it does not recognize the novelty of the strategy. This novelty relates to the biology of a regressing solid tumor which is a major challenge in terms of mechanisms and impact on local treatment strategies. Neoadjuvant chemotherapy is similarly precise but also recognizes the novelty of the challenge that is the fact that it's an idea whose time has come.(1)

The next slide represents a mature study performed at the Dana-Farber Cancer Institute wherein survival is presented as a function of whether patients achieved a complete remission, a partial response, or no response to neoadjuvant chemotherapy prior to local treatment.(2) As is true for almost all studies, patients achieving a complete response had a far superior survival and this was true even after multi-variant analysis and adjustment for other prognostic factors. While the role of neoadjuvant chemotherapy generally in head and neck cancer is controversial, it seems reasonable to conclude at the present time that the minority of patients who achieve complete remission in fact have improved cure rates. This is not surprising since it is almost axiomatic in chemotherapy that an initial complete response to systemic treatment is associated with improved cure rates. In Figure 3 the data for Hodgkin's Disease and MOPP chemotherapy is presented. The patients achieving complete response do very well in terms of survival, whereas patients achieving partial response do very poorly and only minimally better than patients who achieve no response.

The above information impacts in a major way on experimental design for neoadjuvant chemotherapy in head and neck cancer. (Figure 4) If CR's only effect survival than the CR rate must be greater than 20% to see an anticipated, greater than 20% improvement in survival in a comparative study. Thus to go from a control of 30 to greater than 50% survival in a Phase III controlled study would require almost 200 patients. On the other hand, the CR rate of over 40% would require a much more managable number of patients. Given the above, the choices are to proceed now with comparative studies, and many in fact are ongoing. Such studies may stabilize current knowledge but will not advance it. The other choice is to focus on Phase I and II studies designed to improve the complete response rate and later to proceed to a comparative study. This is what we have chosen to do and will be the focus of my presentation.

In Figure 5 are presented some of the opportunities for improving neoadjuvant chemotherapy for head and neck cancer. Historically improving cancer treatment by identifying better new agents, doses, and schedules has been critical. Rather than deal with each of these choices, I will focus on the choice of local treatment, leucovorin modulation of fluorouracil, fluosol, and drug resistance.

Figure 6. There is a major need and opportunity to acquire knowledge concerning biology of tumor regression from chemotherapy. This is a new area for research and such knowledge has major implications for the choice of local treatment. (Figure 6) The 2 extremes of the biology of tumor regression may be referred to as centripital and rarefaction. With centripital regression the tumor margins contract but density in terms of tumor cells remains the same. This should make surgery far more effective but would also allow for reducing field sizes for radiotherapy. The other extreme is rarefaction regression wherein the tumor size remains the same but tumor cell density decreases. Clinically, such a patient may be called an excellent response because the tumor will soften. However, if the tumor was inoperable initially, it would remain inoperable. Such rarefaction, while it would not decrease field sizes for radiotherapy, it should increase relative vascularity, therefore, decrease hypoxia and make radiotherapy more effective. In Figure 7 is presented semi-quantitative data obtained by Boheim indicating that poorly differentiated head and neck cancer tends to regress by rarefaction whereas more well differentiated lesions regress centripitally. It is proposed that careful quantitative pathology and clinical trial data be obtained to define this problem more precisely and particularly to define its correlates with marginal involvement and with duration of control after local treatment.

Fluorouracil is one of the mainstays of the chemotherapy of head and neck cancer. A major advance in the use of fluorouracil relates to modulation by leucovorin. (Slide 8) Fluorouracil is converted by a series of enzymatic steps to FDUMP which is an inhibitor of the enzyme thymidylate synthatase. This enzyme has an allosteric site to which 5,10 methylene tetrahydrofolate, the major product of leucovorin, binds. Such binding leads to a conformational change in the enzyme, with a change in the substrate site such that FDUMP becomes a much better fit with a greater and particularly a more prolonged degree of inhibition of the enzyme. Moreover, this effect is stoichiometric, that is, the greater the concentration of the tetrahydrofolate, the greater the degree of inhibition by FDUMP. This modulation of the FU effect by leucovorin occurs at an enzymatic, a subcellular, a cellular, and an *in vivo* level and now has been extended to the clinic. This effect should be even greater for FUDR which is closer to thymidylate synthetase and subject to fewer enzymatic chances to resistance. Not surprisingly it is in metastatic colorectal cancer that FU plus leucovorin has been studied most vigorously and four randomized comparative studies are presented in Figure 9.(3) All of these studies indicate a significantly improved response rate for FU plus leucovorin. We have initiated a Phase I study of fluorouricil plus leucovorin in combination with cisplatin in patients with head and neck cancer. Preliminary results suggest excellent tumor responsiveness but an increase in mucosal toxicity.

Another approach to improving neoadjuvant chemotherapy relates to fluosol. Figure 10. Fluosol consists of perfluorocarbon colloid particles which have been demonstrated *in vivo* including in man to be red blood cell substitutes, that is, they can on and off load oxygen. Most particularly, they have 1% the volume of red blood cells and therefore can penetrate hypovascular areas such as in solid tumors. This improves the PO_2 in solid tumors and thus has the potential for increasing the effectiveness of radiotherapy, particularly, and, it turns out, chemotherapy as well. In Figure 11, fluosol plus oxygen breathing in animals bearing transplanted tumors markedly improves the antitumor effect of x-ray but also for a number of chemotherapeutic agents. This includes some chemotherapeutic agents such as the nitrosoureas, where oxygen is not known to be essential for cytotoxicity. It is possible that fluosol's effect for these agents relates to an increase in cytokinetic activity of the tumor. Fluosol may assist in carrying the drug into the tumor. Whatever the mechanism, the experimental results are promising, and fluosol is currently in clinical trial, both with respect to the potential capacity for improving local radiotherapy for head and neck cancer and for improving the effect of alkylating agents in the treatment of solid tumors.

The molecular and cell biology of drug resistance for the real clinical world is an important area for research. It is possible to establish most human squamous cell carcinomas of the head and neck in culture by using appropriate techniques such as an irradiated 3T3 feeder layer. We have established a large number of cell lines and have produced drug resistance by selection pressure _in vitro_. These studies are interesting with respect to their implications for the chemotherapy of head and neck cancer. For methotrexate, we have found that for increasing levels of drug resistance, the first molecular change is a decrease in drug transport following by a decreased capacity in polyglutamation and subsequently only at higher levels of resistance by an increase in the target enzyme due to gene amplification.(5) Since it is only low levels of drug resistance that are probably important clinically, we had hoped that the aforementioned data would generalize, that is, the low levels of drug resistance would relate prominantly to transport. Accordingly, we produced low levels of resistance to some 4 head and neck cell lines and analyzed them for mechanisms. It was found that drug resistance to methotrexate was multifactorial not only between cell lines but within cell lines. Thus depending upon the cell line, drug transport, polyglutamation, and increase in the target enzyme were variably important. Of even greater interest was the fact that within specific cell lines it was common for more than 1 mechanism to be involved in resistance.(6) This was a disappointment in terms of potential for treatment, but probably represents the real world in terms of clinical resistance and must be addressed. Similarly, for human squamous cell carcinoma made 12 fold resistant to platinum, we found that this line had a decreased capacity to transport cisplatin, an increase in glutathione transferase which may complex with an inactivate cisplatin, an increase in methalothionine which may do the same, and a possible increase in DNA repair.(7) Thus again, in the clinical world of drug resistance, multifactorial factors may dominate.

Can we do something about drug resistance? We can and have for antimicrobial drug resistance. The potential for preventing or exploiting drug resistance is real (Fig. 12). For methotrexate resistance due to a decrease in transport, lipid soluble antifoles such as trimetrexate are in clinical trial. Leucovorin could modulate FU resistance as already discussed. Cyclophosphamide resistance has recently been described to increase in activation by the enzyme aldehyde oxidase which can be inhibited by disulfiram. For many drugs wherein gene amplification is a mechanism of resistance, the use of high dose intermittent therapy should and does experimentally prevent the development of gene amplification. Finally, multidrug resistance can be circumvented at least experimentally by calcium agents such as calcium channel blockers. In short, advances in cell biology make it possible to study *in vitro* the majority of human head and neck cancers and molecular pharmacology should make it possible in the near future to identify responsiveness and to understand and perhaps exploit or prevent drug resistance.

REFERENCES

1) Frei E. III. Clinical cancer research: An embattled species. 50: 1979-1982.

2) Clark, J.R., Fallon, B.G., Frei E. III. Induction chemotherapy as an initial treatment for advanced head and neck cancer: A model for the multi disciplinary treatment of solid tumors. In: Important Advances in Oncology 1982. Editors, DeVita, Hellman, and Rosenberg. Lippincott, Philadelphia. 1987. p.175.

3) Erlichman, C., Fine, S., Wong, A., et al. A comparison of fluorouracil and folinic acid versus fluorouracil in

metastatic colorectal carcinoma. Proc. ASCO 8:82, 1986, (abstract #319).

4) Teicher, B.A., Holden, S.A., Jacobs, J.L. Aproaches to defining the mechanism of advancement of fluosol with carbagen of nelphelan antitumor activity. Cancer Research 47: 513, 1987.

5) Frei E. III., Rosowsky, A., Wright, J.E., et al. Development of methotrexate resistance in a human squamous cell carcinoma of the head and neck in culture. Proc. Natl. Acad. Sci. 81: 873, 1984.

6) Rosowsky, A., Wright, J.E., Cucchi, C., et al. Phenotypic heterogeneity in cultured human head and neck squamous cell carcinoma lines with low level methotrexate resistance. Cancer Research 45: 6205, 1985.

7) Teicher, B., Holden, S., Kelley, M.J., et al. Characterization of a human squamous cell carcinoma cell line resistant to cisplatin. Cancer Research 47: 388, 1987.

Figure 1

Term	Comments
Anterior chemotherapy.	Too broad. Imprecise.
Proto chemotherapy.	Too broad. Imprecise.
Induction chemotherapy.	Old term. Restricted meaning.
Upfront chemotherapy.	Trivial. Too broad.
Preoperative chemotherapy.	Too restricted.
Adjuvant chemotherapy.	Precise. Accepted.
Proto adjuvant chemotherapy.	Precise. Does not recognize novelty.
Neoadjuvant chemotherapy.	Precise. Recognizes novelty.

Figure 2

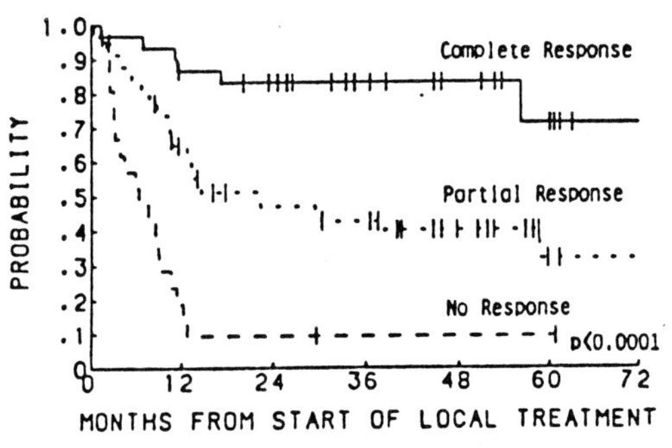

Response	Failed/Total
Complete	6/30
Partial	33/59
None	19/21

Figure 3

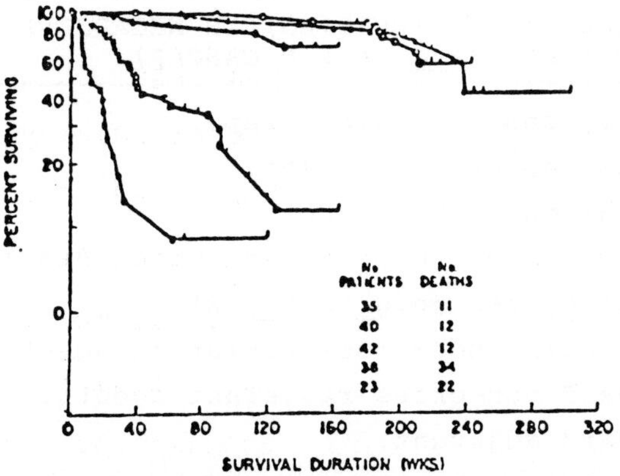

Effect of remission and maintenance treatment on survival. CR = complete remission; (|) = to date of last follow-up examination.

Figure 4

Head and Neck Cancer: Experimental Design Problems

Premises

1) For NeoA chemo only a CR (particularly CR_p) affects survival. (H & N, all tumors).
2) In a comparative study a > 20% increase in survival is the objective.

∴ NeoA Ch. CR rate must be > 20%.

To go from a 30 to a 50+% survival (cure) in a Phase III controlled study with a= < 0.05 and b=80%, 92 x 2 patients would be required.

A CR rate of 40+% (projects increase in survival 40%) would require 23 x 2 patients.

Therefore: choices

1) Big Phase III studies. Stablize but no advance.
2) Phase I-II studies designed to ↑ CR rate.

Figure 5

CHALLENGES (OPPORTUNITIES) IN NEOADJUVANT CHEMOTHERAPY (e.g. H & N CANCER)

- Surgery and/or radiotherapy.
- Agents, doses, schedules.
- Modulation (LCV for FU).
- Midcycle non-myelosuppressive agents (Mtx/Lcv) (PFM)
- No. of cycles (e.g. 3 vs. 2).
- Alternating non-cross resistant agents.
- Standard non-cross resistant agents.
- Standard adjuvant.
- Synchronous chemo & rad.
- Fluosol (with RT) with chemo.
- Drug resistance.

Figure 6

TUMOR CYTOREDUCTION WITH NEOADJUVANT CHEMOTHERAPY

Nature of Regression	Pre-Chemo	Post-Neo-Adjuvant Chemo	Potential Impact on Local Therapy		
			Surg	RadioT.	Best Might Be
Centripetal	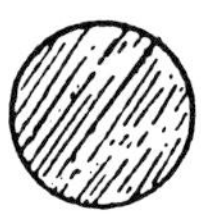		↓	↓ field size	S only
Rarefaction	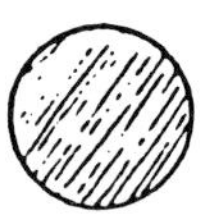	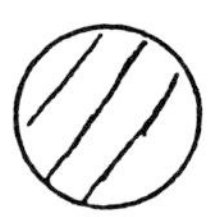	No Change	↓ rads	R only

Figure 8

TMP Synthetase. FU and LCV.

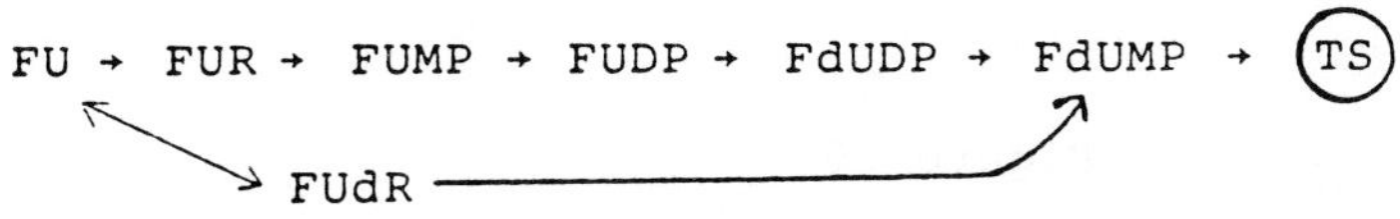

TS = TMP Synthetase

• = Allosteric site for 5,10m 4HF

Conformational change

Increase in duration of ↓ of TS by FdUMP

Stoichometry

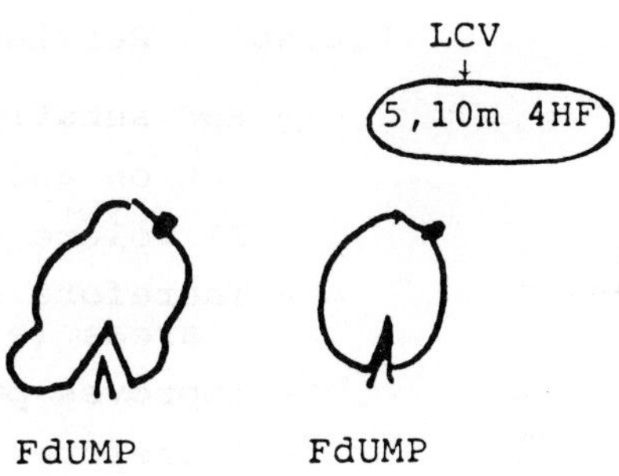

Figure 9

FU/LCV

Colorectal Cancer. FU + LCV Randomized Studies.

	Response To FU	FU + LCV	
Erlichman	6%	37%	
Doroshow	15%	45%	
Petielli	11%	44%	
GITSG	10%	LD LCV 19%	HD LCV* 29%

* 500 mg/M^2 iv over 2 hrs.

Toxicity

Figure 10

Fluosol = Perfluoro colloid particles

- RBC substitute.
- Can on and offload O_2.
- 1% volume of RBC.
- Therefore can penetrate hypovascular areas (e.g. solid tumors).
- Improves pO_2 in solid tumors. (Sang).
- Therefore increases effectiveness of RT and some chemotherapy.

Figure 11

Flousol - perfluorocarbon

- Can on and offload O^2 + CO_2.
- RBC substitute.
- Colloid particles 1% size of RBC.
- Therefore enter solid tumors more effectively than RBC.
- Fluosol + O^2 breathing↑ po_2 in hypoxic solid tumors (exp.).
- Fluosol + O^2 ↑ response 3-5x of RT in mouse solid tumors.
- Fluosol + O^2 ↑ 5x response of solid tumors to Alk. agents and adriamycin.

Figure 12

Cisplatin resistance in H & N cancer

SCC 25/plat.	12x resistant
Membrane transport	↓ x 3
GSH	-
GST	↑ x 3
Metallothionine	↑ x 2
DNA repair	? ↑
Multifactorial	

Neo-Adjuvant Chemotherapy. Ed. Cl. Jacquillat, M. Weil, D. Khayat. Colloque INSERM/John Libbey Eurotext Ltd. © 1988. Vol. 169, pp. 275-280.

Present concept and status of adjuvant chemotherapy in patients with locally advanced head and neck cancer

M. Al-Sarraf

Division of Hematology and Oncology, Wayne State University and Harper-Grace Hospitals, Detroit, Michigan 48201, USA

ABSTRACT

The results of standard therapy of surgery and/or radiotherapy in patients with locally advanced head and neck cancer are poor and not acceptable. High overall and complete response rates to cisplatin based chemotherapy when given as the initial treatment, were reported in these patients. This led to incorporation of these active combination as part of combined modality therapy. Before investigating the efficacy of chemotherapy in randomized trials, it is important to answer conceptual questions related to the use of chemotherapy in these studies. These are: 1. what is the best combination chemotherapy? and the number of courses to be given? 2. the timing and sequence of chemotherapy as part of combined modality treatment? 3. when to include chemotherapy as part of these combined treatments? Also, the identification of prognostic factors that may influence the outcome, the compliance of patients, the number of patients needed in phase III study, and the percent differences expected between the arms of the randomized trial, are important factors in the design of these studies. Failure to follow these important concepts may lead to negative randomized trials and premature abandonment of a possible effective mode of therapy.

KEYWORDS

Head and neck cancer, chemotherapy, combined modality therapy, study design, prognostic factors

INTRODUCTION

Cancer of the head and neck may be the most common malignant tumor in the world. Although in the United States and Western Europe this type of cancer is rather uncommon (5%). Because of the location of these tumors, the recent progress in their treatment and the combined modality approach and team effort, led to a great increase in interest than its incidence might suggest.

Table 1. Complete and overall response rates to Cisplatin containing regimen

Agent(s)	No. of Patients	% Response CR Range	CR Total	Overall Range	Overall Total
C	80	0-4	1	3.5*-4.0	28
CB	506	0-19	7	37-81	49
CB (V or O)	396	0-32	16	58-93	74
CMB	440	0-33	19	46-89	67
CBM (V or O)	227	0-35	21	48-86	67
CF (I)	442	13-54	34	38-100	77
Other	337	4-36	23	64-100	74

*32% of patients had improved disease.
C= Cisplatin, B= Bleomycin, V= Vinblastine, O= Oncovin, M= Methotrexate, F=5-Fluorouracil, I=Infusion

The majority of the cases (70%-80%) may present with locally advanced disease. Inspite of the high clearance rate with definitive therapies, the disease free and overall survivals are poor and unacceptable. The majority (>70%) of the failure are at the local and/or regional level (Vikram, 1984, 1984a). To improve on these results, many attempts have been investigated and continue to be tested to improve the delivery and the effectiveness of radiotherapy (Marcial, 1988). Recent advances in the treatment of patients with locally advanced head and neck cancer include the development of improved and active chemotherapy regimens (Al-Sarraf, 1984, 1987, 1988).

CONCEPTS OF ADJUVANT CHEMOTHERAPY

Active combination chemotherapy have been increasingly incorporated as part of the definitive treatments in patients with locally advanced head and neck cancer (Al-Sarraf, 1984, 1987, 1988). Chemotherapy is usually administered before local treatments of surgery and/or radiotherapy. This was done to investigate the effectiveness, and side effects of these agents, and to test the feasibility of the combined modality therapy. Few randomized studies have been attempted and being conducted mostly on the cooperative group level to investigate the efficacy of these chemotherapy or for the purpose of organ preservation. Continued intensive efforts are underway to improve on the effectiveness and the safety of these cytotoxic drugs (Ensley, 1988). It is important that before we activate phase III randomized studies to investigate the efficacy of adjuvant chemotherapy in these patients, we answer important conceptual questions related to study of chemotherapy as part of combined modality treatment.

The Best Chemotherapy

Before studying the value of effective chemotherapy as an adjuvant treatment with the present definitive therapy in patients with locally advanced head and neck cancer, it is essential to identify and to use our best chemotherapy regimen available. The question is how do we define the most active combination of cytotoxic agents? and how to define the best adequate chemotherapy? When the activity chemotherapy was investigated in these patients they were given as the initial (proto) treatment. Most of these patients had unresectable and/or inoperable disease. The most common combinations were investigated was cisplatin based combination (Table 1) (Al-Sarraf, 1987). The results were reported in overall and clinical complete response rates. It is important to emphasize here the various prognostic factors that may influence the response rate and especially the complete response rate to these induction chemotherapies (Table 2) (Al-Sarraf, 1984, 1987, 1988).

Table 2. Prognostic factors that influence the response to chemotherapy and/or survival

I. Stage
  A. Stage III vs Stage IV
  B. Actual T and N staging
II. Site (and sub-sites)
III. Tumor Morphology
IV. Patients Performance Status
V. Associated disorders
VI. Number of primary sites
VII. Response to initial chemotherapy
VIII. Type of response to chemotherapy
  A. CR vs <CR
  B. Clincial CR vs Histological CR
IX. Type of chemotherapy
X. Other

The most important of these prognostic factors is the T and N stage of the head and neck cancer, and especially the degree of the nodal involvement. It was found that patients with overall and complete responses to initial chemotherapy had improved survival as compared to non-responders, regardless of the sequence and the type of the definitive treatments. And even more important is the significant improvement of the overall survival for those patients with histologically complete clearance of the cancer based on the evaluation of the resected surgical specimen (Al-Kourainy, 1987). It seemed that the combination of cisplatin and 120 hour infusion of 5-fluorouracil (5-FU) produced the better range and average of complete response rates reported so far, regardless of the T and N stages of the cancer. Attempts to add other active agents like methotrexate, bleomycin, vinblastine, etc. to the combination of cisplatin and 5-FU infusion did not improve on the complete response rate, but increased the side effects to these agents (Al-Sarraf, 1987).
It is important to mention that the time when clinical complete response was achieved in relation to the number of courses of chemotherapy was critical in determining the incidence of histological complete response rate and possible influence on overall survival. A clinical complete response, occurring after one course of chemotherapy when additional courses are planned, has a more favorable prognostic factor than clinical complete response occurring at the end of the last planned course of chemotherapy.

Timing and Sequence of Chemotherapy

As important as the selection of our best chemotherapy to be used in clinical trials, the timing and sequence of active chemotherapy as part of definitive treatments is important and needs to be investigated. This led us as early as 1982 to study the feasibility of effective chemotherapy post-surgery followed by radiotherapy (Al-Sarraf, 1982) and concurrent cisplatin and total radiotherapy in unresectable cancer (Al-Sarraf, 1987a). This simultaneous chemo-radiotherapy was found to be very effective at the cooperative group level. In patients with resectable and those with unresectable and/or inoperable disease, many possible timings of chemotherapy can be designed for further study:

1. Induction (proto), before surgery and post-op radiotherapy
2. Chemotherapy post-surgery
3. Chemotherapy following surgery and post-op radiotherapy
4. Chemotherapy before radiotherapy
5. Chemotherapy post-radiotherapy
6. Chemotherapy combined with concurrent radiotherapy
7. Combination of the above

The activity of our best chemotherapy was tested against gross, mostly unresectable lesions, and should be as effective against microscopical cancer. Also, up to 30% overall and up to 50% of patients with complete response to chemotherapy refused our best therapy, surgery. To shrink gross disease, especially less than histological complete response, and then perform radical surgical resection may not change our overall results vs performing adequate surgery first without additional initial treatment of radiation or chemotherapy. Because of the above and many other factors, we believe that if surgery is planned, then chemotherapy should be given post definitive therapy. This could be done as post-surgery followed by radiotherapy, which is being investigated by the Head and Neck Cancer Intergroup in the United States. Or combined with concurrent post-op. radiotherapy, which being investigated at Wayne State University, Detroit, Michigan, USA. Also, recent evidence supports the addition of a certain number of courses of chemotherapy post-definitive treatments, especially for those who initially responded to the same induction chemotherapy (Adjuvant, 1987, Ervin, 1987).

In patients with inoperable or unresectable cancer, the best therapy is concurrent cisplatin with radiotherapy. Additional chemotherapy needs to be administered either before or after the combined chemo-radiotherapy.

When to Use Adjuvant Chemotherapy

The significant improvement in survival was observed only in patients with clinical complete response and especially those with histological complete response to chemotherapy (Al-Kourainy, 1987). This means to observe statistical differences in our randomized phase III trial, investigating the efficacy of this chemotherapy, we have to utilize the best combination chemotherapy that is known to produce the highest possible clinical and histological complete responses. Also, these chemotherapy have to be given in adequate number of courses to achieve such results. In testing the efficacy of adjuvant chemotherapy pre-maturely, or in less than adequate courses, may lead to negative trials and to early abandonment of a possible effective mode of treatment.

Organ Preservation

The main goal of investigating adjuvant chemotherapy as part of multimodality treatment in patients with locally advanced head and neck cancer is to improve on the present results of cure rate and overall survival. Quality of life and reduction in the unacceptable functional and cosmetic sequelae of the definitive therapy especially radical surgical resection, is an important goal that need to be studied. This usually done after the efficacy of adjuvant chemotherapy have been proven. Since these trials may take many years, many investigations are underway already to minimize the surgical resection at the institutional level (Ensley, 1984, Jacobs, 1987) and on the national multi-institutions is being carry out by the Veterans Administration Laryngeal Cancer Group.

POSSIBLE REASONS FOR NEGATIVE RANDOMIZED TRIALS

In studying the efficacy of adjuvant chemotherapy following the proper concepts that may influence the results of these combined modality therapy are important to ensure good and acceptable results of these trials. Few randomized phase III studies have been conducted especially on the cooperative group level. Most of these trials have been negative so far, this is due to many reasons and especially some or all of the following:

1. Small number of patients included
2. No or poor stratification to important prognostic factors
3. Inadequate definition of staging systems, especially T4 and N3 to adequately stratify patients

4. Poor design and/or concept
5. Compliance problem
6. Poor choice of chemotherapy (ineffective)
7. Number of courses of chemotherapy given (inadequate)
8. High incidence of second primary cancer and/or high rate of death from unrelated causes

REFERENCES

Vikram, B., Strong, E.W., Shah, H.P, Spiro, R. (1984): Failure at the primary site following multimodality treatment in advanced head and neck cancer. Head and Neck Surg. 6, 720-723.

Vikram, B., Strong, E.W., Shah, H.P., Spiro, R. (1984a): Failure in the neck following multimodality treatment for advanced head and neck cancer. Head and Neck Surg. 6, 724-729.

Al-Sarraf, M. (1984): Chemotherapy strategies in squamous cell carcinoma of the head and neck. CRC Crit. Rev. Oncol. Hematol. 1, 323-355.

Al-Sarraf, M. (1987): Chemotherapy strategies in squamous cell carcinoma of the head and neck. Cancer Metas. Rev. 6, 181-198.

Al-Kourainy, K., Kish, J.A., Ensley, J.F., et al (1987): Achievement of superior survival for histologically negative vs histologically positive clinically complete responders to cis-platinum combination in patients with locally advanced head and neck cancer. Cancer 59, 233-238.

Al-Sarraf, M., Pajak, T.F., Marcial, V.A., et al (1987a): Concurrent radiotherapy and chemotherapy with cisplatin in in-operable squamous cell carcinoma of the head and neck. RTOG study. Cancer 59, 259-265.

Adjuvant chemotherapy for advanced head and neck squamous carcinoma: Final report of the head and neck contract program (1987). Cancer 60, 301-311.

Al-Sarraf, M., Kinzie, J., Jacobs, J., et al. (1982): New way of giving chemotherapy as part of multi-disciplinary treatment for patients with head and neck cancers. Preliminary report. Proc. AACR 23, 134.

Jacobs, C., Goffinet, D.R., Goffinet, L., et al. (1987): Chemotherapy as a substitute for surgery in the treatment of advanced resectable head and neck cancer. Cancer 60, 1183-1187.

Ervin, T.J., Clark, J.R., Weichselbaum, R.R., et al. (1987): An analysis of induction and adjuvant chemotherapy in the multidisciplinary treatment of squamous-cell carcinoma of the head and neck. J. Clin. Oncol. 5, 10-20.

Ensley, J.F., Jacobs, J.R., Weaver, A., et al. (1984): The correlation between response to cis-platinum combination chemotherapy and subsequent radiotherapy in previously untreated patients with advanced squamous cell cancers of the head and neck. Cancer 54, 811-814.

Al-Sarraf, M. (1988): Head and neck cancer: chemotherapy concepts. Sem. Oncology (in press).

Ensley, J.F., Kish, J.A., Tapazoglou, E., et al. (1988): An intensive five course alternating combination chemotherapy induction regimen employed in patients with advanced unresectable head and neck cancer. J. Clin. Oncol. (in press).

Marcial, V.A., Pajak, T.F., Kramer, S., et al. (1988): Radiation Therapy Oncology Group (RTOG) studies in head and neck cancer. Sem. Oncol. (in press).

Résumé

La chimiothérapie des tumeurs tête et cou localements avancées: "present concept and status"
La confirmation des taux de résponses très élévées par traitement chimiothérapeutipue, surtout les combinaisons sur base de Cisplatine et en cas de traitement initiel dans des patients atteints de cancer tête et cou localement avancé, était le facteur principal de l'intégration de ces drogues dans des combinaisons de différentes modalités thérapeutiques. Avant d'activer des études randomisées phase III, il est important de répondre aux questions conceptuelles et importantes qui se posent en relation avec l'utilisation de la chimiothérapie dans des combinaisons de différentes thérapies. Elles sont: 1. Quelle est la meilleure combinaison chimiotherapique et quel est le nombre de cycles optimal . Combien de cycles à ajouter après avoir atteint la meilleure résponse. 2. Comment intégrer la chimiothérapie dans le plan thérapeutique; comment faire le "timing and sequencing" dans le cas d'une tumeur opérable ou inopérable. 3. A quel moment faut-il combiner la chimiothérapie avec autres traitements. Quel taux de résponses complètes cliniques et histologiques est suffisant pour introduire ces drogues dans des études de phase III. La négligeance de ces "concepts" importants pourrait être la cause d' un abandon précoce d'une modalité de traitement, peut-être efficace.

Neo-Adjuvant Chemotherapy. Ed. Cl. Jacquillat, M. Weil, D. Khayat. Colloque INSERM/John Libbey Eurotext Ltd. © 1988. Vol. 169, pp. 281-285.

Laryngeal and pharyngeal carcinomas treated by association of induction chemotherapy and laryngeal conservative surgery

H. Laccourreye*, D. Brasnu*, P. Bonfils*, V. Bassot* and Cl. Jacquillat**

** Service d'ORL et de Chirurgie Cervico-Faciale, Hôpital Laënnec, 42, rue de Sèvres, 75007 Paris, France*
*** Service d'Oncologie Médicale, Hôpital de la Salpétrière, 47, boulevard de l'hôpital, 75651 Paris Cedex 13, France*

.SUMMARY

The aim of this study was to analyze the results of the association of chemotherapy and laryngeal conservative surgery for 185 patients with laryngeal or pharyngeal cancers. The main results are : (i) Tumor clinical regression after initial chemotherapy was higher than 50% for 79% of the patients : (ii) Histopathological study of the specimen showed residual tumor or complete response to chemotherapy for 55% of the patients : (iii) the actuarial 3-year survival rate for all patients was 81% ; (iv) the surgical procedure initially planned (i.e., total laryngectomy) was modified in 23 cases. Since quantitative appreciation of tumor response seems to be difficult, this modification of the surgical procedure initially planned must be done prudently.

.MOTS CLES

Neoadjuvant chemotherapy : chimiothérapie néo-adjuvante
Laryngeal conservative surgery : chirurgie partielle laryngée

.INTRODUCTION

The role of chemotherapy as initial treatment of Head and Neck cancer has yet to be legitimized. Many studies were reported concerning induction chemotherapy in unresectable squamous cell carcinomas of the upper aero-digestive tract (1,2). But, chemotherapy as an adjuvant to a laryngeal conservative surgery has not been reported. In this study, the use of the association of chemotherapy and laryngeal conservative surgery for patients with pharyngeal or laryngeal cancers was undertaken with three major objectives : (i) the first was to determine the tumor response to neo-adjuvant chemotherapy ; (ii) the second was to determine whether a response to induction chemotherapy could modify the surgical procedure initially planned ; and (iii) the third one was to determine whether local surgical treatment following neo-adjuvant chemotherapy was capable of controlling either local and regional disease or distant micrometastases.

.METHODS

Patients:
One hundred and eighty-five patients were included in this study. All patients were staged retrospectively according to the 1987 UICC classification. Distribution according to primary site, and T status is presented in Table 1.

Table 1. Distribution by primary site, T status.

PRIMARY SITE	T1	T2	T3	T4
glottic cancer	13	21	7	2
supraglottic cancer	7	16	25	0
vallecula	4	11	12	0
pyriform sinus cancer	9	20	3	0
laryngeal margin cancer	6	24	5	0

Of note, 71,4% (132) were classified as NO; 13% (24) as N1; 6,5% (12) as N2a; 0.5% (1) as N2b; 3.8% (8) as N2c; 4.8% (9) as N3 at presentation.

Treatment:
All patients received as initial treatment a multiple agents chemotherapy. From 1981 to 1985, all patients were treated by the following protocol at three weeks intervals : cisplatinum 100mg/m2, D1; fluoro-5-Uracile: 1 g/m2, D1-D4 (continuous infusion); Bleomycin: 15 mg, D1; 7,5 mg, D2-D4, Since 1985, patients received : cisplatinum 25 mg/m2, and fluoro-5-uracile : 1g/m2, D1-D2 (continuous infusion).
Conservative surgery consisted of either supracricoid partial laryngectomy or supraglottic laryngectomy for laryngeal cancers, and either supraglottic laryngectomy extended to the base of the tongue, or supra-cricoid hemi-pharyngo-laryngectomy for pharyngeal cancers. Bilateral modified neck dissection was carried out for supraglottic, laryngeal margin, and vallecula cancers. Ipsilateral radical neck dissection was performed for pyriform sinus and lateral margin carcinomas. Only 84 patients received post-operative radiation therapy : 50 Gy by external "CO60" beam to the primary and to both cervical lymph node chains.

.RESULTS:

1. Tumor response after neo-adjuvant chemotherapy
Tumor responses after initial chemotherapy are expressed in Table II and Table III according to T status.

Table II. Tumor clinical regression versus T status.

Tumor response	T1+T2		T3+T4	
less than 50%	25	19%	15	28%
more than 50%	8	44%	27	50%
Complete Response	48	37%	12	22%

Table III. Histopathological tumor response according to T status.

Tumor response	T1+T2	T3+T4
no response	54 (30%)	29 (15%)
residual tumor	46 (24%)	20 (11%)
Complete Response	31 (17%)	05 (03%)

2. Modification of the surgical procedure initially planned after chemotherapy.

In twenty-three cases (12.4%), the surgical procedure initially planned was modified because of good response to neo-adjuvant chemotherapy. In these cases, the T status was always T3, and the initial surgical indication was always a total laryngectomy. In this series, 17 patients have been followed for time varying from 5 months to 5 years (mean value : 1 year,9 months), and are alive without cancer. In three cases, subjects died of intercurrent disease free of cancer. Three patients died with cancer : second primary cancer (one case), nodal recurrence (one case), and local recurrence (once case).

3. Survival:

The actuarial 3-year survival rate for all patients was 81%. Survival according to the primary site is expressed in Table IV.

Table IV. Actuarial 3-year survival according to primary sites.

PRIMARY SITE	3-year survival	number of cases
glottic cancer	87%	43
supraglottic cancer	78%	48
vallecula cancer	83%	27
pyriform sinus cancer	89%	32
laryngeal margin cancer	71%	35

3-year actuarial survival rate of T2 pharyngeal carcinomas was 84% (n=55 cases).

4. Local and nodal recurrences:
Among 91 patients with laryngeal carcinomas, only two patients had a local recurrence (2.2%), and only one of them needed a total laryngectomy. No nodal reccurence occured. Among 94 patients with pharyngeal cancer, two local recurrences (2.1%) and 2 nodal recurrences (2.1%) occured.

5. Distant metastases and second primary cancer:
Distant metastases and second primary cancer for patients with laryngeal or pharyngeal carcinoma is expressed in Table V.

Table V. Metastases and second primary cancer versus primary site.

PRIMARY SITE	Distant Metastases	Second primary Cancer
larynx	4 (4.4%)	1 (1.1%)
pharynx	12 (12.8%)	8 (8.5%)

.DISCUSSION

The intent of this study was to analyze the role of neo-adjuvant chemotherapy in the treatment of patients with tumors that could be treated by laryngeal conservative surgery.
The first objective was to determine the tumor regression. Such regression occurred in 80% of patients, with complete clinical response in 33%. These rates were more important for T1 and T2 tumors than for T3 or T4 tumors. Histopathological responses were present in only 55% of patients (residual or absence of tumor), with complete histological response in 20%. This discrepancy could be explained by the difficulty of quantative evaluation of the clinical regression.
The second objective was to determine whether chemotherapy could modify the surgical procedure initially planned. This surgical procedure (i.e., total laryngectomy) was modified in 23 cases. Among these 23 cases, only one patient had a local recurrence (4%). Moreover, in 6 cases, no cancer was found on the histopathological examination of the specimen (25%). However, since quantative evaluation of tumor response seems to be difficult, this modification of the surgical procedure initially planned must be carefully done.
The third objective of this study was to determine whether local surgical treatment (i.e., laryngeal conservative surgery) following neo-adjuvant chemotherapy was able to control either local and regional disease or distant micrometastases. The actuarial 3-year survival rate varied between 78% (supraglottic cancer treated by supraglottic laryngectomy) and 89% (pyriform sinus treated by hemi-pharyngo-laryngectomy). The rate of distant metastases was not higher as compared to other series. It could be related to the action of neo-adjuvant chemotherapy. This hypothesis needs to be precised by other studies. These data have to be compared to results obtained with series of patients treated by association of chemotherapy and radiation.

.REFERENCES

1. BRASNU et al., 1988, Les cancers inopérables des voies aéro-digestives supérieures. L'intérêt de la chimiothérapie. Nouvelle Presse Médicale, in press.
2. ERVIN, T.J., CLARK, J.R., WEICHSELBAUM, R.R., et al., : An analysis of induction and adjuvant chemotherapy in the multidisciplinary treatment of squamous-cell carcinome of the head and neck. J. Clinical Oncol. 5, 10-20.

Résumé

Le but de cette étude a été d'analyser l'apport de la chimiothérapie à base de 5 FU et Cisplatinum dans le traitement de cancers du larynx et du pharynx traités par chirurgie partielle laryngée (185 cas). Les principaux résultats exposés sont : (1) une régression tumorale appréciée cliniquement de plus de 50% dans 79% des cas tandis qu'une régression histologique majeure n'a été retrouvée que dans 55% des cas ; (2) une survie actuarielle globale est de 81% à 3 ans, survie variant de 71% à 89% suivant la localisation initiale ; (3) dans 23 cas (12,4%), l'indication chirurgicale initiale était une laryngectomie totale, indication modifiée après chimiothérapie en chirurgie partielle laryngée. Dans ces derniers cas, une grande prudence doit être de règle dans la modification de l'indication initiale.

Neo-Adjuvant Chemotherapy. Ed. Cl. Jacquillat, M. Weil, D. Khayat. Colloque INSERM/John Libbey Eurotext Ltd. © 1988. Vol. 169, pp. 287-294.

Strategy of combining chemotherapy and radiotherapy in advanced head and neck cancer

Asit J. Choksi, Isaiah W. Dimery, Alan Kramer and Waun K. Hong

The University of Texas System Cancer Center, M.D. Anderson Hospital and Tumor Institute, Head/Neck and Thoracic Medical Oncology, 1515 Holcombe Boulevard, Box 80, Houston, Texas 77030, USA

ABSTRACT

Five-year survival for patients presenting with stage III or IV cancer of the head and neck who undergo standard treatment (surgery, radiotherapy or both) ranges from 0% to 60%. Therefore, an approach utilizing chemotherapy prior to local treatment has been vigorously pursued over the last decade.

This paper addresses the following issues: 1) treatment strategies of various combinations of chemoradiotherapy, 2) status of sequential and simultaneous chemoradiotherapy, 3) potential obviation of surgery by chemoradiotherapy, and 4) ongoing clinical trials of chemoradiotherapy combinations in the United States.

INTRODUCTION

Early-stage head and neck cancer can be cured with radiotherapy or surgery. Traditionally, patients who present with locally advanced lesions are treated with surgery ± radiotherapy if lesions are resectable, and with radiotherapy alone if lesions are unresectable. Of those patients, 50% to 60% develop local recurrence and 20% to 30% develop distant metastases.[1] Five-year survival ranges from 0% to 60%.[2] Many patients will also develop functional and cosmetic disabilities as a result of radical surgery or loco-regional recurrence. Thus, incorporation of an additional modality, such as chemotherapy, into the standard treatment has been vigorously pursued over the last decade.

The reason for combining chemotherapy and radiotherapy is to utilize chemotherapy as both a radiosensitizer and a cytotoxic agent to achieve the objectives of better local tumor control, possible elimination of surgery, and control of distant micrometastases, with the further results of improved quality of life and better survival.

Three treatment strategies of combinations of chemotherapy and radiotherapy have been under investigation for many years: 1) *sequential* chemotherapy followed by radiotherapy, 2) *simultaneous* chemotherapy and radiotherapy, and 3) *interdigitating*, or alternating chemotherapy with radiotherapy.

SEQUENTIAL CHEMORADIOTHERAPY

In sequential chemoradiotherapy, radiotherapy is administered after 2 or 3 courses of chemotherapy. The major advantages of this approach are: 1) that a decrease in tumor size possibly eliminates the hypoxic cell subpopulation, making the tumor more radiosensitive, 2) the ability to monitor a sequential response pattern of the tumor, 3) that drug concentration in tumor cells may remain high enough to function as a radiosensitizer during radiotherapy, 4) that administration of standard or higher doses of chemotherapy still allows full-course radiotherapy with curative intent, and 5) that unresectable tumor may become resectable after chemotherapy. The approach has a few disadvantages: 1) the radiosensitization effect is much less compared to simultaneous chemoradiotherapy; 2) patients may refuse radiotherapy after a good response to chemotherapy; 3) duration of therapy is prolonged; and 4) nonresponders to chemotherapy may have increased tumor burden at initiation of local treatment.

Randomized trials comparing sequential chemoradiotherapy to radiotherapy alone have not shown any significant benefit (Table 1).[3-8] However, all these trials have used single agents or ineffective regimens. Recently, many nonrandomized trials have shown promisingly high local control rates (Table 2).[8-22] A few trials have demonstrated that patients achieving complete or near-complete response do well with radiotherapy without radical surgery.[23-27]

Table 1. Randomized Trials of Sequential Chemotherapy and Radiotherapy versus Radiotherapy Alone

Study	Regimen	Total No. Patients	Overall Survival Benefit
Von Essen, 1968	MTX, IUDR, 5-FU	100	No
Knowlton, 1975	MTX	96	No
Lustig, 1976	MTX	75	No
Fazekas, 1980	MTX	638	No
Stell, 1983	Price-Hill regimen	86	No
Szpirglas, 1987	PVB + Dox	114	Yes (?)

Table 2. Sequential Chemotherapy and Radiotherapy in Advanced Head and Neck Cancer

Study	Regimen	Total No. Patients	Complete Response Rate
Randolph, 1978	PB	18	33%
Glick, 1980	PB	25	48%
Figueroa-Velles, 1982	VBM	37	46%
Tannock, 1982	PBM	30	40%
Schaeffer, 1983	CDDP	28	39%
Coughlin, 1984	PB	23	57%
Ensley, 1984	PVB or PF	79	66%
Hong, 1984	CDDP ± Bleo	39	61%
Kukla, 1984	PVB	19	42%
Adelstein, 1985	PBM	12	50%
Rosso, 1985	VBM	45	58%
Hill, 1986	Price Hill regimen	199	69%
Haines, 1987	PB	21	81%
Szpirglas, 1987	PVB + Dox	56	41%
Zidan, 1987	PBM	29	66%

Jacobs et al[27] treated 30 patients with 3 cycles of CDDP plus 5-FU, followed by re-endoscopy and biopsy. Twelve patients who achieved a pathologic complete response at the primary site received only radiotherapy; at 2 years, relapse-free survival and overall survival for these 12 patients were 60% and 70%. For all patients in the study, relapse-free survival and overall survival were 52% and 53%. Thus, it was shown that elimination of surgery with treatment by radiotherapy alone does not compromise survival in patients who achieve pathologic complete response.

This approach is now being tested by the Veterans Administration Cooperative Laryngeal Study Group in a randomized fashion in patients with stage III or IV operable laryngeal carcinoma (Fig. 1).[28] Responders in the chemotherapy arm are treated with radiotherapy and if found to have NED after treatment are followed without surgery. Patients with residual disease after radiation therapy undergo salvage surgery. Preliminary results are very encouraging. Of 76 patients on the chemotherapy arm, 67 were evaluable for tumor response. Objective response rates were: complete response, 33%, partial response, 46%. Histologic complete response of the primary tumor was seen in 37%. At the last report on the 76 patients on the chemotherapy arm, 33 were with NED of the larynx, 21 required salvage surgery, 18 were on chemotherapy or radiotherapy, 4 had died, and 1 had withdrawn from the study.

Figure 1.
Veterans Administration Cooperative Laryngeal Cancer Study Schema

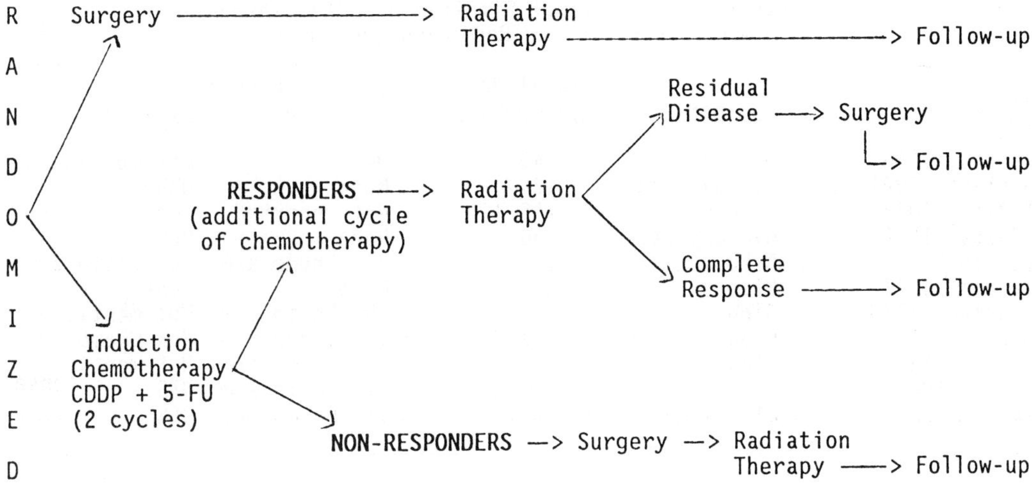

SIMULTANEOUS CHEMORADIOTHERAPY

Major advantages of simultaneously administered chemotherapy and radiotherapy are: 1) Chemotherapy can function much better as a radiosensitizer, resulting in a synergistic effect on the local tumor. 2) Radiotherapy can reduce tumor volume, leading to increased cell proliferation and chemosensitivity. 3) Duration of treatment is usually not prolonged. However, there are some disadvantages: 1) There is more toxicity from concomitant administration of chemoradiotherapy. 2) Compromised chemotherapy doses may not be enough to control distant metastases. 3) Surgery may be more difficult after a full curative dose of radiotherapy has been administered with chemotherapy.

Randomized trials of simultaneous chemoradiotherapy versus radiotherapy alone have reported better response rates in the chemoradiotherapy arm, although only 3 trials have reported survival benefit (Table 3).[29-39] Two of these trials report benefit only in oral cavity cancer patients. However, none of these trials have used CDDP. CDDP is one of the most active agents in head and neck cancer; it also has been reported to have radiosensitizing properties.[40-42] Cisplatin may interfere with repair of sublethal and potentially lethal radiation damage, act as a hypoxic cell radiosensitizer, and enhance radiation cytotoxicity.

Nonrandomized trials using CDDP ± 5-FU and radiotherapy have reported encouraging results (Table 4).[43] **Taylor et al**[44] treated 34 patients which had advanced head and neck cancer with a planned 7 cycles of radiation at 2 Gy/day, days 1 through 5, combined with CDDP at 60 mg/m^2 on day 1, and 5-FU at 800 mg/m^2 over 24 hours, days 1 through 5. Cycles were repeated every 14 days and were modified for hematologic and mucosal toxicity. All 34 patients had a major response with a complete response rate of 59%. Using Kaplan-Meier estimates, the 75% survival was 16 months, and the 50% survival 38 months for all 34 patients. Taylor's group has initiated a randomized trial of sequential chemoradiotherapy versus simultaneous chemoradiotherapy.

Another important ongoing trial has been initiated by the Head and Neck Intergroup comparing cisplatin plus radiotherapy versus radiotherapy alone. Results of these trials are not yet available.

Table 3. Randomized Trials of Simultaneous Chemotherapy Plus **Radiotherapy Versus Radiotherapy Alone**

Study	Regimen	Total No. Patients	Benefits: Response	Survival
Condit, 1968	MTX	40	None	Not mentioned
Stefani, 1971	Hydroxyurea	126	None	None
Gollin, 1972	5-FU	155	Not reported	Yes-Chemo arm
Hussey, 1975	Hydroxyurea	40	None	None
Lo, 1986	5-FU	136	Yes-Chemo arm	Yes-Chemo arm
Cachin, 1977	Bleo	224	None	None
Kapstad, 1978	Bleo	32	Yes-Chemo arm	Not mentioned
Shanta, 1980	Bleo	117	Yes-Chemo arm	Yes-Chemo arm
Morita, 1980	Bleo	45	Yes-Chemo arm	Not mentioned
Papac, 1987	MTX	120	Yes-Chemo arm	DFS
Fu, 1987	Bleo + MTX	104	Yes-Chemo arm	DFS

Table 4. Nonrandomized Simultaneous Chemoradiotherapy with CDDP ± 5-FU

Study	Regimen	Total No. Patients	Complete Response: No.	Rate
Slotman, 1986	CDDP	18	13	72%
Al-Sarraf, 1987	CDDP	124	86	69%
Crispino, 1987	CDDP	19	10	53%
Wendt, 1987	PF + FA	60	45	75%
Taylor, 1987	PF	34	20	59%
Wheeler, 1987	CDDP High-dose	18	17	94%

INTERDIGITATING CHEMORADIOTHERAPY

Interdigitating chemoradiotherapy is another interesting approach. The mathematical model developed by **Goldie and Coldman** relates the drug sensitivity of heterogeneous tumor to its own mutation rate toward phenotypic drug resistance. The implication of this theory is that the most effective therapy to circumvent the problems of heterogeneous tumor cell population and drug resistance is either a combination of all active agents given simultaneously as initial therapy or the administration of alternating non-cross-resistant regimens.[45] It has also been shown in vitro that cell lines, when made resistant to chemotherapeutic agents by stepwise incubation with the drug, become resistant to radiotherapy.[46] Thus, the attenuation of chemotherapy with radiotherapy (one of the most effective cytotoxic agents in cancer therapy) reduces emergence of drug- and radio-resistant clones. It also combines most of the advantages of sequential and simultaneous chemoradiotherapy, resulting in better tolerance and improved local control, and at the same time possibly eliminating distant micrometastases. A trial with this approach is being initiated at M. D. Anderson Hospital (Fig. 2).

Figure 2.

One course of treatment:

Chemotherapy	REST	**Radiotherapy**	REST
Days 1-5	Days 6-13	Days 14-18	Days 19-28
CDDP 100 mg/m2 Day 1		3.2 Gy/day	
5-FU 1000 mg/m2 Days 1-5		16.0 Gy total	

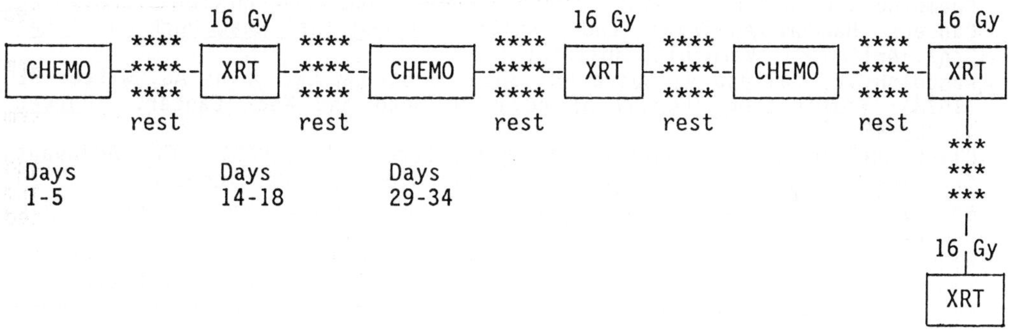

CONCLUSION

Treatment strategies using sequential, simultaneous, or interdigitating chemotherapy and radiotherapy have been studied in the past decade and are still under investigation. No firm conclusions are available as to which strategy is most effective. Optimal scheduling of chemotherapy and radiotherapy may differ for different combinations of chemotherapy and radiotherapy. Because of no improvement in survival with current chemoradiotherapy combinations compared with radiotherapy alone, it is important that radiotherapy alone or radiotherapy with surgery continue to be used as standard treatment in future randomized trials of various combinations of chemotherapy and radiotherapy in advanced head and neck cancer.

ABBREVIATIONS

Abbreviations used: **Bleo**, bleomycin; **CDDP**, cisplatin; **DFS**, disease-free survival; **Dox**, doxorubicin; **FA**, folinic acid; **5-FU**, 5-fluorouracil; **IUDR**, iododeoxyruidine; **Mito-C**, mitomycin C; **MTX**, methotrexate; **NED**, no evidence of disease; **PB**, cisplatin + bleomycin; **PVB**, cisplatin + vincristine + bleomycin; **PBM**, cisplatin + bleomycin + methotrexate; **PF**, cisplatin + 5-fluorouracil; **VBM**, vincristine + bleomycin + methotrexate; **XRT**, radiation therapy.

REFERENCES

1. Hong WK, Bromer R (1983): Chemotherapy in Head and Neck Cancer. N Engl J Med 308(2):75-79.
2. Wolf G (1984): An Overview of Preoperative Chemotherapy: Where Do We Go From Here? Am J Otolaryngol 5:77-79.
3. von Essen CF, Joseph LBM, Simon GT, Singh AD, Singh SP (1968): Sequential Chemotherapy and Radiation Therapy of Buccal Mucosa Carcinoma in South India. Forty-ninth Annu Meet of Am Radiol Soc, Ontario, Canada, pp 530-540.
4. Knowlton AH, Percarpio B, Bobrow S, Fischer JJ (1975): Methotrexate and Radiation Therapy in the Treatment of Advanced Head and Neck Tumors. Radiology 116:709-712.
5. Lustig RA, DeMare PA, Kramer S (1976): Adjuvant Methotrexate in the Radiotherapeutic Management of Advanced Tumors of the Head and Neck. Cancer 37:2703-2708.
6. Fazekas JT, Sommer C, Kramer S (1980): Adjuvant Intravenous Methotrexate or Definitive Radiotherapy Alone for Advanced Squamous Cancers of the Oral Cavity, Oropharynx, Supraglottic Larynx or Hypopharynx. Int J Radiat Oncol Biol Phys 6:533-541.
7. Stell PM, Dalby JE, Strickland P (1983): Sequential Chemotherapy and Radiotherapy in Advanced Head and Neck Cancer. Clin Radiol 34:463-467.
8. Szpirglas H, Lacoste JP, Marneur M, Nizri D (1987): Neo-Adjuvant Chemotherapy Before Radiotherapy in Oral and Oropharyngeal Advanced Cancers. Randomized Trial: End Results. Second Intl Head Neck Oncol Res Conf, Arlington, Virginia, Abstract 1.3.
9. Randolph VL, Vallejo A, Spiro RH, Shah J, Strong EW, Huvos AG, Wittes RE (1978): Combination Therapy of Advanced Head and Neck Cancer. Cancer 41:460-467.
10. Glick JH, Marcia V, Richter M, Velez-Garcia E (1980): The Adjuvant Treatment of Inoperable Stage III and IV Epidermoid Carcinoma of the Head and Neck With Platinum and Bleomycin Infusions Prior to Definitive Radiotherapy: An RTOG Pilot Study. Cancer 46:1919-1924.
11. Figueroa-Valles NR, Marcial VA, Velez-Garcia E, Cintron J, Vallecillo LA (1982): Multidrug Chemotherapy (Vincristine-Bleomycin-Methotrexate) Followed by Radiotherapy in Inoperable Carcinomas of the Head and Neck. Am J Clin Oncol (CCT) 5:399-404.
12. Tannock I, Cummings B, Sorrenti V, and the ENT Group (1982): Combination Chemotherapy Used Prior to Radiation Therapy for Locally Advanced Squamous Cell Carcinoma of the Head and Neck. Cancer Treat Rep 66(6):1421-1424.
13. Schaeffer SD, Middleton R, Reisch J, Frenkel EP (1983): *Cis*-Platinum Induction Chemotherapy in the Multi-Modality Initial Treatment of Advanced Stage IV Carcinoma of the Head and Neck. Cancer 51(12):2168-2174.
14. Coughlin CT, Grace M, O'Donnell JF, LeMarbre JP, Morain WD, Geurkink NA, McIntyre OR (1984): Combined Modality Approach in the Management of Locally Advanced Head and Neck Cancer. Cancer Treat Rep 68(4):591-597.
15. Ensley JF, Kish JA, Jacobs J, Weaver A, Crissman J, Al-Sarraf M (1984): Incremental Improvements in Median Survival Associated with Degree of Response to Adjuvant Chemotherapy in Patients with Advanced Squamous Cell Cancer of the Head and Neck. Adjuvant Therapy of Cancer IV, SE Jones and SE Salmon eds, pp 117-125. Grune & Stratton, New York.

16. Hong WK, Popkin J, Bromer R, Shapshay S, Hoffer S, Willett B, Strong MS, Vaughan C, Katz A, Fofonoff S, Amato D (1984): Adjuvant Chemotherapy as Initial Treatment of Advanced Head and Neck Cancer: Survival Data at Three Years. Adjuvant Therapy of Cancer IV, SE Jones and SE Salmon eds, pp 127-133. Grune & Stratton, New York.
17. Kukla LJ, Mantravadi RVP, Applebaum EL, McGuire WP (1984): Preirradiation Chemotherapy for Advanced Head/Neck Carcinoma. Arch Otolaryngol 110:78-81.
18. Adelstein DJ, Hines JD, Sharan VM, Streeter RR, Earle AS, Haria CD, Carter SG, Shah AC, Vlastou C, Damm C (1985): Combination Chemotherapy Prior to Definitive Local Therapy in Squamous Cell Carcinoma of the Head and Neck. Oncology 42:80-85.
19. Rosso R, Merland M, Scarpati D, Grimaldi A, Bonelli L, Barbieri A (1985): Combined Polychemotherapy and Radiotherapy in Advanced Inoperable Squamous Cell Carcinoma of the Head and Neck. Head Neck Surg 8:74-77.
20. Hill BT, Price LA, MacRae K (1986): Importance of Primary Site in Assessing Chemotherapy Response and 7-Year Survival Data in Advanced Squamous-Cell Carcinomas of the Head and Neck Treated with Initial Combination Chemotherapy without Cisplatin. J Clin Oncol 4:1340-1347.
21. Haines I, Bosl G, Pfister D, Spiro R, Gerold F, Sessions R, Shah J, Strong E, Vikram B, Harrison L (1987): Very-High-Dose Cisplatin with Bleomycin Infusion as Initial Treatment of Advanced Head and Neck Cancer. J Clin Oncol 5(10):1594-1600.
22. Zidan J, Kuten A, Cohen Y, Robinson E (1987): Multidrug Chemotherapy Using Bleomycin, Methotrexate, and Cisplatin Combined with Radical Radiotherapy in Advanced Head and Neck Cancer. Cancer 59:24-26.
23. Krasnow SH, Cohen MH, Johnston-Early A, Citron ML, Fossieck BE, Mauk CM, Yenson A, Banda FP, Lunzer S, deFries HO (1984): Combined Therapy for Stage III-IV Head and Neck Cancer: Preliminary Results. J Clin Oncol 2(7):804-810.
24. Ervin TJ, Weichselbaum RR, Fabian RL, Miller D, Norris CM, Ponser MR, Rose C, Lockhart P, Tuttle SA, MacIntyre JM, Frei E III (1984): Advanced Squamous Carcinoma of the Head and Neck. Arch Otolaryngol 110:241-245.
25. Greenberg B, Ahmann F, Garewal H, Koopmann C, Coulthard S, Berzes H, Alberts D, Shimm D, Slymen D (1987): Neoadjuvant Therapy for Advanced Head and Neck Cancer with Allopurinol-Modulated High Dose 5-Fluorouracil and Cisplatin. Cancer 59:1860-1865.
26. Kadish SP, Cohen N, Conway HW, Sherman DM, Schwartz JH, Strauss GH, Ricciardi PA (1987): Induction Chemotherapy and Full Course Irradiation for Advanced Head and Neck Cancer: A Non-Operative Approach with Results Comparable to Surgical Series. Second Intl Head Neck Oncol Res Conf, Arlington, Virginia, Abstract 1.5.
27. Jacobs C, Goffinet DR, Goffinet L (1987): Chemotherapy as a Substitute for Surgery in the Treatment of Advanced Resectable Head and Neck Cancer. Cancer 60:1178-1183.
28. Hong WK, Wolf GT, Fisher S (1987): A New Strategy to Preserve the Larynx in the Treatment of Advanced Laryngeal Cancer: Preliminary Report (Abstract 509). Proc Am Soc Clin Oncol 6:130.
29. Condit PT (1968): Treatment of Carcinoma with Radiation Therapy and Methotrexate. Mo Med 65:832-835.
30. Stafani S, Eells RW, Abbate J (1971): Hydroxyurea and Radiotherapy in Head and Neck Cancer. Radiology 101:391-396.
31. Gollin FF, Ansfield FJ, Brandenburg JH, Ramirez G, Vermund H (1972): Combined Therapy in Advanced Head and Neck Cancer: A Randomized Study. Am J Roentgenol 114(1):83-88.
32. Hussey DH, Abrams JP (1975): Combined Therapy in Advanced Head and Neck Cancer: Hydroxyurea and Radiotherapy. Prog Clin Cancer 6:79-86.
33. Lo TCM, Wiley AL, Ansfield FJ, Brandenburg JH, David HL, Gollin FF, Johnson RO, Ramirez G, Vermund H (1975): Combined Radiation Therapy and 5-Fluorouracil for Advanced Squamous Cell Carcinoma of the Oral Cavity and Oropharynx: A Randomized Study. Am J Roentgenol 126(2):229-235.

34. Cachin Y, Jortay A, Sancho H, Eschwege F, Madelain M, Desaulty A, Gerard P (1977): Preliminary Results of a Randomized E.O.R.T.C. Study Comparing Radiotherapy and Concomitant Bleomycin to Radiotherapy Alone in Epidermoid Carcinomas of the Oropharynx. Eur J Cancer 13:1389-1395.
35. Kapstad B, Band G, Rennaes S, Dahler A (1978): Combined Preoperative Treatment with Cobalt and Bleomycin in Patients with Head and Neck Carcinoma--A Controlled Clinical Study. Int J Radiat Oncol Biol Phys 4:85-89.
36. Shanta V, Krishnamurthi S (1980): Combined Bleomycin and Radiotherapy in Oral Cancer. Clin Radiol 31:617-620.
37. Morita K (1980): Clinical Significance of Radiation Therapy Combined with Chemotherapy. Strahlentherapie 156:228-233.
38. Papac RJ, Weissberg JB, Son YH (1987): Prospective Randomized Trial of Radiation Therapy (RT) ± Mitomycin C (MC) in Head and Neck Cancer. Proc Am Soc Clin Oncol Abstract 492, 6:126.
39. Fu KK, Phillips TL, Silverberg IJ, Jacobs C, Goffinet DR, Chun C, Friedman MA, Kohler M, McWhirter K, Carter SK (1987): Combined Radiotherapy and Chemotherapy with Bleomycin and Methotrexate for Advanced Inoperable Head and Neck Cancer: Update of a Northern California Oncology Group Randomized Trial. J Clin Oncol 5:1410-1418.
40. Richmond RC, Powers EL (1976): Radiation Sensitization of Bacterial Spores by *cis*-Dichlorodiammineplatinum (II). Radiat Res 68:251-257.
41. Douple EB, Richmond RC (1979): Radiosensitization of Hypoxic Tumor Cells by *cis*- and *trans*-Dichlorodiammineplatinum (II). Int J Radiat Oncol Biol Phys 5:1369-1372.
42. Douple EB, Richmond RC (1978): Platinum Complexes as Radiosensitizers of Hypoxic Mammalian Cells. Br J Cancer 37(Suppl III):98-102.
43. Choksi AJ, Dimery IW, Hong WK (1988): Adjuvant Chemotherapy of Head and Neck Cancer: The Past, the Present, and the Future. Semin in Oncol (in press).
44. Taylor SG, Murthy AK, Showel J, Caldarelli DD, Hutchinson JC Jr, Holinger LD, Witt TR, Hoover S (1987): Treatment of Advanced Head and Neck Cancer with Concomitant Radiation and Chemotherapy. Second Intl Head Neck Oncol Res Conf, Arlington, Virginia, Abstract 1.1.
45. Goldie JH, Coldman AJ, Gudauskas GA (1982): Rationale for the Use of Alternating Non-Cross-Resistant Chemotherapy. Cancer Treat Rep 66:439-499.
46. Louie KG, Behrens BC, Kinsella TJ, Hamilton TC, Grotzinger KR, McKoy WM, Winkler MA, Ozols RF (1985): Radiation Survival Parameters of Anti-Neoplastic Drug-Sensitive and -Resistant Human Ovarian Cancer Cell Lines and Their Modification by Buthionine Sulfoximine. Cancer Res 45:2110-2115.

Résumé

La survie à 5 ans des malades porteurs de stade III ou IV de cancer de la tête et du cou qui subissent des traitements standard (chirurgie-radiothérapie ou les deux) varie entre 0 % et 60 %. C'est pourquoi, une approche utilisant une chimiothérapie avant un traitement local a été poursuivi vigoureusement durant les 10 dernières années. Cet article traite des problèmes suivants : stratégie thérapeutique des différentes combinaisons de chimio-radiothérapie, état actuel de l'association séquentielle ou simultanée de chimio-radiothérapie, possibilités éventuelles d'éviter la chirurgie par la chimio-radiothérapie et les essais cliniques d'associations chimio-radiothérapiques en cours aux Etats-Unis.

Neo-Adjuvant Chemotherapy. Ed. Cl. Jacquillat, M. Weil, D. Khayat. Colloque INSERM/John Libbey Eurotext Ltd. © 1988. Vol. 169, pp. 295-299.

Unresectable cancers of the upper aero-digestive tract. Results of neo-adjuvant chemotherapy

D. Brasnu*, V. Bassot*, M. Menard*, A. Fabre*, F. Janot*, Cl. Jacquillat** and H. Laccourreye*

* *Service d'ORL et de Chirurgie Cervico-Faciale, Hôpital Laënnec, 42, rue de Sèvres, 75007 Paris, France*
** *Service d'Oncologie Médicale, Hôpital de la Salpétrière, 47, boulevard de l'hôpital, 75651 Paris Cedex 13, France*

.RESUME:
One hundred and eighty five unresectable squamous cell carcinomas of the Upper aerodigestive tract treated between 1980 and 1986 at our institution were retrospectively analyzed. All the patients of the series received neo-adjuvant chemotherapy. The overall tumor response rate was 38% and 15% were evaluated as Complete Clinical Responders. Lethal toxicity after chemotherapy occurred at the rate of 5.9%. One hundred and thirty nine primaries were unresectable as compared to only 17 cervical lymph nodes and 18 primary and cervical nodes. Thirty nine patients (22.4%) became resectable after neo-adjuvant chemotherapy. Disease free survival of complete responders was statistically higher than was for partial and non-responders (at 2-year respectively : 51%, 14% and 8%). Survival of complete responders treated either by radiation therapy or surgery was similar. Survival of partial responders was highter after surgery (34%) than after radiation (17%) and local and regional reccurences occurred less frequently after surgery (67%) than radiation therapy (83%). This study emphasizes that chemothery improved resectability of unresectable Head and Neck Cancer. A less radical surgical procedure than initially planned could be performed in order to decrease the local and regional failure rate for non and partial responders. In other words, the surgical resection could be limited and not based on the initial volume of the tumor before initiation of chemotherapy.

.MOTS CLES:

Head and Neck Tumor	Tumeurs de la Tête et du cou.
Unresectable cancers	Cancers inopérables.
Neo-adjuvant chemotherapy	Chimiothérapie neo-adjuvante.

.INTRODUCTION:

Unresectable Head and Neck Cancers have a very poor prognosis with median survivals ranging from 10 to 16 months (1). The role of surgery after induction chemotherapy is not yet precisely defined.

Norris and associated reported in 1986 a very interesting study with encouraging results of surgical resection after induction chemotherapy (2).
As early as 1970, induction chemotherapy was routinely employed at our institution for all upper aerodigestive tract cancers in order to reduce the tumor volume, to improve local and regional prognosis and to eradicate the subclinical distant metastases and second primary cancers (3). In 1980 Cisplatinum was associated with Bleomycin and Methotréxate and three courses were systematicaly given. Fluoro 5 Uracile in continuous infusion was then administered instead of Methotrexate as in Al Saraf's report (4). More recently a protocol associating Cisplatinum and 5 FU administred in continuous infusion was employéd (5) with an overall response rate of 61% in resectable head and neck cancers. This experience alows us to evaluate the effects of neo-adjuvant chemotherapy on the unresctable head and neck cancers which represent a specific population and remain a major challenge for the head and neck surgeon.

.MATERIAL AND METHODS:
One hundred and eighty five previously untreated unresectable squamous cell carcinomas of the upper aerodigestive tract treated between 1980 and 1986 were retrospectively analyzed. All of them received as initial treatment a multiple agents induction chemotherapy. After completion of chemotherapy and depending on the response to chemotherapy they were treated either by surgical resection and post operative radiation or radiotherapy alone or chemotherapy as single treatment.
The criteria of unresectability which have been adopted were as following :
- Primary site and/or cervical lymph nodes macroscopically unresectable.
- Surgical resection technically possible but microscopically insufficient .
- Surgical resection technically possible but debilitating and functionnaly inacceptable (for instance a simultaneous total glossectomy and total laryngectomy).

In order to select a homogenous population we have adopted the following criteria of exclusion :
- Multiple simultaneous primary carcinomas
- Local or regional recurrences
- Field cancerization
- Nasopharynx and paranasal sinus cancers
- Patients with distant metastases
- Metastatic cervical lymph nodes of unknown origin.

One hundred and thirty nine primaries were evaluated as unresectable as compared with only 17 cervical nodes and 18 were unresectable locally and regionally.
All the patients of the series were treated by multiple agents induction chemotherapy ; eleven patients died during or after completion of chemotherapy. The death rate secondary to chemotherapy administration was 5.9% and is acceptable in regards to the poor prognosis of these patients. The overall response rate of our series to neo-adjuvant chemotherapy was 38%. 15% of patients were evaluated as complete clinical responders.
Three groups according to the locoregional treatment employed after completion of neo-adjuvant chemotheapy can be retrospectively selected : the surgical group (n=39); patients

treated by radiation therapy alone (n=89) and the third group wihich consists of patients treated by chemotherapy as single treatment without surgery or radiotherapy (n=41).
The repartition according to the TNM UICC classification is presented in table 1.
Failure free survival curves according to response to chemotherapy are shown in figure 1.
Local an regional failures according to the treatment eomployed are respectively presented in table 2.

.RESULTS AND DISCUSSION:
At 2-year, survivals for complete responders were higher than survivals for partial and non responders : survival rates were respectively 51%, 14% and 8%. This improvement of survival can be correlated with a decrease of local and regional failures secondary to induction chemotherapy as reported by other authors (2, 3, 6,).

Table 1 (TN Repartition).

	n	%
T1	1	0.5
T2	4	2.4
T3	23	13.2
T4	146	83.9
N0	41	23.6
N1	73	41.9
N2	27	15.5
N3	33	19

Table II.
Locoregional recurrences according to the tretment and responses to chemotherapy at 24 months.

	C+RT		C+S		C	
TR=0	53/56	95%	13/22	59%	19/19	100%
PR	15/18	83%	8/12	67%	4/4	100%
CCR	2/8	25%	0/5	0	2/4	50%

Thirty unresectable primary sites became resectable after induction chemotherapy (21%) and 7 regional matastatic cervical nodes initially considered as unresectable (41%) and only 2 unresectable primary sites and cervical lymph nodes (11%). If the cervical lymph nodes were in our series less frequently a criteria of surgical unresectability than the primary site, they became after neo-adjuvant chemotherapy more frequently resectable than the tumor.

The analysis of the results of our series demonstrates that a surgical resection enhanced significantly survivals and decreased local and regional failures for non responders (including less than 50% reduction of tumor volume). This conclusion can be probably drawn for the partial responders (more than 50% reduction of tumor volume). After radiation therapy alone on partial and non responders survivals were lower and local and regional recurrence rates were higher. A surgical treatment should be therefore prefered to radiotherapy when surgical resection became possible for patients who did not or partially respond to chemotherapy. There was not statistically significant difference in term of survival and local and regional failure between surgical treatment and radiation therapy for complete responders.
This study suggests that for unresectable head and neck cancers chemotherapy probably improves resectability. A less radical surgical procedure than initially planned could be performed in order to decrease the locoregional failure rate for non and partial responders. In other words, the surgical resection could be limited and not based on the initial volume of the disease before initiation of chemotherapy; a debilitating surgery could therefore be avoided. Surgery should be completed by post-operative radiation in order to enhance local and regional control. These conclusions modified the oncologic dogma of the head and neck cancers but have to be interpreted prudently. Futher investigations are necessary to confirm these hypotheses.

.REFERENCES:

1. VOGEL S.EE, LERNER H., KAPLAN B.H. et al. : Failure of effective initial chemotherapy to modify the course of stage IV squamous cancer of the Head and Neck. Cancer, 50 : 840-844, 1982.
2. NORRIS C.H., CLARK J.R., FREI E et al. : Pathology of Surgery after induction Chemotherapy : an analysis of resectability and locoregional control. Laryngoscope, 96 : 292-302, 1986.
3. LACCOURREYE H., HAGUET J.F., Bleomycin as a complement in the treatment of pharynx and larynx carcinomas : a three-year assessment. Gann Monograph on Cancer Research, 19 : 171-175, 1976.
4. AL SARRAF M., DRELICHMAN A., PEPPARD S. et al. : Adjuvant Cisplatinum and 5 Fluoro uracil 96 hour infusion in previously untreated epidermoid cancers of the Head and Neck. Proc. ASCO, 22 : 428. 1981.
5. BASSOT V., BRASNU D., LACAU ST GUILY J. et al. : Chimiothérapie d'induction des cancers des V.A.D.S par perfusions continues associant Cisplatinum (C), 5 FU (F), Bléomycine (B) ou C.F. Ann oto-laryng., 103 : 73-76. 1986.
6. WEICHSEL BAUM R.R., CLARK J.R., MILLER D. et al. : Combined mobility treatment of head and neck cancer with Cisplatin, Bleomycin, Methotrexate. Leucoverin chemotherapy. Cancer, 55 : 2149-2155, 1985.

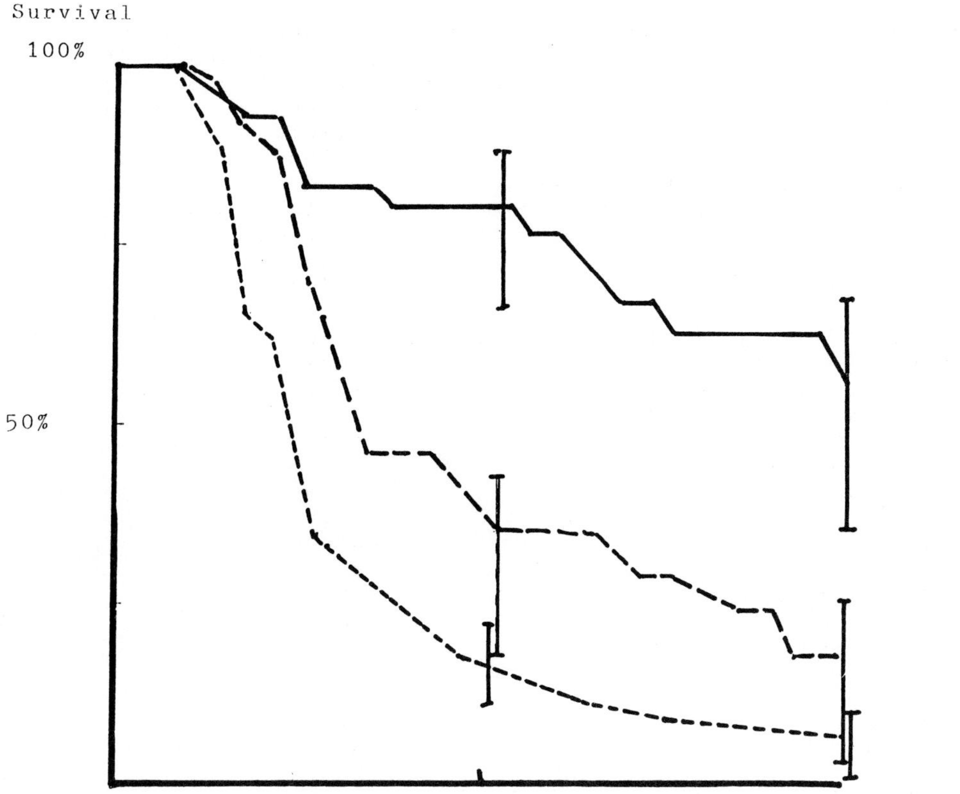

Fig 1 : Failure Free Survivals.

Complete responders
Partial responders
Non responders

Résumé

185 carcinomes épidermoïdes inopérables des V.A.D.S. traités entre 1980 et 1986 ont été analysés rétrospectivement. Tous les patients ont reçu une chimiothérapie néo-adjuvante avec un taux global de répondeurs de 38% dont 15% de répondeurs cliniques complets. Au total 39 patients soit 22% ont été rendus opérables par la chimiothérapie néo-adjuvante. La survie sans récidive des répondeurs cliniques complets à 2 ans est statistiquement supérieure à celle des répondeurs partiels et nuls (respectivement 51%, 14% et 8% pour p 0,001. Chez les répondeurs complets il n'y a pas de différence en terme de survie entre la radiothérapie et la chirurgie . Chez les répondeurs partiels, la survie est meilleure après chirurgie 34% contre 17% après radiothérapie et les échecs locorégionaux moins fréquents 67% contre 83 après radiothérapie. Cette étude souligne l'importance de la réponse à la chimiothérapie néo-adjuvante comme critère pronostique. Cette chimiothérapie a augmenté l'extirpabilité introduisant la notion nouvelle d'une chirurgie du reliquat et a amélioré le pronostic locorégional tout en évitant une chirurgie mutilante.

Head and neck II

Voies aérodigestives II

Neo-Adjuvant Chemotherapy. Ed. Cl. Jacquillat, M. Weil, D. Khayat. Colloque INSERM/John Libbey Eurotext Ltd. © 1988. Vol. 169, pp. 303-308.

Induction combination chemotherapy without cisplatin followed by radiotherapy without radical surgery as definitive treatment for advanced laryngeal cancer

Bridget T. Hill*, Len A. Price*** and Sharon Love**

** Cellular Chemotherapy Laboratory and ** Research Computer Unit, Imperial Cancer Research Fund, London WC2A 3PX, and *** 111 Harley Street, London W1N 1DG, England, UK*

ABSTRACT

Two hundred and eight patients with advanced, previously untreated tumours at different sites within the head and neck region were eligible for this study designed to evaluate the impact of two courses of non-cisplatin-containing Schedule A chemotherapy prior to definitive local therapy on complete remission (CR) rate and survival. Toxicity associated with Schedule A was minimal, with 100 per cent patient compliance. Tumour site proved significant in determining chemotherapy response ($p<0.001$), overall survival ($p<0.002$) and relapse-free survival (RFS). Detailed subset analyses were possible in this large series and we now report on 73 patients with laryngeal carcinomas: 61 per cent responded to this initial chemotherapy, 51 patients then had radiotherapy (DXT) only, 14 had DXT plus salvage surgery, whilst 7 had total laryngectomies and post-operative DXT and their respective final CR rates were 79, 73 and 86 per cent. Compared with the entire group of 208 patients, those patients with tumours of the larynx had significantly better overall survival ($p=0.0014$) and RFS ($p=0.004$) figures. Chemotherapy responders lived significantly longer than non-responders (medians of 71 versus 40 months) and patients achieving a final CR had a median survival of 7 years. Survival and RFS figures in patients receiving DXT only without surgery, were not significantly different from those who underwent total laryngectomies plus post-operative DXT. These retrospective analyses suggest that this initial chemotherapy followed by definitive radiotherapy may eliminate radical surgery, so preserving the larynx in patients with advanced disease.

KEY WORDS

Initial chemotherapy; non-cisplatin-containing drug combination; advanced squamous cell laryngeal carcinomas; predictive factor; eight year survival data.

INTRODUCTION

We have reported previously that in a large series of 208 patients with untreated advanced squamous cell carcinomas of the head and neck the use of two courses of a four drug combination (Schedule A) of vincristine, 5-fluorouracil, methotrexate and bleomycin given together with hydrocortisone, as initial treatment prior to local therapy appeared of significant benefit in prolonging good quality life for patients with tumours at certain sites but not at others, within the head and neck region (Hill et al., 1986a and 1986b; Hill and Price, 1987). We now present a detailed report on the subset of 73 patients with laryngeal carcinomas, providing details of response rates, overall survival and relapse-free survival after a median follow-up of eight years, and identifying significant predictive factors associated with increased response rates and increased survival.

PATIENTS AND METHODS

73 patients with advanced, histologically-proven, previously untreated, squamous cell carcinoma of the larynx were eligible for these retrospective analyses. 61 patients were male and 12 female, with an age range of 37 to 76 years (median 59 years). There were 17 patients with Stage IV and 34 with Stage III disease. The 22 patients with Stage II tumours (T2NO) were considered 'bad risks', for example, because of extension to an adjacent site or the involvement of two sites. There was a preponderance (59 per cent) of poorly differentiated tumours.

Patients were scheduled to receive two courses of Schedule A as initial treatment on days 1 and 14. The drugs were given as follows: Vincristine, 2mg iv at zero hours; bleomycin, 60mg infused from 12 to 18 hours; methotrexate, 100mg iv at 12, 15 and 18 hours; 5-fluorouracil, 500mg iv at 18 hours; hydrocortisone, 500mg iv at 12 and 18 hours; and folinic acid, 15mg orally at 26, 32, 38 and 44 hours. Full details of this protocol have been provided previously (Hill et al., 1986b). On day 28 patients were assessed for chemotherapy response and 'curative' local treatment was initiated. 51 patients had radiotherapy only with approximately 65Gy given over 6 to 7 weeks as 10Gy over five days per week, as detailed earlier (Price et al., 1983). 14 patients had similar radiotherapy but to a total dose of only 40Gy and then went on to surgery, whilst 7 patients electively had total laryngectomies followed by post-operative radiotherapy.

Standard definitions of response were used (see Hill et al., 1986a). Response to initial chemotherapy was assessed in 67 patients, the six exceptions being: 3 patients had inadequate tumour measurements, 2 commenced surgery after the first course and 1 patient died following a protocol violation. Response to local therapies was assessed in 72 patients. Response rates were compared using the Chi-squared test. Survival was calculated by a product-limit and compared using the Mantel test. The Cox regression model was used in multivariate analysis.

RESULTS

Response to initial chemotherapy

Of the 67 patients assessed for response to two courses of initial Schedule A chemotherapy, 41 (61 per cent) responded (at least a partial response) and 26 were classified as non-responders, although 6 of these patients had a minimal 20 to 30 per cent response. As shown in Table 1 chemotherapy response rates for the different anatomical sites within the laryngeal region were not significantly different. Response rates to initial chemotherapy were not significantly influenced by disease stage (see Table 1), T stage or nodal status, age or sex. Response by histologic grade was 78 and 71 per cent for well and moderately differentiated tumours but only 55 per cent for poorly differentiated lesions. The overall data set were used to attempt to identify prognostic factors for chemotherapy response using logistic regression. Site, stage, T and N classification, age, sex and histologic grade were tested and none was predictive of chemotherapy response.

Toxicities

Provided the standard medical precautions (see Price and Hill, 1982) were always observed, the toxicity associated with Schedule A chemotherapy was minimal, as detailed earlier (Hill et al., 1986b). 63 per cent of patients had no side-effects at all. In the remaining 27 patients, there were 5 incidences of mucositis, 8 of skin rashes, 2 of alopecia, 6 of nausea and vomiting and 5 cases of malaise or lethargy: These symptoms were all described as mild. There was one treatment-related death resulting from a protocol violation since the patient with known impaired renal function (creatine clearance of 70mL/min) did not receive a prolonged folinic acid rescue.

Table 1. Response Rates: Analyses by Tumour Site and Stage.

Site or Stage	Response to Initial Chemotherapy			Final Response after Local Therapy		
	*R(%)	NR	NA	CR(%)	RD	NA
All sites	41 (61%)	26	6	58 (81%)	14	1
- supraglottic	17 (55%)	14	5	25 (71%)	10	1
- glottic	19 (66%)	10	1	27 (90%)	3	0
- transglottic	3 (60%)	2	0	4 (80%)	1	0
- subglottic	2	0	0	2	0	0
Stage II	15 (64%)	6	1	19 (90%)	2	1
Stage III	17 (57%)	12	5	25 (86%)	4	0
Stage IV	9 (53%)	8	0	9 (53%)	8	0

* R - responders; NR - non-responders; NA - not assessed;
CR - complete remission; RD - residual disease.

Response to local therapies

Following completion of local therapy patients were classified as being either in final complete clinical remission (CR) or with residual disease. 58 patients (81 per cent) achieved a final CR and 14 were judged still to have residual disease. The CR rate by stage was significantly superior in patients with stage II or III disease, being 90 and 86 per cent respectively, than the 53 per cent noted in stage IV disease (p=0.007). The final CR rate was not significantly different in those patients who responded to initial chemotherapy (83 per cent) compared with those classified as non-responders (74 per cent), unless one excludes the six patients with a minimal response to initial chemotherapy, and then the final CR rate in patients failing to show any response to initial chemotherapy fell to 50 per cent. Both Stage and nodal status were predictive for achieving a final CR, with p values of 0.001 and 0.005 for No and stage II disease respectively.

Survival data

The overall median survival of all patients, treated between January 1975 and June 1982 with a median follow-up of 8 years, was 53 months and 42 per cent of these patients were alive at 8 years. Chemotherapy responders lived longer than non-responders (71 versus 40 months). Patients achieving a final CR had a median survival of 85 months. Overall survival and relapse-free survival (RFS) in patients receiving radiotherapy only, without surgery, were not significantly different from those who had total laryngectomies and radiotherapy (see Table 2). By univariate analysis of all patients with laryngeal tumours the prognostic factors for survival were: Stage p=0.001; site p=0.03; N status p=0.0002 and age p=0.03. Superior survival was evident in patients with stage II or III disease, those with glottic or subglottic lesions, with lower N values and those aged less than 49 years. Multivariate analysis also revealed better survival figures for younger patients (p=0.0076) and those with No or N1 disease (p=0.0001). 25 patients remain alive, 23 without recurrences. 38 patients have died, 28 with disease present, mainly locally and/or regionally. Ten patients have been lost to follow-up: 2 with disease at 3 and 4 months, and 8 disease-free at periods of 4 to 27 months.

Table 2. Median Survival Durations for All Patients.

Local Therapy	Overall Survival (months)
Radiotherapy only	71 ± 31
Surgery and radiotherapy	51 ± 43
	p=0.38

DISCUSSION

In our large series of 208 patients, we showed that it was feasible to obtain a high overall response of 66 per cent to two courses of Schedule A combination chemotherapy used as initial treatment. This result involving treatment over 24 hours and a 2-day stay in hospital, was achieved with minimal toxicity and with minimal interference with the patients' quality of life (Hill et al., 1987). As reviewed earlier (Hill et al., 1984), this lack of toxicity is a significant advantage of Schedule A compared with those side effects of cisplatin-containing protocols, none of which has yet been shown significantly to prolong survival.

We first reported that primary tumour site was a highly significant factor for predicting response to treatment and survival (Hill et al., 1984; Hill et al., 1986a and 1986b): Achievement of a final CR in patients with nasopharyngeal and laryngeal tumours was a good prognostic sign with significantly improved survival (p=0.03), compared with all the other sites in the head and neck region. This significance of site has since been reported by others, for example, the Head and Neck Contracts Program (1987) reported better survival (p>0.001) in patients with laryngeal tumours compared with oral cavity or pyriform sinus sites, whilst Ervin et al. (1987) identified nasopharynx as the favourable site (p=0.02). However, our data also highlighted the fact that response to initial chemotherapy and achievement of a final CR did not automatically translate into survival benefit, since the 80 per cent of patients with oral cavity tumours who responded to initial Schedule A chemotherapy had a median survival of only 22 months (Hill and Price, 1987). This contrasts with the figures of 71 months for all patients reported here with laryngeal carcinomas and of 85 months for those achieving a final CR. These results emphasise the heterogeneity inherent in this group of head and neck tumours and led to our earlier proposal that specific chemotherapy protocols may be required for tumours at different sites (Hill and Price, 1987).

Of major significance, however, in these patients with laryngeal cancer is our observation that neither overall survival nor RFS were compromised in patients who, following initial chemotherapy, achieved a final CR with primary radiotherapy only, without radical surgery. This lends support to preliminary reports from other groups also aiming to reduce the impact of radical surgery in these patients with advanced disease (Clark et al., 1987; Kadish et al., 1987).

In conclusion, these data indicate that the use of two courses of Schedule A combination chemotherapy prior to definitive radiotherapy may provide significant benefit in terms of overall survival and RFS, for patients with advanced laryngeal tumours. This approach which eliminates the need for radical surgery, offers the prospect of preserving the larynx, a factor likely significantly to improve patients' overall quality of life. Clearly randomized, controlled studies are essential to define the role of initial chemotherapy in treating laryngeal cancer and we await with interest results of the Veteran's Administration Co-operative study designed to evaluate whether classic induction chemotherapy can either improve overall survival or substitute for surgery in patients with laryngeal tumours, as described recently (Clark et al., 1987).

ACKNOWLEDGEMENTS

We are indebted to Mr. Henry Shaw and Dr. Vera Dalley for referring patients into this study at the Royal Marsden Hospital, London and to Dr. Ken MacRae, Charing Cross and Westminister Medical School, London for statistical advise.

REFERENCES

Clark, J.R., Fallon, B.G. and Frei, E. III.(1987): Induction chemotherapy as initial treatment for advanced head and neck cancer: A model for the multidisciplinary treatment of solid tumors. In Important Advances in Oncology 1987, eds. V.T. DeVita, S. Hellman & S.A Rosenberg, pp 175-195. Philadelphia: J.B. Lippincott.

Ervin, T.J., Clark, J.R., Weichselbaum, R.R., Fallon, B.G., Miller, D., Fabian, R.L., Posner, M.R., Norris, C.M., Tuttle, S.A., Schoenfeld, D.A., Price, K.N. and Frei, E. III.(1987): An analysis of induction and adjuvant chemotherapy in the multidisciplinary treatment of squamous-cell carcinoma of the head and neck. J. Clin. Oncol., 5, 10-20.

Head and Neck Contracts Program.(1987): Adjuvant chemotherapy for advanced head and neck squamous carcinoma. Cancer, 60, 301-311.

Hill, B.T. and Price, L.A.(1987): The significance of primary site in assessing chemotherapy response and survival in advanced squamous cell carcinomas of the head and neck treated with initial combination chemotherapy without cisplatin: Analyses at nine years. In Adjuvant Therapy of Cancer V, ed. S.E. Salmon, pp 111-118. Orlando: Grune & Stratton.

Hill, B.T., Price, L.A., Busby, E., MacRae, K. and Shaw, H.J.(1984): Positive impact of initial 24-hour combination chemotherapy without cis-platinum on 6-year survival figures in advanced squamous cell carcinomas of the head and neck. In Adjuvant Therapy of Cancer IV, eds. S.E. Jones and S.E. Salmon, pp 97-106. Orlando: Grune & Stratton.

Hill, B.T., Price, L.A. and MacRae, K.(1986a): Importance of primary site in assessing chemotherapy response and 7-year survival data in advanced squamous-cell carcinomas of the head and neck treated with initial combination chemotherapy without cisplatin. J. Clin. Oncol., 4, 1340-1347.

Hill, B.T., Price, L.A. and MacRae, K.(1986b): Predictive factors for tumour response and survival to initial combination chemotherapy without cisplatin in patients with advanced squamous cell carcinomas of the head and neck. In Neo-Adjuvant Chemotherapy, eds. C. Jacquillat, M. Weil and D. Khayat, pp 403-412. London, John Libbey.

Kadish, S.P., Cohen, N., Conway, H.W., Sherman, D.M., Schwartz, J.H., Strauss, G.M. and Ricciardi, P.A.(1987): Induction chemotherapy and full course irradiation for advanced head and neck cancer: A non-operative approach with results comparable to surgical series. In Proc. 2nd Int. Head and Neck Oncology Research Conference, Arlington, Virginia, U.S.A. Abs 1.5.

Price, L.A. and Hill, B.T.(1982): Safe and effective induction chemotherapy without cisplatin for squamous cell carcinoma of the head and neck: Impact on complete response rate and survival at five years, following local therapy. Med. Ped. Oncol. 10, 535-548.

Résumé

208 patients avec des tumeurs avancées non traitées de la tête et du cou sont entrés dans cette étude, destinée à évaluer l'impact de deux cures de l'association chimiothérapie A (ne contenant pas de platine) avec un traitement local définitif avec pour critère la rémission complète et la survie.
La toxicité associée au protocole A a été minime, 100 % de respect du protocole. Le site tumoral a déterminé de façon significative la réponse tumorale ($p < 0{,}001$), la survie globale ($p < 0{,}002$) et la survie sans rechute. Des analyses de sous groupes ont été possibles dans ces grandes séries et nous rapportons les résultats chez 73 malades atteints de carcinome laryngé. 61 % ont répondu à cette chimiothérapie initiale. 51 malades ont alors été traités par radiothérapie seule, 14 par radiothérapie plus chirurgie de rattrapage, tandis que 7 malades ont eu une laryngectomie totale suivie d'une radiothérapie post-opératoire et les taux de rémission complète finaux ont été de 79, 73 et 90 %. Comparés avec le groupe entier de 208 patients, les malades avec tumeur du larynx ont une survie globale meilleure ($p = 0{,}0014$) et une survie sans rechute meilleure ($p = 0{,}004$). Les répondeurs à la chimiothérapie ont une survie significativement meilleure que les non répondeurs (médiane 71 contre 40 mois) et les malades chez lesquels une rémission complète peut finalement être obtenue ont une médiane de survie de 7 ans. La survie et la survie sans rechute des malades recevant uniquement de la radiothérapie sans chirurgie n'ont pas été significativement différentes de ceux qui ont reçu une laryngectomie totale suivie d'une radiothérapie post-opératoire. Une analyse, rétrospective suggère que cette chimiothérapie initiale suivie par une radiothérapie définitive peut éviter une chirurgie radicale conservant ainsi le larynx chez des malades atteints de maladie avancée.

Neo-Adjuvant Chemotherapy. Ed. Cl. Jacquillat, M. Weil, D. Khayat. Colloque INSERM/John Libbey Eurotext Ltd. © 1988. Vol. 169, pp. 309-313.

A randomized study comparing two regimens of induction chemotherapy for locally advanced head and neck cancer

Everett E. Vokes, Ralph R. Weichselbaum, William J. Moran, Azhar M. Awan, Allen G. Tybor, Michael E. Goldman, Richard L. Schilsky, Jacob D. Bitran, Christopher M. Barker, Nathan Scher and William R. Panje

Joint Section of Hematology/Oncology, Department of Radiation Oncology, and Section of Otolaryngology, Head and Neck Surgery, the University of Chicago and Michael Reese Hospital and Medical Center, Chicago, IL, USA

ABSTRACT

We have compared two regimens of induction chemotherapy for previously untreated patients with locally advanced head and neck cancer and performance status of 0-2 (ECOG). Patients were randomized to receive 4 cycles of induction chemotherapy either with methotrexate 120 mg/m^2 followed 24 h later by cisplatin 100 mg/m^2 and a 5 day continuous infusion of 5-fluorouracil at 1000 mg/m^2/day (Arm A), or cisplatin 20 mg/m^2/day 1-5, bleomycin 10 U/m^2/day 3-7 and methotrexate 200 mg/m^2 days 14, 21 alternating with cisplatin 100 mg/m^2 and 5 day continuous infusion 5-fluorouracil at 1000 mg/m^2/day (Arm B). Of 42 patients evaluated for study, 16 were randomized to Arm A, 13 to Arm B; 13 patients were excluded (poor pulmonary function: 7 patients; performance status >3:2 patients; miscellaneous: 4 patients). Arms A and B were well balanced for patient characteristics. On Arm A, 4 of 14 evaluable patients (29%) had a complete response, 8 (57%) a partial response and 2 (14%) had no response; on Arm B, 5 patients (38%) had a complete response, 7 (54%) a partial response, and 1 (8%) no response. After completion of local therapy, 13 patients (Arm A) vs, 11 patients (Arm B) were free of disease. Actuarial one year disease-free survival is 80% (Arm A) vs. 78% (Arm B); actuarial one year overall survival is 85% (Arm A) vs. 70% (Arm B). The differences in response and survival rates were not significant. Chemotherapy-induced myelosuppression was mild to moderate in both arms. The incidence of moderate to severe mucositis was significantly higher on Arm A (28 of 51 evaluable cycles) vs. Arm B (13 of 50 cycles). We conclude that, with efficacy being equal, Arm B can be considered superior based on its lower toxicity. Because of the lack of significant differences in complete response rate, survival, and disease-free survival, and the high incidence of mucositis on Arm A, we have closed the study to further patient accrual.

KEY WORDS: head and neck cancer, induction chemotherapy

INTRODUCTION

Despite high response rates, prolongation of survival of patients with locally advanced head and neck cancer as a direct consequence of the use of induction chemotherapy has not been demonstrated to date (Head and Neck Contracts Program, 1987). Several studies, however, have demonstrated that patients who achieve complete response to induction chemotherapy have improved survival compared to those patients who achieve partial or no response (Jacobs, 1987; Ervin, 1987).

One goal of clinical studies in head and neck oncology, therefore, has to be the definition of more active chemotherapy regimens leading to higher complete response rates. The theoretical model developed by Goldie and Coldman (1982) suggests that early exposure of tumors to multiple drugs may be of critical importance in achieving complete response. Clinically this concept has been successfully applied in the treatment of aggressive lymphomas through the use of sequential non-crossresistant combination chemotherapy (Fisher, 1983). While such non-crossresistant chemotherapy regimens have not been described for head and neck cancer, 2 well defined regimens are available, that are largely composed of different single agents. These include the combination of cisplatin, continuous infusion 5-fluorouracil (5-FU) as described by Jacobs (1987) and the combination of cisplatin, continuous infusion bleomycin, and methotrexate as described by Ervin (1987). Therefore, we decided, to administer these 2 regimens in alternating sequence and to compare the efficacy of this approach in a randomized fashion to that of a regimen previously used at our institution. This regimen consisting of methotrexate, cisplatin and continuous infusion 5-FU (Vokes, in press) has been shown to be active, and provided the institutional experience in multimodality therapy of head and neck cancer.

PATIENTS AND METHODS

This study opened in January of 1986 and was closed in March of 1987. Eligible patients had biopsy proven squamous cell carcinoma of the head and neck or lymphoepithelioma of the nasopharynx. In addition to routine clinical staging procedures, a bone scan and CT-scan of the head and neck were performed. Local tumor extent was further assessed by triple endoscopy and biopsy.

Eligible patients had previously untreated locally advanced Stage III or IV disease. A performance status of ≤ 2 (ECOG), creatinine clearance ≥ 50 mg/min, pulmonary function test showing a CO_2 diffustion capacity of $> 50\%$ of predicted, measurable disease and signed informed consent were also required. Eligible patients were then registered on study, stratified by performance status and T and N stage, and randomized to receive chemotherapy on Arm A or Arm B.

The treatment plan called for 4 cycles of induction chemotherapy on Arm A or B followed by response evaluation using standard response criteria. Local therapy generally consisted of surgery followed by radiotherapy except for those patients who refused surgery or were considered unresectable due to the anatomic location or the local extent of the disease at initial presentation. Such patients received radiation therapy only with curative intent. Two additional cycles of chemotherapy were given to those patients who achieved a partial or complete response to initial chemotherapy and were considered to be free of disease at completion of local therapy.

Chemotherapy on Arm A consisted of methotrexate 120 mg/m^2 given on day 1 with leucovorin rescue on day 2, cisplatin 100 mg/m^2 given as a 6 h infusion on day 2, followed immediately by 5-FU at 1000 mg/m^2/day administered by continuous IV infusion for 5 days. Chemotherapy on Arm B consisted of cisplatin 20 mg/m^2 over 2 hours on days 1-5, bleomycin 10 mg/m^2/day administered as a continuous infusion on days 3-7 and methotrexate 200 mg/m^2 days 14 and 21 with leucovorin rescue on days 15 and 22 for cycles 1 and 3. For cycle 5 cisplatin was administered only on days 1-3 and bleomycin only on days 2-4. For cycles 2,4 and 6, 100 mg/m^2 of cisplatin on day 1 were followed by a 5-day continuous infusion of 5-FU at 1000 mg/m^2/day.

Radiotherapy was delivered by a 4mV or 6mV linear accelerator in daily fractions of 180-200 cGy. Total doses ranged from 66-80 Gy, using electron or interstitial boosts when appropriate. For postoperative radiotherapy, doses were 60 Gy to areas of original gross disease and 45-60 Gy to areas of potential microscopic disease.

RESULTS

Forty-two patients with locally advanced head and neck cancer were evaluated for therapy on this study. Thirteen of these were excluded from enrollment because of poor pulmonary function test (7 patients), a performance status of 3 (2 patients), refusal of randomization (2 patients) and prior malignancy (2 patients). Of the remaining 29 patients, 16 were randomized to Arm A and 13 to Arm B. The patient characteristics for each arm are summarized as follows:

Patient Characteristics

	Arm A 16 patients	Arm B 13 patients
Male :	11	10
Female:	5	3
Age, Median:	51 years	56 years
Range:	(23-68)	(44-70)
Performance Status 0:	8	7
1:	5	6
2:	3	0
Stage III	3	3
Stage IV	13	10

Of 16 patients randomized to Arm A, 2 were unevaluable for response to induction chemotherapy. Of the remaining 14 patients, 4 had a clinical complete response, 8 a partial response and 2 patients had no response. All 13 patients randomized to Arm B are evaluable for response. Five had a clinical complete response, 7 a partial response and 1 patient had no response.

Subsequent local therapy on Arm A consisted of surgery and radiotherapy in 10 patients and of radiotherapy alone in 3 patients. One patient refused local therapy. The one year survival for all patients on Arm A is 85% and the one year disease free survival is 80%. On Arm B local therapy consisted of surgery and radiotherapy in 9 patients, and of radiotherapy alone in 2 patients, while 2 patients refused local therapy. At a median follow-up of 12 months, 2 patients have had disease recurrence, 3 patients have expired. The one year survival for all patients registered in Arm B is 70% and the one year disease free survival is 78%.

Ten patients on each arm were eligible to receive 2 additional cycles of chemotherapy. However, because of cumulative toxicity or patient refusal only 5 patients on Arm A and 6 patients on Arm B received additional chemotherapy.

The toxicities observed during induction chemotherapy were mild to moderate myelosuppression on both arms. Moderate to severe mucositis was significantly more frequent on Arm A (28 of 51 evaluable cycles) than on Arm B (13 of 50 evaluable cycles). A similar pattern was observed during adjuvant chemotherapy where moderate to severe mucositis was observed following 6 of 7 cycles administered on Arm A versus only 1 of 12 cycles on Arm B.

DISCUSSION

In this study we attempted to increase the complete response rate to induction chemotherapy in patients with advanced head and neck cancer by administering 2 different regimens in alternating sequence for a total of 4 cycles prior to local therapy. We speculated that thereby, we would be able to increase the clinical complete response rate to > 50%, which would translate into a larger proportion of patients with prolonged survival.

As the control arm we chose a regimen previously studied at our institution in which we had added methotrexate in a sequential schedule to the combination of cisplatin and 5-FU (Vokes, in press). In our initial study we reported an overall response rate of 94% and a complete response rate of 26% following 3 cycles of this regimen as induction chemotherapy. The response and complete response rate in 16 patients treated with this regimen (Arm A) in this study are almost identical. Disappointingly, however, response and survival rates of 13 patients treated on Arm B are not significantly different from those on Arm A and a significantly increased complete response rate on Arm B (>50%) was not documented. While the addition of many more patients to this study might have revealed an advantage of one chemotherapy arm over the other, it is most likely that the difference would have remained small and clinically insignificant. While the response analysis of this study revealed no significant difference, the comparison of toxicities did show a significantly higher incidence of moderate to severe mucositis on Arm A. The toxicity profile of Arm B, therefore, is favorable compared to Arm A.

This preliminary analysis has led to the closure of this study with few patients entered on each arm. However, we feel that the following conclusions are valid: Response and complete response rates of both regimens tested in this study are not significantly different from each other and comparable to those reported from other institutions with these or similar regimens in pilot projects. With additional patient accrual neither study arm would be likely to result in a significantly increased complete response rate (>50%). At the same time, the toxicity profile supports the use of Arm B over Arm A, although a significant proportion of patients will not be able to receive it because of poor pulmonary function tests. While high overall response rates have consistently been reported using neoadjuvant chemotherapy for locally advanced head and neck cancer, it is disappointing that complete response rates continue to constitute only abot 30%. This is true also for the 2 regimens tested in this study. Therefore, until an independent effect of chemotherapy on survival can be demonstrated, neither regimen can be recommended for use outside of controlled clinical trials.

REFERENCES

1. Ervin TJ, (1987): An analysis of induction and adjuvant chemotherapy in the multidisciplinary treatment of squamous-cell carcinoma of the head and neck. J Clin Oncol 5, 10-20.

2. Fisher RI, (1983): Diffuse aggressive lymphomas: increased survival after alternating flexible sequences of ProMACE and MOPP chemotherapy. Ann Intern Med 98, 304-309.

3. Goldie JH, (1982): Rationale for the use of alternating non-crossresistant chemotherapy. Cancer Treat Rep 66, 439-449.

4. Head and Neck Contracts Program (1987): Adjuvant chemotherapy for advanced head and neck squamous carcinoma. Cancer 60, 301-311.

5. Jacobs JR, (1987): Proto-chemotherapy in advanced head and neck cancer. Head Neck Surg 10, 93-98.

6. Vokes EE, (in press): Sequential methotrexate, cisplatin and 5-fluorouracil in multimodal therapy of locally advanced head and neck cancer. NCI - Monograph, Conference on the Interaction of Radiation Therapy and Chemotherapy, Williamsburg, VA.

Résumé

Nous avons comparé deux traitments de chimiothérapie inductive (CT) pour malades avec cancer localement avancé de la tête et du cou, non traités antérieurement, et avec une condition physique de 0-2 (ECOG). Les malades ont été choisi au hasard, de recevoir un de deux traitements dans 4 cycles de CT: 1) Méthotrexate 120 mg/m^2 suivi 24 heures plus tard de Cisplatin 100 mg/m^2 et une infusion ininterrompue pendant 5 jours de 5-Fluorouracil à une dose de 1000 mg/m^2 par jour (**Traitement A**); 2) Cisplatin 20 mg/m^2 jours 1-5, Bleomycin 10 U/m^2 jours 3-7 et Méthotrexate 200 mg/m^2 le 14ème et 21ème jour, tours à tours avec Cisplatin 100 mg/m^2 et une infusion ininterrompue de 5-Fluorouracil à une dose de 1000 mg/m^2 par jour (**Traitement B**). L'investigation a évalué 42 malades parmi lesquels 16 ont reçu le traitement A et 13 le traitement B. 13 malades ont été exclu pour les raisons suivantes: condition pulmonaire débile:7 cas, condition physique >3:3 cas; causes variées:3 cas. Les charactéristiques des malades étaient bien équilibrées dans chacun de deux traitements. Avec le traitement A, 4 sur 14 évaluables malades (29%) ont achevé une réponse complète; 8 (57%) une réponse partielle; et 2 (14%) n'ont eu aucun résultat. Avec le traitement B, 5 malades (38%) ont achevé une réponse complète, 7 (54%) une réponse partielle, et 1 (8%) n'a eu aucun résultat. Après avoir completé le traitement local, 13 malades (A) contre 11 malades (B) étaient en rémission complète. En général, la survie d'un an sans rechute est 80% (A) contre 70% (B). Les différences en réponse et en survie n'étaient pas importantes entre A et B. La myélosuppression causée par la chimiothérapie se range de benigne à moderée. L'incidence de la mucosité, soit moderée que sevère, était bien plus fréquente avec A (28 sur 51 évaluables cycles) qu'avec B (13 sur 50 cycles). Nous concluons que, l'éfficacité étant égale, le traitement B peut être consideré supérieur dû à la moindre toxicité. En vue de l'absence des différences de grande portée en pourcentage de réponse, en survie générale et sans maladie, aussi bien que du nombre d'incidences de mucosité avec A, nour avons terminé le recrutement des malades dans ce traitement.

Neo-Adjuvant Chemotherapy. Ed. Cl. Jacquillat, M. Weil, D. Khayat. Colloque INSERM/John Libbey Eurotext Ltd. © 1988. Vol. 169, pp. 315-319.

Sequential induction chemotherapy and radiotherapy for advanced nasopharyngeal carcinoma

I.W. Dimery, W.K. Hong, L. Peters, H. Goepfert, K. McCarthy, R. Byers and O. Gullamendegui

University of Texas, M.D. Anderson Hospital and Tumor Institute, Houston, Texas 77030, USA

ABSTRACT

Despite aggressive megavoltage radiotherapy, the treatment of advanced nasopharyngeal carcinoma (NPC) results in a poor 5-year survival with a high propensity for local recurrence as well as distant metastases. A prospective program was therefore initiated designed to administer 3 courses of 5-FU/cisplatin neoadjuvant chemotherapy followed by full dose radiotherapy. Twenty-nine patients (pts) with T4 and/or ≥ N2b stage were treated. After completion of all chemotherapy to 19 pts, 15 (79%) achieved CR. Of those, 1 relapsed in nodal site at 8 months and was surgically resected. At a median follow-up of 2 years for all pts, 6 are dead of disease, 16 (55%) are alive NED and 7 are too early to evaluate concluding that this approach is feasible and therapeutically active in advanced NPC.

INTRODUCTION

Although presenting in an advanced stage, nasopharyngeal carcinoma is treated exclusively by megavoltage radiotherapy with a 5-year survival of 20% to 30% in advanced stage disease (T3, T4, with N+ nodal disease) (1,2). The presence of a chemosensitive tumor (3,4) and a younger patient population with good performance status constructs a more effective model for the demonstration of the benefit of induction chemotherapy/radiotherapy used sequentially to increase local control and decrease distant metastases. At our institution radiotherapy alone results in a cure rate (at 5 years) in early stage (T1-2, N0-2a) disease not less than 70% of cases for WHO III, but decreases to < 50% for WHO I histologies (1). The more prognostically unfavorable (T3-4, ≥ N2b-3b) stages are therefore now treated with chemotherapy followed by full dose radiotherapy in an attempt to increase the overall response, and reduce distant failure.

Our previous experience was heterogeneous in terms of the chemotherapeutic regimens employed and the treating physicians; however, results obtained with sequential chemotherapy/radiotherapy were encouraging when compared with standard radiotherapy alone (5). Whereas, the overall survival was improved in that report, toxicity was not entirely negligible.

Based on this data we are uniformly utilizing 5-FU x 5 days infusion and cisplatin, the combination of which has not been associated with enhanced operative or radiotherapeutic toxicities (6).

METHODOLOGY

All patients seen at M.D. Anderson Hospital with biopsy proven squamous cell carcinoma, T4 or $\geq$ N2b or T4 (any N) with cranial nerve involvement (AJC staging), Zubrod performance status ≤ 2, with normal hematologic and renal function were entered. Pretreatment disease documentation included nasopharyngoscopy and CT scanning. Three courses (Q 21 days) of cisplatin 100 mg/m^2 over 24-hour infusion D1 and 5-FU 1,000 mg/m^2 over 24-hour infusion D1-5 was followed within 3 weeks by radiotherapy: 45 Gy in 25 fractions over 5 weeks to the primary and upper neck, and 50 Gy to lower neck (Cobalt-60) raised to 70 Gy at the primary and nodes through reduced lateral fields with high energy photons or electron-bean fields. Response was quantitated using standard criteria by both physical examination including endoscopy, and radiologically pre-radiotherapy and approximately 6 weeks post-radiotherapy. Survival was calculated by the method of Kaplan and Meier (7).

RESULTS

Patient Characteristics

Twenty-nine patients were entered into this treatment. There were 20 males and 9 females with a median age of 41 years (range: 17-71). Twenty-six were evaluable for response to chemotherapy (2 - too early and 1 - drug related death), and 19 evaluable for radiotherapy (6 - too early and 1 - never treated). The stage at presentation was 3 - T1N2-3 (10%), 4 - T2N2-3 (14%), 7 -T3N2-3 (24%), 2 - T4N0 (6%), and 13 - T4N2-3 (45%). Of the 15 patients with T4 lesions, 9 involved base of skull/clivus only, 2 had intracranial extension with cranial nerve involvement and 4 without cranial nerve involvement. Histologically, 2 (7%) were WHO I, 9 (31%) WHO II, and 18 (62%) WHO III classification.

RESPONSE

Response was analyzed at the primary and nodal site as described in Table 1.

Table 1. Nasopharyngeal Carcinoma

Response to Chemotherapy	Nodal response n = 25	(%)	1° response n = 26	(%)
Complete	12	(48)	4	(15)
Partial	11	(44)	18	(69)
Minor/None	1	(4)	4	(15)
Progression	1	(4)	0	
Response to Radiotherapy	**Nodal response n = 18**	**(%)**	**1° response n = 19**	**(%)**
Complete	16	(88)	14	(74)
Partial	2	(12)	*3	(16)
Minor/None	0		0	
Progression	0		2	(10)

*Maintenance chemotherapy:
2 with PR received 1 and 6 cycles -----> CR

To chemotherapy, a complete response (CR) in the nodal site occurred at a higher frequency as compared to the primary; however, overall response rate was high (92% and 84%); nonetheless, with few progressing on chemotherapy. With radiotherapy, nodal response remained higher (88% vs 74%). Of 3 patients with residual disease at the primary site, 2 received maintenance chemotherapy and attained CR.

A radiological definition and clinical definition of CR did not coincide. After chemotherapy 14 (56%) had no palpable nodes and 10 (30%) no visible tumor at the primary. After radiotherapy, nodal response was unchanged whereas 16 (84%) had no primary tumor clinically.

Overall, of 19 patients who received all treatment, 15 (79%) were CR with 3 (16%) progressing during XRT or by the initial post-treatment visit was bone (WHO III), brain (WHO III), and 1^{0} site (WHO I). Interestingly, the patient progressing in brain and leptomeninges had no radiologic evidence of tumor at the primary.

SURVIVAL

All patients (n = 29) were counted for survival (Figure 1). Sixteen (55%) are alive without disease with 6 (21%) dead of disease. One patient relapsed at 8 months in nodal site and was free of disease following surgery. Seven others are still undergoing treatment. At 2-year follow-up median survival and disease-free survival has not been reached.

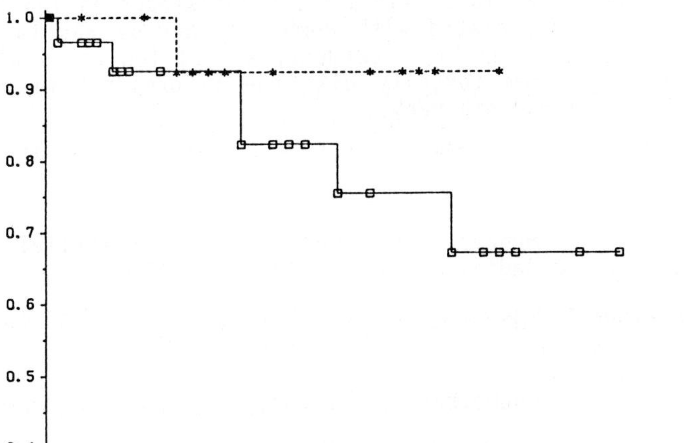

TOXICITY

Other than the usual gastrointestinal toxicity (mild-moderate nausea and vomiting in 97% and mucositis is 59%), weight was maintained or increased in 75%. Hematologically, neutropenia (< 1,500 /mm^3) occurred in 69% without fever of infection. Acute mucosal reaction to radiotherapy occurred in 10/23 (44%) with half requiring parenteral nutrition during treatment and 19 (83%) experiencing a mean loss of 4.9 kg in weight.

DISCUSSION

Although non-randomized, this prospective analysis gives insight into what can be accomplished in this disease entity with sequential therapy, the benefit of which has been challenged (8). Once disease-free, the recurrence rate was quite low; however, the advanced stage resulted in rapid progression/metastases in 3 in close proximity to treatment. It will be interesting as this series matures to evaluate any change in the metastatic pattern as compared to previous studies (9,10). Likewise the development of any chronic toxicities may not be evident for years to come.

We conclude that 1) sequential delivery of chemotherapy and radiotherapy resulted in an overall complete response rate of 79% in advanced T4 and/or N2b disease; 2) overall response including radiotherapy seems to be enhanced using this chemotherapeutic approach; 3) with induction chemotherapy, response at the nodal disease site was superior to that at the primary; 4) at 2 years of follow-up, the median disease-free and overall survival has not been reached; 5) the overall frequency of local and distant metastases is low for this group; 6) the acute toxicity associated with combined therapy was tolerable and did not delay or necessitate stopping treatment; and 7) few cases were observed to have any unusual long-term toxicity with the 5-FU/cisplatin regimen despite delivery of 65-70 Gy of radiotherapy.

REFERENCES

1. Mesic, J.B.(1981): Megavoltage irradiation of epithelial tumors of the nasopharynx. Int J Radiat Oncol Biol Phys 7, 447-453.

2. Haghbin, M.(1985): Carcinoma of the nasopharynx. A 25 year study. Am J Clin Oncol 8, 384-392.

3. Decker, D.A.(1983): Chemotherapy for nasopharyngeal carcinoma. Cancer 52, 602-605.

4. Huang, A.T.(1981): Chemotherapy for nasopharyngeal carcinoma. In: Nasopharyngeal Carcinoma: Cancer Campaign 5, 263-268.

5. Dimery, I.W.(1987): Adjuvant chemotherapy for advanced nasopharyngeal carcinoma. Cancer 60, 943-949.

6. Wolf, G.T.(1987): A new strategy to preserve the larynx in the treatment of advanced laryngeal cancer: Preliminary report. Second International Head and Neck Research Conference (Abstract 1.4).

7. Kaplin, E.L.(1958): Nonparametric estimation from incomplete observations. J Am Stat Assoc 53, 457-481.

8. Tannock, I.(1987): Sequential chemotherapy and radiotherapy for nasopharyngeal carcinoma: Absence of long-term benefit despite a high rate of tumor response to chemotherapy. J Clin Oncol 5, 629-634.

9. Vikram, B.(1985): Patterns of failure in carcinoma of the nasopharynx. I. Failure at the primary site. Int J Radiat Oncol Biol Phys 11, 1454-1459.

10. Vikram, B.(1986): Patterns of failure in carcinoma of the nasopharynx. Failure at distant sites. Head and Neck Surg 8, 276-279.

Neo-Adjuvant Chemotherapy. Ed. Cl. Jacquillat, M. Weil, D. Khayat. Colloque INSERM/John Libbey Eurotext Ltd. © 1988. Vol. 169, pp. 321-325.

Cisplatinum (CDDP) and continuous infusion 5-fluorouracil (5-FU) for the treatment of head and neck cancers

François Demard, Maurice Schneider, Antoine Thyss, Pierre Chauvel, Jacques Vallicioni, José Santini and Cyril Caldani

Centre Antoine-Lacassagne, 06054 Nice Cedex, France

ABSTRACT :

238 patients with advanced squamous cell carcinoma of the upper aero-digestive tract were given 3 courses of chemotherapy (cis-platinum 100 mg/m2 D 1 and 5-Fluorouracil 1000 mg/m2 D2-D6) before any local treatment.The toxicity of this protocol was acceptable as 81 % of the patients were able to receive the scheduled drug dose.An objective response was obtained on the primary tumour in 82.7 % of the cases, including 47.7 % complete responses (CR). 29 % of CR were obtained for nodal metastases. The best results were obtained for tumours of the hypopharynx. After local treatment and at 36 months median follow up, the local control, disease-free interval and survival are higher in chemotherapy responders.

KEY WORDS
HEAD AND NECK CANCER, INDUCTION CHEMOTHERAPY, CISPLATINUM - 5 FLUOROURACIL.

For more than 5 years, the efficacy of CDDP-5 FU combination, has been widely demonstrated in induction chemotherapy of head and neck cancers (Al Sarraf et al 1979 ; Kish et al 1982 ; Lacau Saint Guily et al 1985). Since 1983, we have confirmed these results (Demard et al 1987 ; Thyss et al 1986). The present data concern 238 patients at 36 months median follow-up.

MATERIALS AND METHODS

Patients

A total of 238 patients were entered in the study (199 men and 39 women) ; mean age was 59 years (range 25-82). All patients had histologically confirmed squamous cell tumours of the UADT. None had been treated previously or had metastatic disease. The sites of primary tumours were as follows = 51 oral cavity, 94 oropharynx, 50 larynx,31 hypopharynx, 8 facial sinuses, 4 rhinopharynx. Table 1 lists patients by TNM criteria. The distribution by UICC criteria was as follows = 5 stage I ; 45 stage II ; 119 stage III ; 66 stage IV.

Induction chemotherapy with cis-platinum and 5 fluorouracil
Patient distribution by tumor size and node involvement. Table 1

	T1	T2	T3	T4
N0	5	45	54	10
N1	3	19	43	3
N2	1	2	8	4
N3	5	7	18	8

Induction chemotherapy regimen

A central venous catheter was first inserted for all patients. Treatment consisted in continuous infusion of CDDP 1000 mg/m2 on day 1 followed by 5-Fu 1000 mg/m2 from day 2 to day 6. The protocol called for three courses per patient. The interval between cycles was 15 days (D1 = D22 = D44). Drug doses were reduced 10 % for every 5 years over 70 years of age. 81 % of the patients received three chemotherapy courses, 12 % two courses, and 7 % only one course. After completion of the induction chemotherapy, patients were given local regional treatment : either uni-or bilateral surgical resection, sometimes completed by irradiation (55-65 Gy) or radiotherapy alone (65-75 Gy to the tumour bed and 55-65 Gy to nodal regions)

Evaluation of response

Before treatment, lesions were biopsied during endoscopy under general anesthesia. Response was assessed by multiple biopsies obtained under identical conditions 10 days after the last chemotherapy course. Patients with tumours of the facial sinus were evaluated by computed tomography. Response was defined as complete (CR), partial (PR) with tumour regression over 50 %, or no response (NR). The response of palpable lymph nodes was evaluated with the same criteria by physical examination and ultrasonography.

RESULTS

Results for primary tumours

Response was evaluable for 214 patients. As shown by table 2, an objective response was obtained in 177/214 patients (82.7 %):there were 102 CR (47.7 %), 75 PR (35 %) and 37 NR (17.3 %). Analysis of response as a function of tumour size revealed that a CR was achieved for 71.4 % of T1, 69 % of T2, 34.5 % of T3 and 21 % of T4.

Table 2. Results on the primary tumour.

	Tumour Size					
RESPONSE	T1	T2	T3	T4	Total	%
COMPLETE	10	50	38	4	102	47.7
PARTIAL	3	17	47	8	75	35
NO RESPONSE	1	5	23	8	37	17.3

Results for metastatic lymph nodes (Table 3)

As is often the case, the quality of clinical response was not as good as for primary tumours. Even so, the overall response rate of 83.5 % (including 29 % CR) is particularly high.

Table 3. Results on lymph node metastases.

RESPONSE	N1	N2	N3	Total	%
COMPLETE	24	2	6	32	29
PARTIAL	26	8	26	60	54.5
NO RESPONSE	11	3	4	18	16.5
TOTAL	61	13	36	110	

Results by anatomic site

Table 4 reveals that good results were obtained in all anatomic sites, but the percentage of CR was particularly high for patients with lesions of the hypopharynx (60 %).

Table 4 Results by anatomic site.

	RC		RP		NR	
	Nb	%	Nb	%	Nb	%
ORAL CAVITY	22	50	13	29.5	9	20.5
ORO PHARYNX	40	45	33	37	16	18
LARYNX	19	44	18	42	6	14
HYPOPHARYNX	15	60	7	28	3	12
FACIAL SINUSES	2/8		3/8		3/8	
RHINO-PHARYNX	3/4		1/4		-	

Local control after completion of the treatment.

After induction chemotherapy, 37 patients were treated by surgery alone, 135 by radiotherapy alone, and 45 by surgery followed by radiotherapy. Local control was obtained in 98.7 % of patients in CR after induction chemotherapy, and in respectively 88 and 63.5 % of patients in PR or NR.13 patients died during the treatment program (9 during chemotherapy, 3 postoperatively, 1 during radiotherapy).

Evaluation of the histologic response

82 patients underwent surgery immediately after induction chemotherapy. Histologic examination revealed complete sterilization in only 11 cases/17 who had been clinically classed CR, but also in 5 cases/17 who had been classed PR.

Disease free interval and survival.

After completion of the local regional treatment during the median follow up of 36 months a tumour relapse was observed in respectively 15.6 %, 22.7 % and 35 % of patients who had been clinically classed CR,PR or NR. Both tumoural and lymph node relapses were observed in 16. 6 % of the RC, 26.7 % of the PR, and 37.8 % of the NR. Distant metastases were observed in 4.9 % of the CR, 14.6 % of the PR, and 16.2 % of the NR. Fig 1 Reveals that there was significant difference in survival in favour of patients who achieved a CR or a PR as opposed to non-responders.

Fig . i

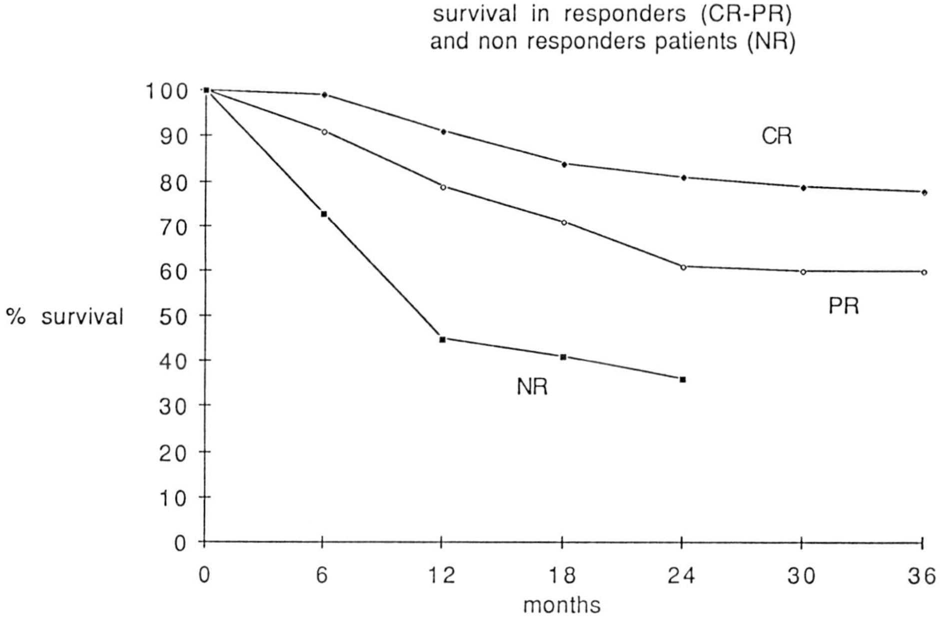

Toxicity.

Most of the patients experienced nausea and vomiting. Severe venous damage has almost entirely been eliminated since a central catheter has been inserted on a routine basis. Haematological toxicity was evaluable for 573 cycles : a severe toxicity (WHO grade III-IV) was observed in only 3% of the cycles. Severe gut toxicity (mucositis and/or diarrhoea) was observed in 9.5 % of the cycles. Other toxic manifestations included asthenia, transient rise in plasma creatinine, coronary spasm in 11 patients. Nine deaths were attributable to the chemotherapy regimen, but most of these patients had significant medical complications = decompensated alcoholic cirrhosis, myocardial infarction, severe arteriosclerosis. At this time, the toxic manifestations of this treatment have been considerably reduced thanks to pharmacokinetic monitoring of the 5-FU AUC on Day 3, which can predict and thereby allow prevention of severe toxicity by reduction of ther drug dose (cf article by G. Milano in this book).

DISCUSSION.

Our results confirm that 3 courses of CDDP-5 FU certainly constitute one of the best induction chemotherapy regimens for head and neck cancer. In 238 patients after a median follow up of 36 months, the response rate on the tumour was 82.7 %, with 47.7 % complete responses. This chemotherapy regimen was more effective on primary tumours than on metastatic lymph nodes, considering the complete responses 47.7 % vs 29 %. The anatomic site of lesions also affected results = more complete regressions were obtained for lesions of the hypopharynx than for other sites. The difference between clinical and histologic evaluation of tumour response warrants mention : minimal histologic lesions were detected in certain patients clinically graded CR, and 5 of the 17 PR patients non longer had histologic lesions. The local control rate, disease-free interval (local regional relapses and distant metastasis) and survival were higher in induction chemotherapy responders than in non-responders. Administration of 3 courses of our regimen proved feasible despite the problem of toxicity, which can be reduced and often predicted by pharmacokinetics studies. Finally, this combination of CDDP-5 FU improves the local control rate, and allows reduction of the need for certain major surgical procedures. This advantage patient confort and functional results is decisive in our opinion, and sufficient to justify use of this induction chemotherapy regimen even through its long term effect remains controversial.

REFERENCES.

Al Sarraf M., AMER MH, VAISHAUPAYONG et Al (1979) : A multi modality therapeutic approach for advanced previously untreated epidermoid cancer of the head and neck Preliminary Report. Int.J. Radiat.Oncol. Biol. Phys,5 :1421-1423

Demard F., Schneider M., Chauvel P., Ramaioli A., Vallicioni J., Santini J :(1987) Chimiotherapie d'induction Platine 5-fluorouracile. Resultats actuels en cancérologie cervico faciale. Ann. Oto. Laryng, 104 :399-406

Kish J., Drelichman A., Jacobs J.R. et al (1982) : clinical trial of cis-platinum and 5-fluoruracil infusions as initial treatment for advanced squamous carcinoma of the head and neck. Cancer Treat.Rep.,66 : 471-474.

Lacau Saint Guily J, Brasnu D, Bassot V (1985) : Chimiothérapie d'induction des cancers des voies aéro-digestives supérieures. Analyse de la réponse tumorale chez 176 malades. Presse Méd.,14 : 1313.

Thyss A., Falewee M.N., Leborgne L., Viens P.,Schneider M., Demard F(1987) : Cardiotoxicité du 5-Fluorouracile. Spasme ou toxicité myocardique directe. Bull. Cancer,74 : 381-385.

Thyss A., Schneider M., Santini J., Caldani C., Vallicioni J., Chauvel P., Demard F. (1986) : Induction chemotherapy with cis-platinum and 5 fluorouracil for squamous cell carcinoma of the head and neck. Br.J. Cancer,54 : 755-760.

Résumé

238 patients atteints de carcinomes épidermoides avancés des VADS ont reçu avant tout traitement local 3 cycles de chimiothérapie associant cis-platinum 100 mg/ m2 au J1 et 5 Fluorouracile 1000 mg/m2 J2 à J6 en perfusion continue. 81 % des patients ont pu recevoir les 3 cycles. Sur la tumeur primitive, on note 87,7 % de réponses dont 47,7 % sont cliniquement complètes. Les résultats sont moins bons sur les adénopathies : 29 % de RC. Les meilleurs résultats ont été obtenus pour les tumeurs de l'hypopharynx. Après les traitements locaux et avec une médiane de survie de 36 mois, le contrôle local, l'intervalle libre et la survie sont supérieurs pour les patients répondeurs à la chimiothérapie.

Neo-Adjuvant Chemotherapy. Ed. Cl. Jacquillat, M. Weil, D. Khayat. Colloque INSERM/John Libbey Eurotext Ltd. © 1988. Vol. 169, pp. 327-332.

Low dose neo-adjuvant chemotherapy in head and neck cancers : anti-tumour activity, prediction of radiotherapy response and influence on survival

Jean-Marie Deneufbourg

Radiotherapy department, University hospital, 66 boulevard de la Constitution, Liège, Belgium

ABSTRACT

184 consecutive patients, all recently diagnosed and previously untreated, received a chemotherapy consisting of bleomycin (10 mg), etoposide (100 mg) and cisplatinum (15 mg) given as single course on days 1,3,5,15,17 and 19. There were 147 males and 37 females, aged 27-91 (mean 58). Oropharynx (68), oral cavity (37), larynx (35) and hypopharynx (25) were the predominant sites. Most tumours were locally advanced (27 T1, 55 T2, 51 T3, 51 T4) with frequent lymph nodes involvement (95 N0, 25 N1, 4 N2, 63 N3). Squamous cell carcinoma was present in 175 cases. A significant anti-tumour activity was obtained :

CHEMOTHERAPY	Patients	Tumour	Nodes
CR	11%	14%	6%
PR	59%	72%	52%
CR + PR	70%	86%	58%

Side-effects were minimal; no hyperhydration programm nor mannitol diuresis was used; chemotherapy was given on an ambulatory mode. Exclusive irradiation was delivered to full dose (TDF 103) in 148 cases with good tôlerance of normal tissues. Chemotherapy response (C+) or non response (C-) influences tumour control after radiotherapy :

RADIOTHERAPY	Patients		Tumour		Nodes	
	C+	C-	C+	C-	C+	C-
Complete control	82%	39%	95%	67%	60%	33%

Short term effects on survival seem encouraging :

SURVIVAL	55 stage III	79 stage IV
2 years rate	60%	50%
3 years rate	50%	30%

Trends exist for a 10-15% benefit as compared to our own historical controls. Predictive neo-adjuvant chemotherapy might be of great value for treatment optimization and individualization.

KEYWORDS

Neo-adjuvant chemotherapy, head and neck cancers, bleomycin, etoposide, cisplatinum.

INTRODUCTION

A study is going on to assess the efficacy and the feasability of chemotherapy before planned radical irradiation or surgery in head and neck cancers with bad prognosis. The main purpose is to obtain a reduction of tumour volume in order to increase radiosensitivity, especially in hypoxic areas, and to ensure a better surgical resection. An effect on occult metastases already present at the time of diagnosis is also anticipated. Prior chemotherapy must not unduly delay the planned radical treatment nor add peculiar complications to irradiation or surgery. Side-effects should be minimal with a good patients compliance.

PATIENTS

184 consecutive patients were enrolled, all recently diagnosed and previously untreated. There were 147 males and 37 females, aged 27 to 91 (mean 58). Karnofsky index was higher than 70. The predominant sites of disease are detailed in Table 1 Staging referring to UICC TNM classification is given in Table 2.

SITES

Oropharynx	68	Tonsil	51
		Base of tongue	13
		Soft palate	4
Oral cavity	37	Floor of mouth	14
		Tongue	13
		Gingiva	6
		Cheek mucosa	3
		Hard palate	1
Larynx	35		
Hypopharynx	25		
Nasopharynx	7		
Nasal cavities	4		
Salivary glands	3		

Table 1.

TUMOUR STAGING

UICC

	N0	N1	N2	N3	
T1	17	4	0	6	27
T2	28	6	1	22	55
T3	22	6	1	22	51
T4	28	9	2	12	51
	95	25	4	62	

All M0

AJC

I	17
II	28
III	56
IV	83

Table 2.

Histology consisted of squamous cell carcinoma in 175 cases (90 well differentiated, 33 moderately differentiated, 31 poorly differentiated and 21 non other specified). There were 8 adenocarcinomas and 1 synovialosarcoma.

TREATEMENT POLICY

All stages of hypopharynx, nasopharynx and oropharynx cancers are treated by chemotherapy prior to exclusive radiotherapy. T3 N3 and T4 larynx receive the same association. Tumours of the oral cavity whatever T ans N are treated by chemotherapy, surgery and post-operative irradiation.

NEO-ADJUVANT CHEMOTHERAPY

A. Agents
A single course chemotherapy regimen associates bleomycin (10 mg), etoposide (100 mg) and cis-paltinum (15 mg) in a 3 hours IV perfusion of one litre normal saline. This low dose chemotherapy is given six times over a three weeks period on days 1,3,5 and 15,17,19. Ancillary support consists of anti-emetics given as needed. No hyperhydration nor forced diuresis was used. This treatment is carried out on an amulatory mode.
B. Response rate
The results are clinically assessed 8 days after the last injection. Response criterias are those in standard use : complete response (CR) in case of tumour dissepearance, partial response (PR) when the product of 2 diameters is reduced by more than 50%, minor response (MR) when the reduction is less than 50%, no response (NR) in case of stable disease or even tumour progression.
An overall response rate of 70% was obtained (CR + PR). As shown in Table 3, primary lesions proved more sensitive than lymph nodes.

T RESPONSE (175 TARGETS)	N RESPONSE (82 TARGETS)
CR = 14%	CR = 6%
PR = 72%	PR = 52%
CR + PR = 86%	CR + PR = 58%
MR = 11%	MR = 32%
NR = 3%	NR = 10%

Table 3.

The response rate differs according to tumour site (floor of mouth, tonsil and tongue tumours showing the maximum of sensitivity) and correlates with the target volume. On the contrary, histological differentiation seems to exert no influence (Table 4).

PARAMETERS OF RESPONSE

1. Tumour site	T°	N°	GLOBAL°
Tonsil	98	70	78
Larynx	66	54	62
Hypopharynx	76	50	61
Floor of mouth	100	40	75
Tongue	92	25	75
Base of tongue	64	33	50

° *per cent major responses (CR + PR)*

2. Target volume	T1	T2	T3	T4	N1	N2
% CR	26	14	19	3	5	0
% PR	53	69	72	69	53	58
% CR + PR	79	83	91	72	58	58

3. Histology	T°	N°
Well differentiated	82	56
Moderately differentiated	83	47
Poorly differentiated	92	59

° *per cent major responses (CR + PR)*

Table 4.

C. Side effects

The side effects remained acceptable without any life-threatening complications. 85% of patients experienced nausea (mild to severe) and 50% had vomiting. Digestive intolerance was maximal on days 1 and 15. A mild hematologic depression - leukopenia and thrombopenia - usually occured. Treatment had to be protracted in 4% of cases by doubling the time interval; etoposide dose was reduced by half in 8% of cases. No renal dysfunction was observed as measured by rise of serum levels of creatinine. No pulmonary side-effects were encountered but 2 transient bronchospasms occured at the time of injection. Alopecia has been noted in 20% of cases, more frequently among women. 2 patients experienced mild cutaneous effects from bleomycin.

RADICAL TREATMENT

The planned radical treatment consisted of exclusive radiotherapy (148 cases) or surgical resection followed by irradiation (22 cases). 14 non-respects of planning included patient refusals of treatment and cases where clinical deterioration prevented further treatment.
The radical treatment was always initiated without undue delay (mean interval of 15 days for radiotherapy and 18 days for surgery). Irradiation was always given to full dose (TDF 103) using a split-course modality. The local tolerance was unchanged as compared to historical controls treated in the same way. No cumulative toxic effects on normal tissues was observed. 92 patients were eligible for a further chemotherapy with monthly courses of high dose methotrexate (3 gm) and leucovorin rescue. The neo-adjuvant chemotherapy did not alter the tolerance to this long term maintenance treatment.

RESULTS

A. Anti-tumour activity

Early assessment indicates that high rates of tumour control were achieved after exclusive radiotherapy. Within one month after the end of irradiation, 88% of primary tumours had totally regressed and the complete regression rate of lymph nodes amounted to 54% (multiple nodes in the same patient being considered as a single target).

B. Prediction of radiotherapy response

A clear-cut correlation exists between chemotherapy and radiotherapy responses. For primary tumours, 95% of complete regressions occur among chemotherapy good responders versus 67% among chemotherapy poor responders. The predictive value of chemotherapy is observed for all stages except for T1 where irradiation controls 100% of cases (graph 1). The same correlations are observed for nodes : 60% of complete regressions occur among chemotherapy good responders versus 33% among chemotherapy poor responders. Subdivision following N1, N2 and N3 shows that poor responders to chemotherapy have only 10% probability of being controlled (graph 2).

C. Influence on survival

The long term benefit is still putative. Stage III patients survival is 57% at 2 years and 48% at 3 years with perhaps a plateau phase. 50% of stage IV patients are still alive at 2 years but only 31% at 3 years and the curve is still going down (graph 3). A comparison is on study with historical controls treated in the same way except for neo-adjuvant chemotherapy. Trends exist for a ten per cent possible benefit.
However more cases and time are needed.

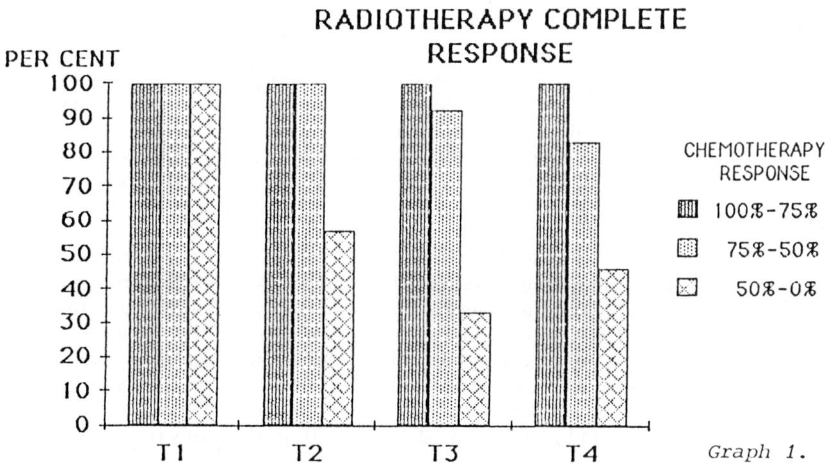

Graph 1.

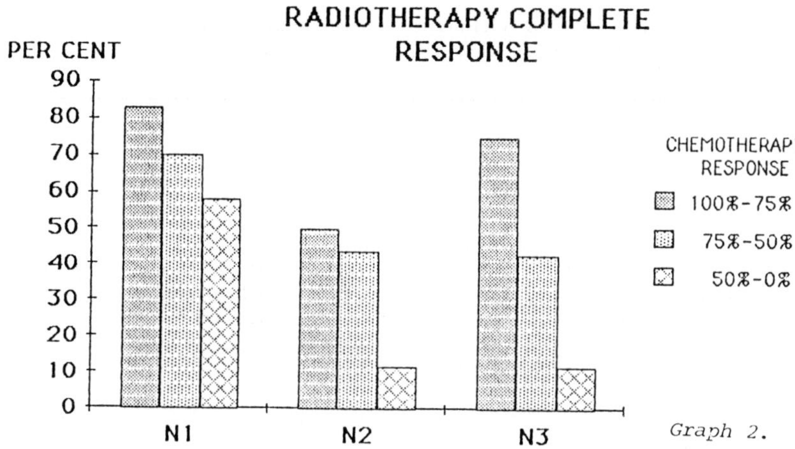

Graph 2.

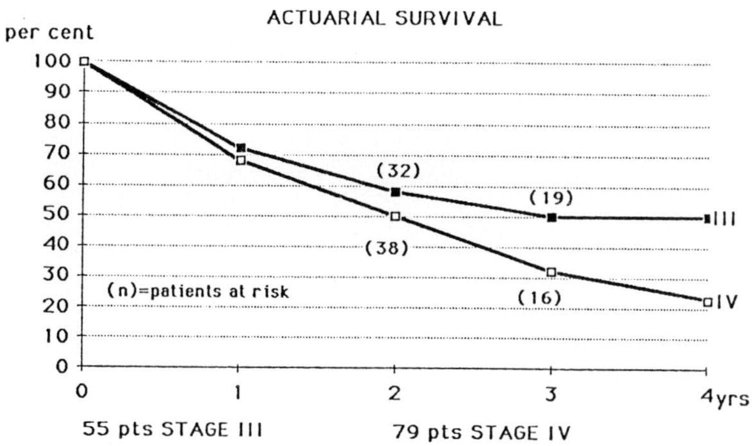

Graph 3.

Résumé

184 patients consécutifs, tous diagnostiqués récemment et sans traitement antérieur ont reçu une chimiothérapie consistant en Bléomycine 10 mg, Vépéside 100 mg, Cis.Platyl 15 mg, donné en une perfusion aux jours 1,3,5, 15,17 et 19. Il y avait 147 hommes et 37 femmes, de 37 à 91 ans (moyenne : 58 ans). Il s'agissait d'oropharynx (68 cas), de la cavité buccale (37 cas), de larynx (35 cas), d'hypopharynx (25 cas), la plupart des tumeurs étaient localement avancées (27 T1, 55 T2, 51 T3, 51 T4) avec envahissement ganglionnaire fréquent (95 N0, 25 N1, 4 N2, 63 N3). Une histologie de cancer épidermoïde a été retrouvée dans 175 cas. Une activité significative anti-tumorale a été obtenue avec une rémission complète chez 11 % des malades avec des effets secondaires négligeables. Une rémission complète après radiothérapie a été observée chez 82 % des malades sensibles à la chimiothérapie et chez 39 % des malades qui étaient résistants. La survie à court terme est encourageante avec 60 % de survie à 2 ans, 50 % de survie à 3 ans pour 55 stades III, 50 % à 2 ans, 30 % de survie à 3 ans pour 79 stades IV.

Par rapport à nos propres contrôles historiques, le bénéfice est de 10 à 15 %.

La valeur prédictive de la chimiothérapie semble d'être de grande valeur pour l'opimisation et l'individualisation du traitement.

Neo-Adjuvant Chemotherapy. Ed. Cl. Jacquillat, M. Weil, D. Khayat. Colloque INSERM/John Libbey Eurotext Ltd. © 1988. Vol. 169, pp. 333-338.

Neo-adjuvant chemotherapy versus alternating chemo-radiotherapy in head and neck cancer

Marco Merlano, Andrea Grimaldi, Marco Benasso, Almalina Bacigalupo, Salvatore Toma, Giovanni Margarino, Alida Santelli*, Renzo Corvo, Mario Roberto Sertoli and Riccardo Rosso

Istituto Nazionale per la Ricerca sul Cancro, Genova, Italy
**Div. ORL, Ospedale S. Martino, Genova, Italy*

SUMMARY

In August '83 we started a phase III study to compare a neo-adjuvant chemotherapy followed by radiotherapy and/or surgery to an alternating chemo-radiotherapy regimen. One hundred sixteen patients entered the study. At the time of the present analysis (November 1987), our data show a statistically significant advantage in terms of response, progression free survival and survival in favour of the alternating program.

Key Words: Head and Neck Cancer - Alternating Chemo-radiotherapy

INTRODUCTION

The prognosis of patients (pts) with advanced squamous cell carcinoma of the head and neck is very dismal.
Inability to achieve loco-regional control has led to various approaches including neo-adjuvant chemotherapy. Few investigators have rejected induction chemotherapy in favour of the theory first presented by Clifford (Clifford, 1976), which claimed that chemotherapy could play a major role if administered alternatively with split-courses of radiotherapy. This concept was later supported by the studies of Looney et al in animal models (Looney, 1979, 1985, 1986).
This report presents the results of a randomized trial comparing an induction chemotherapy followed by definitive local therapy with an alternating regimen of chemotherapy and radiotherapy to determine the best multidisciplinary approach to advanced head and neck cancer.

MATERIALS AND METHODS

Between August '83 and January '87, 116 pts with advanced unoperable stage III (45 pts) and IV (71 pts), M0, previously untreated squamous cell carcinoma of the head and neck entered the

study.
Pts were prospectively randomized into two arms: 55 pts were entered in arm A and 61 in arm B.
Pts' characteristics are shown in table 1.
Arm A consisted of 4 cycles of chemotherapy followed, within 3 weeks, by definitive radiation therapy. In cases of progressive disease during neo-adjuvant treatment, chemotherapy was stopped and pts underwent radical radiotherapy: 65-75 Gy, 2 Gy daily. In arm B 4 cycles of chemotherapy were alternated with 3 courses of radiotherapy, 20 Gy in ten fractions of 2 weeks each. Radiation was administered after the 2nd, 3rd and 4th chemotherapy courses.
Chemotherapy was the same in both arms: Vinblastine 6 mg/m2, followed by Bleomycin 30 mg and Methotrexate 200 mg, 6 hours and 24 hours later respectively. Chemotherapy was repeated every 14 days.

RESULTS

All pts were evaluable for survival (S), while 112 pts were evaluable for toxicity (53 in arm A and 59 in B), since 4 pts refused to start therapy. One hundred five pts were evaluable for response and Progression Free Survival (PFS) (48 in arm A and 57 in B), since 11 pts were unevaluable due to major protocol violation (4 pts), ineligibility (3 pts), or refusal to start therapy (4 pts).
At the end of the treatment we recorded 7 CR and 18 PR in arm A (52% response rate) and 19 CR and 18 PR in arm B (64.9% response rate). The difference observed for CR between arms A and B was statistically significant ($x2=4.9$, $p<.03$). Twenty-one PRs (10 in arm A and 11 in arm B) became operable after treatment. Surgery was performed in all pts, and 18 (7 in arm A and 11 in arm B) were rendered disease-free. The inclusion of these surgical CRs preserves the difference observed between the 2 arms. In fact, after surgery, the response rate was 52% in arm A (14 CR, 11 PR) and 64.9% in arm B (30 CR, 7 PR).
At the time of present analysis (November '87), a statistically significant increase in PFS and S was correlated with the alternating regimen. Median PFS (Fig.1) was 5 months and 7 months in arms A and B respectively ($x2=7.19$, $p<.008$).
Median overall S (Fig.2) was 9 months and 13 months in arm A and B respectively ($x2=4.74$, $p<.03$).
Toxicity was generally accettable; no deaths due to the treatment were detected.Mucositis represented the most serious side effects in arm B: 18 pts (30.5%) suffered grade III-IV (WHO scale) (Miller, 1981) mucosal toxicity, while in arm A only 2 cases (3.8%) were observed.The statistical difference is highly significant ($x2=13.5$, $p<.00004$).
As a consequence of toxicity 2 pts discontinued the treatment in arm A: these pts were fully evaluated as non responders (failure due to toxicity).

DISCUSSION

The aim of this study was to compare sequential chemotherapy and radiotherapy to an alternating program in the multidisciplinary treatment of advanced squamous cell carcinoma of the head and

neck. The purpose of neoadjuvant chemotherapy was to induce a tumor reduction and to control possible micrometastatic disease. The alternating plain, supported by the Goldie and Coldman hypothesis (Goldie, 1979), should reduce the development of double resistant clones and overcome the single-resistant clones.
We used the same drug scheduling and number of courses in both arms, so that the only difference between them was the radiotherapy scheduling.
The analysis of the results showed that alternating treatemnt is associated with a significant increase in the CR rate, PFS and S. The two treatments were satisfactory tolerated, but an impressive mucosal toxicity was observed in the alternating arm. This side effect could be correlated with a toxic synergism between methotrexate and radiotherapy.
Other studies are necessary to confirm our results and to compare the best integration of chemo-radiotherapy to a conventional treatment such as radiotherapy alone.

Tab. 1 - PATIENTS' CHARACTERISTICS

	ARM A	ARM B
Male/Female	46/9	51/10
Median age (range)	59 (34-75)	61 (37-75)
Median P.S. (range)	1 (0-3)	1 (0-3)
Stage III	22	22
Stage IV	33	39
Site of Primary		
Nasopharynx	3	6
Oropharynx	21	34
Hypopharynx	11	7
Oral Cavity	18	11
Larynx (supraglottic)	2	3

REFERENCES

Clifford P.: Perspective in head and neck oncology (James Yeardley Memorial Lecture, March, 1974) (1976): J. Laringol. Otol. 90:221-251.

Goldie J.H., Coldman A.J.: A mathematic model for relating the drug sensitivity of tumors to their spontaneous mutation rate (1979): Cancer Treat. Rep. 63:1727-1733.

Looney W.B., Hopkins H.A., Mac Leod M.S. et al: Solid tumor models for the assessment of different treatment modalities. XII. Combined chemotherapy and radiotherapy: variation of time interval between time of administration of 5-fluorouracil and radiation and its effects on the control of tumor growth (1979): Cancer 44:437-445.

Looney W.B., Goldie J.H., Little J.B., et al: Alternation of chemotherapy and radiotherapy in cancer management. I. Summary of the division of cancer treatment workshop (1985): Cancer Treat. Rep. 69:769-775.

Looney W.B., Hopkins H.A.: Alternation of chemotherapy and radiotherapy in cancer management. III. Results in experimental solid tumor systems and the relationship to clinical studies (1986): Cancer Treat. Rep. 70:141-162.

Miller A.B., Hoogstraten B., Staquet M., et al: Reporting results of cancer treatment (1981): Cancer 47:207-210.

Fig. 1 - PROGRESSION FREE SURVIVAL

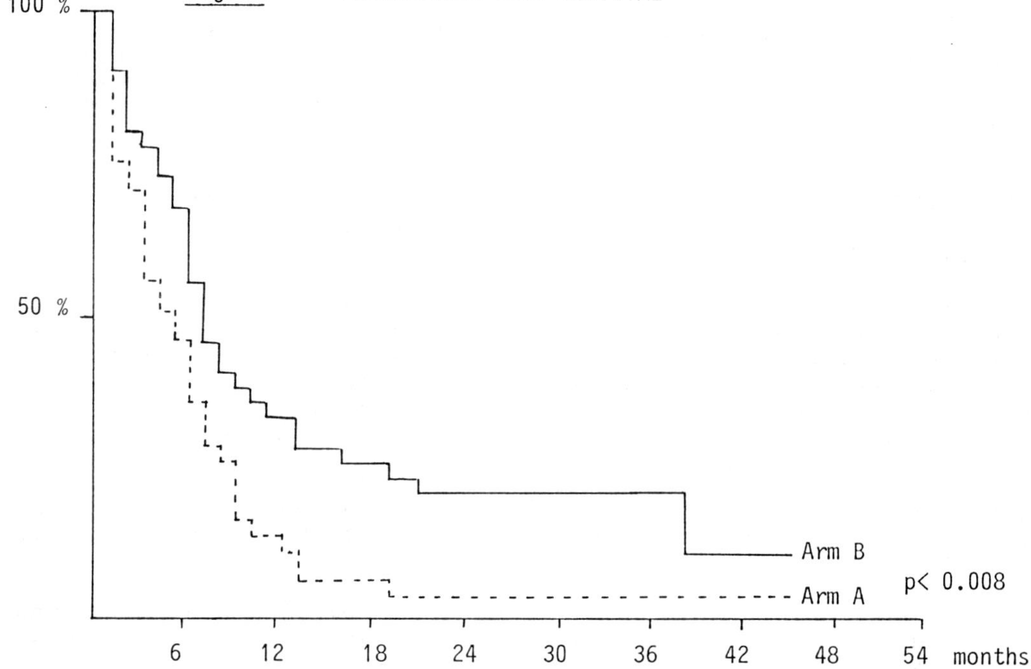

Fig. 2 - SURVIVAL

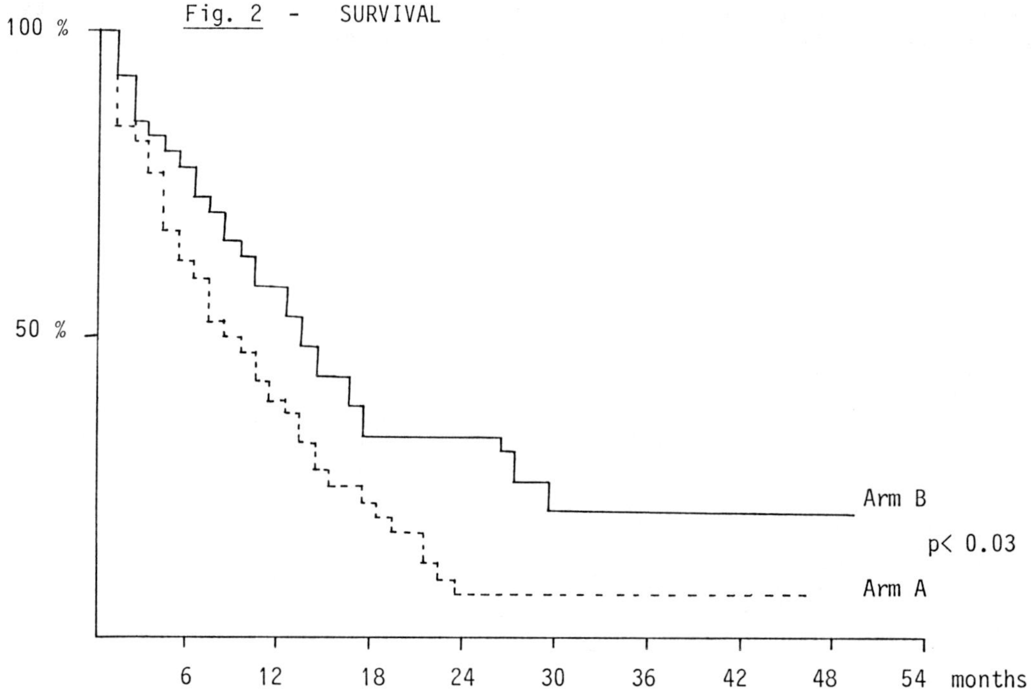

Résumé

Depuis 83 nous avons entrepris une étude de phase III pour comparer la chimiothérapie néoadjuvante suivie par la radiothérapie et par la chirurgie à une alternance de chimio-radiothérapie. 116 patients sont entrés dans cette étude. En novembre 87 nos données montrent un avantage statistiquement significatif en terme de réponse de survie sans rechute de survie en faveur du traitement alterné.

Neo-Adjuvant Chemotherapy. Ed. Cl. Jacquillat, M. Weil, D. Khayat. Colloque INSERM/John Libbey Eurotext Ltd. © 1988. Vol. 169, pp. 339-343.

Induction cisplatin-5FU chemotherapy as initial treatment for advanced head and neck squamous cell carcinoma

P. Cappelaere, J.L. Lefèbvre, E. Buisset, B. Prevost, A. Joveniaux, A. Caty, D. Carlier and L. Adenis

Centre Oscar Lambert (Centre de Lutte Contre le Cancer de la Région Nord) (Directeur: Pr. A. Demaille), BP 307, 59020 Lille Cedex, France

SUMMARY

Due to poor results obtained by definitive radiotherapy for advanced head and neck cancer, an initial treatment by chemotherapy combinating cisplatin-5FU appeared suitable. From 1983 through july 1987, 187 patients received such an induction chemotherapy. After completing this initial treatment, 54 percent of patient had a tumour regression of more than 50 percent. Hypopharynx and larynx were the highest response rates primary sites. If histological type, nodal status and number of primaries at first examination had no incidence on tumour response, the local extension had a direct influence on this response. On the other hand, 41 percent of patients had a nodal response of more than 50 percent. Only one patient deceased due to toxicity and 168 patients could undergo loco-regional treatment after chemotherapy. The median survival time was 13.5 months for the overall population, 19 months for responders and 29 months for complete responders to chemotherapy.

INTRODUCTION

Patients with unresectable advanced head and neck squamous cell carcinoma (HNSCC) have a remarkable poor prognosis with a dramatically short survival time. After completing a retrospective study about 2418 successive new HNSCC observed between 1976 and 1980 at Centre Oscar Lambret, we focused this study on 337 unresectable patients treated by definitive radiotherapy with palliative intent, without induction chemotherapy. The median survival time was 9 months, failures above clavicles occurred in 75 percent of cases, and distant metastases in 12 percent of cases.

For such patients, we started in 1983 a new therapeutic management with induction chemotherapy combinating cisplatin and 5FU.

MATERIAL AND METHODS

Were eligible for that study, previously untreated patients :
- with HNSCC, pathologically proven
- evaluable or measurable lesion,

- with advanced locoregional disease, without distant metastases,
- unresectable, the only therapeutic possibility being radiotherapy with palliative intent.

Between january 1983 and july 1987, 187 patients met those criteria :
- 154 with only one HNSCC (85 percent) at admission,
- 28 with multiple HNSCC (the largest one being the index tumour),
- 5 without primary (cervical SCC lymphnode of unknown primary site, CUPS).

The primary site was :

- oral cavity	42 cases (23 percent),
- oropharynx	78 cases (42 percent),
- hypopharynx	38 cases (21 percent),
- larynx	23 cases (12 percent),
- maxillary antrum	1 case,
- unknown (CUPS)	5 cases.

Clinical staging of index tumour according UICC recommandations (1987) was as follows:

	T0*	T1	T2	T3	T4	Total
N0	-	-	8**	26	14	48
N1	-	-	2**	20	9	31
N2a	-	-	3**	8	5	16
N2b	-	-	-	15	4	19
N2c	1	-	2	15	14	32
N3	4	4	4	16	13	41
Total	5	4	19	100	59	187

* patients with CUPS - ** patients with multiple primaries

All patients received induction chemotherapy with, as advocated by AL SARRAF :
- day 1 : cisplatin 100 mg/m^2
- day 1-5 : 5FU 1000 mg/24 h

Most of patients received three cycles (149 patients), 7 received one cycle, 22 two cycles, 6 four cycles and 3 five cycles.

Response criteria were as follows :
. Complete response (CR), the complete disappearance of all clinical evidence of existing disease ;
. Partial response (PR) a > 50 % reduction in the sum of the products of perpendicular measurements of measurable lesions or a major reduction in size of index lesions or evaluable lesions ;
. Stable disease (SD), a < 50 % regression or < 25 % increase in measurable lesions ;
. Progressive disease (PD), a $\geq$ 25 % increase in size of any measurable lesions, appearance of any new lesion, or worsening of an evaluable clinical parameter.

RESULTS

1°) A little more than 1 out 2 patients (54 percent) were responders at the primary site :

For 182 primaries (index tumours)

. complete response	(CR)	: 30/182 (16 percent)
. partial response	(PR)	: 69/182 (38 percent)
. stable disease	(SD)	: 74/182 (41 percent)
. progression	(PD)	: 9/182 (5 percent)

Response rates varied according to primary sites

- . oral cavity : CR + PR = 17/42 (40 percent)
- . oropharynx : CR + PR = 40/78 (51 percent)
- . hypopharynx : CR + PR = 28/38 (74 percent)
- . larynx : CR + PR = 13/23 (57 percent)
- . sinus : CR + PR = 1/1

We did not found statistical differences between well differentiated SCC (CR + PR = 88/161) and poorly differenciated SCC (CR + PR = 11/21).

Local extension had a direct incidence on response rates :

- . T1 : CR + PR = 4/4
- . T2 : CR + PR = 15/19 (79 percent)
- . T3 : CR + PR = 55/100 (55 percent)
- . T4 : CR + PR = 25/52 (48 percent)

But there were no statistical difference for primary response according to nodal status or to number of primaries at first examination.

2°) A little less than 1 out 2 patients (41 percent) were responders in the neck:

For 139 palpable cervical lymphnode at admission :

- . complete response (CR) : 17/139 (12 percent)
- . partial response (PR) : 41/139 (29 percent)
- . stable disease (SD) : 69/139 (59 percent)
- . progression (PD) : 12/139 (9 percent)

- . and 2 initially NO patients developped metastatic cervical nodes during induction chemotherapy

We did not found statistical differences for nodal response according to local extension, nodal extension, nodal size, primary site, histological type or number of primaries.

3°) Notable toxicity occurred in two patients and only one toxicity was lethal (myelosuppression and nephrotoxicity).

4°) The following treatment after chemotherapy was :
- surgery 2 cases
- radiotherapy 149 cases
- both 17 cases
- no treatment 19 cases.

5°) At the last evaluation (february 1988), 99 patients were alive (74 NED) and 88 were deceased (76 due to evolution of index tumour, 2 to evolution of metachronous cancer, 1 to toxicity and 9 due to unknown causes, but without evolution at the last examination).

Local failures occurred in 73 patients, cervical failures in 75 patients and distant metastases in 23 patients, but many patients have a short follow-up.

The median survival time was :
- 13.5 months for overall population,
- 19 months for responders (CR + PR) to chemotherapy,
- 19 months for responders (CR + PR) to overall treatment,
- 29 months for complete responders (CR) to chemotherapy.

DISCUSSION

Induction chemotherapy appears suitable for previously untreated and unresectable head and neck diseases. Response rate is 54 percent at the primary site which improves the effects of following radiotherapy. Nevertheless the survival remains rather low, even if response to chemotherapy has a good predictive value.

REFERENCES

Al Sarraf, M.(1987): Chemotherapeutic management of head and neck cancer. Cancer Metast. Rev. 6, 181-198.

Bassot, V., Brasnu, D., Lacau-St-Guily, J., Fabre, A., Menard, M., Donnadieu, S., Jacquillat, Cl., Laccourreye, H.(1986): Chimiothérapie d'induction dans les cancers des voies aéro-digestives par perfusions continues associant cisplatinum (C), fluoro-5-uracile (F), Bleomycine (B) ou C, F. Ann. Oto-Laryng. (Paris) 103, 73-76.

Cappelaere, P., Lefebvre, J.L., Madelain, M., Adenis, L., Dehaut, Ph.(1986): La chimiothérapie première des carcinomes épidermoïdes des voies aéro-digestives supérieures. A propos d'une étude rétrospective de 239 patients. Neo-Adjuvant Chemotherapy 137, 363-369.

Chauvergne, J., Cappelaere, P., Fargeot P., Meeus, L., Gary-Bobo, J., Klein, T., Clavel, B., David, M.(1987): Chimiothérapie d'induction des carcinomes des voies aéro-digestives supérieures. Résultats d'une étude prospective randomisée avec cisplatine seul ou associé. Bull. Cancer (sous presse).

Clark, J.R., Fallon, B.G., Frei III, E.(1987): Induction chemotherapy as initial treatment for advanced head and neck cancer : a model for the multidisciplinary treatment of solid tumors. In Imp. Adv. Oncol., ed V. De Vita, S. Hellman, S.A. Rosenberg, pp. 175-195, JB Lippincott Comp.

Crissman, J.D., Pajak, T.F., Zarbo, R.J., Marcial, V.A., Al-Sarraf M.(1987): Improved response and survival to combined cisplatin and radiation in non-keratinizing squamous cell carcinomas of the head and neck : An RTOG study of 114 advanced stage tumors. Cancer 59, 1391-1397.

Demard, F., Schneider, M., Chauvel, P., Ramaioli, A., Vallicioni, J., Santini, J.(1987): Chimiothérapie d'induction platine-5 Fluoro-uracile : Résultats actuels en carcinologie cervico-faciale. Ann. Oto-laryng. (Paris) 104, 399-406.

Ervin, J.T., Clark, J.R., Weichselbaum, R.R., Fallan, B.G., Miller, D., Fabian, R.L.(1987): An analysis of induction and adjuvant chemotherapy in the multidisciplinary treatment of squamous-cell carcinoma of the head and neck. J. Clin. Oncol. 5, 10-20.

Forastiere, A.A., Takasugi, B.J., Baker, S.R., Wolf, G.T., Kudla-Hatch, V. (1987): High-dose cisplatin in advanced head and neck cancer. Cancer Chemother. Pharmacol. 19, 155-158.

Haines, I., Bosl, G., Pfister, D., Spiro, R., Gerold, F., Sessions, R.(1987): Very-high dose cisplatin with bleomycin infusion as initial treatment of advanced head and neck cancer. J. Clin. Oncol. 5, 1594-1600.

Jacobs, C., Goffinet, D.R., Goffinet, L., Kohler, M., Fee, W.E.(1987): Chemotherapy as a substitute for surgery in the treatment of advanced resectable head and neck cancer. Cancer 60, 1178-1183.

Kish, J., Drelichman, A., Jacobs, J., Hoschner, J., Kinzle, J., Loh, J., Weaver, A., Al-Sarraf, M.(1982): Clinical trial of cisplatin and 5FU infusion as initial treatment for advanced squamous cell carcinoma of the head and neck. Cancer Treat. Rep. 66, 471-474.

Rooney, M., Kish, J., Jacobs, J., Kinzie, J., Weaver, A., Crissman, J., Al-Sarraf, M.(1985): Improved complete response rate and survival in advanced head and neck cancer after three-course induction therapy with 120-hour 5FU infusion and cisplatin. Cancer 55, 1123-1128.

Tannock, I.F., Browman, G.(1986): Lack of evidence for a role of chemotherapy in the routine management of locally advanced head and neck cancer. J. Clin. Oncol. 4, 1121-1126.

Vignoud, J., Ripoche, D., Bourdin, S., Peuvrel, P., Beauvillain, C., Dumesnil, Y.(1987): Chimiothérapie première dans les cancers épidermoïdes avancés des voies aérodigestives supérieures. Bull. Cancer 74, 695.

Résumé

Compte tenu des mauvais résultats obtenus par la radiothérapie exclusive pour des cancers très avancés de la tête et du cou, il nous est apparu souhaitable de débuter le traitement de tels patients, non traités antérieurement, par une chimiothérapie de type cisplatine-5FU. De 1983 à Juillet 1987, 187 patients ont été traités par ce protocole. A la fin de la chimiothérapie, 54 % des patients avaient une régression de plus de 50 % du volume tumoral. Les sites ayant le mieux répondu sont l'hypopharynx et le larynx. Si le type histologique, l'envahissement ganglionnaire et le nombre de cancers au premier examen n'influent pas, en revanche l'extension tumorale a une nette influence sur le taux de réponses, les tumeurs moins évoluées répondant mieux. D'autre part, 41 % des patients avaient une régression ganglionnaire de plus de 50 %. Seul un patient est décédé d'une toxicité et 168 ont reçu un traitement complémentaire. La médiane de survie est de 13,5 mois pour l'ensemble de la population. Elle est de 19 mois pour les répondeurs de plus de 50 % et de 29 mois pour les répondeurs complets à la chimiothérapie.

Neo-Adjuvant Chemotherapy. Ed. Cl. Jacquillat, M. Weil, D. Khayat. Colloque INSERM/John Libbey Eurotext Ltd. © 1988. Vol. 169, pp. 345-352.

Neo-adjuvant chemotherapy in head and neck cancer

Gordon B. Snow and Jan B. Vermorken

Free University Hospital, de Boelelaan 1117, 1081 HV Amsterdam, The Netherlands

ABSTRACT

Numerous uncontrolled studies have shown that induction chemotherapy is feasible in patients with advanced head and neck cancer. Cisplatinum containing multiple drug regimens have been shown to be highly effective to attain initial tumour shrinkage. It is a general experience that complete responders to chemotherapy do better in the long run than partial responders and no responders. However, almost all randomized controlled studies carried out to this date have failed to demonstrate improved survival in the chemotherapy arm as compared to the control arm. The possible reasons for this are analysed. It might well be that response to chemotherapy predicts for response to further therapy, particularly radiation therapy, while not necessarily contributing to a survival benefit. Accordingly the concept that mutilating surgery may be omitted in patients demonstrating complete response to induction chemotherapy and that radiotherapy may suffice, is very interesting. The possible benefits of neo-adjuvant chemotherapy are being investigated in ongoing randomized studies. At present there is no place for the use of ad hoc induction chemotherapy in the primary treatment of head and neck cancer patients.

KEYWORDS

Neo-adjuvant chemotherapy - Head & Neck Cancer.

INTRODUCTION

Neo-adjuvant or induction chemotherapy has been used in head and neck cancer patients for almost two decades. Although both the overall response and complete response rates to initial chemotherapy have increased impressively in recent years since the introduction of cisplatinum containing multiple drug regimens, disappointingly, the role of neo-adjuvant chemotherapy in head and neck cancer patients has still not been defined. On the basis of a review of the literature and of the experiences gained within the EORTC, the reasons will be analysed why we have sofar failed to do so. Only well designed randomized studies can answer the crucial question whether neo-adjuvant chemotherapy has a role or not in the treatment of head and neck cancer patients. The essential ingredients for such studies will be reviewed. Two such studies, which are ongoing, will be discussed.

REVIEW OF LITERATURE

Uncontrolled studies.

A large number of single arm studies have been carried out adding initial chemotherapy to surgery and/or radiotherapy in the treatment of patients with locally advanced squamous cell carcinoma of the head and neck. The experiences gained allow for three important observations.

Firstly, this type of chemotherapy integrated into combined modality treatment has been shown to be feasible. Neo-adjuvant chemotherapy does not appear to affect wound healing or limit surgical reconstructive techniques. It is essential that the margins of excision after chemotherapy are determined on the basis of the original extent of the tumour before chemotherapy. It has been a general experience that in patients demonstrating complete response to chemotherapy subsequent determination of adequate margins for surgical resection constitutes a difficult problem. The extent of the tumour, therefore, should be recorded on diagrams before the start of chemotherapy as accurately as possible. The evidence on the value of plotting out the extent of the tumour with submucosal injected deposits of Indian ink, is conflicting. Radiation therapy following initial chemotherapy and surgery also does not result in increased adverse effects of radiation. However, a major negative aspect of neo-adjuvant chemotherapy is that it prolongs considerably an already lengthy treatment.

Secondly, high rates of tumour response to chemotherapy can be obtained when multiple drug combinations, primarily consisting of cisplatin, bleomycin, methotrexate or 5-fluorouracil, are being used. Weaver et al (1984) have reported a combination of bolus cisplatin followed by a 5-day infusion of 5 FU to result in overall and complete response rates upto as high as respectively 94% and 55%. These authors have emphasized the importance of the number of cycles of initial chemotherapy: three cycles result in higher complete response rates than one or two cycles of the forementioned regimen. Two-thirds of the patients achieving a complete clinical response demonstrate a complete pathological response on the evidence of multiple biopsies being negative (Jacobs et al, 1987). On the contrary Taylor et al (1985) reported that none of their complete responders were free of histological disease at surgery. In general disease at the primary tumour site responds more favourably then nodal disease. Furthermore response is correlated with tumour stage. A major concern in using induction chemotherapy are the acute toxic effects, including vomiting, mucositis, myelosuppression and renal dysfunction.

Thirdly, improved survival has been demonstrated for patients achieving a complete response to chemotherapy prior to local therapy, compared to patients with a partial response or no response to chemotherapy (Price et al, 1983; Weaver et al, 1984). It has been cautioned, however, that this difference may not result from chemotherapy response, but rather from the selection of a favourable subgroup by the initial chemotherapy (Taylor et al, 1985). In this regard, it is an important observation that patient's response to chemotherapy appears to predict further response to radiotherapy (Ensley et al, 1984).

Randomized controlled studies.

In Table 1 the data on all randomized controlled studies carried out since 1979 using single agent neo-adjuvant chemotherapy are summarized. Only in the study of Arcangeli et al (1983), in which methotrexate was administered by the intra-arterial route, an improved survival was observed in the chemotherapy arm as compared to the control arm. Looking into more detail into this study, a difference in survival was present to a statistically significant degree in oral cavity cancer only. Further analysis of the oral cavity cases shows that the five year survival difference has only significance for stage II patients.

Table 1. Randomized trials with induction chemotherapy (1979-1987)
Single agent chemotherapy trials

Investigator	Year	No.	Agent	Result
Tepmongkol	1979	88	MTX	Negative
Fazekas et al	1980	638	MTX	Negative
Arcangeli et al	1983	142	MTX*	Positive
Taylor et al	1985	95	MTX	Negative
Rentschler et al	1987	60	MTX	Negative

* Intra-arterial administration
MTX= Methotrexate

In Table 2 the data on all randomized controlled studies carried out since 1983 using multiple drug neo-adjuvant chemotherapy are summarized. The overall and complete response rates generally were much higher than in the single agent studies. In spite of this only one out of the eight studies showed a positive result in favour of the chemotherapy arm and again this was the only study in which the drug was given intra-arterially. Importantly three of these studies reported that survival in the experimental arm actually was worse than in the control arm (Kun et al, 1986; Stell et al, 1983; Toohill et al, 1987).

Table 2. Randomized trials with induction chemotherapy (1983-1987)
Combination chemotherapy trials

Investigator	Year	No.	Agent	Result
Stell et al	1983	86	7 drug regimen@	Negative
Richard et al	1984	225	VCR/BLM*	Positive
Schuller et al	1984	101	CBM/VCR	Negative
Stolwijk et al	1985	68	B-CMF/VLB	Negative
Kun et al	1986	83	B-CMF	Negative
Martin et al	1986	60	CBM/F	Negative
Toohill et al	1987	60	CF x2	Negative
H&N Contracts Progr.	1987	443	CB x1	Negative

*=Intra-arterial administration, @=according to Price & Hill, 1977.
VCR=Vincristine, B=Bleomycin (BLM), C=Cyclophosphamide, M=Methotrexate, F=5-Fluorouracil, VLB=Vinblastine.

Some critical comments can be made in regards to the design and the execution of the studies listed in Table 2. In the largest study, the U.S. Head and Neck Contracts Program, a chemotherapy regimen was used that does not meet todays standards of effective chemotherapy, which is reflected in the low overall and complete response rates in this study. In some of the other studies adequate regimens have been used, but the number of patients included usually has been (too) small and the period of observation after treatment (too) short. A major criticism is that all of these studies have included patients with squamous cell carcinoma of various sites within the head and neck, in spite of the fact that the heterogeneity of head and neck cancer at different sites is generally recognized.

ONGOING STUDIES

In this section only two studies which appear to be well designed will be discussed: a European EORTC study, no. 24844 and a North-American study, carried out by the Veterans Administration Cooperative Study Group on Laryngeal Cancer, no. 268 (Hong et al, 1987). These studies have in common that they each address only one or two particular sites of head and neck cancer. EORTC 24844 is a randomized trial of 5-fluorouracil/cisplatin as induction chemotherapy followed by surgery and postoperative irradiation versus surgery and postoperative irradiation alone in the treatment of advanced squamous cell carcinoma of the lateral oropharynx and the lateral posterior oral cavity. In Table 3 the outline of EORTC 24844 is presented, as well as the scheme of induction chemotherapy.

Table 3

EORTC 24844 outline of the study

Stratification

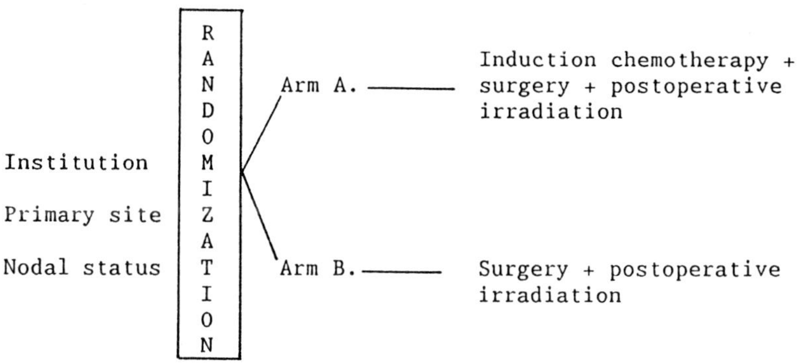

Induction chemotherapy, one cycle:

5-fluorouracil	cisplatin
1000 mg/m2	100 mg/m2
d 1-5 infusion	d 1.

Induction chemotherapy, scheme, depending on evaluation after each cycle:

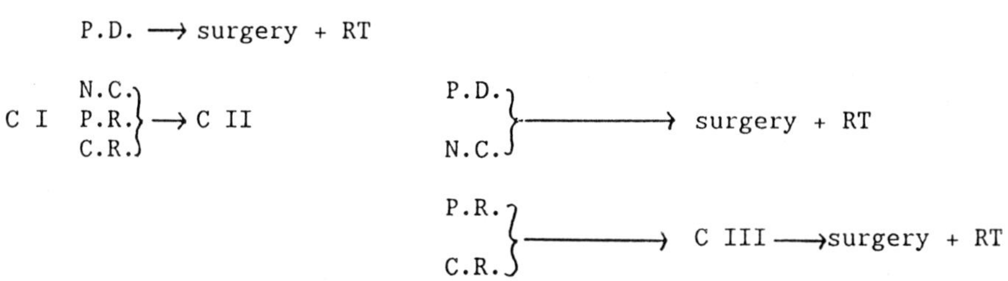

C I = Cycle I
C.R. = Complete remission
P.R. = Partial remission
C III= Cycle II
P.D. = Progressive disease
N.C. = No change
C II = Cycle I

If cycle is repeated this is done after 3 weeks.

The objectives of this study are to compare the duration of disease-free survival, the overall survival and the local regional recurrence rate at 3 years and to compare the morbidity in the two treatment arms. This study then should provide the ultimate answer to the question whether induction chemotherapy added to maximal standard treatment can contribute to survival.

The V.A. study, no. 268, is named: "A new strategy to preserve the larynx in treatment of advanced laryngeal cancer". Actually this study attempts to answer the question whether induction chemotherapy is able to select a subgroup of patients who will do well on subsequent radiotherapy and thus can be spared mutilating surgery. The study is based on the observation that patient's response to chemotherapy might predict further response to radiotherapy (Ensley et al, 1984) and on the hypothesis that it may be feasible in patients with resectable disease who achieve a complete response to induction chemotherapy at the primary site to omit surgery and treat with radiotherapy without compromise in survival (Jacobs et al, 1987). The study scheme is presented in Table 4.

Table 4.

V.A. Study Scheme.

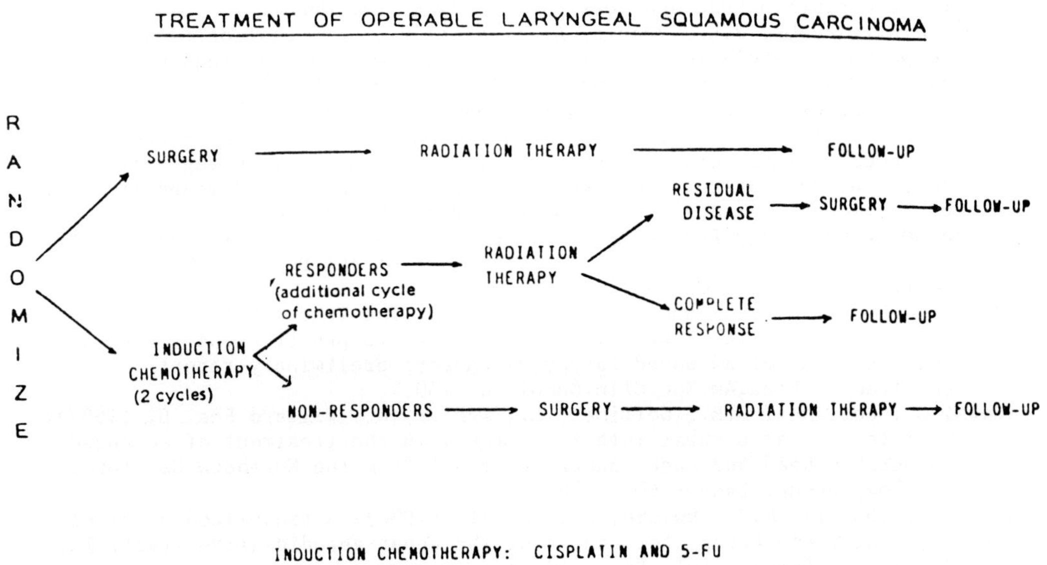

DISCUSSION

In spite of the critisms which can be raised against the design of randomized studies carried out in the past regarding the role of induction chemotherapy in head and neck cancer patients, the pertinent question comes up why initial chemotherapy has been ineffective in these studies in prolonging life, whereas it has been highly effective in shrinking tumours. Both Tannock et al (1986) and Taylor (1987) point to the short duration of response, characteristic of chemotherapy responses in recurrent head and neck cancer, which indicates limited cell kill and the presence of drug-resistant subpopulations. Thus, even in patients who achieve a complete clinical response on chemotherapy, the surviving number of cancer cells is likely to be considerable. As there is no evidence that initial chemotherapy will sterilize the peripheral margins and off-shoots of the tumour leaving viable cells only in the center of the tumour, it is not to be expected that an inoperable patient becomes operable with neo-adjuvant chemotherapy. More benefit might be expected from the combination of induction chemotherapy and radiotherapy, provided that the irradiation fields encompass the original extent of the tumour before chemotherapy and that the radiation dose is not compromised because of the previous chemotherapy. In that case the additional cell kill by chemotherapy might increase the probability of loco-regional cure. The approach to attempt to select via the response to inital chemotherapy a subgroup of patients with advanced head and neck cancer that might benefit from this concept without undergoing mutilating surgery, as actualized in V.A. study no. 268, is indeed very interesting.

REFERENCES

Arcangeli, G., Nervi, C., Righini, R. et al (1983): Combined radiation and drugs: The effect of intra-arterial chemotherapy followed by radiotherapy in head and neck cancer. Radiother.Oncol. 1, 101-107.

Ensley, J.R., Jacobs, J.R., Weaver, A. et al (1984): Correlation between response to cisplatinum-combination chemotherapy and subsequent radiotherapy in previously untreated patients with advanced squamous cell cancers of the head and neck. Cancer 54, 811-814.

Fazekas, J.T., Sommer, C., Kramer, S. et al (1980): Adjuvant intravenous squamous cell cancers of the oral cavity, oropharynx, supraglottic larynx or hypopharynx. Concluding report of an RTOG randomized trial on 638 patients. Int.J.Radiat.Oncol.Biol.Phys. 6, 533-541.

Head and Neck Contracts Program (1987): Adjuvant chemotherapy for advancedhead and neck squamous carcinomas: final report of the Head and Neck Contracts Program. Cancer 60, 301-311.

Hong, W.K., Wolf, G.T., Fisher, S. et al (1987): The Veterans Administration Cooperative Studies Program: a new strategy to preserve the larynx in the treatment of advanced laryngeal cancer: preliminary report (abstract). Proc.Am.Soc.Clin.Oncol. 6, 130.

Jacobs, C., Goffinet, D.R., Goffinet, L., Kohler, M., Willard Fee, E. (1987): Chemotherapy as a substitute for surgery in the treatment of advanced resectable head and neck cancer. A report from the Northern California Oncology Group. Cancer 60, 1178-1182.

Kun, L.E., Toohill, R.J., Holoye, P.Y. et al. (1986): A randomized study of adjuvant chemotherapy for cancer of the upper aerodigestive tract. Int. J. Radiat. Oncol. Biol. Phys. 12, 173.

Martin, M., Mazeron, J.J., Glaubiger, D. et al (1986): Neo-adjuvant polychemotherapy of head and neck cancer: preliminary results of a randomized study. In: Leventhal, B. (ed). Proc.American Society of Clin. Oncol. Grune and Stratton Inc. Orlando, pp. 141.

Price, L.A., MacRae, K., Hill, B.T. (1983): Integration of safe initial combination chemotherapy (without cisplatin) with a high response rate and local therapy for untreated stage III and IV epidermoid cancer of the head and neck: 5-year survival data. Cancer Treat.Rep. 67, 535-539.

Rentschler, R., Wilbur, D.W., Petti, G.H. et al (1987): Adjuvant methotrexate escalated to toxicity for resectable stage III and IV squamous head and neck carcinomas - a prospective randomized study. J. Clin. Incol. 5, 278-285.

Richard, J., Molinari, R., Sancho-Garnier, H. et al (1984): A randomized trial comparing surgery preceded or not by intra-arterial chemotherapy in squamous cell carcinoma of the head and neck. Proceedings of the International Conference on Head and Neck Cancer, Baltimore, pp. 113.

Schuller, D.E., Wilson, H., Hodgson, E. et al. (1984): Preoperative reduction chemotherapy for stage III-IV operative epidermoid carcinoma of the oral cavity, oropharynx, or larynx, phase III: a SWOG study. International Conference on Head and Neck Cancer, Baltimore, abstr. 185.

Stell, P.M., Dalby, J.E., Strickland, P. et al (1983): Sequential chemotherapy and radiotherapy in advanced head and neck cancer. Clin. Radiol. 34, 463-467.

Stolwijk, C., Wagener, D.J.T., van den Broek, P. (1985): Randomized neo-adjuvant chemotherapy trial for advanced head and neck cancer. Neth. J. Med. 28, 347.

Tannock, I.F., Browman, G.: Lack of evidence for a role of chemotherapy in the routine management of locally advanced head and neck cancer. J. Clin. Oncol. 4:1121-1126.

Taylor, S.G. IV, Applebaum, E., Showell, J.L., Norusis, M., Holinger, L.D., Hutchinson, J.C., Murthy, A.K., Caldareli, D.D. (1985): A randomized trial of adjuvant chemotherapy in head and neck cancer. J. Clin. Oncol. 3, 672-679.

Taylor, S.G. (1987): Induction chemotherapy for head and neck cancer. Int. J. Radiat.Oncol.Biol. Phys. 13:779-783.

Tepmongkol, P. (1979). J. med. Ass. Thailand. 62, 17.

Toohill, R.J., Anderson, T., Byhardt, R.W. et al (1987): Cisplatin and fluorouracil as neo-adjuvant therapy in head and neck cancer. A preliminary report. Arch. otolaryngol. Head and Neck Surg. 113, 758-761.

Weaver, A., Fleming, S., Ensley, J., Kish, J.A., Jacobs, J., Kinzie, J., Crissman, J., Al-Sarraf, M. (1984): Superior clinical response and survival rates with initial bolus of cisplatin and 120 hour infusion of 5-fluorouracil before definitive therapy for locally advanced head and neck cancer. Am. J. Surg. 148, 525-529.

Résumé

De nombreuses études non contrôlées ont montré que la chimiothérapie d'induction était faisable chez des malades porteurs de cancer avancé de la tête et du cou. Il a été démontré que des associations médicamenteuses contenant du platine sont très efficaces pour réduire le volume initial de la tumeur. De façon générale, les répondeurs à la chimiothérapie ont un meilleur pronostic que les répondeurs partiels ou les non répondeurs. Cependant, la plupart des études randomisées controlées faites jusqu'à présent n'ont pas démontré une amélioration de la survie la dans le bras chimiothérapie comparé au bras contrôle. Les raisons possibles de ceci sont analysées. Il se peut que la réponse à la chimiothérapie prédise une réponse à une autre thérapeutique en particulier l'irradiation sans contribuer nécessairement à un bénéfice de survie. C'est pourquoi le concept que la chirurgie mutilante peut être évitée chez des malades ayant une réponse complète à la chimiothérapie d'induction et que dans ce cas là la radiothérapie pourrait suffire est très intéressant. Les bénéfices possibles de la chimiothérapie néoadjuvante sont étudiés dans des études randomisées en cours. Actuellement, il n'y a pas de place pour la chimiothérapie d'induction à titre systématique dans le traitement primaire des patients atteints de cancer de la tête et du cou.

Neo-Adjuvant Chemotherapy. Ed. Cl. Jacquillat, M. Weil, D. Khayat. Colloque INSERM/John Libbey Eurotext Ltd. © 1988. Vol. 169, pp. 353-355.

Preliminary results of a randomized study of neo-adjuvant chemotherapy of VDS-CDDP and BLM-5FU-CDDP in the therapy of 72 patients with squamous carcinomas of the head and neck

M. Housset, P. Gomez, A. Botton, M. Ciupa, J. Fabi and F. Baillet

Centre de Traitement des Tumeurs, Hôpital Necker, 149 rue de Sèvres, 75015 Paris, France

SUMMARY

From January 1985 to December 1986, a randomized study of two initial (neoadjuvant) chemotherapy protocols in patients with ENT squamous carcinomas was performed. Group A (n = 42) received Bleomycin, Fluorouracil, Cisplatinum (BLM-5FU-CDDP); and Group B (n = 30) Vindesine and Cisplatinum (VDS-CDDP). The two populations were comparable in tumor location and TNM classification, and an average of two courses was given. Response rates (complete remissions and partial remissions $\geq$50%) were 57% for Group A and 20% for Group B ($p < 0,01$). After loco-regional therapy, complete remissions were 80% for Group A and 57% for Group B ($p < 0,05$). Local relapses in the two groups were similar (A : 44%, B : 41%). Two year survival was 42% in Group A and 26% in Group B. The combination of BLM-5FU-CDDP appears superior to that of VDS-CDDP with improved local control and survival at two years.

KEYWORDS

ENT Squamous Carcinoma, Neoadjuvant, Chemotherapy, Response, Survival.

INTRODUCTION

The place of chemotherapy in the therapy of upper aerodigestive carcinomas remains controversial, with several randomized trials having not shown an increase in survival (2) (4) (6). Nevertheless, the rates of local response induced by neoadjuvant chemotherapy, especially with Cisplatinum (CDDP) are such that this modality is often included in the therapy of ENT carcinomas.
We have performed a randomized study of two chemotherapy protocols. The first, a combination of Vindesine (VDS) and CDDP which was used in our center until 1983 for aerodigestive squamous carcinomas, was compared with the combination of Bleomycin (BLM), Fluorouracil (5FU) and CDDP, which was the most effective reported in the literature.

MATERIALS AND METHODS

From January 1985 to December 1986, patients with ENT squamous carcinomas were randomized into a prospective neoadjuvant chemotherapy protocol : Group A, 42 patients, (BLM 10mg/m2/d, 5FU 750mg/m2/d, from days 1 through 4 in a semi-continous infusion and CDDP 80mg/m2 on day 1) and Group B, 30 patients, (VDS 2,5mg/m2 on days 1, 8, 15 and CDDP 80mg/m2 on day 1). Two cycles at 25 days interval was to be administered prior to loco-regional therapy, decided upon prior to randomization. In case of progression after the first course, the chemotherapy was stopped. In case of response $\geq$50% in the largest tumor diameter, a third course was given.

The two populations were comparable in age, Karnofsky score, tumor localizations and sizes (Table 1).

RESULTS

Follow-up was from 12 to 36 months. There were 24/42 (57%) complete (CR) and partial remissions (PR) in Group A, and 6/30 (20%) CR and PR in Group B ($p < 0,01$). There were no tumor progression during chemotherapy in Group A and 10% in Group B (Table 2).

Loco-regional therapy was either radiotherapy or surgery plus radiotherapy. There was no statistical difference between these two groups. After this loco-regional therapy, 32/40 (80%) of patients in Group A and 17/30 (57%) of patients in Group B achieved clinical CR ($p < 0,05$). For patients in CR, the loco-regional relapse rate in the two groups was identical (44% vs 41%). Deaths in Group A was 15/42 (36%), and 18/30 (60%) in Group B ($p < 0,05$). The 2 year actuarial survival rate was 42% (A) vs 26% (B) ($p = 0,08$), this difference was due to the deaths with loco-regional failures.

DISCUSSION

The combination BLM-5FU-CDDP was significantly superior to that of VDS-CDDP when used as neoadjuvant therapy for carcinomas of the upper aerodigestive tract, with a higher rate of response and improved loco-regional control. We can supposed that the response rate for a loco-regional therapy alone (radiation or surgery plus radiation)would be probably worse or equal than for the Group B. The increased survival rate observed at two years with Group A was due to better loco-regional control.

It should be stated however, that the follow-up period is short, and although the two population were statistically comparable, there was a higher percentage of patients with adenopathy in Group B.

Several trials have shown that the most effective neoadjuvant chemotherapy has been a combination of 5FU and CDDP (1) (2) (3) (5) (7) with response rates of 70-86%. Our study confirms these results, and since the end of 1986 we have stopped this trial.

We have not analysed in this study whether response to chemotherapy could permit modification of loco-regional therapy. Our current objective is to see if less radical loco-regional therapy is possible in the good responders to neoadjuvant chemotherapy.

Table 1 : PATIENTS CHARACTERISTICS

	Group A	Group B
Mean Age (years)	56	54
Mean Karnofsky score	87	85
Mean Tumor Diameter	4,8 cm	5,3 cm
No with adenopathie	20 (48%)	18 (60%)
T location :		
oral cavity	10	10
oropharynx,		
base of tongue	14	13
pharyngo-larynx	12	4
multiple	6	3

Table 2 : RESPONSE TO CHEMOTHERAPY

	Group A (n = 42)	Group B (n = 30)
CR	10 (24%)	2 (6,5%)
PR ⩾ 50%	14 (33,3%)	4 (13%)
PR < 50%	14 (33,3%)	15 (50%)
NR	4 (9,5%)	6 (20%)
Progression of tumor	0	3 (10%)

REFERENCES

1 - Demard F., Schneider M., Chauvel P., Ramaioli A., Vallicioni J., Santini J. : Chimiothérapie d'induction Platine-5 Fluoro-uracile. Résultats actuels en carcinologie cervico-faciale. Ann. Oto-Laryng, Paris, 1987, 104, 399-406.

2 - Haas C., Anderson T., Byhardt R., Cox J., Duncavage J., Grossman T., Haas J., Libnoch J., Malin T., Ritch P., Toohill R. : Randomized neo-adjuvant study of 5-Fluorouracil and cis-platinum for patients with advanced resectable head and neck cancer. Pro. Am. Assoc. Cancer Res. 27 : 185,1986.

3 - Jacobs J.R., Kish J., Ensley J.F., Ahmad R., Weaver A., Crissman J., Al Sarraf M. : Combined modality therapy utilizing a cisplatin combination for effective chemotherapy in patients with previously untreated head and neck cancer. Am. J. Surg., 1986, 152, 451-5.

4 - Martin M., Mazeron J.J., Glaubiger D., Brun B., Langlois A., Feuillade F., Lelièvre G., Stranski W., Vergnes L., Denarnaud J., Peynegre R. Pierquin B. : Neo-adjuvant polychemotherapy of head and neck cancer : Preliminary results of a randomized study. Proc. Am. Soc. Clin. Oncol. 5 : 141, 1986.

5 - Taylor S.G., IV : Head and neck cancer. In Cancer Chemotherapy Annual 1-7, H.M. Pinedo and B.A. Chabner, (Eds). Amsterdam, Elsevier Science Pub. 1979, 1980, 1981, 1982, 1983, 1984, 1985.

6 - Taylor S.G. IV, Applebaum E., Showel J., Norusis M., Holinger L.D., Hutchinson J.C. Jr., Murthy A.K., Caldarelli D. : A randomized trial of adjuvant chemotherapy in head and neck cancer. J. Clin. Oncol. 3 : 672-9, 1985.

7 - Weaver A., Flemming S., Kish J. : Cis-platinum and 5-fluorouracil as induction therapy for advanced head and neck cancer. Am. J. Surg. 144 : 445-8, 1982.

Lung cancers

Cancers du poumon

Neo-Adjuvant Chemotherapy. Ed. Cl. Jacquillat, M. Weil, D. Khayat. Colloque INSERM/John Libbey Eurotext Ltd. © 1988. Vol. 169, pp. 359-364.

Neo-adjuvant chemotherapy of lung cancer : current North American experience

Daniel C. Ihde

NCI-Navy Medical Oncology Branch, National Cancer Institute and Naval Hospital, and Uniformed Services University of the Health Sciences, Bethesda, MD 20814, USA

ABSTRACT

Justification for neoadjuvant chemotherapy differs in small cell (SCLC) and non-small cell (NSCLC) lung cancer, since chemotherapy is obligatory treatment in the former while in the latter surgical resection and chest irradiation are the only potentially curative therapies. With the realization that rare SCLC patients are cured by surgery alone and that relapses at the primary site occur despite radiotherapy, chemotherapy followed by surgery is being actively investigated. Resected patients clearly live longer than other limited stage cases. Prospective studies indicate 18%-37% of limited patients can be surgically resected after chemotherapy response. Markedly better survival results are not obtained with tumor resection after chemotherapy, however, compared to patients of similar tumor extent given chemotherapy or chemoradiotherapy. A current randomized trial should help to clarify this issue. In NSCLC, there are preliminary data on pre-operative chemotherapy or chemoradiotherapy in marginally resectable or unresectable patients, and on chemotherapy prior to definitive irradiation in clearly unresectable cases. A small number of pilot studies suggest possible benefit. Because of many other negative studies and heterogeneity in staging, case selection, and therapy, the role of neoadjuvant chemotherapy in NSCLC is undefined.

KEY WORDS

Small cell lung cancer, non-small cell lung cancer, neoadjuvant chemotherapy, surgical resection, chest irradiation

INTRODUCTION

Neoadjuvant chemotherapy is defined as chemotherapy given prior to definitive locoregional treatment to reduce risk of later distant or local failure or to enable surgical resection to be performed. This paper will review current experience with neoadjuvant chemotherapy of lung cancer, concentrating on North American results.

The justification for neoadjuvant chemotherapy in lung cancer varies depending on the cell type. In small cell lung cancer (SCLC), initial chemotherapy is already standard practice due to its effectiveness and to the almost universal presence of overt or occult distant metastases. In non-small cell lung cancer (NSCLC), the frequency of distant relapse is high after surgery or chest irradiation. Thus, the model of neoadjuvant chemotherapy applies, but the efficacy of available agents is modest. The role of neoadjuvant chemotherapy in currently relevant therapeutic strategies for locoregionally confined lung cancer thus depends upon the cell type. In SCLC, for which chemotherapy with or without chest irradiation is the definitive treatment, surgical resection should be considered the adjunctive modality. Resection can be performed either following or prior to chemotherapy. Surgery and, to a lesser extent, chest radiotherapy, remain the definitive treatments for NSCLC, and effective neoadjuvant chemotherapy would be a valuable adjunctive therapy.

"NEOADJUVANT" CHEMOTHERAPY OF SMALL CELL LUNG CANCER

Several factors have recently led to renewed interest in surgical resection of SCLC. It is now clear that a small number of patients can be cured with surgery alone (Shields, 1982). A superior outcome occurs in patients with limited stage SCLC undergoing surgical resection prior to chemotherapy or chemoradiotherapy (Friess, 1985; Osterlind, 1986; Shepherd, 1983). There is still a high frequency of relapse in the primary site after chemotherapy or chemoradiotherapy. In contrast, after surgery relapse in the primary site is infrequent (Johnson, 1987; Prager, 1984; Shepherd, 1983). Retrospective studies, however, do not suggest major survival impact in resected patients compared to patients with similar disease extent not receiving surgery (Osterlind, 1986; Shepherd, 1984). Several considerations suggest that surgery in limited SCLC might be more effective if performed after initial "neoadjuvant" chemotherapy rather than at diagnosis. Immediate chemotherapy would be administered to systemic disease. Only chemoresponsive patients, those most likely to benefit, would receive surgery. Comprehensive initial preoperative staging procedures could be avoided since chemotherapy would be the first treatment. Finally, after response to chemotherapy, a larger fraction of patients might be surgical candidates.

Little data exist on how often surgical resection of SCLC is possible at diagnosis. Prospective studies by their nature cannot include cases without a preoperative pathologic diagnosis who are discovered only at thoracotomy to have resectable SCLC. A large retrospective analysis of 435 limited stage patients by Osterlind (1986) indicated that 35% could be considered operable at diagnosis. Of 96 patients actually subjected to thoracotomy, only 38% were completely resected. Thus, the estimated resectability rate was 13%. A higher frequency of patients might be suitable for surgical resection after chemotherapy. In prospective studies by Prager (1984), Johnson (1987), and Williams (1987), 20%, 18%, and 37% of limited stage patients beginning chemotherapy were eventually resected.

Findings from studies of surgical resection after initial chemotherapy for limited stage SCLC may be summarized as follows. There is no excessive operative morbidity or mortality. No cancer is present in the resected specimen in 5%-20% of cases, and not surprisingly such patients have better survival (Williams, 1987). Some patients have pathologic evidence of NSCLC in the resected tumor (Baker, 1987; Valdivieso, 1984), and it is conceivable that surgery represents the best treatment for these NSCLC elements. Data from the literature (Williams, 1987) indicate that resected patients have a good prognosis compared to other limited stage SCLC patients, with over 27% disease-free survival. Pathologic mediastinal staging has not usually been performed prior to chemotherapy, although one early report (Meyer, 1984) indicated patients with proven initial mediastinal node involvement derived little benefit from post-chemotherapy resection. Whether surgical resection after chemotherapy can improve survival will be the ultimate measure of its value. Thus far, markedly better survival for all patients beginning chemotherapy with the intent of performing later resection whenever possible has not been apparent (Williams, 1987).

A prospective randomized trial designed to assess the value of surgical resection of localized SCLC after initial chemotherapy is currently being conducted by the Lung Cancer Study Group (Ruckdeschel, J.D.: Personal communication). Patients are randomized to chemoradiotherapy alone versus chemotherapy followed by attempted surgery and postoperative irradiation. Over 150 patients have been entered, and a survival difference between the two plans of therapy is suggested in an early analysis.

The following preliminary conclusions regarding "neoadjuvant" chemotherapy followed by surgery for limited stage SCLC appear justified. Surgical resection is possible in 18% to 37% of cases, possibly a higher fraction than at diagnosis. Marked variation exists in patient selection, criteria for operability and resectability, and duration of preoperative chemotherapy. Resected patients have superior survival compared to other limited stage cases, especially those in whom no residual SCLC is found in the pathologic specimen. Current results are not conclusive regarding survival advantage or definition of subsets of patients most likely to benefit. Results of the large randomized Lung Cancer Study Group trial should clarify some of these points.

NEOADJUVANT CHEMOTHERAPY OF NON-SMALL CELL LUNG CANCER

Because of early discouraging results of chemotherapy of NSCLC both in metastatic disease and as an adjuvant to surgical resection or irradiation, trials of neoadjuvant chemotherapy employing current combination regimens have only recently been initiated. Pilot studies have evaluated administration of chemotherapy prior to both attempted surgical resection and definitive chest irradiation. The revised TNM staging system for lung cancer defines advanced but potentially resectable Stage IIIA cancer as primary tumor extending to the chest wall, diaphragm, mediastinal pleura, pericardium, or within 2 cm of the carina, or as ipsilateral or subcarinal mediastinal node involvement. Patients with more extensive locoregional T or N factors have clearly unresectable Stage IIIB tumors. Despite these new staging definitions, there is still considerable variability among thoracic surgeons in the selection of potentially resectable patients.

Analysis of four recent trials of neoadjuvant combination chemotherapy before attempted thoracotomy in marginally resectable and advanced locoregional NSCLC illustrates this variability (Skarin, 1982; Bitran, 1986; Taylor, 1987; Eagan, 1987). Biopsy proof of either N2 or T3 disease was obtained in 22% to 100% of patients. Three trials incorporated concurrent or sequential radiotherapy into the preoperative regimen. Response rates to chemotherapy or chemoradiotherapy were substantial, ranging from 43% to 64%. Complete resections were carried out in 14% to 85% of patients, with median survival figures of 9 to 30 months roughly correlating with resectability rates. Survival in most cases was not greatly different from anticipated results with surgery or radiation alone.

Additional findings have emerged from these pilot studies. Surgical procedures have been found technically difficult after employment of preoperative chemotherapy with irradiation (Eagan, 1987; Taylor, 1987). Correlation between clinical asssessment of response and pathologic response has sometimes been poor (Taylor, 1987). Up to 23% of resected specimens have been pathologically free of tumor, but in the largest series pathologic status predicted freedom from local recurrence but not from distant metastases (Taylor, 1987).

Patient selection in one provocative neoadjuvant study employing chemotherapy alone relies solely on clinical staging without computed tomography or biopsy of the mediastinum (Gralla, R.J.: these Proceedings). Ipsilateral mediastinal nodes detected by chest X-ray or bronchoscopically have been associated with a 14% resection rate and 6% 3-year survival at Memorial Hospital (New York). Two or three courses of mitomycin, vinblastine or vindesine, and cisplatin in such patients have produced a 73% response rate (17% complete responses) in 41 patients. A 51% complete resection rate was possible, with 8/21 specimens being pathologically negative. Three-year survival is 34%, much better than in historical controls, in this ongoing study.

Most pilot studies of neoadjuvant chemotherapy prior to irradiation in inoperable Stage III NSCLC patients have not yielded promising results. Two representative trials (Fram, 1985; Cox, 1986) with response rates to chemotherapy of 47% and 20% produced median survivals of 9 and 12 months, very similar to many studies with irradiation alone. A recent positive study of Cancer and Leukemia Group B (Green, M.: Personal communication) was restricted to fully ambulatory patients without weight loss. Patients were randomized to receive or not receive 5 weeks of vinblastine and cisplatin before radiotherapy. Over 130 evaluable patients were entered with current median follow-up time of 19 months, and a significant survival advantage for the chemotherapy arm, with an almost doubled median survival, has been observed.

Analysis of available data on neoadjuvant chemotherapy in NSCLC suggests the following preliminary conclusions. Chemotherapy response rates in some studies appear higher than in metastatic NSCLC. The contribution of irradiation to the results of preoperative studies is uncertain, but surgery is sometimes made technically more difficult. Some studies demonstrate pathologic clearance of tumor at operation and suggest an increased resection rate compared to historical experience. Results from most trials are not suggestive of improved survival. A single promising randomized study of pre-irradiation chemotherapy will soon be fully presented. Heterogeneous patient selection, staging procedures, and therapeutic techniques cloud interpretation of most results. Randomized trials in pathologically staged patients are sorely needed. Clearly, the role of neoadjuvant chemotherapy in NSCLC is presently undefined.

REFERENCES

Baker, R.R., Ettinger, D.S., Ruckdeschel, J.D., et al (1987): The role of surgery in the management of selected patients with small cell lung cancer. J. Clin. Oncol. 3, 697-702.

Bitran, J.D., Golomb, H.M., Hoffman, P.C., et al (1986): Protochemotherapy in non-small cell lung carcinoma: An attempt to increase surgical resectability and survival. Cancer 57, 44-53.

Cox, J.D., Samson, M.K., Herskovic, A.M., et al (1986): Cisplatin and etoposide before definitive radiation therapy for inoperable squamous carcinoma, adenocarcinoma, and large cell carcinoma of the lung. Cancer Treat. Rep. 70, 1219-1220.

Eagan, R.T., Ruud, C., Lee, R.E., et al (1987): Pilot study of induction therapy with cyclophosphamide, doxorubicin, and cisplatin and chest irradiation prior to thoracotomy in initially inoperable Stage III M_0 non-small cell lung cancer. Cancer Treat. Rep. 71, 895-900.

Fram, R., Skarin, A., Balikian, J., et al (1985): Combination chemotherapy followed by radiation therapy in patients with regional Stage III unresectable non-small cell lung cancer. Cancer Treat. Rep. 69, 587-590.

Friess, G.G., McCracken, J.D., Troxell, M.L., et al (1985): Effect of initial resection of small cell carcinoma of the lung. J. Clin. Oncol. 3, 964-968.

Johnson, D.H., Einhorn, L.H., Mandelbaum, I., et al (1987): Postchemotherapy resection of residual tumor in limited stage small cell lung cancer. Chest 92, 241-246.

Meyer, J.A., Gullo, J.J., Ikins, P.M., et al (1984): Adverse prognostic effect of N2 disease in treated small cell carcinoma of the lung. J. Thorac. Cardiovasc. Surg. 88, 495-501.

Osterlind, K., Hansen, M., Hansen, H.H., et al (1986): Influence of surgical resection prior to chemotherapy on the long-term results in small cell lung cancer: A study of 150 operable patients. Eur. J. Cancer Clin. Oncol. 22, 589-593.

Prager, R.L., Foster, J.M., Hainsworth, J.D., et al (1984): The feasibility of adjuvant surgery in limited stage small cell carcinoma: A prospective evaluation. Ann. Thorac. Surg. 38, 622-626.

Shepherd, F.A., Ginsburg, R., Evans, W.K., et al (1983): Reduction in local recurrence and improved survival in surgically treated patients with small cell lung cancer. J. Thorac. Cardiovasc. Surg. 86, 498-506.

Shepherd, F.A., Ginsburg, R., Evans, W.K., et al (1984): "Very limited" small cell lung cancer: Results of non-surgical treatment. Proc. Am. Soc. Clin. Oncol. 3, 223.

Shields, T.W., Higgins, G.A., Matthews, M.J., et al (1982): Surgical resection in the management of small cell carcinoma of the lung. J. Thorac. Cardiovasc. Surg. 84, 481-488.

Skarin, A., Veeder, M., Malcolm, A., et al (1982): Chemotherapy prior to radiotherapy and surgery in marginally resectable non-small cell lung cancer. Proc. Am. Soc. Clin. Oncol. 1, 143.

Taylor, S.G., Trybula, M., Bonomi, P.D., et al (1987): Simultaneous cisplatin fluorouracil infusion and radiation followed by surgical resection in regionally localized Stage III non-small cell lung cancer. Ann. Thorac. Surg. 43, 87-91.

Valdivieso, M., McMurtrey, M.J., Farha, P., et al (1984): Prospective evaluation of adjuvant surgical resection in small cell lung cancer. Proc. Am. Soc. Clin. Oncol. 3, 220.

Williams, C.J., McMillan, I., Lea, R., et al (1987): Surgery after initial chemotherapy for localized small cell carcinoma of the lung. J. Clin. Oncol. 5, 1579-1588.

Résumé

La justification conceptuelle de la chimiothérapie néoadjuvante diffère considérablement pour les cancers à petites cellules et pour les cancers non à petites cellules, puisque la chimiothérapie est l'essentiel du traitement dans le premier cas alors que dans le second, l'exérèse chirurgicale et moins souvent l'irradiation thoracique sont les seules interventions potentiellement curables. Eu égard au fait que de rares malades avec des cancers à petites cellules peuvent être guéris par la chirurgie et que les rechutes surviennent au niveau de la tumeur primitive en dépit de la radiothérapie, des programmes de traitement de chimiothérapie suivie par de la chirurgie sont actuellement étudiés. Les données rétrospectives suggèrent que 13 % des malades atteints de stade localisé de cancer à petites cellules du poumon au moment du diagnostic sont des tumeurs qui peuvent être complètement réséquées selon les critères chirurgicaux standarts. Les malades pour lesquels cette résection a pu être faite, survivent plus que les autres stades localisés. Les études prospectives révèlent que entre 18 et 37 % des malades ayant des formes localisées peuvent être traités chirurgicalement après une réponse à la chimiothérapie. La survie est la même que la résection tumorale puisse avoir lieu d'emblée ou après la chimiothérapie, que la chimiothérapie soit donnée avec ou sans radiothérapie. Une étude randomisée actuellement en cours devrait indiquer de façon plus claire le bénéfice de la chirurgie dans les cancers à petites cellules.

Dans les cancers non à petites cellules, les données préliminaires concernent la chimiothérapie néoadjuvante pré-opératoire des stades IIIa non opérables ou d'opérabilité limite, ou non opérable avant l'irradiation. Une étude pilote suggère que la chimiothérapie augmente le taux d'opérabilité des malades avec des formes N2 sur les radiographies du thorax. Une étude randomisée démontre l'amélioration de la survie avec la chimiothérapie donnée avant l'irradiation. Eu égard à beaucoup d'autres études négatives et à une hétérogénéité dans les stades, la sélection des cas et les traitements, le rôle de la chimiothérapie néoadjuvante dans les cancers du poumon non à petites cellules reste à définir.

Neo-Adjuvant Chemotherapy. Ed. Cl. Jacquillat, M. Weil, D. Khayat. Colloque INSERM/John Libbey Eurotext Ltd. © 1988. Vol. 169, pp. 365-370.

A randomized phase II trial of neo-adjuvant chemotherapy in resectable bronchogenic non small cell carcinoma. Short term results

B. Dautzenberg, Cl. Chastang, B. Lebeau, Ph. Allard, D. Coëtmeur, J. Bénichou, M.J. Postal and the GETCB*

** Groupe d'étude et de traitement des cancers bronchiques*
Service de pneumologie, GH Pitié-Salpêtrière, 75651 Paris Cedex 13, France

Summary

In 1985, we started a randomized phase II study to assess the PCV polychemotherapy (cisplatin 100mg/m^2, eldesine 3mg/m^2, cyclophosphamide 600 mg/m^2) in patients with resectable bronchogenic non small cell carcinoma. Patients were randomized to receive either two courses of PCV chemotherapy, surgery and two other courses of PCV chemotherapy or immediate surgery. A staging procedure using CT-scan was performed before randomization for all patients and in addition an identical staging procedure was performed before surgery in the chemotherapy group. The design allowed to compare surgical morbidity and complications, disease free interval and overall survival being secondary criteria.

26 patients (24 males) were randomized, 13 in each group. 11 patients received the two preoperative courses of chemotherapy. A response was observed in five patients (45%) and a progression in four patients (36%). For two patients in the chemotherapy group, curative surgery was cancelled because of progression.

Preoperative staging was in agreement with surgical findings in 75 % of patients for the N classification and in 83 % for the T one. The mean of tumor volume was estimated at 50 ± 52 cm^3 (preoperative staging), 42 ± 40 cm^3 (surgeon) and 54 ±44 cm^3 (pathologist).

The two groups were not different in terms of postoperative care (duration of chest tubing 3.2 versus 3.7 days, temperature at J3 37.4°C in both groups, no death) except for the time spent in surgery units (17 ± 3:days in the chemotherapy group versus 23 ± 8 days in the control group).

Although no death could be related to chemotherapy, it was decided to stop entering new patients in this trial because of the rate of tumor progression in the chemotherapy group.

KEY WORDS
Bronchogenic carcinoma
Néoadjuvant chemotherapy

MOTS CLEFS
Cancer bronchique
Chimiothérapie néoadjuvante

Participating centers:

G.H. Pitié-Salpêtrière	B. Dautzenberg, M-J. Postal, M-S. Richard, Ch. Sors.
Hôtel Dieu	B. Lebeau, J-M. Bréchot
Hôpital Percy	Ph. Allard, D. L'Her
Hôpital de St Brieuc	D. Coëtmeur
Stastistical center (Hôp. St Louis)	Cl. Chastang, J. Bénichou

Neoadjuvant chemotherapy trials in bronchogenic non small cell lung cancer have been sustained on several arguments : (i) after two or three courses of the polychemotherapy regimen, a 40 percent response rate was observed (Gralla et al., 1981), (ii) among responders, chemotherapy could theoretically reduce the volume of the tumor, make the surgical act easier and cure occult micrometastases, (iii) for a quarter of totally resected patients, metastases occur during the first 18 months (Chastang et al., 1986) and since local treatment cannot have an effect on metastases occurence, a general treatment is needed, (iv) preoperative chemotherapy allows to asses the response rate in contrast with postoperative chemotherapy.

The aim of this trial was to study the feasibility of neoadjuvant chemotherapy by studying : (i) the response rate to PCV chemotherapy, (ii) the quality of staging procedures, (iii) the problems in the surgical procedure induced by preoperative chemotherapy, (iv) the overall survival.

MATERIAL AND METHODS

Patients of both sex with pathologically proven non small cell primitive bronchogenic carcinoma needing a curative surgery and without contra indication to chemotherapy were included.
Patients were randomized to receive either immediate surgery or two courses of chemotherapy, surgery and then two other courses of chemotherapy. The PCV chemotherapy consisted of cisplatin 100mg/m^2, cyclophosphamide 600 mg/m^2, eldesine 3mg/m^2 delivered in one day every four weeks. Two identical courses of postoperative PCV chemotherapy were planned for all patients in the chemotherapy group. The staging procedure was performed before randomization in both groups and before surgery in the chemotherapy group. This staging procedure consisted of chest X ray, fiberoptic bronchoscopy, thoracic CT-scan, liver ultrasonography, biologic tests, respiratory function tests and optionally cases abdominal CT scan and bone scan. The tumoral mass was assessed in two or three dimensions on the CT-scan picture. The nodes were considered positive if the smallest diameter was greater or equal to 15 mm.
The judgment critera were response and tolerance of preoperative chemotherapy, operative morbidity and complications, disease free interval and overall survival. The follow-up of patients was quaterly planned.
The sample size was 66 patients and an interim analysis was planned after the inclusion of 33 patients.

RESULTS

Patients characteristics

26 patients were randomized, 13 in each group (table I), 24 were males. The mean age was 55.5 ± 15.5 years (mean ± SD). The Karnofsky index was 89 ± 10 %.

The mean tumoral mass was 55 ± 42 cm^3. According to the TNM classification, 21 out of 26 patients were staged T2 (80 %) and 13 out of 26 patients were staged N1 (50%) . There was no statistical difference between the two groups.

Table I : Patients characteristics at randomization time.

	surgery only (13)	neoadjuvant chemotherapy (13)
male	12	12
age (yrs)	58 ± 12	53 ± 19
weight (kg)	62 ± 11	69 ± 12
Karnofsky index (%)	88 ± 12	91 ± 7
squamous cells	11	11
tumor volume (cm^3)	55 ± 5	55 ± 80
T1	1	0
T2	10	11
T3	2	2
N0	5	3
N1	7	6
N2	1	4

The response to PCV chemotherapy

Only 11 out of 13 patients in the chemotherapy group received the two preoperative courses of PCV chemotherapy, two patients refused the chemotherapy. Between the randomization staging and the preoperative staging, the mean tumoral volume decreased by 14 ± 39.

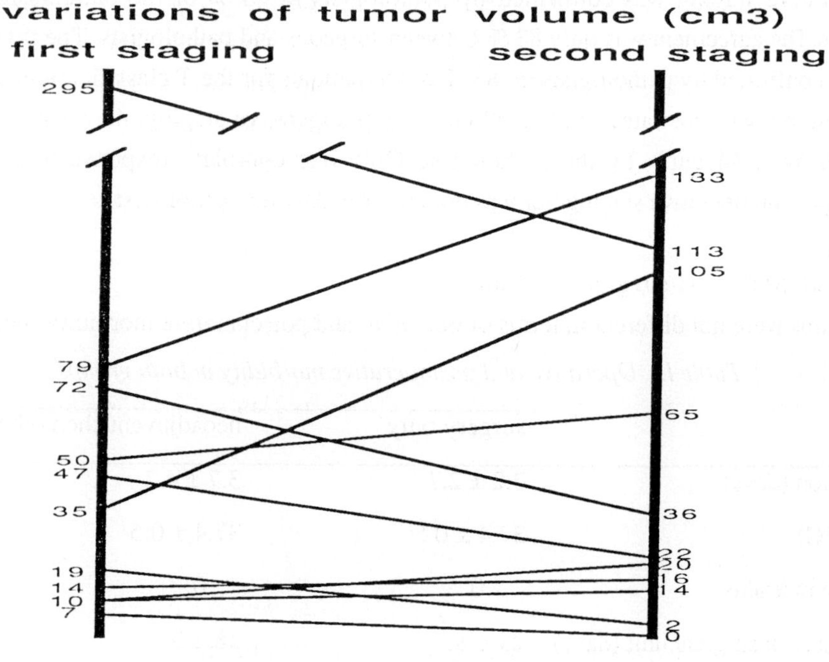

Figure 1: Individual variation of tumoral volume after PCV chemotherapy (volume in cm^3)

A response weither complete or partial was observed in five patients (45%) and a progression greater than 25% in four patients (36%). For two patients in chemotherapy group, surgery was cancelled because of progression. In the two other patients with progression, complete resection was completed. Figure 2 displays an example of progression mode during chemotherapy. Patient entry was stopped because of the occurence of such tumor progression.

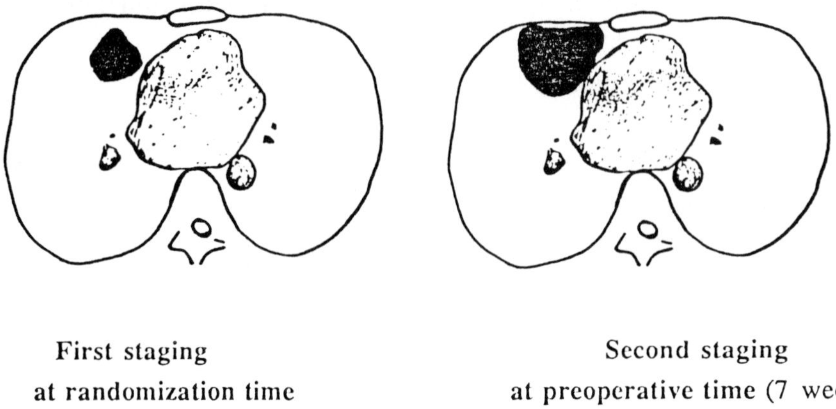

Figure 2 : Example of progression under chemotherapy between the two staging procedures. In spite of disease progression, a complete resection was performed.

The assesment of staging procedures

The preoperative staging was confirmed by pathologists in 75 % of the patients for the N classification.The agreement was only 83 % between surgeons and pathologists. The preoperative staging was confirmed by pathologists in 83 % of the patients for the T classification. The mean of tumor volume was estimated at 50 ± 52 cm3 by preoperative staging, 42 ± 40 cm3 by the surgeon and 54 ± 44 cm3 by the pathologist. Only one complete response was observed according to the preoperative staging but was not confirmed by the pathologist.

The surgical and post-surgical periods

The two groups were not different in terms of operative and postoperative morbidity (table II).

Table II : Operative and postoperative morbidity in both groups.

	surgery only	neoadjuvant chemotherapy
tubing duration (days)	3.2 ± 2.7	3.7 ± 4.3
fever at J3 (°C)	37.4 ± 0.5	37.4 ± 0.5
perioperative mortality	0	0
duration of stay in surgical unit (days)	23 ± 8.	18 ± 3

DISCUSSION

There was a 75 % agreement for the N staging and a 83 % agreement for the T staging between preoperative and surgical findings. For tumor size, the agreement between CT-Scan and pathological staging was good enough to evaluate tumor response to chemotherapy. The neoadjuvant chemotherapy enables, contrary to postoperative chemotherapy, to assess response. Thoracic CT-scan was the main procedure in this staging.

The mean response to PCV chemotherapy using cyclophosphamid in addition to the classical association platine and eldesine was estimated at 45%. This response rate was close to the response rate of previous trials in non resectable bronchogenic carcinoma (Gralla et al., 1981), but the progression rate was surprisingly high (35%). Four cases of progression were observed in the chemotherapy group. Among them, surgery had to be cancelled for two patients. This led us to stop patient entry in this trial.

The neoadjuvant chemotherapy does not make surgery more difficult nor does it influence post surgical recovery. Since our study was only performed on patients with primarly resectable tumor, it was not possible to confirm the bad surgical results often observed after chemotherapy for primarly resectable tumors (Splinter et al., 1986 ; Gralla et al., 1987 ; Stampleman et al., 1987 ; Morere et al., 1985) but in our study chemotherapy was performed only on primarily resectable carcinoma.

More research is needed in order to find a chemotherapy regimen with at least a 60 % response rate and at most a 10 % progression rate among resectable patients. Only then will it be possible to think of planning a phase III trial.

BIBLIOGRAPHY

Chastang Cl, Lebeau B, Benichou J, Fabre Ch, Fichet D, Dautzenberg B, Decroix G. (1986) : Occurence over time of locoregional and metastatic recurrences in resected lung carcinoma. A study from two randomized clinicals trials.
Bull Europ. Physiopath. Resp. 22 : supp. A420

Gralla RJ, Kris MG, Burke MT, Martini N. (1987) : Adjuvant chemotherapy in non-small cell lung cancer
Fifth international conference on the adjuvant therapy of cancer.Tucson Arizona pp 36.

Gralla RJ, Casper ES, Kelsen DP, Braun DW, Dukeman ME, Martini N. Young CW, Golbey RB. (1981) : Cis-platin and Vindesine combination chemotherapy for advanced carcinoma of the lung : A randomized trial investigating two dosage schedules.
Ann. Int. Med. 95 : 414-420.

Morere JF, Israel L, Breau JL, Clavier J, Guillerm D, Zabbé C, Raut Y, Morère P, Nouvet G, Lerebourgs-Pigeonnière G. (1985) : Preoperative chemotherapy in epidermoid bronchogenic carcinoma.
Future trends chemother. 6 : 495-497.

Splinter TA., Kho GS, Frederiksz A, Kate FJ (1986) : Preoperative chemotherapy in non-small cell lung cancer : a pilot study.
INSERM ed Paris 137 : 491-499.

Stampleman LV, Kris MG, Gralla RJ, Martini N, Bruke MT, Kelsen DP, Heelan RT, Kalman LA. (1987) : Complete response in stage III and IV non-small cell lung cancer with chemotherapy or chemotherapy plus surgery : an analysis of treatment in 554 patients.
Proc. Am. Soc. Clin. Oncol. 6: A696.

Résumé

Un essai phase II randomisé de chimiothérapie néoadjuvante dans les cancers bronchiques opérables non à petites cellules. Résultats à court terme.

B. Dautzenberg, Cl. Chastang, B. Lebeau, Ph. Allard, D. Coëtmeur, J. Bénichou, M-J. Postal and the GETCB (Groupe d'étude et de traitement des cancers bronchiques)
Service de pneumologie, GH Pitié-Salpêtrière 75651 Paris Cédex 13 France

En 1985, a débuté un essai de phase II randomisé visant à tester la faisabilité d'un protocole de chimiothérapie préopératoire pour des malades atteints de cancer bronchique non à petites cellules d'emblée opérable. 26 patients ont été randomisés après un premier staging comprenant un scanner thoracique, pour recevoir soit une chirurgie d'emblée (13 patients), soit deux cures de chimiothérapie PCV préopératoires et deux cures de chimiothérapie postopératoires (13 patients). La chimiothérapie PCV comprend 100 mg/m^2 de cisplatinium, 3 mg/m^2 d'eldesine et 600 mg/m^2 de cyclophosphamide. L'étude de la qualité du staging préopératoire a montré 75 % de concordance pour le N et 83 % pour le T entre le staging preopératoire et les constatations opératoires. Les difficultés opératoires et les suites opératoires n'ont pas été différentes dans les deux groupes. Dans le groupe chimiothérapie deux patients ont refusé secondairement la chimiothérapie et ont été opérés. Le taux de réponse est de 45% (5/11) et le taux de progression de 36 % (4/11) , 2 malades de ce groupe en progression n'ont pas pu faire l'objet d'une exerèse, ce qui a conduit à arrêter définitivement l'inclusion.
En conclusion la chimiothérapie preopératoire pour des cancers non à petites cellules peut être évaluée par staging médical. La chimiothérapie ne complique pas l'intervention, mais si un tel essai doit être planifié, il faut une chimiothérapie donnant moins de 10 % de progression, ce qui n'a pas été le cas dans cet essai.

Neo-Adjuvant Chemotherapy. Ed. Cl. Jacquillat, M. Weil, D. Khayat. Colloque INSERM/John Libbey Eurotext Ltd. © 1988. Vol. 169, pp. 371-376.

Résultats à cinq ans d'une chimiothérapie pré-opératoire dans les cancers épidermoïdes bronchiques opérables

J. Clavier*, Cl. Zabbe*, G. Nouvet**, G. Lerebourg-Pigeonnière*, S. Gouva*, N. André*, Ph. David**, Ph. Mondine* et R. Soyer**

* *Service de pneumologie, CHU, 29200 Brest, France*
** *Service de pneumologie, CHU, 76000 Rouen, France*

RESUME

Entre mars 81 et décembre 86, 76 patients porteurs de cancer épidermoïde bronchique opérable ont reçu 2 ou 3 cures de chimiothérapie (27 CisDDP-BLM ; 18 CisDDP-BLM-Mito C ; 31 CisDDP-BLM-5 FU). Le taux de réponse est de 67 % avec 15 % de réponse complète. Le traitement post-opératoire a été variable selon la réponse à la chimiothérapie et les constatations opératoires (24 aucun traitement ; 34 une ou deux cures de chimiothérapie ; 8 radiothérapie ; 10 association chimio-radiothérapie). Plusieurs constatations méritent d'être soulignées : la diminution du nombre de décès par cancer par rapport aux séries de la littérature : 2,6 % la première année, 30 % pour l'ensemble du groupe ; l'augmentation de la médiane de survie chez les répondeurs (44 mois pour les stades I, 38 mois pour les stades II et III), alors qu'elle est comparable aux données de la littérature chez les non-répondeurs ; l'absence de modification du geste opératoire ; l'absence de surmortalité post-opératoire précoce < 30 jours (4 décès : 5,2 %).

MOTS CLEFS

Chimiothérapie pré-opératoire, cancers épidermoïdes bronchiques.

INTRODUCTION

Le pronostic du cancer épidermoïde des bronches est le même aujourd'hui qu'il y a 20 ans (Israël, 1986 ; Belcher et Anderson, 1965 ; Bates, 1981) et reste particulièrement péjoratif puisqu'il est considéré que seul le traitement chirurgical a une quelconque efficacité. Or 25 % seulement des patients sont opérables et moins de 30 % d'entre eux sont vivants 5 ans plus tard, avec une médiane de survie de l'ordre de 24 mois pour les stades I et de 12 à 18 mois pour les stades II et III.

D'autre part 75 à 80 % des malades opérés (Lebeau et coll., 1977 ; Shields, 1983) décèdent soit par récidive, soit par métastase, et cette surmortalité se retrouve plus de 10 ans après l'acte opératoire (Merlier et coll., 1981).

Ceci signifie que malgré son efficacité, le traitement chirurgical ne suffit pas à contrôler la maladie cancéreuse dans la très grande majorité des cas, et qu'il est nécessaire d'intensifier le traitement initial si l'on veut essayer d'améliorer le pronostic. C'est dans ce but que dès 1981 nous avons introduit une chimiothérapie pré-opératoire systématique dans les cancers bronchiques épidermoïdes opérables.

MATERIEL ET METHODES

Entre mars 1981 et décembre 1986, 76 patients (75 hommes et 1 femme) d'un âge moyen de 57 ans (39 - 74) considérés comme opérables d'emblée d'après les données du bilan d'extension et du bilan fonctionnel, porteurs d'un cancer épidermoïde confirmé histologiquement, ont reçu une chimiothérapie pré-opératoire basée sur l'association Cisplatinum (Cis DDP), Bléomycine (BLM), recommandée par L. Israël (Israël et coll., 1981).

Trois protocoles ont été utilisés :

A) Cis DDP : 20 mg/m2/jour pendant 5 jours
BLM : 5 mg/m2/jour pendant 5 jours
en perfusion continue
27 patients (5 stade I, 13 stade II, 9 stade III) ont reçu ce traitement

B) Cis DDP - BLM comme pour le protocole A avec Mitomycine C : 6 mg/m2 à J1
18 patients ont reçu ce traitement

C) Cis DDP - BLM - 5 Fluoro-uracile à la dose de 1 g/m2/jour pendant 4 jours
31 patients ont reçu ce traitement.

29 patients (3A, 8B, 18C) ont reçu 2 cures, 47 patients (24A, 10B, 13C) ont reçu 3 cures en pré-opératoire.
Les cures étaient séparées de 24 jours.
L'intervention chirurgicale a eu lieu en moyenne 25 jours après le dernier jour de la dernière cure (47 lobectomies, 29 pneumonectomies).
Le traitement post-opératoire a été variable : selon les constatations anatomiques opératoires et la qualité de la réponse à la chimiothérapie. La radiothérapie a été réservée aux patients avec un envahissement ganglionnaire ou une recoupe bronchique envahie.

24 patients n'ont reçu aucun traitement après l'intervention ;
chez 34 patients reprise de la chimiothérapie initiale (1 ou 2 cures) ;
chez 8 patients radiothérapie seule ;
chez 10 patients chimiothérapie plus radiothérapie.

Ce protocole s'est précisé avec le temps et actuellement, sauf en cas d'échec de la chimiothérapie en pré-opératoire, nous reprenons systématiquement deux cures en post-opératoire, quelques soient les constatations anatomiques, limitant la radiothérapie aux N2.

LES RESULTATS

La réponse à la chimiothérapie

Nous avons noté 51 (67 %) réponses objectives supérieures à 50 % (appréciées sur la radiologie, la fibroscopie, le scanner thoracique), dont 12 (15 %) réponses complètes confirmées par l'absence de cellules néoplasiques sur la pièce opératoire.

La réponse à chaque protocole est détaillée dans le tableau I.

Tableau I

		NC	RP	RC
A. DDP - BLM	27			
Stade I	5	2	2	1
Stade II	13	5	8	0
Stade III	9	3	3	3
B. DDP - BLM - Mit C	18			
Stade I	4	0	2	2
Stade II	3	0	1	2
Stade III	11	3	7	1
C. DDP - BLM - 5 FU	31			
Stade I	13	5	6	2
Stade II	10	5	5	0
Stade III	8	2	5	1

Tolérance

Pulmonaire

Sur l'ensemble des 76 patients, nous avons noté 8 baisses de la diffusion alvéolo-capillaire sans gêne fonctionnelle importante. Mais nous avons déploré 7 tableaux de fibrose avec malheureusement 6 décès.

Plusieurs causes peuvent expliquer ces accidents :
- l'utilisation de la mitomycine : cet antimitotique potentialise la toxicité de la bléomycine. 5 patients faisaient parti du protocole B.
- l'utilisation de concentration d'oxygène élevée (FiO2 100 %) lors de l'anesthésie. 4 patients ont reçu de telles concentrations.
- la radiothérapie. 5 patients sur les 6 ont reçu 60 gray sur le médiastin.

La suppression de la mitomycine de nos protocoles et la modification des protocoles d'anesthésie avec réduction des concentrations d'oxygène, ont permis de supprimer ces accidents de fibrose aiguës mortelles.

La toxicité hématologique est modérée. Une toxicité de grade III (critère OMS) sur l'hémoglobine, les leucocytes et 2 sur les plaquettes dans le protocole B.

Une toxicité digestive de grade III dans le protocole C.

Mais en aucun cas un problème toxique n'a obligé à retarder ou annuler l'intervention.

Malgré la toxicité pulmonaire survenue 3 à 4 mois après l'intervention pour 4 patients, il n'existe pas dans notre série de surmortalité post-opératoire, puisque 4 patients sont décédés moins de 30 jours après l'intervention (2 embolies pulmonaires, 1 état de choc, 1 oedème aigu du poumon hémodynamique). De même les fistules bronchiques n'apparaissent pas plus élevées que dans les suites chirurgicales habituelles (2 cas sur 76). Il faut donc insister sur le fait que le geste chirurgical n'est ni gêné, ni modifié, par la chimiothérapie pré-opératoire.

La survie

Sur ce groupe de 74 patients (+ 2 perdus de vue), suivis depuis 18 mois et plus, il est difficile de tirer des conclusions précises en raison du petit nombre de patients et du caractère inhomogène des thérapeutiques post-opératoires. Nous pouvons seulement souligner un certain nombre de faits :

- Seulement 17 patients sont décédés moins d'un an après le diagnostic, soit 23 %, ce qui est très inférieur aux chiffres de la littérature. Surtout, parmi ces 17 patients, 2 seulement sont décédés d'une reprise évolutive de leur cancer, soit 2,6 % . Les autres causes de décès en dehors des 4 décès post-opératoires sont :

. 4 fibroses
. 3 pneumopathies
. 1 insuffisance cardiaque
. 2 embolies pulmonaires
. 1 malade décédé de cause inconnue non cancéreuse.

- La médiane de survie des 22 stade I est de 38 mois ; elle atteint 44 mois pour les répondeurs, 29 mois pour les non répondeurs. 13 patients sont encore vivants (59 %).

- Pour les stades II et III, soit 52 patients, la médiane est de 18 mois pour l'ensemble du groupe, mais elle atteint 38 mois pour les 33 répondeurs et 14 mois pour les non répondeurs. 13 patients sur 33 sont vivants chez les répondeurs (dont 2 en rechute) contre 3 sur 19 chez les non répondeurs.

- Enfin, pour l'ensemble des 74 patients suivis, on constate 22 décès par cancer, soit 30 % :

. 4 autres cancers (2 ORL, 1 colique, 1 ovarien)
. 8 métastases (5 cérébrales, 1 osseuse, 1 hépatique, 1 surrénales)
. 8 récidives in situ
. 2 récidives controlatérales.

DISCUSSION

Au moment du diagnostic, le cancer bronchique est dans une très grande majorité des cas une maladie disséminée, puisque le nombre de décès par métastases et/ou reprise évolutive médiastinale atteint 75 à 80 %. Il semble donc nécessaire, pour pouvoir contrôler plus longtemps la maladie, d'associer au traitement loco-régional un traitement général capable d'agir non seulement sur la tumeur primitive, mais surtout sur les micrométastases. L'urgence avec laquelle il faut traiter ces métastases, si l'on veut être efficace, incite à introduire le traitement médical le plus rapidement possible, avant même le geste chirurgical. Notre travail montre que cela est parfaitement possible sans modifier en rien le geste chirurgical.

Cette chimiothérapie n'entraîne pas une surmortalité si l'on évite d'utiliser avec la bléomycine des produits potentialisant sa toxicité pulmonaire (mitomycine, oxygène à forte concentration). L'adjonction d'une chimiothérapie efficace à la chirurgie semble réduire de façon importante le nombre de décès par cancer : 2,6 % la première année, contre 25 à 30 % dans la littérature. 30 % de décès par cancer sur l'ensemble du groupe suivi depuis plus de 15 mois ; là aussi le chiffre est très inférieur aux chiffres retrouvés dans la littérature qui sont de 75 à 80 %. On peut donc penser qu'une chimiothé rapie efficace réduit le risque de développement des micrométastases.

Par ailleurs, il faut souligner l'allongement de médianes de survie de façon globale, mais beaucoup plus nette si l'on regarde celles des répondeurs. Dans la littérature, Israël (1986) et Vincent (Vincent et coll., 1976) rapportent des médianes de 24 et 26 mois pour les stades I, de 18 et 10 mois pour les stades II et III. Ce sont pratiquement les chiffres que nous retrouvons pour les non répondeurs (stade I : 29 mois ; stades II et III : 18 mois). Par contre les répondeurs ont des médianes beaucoup plus importantes (stade I : 44 mois ; stades II et III : 38 mois).

CONCLUSION

Ces résultats sont très encourageants, mais demandent à être confirmés par une étude randomisée qui est débutée depuis le premier janvier 1988.

REFERENCES BIBLIOGRAPHIQUES

Israël, L. (1986) : Cancers épidermoïdes bronchiques. In Cancer Intra-thoracique, éd Flammarion, Médecine Science, pp 71-100.

Belcher, J.R., Anderson, R. (1965) : Surgical treatment of carcinoma of the bronchus. Br. Med. J. 1, 948-954.

Bates, M. (1981) : Surgical treatment of bronchial carcinoma. Am. R. Coll. Surg. Engl. 63, 164-167.

Lebeau, B., Bouguenec, B., Rochemaure, J. (1977) : Pronostic des carcinomes bronchiques épidermoïdes traités chirurgicalement - A propos de 102 cas. Poumon - Coeur 33, 4, 213-218.

Shields, T.W. (1983) : Surgical therapy for carcinoma of the lung. Clin. Chest. Med. 3, 2, 369-387.

Merlier, M., Lebrigand, H., Rojas-Miranda, A., Levasseur, P., Dartevelle, P.(1981): Généralités sur la survie éloignée des exérèses pulmonaires des cancers bronchiques primitifs (anaplasiques exclus). Rev. Fr. Mal. Resp. 9, 493.

Israël L., Aguilera, J., Breau, J.L. (1981) : Traitement des cancers épidermoïdes par bléomycine et platine en administration continue prolongée - Série préliminaire de 80 cas avec 75 % de réponses objectives. Nouv. Pres. Med. 10, 1817-1824.

Vincent, R.G., Hiroshi Takita, Lane, W.W., Gutierrez, A.C., Pickren, J.W. (1976) : Surgical therapy of lung cancer. J.T.C.S. 71, 4, 581-591.

Résumé

Between April 1981 and December 1986, 76 patients (74 evaluable) (22 stage I, 26 stade II, 28 stage III, TNM UICC) with operable squamous cell carcinoma of the lung were given systematic preoperative chemotherapy :

A) Cis DDP - BLM (27 patients)
B) Cis DDP - BLM - Mito C (18 patients)
C) Cis DDP - BLM - 5 FU (31 patients)

29 patients were given 2 preoperative treatment cycles (3A, 8B, 18C), 47 patients were given 3 preoperative treatment cycles (24A, 10B, 13C). The chemotherapy response rate was the same in each protocol. For all patients we noted 67 % responses with 15 % complete responses, no progression was noted. As for tolerance, certain associations with Bleomycin (Mitomycin, pure oxygen during surgery) must be avoided because of increased pulmonary toxicity. Equally, radiotherapy requires careful supervision of respiratory function.

Four results deserve attention : there were only 2 deaths due to cancer during the year following the diagnosis of the disease. There were 22 deaths (30 %) due to cancer for all patients. There was a median rate survival of 28 months with 29 patients still alive. The median rate survival for stage I and stage II - III is higher in responders than in non-responders. These results show : pre-operative chemotherapy is possible in squamous cell carcinoma of the lung, a better control of the disease.

These results have also encouraged us to begin a randomised study to confirm the benefits of preoperative chemotherapy with regard to the survival rate.

Neo-Adjuvant Chemotherapy. Ed. Cl. Jacquillat, M. Weil, D. Khayat. Colloque INSERM/John Libbey Eurotext Ltd. © 1988. Vol. 169, pp. 377-381

Neo-adjuvant chemotherapy for locoregionally advanced non small cell lung cancer

Everett E. Vokes, Jacob D. Bitran, Philip C. Hoffman, Harvey M. Golomb, Ralph R. Weichselbaum, Charles M. Brown, Alex G. Little, Laura Fullem and Jan A. Golick

Joint Section of Hematology/Oncology, Department of Radiation Oncology and Department of Surgery, the University of Chicago and Michael Reese Hospital and Medical Center, Chicago, IL, USA

ABSTRACT

Twenty-seven patients with stage III_{mo} non-small cell lung cancer (NSCLC) were registered on this phase II study. There were 22 males, 5 females; median age was 58 years (range 41-73), performance status was 0:5 patients, 1:17 patients, 2:4 patients, and 3:1 patient. Tumor histology was adenocarcinoma: 12 patients, large cell carcinoma: 6 patients and squamous cell carcinoma: 9 patients. Chemotherapy consisted of vindesine 3.0 mg/m^2 weekly x 6, etoposide 300 mg/m^2 weekly x 6 and cisplatin 120 mg/m^2 on days 1 and 22. Four patients were unevaluable for response. Of 23 evaluable patients, 13 had a partial response while 10 had stable disease or disease progression. The response rate to neoadjuvant chemotherapy is 48% (13/27). Subsequent local therapy consisted of surgery plus radiation therapy in 4 patients and of radiotherapy alone in 14 patients. The radiotherapy dose was 54 Gy to the chest (30 GY prophylactic cranial radiation was given to patients with adenocarcinoma after completion of chest radiation). Five patients did not receive local therapy due to disease progression. Following local therapy 7 patients were considered free of disease, 5 had a partial response and 6 pts had no response. Median time to disease progression from response to neo-adjuvant chemotherapy is 8 months (3-46 months). The median survival for all pts registered on study is 8 months (3 days-48 months). Chemotherapy induced toxicities included moderate myelosuppression (median WBC count nadir: 1900/µl), nausea and vomiting, and occasional ototoxicity, neurotoxicity and wasting syndrome. One patient died from intracerebral hemorrhage due to thrombocytopenia. This trial shows that administration of neoadjuvant chemotherapy to patients with locoregionally advanced NSCLC is feasable and can result in increased response rates compared to patients with metastatic disease. While no effect of the use of chemotherapy on patient survival was apparent in this study, further studies with the goal to identify more active drug combinations are warranted.

KEY WORDS: non-small cell lung cancer, neoadjuvant chemotherapy.

INTRODUCTION

The prognosis for patients with locoregionally advanced non-small cell lung cancer (NSCLC) remains dismal. Five year survival rates of less than 10% have been reported for patients with mediastinal or supraclavicular lymph node involvement (Mountain, 1977; Pearson, 1982). Recently, efforts at improving this prognosis have focused on the combined use of multiple treatment modalities, including surgery, radiotherapy and neoadjuvant chemotherapy.

The concept of neoadjuvant chemotherapy has been applied in locally advanced squamous cell cancer of the head and neck, ostegenic sarcoma, and inflammatory breast cancer. High response rates to initial chemotherapy have been observed in patients with these malignancies suggesting that higher response rates to chemotherapy could also be achieved in patients with NSCLC by administering cytotoxic drugs prior to local therapy. Therefore, in 1983 we decided to study the feasability of administering etoposide, vindesine and cisplatin prior to local therapy to patients with locoregionally advanced NSCLC.

PATIENTS AND METHODS

This study opened in March of 1983 and closed in June of 1985. Initial staging procedures for all patients consisted of a complete history and physical examination, complete blood count, routine serum chemistries, 24 hour urine creatinine clearance, split pulmonary function studies, chest x-ray, a CT-scan of the chest to the level of the adrenals, a bone scan, a liver spleen scan, and a whole body gallium scan. Bronchoscopy was performed in all patients; many patients also had mediastinoscopy to confirm clinically suspicious appearing mediastinal lymph nodes as malignant.

Eligible patients had histologically or cytologically confirmed NSCLC with T_2 or T_3 primaries and mediastinal or ipsilateral supraclavicular lymph node involvement, a performance status of 0-3 (ECOG), and a 24 hour urine creatinine clearance of $\geq$ 50 m/min. All patients were previously untreated and signed informed consent.

The treatment plan called for 2 cycles of chemotherapy followed by response evaluation consisting of a repeat chest x-ray and CT-scan of the chest down to the adrenals. Standard response criteria were applied. Local therapy consisted of surgery followed by radiotherapy when the patient's disease was considered resectable by the attending surgeon; otherwise, radiotherapy alone was administered. Following local therapy, additional cycles of chemotherapy were administered unless prohibited by disease progression or cumulative toxicity.

Chemotherapy consisted of vindesine 3.0 mg/m^2 by IV bolus and etoposide 300 mg/m^2 by IV infusion over 30-45 minutes, both on days 1,8,15,22,29 and 36. Cisplatin 120 mg/m^2 was administered IV over 4 hours on days 1 and 22. Standard hydration and antiemetic schedules were applied.

Radiotherapy was delivered by a 4 mV or 6 mV linear accelerator in daily fractions of 200 cGy for a total dose of 54 Gy. Included in the radiotherapy field were the primary tumor, the ipsilateral hilum, the mediastinum and supraclavicular fossa. Prophylactic cranial irradiation consisting of 30 Gy in 10 fractions was administered to patients with adenocarcinoma who were clinically considered free of disease following completion of local therapy.

RESULTS

Thirty patients were registered on this study. Three of these were found to be ineligible on chart review: one patient had received prior chest irradiation, one patient was found to have progressive metastatic pancreatic adenocarcinoma during cycle 2 as her primary malignancy, and one patient was lost to follow-up. These patients are excluded from subsequent analysis. The patient characteristics of the true study cohort of 27 patients are summarized as follows:

Patient Characteristics

Sex		
Male	:	22 patients
Female	:	5 patients
Age, Median	:	58 years
Range	:	41-73 years
Performance Status		0:5 patients
		1:17 patients
		2:4 patients
		3:1 patient
Histology		
Adenocarcinoma	:	12 patients
Large cell carcinoma	:	6 patients
Squamous cell carcinoma	:	9 patients

Four patients expired prior to completion of 2 cycles of chemotherapy and were not evaluated for response: one patient died of respiratory arrest from compression of his mainstream bronchus by tumor, one patient died of acute pulmonary embolism following cycle 2, one patient of intracerebral hemorrhage while thrombocytopenic from chemotherapy, and one patient of progressive atypical tuberculosis.

Of 23 patients who were evaluated for response, 13 had a partial response while 10 had stable or progressive disease. The overall response rate, therefore, is 48% (13 of 27 patients) or 57% (13 of 23 patients) when considering only those patients who completed neoadjuvant chemotherapy.

Subsequent local therapy consisted of surgery followed by radiotherapy in 4 patients. Fourteen patients received radiotherapy alone, while 5 patients did not receive any local therapy; all five had failed to respond to initial chemotherapy. Overall, 7 patients were considered free of disease at completion of local therapy, including all 4 patients who had undergone surgery.

The median survival for all 27 patients is 8 months (range 3 days-48 months); the median time to disease progression in patients responding to neoadjuvant chemotherapy is 8 months (3-46 months). Overall, 21 patients have died of progressive NSCLC, 5 have died of intercurrent disease (1 of myocardial infarction while clinically free of disease) and 1 patient is alive at 48 months.

The toxicities of this chemotherapy regimen consisted mainly of myelosuppresion (median WBC count nadir: 1900/μl; median platelet count nadir: 120,000/μl). Sporadic renal toxicity, ototoxicity and neurotoxicity were also observed. One patient died of chemotherapy-related intracerebral hemorrhage.

DISCUSSION

The goal of this study was to assess the feasibility of administering 2 cycles of neoadjuvant chemotherapy with vindesine, etoposide, and cisplatin to patients with locoregionally advanced NSCLC. With the exception of one incidence of fatal intracerebral hemorrhage, no severe complications were observed during initial 2 cycles of chemotherapy. Moreover, although 10 of 23 patients evaluable for response had no tumor shinkage or eventual tumor progression while receiving chemotherapy, it is unlikely that the chemotherapy had a negative impact on their survival given the advanced stage of their disease. On the other hand, a response rate of approximately 50% to only 2 cycles of chemotherapy in patients with advanced NSCLC is most encouraging. It compares favorably to response rates achieved in patients with metastatic or recurrent disease (Bitran, 1978) and supports the investigational use of initial chemotherapy. Similarly increased response rates to neoadjuvant chemotherapy in patients with NSCLC have recently been reported by others (Strauss, 1987; Spain, 1987).

Although a prolongation of survival as a result of neoadjuvant chemotherapy in this study is not suggested by our analysis, this study does support further investigation of the concept of neoadjuvant chemotherapy in NSCLC. The goal of such studies will be the definition of more active regimens in this setting and the determination of the optimal number of cycles to be administered.

REFERENCES

1. Bitran, JD (1978): Treatment of metastatic (stage III$_{M1}$) non-oat cell bronchogenic carcinoma with cyclophosphamide, adriamycin, methotrexate, and procarbazine (CAMP). JAMA 240, 2743-2746.

2. Mountain, CFC (1977): Assessment of the role of surgery for control of lung cancer. Ann Thor Surg 24, 365-372.

3. Pearson, FG (1982): Significance of positive superior mediastinoscopy in patients with resectable cancer of the lung. J Thorac Cardiovasc Surg 83, 1-11.

4. Spain, RC (1987): Neoadjuvant mitomycin, cisplatin and infusion vinblastine with reduced pulmonary toxicity in Stage III Non-Small Cell Lung Cancer. In: Adjuvant therapy of Cancer V, , Ed: Salmon SE, Grune & Stratton, Inc., 165-178.

5. Strauss, G (1987): Combined modality therapy for regionally advanced Stage III Non-Small Cell Carcinoma of the lung employing neoadjuvant chemotherapy, radiotherapy and surgery. Proc Fifth Internat Conf. Adj. Ther. Cancer, Tucson, AZ., 18 (Abstr.).

Résumé

Ving-sept malades, stage III (CCNPP) ont participé dans la phase II de cette investigation. Il y avait 22 hommes et 5 femmes, l'âge médian était 58 ans (rang 41-73), la condition physique 0:5 cas, 1:17 cas, 2:4 cas, 3:1 cas. Histologie du tumeur était adénocarcinome:12 cas, cancer à cellule grande:6 cas, et cancer à cellule épidermoïde:9 cas. La chimiothérapie comportait l'administration de Vindesine 3mg/m^2 chaque semaine x 6, Etoposide 300 mg/m^2 chaque semaine x 6, et Cisplatin 120 mg/m^2 le premier et le 22ème jour. 4 malades n'ont pas pu être évalué. Nous avons évalué 23 malades parmi lesquels 13 ont achevé une réponse partielle, tandis que parmi les autres 10, la maladie était stable ou progressive. Le pourcentage de réponse à la chimiothérapie néo-adjuvante est 48% (13/27). La chimiothérapie a été suivi par la thérapie locale comprenant chirurgie et radiothérapie (RT) dans 4 cas, ou seulement RT dans 14 cas. La dose de RT était 54 Gy à la poitrine (malades avec adéno-carcinome ont reçu 30 Gy RT préventive au crâne suivant RT à la poitrine). 5 malades n'ont pas reçu la thérapie locale à cause du progrés de la maladie. A la suite de la thérapie locale, 7 malades étaient en remission, 5 ont achevé une réponse partielle, et 6 n'avaient obtenu aucun résultat. L'intervalle médian entre la réponse à la chimiothérapie néoadjuvante et la progression de la maladie est 8 mois (3-46 mois). La survie médiane pour tous les malades partécipant dans cette investigation est 8 mois (3 jours-48 mois). La toxicité de la CT s'est manifestée avec myélosuppression moderée (nadir du compte médian des leucocytes: 1900/ul), nausée, vomissement, ototoxicité, neurotoxicité, et syndrome ravageur. Le décès d'un malade a été causé par la hémorragie intracérébrale à la suite d'une thrombocytopénie. Cette investigation démontre que l'administration de la chimiothérapie néoadjuvante aux malades avec CCNPP localement/régionalement avancé, est faisable et peut donner meilleurs pourcentages de réponse si on la compare aux malades avec métastases. Bien que l'effet de la chimiothérapie sur la survie des malades n'a pas été demontré dans cette investigation, il est pourtant justifié de l'avancer à bout d'identifier combinaisons de drogues plus effectives.

Mots clef: cancer à cellule non-petite du poumon, chimiothérapie néoadjuvante

Neo-Adjuvant Chemotherapy. Ed. Cl. Jacquillat, M. Weil, D. Khayat. Colloque INSERM/John Libbey Eurotext Ltd. © 1988. Vol. 169, pp. 383-387.

Combined modality treatment for small cell bronchial carcinomas

E. Ulsperger[1], H. Denck[2], M.L. Liao[3], G.M. Salzer[4], W. Schlick[5], A. Lattuneddu[6] and K. Karrer[1] for the ISC-Lung Cancer Study Group

Institute for Epidemiology of Neoplasms of the University, A-1090 Vienna, Austria (1); I. Surgical Dept., Hosp. Lainz and L. Boltzmann Inst. for Clinical Oncology, A-1130 Vienna, Austria (2); Shanghai Chest Hosp., Shanghai, P.R. China (3); II. Surgical Dept. of the Univ., A-6020 Innsbruck, Austria (4); II. Surgical Univ. Clinic, A-1090 Vienna, Austria (5); Ospedale Morgani, I-47100 Forli, Italy (6)

ABSTRACT

In small cell bronchial carcinoma at pTNM stages I and II multimodality treatment including surgery for cure can be accomplished as the treatment of choice. For the pT1-3 N+ M0 stages a pilot ISC study III with neo-adjuvant chemotherapy is performed. From 71 patients from 15 stations of this still ongoing study, 21 are judged to be evaluable per February 1988. They received praeoperative chemotherapy (CT) and surgery, as response was judged, followed by postoperative CT. From these, 11 patients are still alive with a median observation time of 39 month. From these, 5 patients had a complete response, were staged at surgery as ypT0 N0 M0 and showed an observation-time of 36-87 month (mean 51), while 6 patients with partial response were observed for 4-51 months (mean 35). The median survival time of 10/21 patients who already died is 15,4 months (8-26). These patients had only partial response to CT. The results given above seem to justify the continuation of our pilot study III. The feasibility of the protocol was proven by 15 independent departments and therefore we like to invite further groups for cooperation.

KEY WORDS

small cell bronchial carcinoma, chemotherapy, neo-adjuvant chemotherapy, surgery, multimodality treatment

INTRODUCTION

Results of the British Medical Research Council (1973), have been misleading interpreted by diminishing the importance of surgery for SCLC. Various studies and investigations during the past decade emphasized the importance of surgery in SCLC. It is obvious that surgery is the most effective measure to eliminate the whole primary tumor and its regional lymphnodes at once and is related to

patients 24 are still under praeoperative chemotherapy and it is too early for evaluation as yet.
21 patients received surgery for cure according to the protocol after complete or partial response to praeoperative chemotherapy. From these, 10 patients died after a median SVT of 15,4 months (8-26) as given in detail in table 1.

Table 1.
Survay of patients with partial response to CT and surgery for cure

pat.no	c TNM stage	no.cycles praeop.CT	yp T N M	no.cycles postop.CT	SVT months	mean SVT
1	II	2	2 1 0	4	26	
2	II	2	2 1 0	5	23	
3	IIIa	2	2 2 0	3	21	
4	IIIa	2	3 1 0	3	15	
5	IIIa	2	3 0 0	2	14	
6	II	3	3 2 0	5	14	15,4
7	IIIa	3	3 2 0	2	13	
8	IIIa	2	3 1 0	1	12	
9	IIIa	3	3 1 0	1	8	
10	II	2	2 1 0	2	8	

The clinical staging (c TNM) is done at onset of praeoperative chemotherapy consisting of 2 or 3 chemotherapy cycles as given in the table. The pTNM staging performed after surgery is additionally labeled with the prefix "y" in the histopathological determination of the operation specimen of patients under multimodality treatment. The pathologist has to evaluate two parameters: first, the size of the tumor and the absence or presence of tumor positive lymph nodes and second the viability of the tumor cells.
The tumor stage was not changed by the praeoperative chemotherapy. After surgery the chemotherapy cycles are continued as given in the next column. The SVT of each patient is calculated from onset of chemotherapy until date of death.

From the above mentioned 21 evaluable patients receiving surgery for cure after response to CT, 11 are under observation for 4-87 months (mean 39) and given in table 2 in the same sense as shown in table 1.

Patients 11-15 who had cTNM-stages II or IIIa showed complete response after 2-3 CT-cycles, which was veryfied by pathohistological examination where no viable tumor cells were found. It seems encouraging that the median observation time (OBT) of these patients, showing complete response, is 51 months (36-87 months) and that of patients no. 16-21 with partial response to initial CT is 35 months (4-51).
Patient no. 16, observed for 51 months, had tumor positive mediastinal lymph nodes prior to chemotherapy and was staged after surgery as ypT1 N0 M0.

continuation of study III using neo-adjuvant chemotherapy seems to be indicated.

It is of prognostic importance to distinguish between the tumor involvement at diagnosis and the viability of the tumor cells at the pathohistological examination after initial chemotherapy. But the ypTNM staging cannot express if N0 means an involved lymphnode, or a lymph node involved with non viable tumor cells represented only by shadows, which demonstrate a definite proof of the effectiveness of the chemotherapy.

The judgement of the viability of tumor cells, besides the pathohistologoical staging of the operation specimen, in patients, treated by initial multimodality treatment, has to be defined precisely by the local pathologists. This can not be done by the routine examination but should be performed very carefully. This is the objective control for the effectiveness of chemotherapy.

However, even a complete remission determinated by the tumor cell shadows within a necrotic area can not be judged as a definite exclusion of the possibility of recovering of the viability of the tumor cells. Considering this the continuation of the postoperative chemotherapy is indicated, but further experience has to be gathered to conclude the future policy of the length of this treatment as well as wether surgery has to be the first step or if initial chemotherapy has to be administered.

CONCLUSIONS

1. In pTNM stages I and II surgery is the treatment of choice in combination with chemo- and radiotherapy.
2. The N2-patients of ISC study III seem to benefit of surgery after response to chemotherapy.
3. The feasibility of this world-wide cooperation can be seen as an important result, therefore its continuation seems to be not only justified but emphatically indicated.

REFERENCES

Fox, W. (1973): Medical research council comperative trial of surgery and radiotherapy for primary treatment of small cell carcinoma of the bronchus. Ten year follow-up Lancet 2, 63.

George, T.K. (1986): Long-term survival in limited-stage small cell lung carcinoma. Cancer 58, 1193.

Ihde, D.C. (1986): Neo-adjuvant chemotherapy of lung cancer: Preliminary North American experience. Neo-adjuvant chemotherapy 137, 467.

Karrer, K. (1987): Multimodality treatment with surgery in small-cell lung cancer. Int. J. Clin. Pharm. Res. 7, 313.

Karrer, K. (1987): Combined modality treatment after surgery for cure for SCLC at TNM stage I. In Adjuvant Therapy of Cancer V, ed S. Salmon, pp 189. New York: Grune & Stratton.

Meyer, J.A. (1987): Indications for surgical treatment in small cell carcinoma of the lung. Surg. Clin. N. America 67, 1103.

PARTICIPANTS OF THE COOPERATIVE STUDY ISC-III

Country/City	Surgery	Medical Oncology	Radiology	Pathology
A Vienna	H.Denck,N.Pridun	M.Neumann,N.Vetter	G.Alth	H.Hackl
RC Shanghai	O.Wang,Y.Chow	M.Liao,J.Chao	M.Lin	Z.Lin
A Innsbruck	G.M.Salzer,L.Müller	H.Huber	H.Frommhold	G.Mikuz
I Forli	A.Lattuneddu,D.Dell'Amore	A.Galassi,A.Campanini		
A Vienna	E.Wolner,F.Eckersberger	W.Schlick	K.Kärcher	Holzner
RA B.Aires	A.Imposti	M.Bruno,N.Brocato	N.Ruggeri	
I Cosenza		V.Zottola,S.Barbera		G.Gallippi
A Gaisbühel	G.Zimmermann	J.Rothmund,M.Amann	Oser	G.Breitfellner
Jp Kawasaki	H.Osada	M.Koike	M.Endoh	Y.Sodemoto
I Firenze	C.Crisci	N.Nozzoli,S.Nutini	N.Dini,M.Santucci	
SU Moscow	A.Pirogov	N.Perevodchikova,A.Garin		
Jp Toyama	Y.Kusajima	Y.Mizukami	M.Sugihara	N.Takayanagi
RA B.Aires	H.Della Torre	H.Pepe,L.Tabares	M.Filomia	I.Kaufer
I Bologna	P.Sette		L.Cacciari	
D Donaustauf		F. von Bültzingslöwen		
A Vienna	ISC-Study Center: K.Karrer, E.Ulsperger, G.Mann			

per 10.2.1988

Résumé

Dans les cancers à patites cellules bronchiques TNM stades I et II, un traitement combiné incluant une chirurgie peut être considéré comme traitement de choix. Pour les stades T1 à T3 N+ nous avons conduit une étude pilote avec le groupe ISC, avec une chimiothérapie néoadjuvante. 21 des 71 malades entrés dans l'étude sont évaluables en février 88, ils ont reçu une chimiothérapie pré-opératoire, une chirurgie qui a permis de juger de la réponse qui a été suivi d'une chimiothérapie post-opératoire. Parmi ces malades 11 patients sont toujours vivants avec un temps d'observation médian de 39 mois, 5 de ces malades ont eu une réponse complète histologique leur temps d'observation est de 36 à 87 mois (moyenne 51 mois), et 6 malades ayant eu une réponse partielle ont été observés entre 4 et 51 mois (moyenne 35 mois). La survie médiane des 10 malades qui sont morts est de 15,4 mois (8-26). Ces malades n'avaient eu qu'une réponse partielle à la chimiothérapie. L'ensemble de ces résultats justifient la poursuite de notre étude. La faisabilité du protocole a été prouvée par le fait qu'il a pu être suivi par 15 services indépendants.

Neo-Adiuvant Chemotherapy. Ed. Cl. Jacquillat, M. Weil, D. Khayat. Colloque INSERM/John Libbey Eurotext Ltd. © 1988. Vol. 169, pp. 389-395.

Résectabilité des cancers bronchiques non à petites cellules (NSCLC) après chimiothérapie d'induction

S. Gouva*, Cl. Zabbe*, E. Lemarie***, G. Nouvet**, Ch. David** et J. Clavier*

Services de pneumologie, Centres Hospitaliers Universitaires, 29285 Brest, 76000 Rouen**, 37044 Tours***, France*

RESUME

La chimiothérapie réalisée chez des patients porteurs de carcinomes bronchiques non à petites cellules jugés initialement non opérables permet parfois après traitement chez les répondeurs, une chirurgie seconde.
Nous avons rétrospectivement repris 23 dossiers de patients d'âge moyen 50 ans, atteints de NSCLC (19 stade III et 4 stade IV) et répondeurs à une chimiothérapie à base de Cisplatinum (DDP) se répartissant en 20 épidermoïdes et 3 adénocarcinomes. Les patients ont reçu en moyenne 3 cures pré-opératoires, les causes de non opérabilité étaient une extension médiastinale, pariétale, trachéale, ou des lésions métastatiques. Une radiothérapie complémentaire a été réalisée s'il existait sur la pièce d'exérèse des ganglions médiastinaux envahis, une extension pariétale ou une recoupe envahie. Il s'agit de 23 patients répondeurs à la chimiothérapie (une rémission complète, 18 réponses partielles, et 4 réponses inférieures à 50 %). Le geste chirurgical a consisté en 9 pneumonectomies et 14 lobectomies. La toxicité a été modérée. Sur 23 patients, 10 sont décédés dont 3 de récidive locale ou de lésions métastatiques. La moyenne de survie est de 24 mois. 13 patients sont en vie, avec une moyenne de survie de 29 mois. Les chimiothé rapies à base de Cisplatinum permettent d'obtenir un nombre non négligeable de réponses chez les patients porteurs de NSCLC et ainsi permettent dans certains cas une exérèse chirurgicale complète. Notre étude rétrospective le confirme sans pouvoir affirmer qu'il existe un bénéfice de survie pour les patients.

MOTS CLEFS

Carcinomes bronchiques non à petites cellules, chimiothérapie, Cisplatinum.

INTRODUCTION

Le pronostic des cancers bronchiques non à petites cellules reste pour l'ensemble des auteurs corrélé au taux de résectabilité ; les cancers jugés inopérables d'emblée ayant un taux de mortalité très élevé du fait de la diffusion rapide de la maladie cancéreuse.

Certains auteurs (Morere et coll., 1985) ont montré que l'administration, 5 jours consécutifs, d'une chimiothérapie associant le cisplatinum (DDP) et la bléomycine (BLM) permet parfois une exérèse seconde des NSCLC jugés inopérables initialement.

Il n'est cependant pas prouvé qu'une telle chimiothérapie permette d'obtenir une survie prolongée chez ces patients.

MATERIEL ET METHODES

Nous avons repris rétrospectivement 23 dossiers de patients traités entre 1981 et 1987, et opérés secondairement après chimiothérapie. Tous les patients étaient fumeurs, d'âge moyen 50 ans (35-70). Le diagnostic de cancer bronchique a été porté dans tous les cas par fibroscopie bronchique et biopsies (20 carcinomes épidermoïdes et 3 adénocarcinomes).

Les patients ont été jugés inopérables (tableau I) après un bilan d'extension comportant outre la fibroscopie, une radiographie thoracique, un scanner thoracique et cérébral, une scintigraphie osseuse et une échographie hépatique, et inclus dans un protocole d'étude de chimiothérapie.

Tous les patients ont reçu du cisplatinum (DDP) en association à la bléomycine (BLM) pour 19 d'entre eux. Le détail des protocoles figure dans le tableau II.

Tableau I : Causes d'inopérabilité initiale.

Extension intra-médiastinale (N2 +)	12 patients
Atteinte proximale de la bronche souche	3 patients
Envahissement pariétal	3 patients
Métastases	4 patients
. ganglionnaires cervicales	2
. cérébrales	2
Cancer bilatéral	1 patient

Tableau II : Type de chimiothérapie.

DDP - BLM - MTC	4 patients	DDP 20 mg/m2/J1 à J5 BLM 5 mg/m2/J1 à J5 MTC 6 mg/m2 à J1
DDP - BLM	9 patients	DDP 20 mg/m2/J1 à J5 BLM 5 mg/m2/J1 à J5
DDP - BLM - 5 FU	4 patients	DDP 20 mg/m2/J1 à J5 BLM 5 mg/m2/J1 à J5 5 FU 1 g/m2/J1 à J4 continuous infusion)
DDP - BLM - VP 16	1 patient	DDP 20 mg/m2/J1 à J5 BLM 5 mg/m2/J1 à J5 VP 16 300 mg/m2/J1 à J3
DDP - BLM - VDN	1 patient	DDP 20 mg/m2/J1 à J5 BLM 5 mg/m2/J1 à J5 VDN 3 mg/m2 à J1
DDP - 5 FU	4 patients	DDP 20 mg/m2/J1 à J5 5 FU 1 g/m2/J1 à J4 (continuous infusion)

Abréviations DDP : cisplatinum
BLM : bléomycine
MTC : mitomycine C
5 FU : 5 fluoro-uracile
VP 16 : Etoposide
VDN : vindésine

Les cures de chimiothérapie ont été effectuées tous les 28 jours. Après une moyenne de 3 cures (2 à 6 ; tableau III) une chirurgie d'exérèse a été décidée du fait de la réponse obtenue sur la tumeur et effectuée en moeynne 29 jours (+ 8) après la fin du dernier cycle (14 lobectomies, 99 pneumonectomies).

Le traitement post-opératoire a tenu compte du TNM résiduel chirurgical. Une radiothérapie de clôture de 60 gray en étalement sur 6 semaines étant réalisée en cas d'envahissement ganglionnaire médiastinal (N2 +), d'extension pariétale ou d'envahissement de la recoupe bronchique à l'examen de la pièce d'exérèse (tableau III).

Tableau III : Détail des traitements

Nombre de cures pré-opératoires J1 = J28	3 patients : 2 cures 12 patients : 3 2 : 4 4 : 5 2 : 6
Type d'exérèse chirurgicale	Pneumonectomies : 9 Lobectomies : 14
Traitements post-opératoires	chimiothérapie (2 cycles) 1 patient chimiothérapie + radiothérapie (2 cycles) 6 patients Radiothérapie 5 patients

RESULTATS

Evaluation de la chimiothérapie :

La réponse médicale a été évaluée avant chaque cycle en tenant compte de la radiographie thoracique, de la fibroscopie bronchique et du résultat des biopsies. Nous la formulons en réponse partielle (RP) en cas de régression > 50 %, réponse minime (Rm) en cas de régression < 50 % et réponse complète (RC) lors de la normalisation radiologique, endoscopique et de biopsies négatives.

La réponse chirurgicale a tenu compte de l'extension des lésions lors de la thoracotomie et de l'examen histologique de la pièce d'exérèse et des ganglions prélevés. Nous avons comparé ces résultats à la réponse médicale.

Nous n'avons retenu lors de cette étude que des patients répondeurs, l'objectif de cette présentation n'est donc pas l'évaluation de la réponse à la chimiothérapie. Nous avons retrouvé 1 RC, 18 RP, et 4 Rm. Cette évaluation est confirmée par l'étude de la réponse chirurgicale dans 18/23 cas. La réponse médicale avait été surévaluée chez 3 patients et sous-évaluée chez deux autres par rapport aux données de la chirurgie.

Etude de la toxicité :

Le tableau résume l'ensemble des complications observées selon la classification de l'OMS. La chimiothérapie d'induction n'a créé aucune difficulté d'exérèse et dans les suites opératoires immédiates (< 30 jours), on note simplement une embolie pulmonaire résolutive.

Trois décès sont imputables au traitement du fait de l'association chimio et radiothérapie. Ils sont observés à 9, 10 et 12 mois par rapport au J1 du traitement.

La toxicité hématologique et digestive reste modérée et toutes les chimiothérapies (101 cycles) ont été administrées à 100 % des doses théoriques aux dates initialement prévues.

Tableau IV : Détail des toxicités imputables au traitement.

Décès	2 fibroses pulmonaires 1 fistule trachéo-oesophagienne		
Complications de la chirurgie	1 embolie pulmonaire réversible		
Toxicité hématologique	Hb :	grade 1 (OMS)	2
		3	1
	GB :	grade 3	1
	plaquettes :	grade 1	1
		grade 2	1
		4	1
Toxicité digestive		grade 1	4
		2	4

Devenir des patients

- Patients décédés : 10 patients sur 23 sont décédés (43 %) après une moyenne de survie de 17 mois (6 - 58 mois). Les causes de décès sont développées dans le tableau V.

- Patients vivants : 13 patients sont vivants (57 %) avec une moyenne de 29 mois + (8 - 73 mois). L'un d'entre eux a présenté à 38 mois une métastase cérébrale qui a pu être traitée (chirurgie + radiothérapie), le patient est en vie à 62 mois +.

Tableau V : Causes de décès (10 patients = 43 %)

Récidives locales ou métastases	3 patients
Complications imputables au traitement	3 patients
Autres causes (non cancéreuses)	4 patients

La survie globale moyenne des patients est de 24 mois (7 - 64).

DISCUSSION

La plupart des cancers bronchiques NAPC sont diagnostiqués à un stade déjà évolué de la maladie et l'on considère que seuls environ 30 % des patients sont opérables lors du diagnostic.

Selon les auteurs, le critère pronostique de survie reste la possibilité d'une exérèse chirurgicale, bien que celle-ci ne soit pas toujours satisfaisante sur le plan carcinologique, comme en témoigne la fréquence des récidives et des métastases dans les deux ans suivants l'exérèse (Merlier et coll., 1981) et la surmortalité liée au cancer au-delà de 15 ans après l'acte chirurgical (Silbert et coll., 1981).

Nous avons préalablement montré qu'une chimiothérapie d'induction était réalisable dans le traitement des cancers bronchiques NAPC opérables (Clavier et coll., 1985 ; Zabbé et coll., 1986) et se justifiait par la stagnation des résultats obtenus dans le traitement de cette maladie par l'association chirurgie - radiothérapie.

La justification d'une chimiothérapie précoce s'appuie sur la nécessité de contrôler, lors de la découverte du cancer, le potentiel de récidives et de métastases d'une tumeur même considérée comme initialement opérable et l'importance d'agir sur de petites tumeurs (Greenspan, 1982 afin d'éviter l'apparition de lignées cellulaires résistantes (Goldie and coll., 1979). Une fraction constante de la masse tumorale étant détruite par chaque chimiothérapie, il paraît logique d'introduire ce traitement avant l'exérèse chirurgicale (Skipper and coll., 1964 ; Papaionnou, 1985).

Beaucoup de cancers bronchiques NAPC sont considérés comme inopérables du fait de l'extension loco-régionale de la maladie. Une chimiothérapie cytoréductrice peut permettre dans certains cas une chirurgie seconde (Morere and coll., 1985) et peut-être une augmentation de la survie de ces patients.

Notre étude rétrospective confirme la faisabilité d'une telle attitude sans augmentation notable du risque thérapeutique. Cette cytoréduction permet l'institution en seconde intention d'un traitmeent loco-régional. Actuellement cette orientation thérapeutique semble intéressente en association avec une radiothérapie (Hiroschitakita and coll., 1986) et semble apporter un bénéfice de survie pour ces patients.

Nous pensons qu'une attitude semblable intègrant une chirurgie après la chimiothérapie puisse apporter un bénéfice thérapeutique pour certains patients présentant une indication opératoire limite du fait de l'extension locale de la tumeur. De plus, elle laisse possible dans tous les cas la décision d'une radiothérapie de clôture soit d'emblée, soit différée en cas de reprise évolutive du cancer.

CONCLUSION

Les chimiothérapies à base de DDP permettent d'obtenir un nombre non négligeable de réponses chez les patients porteurs de cancers bronchiques non à petites cellules.

L'utilisation de telles chimiothérapies en première intention permet chez certains patients une exérèse chirurgicale complète d'une tumeur primitive considérée initialement inopérable.

Notre étude rétrospective le confirme, sans cependant pouvoir affirmer ici qu'il existe un bénéfice de survie pour ces patients.

REFERENCES BIBLIOGRAPHIQUES

Aisner J., Hansen H.H. (1981) : Commentary : current status of chemotherapy for non small cell lung cancer. Cancer Treat. Rep., 65, 979-986.

Belpomme D., Gautier H., Chastang C. (1983) : Cancers bronchiques primitifs inopérables : traitements par combinaisons chimiothérapiques incluant le cis-platinum. Nouv. Pres. Med., 12, 2671-2675.

Bergsagel D.E., Jenkin R.D.T., Pringle J.F. et al. (1972) : Lung cancer : clinical trial of radiotherapy alone VS. Radiothérapie plus cyclophosphamide. Cancer, 30, 621-627.

Classification TNM (1982). UICC Technical reports series, Vol 51 TNM. Classification of Malignant Tumors, Edition 1980, revised 1982.

Clavier J., Zabbé Cl., Raut Y., et coll. (1986) : Chimiothérapie pré-opératoire dans le cancer bronchique épidermoïde. Résultats d'une étude pilote portant sur 60 patients. Neo-adjuvant chemotherapy. Colloque INSERM, vol 137, 473-478.

Cormier Y., Bergeron D., La Forge J., et coll. (198) : Benefits of polychemotherapy in advanced non small cell bronchogenic carcinoma. Cancer, 50, 845-849.

Goldie J.H., Coldman A.J. (1979) : A mathematic model for relating the drug sensibility of tumors to their spontaneous mutation rate. Cancer Treat. Rep., 63, 1727-1733.

Gralla R.J., Casper E.S., Kebsen D.P. (1980) : Vindesine and cisplatin combination chemotherapy in non small cell lung cancer. In Hansen H.H., Dombernosky (Eds) : Abstract I. World Conference on Lung Cancer, 229. Copenhagea Excerpto Medica 1980.

Hansen H.H., Dambernowsky P., Hansen H. et coll. (1979) : Chemotherapy versus chemotherapy plus radiotherapy, in regional small cell lung carcinoma of the lung. A randomized trial. Proc. Am. Assoc. Cancer. Res., 20, 277-280.

Hasley H.F., Marangoudakis S., Ross C.A. et al. (1962) : Combined radiation chemo-therapy for bronchogenic carcinoma. Cancer Chemother. Rep., 16, 467-471.

Hiroshitakita, MD, REGAL A.M., MD, Antkoxiat J.G., MD, Uma N.H. Rao, MD, Nilolaos K., MD, Warren W. Lane (1986) : Chemotherapy followed by lung resection in inoperable non-small cell lung carcinomas due to locally far advanced disease. Cancer, 57, 630-635.

Le Chevalier T., Arriagada R., Baldeynou P. et coll. (1985) : combined chemotherapy (Vindesine, Lomustine, Cisplatin and cyclophosphamide) and radical radiotherapy in inoperable non metastatic squamous cell carcinoma of the lung. Cancer Treat. Rep. 69, 469-472.

Merlier, Le Brigand, Rojas-Mirandas, Levasseur, Dartevelle, Wapler, Pesle, Gharbi, Menella, Serrano, Silbert (1981) : Généralités sur la survie éloignée des exérèses pulmonaires des cancers bronchiques primitifs (anaplasiques exclus). Rev. Fr. Mal. Resp., 9, 493.

Morere J.F., Israël L., Breau J.L., Clavier J., Guillerm D., Zabbé Cl., Raut Y., Morere P., Nouvet G., Lorebours-Pigeonniere G., Gres J.J., David P. (1985) : Pre-operative chemotherapy in epidermoïd bronchogenic carcinoma. Drugs Expt.Clin. Res., 11, 233-235.

Papaionnou A.N. (1985) : Preoperative chemotherapy : advantages and clinical application in stage III. Breast cancer, in Recent Results in Cancer Research, vol 98, Springer Verla. Ed.

Silbert D., Merlier M. (1981) : Mortalité et surmortalité des cancers bronchiques primitifs opérés après dix ans de survie. Rev. Fr. Mal. Resp., 9, 521.

Skipper H.E., Schabel F.M. Jr, Wilcox W.S., (1964) : Experimental evaluation of potential anticancer agents. XIII : on the criteria and kinetics associated with "curability" of experimental leukemia. Cancer Chemoth. Rep., 35, 1-111.

Zabbé Cl., Khayat D., Gouva S., Kerbourc'H J.F., Jacquillat Cl., Clavier J. (1986) : Cisplatine, Bléomycine et 5 Fluoro-Uracile (CBF) en traitement pré-opératoire du cancer bronchique épidermoïde.Neo-Adjuvant chemotherapy. Colloque INSERM, vol 137, 501-506.

Résumé

We know that the only efficient treatment in non small cell lung carcinoma (NSCLC) is surgery. So it seems important to increase the number of operable patients.
23 patients with initialy inoperable NSCLC (19 stage III, 4 stage IV) were operated on after chemotherapy with cisplatinum. On average, each patient was operated on after 3 courses of chemotherapy.
We noted 1 complete response
18 partial responses > 50 %
4 minor responses
Surgery consisted of 9 pneumonectomies and 14 lobectomies. Toxicity was moderated.
Results : 10 patients died (due to metastasis or local recurrence in 3 cases)
13 patients are still alive and disease free.
The survival median rate is 24 months for all patients, 29 for alive patients.
We conclude that it seems logical to systematically use chemotherapy in previously unoperable cases to initially try to decrease the dimension of the tumor and to allow surgery, therefor making treatment possible for a greater number of patients and perhaps improving prognosis for some of them.

Urology I

Urologie I

Neo-Adjuvant Chemotherapy. Ed. Cl. Jacquillat, M. Weil, D. Khayat. Colloque INSERM/John Libbey Eurotext Ltd. © 1988. Vol. 169, pp. 399-403.

Upfront chemotherapy in invasive transitional cell carcinoma of the bladder : some considerations about the goals of upfront chemotherapy and the value of the response of the primary tumour

T.A.W. Splinter

Dept. of Medical Oncology, University Hospital Dijkzigt, 3015 GD Rotterdam, The Netherlands

ABSTRACT

The two major items for research in upfront chemotherapy of invasive transitional cell carcinoma of the bladder (TCCB) are local tumor control plus bladder preservation and secondly improvement of survival. These goals should be investigated in different and separate trials. From several studies data become available to indicate that the response of the primary tumor may have a strong prognostic value i.e. especially the prognosis of the non-responder seems to be very poor. Such data may become a very strong argument to use different kinds of loco-regional therapy in responding- and non-responding patients.

KEYWORDS

invasive transitional cell carcinoma of the bladder, upfront chemotherapy.

INTRODUCTION

Recently it has been shown that several Cisplatin based chemotherapy regimes can induce major responses in 50 percent or more of patients with advanced transitional cell carcinoma of the bladder (TCCB) (Carmichael, 1985; Harker, 1985; Hrushesky, 1987; Sternberg, 1986; Stoter, 1987). Interestingly a complete response (CR) rate according to WHO-criteria of approx. 25 percent is observed in all these studies and a median survival for complete responders of 18 (Stoter, 1987) to more than 36 months (Sternberg, 1986). An important observation is the lack of a survival difference between patients with a partial remission or no change (Hrushesky, 1987; Stoter, 1987), which suggests that an improvement of survival is probably achieved only in case of a CR. These results have raised much enthusiasm to try and improve the 10 - 45 percent five-year survival of patients with invasive TCCB (Whitmore,1979; Skinner, 1984) with chemotherapy. Unanimously all over the world the choice was made to use chemotherapy upfront. One reason may have been that Einstein (1984) have shown that after a cystectomy even Cisplatin alone was badly tolerated. The most important reason probably is that most investigators want to kill two birds with one stone i.e. killing micrometastases and preserve the bladder, which is methodologically very difficult to investigate in one trial. Several studies on chemotherapy in invasive TCCB have now been published or are in press, which have shown that this kind of treatment is feasible and can induce downstaging even to pathological complete remissions (Raghavan,

1985; Meyers, 1985; Denis, 1986; Veronesi, 1986; Fossa, 1987; Vogelzang, 1987; Fagg, 1984; Kaye, 1985; Maatman, 1986; Lee, 1987; Simon, 1986; Bukowski, 1987; Clyne, 1983; Logothetis, 1985; Scher, 1988; Splinter, 1988). All these studies were non-randomized phase II studies and can therefore never answer the question whether the survival of the patients is improved. As shown by the contributions to this conference a lot more phase II studies will follow, which probably will not add much to the already available knowledge. Instead there is a great need for cooperative studies to investigate whether and how upfront chemotherapy may lead to bladder preservation and at least the same survival as achieved by radical surgery. Secondly it should be investigated whether upfront chemotherapy may improve survival.
Since these goals of upfront chemotherapy should be tested in different and separate trials with different endpoints, I want to introduce the following definitions of upfront chemotherapy.

SUBJECTS AND METHODS

Definitions of the different goals of upfront chemotherapy

I Neoadjuvant chemotherapy is upfront chemotherapy, aimed at killing micrometastases. The method to prove its efficacy is a randomized phase III trial, in which chemotherapy is added to standard locoregional treatment. The endpoint is survival .

II Additional chemotherapy is upfront chemotherapy to improve resectability and/or response to radiotherapy, aimed at local tumor control and organ preservation. The method to prove its efficacy is a phase II or probably a randomized phase II trial. The endpoint is local tumor control.

III Definitive chemotherapy is upfront chemotherapy as the main treatment, aimed at cure of the primary tumor and micrometastases. Endpoints are local tumor control and survival. Other treatment modalities are either adjuvant or additional.

Value of the response of the primary tumor to upfront chemotherapy

By using upfront chemotherapy and measuring the response clinically and/or pathologically the distinction is introduced of responders and non-responders. As expected the behaviour of the doctor and/or the patients is influenced by this distinction and may make a consistent performance of a study difficult.

Table 1. EORTC 30851: DEFINITIVE RESPONSE AFTER CHEMOTHERAPY (N = 51)

pCR 6	pPR 3	pSD 22		61%
cCR 8	cPR 5	cSD 2	cPD 5	39%
27,5%	15,5%	57%		

In table I the response of the primary tumor to a combination of Cisplatin and Methotrexate, as observed in the ongoing EORTC-study 08825 is shown. Sixty percent of the patients were pathologically evaluated and 40 percent only clinically. Of the pathologically evaluated patients 29 percent had a major response and of the clinically evaluated patients 65 percent had a major response. The difference seems to indicate that the responsible urologist is obviously making a subjective choice concerning the type of locoregional treatment in favour of no cystectomy in non-responders.
In 1986 20 patients with invasive TCCB, who had been treated with Cisplatin and Methotrexate followed by a radical cystectomy, were randomly selected. There were

10 patients with a pathological CR or PR (responders) and 10 patients with unchanged invasive cancer (non-responders). Median follow-up of the responding patients is 18 months (range 15 - 24) and of the non-responding patients 17 months (range 10 - 37). Of the responders 7 patients have NED, 1 died, 2 relapsed. Of the non-responders 3 have NED, 7 died. All patients died of malignant disease.
At the recent Heinrich Warner Symposium on bladder cancer the updated results on upfront chemotherapy were presented by Herr from Memorial Sloan Kettering Cancer Center in New York, Denis from Antwerp and Freiha from Stanford University. Herr presented 30 pathologically evaluated patients. Nine patients had a pCR and the remaining 21 patients were made tumor free by radical cystectomy. All 9 patients were NED, 12 of the remaining 21 patients were dead. No information was available on duration of follow-up. Denis showed 24 pathologically evaluated patients with a follow-up of 18 - 48 months. Eleven of 14 patients with a major response were NED and 9 of 10 non-responding patients had died. Freiha, who had used upfront chemotherapy in patients with T4 and/or N+ bladder cancer, presented 36 pathologically evaluated patients. All 24 non-responders had died, whereas 11 of 12 responders were still alive. These preliminary data seem to indicate that non-responders have a very poor prognosis. Therefore in the future, when the data about the fate of the non-responding patients are larger and more mature, the subjective choice of the urologist for the type of locoregional treatment after upfront chemotherapy may have to be changed drastically. These data will also be very important for the design of future trials to investigate the efficacy of upfront chemotherapy as neoadjuvant - or additional chemotherapy.
The EORTC-GU group has therefore decided to continue the ongoing phase II study in order to learn more about the prognosis of responders and non-responders before embarking on a randomized trial.

CONCLUSIONS

The different goals of upfront chemotherapy in invasive TCCB should be investigated in different and seperate trials with different endpoints.
The probably strong relationship between the response of the primary tumor and survival may become a very strong argument to use different kinds of locoregional therapy in responding- and non-responding patients.
N.B.
Better survival of responders does not prove the efficacy of upfront chemotherapy!

REFERENCES

Bukowski RM, Montie JE, Pontes EJ (1987): Neoadjuvant chemotherapy of locally advanced transitional cell carcinoma of the bladder. Results of a phase II trial and follow up. ASCO Proc 6, 108.

Carmichael, J, Cornbleet MA, MacDougall RM, Allan SG, Duncan W, Chrisholm GD, Smyth JF (1985): Cisplatin and Methotrexate in the treatment of transitional cell carcinoma of the urinary tract. Br J Urol 57: 299 - 302.

Clyne CHC, Jenkins JD, Smart CJ, Guthrie J, Buchanan RB (1983): A trial of adjuvant chemotherapy for stage T_3 bladder tumors. J Urol 129, 736 - 737.

Denis L, Hendrickx G, Keuppens F (1986): Preoperative chemotherapy $T_{3/4}$ N_x M_0 bladder cancer. J Urol 135, 222A

Einstein A, Shipley W, Coombs J, Cummings K, Hawkins I, Prout G (1984): Randomized controlled trial of Cisplatin (DDP) following preoperative radiotherapy plus radical cystectomy (RT + R Cy) for invasive bladder carcinoma: a national bladder cancer collaborative group. A (NBCCGA) study. ASCO Proc 3: 154.

Fagg SL, Dawson-Edwards P, Hughes MA, Latief TN, Rolfe EB, Fielding JWL (1984): Cis-diammine dichloroplatinum (DDP) as initial treatment of invasive bladder cancer. Br J Urol 56, 296 - 300

Harker WG, Meyers FJ, Freiha FS, Palmer JM, Shortliffe LD, Hanningan JF, McWhirter KM, Torti FM, (1985): Cisplatin, Methotrexate and Vinblastine (CMV): an effective chemotherapy regimen for metastatic transitional cell carcinoma of the urinary tract. A Northern California Oncology Group Study. J Clin Oncol 3, 1463 - 1470.

Hrushesky WJM, Roemeling RV, Wood PA Langevin TR, Lange P, Farley E (1987). High-dose intensity systemic therapy of metastatic bladder cancer. J Clin Oncol 5, 450 - 455.

Kaye SB, MacFarlane JR, McHattie I,Hart AJL (1985): Chemotherapy before radiotherapy for T_3 bladder cancer. A pilot study. Br J Urol 57, 434 - 437.

Lee ML, Bukowski RM, Montie JE, Pontes R, Ganapathi R, Budd GT (1987): Adjuvant M-VAC with intra-arterial (I.A.) Cisplatin (CDDP) in locally advanced transitional cell carcinoma of the bladder. AACR Proc 28, 191.

Logothetis CJ, Samuels ML, Selig DE, Wallace S, Johnson DE (1985): Combined intravenous and intra-arterial Cyclophosphamide, Doxorubicin and Cisplatin (CISCA) in the management of select patients with invasive urothelial tumors. Cancer Treat Rep 69, 33 - 38.

Maatman TJ, Montie JE, Bukowski RM, Risius B, Geisinger M (1986): Intra-arterial chemotherapy as an adjuvant to surgery in transitional cell carcinoma of the bladder. J Urol 135, 256 - 260.

Meyers FJ, Palmer JM, Freiha FS,Harker EG, Shortliffe LD, Hannigan J, McWhirter K, Torti FM (1985): The fate of the bladder in patients with metastatic bladder cancer treated with Cisplatin, Methotrexate and Vinblastine: a Northern California Oncology group study. J Urol 134, 1118 - 1121.

Raghavan D, Pearson B, Duval P Rogers J, Meagher M, Wines R, Mameghan H, Boulas J, Green D (1985): Initial intravenous cisplatinum therapy: improved management for invasive high risk bladder cancer? J Urol 133, 399 - 402.

Scher H, Yagoda A, Herr H. Sternberg C, Bosl G, Morse M, Sogani P, Watson R, Dershaw DD, Reuter V, Geller N, Hollander P, Darracott Vaughan Jr. E, Whithmore W, Fair W (1988): Neo-adjuvant M-VAC (Methotrexate, Vinblastine, Adriamycin and Cisplatin): effect on the primary bladder lesion. J Urol. In press.

Simon SD, Srougi M. (1986): Systemic M-VAC chemotherapy for primary treatment of locally invasive transitional cell carcinoma of the bladder (TCCB): A pilot study. ASCO Proc 5, 111.

Skinner DG, Lieskovsky G (1984): Contemporary cystectomy with pelvic node dissection compared to preoperative radiation therapy plus cystectomy in the management of invasive bladder cancer. J. Urol 131, 1069 - 1072.

Splinter TAW, Schröder FH, Denis L, Newling D, Jacqmin D, Hall RR, de Pauw M for the EORTC-GU Group (1988a): A phase II study of neoadjuvant chemotherapy in T_{3-4} N_{0-x} M_0 transitional cell carcinoma of the bladder. A preliminary analysis. Eur Urol. In press.

Splinter TAW, ten Kate FJW, Schröder FH, Denis L, Newling D, Jacqmin D, Hall RR, de Pauw M (1988b): Neoadjuvant chemotherapy in T_{3-4} N_{o-x} M_o transitional cell carcinoma of the bladder. Problems of clinical and pathological evaluation of response. In Schröder FH etal (eds): "Progress and Controversies in Urological Oncology II," New York: Alan R. Liss Inc., In press.

Sternberg CN, Yagoda A, Scherr HI, (1988): M-VAC: Methotrexate (MTX), Vinblastine (VLB), Adriamycin (ADM) and Cisplatin (DDP) for metastastic and node positive carcinoma of the urothelium. Workshop on the treatment of advanced bladder cancer, Erice, Sicily. In press.

Stoter G, Splinter TAW, Child JA, Fossa SD, Denis L, Boven E, van Oosterom AT, de Pauw M, Sylvester R (1987). Combination chemotherapy with Cisplatin and Methotrexate in advanced transitional cell cancer of the bladder. J Urol 137, 663 - 667.

Veronesi A, Galligioni E, Lo Re G, Sorio R, Saracchini S, Francini M, Merlo A, Dal Bo V, Monfardini S (1986): Combination chemotherapy with Fluorouracil, Adriamycin, Cisplatinum and Vm-26 in advanced transitional cell carcinoma of the urinary tract. Eur J Cancer Clin Oncol 22, 1457 - 1460.

Vogelzang NJ, Chodak GW, Awan AM, Ruane M, Straus FH, Schoenberg HW (1987): Neoadjuvant chemotherapy for locally invasive transitional cell carcinoma of the bladder (TCCB). AACR Proc 28, 204

Whitmore WF, (1979): Management of bladder cancer. Curr Probl Cancer 4: 1 - 48.

Résumé

Les deux objets de recherche de la chimiothérapie d'emblée dans les cancers transitionnels invasifs de la vessie sont le contrôle de la tumeur locale avec conservation de la vessie et en second lieu l'amélioration de la survie. Ces buts devraient être étudiés dans des études différentes et séparées. A partir de différentes études nous commençons à avoir des documents qui montrent que la réponse à la tumeur primaire peut avoir une forte valeur pronostique et en particulier le pronostic des non-répondeurs semble très mauvais. Ces données peuvent devenir un argument très fort pour utiliser différentes sorte de traitements loco-régionaux selon qu'il s'agit de malade répondeur ou non-répondeur.

Neo-Adjuvant Chemotherapy. Ed. Cl. Jacquillat, M. Weil, D. Khayat. Colloque INSERM/John Libbey Eurotext Ltd. © 1988. Vol. 169, pp. 405-409.

Pilot phase II trial of pre- and postoperative cisplatin, methotrexate and vinblastine in infiltrating bladder cancer : preliminary results

J.P. Droz, M.B. Azab, J.M. Caillaud, M. Ghosn, B.H. Court, J.L. Perrin, J.P. Travagli and P. Wibault

Institut Gustave-Roussy, 94805 Villejuif, France

ABSTRACT

From 9.1986 to 12.1987, 28 patients (pts) with infiltrating bladder cancer were treated by chemotherapy (CT) and radical surgery (RS) with bilateral pelvic lymph node dissection ± radiotherapy (RT). Sex distribution was 26 M/2F, mean age was 60 years (range 42-71). All pts had transitional cell carcinoma with muscular invasion after the pretreatment work-up. CT consisted of 2 pre-operative (OP) and 4 post OP courses of cisplatin (C) 70 mg/sqm d1, methotrexate (M) 30 mg/sqm D1, 15 and vinblastine (V) 3 mg/sqm d1, 15 Q 4 weeks. Until 12.1987, 26 pts received the pre OP CT while 2 pts are still ongoing. 23 pts were submitted to RS. The pathologic staging showed no tumor in 8 pts, stage A in 3 pts, B in 8, C in 2 and D1 in 2. Thus 11/23 pts (48 %) were downstaged. 15/23 pts (65 %) had evidence of fibrosis. Of the 23 operated pts, 11 completed the post OP CT of whom 3 pts also received 45 Gy whole pelvis RT between the second and the third post OP cycles due to perivesical fat infiltration. 6/28 pts discontinued the protocol : 1 pt refused surgery, 1 was lost to follow up, 1 died of acute hepatitis before surgery, 1 had an important post OP morbidity, 1 had an early post OP death and finally 1 pt was taken off study due to protocol violation. All remaining 22 pts are still alive with no evidence of disease except for one pt who died of an important peritoneal recurrence with intestinal fistula on top of radiation enteritis. CT was well tolerated with only 1 pt experiencing a grade 4 toxicity however 2 of the 3 pts who received post OP RT developed radiation enteritis.

We concluded that pre OP CT is effective in downstaging infltrating bladder cancer with minimal toxicity. Post OP CT ± RT is feasible but its effect on the overall and disease free survival rates is still to be evaluated with longer follow up.

KEYWORDS

Bladder cancer, Neoadjuvant chemotherapy, Clinical trial, Cisplatin, Methotrexate, Vinblastine.

INTRODUCTION

Bladder cancer is a common malignancy in a population of patients in the fifth to seventh decades and the standard treatment of invasive forms is still radical surgery with or without radiotherapy. The main histological type of bladder cancer in western countries is urothelial transitional cell carcinoma and the depth of penetration into the bladder wall can be staged according to the Jewett-Marshall classification (Marshall, 1952). In stage B and C the 5-year survival rate is around 30 % - 50 % after radical surgery with or without preoperative radiotherapy ((Blandy, 1980 ; Montie et coll., 1984). Modern regimens of chemotherapy (CT) as CISCA (Logothetis et coll., 1985), CMV (Harker et coll., 1985), and M-VAC (Sternberg et coll., 1985) have shown a high objective response rate (50 % - 70 %). The introduction of preoperative CT could decrease the risk of local recurrence and/or distant metastases after radical surgery. Furthermore, regimens with high complete remission rate like M-VAC combined or not with radiotherpy could eventually permit bladder conservation. We hereby report the preliminary results of a multimodality treatment protocol for invasive bladder cancer using pre- and postoperative CT.

PATIENTS AND METHODS

From September 1986 to December 1987, 28 pts were included in this pilot study. Patients were 26 males and 2 females with a mean age of 60 years (range 42-71). Initial work-up included cystoscopy with multiple biopsies, IVP, abdominal and pelvic CAT scan, chest X-ray, hematologic and blood chemistry profiles. All pts had a histologically proven urothelial bladder carcinoma with muscular infiltration, one pt had enlarged pelvic lymph nodes on the pretreatment scan. Other criteria of eligibility included age <75 years, performance status ≤ 2, serum creatinine level <120 micmol/l and normal blood counts.

Treatment protocol consisted of two preoperative and four postoperative cycles of cisplatin (C) 70 mg/sqm day 1 with over hydratation and forced diuresis, methotrexate (M) 30 mg/sqm days 1 and 15, vinblastine 3 mg/sqm days 1 and 15 every 4 weeks. Chemotherapy was administered when white blood counts were more than 2000/mm^3 and platelets more than 100.000/mm^3. Radical surgery was prostatocystectomy in men, anterior pelvectomy in women, in both cases associated with bilateral pelvic lymph node dissection. Radiotherapy was indicated only in patients with stage C or D1, 45 Gy in 18 fractions over 4 weeks and a half were given to the whole pelvis between the 2nd and 3rd postoperative CT cycles. Patients finishing the treatment were followed every 2 months with clinical, radiological and biological examinations.

RESULTS

Treatment actually received in the preoperative period is shown in Table I.

Table I. Preoperative treatment in 28 pts with invasive bladder cancer

2 pts	On going preoperative CT
1 pt (4 CMV)	Refused surgery
1 pt (2 CMV)	Lost to follow up
1 pt (2 CMV)	Died of acute hepatitis before surgery
23 pts (2 CMV)	Submitted to radical surgery

Results of pathologic staging are shown in Table II.

Table II. Pathologic staging in 23 operated pts with invasive bladder cancer

8 pts	No residual tumor
3 pts	p stage A
11/23 (48 %)	downstaging
8 pts	p stage B
2 pts	p stage C
2 pts	p stage D1
15/23 (65 %)	Post chemotherapy fibrosis

The evolution of the 23 operated patients is given in Table III.

Table III. Post operative treatment in 23 operated pts with invasive bladder cancer

1 pt (2 CMV)	Refused further CT
3 pts (no CT)	1 postoperative death
	1 postoperative morbidity
	1 protocol violation
9 pts (on going CT)	
10 pts (4 CMV)	of whom 3 had radiotherapy

The mean follow up is 7 months (range 1 - 15m). One patient had a peritoneal relapse, none developed distant metastases. Twenty four pts are alive with no evidence of disease, one pt was lost to follow up and 3 pts died (1 acute hepatitis, 1 postoperative complication, 1 peritoneal relapse with intestinal fistula and radiation enteritis). The major side effects of treatment are shown in Table IV.

Table IV. Treatment complications

Chemotherapy		
Nausea - vomiting (grade 2 - 3)	28/28	100 %
Mucositis (grade 1 - 2)	5/28	18 %
Neutropenia (grade 1, 2 and 4)	3/28	11 %
Neuropathy (grade 1)	2/28	7 %
Acute viral hepatitis	1 pt	
Surgery		
(Enterocystoplasty : 7, Bricker : 11, Ureterostomy : 4, Coffey : 1)		
Impotence	20/20 (3 operated pts were females)	
Nocturnal incontinence	7/7	
Diurnal incontinence	0/7	
Septicemia and Renal failure	1/23	
Death (septicemia)	1/23	
Radiotherapy		
Radiation enteritis	2/3	

DISCUSSION

About 50 % of pts with stages B and C bladder cancer will develop distant metastases within 2 years after local treatment. Survival is even worse for stage D1 pts. Modern multiagent CT regimens have shown a high rate of complete remission in advanced or metastatic bladder cancer. In one study 50 % of complete responses were confirmed by cystectomy (Sternberg et coll., 1985). The M-VAC regimen was used as a neoadjuvant CT with encouraging preliminary results since 33 % of pts had a pathologic complete response (Scher et coll., 1987). Similar promising results of neoadjuvant CT were obtained using cisplatin (Raghavan, 1985) or CMV regimen (Meyers et coll., 1985). Our preliminary results are in accordance with those reported in the literature. Downstaging was observed in 11/23 pts (48 %) of whom 8 pts had a pathologic complete response (35 %). However more follow up and randomized studies are needed to prove the beneficial influence of this approach on the overall and disease free survival rates of pts with invasive bladder cancer.

CONCLUSION

A multimodality treatment program with pre- and postoperative CT for invasive bladder cancer is feasible. Preoperative CMV regimen is effetive and produces 48 % of downstaging with acceptable toxicity. Postoperative radiotherapy may have to be re-evaluated in this protocol due to important toxicity in this preliminary evaluation, however the number of pts who received radiotherapy is very small. It should be pointed out that only randomized clinical trials with long term follow up will determine the place of neoadjuvant CT in the treatment arsenal of invasive bladder cancer.

REFERENCES

Blandy, J.P. ; England, H.R. ; Evans, S.J.W. et coll. (1980) : T3 bladder cancer. The case for salvage cystectomy. Br J. Urol 52, 506-510.

Harker, W.G. ; Meyers, F.J. ; Freiha, F.S. et coll. (1985) : Cisplatin, Methotrexate, and Vinblastine (CMV) : an effective chemotherapy regimen for metastatic Transitional cell Carcinoma of the urinary treat. J. Clin. Oncol. 3, 1463-1470.

Logothetis, C. ; Samuels, M.L., Ogden, S. et coll. (1985) : Cyclophosphamide, doxorubicin and cisplatin chemotherapy for patients with locally advanced urothelial tumors with or without nodal metasases. J. Urol. 134, 460-464.

Marshall, V.F. (1952) : The relation of the preoperative estimate to the pathologic demonstration of the extent of vesical neoplasms. J. Urol. 68, 714-721.

Meyers, F.J. ; Palmer, J.M. ; Freiha F.S. et coll. (1985) : The fate of the bladder in patients with metastatic bladder cancer treated with cisplatin, methotrexate and vinblastine : A Northern California Oncology Group Study. J. Urol. 134, 1118-1121.

Montie, J.E. ; Straffon, R.A. & Stewart, B.H. (1984) : Radical cystectomy without radiation therapy for carcinoma of the bladder. J. Urol. 131, 477-482.

Raghavan, D. (1985) : First line intravenous cisplatinum for invasive clinically nonmetastatic bladder cancer. In Genitourinary cancer, ed M.B. Garnick, pp 193-207. New York, Churchill Livingstone.

Scher, H. ; Reuter, V. ; Sternberg, C. et coll. (1987) : Pathologic response to M-VAC (Methotrexate, Vinblastine, Adriamycin and Cisplatin) in urothelial tract tumors. Proc. Am. Soc. Clin. Oncol. 6, 105.

Sternberg, C.N. ; Yagoda, A. ; Scher, H.I. et coll. (1985) : Preliminary results of M-VAC for transitional cell carcinoma of the urothelium. J. Urol. 133, 403-407.

Résumé

Du 9.1986 au 12.1987, 28 pts présentant un cancer infiltrant de la vessie sont inclus dans un essai pilote non randomisé de combinaison d'une chirurgie radicale avec curage ilio-obturateur bilatéral, d'une chimiothérapie (CT) pré- et post-opératoire (OP) ± une irradiation. La CT comportait 2 cycles pré OP et 4 cycles post OP de cisplatinum (C) 70 mg/m^2 J1, méthotrexate (M) 30 mg/m^2 J1, 15, vinblastine (V) 3 mg/m^2 J1, 15 à effectuer toutes les 4 semaines. La radiothérapie (RT) était réservée uniquement aux stades pathologiques C et D1 à une dose de 45 Gy en 4 semaines et demie sur le grand pelvis entre le 2ème et 3ème cycle de la CT post OP. Après un bilan initial par cystoscopie avec biopsies multiples, urographie intraveineuse et scanner abdomino-pelvien tous les malades avaient un cancer de la vessie à cellules transitionnelles infiltrant au moins le muscle vésical. Les malades se répartissaient en 26 hommes et 2 femmes d'âge moyen 60 (42-71 ans). Jusqu'au 12.1987, 26 pts avaient reçu la CT pré OP, 2 pts étaient en cours. 23 pts ont été opérés. Les stades pathologiques étaient : pas de tumeur chez 8 pts, stade A : 3 pts, stade B : 8 pts, stade C : 2 pts, stade D1 : 2 pts. Un effet dit de "downstaging" est donc observé chez 11/23 (48 %) des malades. Une fibrose post-chimiothérapique a été constatée chez 15 pts (65 %). Parmi les 23 malades opérés, 11 avaient fini la CT post OP dont 3 avaient reçu de la RT. 6 malades sur 28 n'ont pas poursuivi le protocole : 1 pt a refusé la chirurgie, 1 pt est perdu de vu, 1 pt est décédé d'une hépatite aiguë avant la chirurgie, 1 pt a eu une morbidité post OP importante (septicémie et insuffisance rénale), un décès post OP et un malade exclu en raison d'une violation du protocole. Les 22 autres malades sont toujours vivants sans rechute sauf 1 malade décédé d'une rechute péritonéale avec une fistule intestinale est un grêle radique. La CT était bien tolérée. Néanmoins tous les malades avaient des nausées et vomissements grade 2-3 (100 %) ; 5/28 (18 %) avaient une mucite grade 1-2 ; 3/28 (11 %) avaient une neutropénie grade 1, 2 et 4 ; et 2 pts (7 %) avaient une neuropathie grade 1. Deux des trois malades irradiés ont développé un grêle radique.

Nous avons conclu que la CT pré OP est efficace (48 % de "downstaging") dans les cancers infiltrants de la vessie. La CT ± RT post OP est faisable mais un recul suffisant est nécessaire pour juger son effet sur la survie globale et la survie sans rechute.

Neo-Adjuvant Chemotherapy. Ed. Cl. Jacquillat, M. Weil, D. Khayat. Colloque INSERM/John Libbey Eurotext Ltd. © 1988. Vol. 169, pp. 411-416.

Neo-adjuvant chemotherapy of invasive bladder cancer by combination of cisplatin and VM 26

P. Chauveau, J.Y. Soret, J.L. Verine and V. Lepinard

Service d'Urologie, CHU, 1 avenue de l'Hôtel Dieu, 49033 Angers Cedex, France

SUMMARY

38 patients with invasive bladder cancer Nx/Mo were treated by neoadjuvant combination of cisplatin 100 mg/m2 and VM 26 60 mg/m2 followed by radical cystectomy (20 patients), partial cystectomy (7 patients) or trans uretral resection (11 patients). The protocol was well tolerated. An objective response histologically proven was noted in 20 patients (53 %) and 8 (21 %) of this 20 patients had a complete response. The 3-year actuarial survival rate was 51 % with a significant difference (p < 0,001) between responders (81 %) and non-responders (25 %).

KEY-WORDS

Bladder, Cancer, Neoadjuvant chemotherapy

INTRODUCTION

Treatment of infiltrating bladder cancer by radical cystectomy with or without preoperative radiotherapy yields actually the most important overall 5-year survival rate of 40 to 50 per cent (only 10 per cent in case of lymph node metastasis) (Whitmore et coll., 1984). Pelvic recurrence rate is less than 10 per cent but nearly 50 per cent of patients die within 2 years of diagnosis by development of distant micrometastasis (Prout et coll., 1979).

Thus localised bladder cancer must be considered as a potential systemic disease. Use of a neoadjuvant chemotherapy seems logical under two conditions : 1) proven efficacy on metastatic bladder cancer (Table I) : cisplatin is considered to be the most active single agent with overall response rates of 30 to 50 per cent (Yagoda, 1984) 2) acceptable toxicity : only 50 per cent of patients are affected in theory and radical pelvic surgery do not be delayed or compromized.

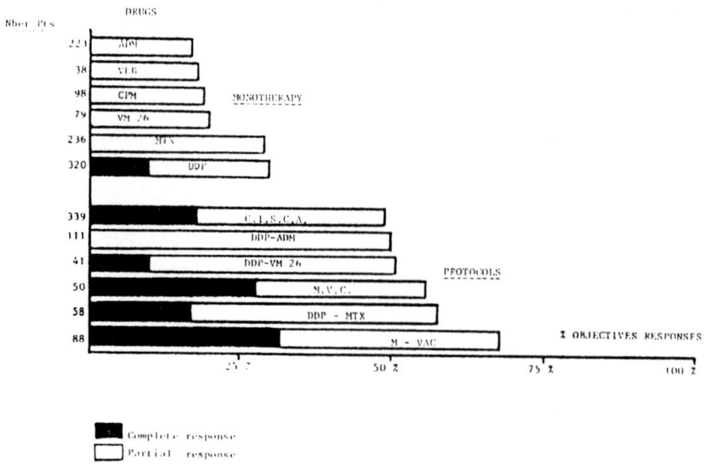

Table I : Results of chemotherapy on metastatic bladder cancer

PATIENTS AND METHODS

38 evaluable patients were entered in this consecutive and homogenous series. There were 32 men and 6 women aged between 52 and 82 years (mean 66) (Table II). All patients had biopsy-proved invasive transitional cell carcinoma (1 grade II and 37 grade III) without evidence of distant metastasis (Nx/Mo). According to the classification of the UICC, 9 patients had stage T1, 17 had stage T2, 11 had stage T3 and 1 had stage T4.

Pre-treatment assessment included physical examination and cystoscopy under anesthesia with a more or less complete biopsy or transurethral resection (TUR) of the tumors, plus randomized biopsies of the bladder, chest X-ray and intravenous urography (IVP). Lymphography, liver ultra-sonography, bone scan and CT scan of the abdomen and pelvis were done inconstantly. Criteria of exclusion included : low performance status, white blood count < 4,000/mm3, platelet count < 100,000/mm3 and serum creatinine level > 120 µmol/l.

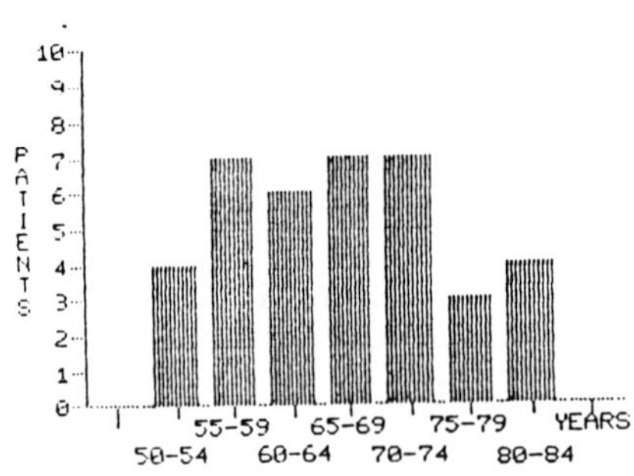

Table II : Age of patients

The chemotherapeutic regimen consisted of two cycles (27 patients) or three cycles (11 patients) of cisplatin (100 mg/m2 day 1) and VM 26 (60 mg/m2 day 2) of 28 days.

One month after the last cycle, assessment of response, according to the WHO criteria, were founded upon comparison between clinical (T) and pathologic (pT) staging, achieved by radical cystectomy with bilateral ilio-obturator lymphadenectomy (20 patients), by partial cystectomy with lymphadenectomy (7 patients), by biopsies or TUR of residual bladder lesions (11 patients).

RESULTS

RESPONSE :

Objective response was noted in 20 patients (53 %) : 8 patients (21 %) achieved a complete response with total disappearance of all lesions including a "target" tumor (in vivo marker), 6 patients achieved a partial response with tumor size decrease ⩾ 50 % and/or down staging, and 6 patients achieved a complete but "relative" response defined by absence of tumor reappearance after complete initial TUR.

SURVIVAL :

No patients were lost to follow up (mean follow up 32 months). The 3-year survival rate calculated by the kaplan-Meier method was 51 % with a very significant difference ($p < 0{,}001$ according to the Logrank Test) between responders (81 %) and non-responders (25 %) (Table III). The 3-year survival rate was 61 % for patients treated by radical cystectomy and 40 % for patients treated by conservative methods (non significant difference) (Table IV).

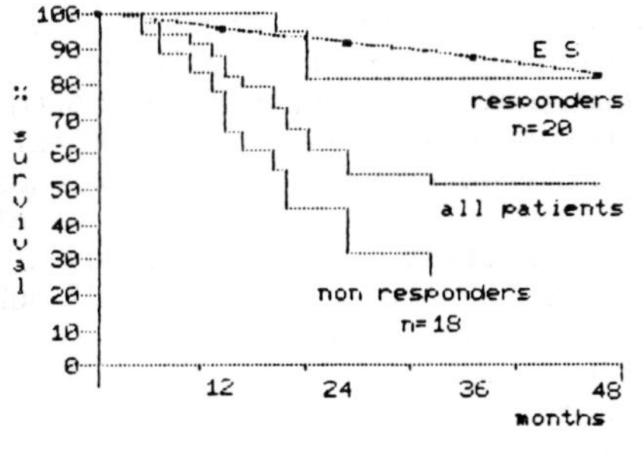

Table III : Actuarial survival related to response

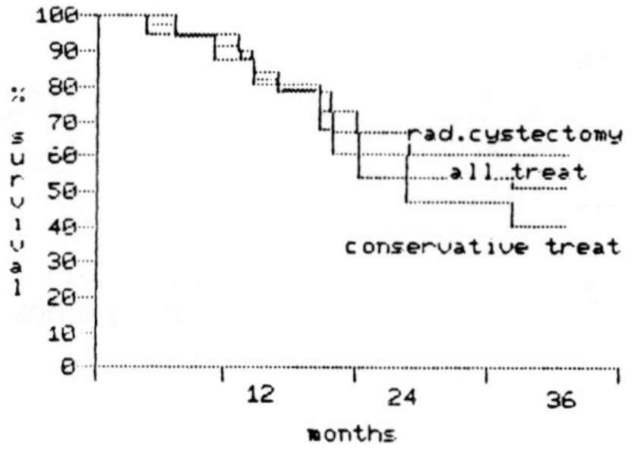

Table IV : Actuarial survival related to surgical treatment

TOXICITY :

The treatment was specially well tolerated, even for elderly patients (Table V). Side effects were more frequent among patients who presented a radiological ureteral obstruction (9/12). There was no deaths related to treatment and no added surgical morbidity (22 % at 1 month and 11 % between 1 and 3 months).

SIDE EFFECTS	Nber Pts
Mortality	0
Major accident	0
Néphrotoxicity (100 < creat < 200 µmol/l)	7
Leucopenia (2,000 < WBC < 4,000/mm3	4
Thrombopenia (50,000 < platelets < 100,000/mm3)	1
Severe Nausea and Vomiting	11
Diarrhoea	7
Alopecia	1
Auditory	0
Peripheric Neuropathy	0
Change or Stop in the protocol	2

Table V : Toxicity

DISCUSSION

Efficacy of this protocol is demonstrated by a 53 % response rate with a 21 % complete response rate. These results seems to confirm the synergism between cisplatin and VM 26 as described in vitro by Burchenal et coll. (1978). Absence of toxicity is the second important result for those patients candidate to extended exeresis. This regimen realised an interesting compromise between efficacy and tolerance with regard to protocols more effective but highly toxic as M-VAC (Sternberg et coll., 1985) or combination Cisplatin-Methotrexate (Oliver et coll., 1986).

It is important to emphasize the difficulties in accurately defining response for localised non measurable bladder cancer. With regard to surgical staging, CT scan is inadequate for assessment of response on the primitive tumor site as on the pelvic lymph nodes. Objectivity of response must be supported by histological downstaging (Table VI) and macroscopic disappearance of a "target" bladder tumor deliberately preserved at initial endoscopic evaluation. Under these conditions, objective response may indicate an adjuvant post operative chemotherapy.

AFTER Chemotherapy / BEFORE	pT0	pTis / pTa	pT1	pT2	pT3	pT4	N+
T1 (n=9)	3	3	3				
T2 (n=17)		3	3	2	5	2	2
T3 (n=11)	3	3	1		3		1
T4 (n=1)							1

(shaded) downstaging

Table VI : Downstaging induced by chemotherapy

Improvement in operability of some locally unresectable bladder cancer showed the importance of a meticulous restaging at critical intervals. In this cases, radical cystectomy must be performed without delay and before relapse which generally occurs after 6 months of remission (Yagoda, 1980).

Response to neoadjuvant chemotherapy is of prognostic value and divided 2 groups : G I of responders with good prognosis (3-year actuarial survival rate of 81 %) as opposed to G II of non-responders with poor prognosis (3-year actuarial survival rate of 25 %)

At long-term, efficacy of this neoadjuvant chemotherapy has still to be demonstrated since the survival data are no better than those which might be achieved by radical cystectomy alone (Skinner et coll., 1984). Survival of responders group seems promising but, for the moment, efficacy of chemotherapy is insufficient to avoid the radical cystectomy which remains the basic treatment of bladder cancer.

REFERENCES

Burchenal (J.H.), Kalaher (K.), Lokys (L.), Gale (G.) (1978) : Studies of cross resistance synergistic combinations and blocking of activity of platinium derivatives. Biochimie. 60, 961-965.

Oliver (R.T.D.), Kwok (H.K.), Highman (W.J.), Waxman (J.) (1986) : Methotrexate, Cisplatin and Carboplatin as single agents and in combination for metastatic bladder cancer. BR. J. Urol., 58, 31-35.

Prout (G.R.), Griffin (P.P.), Shipley (W.V.) 1979 : Bladder carcinoma as a systemic disease. Cancer, 43, 2532-2539.

Raghavan (D.), Pearson (B.), Duval (P.), Rogers (J.), Meagher (M.), Wines (R.), Mameghan (H.), Boulas (J.), Green (D.) (1985) : Initial intravenous cisplatinum therapy : improved management for invasive high risk bladder cancer ?. J. Urol. (Baltimore), 133, 399-402.

Richard (F.), Botto (H.), Plougastel (M.L.), Camey (M.) (1986) : Chimiothérapie néo-adjuvante associée à la cysto-prostatectomie radicale dans les tumeurs urothéliales de vessie. Colloque INSERM, John Libbey Eurotext, 137, 705-709.

Skinner (D.G.), Lieskovsky (G.) (1984) : Contemporary cystectomy with pelvic node dissection compared to pre-operative radiation therapy plus cystectomy in management of invasive bladder cancer. J. Urol. (Baltimore), 131, 1069-1078.

Sternberg (C.N.), Yagoda (A.), Scher (H.I.), Watson (R.L.), Ahmed (T.), Weiselberg (L.R.), Geller (N.), Hollander (P.S.), Herr (H.W.), Sogani (P.C.), Morse (M.J.), Whitmore (W.F.) (1985) : Preliminary results of M. VAC (Methotrexate Vinblastine, Doxor ubicine and Cisplatin) for transitional cell carcinoma of the urothelium. J. Urol. (Baltimore), 133, 403-407.

Whitmore (W.F.), Batata (M.A.) (1984) : Status of integrated irradiation and cystectomy for bladder cancer. Urol. Clin. N. AMER., 11, 4, 681-691.

Yagoda (A.) (1980) : Chemotherapy of metastatic bladder cancer. Cancer, 45, 1879-1888.

Yagoda (A.) (1984) : Progress in chemotherapy for cancers of the urothelium. Urology, 23, supl. 4, 118-123.

Résumé

38 patients porteurs d'un carcinome vésical infiltrant localisé Nx/Mo ont reçu une association néoadjuvante de cisplatine 100 mg/m2 et VM 26 60 mg/m2 avant la cystectomie totale (20 patients), la cystectomie partielle (7 patients) ou la résection transurétrale (11 patients). La tolérance a été excellente. La comparaison histologique montre 20 réponses objectives (53 %) dont 8 réponses complètes (21 %). La survie globale calculée à 3 ans est de 51 % avec une différence très significative ($p < 0{,}001$) entre les "répondeurs" (81 %) et les "non-répondeurs" (25 %).

Urology II

Urologie II

Neo-Adjuvant Chemotherapy. Ed. Cl. Jacquillat, M. Weil, D. Khayat. Colloque INSERM/John Libbey Eurotext Ltd. © 1988. Vol. 169, pp. 419-423.

Neo-adjuvant M-VAC (methotrexate, vinblastine, adriamycin and cisplatin) : for muscle infiltrating bladder cancer

Howard Scher[1], Harry Herr[2], Cora Sternberg[1], George Bosl[1], Michael Morse[2], Pramod Sogani[2], Robin Watson[3], D. David Dershaw[3], Victor Reuter[4], Tracy Curley[1], E. Darracott Vaughan Jr.[5], Willet Whitmore[2], William Fair[2] and Alan Yagoda[1]

(1) Solid Tumor Service, Department of Medicine, (2) Urology Service, Department of Surgery, (3) Department of Medical Imaging, (4) Department of Pathology, Memorial Sloan-Kettering Cancer Center, 1275 York Avenue, New York, N.Y. and (1) Department of Medicine, (5) Division of urology, Department of Surgery, New York N.Y., USA

ABSTRACT

Seventy-one patients with invasive (T2-4NoMo) bladder cancer were given 1-6 (median 3) M-VAC cycles neo-adjuvantly in a pilot phase II evaluation. Pretreatment evaluation included TURB, CT scan and/or sonogram and urinary cytology. Response was noted by a) TURB (To) in 48%, b) cytology in 54%, and c) TURB with other non-invasive procedures in 21% of cases. Twenty-three patients did not have surgical staging, 12 were clinical To; 7 Tis and 4 ≥ T2. Six have required salvage surgery for muscle infiltrating disease, of whom 2 were unresectable. Forty-seven patients had pathological staging: 29 had radical cystectomy, 13 had partial cystectomy and 5 were found to be unresectable. One additional patient died in clinical complete remission ($_C$CR) with no disease at autopsy (PO). Overall, 12 (26%) cases were PO (95% confidence limits 13-38%), 4 had Pis, 1 P1 and 25 residual muscle infiltrating disease. A correlation of clinical and pathologic staging techniques showed that 40/51 (78%) were correctly staged; 7 were clinically understaged and 4 were overstaged. With a median follow-up is 16 months, range 2 to 34+, 18 (25%) are alive with no evidence of disease and a functional bladder; yet one-third of those who had residual disease at surgery that was completely resected have relapsed with metastatic disease. M-VAC can produce significant T-P downstaging and in selected cases bladder preservation may be possible. Based on these data, a prospective randomized trial of M-VAC alone vs. M-VAC plus radiation therapy has been initiated with an endpoint of bladder preservation.

INTRODUCTION

Five year survival for muscle infiltrating bladder tumors range from 10-45%, irrespective of treatment modality,[1,2] with most patients succumbing to metastatic disease. The strategy of chemotherapy as initial therapy provides an in vivo marker of chemosensitivity, where full doses of chemotherapy can generally be used which may be more effective against occult micrometastases. Non-responders can also be considered for alternative treatment. If complete local control is achieved, patients may be spared radical surgical procedures, and possible criteria for bladder preservation can also be identified. Recognizing the poor prognosis of invasive bladder cancer, coupled with the experience using M-VAC (methotrexate, vinblastine, adriamycin, cisplatin) in patients with M+ or N3-4 bladder tumors,[3,4] led to the investigation of M-VAC as initial therapy (neo-adjuvant chemotherapy) in patients with muscle infiltrating tumors.[5]

MATERIALS AND METHODS

Seventy-one patients with T2-4N0M0 bladder tumors received 1-6 (median 3) M-VAC cycles. Entry required adequate hematologic and renal function (creatinine clearance > 55 ml/min/1.73 M^2). Pretreatment evaluation included a bimanual examination under anesthesia, cystoscopy and biopsy, abdominal and pelvic CT scan and/or transabdominal ultrasound, and urine cytology. M-VAC chemotherapy was administered as previously described.[2] Therapeutic efficacy was evaluated by sequential changes in T category, assessed by cystoscopy and biopsy, non-invasive tests (CT scan, ultrasound), urine cytology, and surgical/pathological P evaluation (radical or partial cystectomy or laparotomy with biopsy via the peritoneal aspect of the bladder at the estimated site of the original tumor, and nodal excision, in a few cases selected lymph node dissection). All procedures were not performed in all 71 cases, thus the number evaluable for each parameter varies.

Response criteria incorporated designations suggested by the First International Consensus Development Conference.[6,7] Clinical complete remission ($_C$CR) was defined as the complete disappearance of all evidence of disease by physical examination, normalization of a previously abnormal CT scan and/or transabdominal ultrasound, negative cystoscopy and biopsy, and negative urinary cytology. For assessment of T category only downstaging to T0/Tis was considered significant. In cases where the TURB found no tumor (T0), but non-invasive staging (CT scan and/or transabdominal ultrasound) revealed bladder wall thickening, the patient was classified as a clinical partial remission ($_C$PR). Any response less than complete or partial was classified as incomplete (IR).

The presently accepted standard therapy of T_{2-4} bladder tumors is radical cystectomy, with or without radiation therapy and patients were advised to undergo cystectomy. Since some patients refused surgery because of improvement in clinical symptomatology, and a reluctance of having an ileal conduit with compromise in quality of life, laparotomy with selective lymph node dissection and biopsy of the serosal surface of the bladder was recommended. If residual disease was documented and completely resected, two additional M-VAC cycles were advised. Durations of response and survival were measured from initiation of chemotherapy.

Patient characteristics are outlined in Table 1. Three patients had disease completely resected prior to M-VAC and are not considered for response evaluation. By transurethral resection alone, 48% (32/66) were T0 and 14% (9/66) had Tis, while 54% had normalization of an initially abnormal urinary cytology. When all parameters of response (cystoscopic, cytologic and non-invasive studies) were considered only 21% (14/66) achieved complete ($_c$CR) and 39% (26/66) a partial remission ($_c$PR). The overall response rate [CR+PR] was 60% (95% confidence intervals 49-72%).

Twenty-three patients (12 T0, 7 Tis and 4 ≥ T2 disease) did not undergo surgical restaging immediately after M-VAC. Of 12 with T0, 7 remain disease-free, 1 is receiving intravesical BCG for recurrent CIS at 26 months, 1 died of metastatic disease at 12 months, and 3 required radical cystectomy for new invasive tumors at 23, 24, and 29 months respectively. For those with Tis, 3 are alive with positive cytology at 7, 18 and 22 months respectively, 3 have died of metastatic disease, and 1 remains disease-free after treatment with intravesical BCG at 15 months. Of 4 with residual muscle infiltrating tumors, 3 underwent salvage cystectomy at 11, 12 and 18 months, and 1 is alive with invasive disease at 18 months. For all 23 cases, 6 had salvage cystectomy performed at a median of 21 months (range 11-29) after chemotherapy.

Forty-eight patients had pathological evaluation of the bladder after chemotherapy including one $_c$CR patient who died of a pulmonary embolus after 3 cycles of chemotherapy and was found to have no disease (PO) at autopsy. Of the remaining 47, 29 had a radical cystectomy, 13 partial cystectomy and 5 were unresectable. Overall, 12 (26%) (95% confidence intervals 13-38%) [7 partial and 5 radical cystectomy] were P0, 4 [3 partial and 1 radical] had Pis, 1 had P1 and 25 had residual muscle infiltrating disease [2 partial and 23 radical].

A correlation of the clinical and pathologic responses for all 54 patients is shown in Table 2. Overall 40/51 (78%) were correctly staged and 7 were understaged. Two $_c$CR cases were understaged, one had microscopic P1 disease and the second microscopic disease in a lymph node with a negative bladder. The most difficult group to accurately assess were those in the $_c$PR category, where only 5/13 (38%) were correctly staged. Clinical overstaging was due to persistence of radiographic abnormalities by CT scan and/or transabdominal ultrasound that could not distinguish necrosis, fibrosis and post-operative changes from viable tumor.

Toxicities were similar to that previously reported.[5] The primary toxicity was hematologic which was reversible. One patient, however, died in clinical CR with no disease at autopsy.

With a median follow-up of 16 months (range 2-34+ months), thirty-eight (54%) are alive and free of disease, including 18 (25%) with a functional bladder. Eighteen patients have died, 17 with metastatic disease, and 15 are alive with disease including 7 with localized bladder tumors, 6 with regional nodal disease and 2 with positive margins following salvage cystectomy.

DISCUSSION

The preliminary conclusions from this pilot phase I-II study suggest that M-VAC induces significant tumor regression of invasive bladder tumors, but may not be as efficacious for a) existing T_{is}, b) preventing the development of future *de novo* T_{is} or c) invasive tumors elsewhere in the urothelium, and d) non-transitional cell components. At present, with a median follow-up of 16 months, 18 (25%) are currently alive with a functional bladder suggesting that bladder preservation is a realistic endpoint for future clinical trials. The additional observation of a high rate of relapse in non-responding patients raises the question of the utility salvage surgery. While selected patients can preserve the bladder, the development of new invasive tumors bodes for a poor prognosis; 4/12 T0 cases have developed new muscle infiltrating tumors. Based on these data, a randomized prospective trial comparing M-VAC alone vs. M-VAC plus sequential radiation therapy with an endpoint of bladder preservation has been initiated.

REFERENCES

1. Whitmore, W.F.: Management of bladder cancer. Curr Prob Cancer 4: 3, 1979.
2. Skinner, D.G. and Lieskovsky, G.: Contemporary cystectomy with pelvic node dissection compared to preoperative radiation therapy plus cystectomy in management of invasive bladder cancer. J Urol 131: 1069, 1984.
3. Sternberg, C., Yagoda, A., Scher, H., Watson, R., Ahmed, T., Weiselberg, L., Geller, N., Hollander, P., Herr, H., Sogani, P., Morse, M. and Whitmore, W.: Preliminary results of M-VAC (methotrexate, vinblastine, doxorubicin and cisplatin) for transitional cell carcinoma of the urothelium. J Urol 133: 403, 1985.
4. Sternberg CN, Yagoda A, Scher HI, Watson RC, Herr HW, Morse MJ, Sogani PC, Vaughn ED, Bander N, Weiselberg LR, Geller N, Hollander PS, Lipperman R, Fair WR, Whitmore WF: M-VAC (Methotrexate, vinblastine, adriamycin and cisplatin) for advanced transitional cell carcinoma of the urothelium. J Urol (in press).
5. Scher H, Herr H, Yagoda A, Sternberg C, Bosl G, Morse M, Sogani P, Watson R, Dershaw D, Reuter V, Geller N, Hollander P, Vaughn ED, Whitmore WF, Fair WR: Neoadjuvant M-VAC: Effect on the primary bladder lesion. J Urol (in press).
6. Yagoda, A.: Progress in the treatment of advanced urothelial tract tumors. J Clin Oncol 3: 1448, 1985.
7. Van Oosterom, A.T., Akaza, H., Hall, R., Hirao, Y., Jones, W.G., Matsumara, Y., Raghavan, D., Tannock, I.F. and Yagoda, A.: Response criteria phase II/phase III invasive bladder cancer. In: Denis, L., Nijiim, T., Prout, G., Schroder, F.H.: EORTC Genitourinary Group Monograph 3: Developments in Bladder Cancer. New York, Alan R. Liss, Inc., 1986, 301-310.

TABLE 1: PATIENT CHARACTERISTICS

NO. PATIENTS	71	
AGE, YRS, MEDIAN (Range)	62	(35-78)
SEX, MALE:FEMALE	63:8	
KPS, MEDIAN (Range)	80%	(60-90)
PRE M-VAC CLINICAL STAGE:		
T4	14	(20%)
T3	46	(65%)
T2	10	(14%)
Tis	1	(1%)
RESECTED AT START:	3	(4%)
PATHOLOGY:		
Transitional cell	64	(90%)
Transitional cell + adenocarcinoma	2	(3%)
Transitional cell + prostatic adenocarcinoma	2	(3%)
Transitional cell + squamous cell	2	(3%)
Small cell	1	(1%)

TABLE 2: CORRELATION OF CLINICAL VS. PATHOLOGIC RESPONSE

Clinical Response	Pathological Response No.	$_pCR$	$_pPR$	$_pIR$
$_cCR$	10	8	2	0
$_cPR$	13	3	5	5
$_cIR$	28	0	1	27
TOTAL	51	11	8	32

Dr. Scher and Dr. Sternberg are recipients of American Cancer Society Career Development Awards. Supported by NIH Grant CA-05826, and the Isadore Komanoff and Solid Tumor Service Funds.

Neo-Adjuvant Chemotherapy. Ed. Cl. Jacquillat, M. Weil, D. Khayat. Colloque INSERM/John Libbey Eurotext Ltd. © 1988. Vol. 169, pp. 425-429.

Transurethral resection (TUR) plus adjuvant systemic chemotherapy as the initial treatment for infiltrating bladder tumors (pT2 – T4N × M0)

H. Quintens*, J. Amiel*, A. Thyss**, M. Schneider** and J. Toubol*

** Hôpital Pasteur and ** Centre Antoine-Lacassagne, 06 Nice, France*

ABSTRACT

TRANSURETRAL RESECTION (TUR) AND NEOADJUVANT CHEMOTHERAPY AS PRIMARY TREATMENT FOR pT2-pT4, Nx, M0 BLADDER CANCER

From Sept. 83 to Sept. 86, 20 patients (pts), mean age 65 yr, with a muscle-infiltrating bladder tumor would normally have been treated by total cystectomy. Pts were staged by intravenous urography, pelvic and abdominal CT, physical examination under general anesthesia, and deep TUR, then given neoadjuvant chemotherapy: cisplatinum and 5-FU. Courses were given every 28 days. Results were evaluated after the 3rd and 6th courses by CT, IVP and TUR. 9 pts had a histologically confirmed complete response (pCR: 6 pT2, 2 pT3, 1 pT4). Median follow-up in Jan. 1988 was 30 mo. (17-52). This protocol was objectively active and well tolerated, even by elderly pts. Problems remain concerning pCR pts: (1) the respective roles of chemotherapy and TUR on the outcome ; (2) prevention of recurrence (5/9 pCR).

KEYWORDS
Bladder cancer, neo-adjuvant chemotherapy, transurethral resection (T.U.R.)

INTRODUCTION

The results of combined radiotherapy-surgical treatment of infiltrating and focal bladder cancers (pT2-T4NxM0) are disappointing: survival in the best series is approximately 50% at 5 years. The limitations of locoregional treatment can be partly explained by the fact that at the time of surgery, certain patients already have metastases that will ultimately cause death. Infiltrating bladder cancer (pT2-pT4) thus rapidly appears to be a generalized pathology. The initial treatment must therefore simultaneously include local tumor control and systemic treatment.

PATIENTS AND METHODS

From Sept. 83 to Sept. 86, 20 patients (pts) with an urothelial tumor infiltrating the bladder muscle (pT2-pT4) and focal in nature (NxMO) would generally have been treated by total cystectomy. These pts included 3 women and 17 men with a mean age of 65 yr (range 37-80). These 20 pts were given an initial treatment combining TUR and neo-adjuvant chemotherapy (NEO-AD).

The initial workup included intravenous urography (IVU), abdominal and pelvic computed tomography (APCT), physical examination under general anesthesia and deep TUR of the bladder tumor. Upon completion of the workup, the degree of tumor infiltration and the absence of metastases (M0) were determined. Pelvic lymph node involvement could not be determined accurately because no nodes were sampled.

The associated chemotherapy consisted in Cisplatin (DDP) and 5-Fluorouracil (5-FU): Day 1 DDP 100 mg/m2, days 2-6 5-FU 1000 mg/m2. Drug doses were reduced in cases of renal insufficiency and after 70 years of age (10% dose reduction for every 5 yr increment). Courses were spaced 28 days apart. Results were reevaluated (IVU, APCT, TUR) after the first three courses and after the sixth course.

The histologic distribution of the 20 pts treated was 8 pT2, 5 pT3a (1 N+ on APCT), 5 pT3b (1 N+ on APCT), 2 pT4.

RESULTS

The simple definitions used for responses were as follows:
- complete response (pCR) : disappearance of all histologically confirmed tumor (by TUR)
- partial response (pPR) : reduction of at least 50% in tumor volume
- failure: lesion stabilization or progression or nonsignificant tumor regression.

One death occurred due to septicemia after the third course (pT2). The chemotherapy for the 19 other pts never had to be interrupted for renal or hematologic complications. However, all pts had digestive tract problems, usually minor in nature, with nausea and vomiting being the most prevalent. There were 3 cases of severe mucitis.

After the 3rd course, the response was evaluable in 19 pts: 4 failures (3 pT3, 1 pT4), 6 pPR (1 pT2, 5 pT3), 9 pCR (6 pT2, 2 pT3, 1 pT4).

All 19 evaluable pts received 6 courses. Analysis of results after the 6th course revealed that the initial response was maintained and remained unchanged. Pts who achieved a pPR never achieved a pCR even after 3 additional courses.

After the 6 courses, the therapeutic approach was adapted as a function of the tumoral response:
- for pts who achieved a pCR, we deliberately chose abstinence from therapy but performed regular follow-up examinations. Ulterior treatment was given only if tumor recurrence was detected.
- in the other cases, the systemic treatment was abandonned and a locoregional treatment (conservative when possible) combining radiotherapy and surgery was used to obtain local control of the bladder tumor.

In Jan. 1988, median survival was 30 months (range 16-52). Of the 9 initial CR:
- 4 pts never presented any ulterior recurrence (3 pT2 with follow-ups of 52, 25 and 18 mo. and 1 pT3 with a follow-up of 33 mo.)
- 2 pts (1 pT2, 1 pT3) developed a superficial bladder recurrence (pT1) during the first year of follow-up and were treated by TUR and intra-vesical BCG. These two pts are currently tumor-free with follow-ups of 40 and 52 mo.

- 3 pts developed an infiltrating bladder recurrence: 2 pT3 tumors (in two pts initially pT2) and one pT4 tumor (in a pt initially pT4). One pt (pT3) was treated by total cystectomy, and is currently alive with a follow-up of 42 mo. The other two pts had contraindications to surgery and were treated by radiotherapy; they died at 36 and 26 mo. respectively.

As concerns the other pts (failures or PR), the prognosis is not very good:
- of the 6 pts who achieved a PR, 4 died after an average of 16 mo. despite partial (3 cases) or total (1 case) cystectomy. The other two pts, initially classed pT3, are alive respectively 16 mo. after a total cystectomy and 19 mo. after a partial cystectomy.

When chemotherapy fails (4 cases: 3 pT3, 1 pT4), conventional therapy was used: total cystectomy in the one case where it was possible (pT3) and pelvic irradiation in the other cases. Despite such treatment, the course was rapidly fatal, with all pts dying after an average of 12 mo.

COMMENTS

Analysis of our results leads to the following remarks:

1. This neo-adjuvant chemotherapy protocol produced nearly 50% pCR after the third course.
2. The initial response obtained after the 3rd course is maintained but unchanged by 3 additional courses. This observation prompted us to now give only 3 courses.
3. Tolerance of treatment was good because the chemotherapy never had to be interrupted. This tolerance and the brief time required for the initial treatment do not prevent "in fine" radio-surgical treatment in cases of failure or PR
4. Disease recurrence after a pCR raises two questions:
- should maintenance chemotherapy be given, and if so at what doses and for how long?
- should total cystectomy + nodal sampling be performed as a matter of principle?
Today, we systematically offer pCR pts 3 additional courses (total of 6 courses) and do not remove the bladder.
5. The poor results of nonresponders (failures or pPR) suggest that chemotherapy selects the "good cases". It is impossible to know whether the time interval required for chemotherapy between diagnosis and radio-surgical treatment has an adverse influence.
6. Our 9 pCR pts included 6 of the 8 pts initially classed pT2 and only 3 of the 12 pts initially classed pT3, pT4.This requires investigation of the respective roles of TUR and chemotherapy in the obtainment of these pCR.

DISCUSSION

Use of chemotherapy for the treatment of advanced bladder tumors (N+ and M+) has been found effective in certain series, and complete clinical responses have been observed, although at the cost of significant toxicity, namely with the M-VAC protocol (1). These results led us in 1983 to offer chemotherapy in the initial treatment schedule for focal infiltrating tumors (pT2-T4NxM0).

Three reasons prompted adoption of first-line, neo-adjuvant chemotherapy:
- the hope of obtaining a reduction in tumor volume that would allow conservation of the bladder in certain cases
- better patient tolerance of the chemotherapy before surgical "aggression"
- greater efficacy of systemic treatment when given immediately after diagnosis.

Selection of the DDP-5-FU combination was based on:
- demonstration of its efficacy in other disease sites, and namely head and neck cancers (2)
- the superiority of DDP as compared to other drugs for urothelial tumors (1)
- better tolerance of this combination than of M-VAC

In 1988, it is difficult to define the role that should be played by an association of neo-adjuvant chemotherapy and TUR for the treatment of pT2-T4NxM0 pts. Few studies have been published, the follow-up is still short, and numerous protocols have been tested, some of which include radiotherapy. Furthermore, evaluation of CR varies from one author to another, from a simple clinical complete response (cCR) to histopathologic complete response (pCR) which can lead to total cystectomy as a matter of principle.

In this series, definition of pCR was based on repeat endoscopic biopsies. While this procedure may not be as precise as examination of a cystectomy specimen, at least it has the advantage of avoiding systematic multilation, which is, after all, the aim of our therapeutic approach.

This attitude certainly causes us to overestimate the true incidence of initial pCR, which was close to 50%, and partly explains the infiltrating recurrence we observed. However, other factors also warrant consideration:
- chemotherapy was stopped after 6 courses. Because no disease recurrences (infiltrating or not) were noted during treatment, the possible need for maintenance chemotherapy must be considered.
- in 2 out of 3 cases, the infiltrating disease recurrence was at a distance from the initial site; this pleads in favor of resection as a principle when the initial tumor is associated with an extensive in situ lesion or histologically mixed lesions (1). However, in our 3 cases, we did not re-utilize chemotherapy.

Hall (3) reported on a series of pts treated by TUR + cisplatin and methotrexate, and obtained results similar to ours. In a study comparing TUR + chemotherapy to chemotherapy alone, he found that 79% of pts were tumor-free at 1 yr in the group that had received chemotherapy + TUR versus only 13% of the pts in the other group. These few cases tend to show that the association of TUR and chemotherapy is effective whereas chemotherapy alone gives poor results.

CONCLUSION

Use of a combination of TUR and neo-adjuvant chemotherapy (5-FU-CIS) for T2-T4NxM0 bladder tumors gives results comparable to those of traditional cystectomy-radiotherapy associations as far as local control is concerned, but also preserves bladder function and thus improves patient comfort. Average survival at 5 years is not evaluable, but seems very close to that obtained with cystectomy.

It is still too soon to affirm that this new approach is a reliable alternative to cystectomy for infiltrating bladder tumors. Only a randomized study on a large population with a long follow-up period can provide a valid answer. Even so, this type of treatment seems to have an effective role in the selection of pts who can hope to achieve a cure while conserving their bladder with minimal risks of morbidity.

REFERENCES

1. Sternberg C.N. et al. (1987) Oncology 1: 41-49
2. Schneider M et al. (1986) Brit J Cancer 54: 755-760
3. Hall R.R. (1986) in Yagoda A. (ed.) Bladder cancer. Future directions for treatment. New York, John Wiley and Sons, pp 117-122

Résumé

De sept. 83 à sept. 86, 20 patients (pts), âge moyen 65 ans, auraient dû être traités par cystectomie totale pour une tumeur infiltrant le muscle vésical. Ces patients ont eu un bilan initial comprenant un examen clinique sous anesthésie générale, un scanner, une urographie et une résection (RTU) profonde puis une chimiothérapie néo-adjuvante : CISPLATINE et 5-FU. Six cycles ont été réalisés, espacés de 28 jours, un bilan identique (cf supra) a été réalisé au décours du 3ème et du 6ème cycle. 9 patients ont eu une réponse complète confirmée histologiquement (pCR) (6 pT2, 2 pT3, 1 pT4). En janvier 1988, la médiane de survie est de 30 mois (17-52 mois). Notre protocole est objectivement actif et bien toléré même chez les sujets âgés. Le problème demeure concernant les pCR : (1) rôles respectifs de la chimiothérapie et la résection, (2) la prévention des récidives (5/9 pCR).

Neo-Adjuvant Chemotherapy. Ed. Cl. Jacquillat, M. Weil, D. Khayat. Colloque INSERM/John Libbey Eurotext Ltd. © 1988. Vol. 169, pp. 431-435.

Tumeurs infiltrantes de vessie : réponse locale à la chimiothérapie systémique à base de platine

L. Boccon-Gibod**, S. Adjiman*, P. Beuzeboc*, M. Zerbib* et A. Steg*

Clinique Urologique de l'Hôpital Cochin et Service d'Urologie de l'Hôpital Bichat**, Paris, France*

RESUME

16 patients (pts), atteints de cancers urothéliaux infiltrants de vessie, ont été soumis, de première intention à une chimiothérapie à base de Platine, vessie en place. (M-VAC ou CDDP + MTX). 11 pts présentaient des lésions T1 à T4, N+, MØ ou M+; 5 pts des lésions T1, T2, NØ, MØ. Le but de l'étude était d'apprécier l'effet de la chimiothérapie sur la lésion vésicale. Nous avons observé deux réponses complètes (RC), six réponses partielles (RP), huit pts sont non-répondeurs (NR). Toutes les RC avaient eu des résections complètes, de même que 5 des 6 RP. Les pts NR avaient eu, en majorité, des résections incomplètes. Les résultats actuels sont décevants et font se poser la question de l'efficacité d'une éventuelle chimiothérapie néo-adjuvante.

Protocole :

M-VAC	MTX	40 mg	J1, J15, J22
	VLB	5 mg	J2, J15, J22
	ADM	40 mg	J2
	CDDP	125 mg	J2
CDDP + MTX	MTX	40 mg	J1 – J8
	CDDP	125 mg	J2

Mots Clefs / Key Words :

- Chimiothérapie néo-adjuvante; tumeur de vessie
- Neo-adjuvant Chemotherapy; Bladder Cancer

INTRODUCTION :

Le traitement des tumeurs infiltrantes de vessie a un double but : contrôler et traiter la lésion vésicale et prévenir ou modifier l'évolution de la maladie générale. Le contrôle local est obtenu, généralement, par la chirurgie seule ou associée à la Radiothérapie. La Chimiothérapie systémique demeure le seul traitement permettant d'espérer modifier l'évolution de la maladie néoplasique quand elle a diffusé (N+ ou M+).

En utilisant la Chimiothérapie de première intention chez des patients porteurs de lésion vésicale infiltrante, indemnes de métastases cliniquement décelables, on peut espérer lutter contre les micro-métastases présentes dès le diagnostic, diminuer les risques de récidive locale ou l'apparition ultérieure de métastases à distance. Plusieurs protocoles de Chimiothérapie "néo-adjuvante" utilisant le Cis-Platine seul ou combiné à d'autres agents chimiothérapiques, ont déjà été publiés à ce jour, avec des résultats qui semblent prometteurs (HALL 1984, PEARSON & RAGHAVAN 1985, STRERNBERG & YAGODA 1986, et RAGHAVAN 1987).

Nous présentons ici les résultats d'une série de 16 patients atteints d'une tumeur de vessie infiltrante et traités de première intention par une Chimiothérapie à base de Cis-Platine. Le but de l'étude était d'apprécier l'effet de la Chimiothérapie sur la lésion vésicale et de préciser les possibilités d'une éventuelle Chimiothérapie "néo-adjuvante".

MALADES ET METHODES :

Seize patients âgés, en moyenne de 63 ans, atteints de cancers urothéliaux infiltrants de vessie (âges extrèmes : 45-78 - 13 hommes-3 femmes), ont été soumis, de première intention, à une Chimiothérapie, vessie en place (Clinique Urologique de L'Hôpital COCHIN - Service du Professeur STEG). La Chimiothérapie était motivée 11 fois par l'extension loco-régionale, la présence d'un envahissement ganglionnaire ou de métastases à distance, contre-indiquant l'exérèse vésicale (11 tumeurs pT1 à pT4, N+ (9), MO ou M+ (2). 5 fois la Chimiothérapie a été choisie de première intention dans le cadre d'un essai clinique d'alternative à l'exérèse (5 tumeurs pT1 à pT2, NO, MO).

Le bilan d'extension initial a toujours compris un examen clinique, une radiographie thoracique, une urographie intra-veineuse, un scanner abdomino-pelvien, une lymphographie pédieuse bilatérale avec cyto-ponction systématique, des touchers pelviens sous anesthésie et une résection trans-uréthrale profonde de la tumeur, avec biopsies des zones optiquement saimes (cartographie vésicale).

La résection est considérée comme complète dans 8 cas (pT1 et pT2), dans 8 cas la tumeur dépassant les possibilités de résection complète, avec 5 fois la présence d'une masse pelvienne perceptible. La Chimiothérapie a été instituée de un à deux mois après la résection initiale et deux types de protocoles ont été utilisés.

- Le protocole M.VAC (8) (Fig.) a été utilisé chez 10 patients. Tous étaient porteurs de lésions pT1 à pT4, N+, MO, ou M+, parmi lesquels 5 avaient eu une résection complète avant mise en route de la Chimiothérapie.

- Le protocole Cis-Platine et Methotrexate (CDDP + MTX) (2, 10) (Fig.) a été utilisé chez 6 patients : un seul était porteur d'une lésion pT4, les 5 autres, de lésions pT1, pT2, NO, MO dont 3 avaient eu une résection complète.

TOXICITE :

Aucun décès n'a été rapporté à la Chimiothérapie. Nausées et vomisssements sont les effets secondaires les plus fréquemment rencontrés. 4 patients ont présenté des mucites peu sévères; 2 patients une leucopénie modérée dont l'une a obligé au report d'un cycle. Un patient a développé une neuropathie sensitive des membres inférieurs, attribuée au CDDP.

EVALUATION DES RESULTATS :

Tous les patients ont été réévalués après 3 cycles :

- 3 ont eu une cysto-prostatectomie après 3 cycles,
- Pour 3 patients la chimiothérapie a été arrêtée après 3 cycles devant l'absence d'efficacité du M-VAC.
- 10 patients ont eu des cycles complémentaires (1 à 3) au terme desquels 3 ont eu une cysto-prostatectomie et 7 ont finalement été traités par chimiothérapie exclusive.

La réponse locale a été appréciée par un examen clinique et endoscopique sous anesthésie, avec résection de toute tumeur visible, biopsies systématiques des zones optiquement saines (10 cas) et dans 6 cas, examen de la pièce de cystectomie.

La réponse complète est définie par l'absence de toute formation tumorale y compris C.I.S (2 patients).

La réponse partielle est une amélioration du stade anatomique (6 patients).

La stabilisation ou la progression malgré la Chimiothérapie sont considérées comme des non-réponses (8 patients).

Les différents degrés de réponses ont été comparés avec le type de Chimiothérapie employée et le caractère complet ou incomplet de la résection initiale, directement en rapport avec le volume tumoral et le degré d'infiltration.

Les résultats sont les suivants :

- 2 patients ont été considérés comme ayant une réponse locale complète (dysplasie légère ou absence de toute lésion). Les patients ont été traités par le M.VAC. Cependant, chez les 2 patients, la maladie néoplasique a poursuivi son évolution, entraînant l'apparition de métastases dont l'un des patients est décédé.
- 6 patients ont eu une amélioration du stade anatomique (2 traités par le M.VAC et 4 par le CDDP + MTX).
- Enfin, 8 patients sont non-répondeurs (6 traités par le M.VAC, et 2 par le CDDP + MTX).

Le caractère complet ou incomplet de la résection initiale est déterminant pour l'interprétation des résultats : toutes les réponses complètes avaient eu une résection complète. Il en est de même de 5 des 6 patients à réponse partielle. Les patients ayant eu une résection incomplète (8 patients) sont, en majorité, non-répondeurs (7 patients), un seul a une réponse partielle.

DISCUSSION :

Récemment, certaines études ont mis en avant le rôle de la Chimiothérapie seule ouassociée à la Radiothérapie, avec, pour but, le contrôle local des tumeurs de vessie (1, 2, 4, 5, 7). Les résultats rapportés restent variables d'une publication à l'autre et sont difficiles à comparer, du fait de l'hétérogénéité des séries, de la variabilité des protocoles, et des critères d'évaluation des patients. En particulier, le caractère complet ou incomplet de la résection initiale, permettant de juger, précisément de l'existence d'une tumeur résiduelle avant mise en route de la Chimiothérapie, n'apparait que rarement. Certains résultats paraissent prometteurs (jusqu'à 60 % de réponses complètes), alors que pour d'autres les pourcentages de réponses complètes sont très faibles (3, 6, 9).

La qualité de l'évaluation avant et au terme de la Chimiothérapie est capitale. L'étendue de la résection initiale et l'établissement d'une cartographie vésicale par des biopsies multiples, modifie fondamentalement l'interprétation des résultats quant à l'efficacité de la Chimiothérapie, notamment chez les patients ayant eu une résection complète initiale.

Chez ces patients, le moment de la réévaluation est déterminant, seule l'apparition d'une récidive et son délai de survenue permettent de juger de l'efficacité de la Chimiothérapie.

Une réévaluation précoce d'une lésion complètement réséquée interdit de conclure quant à l'efficacité de la Chimiothérapie (6, 9).

Dans notre série, les 2 patients considérés comme ayant eu une réponse complète avaient eu une résection complète, alors qu'aucun des patients ayant eu une résection incomplète n'a eu de réponse complète. Les explorations morphologiques, la cytologie et l'aspect endoscopique ne sont pas suffisants pour apprécier la réponse locale. Certains patients présentent une muqueuse optiquement saine à la cystoscopie sans anomalie à la cytologie urinaire, mais la résection démontre la présence de tumeur évolutive, comme c'est le cas, trois fois, dans notre série (3, 9, 11).

Dans de nombreuses publications, la réponse complète reposesur les constatations des explorations endoscopiques et morphologiques, sans prélèvement histologique, ce qui ne permet pas d'affirmer l'absence de toute tumeur au moment de l'évaluation (8, 9, 11).

Il apparait donc, malgré l'hétérogénéité des groupes de patients, les types de protocoles utilisés, et des critères d'évaluation, que la Chimiothérapie systémique n'a pas, à ce jour, démontré d'efficacité spectaculaire sur la lésion vésicale. Les résultats actuels sont discordants, et mettent en question l'intérêt de l'utilité éventuelle d'une Chimiothérapie néo-adjuvante.

B I B L I O G R A P H I E

1 - FAGG J.L., EDWARDS P., HUGHES M.A., LATIEF T.N., ROLFE E.B., FIELDING J.W.L.
Cis-Diammisedichloro-Platinium (CDDP) as initial treatment of invasive bladder cancer.
Brit. J. Urol. 1984, 56, 246-300.

2 - HALL R.R., NEWLING W.N., RAMSDEN P.D & Al.
Treatment of invasive bladder cancer by local resection and high dose of methotrexate.
Brit. J. Urol. 1984, 56, 668-672.

3 - NEEDLES B., YAGODA A., SOGANI P., GRABSTALD H., WHITMORE W.F.
Intra-venous cis-platin for superficial bladder tumors.
Cancer 1982, 1722-1723.

4 - PEARSON B.S., RAGHAVAN D.
First live intra-venous cis-platin for deeply invasive bladder cancer : update on 70 cases.
Brit. J. Urol. 1985, 57, 690-693.

5 - RAGHAVAN D., PEARSON B., DUVAL P. & Al.
Initial intra-venous cis-platinium therapy : improved management for invasive high risk bladder cancer ?
J. Urol. 1985, 133, 344-403.

6 - RAGHAVAN D.
Pre-emptive (neo-adjuvant) intra-venous chemotherapy for invasive bladder cancer.
Brit. J. Urol. 1988, 61, 1-8.

7 - SCHER H.I., YAGODA A., STERNBERG C. & Al.
Neo-adjuvant M.VAC in transitionnal cell carcinoma of the urothelium.
Proc. Am. Soc. Clin. Oncol. 1986, 5, 108.

8 - STERNBERG C., YAGODA A., SCHER H. & Al.
Preliminary results of methotrexate, Vinblastine, Adriamycine and cis-platin (M.VAC), in advanced urothelial tumors.
J. Urol. 1985, 133, 403-407.

9 - STERNBERG C., SCHER H.I.
Advances in the treatment of urothelial tract tumors.
Urol. Clin. North. Am. 14, 2, 373-387.

10 - STOTER G., SPLINTER TAN, CHILD J.A., FOSSA S.D., DENIS L. VAN OOSTEROM A.T., DE PAUW M., SYLVESTER R. for EORTC.
Combination chemotherapy with cis-platin and methotrexate in advanced transitionnal cell cancer of the bladder.
J. Urol. 1987, 137, 663-667.

11 - WHITMORE W.F.
Chemotherapy for bladder cancer.
J. Urol. 1985, 134, 1181-1182.

Résumé

16 patients (pts) with invasive bladder cancer were treated primiraly "bladder in place", with chemotherapy. (M-VAC, CDDP + MTX). There were 11 with T1 to T4, N+, MØ, M+; 5 with T1, T2, NØ, MØ. The aim of the study was to appreciate the response of bladder lesions to chemotherapy. 2 had complete response (CR), 6 partial response (PR) and 8 no-response (NR). Pts with complete responses and partial responses were found to have complete resection before chemotherapy. Unresectable lesions were associated with NR pts. The results did not show a significative improvement and they question the role of neo-adjuvant chemotherapy.

Urology III

Urologie III

Neo-Adjuvant Chemotherapy. Ed. Cl. Jacquillat, M. Weil, D. Khayat. Colloque INSERM/John Libbey Eurotext Ltd. © 1988. Vol. 169, pp. 439-443.

Chimiothérapie pré-opératoire dans le traitement des tumeurs vésicales infiltrantes : à propos de 22 cas

C. Rudelle*, P. Léandri*, G. Rossignol*, L. Gabay*, J.R. Gautier*, J. Caissel* et J.P. Droz**

** Clinique Saint-Jean-Languedoc, 31077 Toulouse Cedex, France*
*** Institut Gustave Roussy, 94805 Villejuif Cedex, France*

RESUME

De janvier à novembre 1987, 22 patients présentant une tumeur vésicale infiltrante ont été traités par une association chimiothérapie-chirurgie. Après bilan biologique et urologique : cystoscopie, N.U.T., scanner, échographie pelvienne, ce cycle comprend à J1 l'injection de Vinblastine (VBL) 3 mg/m2 IV, Methotrexate (MTX) 30 mg/m2 IV et Cisplatinum (PLAT) 70 mg/m2 ; à J15 : VBL et MTX. A J 28, une cystectomie radicale (CR) avec évidement ganglionnaire iliaque et obturateur est programmée. Elle est encadrée par une Normo Nutrition Parentérale commencée à J25 et précédée d'un nouveau bilan biologique et d'une cystoscopie. 22 patients de sexe masculin, agés de 36 à 75 ans, ont suivi ce protocole. Il s'agissait de tumeurs urothéliales infiltrantes de stade T2 (10), T3A (4), T3B (6) et T4 (2). L'intervention a été 18 fois une CR. 4 fois l'importance des lésions ganglionnaires n'a pas permis de CR. La chimiothérapie a permis de soulager les douleurs pelviennes de 4 patients sur 6 ; la cystoscopie préopératoire objectivait une diminution des lésions tumorales 4 fois et la disparition des lésions, 8 fois. Les effets toxiques ont été mineurs et dominés par des vomissements à J1 (45 % des cas). Notre technique opératoire et notre réanimation n'ont jamais été modifiées. L'étude histologique a montré 16 tumeurs résiduelles ; 6 fois, il n'y avait plus de tumeur vésicale. Ce protocole de chimiothérapie préopératoire est très bien toléré et présente une efficacité clinique et histologique certaine (25 % de réponses complètes).

MOTS CLEFS

Tumeurs infiltrantes de vessie - Association Chimiothérapie-Chirurgie - Normo-nutrition parentérale - Méthotrexate - Vinblastine - Cisplatinum - Histologie.

INTRODUCTION

Parmi les malades opérés de tumeurs vésicales à la CLINIQUE SAINT JEAN LANGUEDOC à TOULOUSE entre janvier et novembre 1987, nous avons isolé 22 patients porteurs de tumeur vésicale infiltrante et traités par une association chimiothérapie-chirurgie. Notre propos, puisque notre recul n'est pas encore suffisant pour estimer leurs chances de survie à long terme, était d'envisager les effets objectifs et immédiats, cliniques et biologiques, du cycle de chimiothérapie pré-opératoire et de comparer l'histologie de la première biopsie vésicale aux résultats de l'examen anatomopathologique de la pièce opératoire. Notre souci étant par ailleurs de savoir si ce traitement n'était pas de nature à alourdir notre protocole antérieur.

MATERIEL ET METHODES

Les 22 patients agés de 36 à 75 ans étaients atteints de tumeurs urothéliales infiltrantes : 10 pT2, 4 pT3A, 6 pT3B, et 2 pT4, déterminées après résection biopsique. Nous avons choisi un protocole de chimiothérapie inspiré des travaux de PROUT, de YAGODA et du NORTHERN CALIFORNIA ONCOLOGY GROUP. Les modalités d'administration et le protocole définitif ont été établis grâce à la participation du GROUPE D'ETUDE THERAPEUTIQUE DES CANCERS DE VESSIE (DROZ J.P., VALLANCIEN G. et PRAPOTNICH D.).

Le cycle de chimiothérapie préopératoire débute à J1 par l'injection intraveineuse directe de :
- VINBLASTINE : 3 mg/m2
- METHOTREXATE : 30 mg/m2
- CISPLATINUM : 70 mg/m2

Ces injections sont assorties d'un remplissage liquidien (4 litres/24 h.) et d'une couverture neuro végétative classique par METOCLOPRAMIDE, CHLORPROMAZINE et CHLORAZEPATE DIPOTASSIQUE.

Un bilan urologique : cystoscopie, néphro-urotomographie, scanner, échographie pelvienne et un bilan biologique précèdent ce premier cycle. Le bilan biologique comprend un bilan électrolytique sanguin et urinaire, une calcémie, une formule numération sanguine avec comptage des plaquettes, une vitesse de sédimentation, un dosage des phosphatases alcalines et des gamma GT. Le patient reste hospitalisé 48 heures pour la réalisation de ce bilan et la première séance de chimiothérapie. 15 jours plus tard, il reçoit une dose identique de VINBLASTINE soit 3 mg/m2 et de METHOTREXATE, 30 mg/m2. Un bilan sanguin est pratiqué la veille, les doses pouvant être modifiées selon l'évolution de la créatininémie ou de la formule sanguine.

Trois jours avant la date programmée pour l'intervention, le malade subit un nouveau bilan biologique et urinaire : cystoscopie, échographie. Parallèlement, est mise en route une normonutrition parentérale qui sera poursuivie en post-opératoire. Associée aux désinfectants intestinaux et à un régime sans résidus, elle assure une meilleure préparation des anses intestinales pour l'entérocystoplastie et simplifie les suites opératoires.

Elle est délivrée par l'intermédiaire d'un catheter jugulaire interne ou sous clavier, placé par dénudation et tunnellisé. La solution nutritive, ternaire, apportant 2 000 à 2 200 calories pour 2 000 ml est infusée par une pompe à débit constant, elle peut être modulée en fonction des besoins énergétiques ou hydro-électrolytiques du malade.

RESULTATS

La chirurgie réalisée est une cystectomie radicale avec évidement iliaque et obturateur. Nous avons pu réaliser cette intervention 18 fois, dont 16 vessies de remplacement avec entérocystoplastie type CAMAY, 1 BRICKER, 1 cystectomie avec U.C.B. 4 fois, l'importance des lésions ganglionnaires, vérifiées extemporanément, n'ont pas permis de chirurgie radicale, nous avons du limiter l'intervention dans deux cas à un évidement ganglionnaire isolé, dans deux autres cas, nous l'avons complété par une cystectomie partielle ou une U.C.B. sans cystectomie. Les effets toxiques ont été mineurs.

On a pu observer quelques nausées (8 %), quelques diarrhées et des poussées hypertensives (8 %). Les vomissements présents chez 45 % des malades lors de la première séance, malgré l'administration préventive de METOCLOPRAMIDE et de CHLORPROMAZINE sont vraisemblablement imputables au CYSPLATYL, en effet on ne les retrouve pas lors de la deuxième séance, à J15. Ils ont été assez bien tolérés.
Sur le plan hématologique, une chute transitoire de l'ordre de 15 à 20 % des plaquettes a été constatée après chaque séance, la "restitutio ad integrum" étant de règle lors du bilan suivant, quinze jours plus tard. Nous n'avons observé aucune altération de la fonction hépatique ou rénale.
L'amélioration clinique a été immédiate chez 4 patients sur 6 qui ont été soulagés de leurs douleurs pelviennes.
La cystoscopie préopératoire objectivait une diminution des lésions tumorales 4 fois et leur disparition 8 fois.
L'étude histologique des pièces ou des prélèvements per-opératoires a montré 16 tumeurs résiduelles.

	HISTOLOGIE INITIALE	HISTOLOGIE APRES INTERVENTION
pT1	0	2
pT2	10	5
pT3A	4	1
pT3B	6	2
pT4	2	6
pTa	0	6 (3 pT2, 2 pT3A, 1 pT3B)

DISCUSSION

Dans 6 cas, on n'observait plus de tumeur vésicale infiltrante. Hormis les 4 malades de stade avancé pour lesquels nous avons choisi des solutions palliatives, nous avons noté une regression sensible de l'extension tumorale dans tous les prélèvements. Dans 25 % des cas, la disparition de la tumeur infiltrante signe l'efficacité de ce protocole. Ces résultats sont comparables à ceux des équipes utilisant cette association MTX-VBL-PLAT, en particulier le Northern California Oncology Group (21 % de CR) ou l'EORTC Urological Group (23 %). La tolérance est excellente et supérieure à celle des protocoles associant d'autres substances cytotoxiques.

CONCLUSION

Nous avons voulu, encouragés par ces premiers résultats objectifs, publier ce travail préliminaire. Notre protocole ultérieur comprend cinq cycles post-opératoires mensuels, débutant 6 semaines après l'intervention. Nous souhaitons trouver des résultats à long terme confirmant cette efficacité de l'association chimiothérapie C.M.V. - chirurgie radicale dans le traitement des tumeurs infiltrantes de la vessie.

REFERENCES BIBLIOGRAPHIQUES

Ahmed, T., Yagoda, A., Needles, B. et al. (1985) : Vinblastine and Methotrexate for Advanced Bladder Cancer. J. Urol. 133, 602-604.
Camey, M., Leduc, A. (1979) : L'Entérocystoplastie après Cystoprostatectomie Totale pour Cancer de Vessie. Indications, Technique Opératoire, Surveillance et Résultats sur quatre vingt sept cas. Ann. Urol., 13, n°2 : 114-123
Cora, N. et al. (1987) : Urothelial Tract Tumors. Urologic Clin. of North Am. vol. 14, n° 2
Daniels, J.R. : Chemotherapy of Carcinoma of the Bladder. In Skinner and Lieskovsky, Diagnosis and Management of Genito-Urinary Cancer.WB Saunders (ed) 1988. 17 : 313-322
De La Pena, J. : Cisplatinum plus Cystectomy vs Cystectomie Alone in Invasive Bladder Cancer. Preliminary Results of a Rrandomized Multicentre Study. International workshop in Urology. Cannes - 1987
Denis, L.J. : Preoperative Chemotherapy in T3/T4 NxMo Bladder Cancer. International Workshop in Urology. Cannes - 1987
Droz, J.P., Amiel, J.L., Cukier, J., Beurton, D., Dufour, B., Pascal, B. (1982) : Chimiothérapie Adjuvante dans le Traitement des Cancers Infiltrants de la Vessie. 25 cas. J. Urol. Nephrol., 88, n°6 : 369-373.
Hall, R.R., Newling, D.W.W., Ramsden P.D., et al (1984) : Treatment of Invasive Bladder Cancer by Local Resection and High Dose Methotrexate. Br.J.Urol., 56 : 668-672.
Hillcoat, B.L., Rahhavan, D., The Australian Bladder Cancer Study Group (1986) : A Randomized Comparison of Cisplatin (C) versus Cisplatin and Methotrexate (C + M) in Advanced Bladder Cancer. Proc Am Soc Clin Oncol, 5 : 426
Ingargiola, G.B. : Upfront Chemotherapy Before Definitive Treatment for Deeply Infiltrating Bladder Cancer. International Workshop in Urology. Cannes 1987.
Kaye, S.B., McWhinnie, D., Hart, A. et al (1984) : The Treatment of Advanced Bladder Cancer with Methotrexate and Cisplatinum-A Pharmacokinetic Study . Eur. J. Cancer Clin. Oncol., 20 : 249-252.
Natale, R.B., Grossman, H.B., Crawford, E.D., et al (1986) : Combination Cisplatin and Dichloromethotrexate in Advanced Bladder Cancer : a Southwest Oncology Group (SWOG) Study : Proc Am Soc Clin Oncol, 5 : 104
Natale, R.B., Yagoda, A., Watson, R.C., et al (1981) : Methotrexate : an Active Drug in Bladder Cancer. Cancer 47 : 1246-1250.
Prout, G.R.JR (1977) : Bladder Carcinoma and a T.N.M. System of Classification. J. Urol., 117 : 583-590
Stoter, G., Fossa, S.D., Klein, GGM, et al (1985) : Combination Chemotherapy with Cisplatin (DDP) and Methotrexate (MTX) in Advanced Bladder Cancer : an EORTC Phase II Study. Proc Am Soc Clin Oncol, 4 : 106
Terry, W. (1988) : Nutritional Support of the Urologic Patient. In Diagnosis and Management of Genito-Urinary Cancer-WB Saunders (ed) 39 : 582-594.

Résumé

Between Januar and November 1987, 22 patients with infiltrating carcinoma of the bladder were treated by surgery with adjunctive chemotherapy. We analised objective effects of preoperative chemotherapy, operatory incidence, toxicity and histology before and after surgery. Chemotherapy starts at J1 with injection of Vinblastine, 3 mg/m2, Methotrexate 30 mg/m2 and Cisplatinum 70 mg/m2 after urologic and biological assessment, then continues at J15 with Vinblastine and Methotrexate at same doses. Radical cystectomy is performed at J28 with lymphadenectomy, surrounded by pre operative nutritionnal support started at J25. 22 male patients (36-75 age range) were suffering from urothelial infiltrating tumors, category T2 (10), T3A (4), T3B (6) or T4 (2). 18 allowed radical surgery, 4 had too important nodal involvement. Chemotherapy relieved pelvic pain in 4 patients on 6. Preoperatory cystoscopy objectived 4 reductions of tumoral lesions and 8 disappearance. Toxic side effects were minors, dominated by vomiting at J1 (45 % cases). Never we had to modify our operatory technic or post-operative management. Histology showed 16 residual tumors and for six patients no more tumor. Such preoperative chemotherapy is well tolerated and its histological and clinical efficacity certain, with 25 % complete reponses.

Neo-Adjuvant Chemotherapy. Ed. Cl. Jacquillat, M. Weil, D. Khayat. Colloque INSERM/John Libbey Eurotext Ltd. © 1988. Vol. 169, pp. 445-453.

Short term efficiency of neo-adjuvant chemotherapy (CAP) in treatment of transitional cell bladder carcinoma

F. Trifard, Y. Chrétien, X. Vallantin, A.T. Lachand, M. Housset, C. Collet and B. Dufour

Department of Urology B, Hôpital Necker, 149 rue de Sèvres, 75743 Paris Cedex 15, France

22 patients with bladder carcinoma (T 2,Mo) received 2 or 3 courses of systemic chemotherapy (CPM 600 mg/m2, ADM 60 mg/m2, cisplatinum 100 mg/m2) prior to total or partial cystectomy.
Response rate was appreciated on the pathologic findings of these 22 bladders surgically removed :

Tumor progression	5/22	(23 %)
Tumor stability	8/22	(36 %)
Partial remission (more tan 50 %)	3/22	(14 %)
Complete remission (PTo)	4/22	(18 %)
PTo after complete TUR	2/22	(9 %)

The long term purpose of that trial was to improve survival, lessening the rate of metastatic reccurence.
The follow up is still too short to allow any conclusion on survival but these preliminary results showed :

. The high rate of tumor progression
. The clinical under-staging of bladder cancer.

That is the reason why, despite the fact we removed 6 bladders free of tumor, we think that cystectomy remains the most efficient treatment.

Radical surgery and/or radiation therapy is the currently accepted treatment for bladder cancer.
The five year survival of T 3 is actually about 40 to 50 per cent.
Most of patients die of metastatic reccurence. That is why further progress requires an effective systemic therapy which ca ndestroy occult metastases.
We know that chemotherapy can produce objective tumor responses on measurable metastases. But, the drugs used for adjuvant chemotherapy did not substantially improve survival
We hope that neoadjuvant chemotherapy will be able to do it.
This is a prospective study of 22 patients with transitional cell carcinoma of the bladder. They received two or three courses of :
Cisplatinum 100 mg/m2, cyclophosphamide 600 mg/m2 and Doxorubicin 60 mg/m2, prior to total or partial cystectomy.
Pathologic findings of theses 22 bladders allowed us to appreciate the exact response rate of that treatment. We report here the preliminary results.

MATERIAL

22 patients were included, 21 males and 1 female. They were 40 to 72 years old (mean age 59,2).
Tumors were assessed by :
. Examination under general anesthesia, cystoscopy, resection as complete as possible,
. Chest X ray, IVP, CT Scan, Ultrasound and sometimes percutaneous node biopsy,
The clinical stages were :

16 T 3   6 T 2

17 No   4 N "doubtful" 1 N+

METHODS

1. Chemotherapy was given intravenously with hydratation using mannitol and saline.
Each patient received two treatments at 4 weekly intervals.
4 Weeks after the second treatment response was assessed by cystoscopy, biopsy, CT Scan.
If there were a response, a third treatment was given.
2. Surgery was performed two or three weeks after the last treatment.
It always began by lymphadenectomy with pathologic examination of frozen sections.
In case of bulky, nodal involvment (N3, N4) no radical cystectomy was performed.
In the other cases, radical or partial cystectomy was performed.

RESULTS

1. Tolerance was good.
Only one patient had severe leucopenia with scepticemia after the third treatment.
2. We performed

	18	radical cystectomy
	3	partial cystectomy
	1	lymphadenectomy alone

There was no operative mortality.
We had serious operative morbidity in 4 patients.
3. Response rate
Clinical staging widely underestimated nodal and bladder involvment as shown on table n° 1

It has ignored 3 resistances ant 3 partial responses.
Response was classified in five different types :

1° Tumor progression	5/22	(23 %)
2° tumor stability	8/22	(36 %)
3° partial remission (more than 50 %)	3/22	(14 %)
4° total remission	4/22	(18 %)
5° PTo after complete TUR	2/22	(9 %)

4. Survival

The follow up is too short (Maximum 26 months) to allow any conclusion on survival.
Actually, 7 patients died of their tumor and 2 are alive with recurrence.
None of them had responded to the treatment.

DISCUSSION

Response rate (7/20 = 35 % including 20 % of complete response) is similar to the response rate obtain by CAP on metastatic urothelial cancer (table 2).
Most of trials on neoadjuvant chemotherapy are still under study and published results are few. (Table 3).
Response rate is better in all series but it is judged on clinical staging except for two (8 , 9).
Clinical staging, even assessed by CT Scan and biopsy, dramaticaly under-estimates tumor extension as shown on table
That is why we think that cystectomy is the only way to appreciate tumor spreading.
5 patients (25 %) had tumor progression under treatment.
Cystectomy was performed 4 months after the diagnosis.
Prognosis of such tumors is, of course, discouraging what ever the treatment may be.
But, we think that we cannot leave such patients "untreated" such a long time.

The result lead as to conclude that :

1° The preoperative period must not be so long and treatment must be more effective.
So we started another study using a combination of radio thérapy and chemotherapy as initial treatment (45 gy + 5 FU. DDP)

2° We think that cystectomy remains the only actual treatment of bladder carcinoma, even if we sometimes remove bladders free of tumor.
Conservative treatment is very fascinating.
The first results of JACKSE (11) seems encouraging (80 % complete remission rate after full dose radiation and chemotherapy) but requires a longer follow up.
We hope that conservative treatment will be the treatment of tomorrow but today, we must keep performing cystectomies.

TABLE 1

	T N M initial	T N M after chemotherapy	pT N M
TO	0	11	6
T1	0	1	0
T2	6	2	3
T3	16	8	12
T4	0	0	1
NO	17	18	16
N?	4	4	/
N+	&	0	6

TABLE 2

CAP for metastatic urothelial cancer

AUTHOR	Pts	CR	PR	CR+PR
CAMPBEL (1)	19	-	-	33%
TRONER (2)	25	-	-	38%
SCHWARTZ (3)	28	7 %	39 %	46%
Al. SARRAF (4)	36	14 %	28 %	42%

TABLE 3

NEOADJUVANT CHEMOTHERAPY FOR BLADDER CANCER

AUTHOR	DRUGS	PTS	PR	CR	PR+CR
FAGG (5)	DDP	17	66%	0	65%
RAGHAVEN (6)	DDP	50	_	_	60%
MEYERS (7)	MVC	17	_	65%	65%
SOLOWAY (8)	MVAC	6	50%	33%	88%
SORET (9)	VM26 DDP	28	18%	32%	50%
QUINTENS (10)	DDP-SFU	21	43%	38%	81%

R E F E R E N C E S

1. CAMPBELL L., BAKER L.H., OPIPARI M. A.L. SARRAF M.
Phase II trial with cap in the treatment of urothelial transitional cell carcinoma.
Cancer treat Rep 65:897 (1981)

2. TRONER M.B. HEMSTREET GP : CAP in the treatment of urothelial malignancy : a pilot study of the southeastern cancer study group
ibid §(: 29 (1981)

3. SCHAWARTZ S. et col.
Phase II trial of segmentially administered cCAP for urothelial tract tumors
J. Urol. 130 : 681 51983)

4. A.L. SARRAF M. et Col.
Phase II trial of CAP versus amaserine in patients with transitional celle carcinoma of the urinary bladder.
Cancer treat Rep 69 : 189 (1985)

5. Fagg S.L. et col.
Cis-diamminedichloroplatinum as initial treatment of invasive bladder cancer
Br. J. Urol. 56 : 296 (1984)

6. RAGHAVAN D. et col.
Initial intravenous cisplatinum therapy : improved managment for invasive hig risk bladder cancer ?.
J. Urol. 133 : 399 (1985)

7. MEYERS F. J. et Col.
The fate of the bladder in patients with metastatic bladder cancer treated with cisplatin, methotrexate and vinblastine : a NCOG study
IBID 134 : 1 1118 (1985)

8. SOLOWAY M.S.
Is there a role for induction therapy for locally advanced bladder cancer
UROLOGY vol. 29 n°6 577 (1985)

9. SORET J.Y. et Col.
Chimiothérapie néoadjuvante des tumeurs vésicales infiltrantes localisées par l'association cysplatine VM 26.
Communication au Congrès Français d'Urologie Nov. 1987

10. Quinters et Col.

Communication au Congrès Français d'Urologie Nov. 1987

11. JAKSE G., FORMMTOLD H. , MARBERGER H.
Combined cisplatinum and radiation thérapy in patients with stages PT3 and PT4 bladder cancer : a pilot study
IBID 129 : 502 (1983)

Résumé

25 malades atteints de cancers de la vessie (T2 M0) ont reçu 2 ou 3 cures de chimiothérapie systémique (Endoxan 600 mg/m2 - Adriamycine 60 mg/m2 Cis-Platyl 100 mg/m2) avant cystectomie totale ou partielle.
Le taux de réponse a été apprécié sur l'histologie. Régression tumorale 23 %, stabilité tumorale 36 %, rémission partielle 14 %, rémission complète 18 %. Le but de cette étude était d'améliorer la survie, de diminuer le taux des rechutes métastatiques. Le recul est trop court pour permettre une conclusion. Les résultats préliminaires montrent un taux élevé de progression tumorale, la mauvaise appréciation du stade des cancers de la vessie d'après la clinique, c'est la raison plus laquelle en dépit du fait que nous avons 6 vessies où il n'y avait plus de tumeur, nous pensons que la cystectomie demeure le traitement le plus efficace.

Neo-Adjuvant Chemotherapy. Ed. Cl. Jacquillat, M. Weil, D. Khayat. Colloque INSERM/John Libbey Eurotext Ltd. © 1988. Vol. 169, pp. 455-457.

Presurgery chemotherapy (CT) in locally advanced bladder carcinoma : a feasible and possibly effective approach

M. Francini**, A. Veronesi*, V. Dal Bo**, A. Merlo**, G. Carmignani***, G. Lo Re*, A. Carbone, M.D. Magri*, R. Talamini and S. Monfardini*

**Div. Medical Oncology, **Div. Urology, Div. Pathology, Div. Epidemiology, Centro di Riferimento Oncologico, Aviano, ***Urologic Clinic, Trieste, Italy*

From June 1982 to September 1984, occasional patients (pts) with locally advanced bladder carcinoma were treated with combination CT (Adriamycin 50 mg/mq, Cisplatin 50 mq on day 1 and Fluorouracil 500 mg/mq and Teniposide 100 mg/mq on day 1 and 8, every 21 days) followed by radical cystectomy within a phase II CT study (1). Of the 6 pts treated, 4 responded to CT (2 complete remission, 2 partial remission). No evidence of disease or neoplastic microfocus were found in the resected specimen of 4 pts (2 treated with a short course of preoperative radiotherapy). These results prompted a prospective study of presurgery CT in locally advanced bladder carcinoma, which was started in October 1984. Criteria of eligibility included histologically proven transitional cell carcinoma of the bladder, age less than 75 years, PS greater than 70, T3b-T4, N0-4,M0 disease after CT scan, lymphangiography and TUR, no previous treatment.
Planned treatment consisted in 3 cycles of CT as above, followed by radical cystectomy. If radical cystectomy was not feasible due to age or general status, extensive check TUR was planned after 3 cycles of CT. Until December 1987, 28 pts have been entered into the study. Pt characteristics include M/F ratio 25/3, median age 61 years (42-75), median PS 100 (70-100), T3b in 26 pts, local relapse in 2, NX in 5 pts, N0 in 16, N+ in 7.
Response to CT is reported in Table 1. Response rate was 80%. Toxicity is reported in Table 2. CT was reasonably well tolerated and it was possible to administer a high percentage of the theoretical dose (88% for Fluorouracil, 99% for Adriamycin, 90% for Cisplatin and 88% for Teniposide).
Out of the 25 pts who have completed CT, 2 refused surgery (1 was operated later on, the other is disease free at 2 years with CT only), 1 received radiation therapy, 1 died for unrelated causes immediately before surgery, 1 is awaiting surgery. Nineteen pts were operated as planned (radical cystectomy in 13, TUR in 3, palliative surgery in 2, exploratory laparotomy with no evidence of disease in 1). Clinico-pathological correlations are shown in Table 3. Five out of 19 pts were found to be histologically tumour free. Three year actuarial survival (all eligible pts) is 45%.

In conclusion, the CT-surgery approach is feasible and may be useful in this poor risk group of pts.

Table 1

RESPONSE TO CT

n. of pts : 28
n. of pts evaluable for response to CT: 25
Reasons for inevaluability:
early death in 2 pts, 1 pt still undergoing CT

Response:			
	CR	5	78%
	PR	15	
	STAB	3	
	PRO	2	

Table 2

TOXICITY (WHO) (27 PTS)

	0	1	2	3	4
Bone Marrow	10	1	9	2	5
Creat.	23	4	–	–	–
N V	4	4	13	2	4
Hair Loss	6	4	8	9	–
Infection	21	1	–	5	–

Table 3

CLINICO-PATHOLOGICAL CORRELATIONS

CLINICAL	PATHOLOGICAL
4 CR	RO= 3(1*) R2= 1
12 PR	RO= 2(1*) R1= 4 R2= 6(1*)
2 STAB	R2=2
1 PRO	R2=2

* TUR

RO= no evidence of disease
R1= microscopic evidence of disease
R2= macroscopic evidence of disease

Reference

A. Veronesi, E. Galligioni, G. Lo Re et al: Combination chemotherapy with Fluorouracil, Adriamycin, Cis-Platinum and VM26 in Advanced Transitional Cell carcinoma of the Urinary Tract. Eur J Cancer Clin Oncol 22: 1457-1460, 1986.

Neo-Adjuvant Chemotherapy. Ed. Cl. Jacquillat, M. Weil, D. Khayat. Colloque INSERM/John Libbey Eurotext Ltd. © 1988. Vol. 169, pp. 459-463.

Alternating chemotherapy and radiotherapy treatment in patients with infiltrating bladder cancer

R. Rosso, M. Venturini, A. Michelotti, M. Merlano, D. Scarpati, G. Martorana, A. Curotto and L. Giuliani

Istituto Nazionale per la Ricerca sul Cancro e Clinica urologica dell'Università, Viale Benedetto XV, 10, 16132 Genova, Italia

ABSTRACT

Thirty-two patients with infiltrating bladder cancer (T2-T4) were treated with one course of alternating chemo-radiotherapy before radical cystectomy(Group A 20 patients) or two courses as definitive procedure(Group B 12 patients). One course consisted of: Cisplatin 20 mg/m^2 iv and 5-Fluorouracil 200 mg/m^2 iv for 5 consecutive days, the first and the fourth weeks; Radiotherapy is given at the dose of 200 cGy daily for 5 consecutive days the second and the third weeks. At the seventh week a second course of the same integrated therapy was repeated in Group B. Results. Group A: 15 patients underwent radical cystectomy. Six (40%) patients had a pathological(p) Complete Response (CR). Two (13.3%) patients p-Partial Response (PR) and seven (46.6%) patients p-No Responders were rendered disease free by surgery. Five patients avoided either the second course and cystecto my because age (3 patients), vascular obliteration (1) and enteritis (1). Actuarial survival is 71% at 26 months. Group B: 12 patients had 2 courses of therapy. All obtained clinical CR. Two patients locally relapsed at 9 and 11 months respectively. They underwent radical cystectomy and they are still alive, and disease free. The median follow-up of this group is 12.5 months (10 - 17). Toxicity. All 32 patients were evaluable for toxicity after the first course: no grade IV toxicity was observed; patients received full planned dose of radiotherapy (20 Gy), 97% of Cisplatin dosage and 93% of 5-Fluorouracil. Significant increase in haematological toxicity was observed in Group B : two patients had grade IV, and 5 patients grade III. All patients (12) received the total dose of radiotherapy(40 Gy) but 91% of Cisplatin and 78% of 5-Fluorouracil.
The high pCR and cCR obtained in patients of Group A and Group B respectively appears a promising result, even if a longer follow-up and a larger number of patients is required to draw any conclusion.

KEY WORDS

Bladder Cancer, Chemo-radiotherapy, Alternating Schedule, Neoadjuvant

INTRODUCTION

Carcinoma of the bladder accounts for 2% of all malignant solid tumors. Although the disease is localized, at the time of initial diagnosis, in 90% of the patients, 4 out of 5 radically treated patients will relapse (Richie et al 1985). Currently, preoperative radiotherapy has entered into clinical practice. Altough several reports indicate a benefit for combined treatment, there is no conclusive evidence that preoperative radiotherapy exceeds radical cystectomy or radical radiotherapy alone. Despite the progress in local control, more than 50% of patients with infiltrating bladder cancer (T2 - T4) will develop distant metastases and only about 30% of patients will alive at 5 years.

Various clinical trials suggest that bladder cancer is a chemoresponsive tumor, with a 50% - 70% of objective response in metastatic disease (Yagoda, 1987).

Therefore, combining chemotherapy and radiotherapy might improve the results achieved by either modality alone (local and remote control, synergistic interaction).

This paper reports the results obtained with a combination of chemotherapy and radiotherapy employed either as neoadiuvant treatment (Group A) or as definitive procedure (Group B).

PATIENTS AND METHODS

The study includes patients with biopsy proven infiltrating bladder cancer (T2 - T4), without metastatic disease, with performance status 0-2 (ECOG scale), normal renal, cardiac and liver function. All patients had no previously treatment with systemic chemotherapy or radiotherapy. Patient characteristics are listed in table 1. The initial evaluation included: history and physical examination, complete laboratory diagnostic studies, excretory urogram, chest-X-ray, bone scan and abdominal computerized tomography (CT). The local extent is evaluated by CT, cystoscopy and transuretral resection (TUR). Initially,patients entered the study if they were elegible for radical cystectomy. However, because of striking responses seen in the first 10 patients, a second group of selected patients (complete TUR, absence of ureteral obstruction and absence of node involvement) or patients refusing cystectomy, were treated with two courses of integrated therapy.

Therefore, treatment plan consisted of one course of chemo-radiotherapy as neoadjuvant therapy before radical cystectomy (Group A 20 patients) or two courses, shared by two weeks, without surgery (Group B 12 patients).

One course included two cycles of chemotherapy(weeks 1 and 4) and one cycle of radiotherapy(weeks 2 and 3).
Chemotherapy consisted of Cisplatin 20 mg/m^2 and 5-Fluorouracil 200 mg/m^2 iv for 5 consecutive days every 3 weeks).
Radiotherapy was administered with cobalt 60,four fields encompassing the whole pelvis. Each cycle consisted of 20 Gy in ten fractions of 200 cGy each, in two weeks.
Cisplatin was given with short hydratation and forced diuresys. Antiemetic therapy was undertaken at the physician's discretion.
A clinical Complete Response (cCR) was defined as a disappearance of all detectable tumor. A clinical Partial Response (cPR) as a persistence of tumor with a superficial stage (Ta-T1-Tis). No response cases (cNR) were considered as those situations different from the above. Pathological (p) category indicates only surgical staging.

Toxicity has been recorded according to WHO criteria.

RESULTS

Group A. Fifteen patients underwent radical cystectomy. Eight (53%) patients had a p-Objective response (40% pCR an 13% pPR).The patients (2/15 pPR, 6/15 pNR) who did not achieve a pCR were rendered disease free by surgery.
Five patients, cCR, after the first course, avoided either the second course and cystectomy because of age (3 patients), vascular oblitera tion (1) and enteritis (1).
Six patients died. Three resected patient died because of surgical complication; other two resected patients died because of disease progression. One additive patient, previously non-resected, died due to other, tumor free.
Actuarial survival in group A is 71% at 26 months.

Group B. Twelve patients had two courses of therapy. All obtained cCR. Two patients locally relapsed at 9 and 11 months respectively. They underwent radical cystectomy and they are still alive, and disease free. The median follow-up of this group is 12.5 months (range 10 - 17).

TOXICITY

All 32 patients were evaluable for toxicity after the first course. No grade IV toxixity was observed. All patients received 100% of the planned dose of radiotherapy(20 Gy), 97% of Cisplatin dosage and 93% of 5-Fluorouracil.
Significant increase in haematological toxicity was observed in 12 patients who received the second course of therapy. These patients received the total planned dose of radiotherapy (40 Gy), 91% of Cisplatin and 78% of Fluorouracil dose.
Other side effects are reported in table 2.

CONCLUSIONS

In literature, the pathological Complete Response rate after an induction treatment ranges between 18% - 27% when only chemotherapy is employed (Bukowsky,1987; Scher,1987). The preoperative radiotherapy offers only 3% - 5% of pCR at the dose of 20 Gy (Herr,1985; Whitmore 1977). The combined treatment (chemotherapy and radiotherapy) is able to achieve a pCR rate of 27% (Herr, 1983; Torti,1986).

In light of these consideration, it is of interest that 40% of patients, who underwent radical cystectomy, were pathologically disease free after only one course of chemo-radiotherapy.

Although the number of patients is small , our study suggests that the alternating treatment is a feasible innovative therapy for infiltrating bladder tumor, as neoadjuvant therapy. A randomized trial is in progress to verify the real utility of this treatment to improve the survival (neoadjuvant therapy and cystectomy versus cystectomy alone) of these patients.

The results obtained in group B show that the proposed treatment is feasible with an acceptable toxicity and that it does not preclude a salvage cystectomy if required. However, a longer follow-up and a larger number of patients is required to determine the role of this integrated therapy in avoiding surgery.

Table 1. PATIENT CHARACTERISTICS

	GROUP A	GROUP B
No. PATIENTS	20	12
SEX (Male:Female)	19:1	12:0
MEAN AGE (years)	62	66
CLINICAL STAGE :		
Tumor extent		
T2	9	10
T3	9	1
T4	2	-
Tx	-	1
Node Involvement		
N-	12	12
N+	8	-
Tumor Grade		
G1	2	-
G2	8	8
G3	10	4

Table 2. TOXICITY

GRADE	1	2	3	4	1	2	3	4
White Blood Cells	8	8	4	-	3	4	3	1
Platelets	4	6	-	-	2	1	2	1
Hemaglobin	6	1	-	-	3	-	-	-
Creatinine	3	-	-	-	1	-	-	-
Fever	1	-	-	-	1	-	-	-
Bladder	2	3	1	-	2	1	1	-
Stomatitis	-	-	-	-	2	-	-	-
Diarrhea	4	2	-	-	1	2	-	-
Nausea & Vomiting	8	24	-	-	3	9	-	-
	number of patients							
	FIRST COURSE +				SECOND COURSE ++			

The toxicity is referred to
+ the first course of chemo-radiotherapy (32 patients)
++ the second course of chemo-rdaiotherapy (12 patients)

REFERENCES

Bukowsky, R.M.(1987): Neoadjuvant chemotherapy of locally advanced transitional cell carcinoma of the bladder. Results of a phase II trial and follow-up. Proc. Am. Soc. Clin. Oncol. 6, 108 (C 424).

Herr, H.W.(1983): Planned preoperative cisplatin and radiation therapy for locally advanced bladder cancer. Cancer 52, 2205-2208.

Herr, H.W.(1985): Preoperative irradiation with and without chemotherapy as adjunct to radical cystectomy. Urology 25, 127

Richie, J.P.(1985): Cancer of bladder. In Cancer Practice & Principles of Oncology, 2nd edn, ed V.T.De Vita Jr. pp 915-928. Philadelphia: Lippincott Company.

Scher, H.(1987): Pathologic response to M-VAC (methotrexate,vinblastine,adriamycin and cisplatin) in urothelial tract tumors. Proc. Am. Soc. Clin. Oncol. 6, 105 (C 410).

Torti, F.M.(1986): Effect of preoperative cisplatin (CDDP) and radiation therapy (XRT) on downstaging of invasive bladder cancer: a NCOG study. Proc. Am. Soc. Clin. Oncol. 5, 103 (C 401).

Whitmore, W.F.(1977): A comparative study of two pre-operative radiation regimens with cystectomy for bladder cancer. Cancer 40, 1077-1086.

Yagoda, A.(1987): Chemotherapy of urothelial tract tumors. Cancer 60, 574-585.

Résumé

32 malades porteurs de cancer de la vessie infiltrant (T2, T4) ont été traités par une cure alternant radio-chimiothérapie avant une cystectomie radicale (groupe A 20 malades), ou deux cures (groupe B : 12 patients). Une cure a consisté en Cis.Platyl 20 mg/m2 I.V. et 5 Fluoro-uracile 200 mg/m2, IV, 5 jours consécutifs, la 1ère et 4ème semaine. La radiothérapie a été donnée à la dose de 200 CGY tous les jours pour 5 jours, la 2ème et la 3ème semaine. A la 7ème semaine, une deuxième cure de la même association a été répétée pour le groupe B.

Résultats : groupe A : 15 malades ont subi une cystectomie radicale , 6 (40 %) ont eu une réponse histologique complète, 2 une réponse partielle et chez 7 (46,6 %) non répondeurs histologiques, la tumeur a pu être enlevée par la chirugie. Chez 5 malades, la deuxième cure ou la cystectomie n'ont pas pu être pratiquées en raison de l'âge 3 malades, d'oblitération vasculaire (1), d'une entérite (1 malade). La survie actuarielle est de 71 % à 26 mois. Dans le groupe B 12 malades ont eu 2 cures de ce traitement combiné ils ont tous une rémission clinique complète, 2 malades ont rechuté localement à 9 et 11 mois, ils ont subi une cystectomie radicale et sont toujours vivants sans tumeur. Le recul médian de ce groupe est de 12,5 mois (10-17 mois). Les 32 malades ont été évaluables pour la toxicité après la 1ère cure. Aucune toxicité de grade IV n'a été observée. Les malades ont pu recevoir la dose de radiothérapie prévue (20 gy), 97 % de la dose de platine et 93 % de la dose de 5.Fu. Une augmentation significative de la toxicité hématologique a été observée dans le group B. Chez deux malades la toxicité a été de grade IV, chez 5 malades de grade III. Tous les malades ont reçu la dose complète de radiothérapie (40 gy), seulement 91 % de la dose de platine et 78 % de la dose de 5. Fu.. Le taux élevé de rémission complète et de rémission partielle observée dans le groupe A et B, paraissent des résultats prometteurs même si un plus long recul et un plus grand nombre de patients est nécessaire pour conclure.

Pediatrics, bones and soft tissue sarcomas

Tumeurs de l'enfant, sarcomes des os et des tissus mous

Neo-Adjuvant Chemotherapy. Ed. Cl. Jacquillat, M. Weil, D. Khayat. Colloque INSERM/John Libbey Eurotext Ltd. © 1988. Vol. 169, pp. 467-471.

Pre-operative chemotherapy as first treatment in children with Wilms' tumour. Results of the SIOP nephroblastoma, trials and studies

P.A. Voûte, J.F.M. Delemarre, M.F. Tournade, J. de Kraker, J. Lemerle, J.M.V. Burgers, H. Perry, M. Carli and P. Bey (for the SIOP Nephroblastoma Committee)

SIOP Nephroblastoma Trial and Study Office, Spinozastraat 51, 1018 HJ Amsterdam, The Netherlands

A Wilms' tumour or nephroblastoma is the most frequently found malignant tumour of the kidney in childhood. In 1899 the tumour was described by Wilms as a mixed tumour derived from embryonal kidney tissue. In a nephroblastoma epithelial as well as non-epithelial components can be found. The tumour is mostly diagnosed in children under the age of 8, although sporadic cases in young adults are found. Progress in treatment of cancer can be clearly illustrated in patients with nephroblastomas. With only one surgical intervention in the beginning of the century a cure rate of 8% was reported With better facilities the cure rate with only surgical intervention was 30% (Ladd, 1941). This was in a period without the possibility of blood transfusions, infusions or simple anaesthesia. When radiotherapy was added to the tumourbed after surgery, 40% of the children were cured (Sutow, 1970). Adding actinomycin D to the treatment with surgery and radiotherapy brought the cure rate to 50% (Wolff, 1968). These better cure rates were achieved in the period that better pre- and postoperative care became available, it is difficult to determine which factor, more intensive therapy or better care, was responsible for the better results. A drastic improvement in the prognosis of the children with a Wilms' tumour occurred when a combination chemotherapy, vincristine and actinomycin D was given. Cure rate reached 80%. Systematic treatment research was initiated in large cooperative studies, in the United States by the 'National Wilms' Tumor Studies' (NWTS) and in Europe international studies were conducted by the International Society of Paediatric Oncology (SIOP). Opinions concerning the primary treatment of a child with a nephroblastoma differ. In the United States the immediate excision is advocated and in Europe a preoperative treatment. Both studies used the same staging system, developed by the NWTS, which later has been translated in the TNM classification for Wilms' tumours (Spiesse, 1985).

In 1971 the first SIOP nephroblastoma study started comparing preoperative radiotherapy to immediate surgery and a single course of actinomycin D to multiple courses. 42 clinics from 14 countries in Europe participated. 397 patients were included in this study. It was concluded that preoperative treatment prevented tumour rupture during surgery and that preoperative treatment therefore was advisable. There was no difference between the group receiving one course actinomycin D versus multiple courses (Lemerle, 1976). Patients who still developed metastases were treated with actinomycin D, vincristine and lungirradiation.

A 2nd study started in October 1974. A comparison between 6 months and 15 months combination chemotherapy with actinomycin D and vincristine was studied. It seemed that 6 months maintenance chemotherapy was as good as 15 months with a recurrence free survival of 78% and a total survival of 85% (fig.1). Following the results of the NWTS 2 study and the SIOP results it was clear that patients with a stage I tumour did not need radiotherapy.

A next study (SIOP 5) compared preoperative combination chemotherapy to preoperative radiotherapy. In this SIOP study 407 patients were included. The recurrence free survival of the two groups of patients in trial was respectively 74% and 64% (fig.2). The survival per stage was stage I 90%, stage II 82%, stage III 67% at 6 years. In this study 44% of the patients were stage I who did not need any radiotherapy (Lemerle, 1983). At this moment it seemed necessary to add another clinical stage, because of the difference between survival rates in stage I and II compared to III. Stage II was split in stage II with negative lymphnodes (II N-) and with positive lymphnodes (II N+).

In the fourth SIOP Wilms' tumour study (SIOP 6) preoperative chemotherapy for 4 weeks with actinomycin D and vincristine was given. In stage I maintenance chemotherapy was randomised between 3 months and 6 months. Stage II N- were randomised in postoperative radiotherapy or not. Stage II N+ & stage III randomised in two different chemotherapy protocols. In December 1987 866 patients with a Wilms' tumour have been registered both in the study and the trial. Repartition of postoperative stages in 849 evaluable patients was

	N	%
stage I	355	42
stage II	231	27
stage III	115	14
stage IV	108	12
stage V	40	5
total	849	

431 patients were included in the three randomised trials: stage I 257, stage II N- 108, stage II N+ and stage III 66. The survival in the three groups is respectively 93%, 88%, 83% (fig.3). Until now there appears no great difference between 3 months and 6 months chemotherapy in stage I. The survival in stage II N- is not different for the two arms (fig.4). There were slightly more local recurrences in the non radiotherapy group, but this did not influence the survival.

It can therefore be concluded that in the patients with a non metastatic Wilms' tumour 82% donot need radiotherapy if they are treated with chemotherapy before surgery.

CONCLUSION

From the different SIOP studies it is concluded that:

1. Chemotherapeutic treatment before surgery is necessary.
2. Radiotherapy is not necessary in ± 80% of the patients.
3. Clinical trials in Wilms' tumour patients have to be continued to determine how treatment can be further reduced.
4. Patients with a Wilms' tumour can be cured and live a normal life with a life expectancy comparable to children of their age group without a nephroblastoma.

Following these conclusions it was decided to start a new study (SIOP 9) with the most important question if a prolonged preoperative chemotherapy treatment could enlarge the number of patients in stage I and stage II N-, to diminish further the number of patients needing radiotherapy. The patients with a stage II N+ and stage III or with an unfavourable histology after preoperative chemotherapy will receive a more intensified chemotherapy adding epirubicin and ifosfamide. This study started the 1st of January 1988 and will be followed by most of the European Centres.

REFERENCES

Ladd, W.E., White, R.R.(1941): Embryoma of the kidney (Wilms' tumour). Jama 117:1858.

Lemerle, J., Voûte, P.A., Tournade, M.F., Delemarre, J.F.M., Jereb, B., Åhström, L., Flamant, R., Gerard-Marchant, R.(1976) Preoperative versus postoperative radiotherapy, single versus multiple courses of actinomycin D, in the treatment of Wilms' tumor. Preliminary results of a controlled clinical trial conducted by the International Society of Paediatric Oncology (SIOP). Cancer 38:647-654.

Lemerle, J., Voûte, P.A., Tournade, M.F., Rodary, C., Delemarre, J.F.M., Sarrazin,D., Burgers, J.M.V., Sandstedt, B., Mildenberger, H., Carli, M., Jereb, B., Moorman-Voestermans, C.G.M.(1983): Effectiveness of preoperative chemotherapy in Wilms' tumor: results of an International Society of Paediatric Oncology (SIOP) clinical trial. J.Clin.Onc.1:604-609.

Spiesse, B., Hermanek, P., Scheibe, O., Wagner, G.(eds) (1985): UICC TNM atlas: illustrated guide to TNM, pTNM classification of malignant tumours. 2nd ed. (Springer Berlin Heidelberg New York Tokyo).

Sutow, W.W., Gehan, E.A., Heyn, R.M., Kung, F.H., Miller, R.W., Murphy, M.L., Traggis, D.G.(1970): Comparison of survival curves, 1956 versus 1962, in children with Wilms' tumor and neuroblastoma. Pediatrics 45:800-811.

Wilms, M. (1899): Die Mischgeschwülste der Niere. Arthur Georgi Verlag Leipzig.

Wolff, J.A., Krivit, W., Newton, W.A., D'Angio, G.J.(1968): Single versus multiple dose Dactinomycin therapy of Wilms' tumor. N.Engl.J.Med.279:290-294.

Nephroblastoma clinical trial SIOP No.9. A therapeutic trial and prospective study. International Society of Paediatric Oncology December 1987.

Fig. 1 SIOP 2 SCHEDULE PATIENTS N = 138

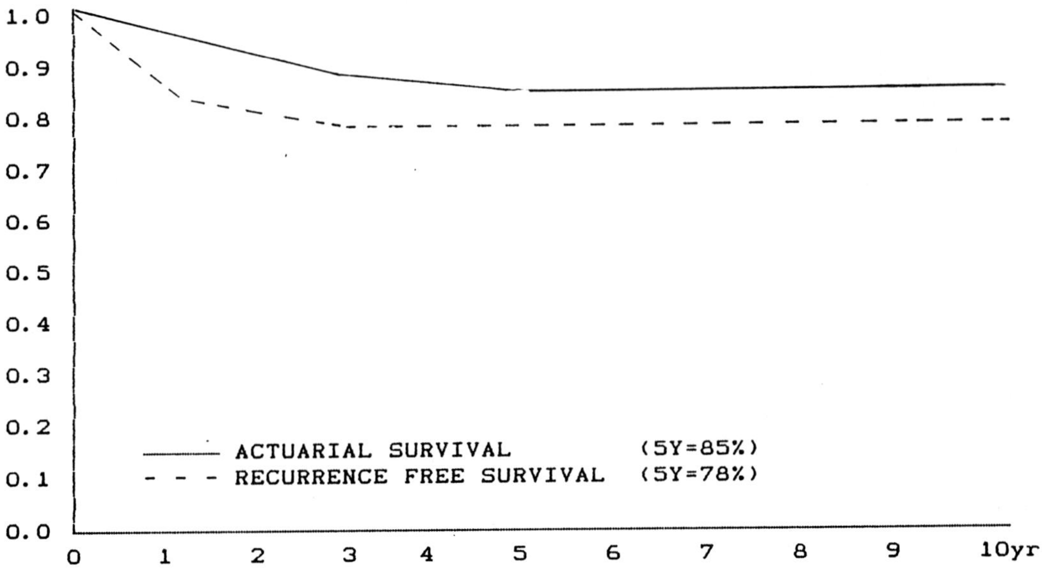

Fig. 2 SIOP 5 TRIAL PATIENTS N = 163

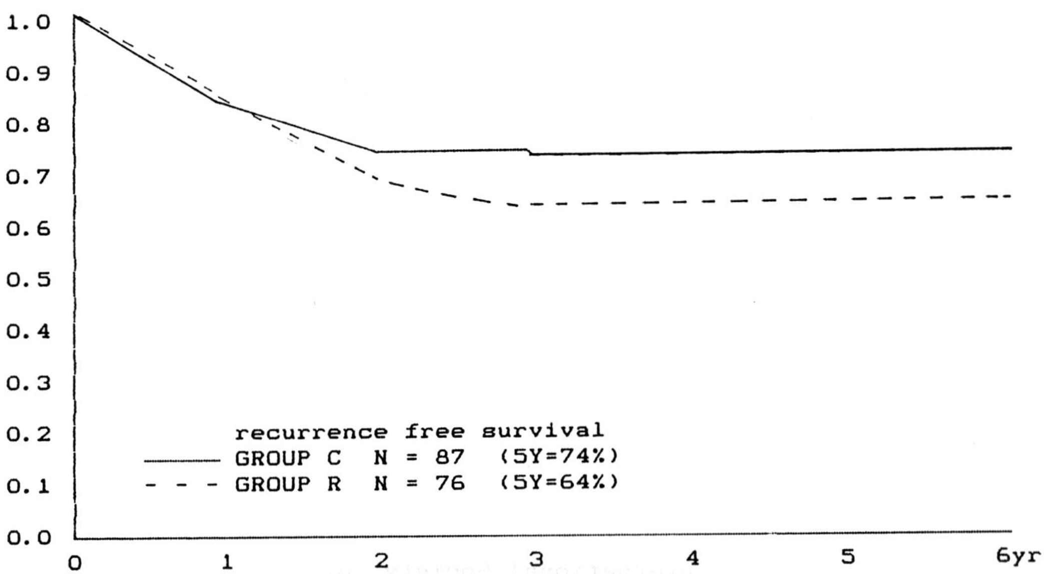

Fig. 3 SIOP 6 RANDOMISED TRIAL PATIENTS N = 431

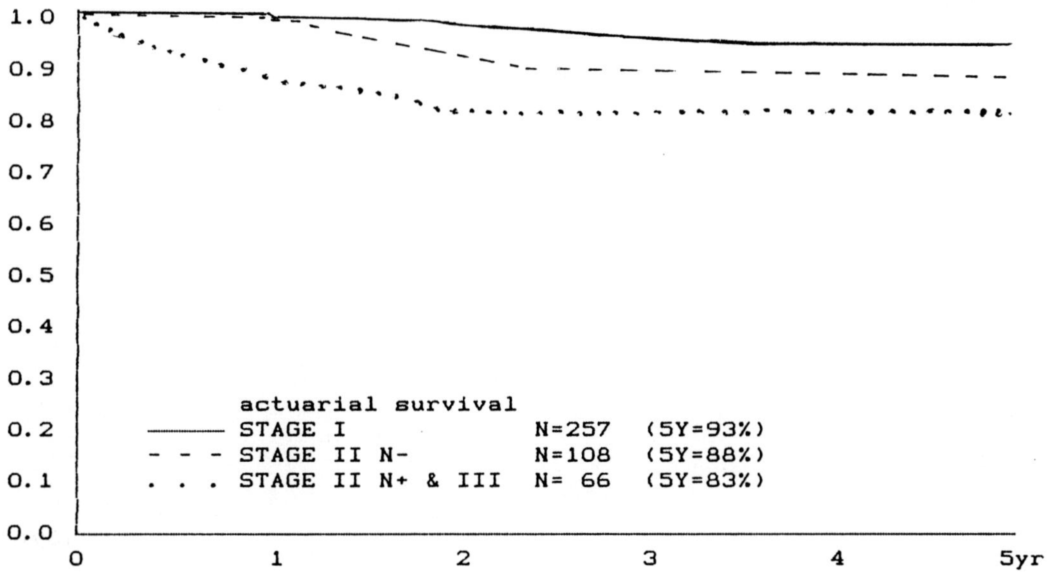

Fig. 4 SIOP 6 TRIAL PATIENTS STAGE II N- N = 108

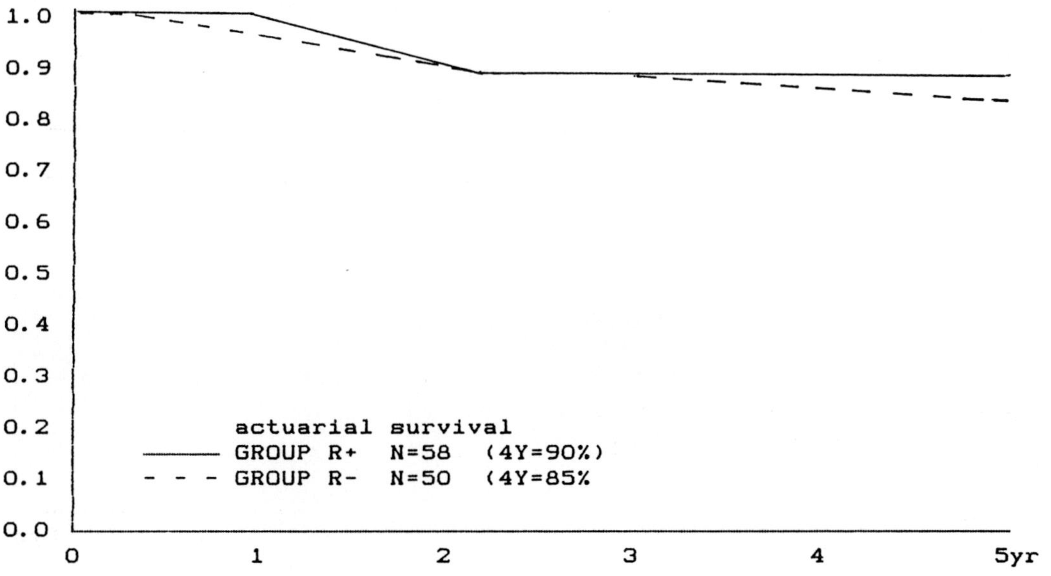

Neo-Adjuvant Chemotherapy. Ed. Cl. Jacquillat, M. Weil, D. Khayat. Colloque INSERM/John Libbey Eurotext Ltd. © 1988. Vol. 169, pp. 473-478.

Protochemotherapy of non-testicular malignant non-seminomatous germ cell tumors (NSGCTs) in children and adolescents : results of the GPO-trials MAKEI 83/86

U. Göbel[1], G. Calaminus[1], R.J. Haas[2], J. Engert[3], J.P.M. Bökkerink[4], H. Gadner[5], H. Jürgens[1] and D. Harms[6] (for the GPO-MAKEI study group)

[1]*Abt. Pädiatrische Hämatologie und Onkologie der Universität Düsseldorf, FRG*
[2]*Abt. Pädiatrische Hämatologie und Onkologie der Universität München, FRG*
[3]*Kinderchirurgische Klinik der Universität Bochum, FRG*
[4]*Sint Radboudziekenhuis, Universiteit Nijmegen, Niederlande,*
[5]*St. Anna Kinderspital, Wien, Österreich*
[6]*Institut für Paidopathologie der Universität Kiel, FRG*
Supported by BMFT-grant n° 01 ZP 850 12

Address for reprints:

Prof. Dr. U. Göbel
Zentrum für Kinderheilkunde
der Universität
Abt. für Hämatologie und Onkologie
Moorenstr. 5
D-4000 Düsseldorf, FRG

SUMMARY

In the 1983 opened trial 66 evaluable protocol patients (pts.) with extracranial NSGCT's had been registered. With respect to the therapy regimen these pts. can be divided into 3 groups:

Group A: pts. with completely resected NSGCT's received 4 courses of vinblastine 3 mg/m², days 1+2, bleomycin 15 mg/m², days 1-3, and cisplatinum 20 mg/m² (with mannitol diuresis), days 4-8 (VBC).

Group B: pts. with incompletely resected malignant NSGCT's received after surgery 4 courses of VBC. Following second-look surgery chemotherapy is continued with 4 courses of VP16 100 mg/m², days 1-3, ifosfamide 1.500 mg/m² (with mesna uroprotection), days 1-5, and cisplatinum 20 mg/m², days 1-5 (VPIC).

Group C: pts. with extensive NSGCT's diagnosed by biopsy received protochemotherapy consisting of 4 courses of VBC prior to definitive surgery followed by 4 courses of VPIC.

Results:

Group A: 16/17 pts. remained disease-free (92 ± 7 %).
Group B: 18/26 pts. remained disease-free (66 ± 10 %).
Group C: 22/23 pts. remained disease-free (95 ± 4 %).

Germ cell tumors originate from primitive germ cells. In infancy and childhood they may be located within the gonades as well as outside the gonades, e.g. in the saccrococcygeal or pineal region, the mediastinum or other sites. The different histological entities may be malignant, potentially malignant or benign. In mixed germ cell tumors the prognosis depends on the most malignant part; therefore the most malignant part and not the quantitative distribution must be considered the predominant histology.

Histology, tumor site, and tumor stage have been reported to be of prognostic value. Therefore, 1983 the cooperative prospective trial for non-testicular germ cell tumors (MAKEI 83) of the German Society of Pediatric Oncology (GPO) was started, where the treatment was stratified according to these different risk factors (6). In 1986 the protocol was supplemented with special treatment guidelines for dysgerminomas and intracranial sites (MAKEI 86).

The two aims of the study are to increase the formerly poor prognosis of malignant germ cell tumors in infancy and childhood, and to avoid mutilation from radical surgery in extended tumors. For instance, out of 23 young girls with yolk sac tumor of the vagina, summarized by KOHORN et al. (8), only 9 were long-term survivors, only 2 of those did not undergo radical hysterectomy and vaginectomy. Therefore, the treatment strategy (fig. 1) employs primary tumor resection only in localized disease, followed by 4 courses of adjuvant chemotherapy consisting of vinblastine, bleomycin, and cisplatinum (VBC). In extended ovarian and all extragonadal tumors, additional chemotherapy is administered, consisting of VP16, ifosfamide, and cisplatinum (VPIC).

In cases of incompletely resected tumors, second-look surgery is mandatory. However, in patients with localized disease of essential organs or bulky disease, protochemotherapy is given to avoid unneccessary organ loss and to allow complete tumor resection in these poor prognostic patients.

This analysis is focused on patients with malignant NSGCT's of non-testicular and extracranial origin.

Fig. 1 TREATMENT STRATEGY

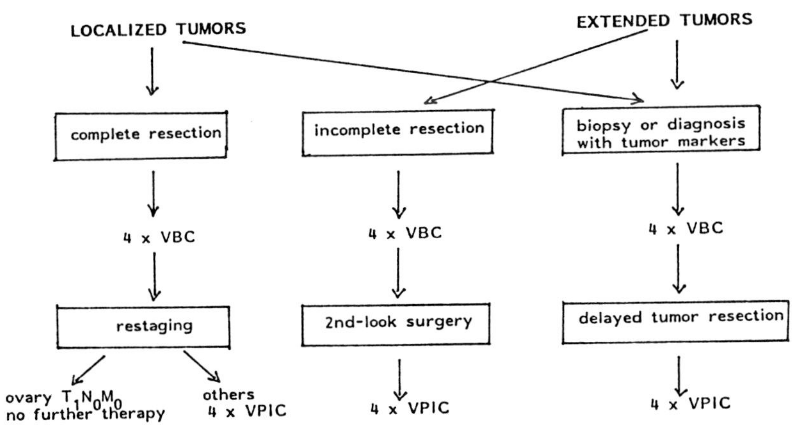

CHEMOTHERAPY FOR MALIGNANT NSGCT's

Vinblastine, 3 mg/m², days 1 and 2 i.v., is given combined with bleomycin 15 mg/m², days 1-3, as continuous infusion. Thereafter cisplatinum 20 mg/m², days 4-8, with mannitol diuresis is administered. This combination (VBC) is repeated four times in non-testicular germ cell tumors every 3 weeks; the cumulative bleomycin dose is limited to 180 mg/m².

VP16 is combined with cisplatinum and ifosfamide in the following schedule: VP 16 100 mg/m², days 1-5, ifosfamide 1,5 g/m², days 1-5, with mesna uroprotection, and cisplatinum 20 mg/m², days 1-5, with mannitol diuresis. This chemotherapy (VPIC) regimen is repeated four times in disseminated ovarian or extragonadal tumors every 3 weeks with careful monitoring of blood counts and renal function.

TREATMENT STRATEGY (Fig. 1)

The diagnosis of malignant NSGCT's is obtained by biopsy, or tumor resection, or clinically in advanced diseases with elevated tumor markers (AFP above 1000 ng/ml or βHCG above 100 ng/ml).

Ovarian tumors are staged according to the UCC-classification. The staging of extragonadal primaries is made according to staging systems applied in soft tissue sarcomas.

According to the relatively low incidence of mNSGCT's in infancy and childhood, patients are classified into two risk groups: The low risk group consists of all girls with ovarian tumors stage T_1, where four courses of VBC are administered.

The high risk group consists of ovarian tumors UCC stage T_2 - T_3 and all extragonadal primaries. After histological or clinical diagnosis, four courses VBC are administered, followed by second-look surgery or tumor resection. In sacrococcygeal germ cell tumors, enbloc resection of tumor and coccyx is mandatory.

Following surgery, four courses of VPIC are administered. With respect to the high cumulative dose of cisplatinum and the increased myelotoxicity of VPIC, strict guidelines for monitoring of blood counts and renal function are to be followed by all participating institutions.

CLINICAL DATA

Between January 1983 and September 1987, 66 protocol patients with mNSGCT's were registered. At the time of this analysis (February 1988) all patients were more than 4 months on treatment and had undergone initial respectively delayed tumor resection.

The age of the patients ranged between 1 month and 20 years, medium age 3 years. Fifty-eight cases were girls and only 8 boys.

The predominant histology was yolk sac tumor in 54 cases, embryonal carcinoma in 11 cases, and chorioncarcinoma in 1 case. The histology was reviewed by a panel of pathologists (Prof. Dr. D. Harms, Institut für Kinderpathologie, Kiel; Prof. Dr. H. Löhrs, Institut für Pathologie, Lübeck; Prof. Dr. H. Müntefering, Institut für Kinderpathologie, Mainz; Prof. Dr. F. Städtler, Institut für Pathologie, Bremen).

RESULTS

Ovarian NSGCT's (23 pts.) were mostly confined to the primary site (14 pts.) despite tumor size up to 17 cm in diameter and were therefore primarily resected. Genito-urinary tumors (5 pts.) have been treated with protochemotherapy to avoid vaginectomy. Sacrococcygeal (29 pts.) and mediastinal (5 pts.) and head and neck (1 pt.) tumors with regional extension mostly had initial surgery, whereas patients with extensive tumors and apparent metastases received protochemotherapy. Therefore, according to surgical treatment, the results can be classified according to three different groups:

Group A: Patients with localized disease and incomplete tumor resection: 1 of 17 patients relapsed.

Group B: Patients with regional disease and incomplete tumor resection: 7 of 26 patients failed; 1 died of septicemia.

Group C: Patients with protochemotherapy and delayed tumor resection: none of the 23 patients relapsed; 1 died of septicemia.

Life-table analyses according to Kaplan-Meier of these three groups of patients resulted at 61 months in an event-free survival of 92 (± 7 %) (Group A), resp. 66 (± 10 %) (Group B), resp. 95 (± 4 %) (Group C) (fig. 2). The difference between group A, resp. group C and group B is statistically significant ($p \geq 0.03$).

Fig. 2 EVENT-FREE SURVIVAL OF EXTRACRANIAL MALIGNANT NSGCTs

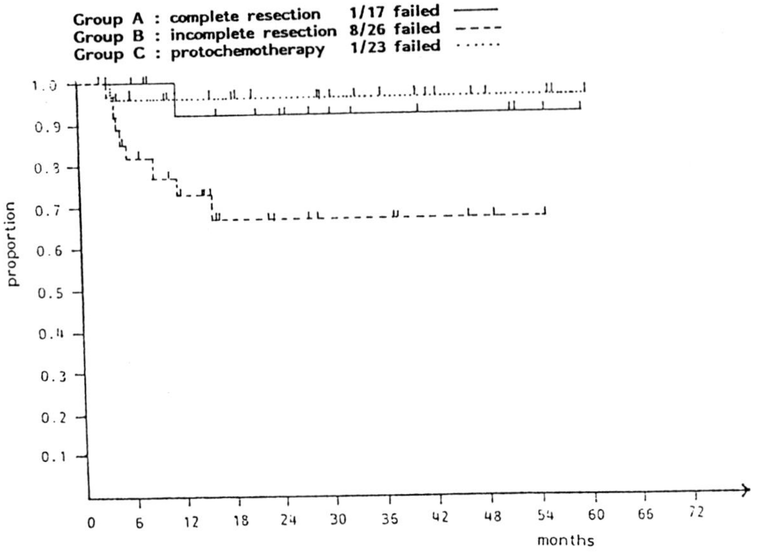

The relapses occured in 3/23 ovarian and 5/29 sacrococcygeal NSGCT's. Age at diagnosis, initial tumor stage, and predominant histology were without apparent influence. As local recurrences occured in 6 out of 8 relapse patients, incomplete tumor resection seems of significant value. Only 2 patients presented with distant metastases without local recurrence resembling resistance to chemotherapy.

Chemotherapy associated toxicity following the VBC-courses was moderate and included two patients with mild pneumopathy, whereas following VPIC, pronounced myelosuppression was seen in one third of the patients. Two of these patients have died during episodes of septicemia. Cisplatinum associated toxicity included transient nephropathy (11 pts.), ototoxicity (4 pts.), and neuropathy (2pts.).

DISCUSSION

In the past malignant germ cell tumors had a very poor prognosis and caused about 3 % of death from malignancy in infancy and childhood. Combined treatment consisting of surgery and chemotherapy, including vincristine, actinomycin D, and cyclophosphamide (VAC) plus/minus adriamycin in high dosages led to a long-term remission rate in about half of the patients with malignant non-testicular NSGCT's (4,10).

The original EINHORN regimen including vinblastine, bleomycin, and cisplatinum proved very effective in adults with testicular cancer, was used successfully in infants and children, but was associated with an increased risk of pulmonary fibrosis (2,3,6). Therefore VBC was used only for poor responders (4,9) or after prolonged intervals alternating with VAC (1).

In the 1982 resp. 1983 GPO protocols for testicular (7) and non-testicular germ cell tumors (6), the original EINHORN protocol was modified to abandon the increased risks of bleomycin toxicity in infancy and childhood in the following manner: Only half of the vinblastine dose was given, bleomycin was given as continuous infusion and restricted in its cumulative dose to 180 mg/m^2, and cisplatinum was administered days 4-5 after the bleomycin infusion, days 1-2, to avoid diminished bleomycin excretion as a result of distal renal tubular dysfunction from cisplatinum.

In poor prognostic patients, additional chemotherapy was given after second-look surgery or delayed tumor resection, consisting of VP16, ifosfamide, and cisplatinum.

This treatment has been proven successful in a recent comparison of protocol and non-protocol patients of MAKEI 83: the event-free survival of protocol patients was 78 (± 6 %) against 40 (± 19 %) in non-protocol patients (5).

In the Childrens' Cancer Study Group, in which 89 evaluable patients with similar histology and tumor site are included and VBC and VAC were given in an alternatend manner, long-term relapse- free survival was 47 % at five years. MANN et al. (9) summarized the treatment results of 52 children with non-testicular GCT's, of whom 39 survived after combined treatment with "high-dose VAC" plus adriamycin, VBC or bleomycin, VP16 and cisplatinum as salvage therapy.

Therefore cisplatinum based combination chemotherapy has been shown to be most effective in infants and children instead of reduced doses of vinblastine and bleomycin. In these regimens long-term survival was independent from initial metastases or primary tumor site (1).

As shown by this evaluation, long-term survival may be further increased by protochemotherapy in advanced tumor states. Local tumor control seems to be a major problem in patients with incomplete primary tumor resection instead of second-look surgery, compared to patients with protochemotherapy and delayed surgery.

The reason for the significant difference in event-free survival in patients with initial incomplete tumor resection and delayed surgery is unknown, as chemotherapy and time to definitive tumor resection are similar in both groups. It can only be speculated that altered vessel support after incomplete tumor resection may diminish efficiacy of chemotherapy resulting in an increased risk for tumor resistance in residual tumor cells.

In conclusion, protochemotherapy in infants and children with malignant NSGCT's will be strengthened in future. Furthermore, with respect to the high remission rate and two toxic deaths (3 %), a reduction in chemotherapy has to be considered for the ongoing 1989 trial.

References

1. Ablin, A.; Krailo M.; Ramsay, N.; Isaacs, H.; Raney, B.; Adkins J.; Hays D.; Leikin, S.; Benjamin, D.; Hammond, D.: Biologic characteristics and response to therapy in 89 patients with malignant germ cell tumors (MGCT): A Childrens Cancer Group (CCG) study. SIOP XIX Meeting (1987) Abstr. p. 10
2. Beddis, I.R.; Noblett, H.; Mott, M.G.: Effective chemotherapy for metastatic malignant saccrococcygeal tumour. Med Pediatr Oncol 12 (1984) 231

3. Cangir, A.; Starbing, K.A.; Howkins, E.P.; Ragab, A.H.; Land, V.J.: Combination chemotherapy with vinblastine sulfate (VLB) and bleomycin (BLEO) infusion in children with recurrent metastatic tumors. AACR/ASCO 1 (1982) 172, Abstr. C-669
4. Flamant, F.; Hartmann, O.; Kalifa, C.; Patte, C.; Caillaud, J.M.; Lemmerle, J.: Review of a series of 82 non seminomatous germ cell tumors (ns GCT) treated in the same center between 1978 and 1984. XIX. SIOP meeting (1987) Abstr p. 61
5. Göbel, U.; Calaminus, G.; Haas, R. J.; Jürgens, H.; Niethammer, D.; Ritter, J.; Spaar, H. J.; Harms, D.: Combination chemotherapy in malignant non-seminomatous germ cell tumors (mNSGCTs): Results of a cooperative study of the German Society of Pediatric Oncology (GPO) (MAKEI 83). Cancer Chem Pharm (in press)
6. Göbel, U.; Haas, R. J.; Harms, D.; Janka, G.; Brämswig, J.; Jürgens, H.; Weißbach, L.; Faber, P.; Müller, E.: Behandlungsstrategie für nicht-testikuläre maligne Keimzelltumoren bei Kindern und Jugendlichen - Konzept der kooperativen Therapiestudie MAKEI 83 der GPO. Klin Pädiat 195 (1983) 201
7. Haas, R.J.; Brämswig, J.; Göbel U.; Harms, D.; Janka, G.; Weißbach, L.: Maligne Hodentumoren bei Kindern und Jugendlichen: Konzept der kooperativen Therapiestudie MAHO 82 der GPO. Klin Pädiat 195 (1983) 196
8. Kohorn, E. J.; McIntosh, S.; Bernard, L.; Knowlton, A. H.; Merino, N.: Case reports. Endodermal sinus tumor of the infant vagina. Gyn Oncol 29 (1985) 196
9. Mann, J. R.; Pearson, D.; Barrett, A.; Raafat, F.; Barnes, J. N.; Wallendszus, K. R.: UKCCSG malignant germ cell tumours - treatment results. XIX. SIOP meeting (1987) Abstr p. 57
10. Sartain, P.; Ducore, J.M.; Buchanan, G.R.: Yolk sac tumors (YST) in childhood: Primary treatment with chemotherapy. AACR/ASCO 1 (1982) 104, Abstr. C404

Neo-Adjuvant Chemotherapy. Ed. Cl. Jacquillat, M. Weil, D. Khayat. Colloque INSERM/John Libbey Eurotext Ltd. © 1988. Vol. 169, pp. 479-483.

Neo-adjuvant chemotherapy in malignant non-seminomatous germ cell tumors (NSGCTs) of the mediastinum in children and adolescents

G. Calaminus*, R.J. Haas, F. Berthold, U. Bode, P. Gutjahr, M. Neidhardt, W. Sternschulte, J. Treuner and U. Göbel*

** Universitäts-Kinderklinik, Moorenstr. 5, D-4000 Düsseldorf, FRG*

Abstract

The prognosis of children and adolescents with high malignant NSGCTs has improved significantly with combination chemotherapy. Between January, 1st 1983 and February, 1st, 1988 66 protocol patients with extragonadal sites were entered into the Cooperative Germ Cell Tumor Trial (MAKEI 83/86) of the German Society of Pediatric Oncology (GPO). The disease-free survival was 83 % (± 5 %) at 61 months (Kaplan-Meier). 5/66 patients presented with mediastinal NSGCTs, which was previously considered as a poor prognostic site.
After biopsy 3 protocol patients received as neo-adjuvant chemotherapy 4 courses of vinblastine 3 mg/m^2 days 1+2, bleomycin 15 mg/m^2 days 1-3 and cisplatinum 20 mg/m^2 days 4-8 followed by 2nd-look surgery, where no residual tumor was found (3 pts.). 2 patients had received the same regimen after incomplete resection. At 2nd-look surgery residual tumor was completely removed. Thereafter chemotherapy was continued with 4 courses of VP 16 100 mg/m^2 days 1-3, ifosfamide 1.500 mg/m^2 with mesna uroprotection days 1-5 and cisplatinum 20 mg/m^2 days 1-5. On Febr. 1st, 1988, 4/5 protocol patients were off therapy and disease-free. The remaining protocol patient is still on therapy. These results are encouraging considering the form e rly poor prognosis of this primary site.

keywords:

neoadjuvant chemotherapy, malignant mediastinal NSGCTs, VBC, VPIC

Introduction

Primary malignant tumors of the lungs, bronchi or diaphragm are extremely rare in children. The mediastinum is the commonest site of intrathoracic tumors in this age group (6).
This region can be devided in two parts: the anterior and the posterior part, each of which is closely related to a particular group of tumors.

Non-Hodgkin lymphomas are the commenest mediastinal tumors in the anterior region followed by Hodgkin' s disease and germ cell tumors. All other listed entities should be notified as very rare tumors in this location (Fig. 1).

Fig. 1

DIFFERENTIAL DIAGNOSIS OF MEDIASTINAL TUMORS IN CHILDREN

ANTERIOR MEDIASTINUM	POSTERIOR MEDIASTINUM
- Non Hodgkin Lymphomas	- Sympathicoblastomas
- Hodgkin's Disease	- Neurofibrosarcoma
- Germ Cell Tumors	- Soft Tissue Sarcomas
- Thymoma	- Germ Cell Tumors
- Soft Tissue Sarcomas	- Paraganglioma
- Neurofibroma	- Neurofibroma

It was shown in clinical studies that half of the germ cell tumors of this location are malignant (9).

Malignant mediastinal germ cell tumors appear to have a poor prognosis even with modern chemotherapeutic approaches.
Martini et al. 1973 showed that in adults only 30 % of all patients with malignant mediastinal GCTs could be cured with adjuvant chemotherapy. In children the results showed a 40 % remission rate for these tumor entities (7, 5).

In 1983 the German Society of Pediatric Oncology started a cooperative trial for non-testicular germ cell tumors (MAKEI 83/86).
Between Jan. 1st, 1983 and Febr. 1st, 1988 153 protocol patients were registered (table 1). 66 of these patients had malignant germ cell tumors localized in extracranial sites, such as YST, embryonal carcinoma, chorioncarcinoma or teratocarcinoma. The event-free survival was 83 ± 5 % at 61 months. 5 of these patients presented with mediastinal malignant non-seminomatous GCTs.

Table 1 TUMOR SITE AND DIGNITY OF GCTs IN 153 PROTOCOL PATIENTS

	benigne	malignant
ovary	26	36
sacrococcyx	31	29
mediastinum	1	5
intracranial	1	12
genito-urinary	-	7
other	3	2
#pts	62	91

Patients and methods

5 patients with malignant mediastinal GCTs were entered into the GPO-study of malignant non-testicular GCTs. All patients had clinical symptoms at time of diagnosis such as cough, dyspnoea and chest pain. The ages ranged between 2 to 15 years with a median age of 7 years. Patients characteristics are shown on table 2.

Table 2 PATIENTS' CHARACTERISTICS

case	age/sex	TNM	tumormarker $_1$-F	β-HCG	histology YST	EC	CH	Germ	delivered therapy	state
protocol patients										
1	2 / F	$T_2N_1M_0$	120	n. d.	+				biopsy, 4 VBC, delayed surgery, 4 VPIC	30+
2	15 / M	$T_2N_0M_1$	49853	1288	+	+	+		biopsy, 4 VBC, delayed surgery, 4 VPIC	17+
3	3 / F	$T_2N_0M_0$	66000	-	+				biopsy, 4 VBC, delayed surgery, 4 VPIC	16+
4	4 / F	$T_2N_1M_0$	4270	1	+				incomplete resection 4 VBC, 2nd-look, 4 VPIC	14+
5	15 / M	$T_2N_0M_1$	175	14	+	+	+	+	incomplete resection 4 VBC	on therapy

All patients were staged according the TNM-system. All of these children showed T_2-tumors. Elevated tumormarkers were seen in each case. Most of the patients presented with metastases at the time of diagnosis. Histological review revealed 3 pure YSTs and 2 mixed GCTs, also with areas of yolk sac tumor.

All patients were treated according to the following therapy regimen Fig. 2).

Fig. 2

MAKEI 83/86 TREATMENT STRATEGY

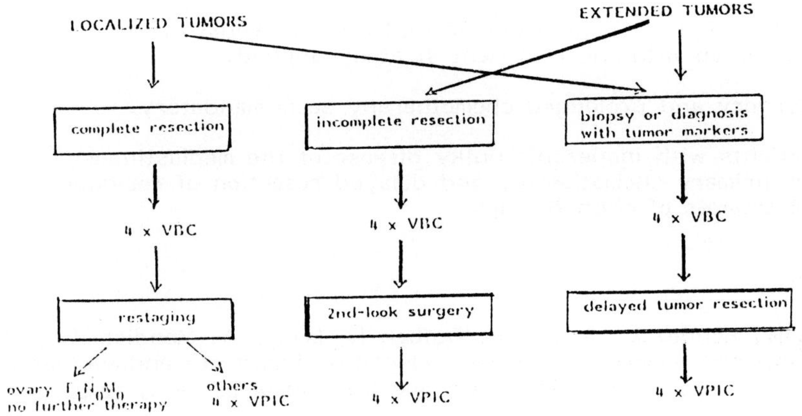

2 patients received primary incomplete resection. Followed by adjuvant chemotherapy consisting of 4 courses vinblastine 3 mg/m^2 days 1+2, bleomycin 15 mg/m^2 days 1-3 and cisplatinum 20 mg/m^2 days 4-8 with mannitol diuresis. After 2nd-look surgery 4 courses of VP 16 100 mg/m^2 days 1-3, ifosfamide 1.500 mg/m^2 days 1-5 (with mesna uroprotection) and cisplatinum 20 mg/m^2 days 1-5 with mannitol diuresis were administered. 3 patients underwent biopsy first and received as protochemotherapy 4 courses of VBC, afterwards the tumor was completely removed and 4 courses of VPIC were added.

Toxicity:
All patients showed a depression of the hemopoetic system, especially following the combination of VP 16, ifosfamide and cisplatinum. Transient nephropathy occurred in 3 patients. 2 patients showed paresthesia of hands and legs. Ototoxicity was seen in 1 patient.

Discussion

The non-seminomatous germ cell tumors are known to be relatively resistant to therapy (12). First Li et al. (8) and Samuels et al. (11), and later Einhorn and Donohue achieved major progress in the treatment of non-seminomatous testicular carcinoma in adults (3, 2).
In 1983 the German Society of Pediatric Oncology (GPO) started a cooperative trial for non-testicular germ cell tumors basing on a modified Einhorn-protocol using the combination therapy of VBC added with the therapy regimen of VPIC (4).
This therapy regimen led to an event-free survival of 83 ± 5 % at 61 months for children with extracranial malignant NSGCTs.

Malignant mediastinal NSGCTs are rare tumors in children, which appear mostly in the anterior mediastinum. Local recurrents and local invasion of major structures of the thorac such als lung, pleura, pericardium and chestwall are major features (10).

Despite chemotherapy regimens using VBC the prognosis of children with these tumor entities ranged under 50 % (1).

The results of our study show an improved prognosis for the mediastinal malignant germ cell tumors.

Conclusions:

- The prognosis of malignant non-testicular GCTs of the mediastinum is considerably improved with the treatment strategy applied.

- Second-look surgery and prolonged chemotherapy seem mandatory.

- Particularly patients with inoperable bulky disease of the mediastinum benefitted from primary chemotherapy and delayed resection of residual disease after 4 courses of chemotherapy.

References:

1. Cortês Funes H, Mendez M, Alonso E, Quiben R, Manas A, Mendiola C (1981) Mediastinal germ cell tumors treated with cisplatin, bleomycin and vinblastine (PVB). Proc Amer Ass Cancer Res Amer Soc Clin Oncol 22, 474, Asco Abstr. C-553

2. Einhorn LH, Donohue JP (1977) Cis-Diamminedichloroplatinum, vinblastine and bleomycin combination chemotherapy in disseminated testicular cancer. Ann Intern Med 87:293-298
3. Einhorn LH, Donohue JP (1977) Improved chemotherapy in disseminated testicular cancer. J Urol 117:65-69
4. Göbel U, Haas RJ, Harms D, Janka G, Brämswig J, Jürgens H, Weißbach L, Faber P, Müller (1983) Behandlungsstrategie für nichttestikuläre maligne Keimzelltumoren bei Kindern und Jugendlichen - Konzept der kooperativen Therapiestudie MAKEI 83 der GPO Klin Pädiatr 195, 201
5. Hawkins PE, Finegold MJ, Hawkins HK, Krischer JP, Starling KA, Weinberg A (1986) Nongerminomatous malignant germ cell tumors in children (A review of 89 cases from the Pediatric Oncology Group, (1971-1984) Cancer 58:2579-2584
6. Heimburger IL, Battersby JS (1965): Primary mediastinal tumors of childhood. J Thorac Cardiov Surg 50:92
7. Hoesel van QGC, Pinedo HM (1980) Complete remission of mediastinal germ-cell tumors with cis-Dichlorodiammineplatinum (II) combination chemotherapy. Cancer Treat Rep 64:319-321
8. Li MC, Whitmore WF, Golbey R (1960) Effects of combined drug therapy on metastatic cancer of the testis. JAMA 174:1291-1299
9. Mahour GH, Landing BH, Wolley MM (1978) Teratomas in children: Clinicopathologic studies in 133 patients. Z Kinderchir, Band 23
10. Martini N, Golbey RB, Haydn SJ, Whitmore WF, Beattie EJ (1974) Cancer Vol 33:263-269
11. Samuels ML, Hologe PY, Johnson DE (1975) Bleomycin combination chemotherapy in the management of testicular neoplasia. Cancer 36: 318-326
12. Wychulis AR, Payne WS, Clagett OT (1971) Surgical treatment of mediastinal tumors: a 40 year experience. J Thorac Cardiovasc Surg 62:379-392

Résumé

Les tumeurs médiastinales sont relativement rares chez les enfants. La plupart de ces tumeurs intéressent la partie antérieure du médiastin. La maladie de Hodgkin et les lymphomes non hodgkinien sont les malades les plus fréquentes suivies par les tumeurs germinales. La moitié des tumeurs germinales doit être considérée comme maligne. En fonction de leur localisation et de leur stade, ces tumeurs étaient autrefois considérées comme de mauvais pronostic même avec les associations chimiothérapies. En 1983 la Société Allemande de Pédiatrie Oncologique a débuté un protocole coopérateur pour les tumeurs germinales. Entre le 1er janvier 1983 et le 1er février 1988, 66 patients sont entrés dans un protocole de localisations primaires extra-gonadiques. Leur survie est de 83 ± 5 % à 61 mois, 5 de ces malades ont eu des tumeurs médiastinales germinales non séminomateuse. Après traitement 4 sur 5 de ces malades sont sans traitement et sans rechute (30+, 16+, 17+, 14+ mois) les autres malades sont toujours en traitement. Le pronostic des tumeurs germinales du médiastin non séminomateuse est considérablement amélioré par la stratégie décrite.

Neo-Adjuvant Chemotherapy. Ed. Cl. Jacquillat, M. Weil, D. Khayat. Colloque INSERM/John Libbey Eurotext Ltd. © 1988. Vol. 169, pp. 485-489.

Chemosensitivity of osteogenic sarcomas : histological evaluation

G. Contesso, M.J. Terrier-Lacombe, F. Bertin, J. Genin, G. Missenard, J. Dubousset, M. Spielmann and C. Kalifa

Institut Gustave-Roussy, 94805 Villejuif Cedex, France

Histologic examination remains at the present time one of the least subjective methods of evaluating the efficiency of chemotherapy (CT) on osteogenic sarcomas (OS). However this requires a well trained team working in collaboration with the radiologists, the orthopedists and the chemotherapists.

The large recruitment of patients with OS at the Institut Gustave-Roussy (IGR) has permitted the histologic (2) (3) evaluation of a large number of specimens of this tumor after CT.

MATERIALS AND METHODS

Between 1982 and 1986 on about 200 surgical specimens post-CT OS were analysed in the pathology department of IGR, of which 133 (32 amputations or disarticulations, and 101 "en bloc" resections : (76 %)) were evaluable for chemosensitivity. The initial diagnosis was made on surgical biopsy which in most cases confirmed the radiologic impression, and the patients treated according to the protocol then in use by several courses of CT, before surgery.

Eighty one were male and 52 female (M/F = 1.55). 23 % of patients were of Maghrebian origin and 8 % Italian. The median age was 15.3 years (4 to 53 years). Two thirds were treated by pediatric oncologists and one third by adult oncologists. In 72 cases this involved the femur, usually the lower portion ; 31 cases the tibia, usually the upper portion ; 20 cases the humerus, 7 cases the fibula, 2 cases the radius and 1 the iliac bones.
The histological subtype of OS (4) (10) was evaluated on the initial biopsy before any therapy. It took into account the degree of differentiation of the sarcoma and the special types encountered.

A precise protocol of examination and dissection was always carried out (3) (6) on the operative specimen after CT. The margins of the specimen were first evaluated for adequacy and the surgeon informed (5) (7) (the proximal and distal bone marrow in cases of resection and/or amputation, staged specimens to transect the scar of the original biopsy, specimens from the principal vasculonervous trunk to look for thrombosis or emboli and any abnormal zone in the soft tissue surrounding the tumor). The tumor was separated from the surrounding soft tissue, and a large section then performed along the axis of the largest diameter. Generally the best plane of dissection was determined with the aid of the radiologist by RX, CT scans and MRI scans. The slice of approximately 3 mm in thickness was X-rayed and photographed, then decalcified in an acid bath into which carbon electrodes were inserted. The time of decalcification was variable according to the thickness and hardness of the slice : usually this did not exceed 8 days (2-10). The slice was then washed thoroughly and totally sectioned in a grill-like fashion into squares of 2 cm length. Each square was noted on a traced design of the tumor radiograph and numbered (Fig 1). These were placed into cassettes, fixed in Bouin's solution for 48 hours, dried, embedded in paraffine, sectioned at about 4 mu, mounted and stained with Hemalun, Erythrosin and Safranin ; then the slides were evaluated for the percentage of "viable cells" compared to the total tumor surface, and this was related to the described design. A mean of all the tumor zones was taken (Fig. 1). The tumor was classified according to the method proposed by Huvos and Rosen (6) (9) : Grade I or $\gg$95 % viable cells to Grade IV where there are no viable cells seen, passing Grade IIa (94-50 %), IIb (49-5 %) and III ($<$5 % viable cells). Grades III and IV are considered as "good responders" (G.R.), with the others considered as "bad responders" (B.R.).
Once all the results were tabulated, the diagrams were sent to the clinician to undertake postoperative CT according to the then current protocol, and to the radiologist to compare his imagings and the actual tissue obtained (Cf Figure 1).

RESULTS

Regarding the classification of this series according to the grades of chemosensitivity : 7 cases were grade I, 31 were IIa, 41 were IIb, 31 were III and 23 were IV, thus 54 of 133 cases (40 %) were "good responders".
We looked at the possible relationship between the type of chemotherapy protocol used and the number of G.R. Whether protocol 04, T10 of Rosen, or the "other" protocols were used, the degree of G.R. was essentially the same, 36 %, 43 % and 40 % respectively.
There appears to be however, a relationship between young age and an increased number of G.R. (Cf table 1) : 46 % before age 16 years vs 32 % after this age (p=0.05).
There also appears to be a relationship between the site of the tumor and degree of good response (Cf figure 2) : 44 % and 48 % for femoral and tibial primaries vs 23 % for all "others" (p=0.05).
The histologic subtype of OS also had an effect on the degree of G.R. (Table 1). The anaplastic and telangectatic forms have a G.R. rate of 52 %, whereas the well differentiated forms, mainly "chondroblastic" and "fibroblastic" O.S. had a G.R. of 29 %, and the "common type" or pleomorphic 41 %. These numbers although not at this time significant, are suggestive of more chemosensitivity of the more anaplastic type, like shown for the different localizations.
A strong relationship was found between the tumor surface area (measured by caliper) and the degree of G.R. This was 28 % for tumors $>$ 40 cm^2 vs 52 % for those of smaller dimentions.
Regarding the correlation of clinical course, the number of relapses are significantly less (p=0,001) in the group of G.R. : shown by log rank test, a 2 and 3 year DFS is respectively 66 and 54 % for B.R. and 85 and 81 % for G.R. (after exclusion of 10 metastatic patients at the first consultation).

DISCUSSION AND CONCLUSION

This study is not intellectually satisfying to the pathologist as it is quite subjective ; indeed the differentiation of "viable" or "non viable" tumor cells is some times difficult and this classification does not take in count the evaluation of the initial tumor on biopsy wich could have had zone of spontaneous necrosis in IGR study of 206 OS : 54 % were necrosis areas (19 %++ and 35 %+) . Additionally not only will the same pathologist not always give a similar response at a different time and other pathologists may also give varying values. It is for this reason that it is desirable to standardize the classifications, taking into account not only the overall percentage of necrosis but also the isolated or multiple nests of "viable" cells and to be able to tell which cells are viable on a strictly histologic basis. Some teams claim to be able to perform the analysis on fine needle biopsy specimens (1) (8). However, the heterogenicity of OS is well known, and the Bologna team has shown the patchy localization of florid cells, which would appear to make this technique very risky (8).

It is for this reason that we have a close relationship with the medical imagery department of IGR to relate the immediate pre-operative MRI scans obtained with the histologic chart that we develop retrospectively. Hopefully this will allow the most precise assessment of CT efficacy, even prior to surgery. Possible in the future we will be able, with other evaluation, to predict the maximum effect of the drugs and the subsequent best time for surgery. This will require however, an appropriate hospital management with synchronization of various teams, beds, and materials such as prostheses.

Nr 210095

Fig.1 O.S. R. TIBIA post CT.

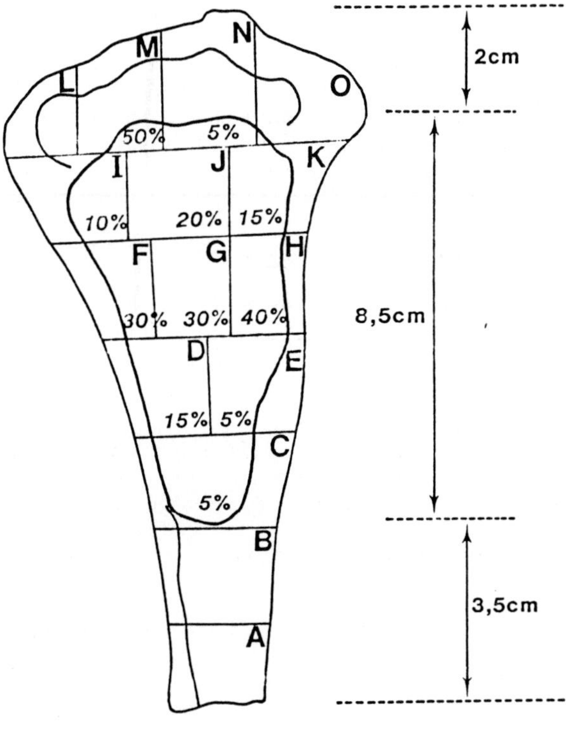

20% VIABLE CELLS = BAD RESPONSE

Table 1. Histological chemosensitivity according to characteristics of OS (IGR 1982-86)

characters	n^r	% good histological response (Gr III + IV)		Comparison
<u>age</u>				
0 10 y.o.	19	47 %	46 %	p=0,05
11 15 y.o.	61	46 %		
16 20 y.o.	37	32 %	32 %	
>20 y.o.	16	31 %		
<u>histological subtype</u>				
well diff O.S. fibroblastic O.S. chondroblastic O.S.	24	29 %		NS
common type O.S. pleomorphic O.S.	88	41 %		
anaplastic O.S. telangiectatic O.S.	21	52 %		
<u>T. surface</u>				
< 40 cm2	71	52 %		p < 0,01
> 40 cm2	62	28 %		

REFERENCES

Ayala, A.G., Raymond, A.K. (1984) : The pathologist's role in the diagnosis and treatment of osteosarcoma in children. Hum. pathol. 15, 258-66.

Contesso, G., Zafrani, B., Mazabrad, A., Lacombe, M.J., Zemoura, L., Genin, J., Missenard, G., Dubousset, J. (1987) : Place de l'anatomopathologiste dans le traitement des sarcomes ostéogènes. Rev. Chir. Ortho. 73, 301-306.

Costa, J., Contesso, G., Remagen, W. (1985) : Anatomie pathologique de l'ostéosarcome de l'enfant et de l'adolescent. Chir. Pédiatr. 26, 226-32.

Dahlin, D.C. (1978) : Bone tumors : general aspects and data on 6221 cases. 3e ed. C.C. Thomas Springfield Illinois U.S.A. 226-73.

Dubousset, J., Missenard, G., Genin, J. (1985) : Traitement chirurgical conservateur des sarcomes ostéogènes des membres. Techniques et résultats fonctionnels. Rev. Chir. Ortho. 71, 435-50.

Huvos, A.G., Rosen, G., Marcove, R. (1977) : Primary osteogenic sarcoma : pathologic aspects in 20 patients after treatment with chemotherapy en bloc resection and prothetic bone replacement. Arch. Pathol. 101, 14-18.

Missenard, G., Dubousset, J., Genin, J., Contesso, G. (1986) : Confrontation anatomo-clinique pré et post-opératoire : à propos de 30 résections conservatrices pour sarcome ostéogène. Rev. Chir. Ortho. 72, 477-83.

Picci, P., Bacci, G., Campanacci, M., Gasparini, M. et al. (1985) : Histologic evaluation of necrosis in osteosarcoma induced by chemotherapy regional mapping of viable and non viable tumor. Cancer 56, 1515-21.

Rosen, G., Caparos, B., Huvos, A. et al. (1982) : Preoperative chemotherapy in osteogenic sarcoma. Cancer 49, 1221.

Trifaud, A., Mazabraud A., Jasmin, C. (1980) : Tumeurs malignes primitives de l'os : les sarcomes ostéogènes. Encyclopédie médico-chirurgicale, Paris, 4030D10, 11, 1-6.

Résumé

Une série de 133 pièces opératoires de sarcomes ostéogènes après chimiothérapie première (101 résections et 32 amputations ou désarticulations) a été analysée dans le laboratoire d'anatomie pathologique de l'Institut Gustave-Roussy de 1982 à 1986. L'évaluation de la chimiosensibilité a été jugée sur des prélèvements "en grille" pratiqués sur une grande tranche tumorale d'après le % de cellules "viables" (CV). 54 cas avaient moins de 5 % de CV et ont été jugés "bons répondeurs" (BR). Le taux de BR est significativement lié à l'âge des malades (p=0,05) et à la surface tumorale (p=0,01). Il semble plus important pour les formes anaplasiques (52 %) que bien différenciées (29 %). Il est de plus fortement lié à la survie globale ($p < 0,005$) et à la survie sans rechute (p=0,001).

Neo-Adjuvant Chemotherapy. Ed. Cl. Jacquillat, M. Weil, D. Khayat. Colloque INSERM/John Libbey Eurotext Ltd. © 1988. Vol. 169, pp. 491-498.

Osteogenic sarcoma in children less than ten years of age : the dramatic effect of neo-adjuvant chemotherapy upon survival

Gerald Rosen[1], Anita Nirenberg[2], Brenda Caparros-Sison[2] and Ralph Marcove[3]

[1]*Cedars-Sinai Comprehensive Cancer Center, 8700 Beverly Boulevard, Los Angeles, California 90048, USA*
[2]*1275 York Avenue, New-York, New-York 10021, USA*
[3]*517 East 71st Street, New-York, New-York 10021, USA*

ABSTRACT

Osteogenic sarcoma occurring in children less than ten years of age is usually a highly malignant tumor. Indeed, historical and concurrent cases treated at the Mayo Clinic report a relapse-free survival at 2 years of only 20% for this group of patients, in spite of the fact that they have reported a better survival overall for osteogenic sarcoma patients of all ages. This report describes the results of aggressive neoadjuvant chemotherapy in the treatment of patients less than ten years of age with osteogenic sarcoma of an extremity. From mid-1976 through 1983, when children were treated with chemotherapy on the T-7, T-10, and T-12 protocols which incorporated high dose Methotrexate at the dose of 12 grams/m^2 given with Leucovorin rescue, 29 patients less than ten years of age were treated. Although the dose of Methotrexate called for on these protocols was 12 grams/m^2, a minimum dose of 10 grams total dose was used for all patients, having recognized the low response rate to high dose Methotrexate in this high risk group of patients. At a median time of 9 years, 72% of these patients remain relapse-free survivors. In addition, 79% are surviving (median 9 years) all of them now currently free of disease. The use of aggressive neoadjuvant chemotherapy as called for in these protocols resulted in far superior survival than had been reported by the Mayo Clinic. The two year relapse-free survival and survival in the treated group of patients reported here was 86% and 96% respectively, compared to 20% and 26% respectively reported by the Mayo Clinic. Aggressive neoadjuvant chemotherapy in younger patients with osteogenic sarcoma has lead to a dramatic increase in their overall survival.

Address for Reprints: Gerald Rosen, M.D., Medical Director, Cedars-Sinai Comprehensive Cancer Center, 8700 Beverly Boulevard, Los Angeles, CA 90048.

Introduction

The value of adjuvant chemotherapy in the treatment of primary osteogenic sarcoma has now been firmly established by many investigators throughout the world (1,2,3). Without question, chemotherapy for primary osteogenic sarcoma has been shown to increase the survival rate dramatically.

The once recent controversy over the role of chemotherapy in osteogenic sarcoma was primarily fostered by studies at the Mayo Clinic which indicated that now the disease may have a better prognosis than had been historically recorded. In a widely publicized report from the Mayo Clinic (4), investigators tried to show that the cure rate with surgery alone had risen to the vicinity of close to 40% in a small group of patients compared to a similar cure rate for patients treated with adjuvant chemotherapy at the Mayo Clinic. Although that study has since been faulted by the fact that the control patients contained primary tumors of low grade histology, and the chemotherapy may not have been optimally administered, some investigators still point to that publication as a justification to consider adjuvant chemotherapy for osteogenic sarcoma "experimental".

In a less widely distributed publication from the Mayo Clinic (Mayo Clinic Proceedings) published in 1985, Taylor, et al, review the same trends in survival for patients with osteogenic sarcoma and concluded that even in patients surgically treated at the Mayo Clinic the cure rate for osteogenic sarcoma under the age of ten years has not improved, and indeed, the survival of patients less than ten years of age with osteogenic sarcoma was approximately 20%, or as dismal as other investigator's historical controls had indicated (5). The lack of better dissemination of this finding, and the inability of other investigators running controlled trials to recognize this fact, was tantamount to scientific negligence on their part by including children less than ten years of age in randomized no treatment trials that were supposedly based upon the Mayo Clinic's data of increased survival for "all" patients with osteogenic sarcoma in recent years (3,4).

In addition, the Mayo Clinic's admission that osteogenic sarcoma under the age of ten years has a dismal prognosis, it has long been the observation of other established investigators in the field that even with optimal chemotherapy, children less than ten years of age do not have as good a survival (and response to chemotherapy when given preoperatively) as do older patients.

This observation was recently made by this author twelve years ago. In 1976, when it was apparent that younger patients did not respond as well to pre-operative chemotherapy with high dose Methotrexate and Leucovorin rescue. In 1976, the T-7 chemotherapy protocol was created specifically to address this point, and the dose of high dose Methotrexate for younder children was raised to 12 grams/m^2. At this dose level, some of the younger children, i.e., those that have not achieved their complete linear growth, seemed to respond better. However, very young children, i.e., those below ten years of age, still did not seem to have as high a response rate to preoperative chemotherapy with high dose Methotrexate. Until this point in time, the recent controversy over the role of chemotherapy in osteogenic sarcoma has precluded us from making suggestions that patients under the age of ten have an even higher dose of Methotrexate, and the dose of 12 grams/m^2 has prevailed for all children, and over the past 12 years coupled with other combination chemotherapy, this seemed to improve the prognosis for this high risk group of patients.

This report summarizes our experience in treating children less than ten years of age with pre and postoperative chemotherapy, or postoperative chemotherapy including high dose Methotrexate at the dose of 12 grams/m^2 as the minimum dose on the T-7, T-10 and T-12 protocols, which were in effect from mid-1976 through the end of 1983.

Patients

The patients reported in this study were all aged less than ten years of age. They presented with osteogenic sarcoma of an extremity, and all tumors were of high grade histology. The pathologists at the Memorial Sloan-Kettering Cancer Center used a grading system of Grade I-IV/IV. All patients reported there had their biopsy read as Grade III or IV at open biopsy. Patients presenting with either pulmonary, bone or lymph node metastases were not included. The 29 patients were treated from mid-1976 through 1983 on the T-7, T-10 and T-12 protocols which were in existence for the treatment of osteogenic sarcoma at that time. The eligibility criteria are summarized in Table 1.

OSA - AGE LESS THAN 10 YEARS OLD

TABLE 1 - THE PATIENTS

- AGE 0 TO 9 YEARS OLD
- OSTEOGENIC SARCOMA OF AN EXTREMITY
- HIGH GRADE (III-IV/IV) HISTOLOGY
- MUSCULOSKELETAL STAGE IIB
- NO METASTESES AT DIAGNOSIS
- TREATED FROM MID-1976 THROUGH 1983 (T-7, T-10, and T-12 PROTOCOLS)

Table 1

The patient's age ranged from 2.8 to 9 years, with a median age of 8 years old. Of the 29 patients, 18 were male and 11 female, making the male to female ratio 1.6:1.0.

The site of the primary tumors in the 29 patients included femur-13; tibia-8; and humerus-8. The combination of femur and humerus lesions equalled 21 of the 29 tumors or 72% of the lesions. Both femur and humerus lesions in this group of patients has been noted to have a poor prognosis as well (5).

Methods

The T-7, T-10, and T-12 chemotherapy protocols have been extensively published before (6,7,8). During the early phases of the T-7 chemotherapy protocol, not all younger patients were referred for preoperative chemotherapy, and 7 patients were referred following amputation. These patients were included since they were placed on the chemotherapy protocol as postoperative adjuvant chemotherapy. All patients treated on the T-10 and T-12 protocol had preoperative chemotherapy with the exception of a 6 year old girl who had a pathologically fractured, bleeding tumor amputated prior to starting chemotherapy. This patient was given postoperative high dose Methotrexate and Platinum and Adriamycin as were non-complete responding patients to preoperative high dose Methotrexate. Postoperative chemotherapy for all patients on the T-7 protocol regardless of the response to preoperative chemotherapy was identical. The one major exception in the treatment of this group of patients was the fact that although the dose of high dose Methotrexate was supposed to be 12 grams/m^2, it had long been recognized that younger children did not respond as frequently, and it was thought that a minimum or threshhold dose of Methotrexate of 10 grams (total dose) was necessary to obtain a response in any patient. Therefore, if the patient's surface area did not dictate a dose of 10 grams/m^2, the starting dose of Methotrexate was arbitrarily escalated to that level. In addition, patients who did not appear to havetheir primary tumor respond to that dose of Methotrexate had the dose of Methotrexate further escalated to 12 grams (total dose) in subsequent treatments.

Results

Pre-Operative Chemotherapy

The results of preoperative chemotherapy, although evaluated clinically, roentgenographically, and by careful evaluation of serial bone and gallium scans, are reported here in terms of the histologic response to preoperative chemotherapy as judged by thorough analysis of the resected operative specimen.

Although many patients had excellent clinical response, and a great deal of tumor necrosis noted on histologic evaluation of the resected specimen, only those patients that had no viable tumor demonstrable in all of the histologic sections of their specimen, or only microscopic clusters of individual cells, were called good responders. Those patients demonstrating almost complete tumor necrosis but yet having areas consisting of confluent microscopic high power fields full of tumor cells (even though this represents only less than 5% of the tumor mass) were still considered poor responders.

Of the 22 patients who underwent preoperative chemotherapy, six or only 27% were judged to be good or complete responders to preoperative chemotherapy. This compares less favorably to the results from the recent T-10 and T-12 protocols where patients of all ages had an overall response rate of 49% and 45% respectively.

Disease-Free Survival and Overall Survival

Twenty one of the 29 patients (72%) remained continuously free of disease without evidence of relapse at the time of this writing, which is a follow up period of from 57 to 141 months (median time 106 months) from the start of chemotherapy. Of the 8 patients that relapsed, two were rendered free of disease and continue to survive without any evidence of disease, making the proportion currently surviving without any evidence of disease 23 of 29 patients (or 79%) at the same follow up period of time, 57 to 141 months (median 107 months).

OSA LESS THAN 10 YEARS OLD
TABLE 2 - RESULTS

PROPORTION SURVIVIVG
CONTINUOUSLY DISEASE-FREE
21/29 (72%) at 57-141 MONTHS (MED. 106)

PROPORTION SURVIVING
(ALL CURRENTLY DISEASE-FREE)
23/29 (79%) AT 57-141 MONTHS (MED. 107)

Table 2

Thus, the median survival with 23 of 29 patients (79%) at almost 9 years (Table 2) demonstrates that chemotherapy in this high risk group of patients can produce results equal to if not superior to those reported for all age groups with similar aggressive chemotherapy.

OSA LESS THAN 10 YEARS OLD
ACTUARIAL SURVIVAL

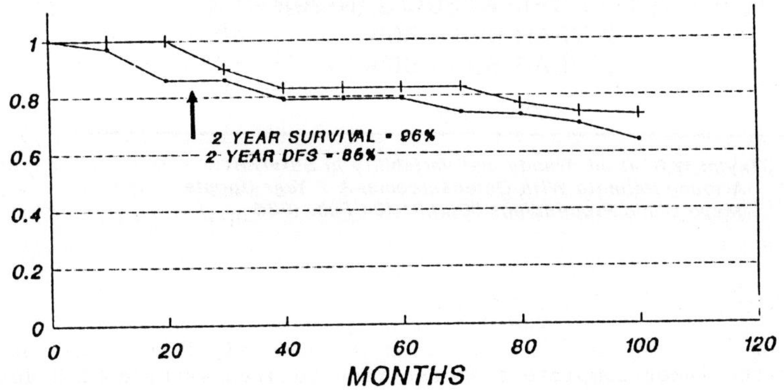

Figure 1

Fig. 1: Survival statistics for children less than ten years old treated with aggressive chemotherapy for osteogenic sarcoma. The 9 year (median) relapse-free survival is 72% and the 9 year (median) survival is 79%. All surviving patients are currently disease-free. The 2 year relapse-free survival (86%) is significantly better than that reported for similar patients at the Mayo Clinic (20%) who did not receive neoadjuvant chemotherapy (Table 3).

Discussion

The results reported here demonstrate the advantage of aggressive chemotherapy in the younger age group patient. In addition to documentation of the poor prognosis for patients under ten years of age with osteogenic sarcoma by the Mayo Clinic (5), it has long been the observation that this group of patients had a poor prognisis with surgery alone. The additional data from the Mayo Clinic documents that the prognosis for this age group patient has not significantly changed over the past few decades, and is equal to that of historical controls. They reported a two year disease-free survival of only 20% in patients less than ten years of age presenting with osteogenic sarcoma. In addition, their two year overall survival including patients that were alive with metastases was only 26%. The cohort of patients reported by the Mayo Clinic was equal to 25 in number, and the superior difference in survival reported in our 29 patients is obviously statistically significant (Table 3). We leave it to the reader who is an avid student of statistics to calculate the "P" value.

OSA LESS THAN 10 YEARS OLD

TABLE 3 - CHEMO. vs. MAYO CLINIC RESULTS

MAYO CLINIC REPORTED RESULTS (N=25): *
2 YEAR DFS = 20%
2 YEAR SUR.= 26%

T-7; T-10; T-12 RESULTS (N=29):
2 YEAR DFS = 86%
2 YEAR SUR.= 96%

P = .00?

Taylor, W.F. et. al. Trends and Variability in Survival Amoung Patients With Osteosarcoma: A 7 Year Update Mayo Clinic Proceedings:60(2);91-104 Feb. 1986

Table 3

The reason for the lower complete response rate to preoperative high dose Methotrexate with Leucovorin rescue in this group of patients may ineeed be that younger patients metabolize Methotrexate differently than adults. We have long made the observation that children given identical doses (per meter squared) of Methotrexate tend to have lower serum levels of Methotrexate 24 hours after the dose is administered. This may be due in part to the fact that children have better renal clearance of high dose Methotrexate, or indeed, they tend to be treated more vigorously with fluid hydration following a dose of high dose Methotrexate. Whatever the reason, it is suggested that further studies make provisions for children less than ten years of age by increasing the dose of high dose Methotrexate still further.

In 1976, we recommended an increased dose of Methotrexate to 8 grams/m^2 for fully grown adults and to 12 grams/m^2 for the usual adolescent patient who has not yet achieved his complete linear growth. Perhaps further dose adjustment for children less than ten years of age who classically do not respond well to preoperative chemotherapy with high dose Methotrexate should be to the dose of 18 grams/m^2. Because the number of patients less than ten years of age that are seen with primary osteogenic sarcoma is quite low it would take inordinately long to complete a randomized study at two different dose levels for this small subgroup of patients. Therefore, this author recommends the empiric use of a higher dose of high dose Methotrexate for the preoperative treatment of children with osteogenic sarcoma that are less than ten years of age.

BIBLIOGRAPHY

1) Rosen, G. Preoperative (Neoadjuvant) chemotherapy for osteogenic sarcoma: a ten-year experience. Orthopedics 8:(5), 659-664, 1985.

2) Eilber, F, Giuliano, A, Eckardt, J, et al. Adjuvant chemotherapy for osteosarcoma: a randomized prospective trial. J. Clin. Oncol. 5 (1): 21-26, 1987.

3) Link, MP, Goorin, AM, Meiser, AW, et al. The effect of adjuvant chemotherapy on relapse-free survival in patients with osteogenic sarcoma of the extremity. N. Eng. J. Med. 314: 1600-1606, 1986.

4) Edmonson, JH, Green, SJ, Gilchrist, GS, et al. A controlled pilot study of high dose Methotrexate as post-surgical adjuvant treatment for primary osteosarcoma. J. Clin. Oncol. 2 (3): 152-156, 1984.

5) Taylor, WF, Ivins, JC, Pritchart, DJ, et al. Trends and variability in survival among patients with osteogenic sarcoma: a 7 year update. Mayo Clinic Proc. 60 (2): 91-104, 1985.

6) Rosen, G, Marcove, RC, Caparros, B, et al. Primary osteogenic sarcoma: the rationale for preoperative chemotherapy and delayed surgery. Cancer 42: 2163-3177, 1979.

7) Rosen, G, Caparros, B, Huvos, AG, et al. Preoperative chemotherapy for osteogenic sarcoma: selection of postoperative adjuvant chemotherapy based on the response of the primary tumor to preoperative chemotherapy. Cancer 49: 1221-1230, 1982.

8) Rosen, G, and Nirenberg, A. Neoadjuvant chemotherapy for osteogenic sarcoma: A five year follow up (T-10) and preliminary report of new studies (T-12). In: Primary Chemotherapy in Cancer Medicine, pp 39-51. Alan R. Liss, Inc. (N.Y.), 1985.

Résumé

Les sarcomes ostéogéniques des enfants de moins de 10 ans sont généralement une tumeur très maligne. En fait, le rapport historique et actuel de la Mayo Clinic rapporte pour ce groupe de malades une survie sans rechute à 2 ans de 20 %, bien qu'il ait été rapportée une survie meilleure pour l'ensemble des sarcomes ostéogéniques. Cet article décrit les résultats d'une chimiothérapie aggressive chez des malades de moins de 10 ans atteints d'ostéosarcome ostéogénique d'une extrémité de 1976 à 1983. 29 enfants de moins de 10 ans ont été traités par les protocoles T7, T10, T12, qui incomporaient de fortes doses de Méthotrexate 12gr/m2 avec acide folinique. Bien que la dose de Méthotrexate était fixée à 12 gr/m2, une dose minimum de 10 gr parfois augmentée à 12 gr a été donnée même si la surface de l'enfant n'appelait pas cette dose, car il a été observé un taux de réponse plus faible chez ces enfants, qui métabolisent peut être le Méthotrexate différemment. Il est possible qu'il faille encore chez ces enfants augmenter la dose jusqu'à 18 gr/m2. Quoiqu'il en soit, la survie sans rechute et la survie de ce groupe sont de 86 % et de 96 % comparées à 20 % et à 26 % pour le groupe de la Mayo Clinic non traité. Ainsi la chimiothérapie néoadjuvante chez les petits enfants atteints de sarcome ostéogénique a conduit à une augmentation dramatique de la survie globale.

Neo-Adjuvant Chemotherapy. Ed. Cl. Jacquillat, M. Weil, D. Khayat. Colloque INSERM/John Libbey Eurotext Ltd. © 1988. Vol. 169, pp. 499-507.

Osteogenic sarcoma in adults : the value of neo-adjuvant chemotherapy

Gerald Rosen[1], Ralph Marcove[2], Adrienne Cacavio[3], Frederick Eilber[4] and Jeffrey Eckardt[5]

[1]*Cedars-Sinai Comprehensive Cancer Center, 8700 Beverly Boulevard, Los Angeles, California 99048, USA*
[2]*517 East 71st Street, New-York, New-York 10021, USA*
[3]*1275 York Avenue, New-York, New-York 10021, USA*
[4]*UCLA School of Medicine, Division of Surgical Oncology, Factor Building : 9-666, Los Angeles, California 90024, USA*
[5]*UCLA School of Medicine, Division of Orthopedic Surgery, Center for Health Sciences : A6-164, Los Angeles, California 90024, USA*

OSTEOGENIC SARCOMA IN ADULTS: THE VALUE OF NEOADJUVANT CHEMOTHERAPY

ABSTRACT

From 1974 through 1983, 42 adult patients with fully malignant (histologic grade III-IV/IV) were treated by the author (G.R.) with preoperative and postoperative adjuvant chemotherapy. The outcome of treatment was compared to a concomittantly treated group of patients who were seen at U.C.L.A., and were randomized to receive no postoperative adjuvant chemotherapy.

Patients in the treatment group were treated on four successive chemotherapy protocols in use during the study period (T-4, T-7, T-10, and T-12). The overall survival of the 12 control patients was only 25% (17% relapse-free survical) compared to an 80% overall survival for the patients treated with chemotherapy (relapse-free survival 67%). Although the control patients received one course of preoperative intra-arterial Adriamycin and radiation therapy to the primary tumor, none of them had the advantage of neoadjuvant chemotherapy to determine the best postoperative treatment for them, and none of them had adjuvant chemotherapy with the two most effective modalities for the treatment of osteogenic sarcoma, namely high dose Methotrexate with Leucovorin rescue, and/or Cisplatinum combined with Adriamycin.

This study demonstrates that fully malignant osteogenic sarcoma in adults untreated with chemotherapy has a very poor prognosis similar to that of highly malignant osteogenic sarcoma that is seen more frequently in children and adolescents. It also demonstrates the dramatic impact on survival of aggressive chemotherapy in adult osteogenic sarcoma. All adults with fully malignant osteogenic sarcoma should be treated with preoperative chemotherapy followed by postoperative adjuvant chemotherapy optimally determined by their response to preoperative chemotherapy with high dose Methotrexate and Leucovorin rescue.

Introduction

In most of the clinical trials utilizing chemotherapy for the treatment of osteogenic sarcoma the arbitrary age cutoff of 21 years has been designated due to the fact that people felt that younger patients with osteogenic sarcoma represented the "classic" disease. The reason for not including older patients was the fact that is is a common held misconception that osteogenic sarcoma in older patients is a more benign disease.

The reason for this misconception is the fact that the histologically low grade, or parosteal osteogenic sarcoma is most common in the third decade of life, and when it occurs it tends to occur in that age group. This group aside, osteogenic sarcoma that occurs in adult patients in the more usual or high grade histology is just as malignant as osteogenic sarcoma occurring in children. In examining the impact of chemotherapy on survival in osteogenic sarcoma in adults, if one looks at only histologically high grade osteogenic sarcoma (by far the most common type) the historical survival in that group is not significantly better than the survival in patients of younger age. Nonetheless, in most trials of chemotherapy for osteogenic sarcoma in the United States patients over 21 have been excluded from these clinical trials based on their age (1,2). This is not only a scientifically erroneous basis for exclusion of patients; it has a practical impact, in that patients over the age of 21 do not have the option of being put on clinical trials to determine the efficacy of chemotherapy in their treatment. Indeed, patients in this category who were covered by state welfare insurance did not have the option of electively choosing adjuvant chemotherapy in their treatment for financial reasons. Therefore it is important to look at the role of chemotherapy in increasing the survival of patients greater than 21 years of age with osteogenic sarcoma.

There was one clinical investigation which was not bounded by age carried out in the United States during the past few years. This was the U.C.L.A. Osteogenic Sarcoma Trial recently reported by Eilber (3). In that trial, all patients were randomized to receive adjuvant chemotherapy according to the Sloan-Kettering T-7 Chemotherapy Protocol or no treatment postoperatively. However, all patients received intra-arterial Adriamycin and radiation therpay to the primary tumor in that study. Nonetheless, the results reported by Eilber for all age groups were significant in favor of adjuvant chemotherapy. This gave us the opportunity to go back and use Eilber's concomittant controls of adult patients who were treated with no postoperative adjuvant chemotherapy from 1973 through 1983 and compare that concurrent group of patients with the patients that were treated (by author G. Rosen) while at the Memorial Sloan-Kettering Cancer Center during the same period of time. This comparison, therefore, does not utilize the highly criticized historical control, but rather patients treated during a same period of time wherein the staging, and surgical expertise, presumably were equal for all patients.

The Patients

The patients, or treatment group included in this study include all patients with osteogenic sarcoma of an extremity, osteogenic sarcoma of high grade histology (III/IV), age greater than or equal to 21 years of age, referred to the senior author (G.R.) for chemotherapy, no metastases at diagnosis, and includes all patients consecutively seen from 1974 when adjuvant chemotherapy was routinely given for all patients referred, through December, 1983. Therefore, the minimum follow up on all patients is approximately 5 years.

Exclusions

There were five adult patients seen during the study period that were excluded. One patient was lost to follow up at 12 months, at which time he was continuously free of any evidence of recurrent or metastatic disease. One patient refused chemotherapy and therefore was not treated. One patient had inadequate renal function and could not receive either high dose Methotrexate or Cisplatinum chemotherapy. Two patients were excluded because of inadequate cardiac function. One of the latter patients had an osteogenic sarcoma of the humerus following irradiation for Hodgkin's Disease. He also had severe cardiomyopathy with a left ventricular ejection fraction less than 20% and could not be treated. This patient died of a myocardial infarction postoperatively. The second patient with inadequate cardiac function had severe cardiomyopathy and emphysema. He was a pulmonary and cardiac cripple who could not undergo chemotherapy. Finally, prior to 1978 many adult patients were treated by the bone service at Memorial Sloan-Kettering Cancer Center and not referred at all for chemotherapy, and those patients are not included in this series.

The Controls

The control patients were consecutively seen at the U.C.L.A. Center for the Health Sciences and presented with osteogenic sarcoma of an extremity. Again, these patients all had tumors with high grade (III/IV) histology. All patients were aged greater than or equal to 21 years and had no metastases at diagnosis. They were all entered on the randomized U.C.L.A. preoperative Adriamycin/Radiation Therapy Protocol during the years 1973 through 1983. All of the control patients had no postoperative adjuvant chemotherapy.

Patient Characteristics

The patients that were treated at Memorial Sloan-Kettering Cancer Center with chemotherapy were aged 21 to 64 years of age. The median age of this group was 28 years. There were 30 males and 16 females with a male:female ratio of 1.9:1.0. Thirty of the 46 patients had femur lesions (65%); 11 (24%) had tibial lesions; and 3 (6.5%) had humerus lesions; and 2 (4.5%) had fibula lesions.

Control Patient Characteristics

The 12 control patients on the U.C.L.A. Protocol were all aged 22 to 75 years, (median = 35 years of age). Eight were male, and the male to female ratio was 2.0:1.0. Seven (58%) had femur lesions, two (17%) had tibia lesions; and three (25%) had humerus lesions.

Treatment

In general, treatment consisted of ablation of the primary tumor either by limb salvage surgery or amputation. The control group had 90 mg total dose of intra-arterial chemotherapy and various doses of radiation therapy given to the primary tumor. The adjuvant therapy group were all treated with chemotherapy according to the T-4 protocol during the interval of 1974 to 1976 (four patients); or the T-7 chemotherapy protocol administered between 1976 and 1978 (ten patients); or the T-10 chemotherapy protocol administered during 1978 through 1981 (sixteen patients); or the T-12 chemotherapy protocol administered from November 1981 through 1983 (sixteen patients). The T-4, T-7, T-10 and T-12 protocols have been extensively published before (4,5,6,7) and basically consisted of chemotherapy with high dose Methotrexate and Leucovorin rescue given at the dose of 8 grams/m^2, and the addition of Adriamycin and Cyclophosphamide (T-4) or Bleomycin, Cyclophosphamide and Vactinomycin, (T-7), or the addition of Cisplatinum and Adriamycin to the former regimen (T-10 and T-12 protocol).

Included in the chemotherapy treatment group are five patients that had questionable CT scans of the chest prior to treatment. All five of these patients proved to have old granulomas or questionable necrotic, metastatic sarcoma at the time of thoracotomy, which was performed following surgery for their primary tumor..

Patients in the treatment group were followed at this period of time from 47 to 155 months (mean follow up time 93+ months).

Results

At a median follow up time of 93 months, 42 patients treated with aggressive chemotherapy had a median survival of 80%. All surviving patients at this time are currently free of disease. The relapse-free survival of the 42 patients was 67%, again at a median time of 93 months (fig. 1).

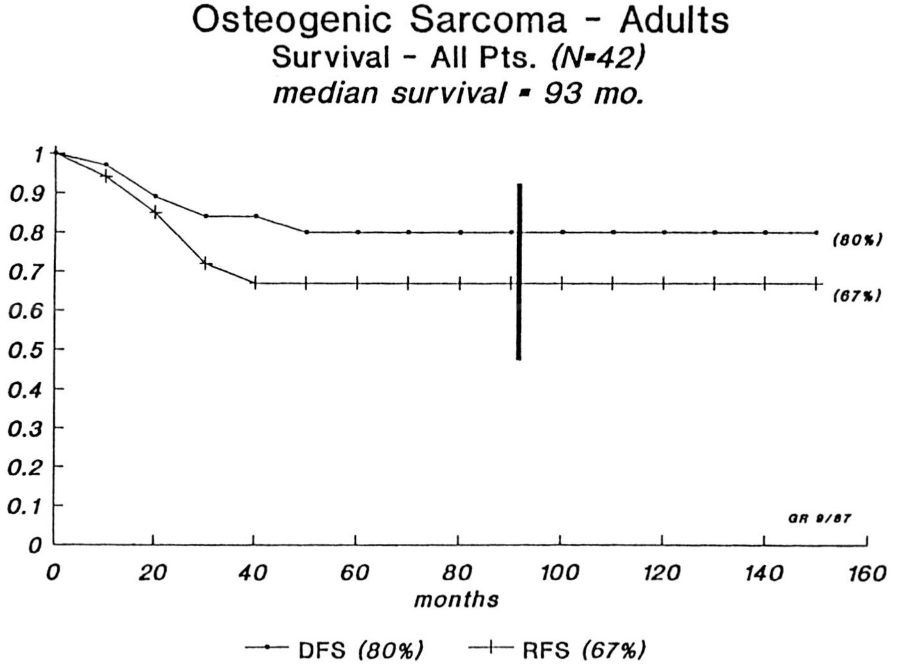

Figure 1

Osteogenic Sarcoma in Adults - Survival for all patients (42) DFS (Are patients currently surviving free of disease); RFT (patients who are surviving who have never relapsed). The relapse-free survival and the current disease-free survival is statistically significantly different from controls (fig. 3). All patients currently surviving are free of disease (at a median time of 93 months).

Of note, of the 42 patients treated with adjuvant chemotherapy, 32 underwent preoperative chemotherapy according to the T-7, T-10 or T-12 chemotherapy protocol. If one looks at the end results by response to preoperative chemotherapy, it can be seen that 84% of the patients having a good response to preoperative chemotherapy with high dose Methotrexate and Leucovorin rescue remain continuously free of relapsing. Of that group, all of the patients that relapsed had solitary relapses which were subsequently removed, and 100% of the patients are currently surviving free of disease. However, of the patients who responded poorly to preoperative chemotherapy with high dose Methotrexate, only 53% of the patients remained continuously free of relapse and only 60% of them were disease-free survivors at a median time of over 7 years (fig. 2).

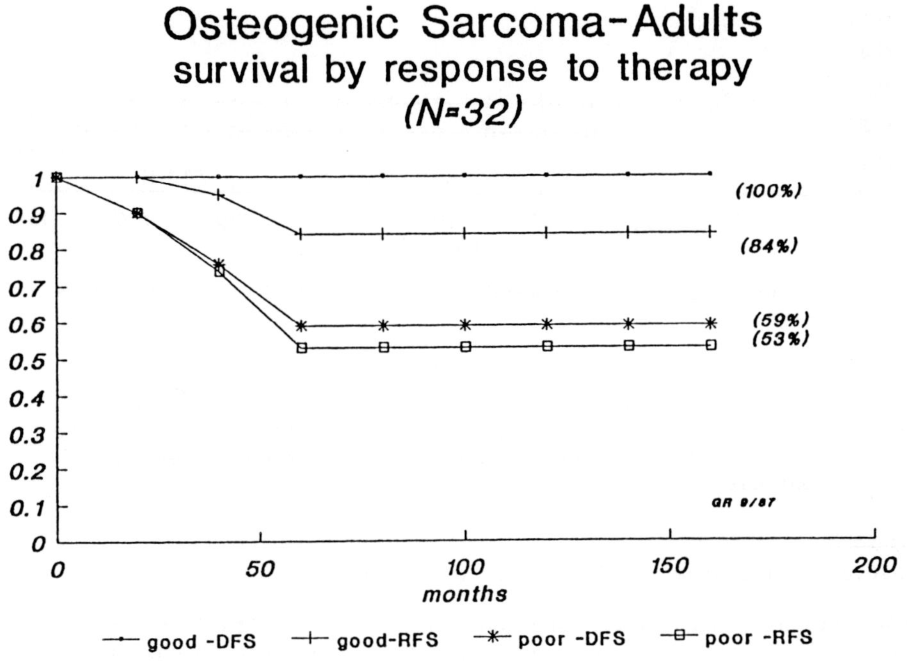

Figure 2

Of the 42 patients reported here, 32 had preoperative chemotherapy. All of those patients achieving a complete response to preoperative chemotherapy are currently surviving free of disease.

If one examines the effect of chemotherapy versus control patients on overall survival, it can be seen that continuous relapse-free survival of all patients treated with chemotherapy was 67% with an overall survival of 80%. All of the patients currently surviving at this time (median greater than 7 years) are currently free of disease and expected to be cured of their disease. Of the control patients that received only preoperative Adriamycin, radiation therapy and no postoperative adjuvant chemotherapy with either high dose Methotrexate with Leucovorin rescue or Cisplatinum, only 25% of the patients are surviving at this time. In addition, only 17% of them were continuous relapse-free survivors. It should be noted that control patients were treated with aggressive surgery and further chemotherapy following their relapse (fig. 3).

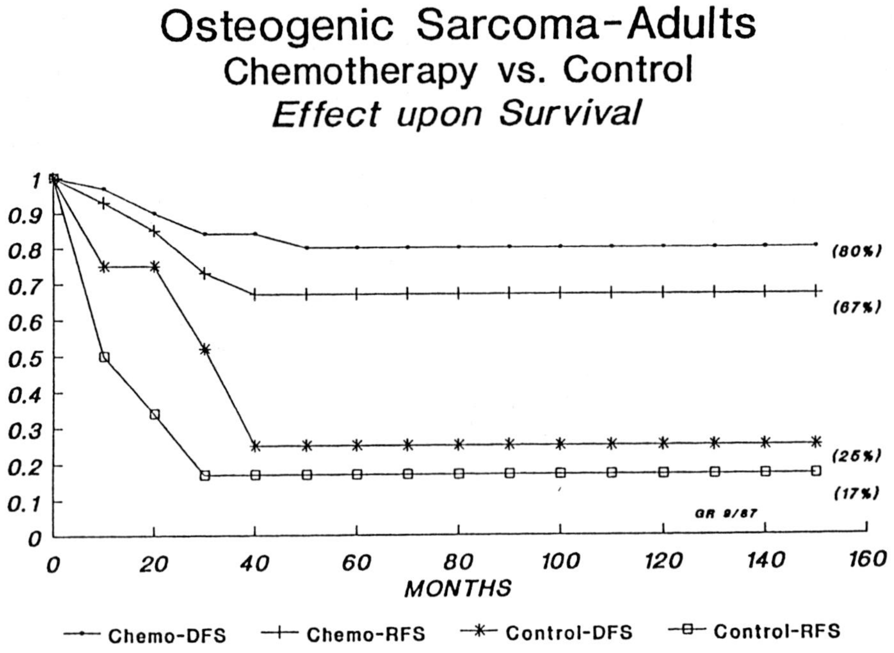

Figure 3

Both the current disease-free survival (DFS) and the overall relapse-free survival (RFS) is significantly improved by the addition of chemotherapy in the treated group versus the controls.

Discussion

The above results draw the following conclusion:

1) Histologically high grade osteogenic sarcoma in adults is a highly malignant disease with a natural history not undifferent from that in children.

2) Chemotherapy has profoundly impacted on the relapse-free survival and survival of adult patients with malignant osteogenic sarcoma.

The misconceptions regarding the benignity of osteogenic sarcoma in adults should be corrected. There is, certainly, a cohort of patients who are greater in age than 21 who develop low grade osteogenic sarcoma in a much higher frequency than do children. However, the majority of osteogenic sarcomas seen in adults are fully malignant lesions which have a very poor prognosis, both historically and by determined concurrent modern controls. Therefore, it is important to realize that when adults present with histologically proven high grade osteogenic sarcoma they are offered aggressive chemotherapy which has now been proven to increase survival dramatically.

If one examines the nine non-surviving patients in the treatment group, it can be seen that some of these patients were even at greater risk for the development of metastases. Indeed, some of them would not have been included in stringently controlled trials, although they were not excluded in this study and make up the nine of 42 patients who did not survive in the treatment group. The patient characteristics of these non-surviving patients are enumerated in Table 1. They include one patient with "small cell" osteogenic sarcoma. This patient would have been excluded from treatment for osteogenic sarcoma by this author at this time since it has become apparently that this particular subvariety of osteogenic sarcoma may indeed be more like a Ewing's sarcoma of bone, and the small cell histology may be a clue to that. This author has subsequently treated several of these patients with chemotherapy similar to that used for a Ewing's sarcoma, with successful outcomes. This may truly be a different disease than the classic osteogenic sarcoma. One 37 year old female with a pathologically fractured tumor had no preoperative chemotherapy because of the advanced stage of her tumor. An additional patient had osteogenic sarcoma of the mid-shaft of the tibia diagnosed during pregnancy. There was over a 10 month delay in starting chemotherapy, and the histology of this tumor was also atypical. Another patient (Patient #9, Table 1) had intrapelvic extension of his tumor with positive para-aortic lymph nodes at the time of diagnosis and subsequent surgery. This patient probably should have been excluded from the treatment group as having metastases, but was included here for the sake of not biasing the study since the positive para-aortic lymph nodes were not documented prior to therapy. Another patient was a 49 year old female who had no preoperative chemotherapy because the biopsy was read as a low grade osteogenic sarcoma. After several months and delay in reviewing the resected specimen, it was obvious that she had a high grade tumor. She was finally placed on postoperative adjuvant chemotherapy (T-12), however, subsequently developed metastases and probably, at this time, has succumbed to her disease. Finally, one patient was a 25 year old male who had a periosteal osteogenic sarcoma. This patient was included in the treatment group because this author has recognized the fact that periosteal osteogenic sarcomas are not the same as paraosteal and, indeed, have a poor prognosis. This patient also succumbed to metastatic pulmonary disease.

OSTEOGENIC SARCOMA IN ADULTS

TABLE 1 - NON-SURVIVORS (N=9)

PT. #	AGE/SEX	SITE	PROTOCOL	SURVIVAL	COMMENT
1	22/M	HUM	T-7	19 MO.	SMALL CELL
2	22/M	TIB	T-7	19 MO.	
3	22/F	FEM	T-10	16 MO.	
4	37/F	FEM	T-10	10 MO.	P.Fx NO PRE-OP
5	32/F	TIB	T-10	27 MO.	PREG/ATYPIC.
6	32/F	FEM	T-10	18 MO.	P,Fx.
7	25/M	FEM	T-12	49 MO.	PERIOSTEAL
8	49/F	FEM	T-12	30 MO.	NO PRE-OP/LBx
9	28/M	FEM	T-12	2 MO.	INTRAPELVIC

P.Fx (PATHOLOGIC FRACTURE),LBx (LOW GRADE BIOPSY)
SEE TEXT.

Table 1

Review of the treatment failures and, of course, of the positive outcome of the treatment group for osteogenic sarcoma in adults leads us to the conclusion that patients with high grade osteogenic sarcoma, regardless of their age, deserve preoperative and/or at least postoperative adjuvant chemotherapy to increase their survival.

The rapidity with which chemotherapy is started in these patients is important, and this author advises immediate preoperative chemotherapy for all patients with fully malignant osteogenic sarcoma. The artificial bias against treating patients greater than 21 years of age with osteogenic sarcoma with chemotherapy should be dispelled, and it should also be recognized that paraosteal osteogenic sarcomas do exist in the adult age group, and these tumors should be excluded from chemotherapy trials because of their low grade nature. However, it should be cautioned that even these low grade tumors deserve adequate and radical surgical resection or removal because a small proportion of these patients that do relapse and die do so because of local recurrence, and evolution of the tumor into a more high grade histology which can lead to metastases. All physicians and investigators involved in the treatment of osteogenic sarcoma should recognize these subtleties of diagnosis and treatment, and all patients with histologically high grade osteogenic sarcoma, regardless of age, should be treated with preoperative and postoperative chemotherapy.

REFERENCES

1) Link, MP, Goorin, AM, Meiser, AW, et al. The effect of adjuvant chemotherapy on relapse-free survival in patients with osteosarcoma of the extremity. N. Eng. J. Med. 314: 1600-1606, 1986.

2) Provisor, A. Childrens Cancer Study Group Protocol #782 (U.S.A.)

3) Eilber, F, Giuliano, A, Eckardt, J, et al. Adjuvant chemotherapy for osteosarcoma: a randomized prospective trial. J. Clin. Oncol. 5 (No. 1): 21-26, 1987.

4) Rosen, G, Murphy, ML, Huvos, AG, et al. Chemotherapy, en bloc resection and prosthetic bone replacement in the treatment of osteogenic sarcoma and guidelines for clinical use. In Pharmanual: A comprehensive guide to the therapeutic use of Methotrexate in osteogenic sarcoma. Editor G. Rosen, pp 47-83, 1984.

5) Rosen, G, Marcove, RC, Caparros, B, et al. Primary osteogenic sarcoma. The rationale for preoperative chemotherapy and delayed surgery. Cancer 43: 2163-3177, 1979.

6) Rosen, G, Caparros, B, Huvos, AG, Kosloff, C, Nirenberg, A, Cacavio, A, Marcove, RC, Lane, JM, Mehta B, Urban, C. Preoperative chemotherapy for osteogenic sarcoma: Selection of postoperative adjuvant chemotherapy based on the response of the primary tumor to preoperative chemotherapy. Cancer 49: 1221-1230, 1982.

Résumé

Le sarcome ostéogénique chez les adultes. Valeur de la chimiothérapie néoadjuvante.

De 1974 à 1983, 42 adultes atteints d'ostéosarcome malins (grade histologique III-IV/IV) ont été traités par l'auteur : chimiothérapie pré-opératoire et post-opératoire. Les résultats de ce traitement ont été comparés à ceux d'un groupe de malades vus dans le même temps à l'UCLA et randomisés pour ne pas recevoir de chimiothérapie post-opératoire. Les malades du groupe traité ont reçu 4 protocoles de chimiothérapie successifs (T4, T7, T10, T12). La survie globale des 12 patients contrôles a été de 25 % (17 % de survie sans rechute) comparée à une survie globale de 80 % pour ces malades traités par chimiothérapie (survie sans rechute 67 %). Bien que les malades contrôle aient reçu une cure d'Adriamycine intra-artérielle, une radiothérapie sur la tumeur, aucun n'a bénéficié de la chimiothérapie néoadjuvante, pour déterminer quel était le meilleur traitement post-opératoire pour eux et aucun d'entre eux n'a bénéficié de la chimiothérapie par les deux traitements les plus efficaces pour les ostéosarcomes soit le Méthotrexate à fortes doses plus acide folinique, et l'association Cis.Platyl et Adriamycine. Cette étude démontre que les sarcomes ostéogéniques des adultes non traités par la chimiothérapie ont un très mauvais pronostic semblable à celui des enfants et des adolescents. Il démontre aussi l'impact dramatique sur la survie d'une chimiothérapie aggressive dans les ostéosarcomes de l'adulte. Tous les adultes avec des sarcomes ostéogéniques totalement malins devraient être traités par une chimiothérapie pré-opératoire, suivie d'une chimiothérapie post-opératoire adjuvante déterminée de façon optimale d'après la réponse des patients à la chimiothérapie pré-opératoire par fortes doses de Méthotrexate et acide folinique.

Neo-Adjuvant Chemotherapy. Ed. Cl. Jacquillat, M. Weil, D. Khayat. Colloque INSERM/John Libbey Eurotext Ltd. © 1988. Vol. 169, pp. 509-513.

Neo-adjuvant chemotherapy in osteosarcoma. Results of a multicentric study in Italy

P. Picci[1*], G. Bacci[2*], M. Campanacci[3*], A. Brach del Prever[4], M. Fiorentini[5], A.M. Mancini[6], M. Avella[3], E. Figus[2*], N. Baldini[1*], M. Mercuri[3*], R. Capanna[3*], R. Biagini[3*] and P. Ruggieri[3*]

*[1]Bone Tumor Center, [2]Department of Internal Medicine, [3]First Orthopaedic Clinic University of Bologna, *Istituto Ortopedico Rizzoli, via Pupilli 1, 40136 Bologna, Italy. [4]Department of Pediatric Oncology, University of Torino, Italy. [5]Department of Oncology, General Hospital of Ravenna, Italy. [6]3rd Department of Pediatric Oncology, University of Bologna, Italy*

KEYWORDS: OSTEOSARCOMA, NEOADJUVANT CHEMOTHERAPY

ABSTRACT

The experience related to 2 studies of preoperative chemotherapy in the treatment of localized osteosarcoma of the extremities is reported. The results of the first study related to 126 consecutive patients, opened in March '83 and closed in September '86, stressed the importance of 1)the use of adriamycin and high dose methotrexate for the control of the disease, 2) the importance of the amount of necrosis induced by the preoperative treatment as prognostic factor, 3) the possibility of conservative surgery in most cases without great risks of local recurrence. Also reported are the encouraging preliminary results of the second study,designed considering the indications obtained with the first study.

INTRODUCTION

In the seventies, the use of adjuvant chemotherapy in localized osteosarcoma gave great improvement in the prognosis of this disease, which increased from 10-15% to 45-50% at a 5 year follow-up.

In the beginning of the eighties it became evident that there was no doubt that this improvement was due to the use of adjuvant chemotherapy, it also appeared evident to us that it was not possible to jump the 50% barrier by modifying the protocols of adjuvant treatment. Moreover, no new drugs on the market appeared to be more effective than those used. For these reasons, in March '83, the Bone Tumor Center of the Istituto Ortopedico Rizzoli of Bologna, in collaboration with the Department of Pediatric Oncology of the University of Torino, the Department of Pediatric Oncology of the University of Bologna and subsequently the Division of Oncology of the General Hospital of Ravenna, designed a study of preoperative chemotherapy in patients with localized osteosarcoma of the extremities.

The aims of the study were: 1) to increase the percentage of limb salvage procedures, 2) to avoid, if possible, the use of adriamycin for its side effects, and 3)to compare in a multidrug treatment the efficacy of high dose of methotrexate versus low doses.

DESIGN OF THE STUDY

Preoperative chemotheray consisted of two cycles of methotrexate(MTX) and two cycles of CDDP. Mtx was given at day 1 intravenously at different doses on a randomized basis: 750 mg/m^2 in half an hour versus 7.5 g/m^2 in a 6-hour infusion. In both cases, citrovorum factor rescue was started 24 hours after the beginning of MTX. CDDP was given intra-arterially in all patietns and at the same dose of 120-150 mg/m^2 in a 72-hour infusion starting on day 6. A second cycle of both drugs was given starting at day 21. Surgery was usually performed after three weeks from the end of chemotherapy.

Surgery was always performed in the same institution (Istituto Ortopedico Rizzoli), by the same surgeons with great expertise in the treatment of bone tumors. The choice between limb salvage procedures or ablative surgery was taken considering the size of the tumor, the involvement of major structures, the efficacy of preoperative treatment in delimiting the tumor, and the residual expected functional activity. In other words, the choice was dictated considering, on one hand, the risk of a local recurrence, and on the other, the residual functional activity remaining to the patient. After surgery, all the specimens were studied by the same pathologist and the necrosis was evaluated on at least two entire sections on the two major diameters of the tumor. Necrosis was graded as "good" if it was greater than 90%; as "fair" if it was between 60 and 90%; and "poor" if it was less than 60%. Postoperatively, the treatment was chosen depending on the grade of necrosis observed:

1. For a "good" necrosis, the same preoperative treatment at the same dose was given intravenously for two cycles.
2. For a "fair" necrosis, adriamycin (ADM), at the dose of 90 mg/m^2 in two or three days was added to the two drugs employed preoperatively. The treatment started with ADM followed after 21 days by MTX and CDDP at the same doses used preoperatively for 3 complete cycles. Another cycle of ADM was given at the end of the treatment. In this way, 360 mg/m^2 of ADM were given in about 6 months.
3. For a "poor" necrosis, the treatment consisted of 5 cycles of ADM with the same modalitites used for "fair" responders, alternated to 5 cycles of BCD (Bleomycin 20 mg/m^2, Cyclophosphamide 750 mg/m^2, Actinomycin-D 0.6 mg/m^2) for about 9 months.

In December 1983, after four early metastases observed in the "good" responders where ADM had not been used, this arm was closed. After this, the "good" responders were also treated with the same schema employed for "fair" responders.

PATIENTS

Until September 1986, 224 patients with osteosarcoma were observed. Eighty patients were excluded, being considered ineligible to the study due to several reasons: metastatic, histological varieties, previous tumor (2 retinoblastomas and 1 leukemia), site not in an extremity, age over 45, refused the protocol.

The remaining 144 patients entered the study and were randomized to receive high or moderate doses of MTX. Preoperative investigations included CT scan of the lesion, and bone scan before and after preoperative treatment. Lung tomograms were performed after preoperative treatment, before surgery. Angiograms were performed before each infusion of CDDP.

Of the 144 randomized patients, 18 are not evaluable for several reasons: 10 patients, after the end of preoperative treatment, refused surgery and were, therefore, sent to other institutions for other treatment; 3 patients, all randomized to receive high doses of MTX developed, after the first MTX, a severe toxicity and therefore changed their treatment; 3 patients started postoperative treatment after 50 days from surgery due to surgical complications, and another one, for the same reasons, was not given any postoperative treatment other than 1 cycle of ADM. Another excluded patient suddenly died due to unknown causes.

The remaining 126 patients are the object of this report. Sixty-six were randomized to receive high doses of MTX and 60 to receive low doses.

RESULTS

Ninety-one patients (72%) were surgically treated with limb salvage procedures and 35 (28%) with amputation or disarticulation. In spite of this high number of limb salvage procedures, only four local recurrences were observed (3 in resected patients and 1 in an amputed patient). Necrosis was evaluated on all 126 specimens. Totally, 52% of the patients showed a "good" necrosis, 36 a "fair" necrosis, and 12 a "poor" necrosis. Differences were noted between the patients treated with high or moderate doses of MTX, but these were not statistically significant; in fact, "good" responders were 62% with higher doses versus 42% with lower doses, "fair" responders were 29% and 43%, and "poor" responders 9% and 15% respectively.

Fifteen patients, all "good" responders (9 treated with high doses of MTX and 6 with the lower doses), were postoperatively treated without ADM. Today, at a median follow-up of 48 months (range 45-54) only four (27%) are continuously disease-free (2 in each of the two groups of MTX), 10 of the remaining 11 patients developed lung metastases after 4-18 months (x=11 months), and another developed a local recurrence due to a skip metastasis erroneously not detected preoperatively, after 29 months. In December 1983, after four of these patients developed early lung metastases, this arm was closed and also the "good" responders were treated with the same postoperative schema employed for "fair" responders. The remaining 111 patients were, therefore, all treated postoperatively with ADM and will be better evaluated now. At a median follow-up of 30 months (range 12-54), 60 patients (61%) are continuously disease-free, 43 (39%) developed distant metastases. Three of these patients developed a contemporary local recurrence (3%). Regarding the doses of MTX, 70% (40/57) of the patients treated with high doses are continuously disease-free versus 52% (28/54) of the patients treated with lower doses. This difference is statistically significant ($p<0.05$).

Analyzing the results in terms of necrosis induced by preoperative chemotherapy, 82% (42/51) of "good" responders are continuously disease-free versus 47% (21/45) of the "fair" responders, and 33% (5/15) of the "poor" responders. The difference between "good" and "fair" responders is statistically highly significant ($p<0.001$), while the difference between "fair" and "poor" responders is not statistically significant.

Our study involves pediatric and adult patients and it is thus correct to evaluate the prognosis with regard to age. Fifty of our patients were 14 or younger, and 34 (58%) are continuously disease-free versus 56% (34/61) of the older patients, ranging from 15 to 45 years. Finally, again no difference in disease-free survival was observed between patients treated by amputation (64%, 21/33) and patients treated by limb salvage surgery (60%, 47/78).

CONCLUSIONS

1. In our study, with the multidrug association and doses we employed, ADM is absolutely necessary.
   Our attempt to avoid this drug for its cardiotoxicity was evaluated in 15 patients only. This attempt revealed to be prognostically negative, only four are disease-free, and this arm of treatment was suddenly closed.
2. Limb salvage is possible and safe. In spite of the very high percentage of limb salvage procedures (73%), only four experienced a local recurrence. It is to be noted that one of these local recurrences was observed after a hindquarter amputation, and that another one was due to a skip metastatsis erroneously not detected during the preoperative staging, but afterwards revealed by the careful examination of the preoperative radio- and angiograms.
3. Our study confirms that "good" responders have a very good prognosis (more than 80%). In our experience, to change postoperative treatment after a "poor" necrosis does not increase the disease-free survival.
4. From our experience, the "breaking point" for the choice of postoperative treatment is 90% necrosis. Our data, in fact, underlines that below this percentage of necrosis, postoperative treatment should be changed or increased, and these variations should not be limited to "poor" responders only.
5. The comparison between high and low doses of MTX seems to indicate a better prognosis using higher doses. Although our results indicate a statistically significant difference, a longer follow-up is necessary to confirm this fact.

SECOND STUDY

At this point there were theoretically two ways to increase prognosis: to know before starting the treatment if the patient will be or not a "good" responder, or to give a more aggressive preoperative treatment to increase the number of "good" responders. Because the first solution is today not yet possible, the second one was chosen.

Based on these conclusions, a new study was opened in September 1986. The aim was to increase the number of "good" responders, giving a more intense preoperative treatment. For this reason, in addition to the previous schema, adriamycin was given intravenously, at the dose of 50-60 mg/m^2, together with the third day of intraarterial cisplatinum . The dose of methotrexate was established in all patients at 8 gr/m^2. A second cycle was repeated on day 28.

Until January '88, 108 new cases of osteosarcoma were diagnosed. 37 cases were excluded due to several reasons: metastases at diagnosis (9 cases), tumor in axial bones (7 cases), osteosarcoma varieties (in Paget disease, parosteal, periosteal) (4 cases), age > 40 years (2 cases), previous chemotherapy (9 cases), other treatments (6 cases). Six more cases started the preoperative treatment which was stopped abruptly for different reasons (haemorrhage from biopsy site - 2 cases, patient refusal - 2 cases, toxicity due to methotrexate - 1 case, or due to cisplatinum - 1 case). Of the remaining 65 cases in the study, 9 are on treatment and have not been operated yet. In the remaining 56 patients, limb saving surgery was performed in 50 cases (89%), rotation plasty was performed in 2 cases (4%) and amputation in 4 (7%). Necrosis was good (> or = 90%) in 47 cases (84%)

and low (<90%) in 9 (16%). It is obviously too early to report results for this second study, but the very high percentage of good necrosis is encouraging us to continue this study. At the 15th of February '88, with a follow-up ranging from 3 to 16 months (x=9 months) only 3 patients developed metastases: 2 between the good responders (4%) and 1 (9%) amongst the poor responders. No patient presented a local recurrence. The postoperative treatment for good responders is the same used in the first study. Poor responders are treated by 3 cycles of adriamycin (45 mg/m^2 in 8 hours for 2 days), ifosfamide (1800 mg/m^2 in 90 minutes for 5 days), methotrexate (8 gr/m^2 in 6 hours) and cisplatinum (120-150 mg/m^2 in 72 hours) given contemporary to VP16 (100 mg/m^2 for 3 days in 1 hour); one more cycle of adriamycin is given at the end of treatment.

Supported in part by a grant from the Italian National Research Council, Special Project "Oncology" N° 87.02810.44, and by a grantfrom Regione Emilia-Romagna, law n°1970 of May 13th, 1986.

This research was carried on amongst the activities of the Interdepartment Center of Cancer Research of the University of Bologna.

Résumé

Cet article rapporte les résultats de deux études de chimiothérapie pré-opératoire dans le traitement des ostéosarcomes localisés aux extrémités.
Les résultats de la première étude portent sur 126 malades consécutifs, traités entre 1983 et septembre 1986. Ils mettent en évidence l'importance de l'Adriamycine et des fortes doses de Méthotrexate sur le contrôle de la maladie, l'importance de la nécrose induite par le traitement pré-opératoire en tant que facteur pronostique, la possibilité d'une chirurgie conservatrice dans la plupart des cas, sans risque important de rechute locale.
Les résultats préliminaires encourageants de la seconde étude qui prend en considération les résultats de la première sont également indiqués.

Neo-Adjuvant Chemotherapy. Ed. Cl. Jacquillat, M. Weil, D. Khayat. Colloque INSERM/John Libbey Eurotext Ltd. © 1988. Vol. 169, pp. 515-520.

Neo-adjuvant chemotherapy for limb osteosarcoma

J. Graham-Pole, R. Saleh, D. Springfield, R. Vander Griend, S. Spanier, N. Dickson, T. Gillespy, R. Hawkins, S. Gross and W. Enneking

University of Florida, Departments of Pediatrics, Orthopedics, and Radiology, Box J-296, JHMHC, 1600 SW Archer Road, Gainesville, Florida, 32610, USA

ABSTRACT

Adjuvant chemotherapy has been shown to significantly increase survival of patients with osteosarcoma (OS). Neoadjuvant chemotherapy (NCT) may further improve this survival. We have studied the effects of NCT, delayed surgery, and adjuvant (ACT) in 36 subjects with OS, on the rate of limb salvage (LSS), extent of histologic necrosis (HN%), complications, and disease-free survival. Patients received 4 courses of NCT (methotrexate, doxorubicin, intravenous or intra-arterial cis-platinum) and 5 courses of the same drugs as ACT.

10 patients have had omissions of NCT and 10 omissions of ACT, due to disease progression, complications, or choice. Significantly more patients completing all NCT underwent LSS, and showed significantly greater HN%, than those not completing NCT. 26 patients (72%) are continuously disease-free a median of 18 (range 5-39) months post-diagnosis. 9 have had disease progression a median of 6 (range 1-15) months post-diagnosis. These results, while encouraging, leave several questions to be resolved in multicenter randomized trials, including the optimal intensity and duration of chemotherapy, the relative effects of NCT + ACT vs ACT alone on disease-free survival, and the prognostic value of HN%.

KEY WORDS

Osteosarcoma, Neoadjuvant, Chemotherapy, Intravenous, Intra-arterial

INTRODUCTION

Adjuvant chemotherapy (ACT) has been shown in randomized studies to significantly increase the likelihood of disease-free survival (DFS) for patients with osteosarcoma (OS) when compared with surgery alone (Link, 1986; Eilber, 1987). Projected survivals from these and from other uncontrolled studies (Winkler, 1984) range from 45% to 68%. Neoadjuvant chemotherapy (NCT) may further improve this outcome to 75%-85%, based on non-randomized studies (Rosen, 1986; Bacci, 1986).

Since October 1984, we have been studying NCT, and asking the following questions: (1) Does NCT allow more limb-salvage surgery (LSS) compared with historical controls? (2) Does NCT improve DFS? (3) Is extent of histological necrosis (HN%) prognostic? (4) Is intra-arterial (IA) more effective than intravenous (IV) cis-platinum (CPDD)? (5) What are the risks involved? This report contains a preliminary analysis addressing these questions.

SUBJECTS

36 consecutive patients with OS affecting a limb diagnosed by incisional or needle biopsy between October 1984 and September 1987 at the University of Florida were entered on this study. There were 21 males, and the median age was 15 (range 6-41) years. Primary sites were the distal femur (12), proximal tibia (11), proximal humerus (8), and other sites (5). Two patients had metastases at diagnosis, and 12 had alkaline phosphatase levels >400 mg/100ml.

METHODS

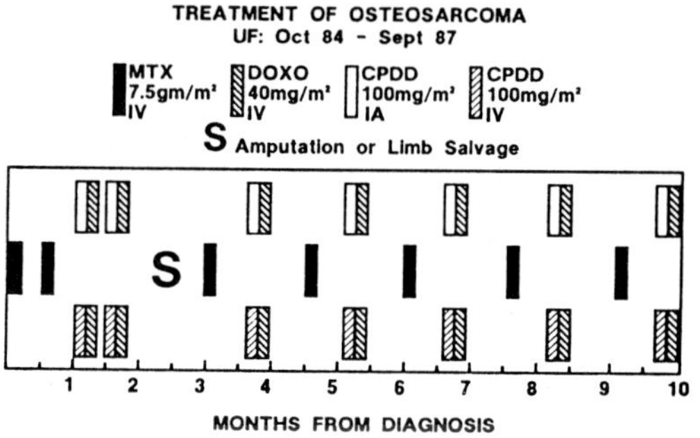

Fig. 1. Treatment Regimen

Figure 1 shows the treatment regimen, consisting of 4 courses of NCT (methotrexate (MTX), cis-platinum (CPDD), doxorubicin (Doxo)), surgery, consisting of either LSS or amputation (AMP) between week 8 and 10, and courses of ACT from approximately week 12 to 36. During NCT, 19 patients received intra-arterial (IA) and 17 intravenous (IV) CPDD. Patients receiving IV CPDD were those diagnosed in the first year of the study (before we adopted the use of IA CPDD), all those aged less than 10 and greater than 30 years, and those who chose not to receive IA CPDD.

MTX was infused over 6 hours in 500 ml/m^2 of 5% dextrose with sodium bicarbonate supplementation, followed by folinic acid 15 mg every 6 hours for 10 doses, with appropriate monitoring of serum MTX levels. Doxorubicin was given by IV bolus injection, and CPDD by infusion over 6 hours IV or over 1 hour IA in 1/2 normal saline with mannitol 10 gm/m^2, and potassium and magnesium supplementation. Hydration at a rate of 3000 ml/m^2/day was maintained before, during, and after MTX and CPDD infusions. IA CPDD was infused into the principle arterial supply of the primary tumor, with angiographic monitoring, using a pulsatile infuser[1] (Wallace, 1984) to increase turbulence and thus rapid admixing of drug within the blood stream.

---

[1]Cook Inc, Bloomington, Indiana, USA

Patients were evaluated and monitored serially with plain radiographs, computer tomography and/or magnetic resonance imaging, radionuclide bone scans, full blood counts, renal, hepatic, cardiac and pulmonary function studies. The study was approved by our Institutional Review Board and informed written consent was obtained from all patients and/or legal guardians.

RESULTS

For comparison, we have separated the patients receiving IV and IA CPDD in this preliminary analysis. To date, 16 subjects have completed all treatment, 5 continue on treatment, and 15 have had part of their NCT and/or ACT omitted, because of disease progression (6), complications (6), or patient choice (3). Complications causing modification or cessation of treatment included reduced glomerular filtration (9), high-frequency hearing loss (3), left ventricular hypokinesia (1), pathological fracture (1), peripheral neuropathy (1), and arteriospasm (2).

Table 1 shows the type of surgery performed in these patients.

Table 1. Type of Surgery

RESULTS: TYPE OF SURGERY

	IV NCT	IA NCT	HISTORICAL CONTROLS
Total Patients	17	19	53
Limb Salvage (%)	8 (47)	12 (63)	16 (30)
Amputation (%)	9 (53)	7 (37)	37 (70)
Patients Completing NCT	13	13	--
Limb Salvage (%)	7 (54)	11 (85)	--
Amputation (%)	6 (46)	2 (15)	--

20 (55%) have undergone LSS, compared with our historical experience of 30% in patients undergoing surgery before we introduced NCT. More patients in the IA than in the IV NCT group had LSS, but this is not yet statistically significant. Regardless of route of administration, however, there were significantly more LSS than AMP among patients completing all 4 NCT courses (X^2=7.15, p<0.01).

Table 2 shows the extent of histologic tumor necrosis (HN%) seen at the time of definitive surgery in 27 fully evaluated patients. Most showed extensive (>80%) necrosis, but we have not so far seen differences between patients receiving IV and IA NCT. Completion of all NCT, however, also correlates significantly with HN% (X^2=10.80, p<0.001).

With a median follow-up of 18 (range 5-39) months, 26 patients (72%) are continuously disease-free, and 3 others are disease-free 9,12, and 22 months after removal of isolated pulmonary metastases (Fig. 2). 7 patients have died, 6 of disease and 1 of sepsis. A diagnostic alkaline phosphatase level <400 mg/100 ml correlates significantly with a higher disease-free survival (DFS) (X^2=5.17, p<0.02). 15 of the 16 patients (94%) who completed all chemotherapy are continuously disease-free, and so far only one patient who stopped treatment early has relapsed. There are no differences yet in these outcomes between the IV and IA NCT groups. Disease progression was documented a median of 6 (1-15) months post-diagnosis.

Table 2. Extent of Histologic Necrosis

RESULTS: HISTOLOGIC NECROSIS

	IV NCT	IA NCT	TOTAL %
Total Patients Evaluated	13	14	27
HN > 80%	7 (54)	8 (57)	15 (56)
HN < 80%	6 (46)	6 (43)	12 (44)
Patients Completing NCT	9	9	18
HN > 80%	7 (78)	7 (78)	14 (78)
HN < 80%	2 (22)	2 (22)	4 (22)

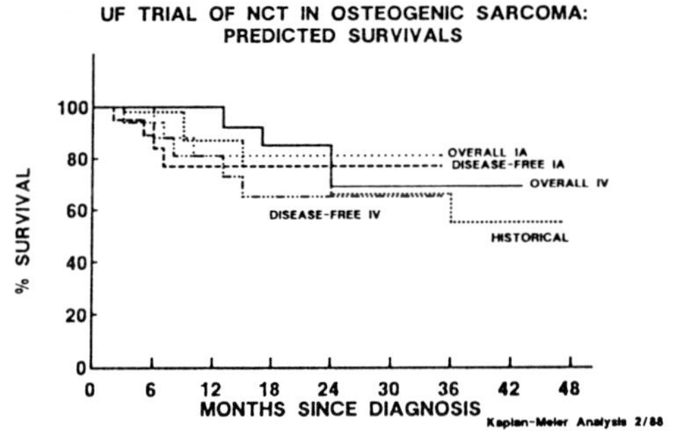

Fig. 2. Predicted Survivals and Disease-free Survivals

Figure 2 is an actuarial analysis of the predicted disease-free and overall survivals of the 36 patients, together with that of 55 on our previous trial of ACT alone (Springfield, submitted, 1988). The overall survivals are currently 81% and 69% for the IA and IV NCT patients respectively, compared with 55% historically.

DISCUSSION

Rosen (1978) introduced NCT for patients with limb OS in the hope of (a) eliminating micrometastases early on; (b) permitting more LSS to be performed; and (c) planning rational ACT on the basis of extent of histologic response at the time of definitive surgery. His results, and those of Jaffe (1985), Bacci (1986), and ourselves, encourage us to think that these hopes may be realized. More patients are undergoing LSS; HN% at the time of surgery is often extensive and can be quantitated (Picci, 1988); and, lastly, there may be an increasing proportion of subjects achieving longterm DFS when compared to recent trials of ACT alone. However, several questions remain. First, the greater number of LSS being performed may reflect developing surgical sophistication, and might be achievable even were definitive surgery still routinely performed at diagnosis. Second, although our patients who completed all their scheduled NCT did have a greater degree of HN% and a greater LSS rate, this at least in part reflects a higher proportion of de novo unfavorable cases (large or more chemoresistant tumors) in the group who did not complete NCT. Lastly, although Rosen (1986) claims that HN% following NCT is useful prognostically, no prospective controlled studies have yet been performed to prove this point.

The current achievement of 70%-80% DFS in our own and other recent series that have combined NCT with ACT is encouraging, when compared with the 45%-68% DFS reported in recent studies of ACT alone (Eilber, 1987; Link, 1986; Winkler, 1984). However, only randomized controlled clinical trials comparing NCT plus ACT with ACT alone will prove if there is any permanent advantage. This will require multicenter cooperation to obtain enough patients to include appropriate stratifications (for example, tumor size, site, patient age, and alkaline phosphatase levels).

Other chemotherapy issues that remain to be defined are the choice of agents, the intensity and duration of their use, and whether or not there is an advantage to IA NCT. Although strongly advocated by others (Jaffe, 1985; Bacci, 1986), it has not been clearly shown by us or them that the increased discomfort and morbidity of IA NCT is justifiable in terms of improved HN%, LSS rate or longterm DFS. As to the duration and intensity of chemotherapy, it is notable that in our series to date the median time to develop disease progression has been 6 months from diagnosis, and that patients not completing chemotherapy because of complications or choice are not faring less well so far. This suggests that the optimal chemotherapy approach may comprise an intensive NCT regimen with a similarly short, intensive ACT course, or even no ACT at all in selected cases. These questions can also be addressed only in large-scale randomized clinical trials.

REFERENCES

Bacci, G.(1986): Sarcomes osteogeniques: et-il possible de raccourcir et de modifier la chimiotherapie postoperatoire selon l'importance de la necrose induite par la traitement preoperatoire? La Presse Medicale 15, 932.

Eilber, F.(1987): Adjuvant chemotherapy for osteosarcoma: a randomized prospective trial. J. Clin. Oncol. 5, 21-26.

Jaffe, N.(1985): Comparison of intra-arterial cisplatinum with high-dose methotrexate and citrovorum factor rescue in the treatment of primary osteosarcoma. J. Clin. Oncol. 3, 1101-1104.

Link, M.P.(1986): The effect of adjuvant chemotherapy on relapse-free survival in patients with osteosarcoma of the extremity. NEJM 314, 1600-1606.

Picci, P.(1988): Histological evaluation of necrosis in osteosarcoma induced by chemotherapy. Cancer (in press).

Rosen, G.(1978): Preoperative (neoadjuvant) chemotherapy for limb preservation. Cancer Treat. Rep. 65, 99-105.

Rosen, G.(1986): Neoadjuvant chemotherapy for osteogenic sarcoma: a model for the treatment of other highly malignant neoplasms. Recent Results in Cancer Research 103, 148.

Wallace, S.(1984): Physioanatomic concepts and radiologic techniques for intra-arterial delivery of therapeutic agents. Cancer Bull. 36, 6-14.

Winkler, K.(1984): Neoadjuvant chemotherapy for osteogenic sarcoma: results of a cooperative German/Austrian study. J. Clin. Oncol. 2, 617-624.

Résumé

La chimiothérapie adjuvante a significativement augmenté la survie des malades porteurs d'ostéosarcomes. La chimiothérapie néoadjuvante améliore encore cette survie. Nous avons étudié les effects de la chimiothérapie néoadjuvante, d'une chirurgie retardée et d'une chimiothérapie adjuvante chez 36 sujets atteints d'ostéosarcomes avec pour critère le taux de préservation du membre, l'étendue de la nécrose histologique, les complications et la survie sans rechute. Les malades ont reçu 4 cures de chimiothérapie néoadjuvante (Méthotrexate-Doxorubicine-Cisplatinum IV ou intra-artériel) et 5 cures semblables en tant que chimiothérapie adjuvante. 10 malades n'ont pas eu une chimiothérapie néoadjuvante complète et 10 malades n'ont pas eu une chimiothérapie complète en raison de la progression de la maladie, des complications ou du choix des malades. Les malades chez lesquels la chimiothérapie néoadjuvante a été complète, ont un taux significativement plus élevé de préservation du membre et de la nécrose histologique 26 patients (72 %) sont en survie sans rechute, avec une médiane de 18 mois après le diagnostic (5 à 39) 9 ont eu une progression de la maladie avec une médiane de 6 mois (1 à 15 mois). Ces résultats bien qu'encourageants laissent plusieurs questions à résoudre pour les essais randomisés multicentres : l'intensité optimale et la durée optimale de la chimiothérapie, l'effet relatif de la chimiothérapie néoadjuvante et de la chimiothérapie adjuvante et la valeur pronostique de la nécrose histologique.

Neo-Adjuvant Chemotherapy. Ed. Cl. Jacquillat, M. Weil, D. Khayat. Colloque INSERM/John Libbey Eurotext Ltd. © 1988. Vol. 169, pp. 521-527.

Chimiothérapie première chez les patients porteurs de sarcomes ostéogènes. Bilan après 5 ans chez 53 patients

L. Belli*, T. Palangie*, E. Garcia-Giralt*, V. Diéras*, V. Mosseri*, J.P. Bataini*, T. Dorval*, M. Jouve*, P. Beuzeboc*, S. Scholl*, A. Livartowski*, E. Courpied**, B. Tomeno** et P. Pouillard*

* *Institut Curie, 75231 Paris Cedex 05, France*
** *Hôpital Cochin, 75014 Paris, France*

RESUME

53 patients âgés de 14 à 59 ans (médiane 22 ans), porteurs d'un sarcome ostéogène des membres ont été traités selon deux protocoles différents. Les 23 patients de la 1ère étude (OS1) ont reçu avant traitement local 1 à 2 cycles de Vincristine (VCR), de Méthotrexate (MTX) à haute dose (7,5g/m2) et Acide Folinique appliqués à 10 jours d'intervalle. Le traitement local se limita à une irradiation exclusive (65 à 72gy) et la chimiothérapie est reprise par application de 6 à 8 cycles mensuels de VCR, MTX, Ac. Folinique et Adriamycine (ADM) 60mg/m2. Le 2ème groupe de 30 patients a reçu avant traitement local 1 à 2 cycles d'ADM (60mg/m2) et Cis-Platinum(100mg) soit par voie I.V. (10 cas) ou intra-artérielle (20 cas). Le traitement local a consisté en une irradiation exclusive (65 à 72 gy) pour 16 patients ; une chirurgie exclusive chez 6 patients, une association irradiation à 30gy et une chirurgie (8 cas). Aux décours, une chimiothérapie mensuelle a été reprise pendant 6 à 8 mois associant ADM, Cis-Platinum et Cyclophosphamide (700mg/m2).
Le taux de survie globale à 5 ans est de 53% et le taux de survie sans récidive de 30%. Ce taux relativement faible est lié à la grande fréquence des rechutes locales chez des patients n'ayant reçu qu'une irradiation pour tout traitement local (53% soit 21/39). Parmi les paramètres pronostiques étudiés, possèdent une signification pronostique significative :
- la taille radiologique de la tumeur ($p = 0{,}003$)
- l'envahissement des parties molles ($p = 0{,}005$)
- les taux sériques initiaux des phosphatases alcalines ($p = 0{,}001$)
  des LDH ($p = 0{,}0001$).

MOTS CLEF

Ostéosarcome, visée conservatrice, chimiothérapie première.

INTRODUCTION

Ce sont certainement les patients porteurs de sarcome ostéogène des membres qui ont le plus bénéficié des stratégies thérapeutiques incluant un programme de chimiothérapie de première intention appliqué avant la mise en oeuvre du traitement local. Le traitement précoce de la maladie métastatique générale a démontré son intérêt en même temps que les circonstances de réalisation du traitement local étaient simplifiées.

La mise en oeuvre d'une telle stratégie pose deux ordres de problèmes : l'un concerne la définition rationelle de la durée optimale d'application de la chimiothérapie avant tout traitement local et l'autre, la définition des paramètres pronostiques susceptibles d'influencer la qualité de la réponse objective au traitement et le pronostic à long terme (Delepine et coll., 1986) (Jaffe et coll., 1985) (Rosen et coll. 1983).

MATERIEL ET METHODES

D'avril 1977 à juillet 1985, 53 patients atteints d'un ostéosarcome des extrémités histologiquement prouvé et non métastasé ont été traités à l'Institut Curie par deux programmes thérapeutiques successifs à visée conservatrice, comportant une chimiothérapie première.
Il s'agit de 35 hommes et 18 femmes, d'âge moyen de 22 ans, avec des extrêmes allant de 14 à 59 ans.
La localisation la plus commune était le fémur (26 cas) suivi par le tibia (15 cas), l'humérus (9 cas), le péroné (2 cas) et le cubitus (1 cas).
Chez 24 patients, la taille radiologique était supérieure à 10cm, atteignant jusqu'à 28cm. 43 patients présentaient un envahissement des parties molles.
Au début du traitement, une scintigraphie osseuse au Technetium 99 a été effectuée chez 37 malades, et un test de captation du Strontium 85, évalué au 8ème jour, chez 42 patients. (tableau I).

Tableau I. Caractéristiques cliniques, radiologiques et isotopiques.
Nbr = 53 patients

AGE MOYEN : 22 ans (14 - 59)
SEXE : 35 ♂ + 18 ♀
SIEGE : 26 fémur
15 tibia
2 péroné
9 humérus
1 cubitus
DELAI DIAGNOSTIC MOYEN : 3 mois (1-9).

CARACTERISTIQUES RADIOL. ET ISOTOP.		Nbr
LONGUEUR	$<$ 7cm	9
	$<$ 10cm	18
	$>$ 10cm	24
CARACTERE	lytique	14
	condensant	12
	mixte	23
ENVAHISSEMENT PARTIES MOLLES	non	10
	douteux	2
	oui	41
REACTION PERIOSTEE	non	13
	douteuse	1
	oui	38
STRONTIUM 85*	$<$ 5	18
	$>$ 5	24
TECHNETIUM 99**	$<$ 5	17
	$>$ 5	20

* Rapport de l'intensité de fixation du Sr 85 au niveau tumoral J8/J1.
** Rapport de l'intensité de fixation du Tc 99 entre la zone tumorale et le point homologue contro-latéral.

Il y avait 7 cas de forme histologique bien différenciée, 11 cas de forme commune, 17 cas avec une composante chondrosarcomateuse, 4 étaient télangiectasiques et 11 anaplasiques.

TRAITEMENT

Les 23 patients ont reçu 1 à 2 cycles d'une association de Vincristine (VCR) 1,2mg/m2 et Méthotrexate 7,5 g/m2 (HD-MTX) suivi d'une administration d'Acide Folinique. Aux décours, un traitement local par irradiation exclusive à 65-72gy était appliqué en 7 semaines. Enfin, ce traitement terminé, 6 à 12 cycles mensuels de VCR, HD-MTX + acide Folinique et Adriamycine (ADM) 60mg/m2 ont été appliqués.
A partir de janvier 1981, le second groupe de 30 patients a reçu 1 à 2 cycles d'ADM 60mg/m2 et Cis-Platinum (DDP) 100mg/m2, administrés par voie intra-veineuse chez 10 d'entre-eux et intra-artérielle chez 20 d'entre-eux.
Parmi les 39 patients qui ont reçu comme traitement local une irradiation exclusive à 65-72 gy, 21 (54%) ont présenté une récidive locale ; en outre, 9 autres patients ont présenté des séquellestrophiques importantes, ayant nécessité chez 2 d'entre-eux une amputation. Une seule récidive locale a été observée chez les 9 patients traités par chirurgie conservatrice.
La signification pronostique de l'ensemble des paramètres cliniques, biologiques et radiologiques analysés est présentée sur le tableau II.

Tableau II : Paramètres pronostiques analysés.

PROTOCOLES OS 1 + OS 2 - nbr = 53

FACTEURS PRONOSTIQUES NON SIGNIFICATIFS ($p > 0,05$)

SURVIE		D.F.I.	
CLINIQUES	: Age Sexe Délai du diagnostic Douleur Impotence fonctionnelle	CLINIQUES	: Age Délai du diagnostic Impotence fonctionnelle
BIOLOGIQUE	: V.S.	BIOLOGIQUE	: V.S.
RADIOLOGIQUES	: Réaction périostée Caractère Technetium 99	RADIOLOGIQUES	: Réaction périostée Caractère Technetium 99
HISTOLOGIQUE	: Sous-groupe	HISTOLOGIQUE	: Sous-groupe

FACTEURS PRONOSTIQUES SIGNIFICATIFS

SURVIE			
FACTEURS	Nbr	DCD	p
BIOLOGIQUES			
PAL < 150	22	4	0,001
> 150	24	16	
LDH < 240	28	7	< 10
> 240	13	12	
RADIOLOGIQUES			
Longueur radiol. < 7cm	9		
< 10cm	18	6	0,003
> 10cm	24	16	
ENVAHISSEMENT PARTIES MOLLES Non	10		0,005
Oui	41	22	
Strontium 85 < 5	18	4	0,02
> 5	24	13	
HISTOLOGIQUES			
Grade nécrose après CT < 50%	5	5	0,01
> 50%	11	2	

D.F.I.			
FACTEURS	Nbr	RECHUTESS	p
BIOLOGIQUES			
PAL < 150	22	10	0,008
> 150	24	21	
LDH < 240	28	15	
> 240	13	12	
RADIOLOGIQUES			
Longueur radiol. < 7cm	9	2	
< 10cm	18	11	0,0006
> 10cm	24	22	
ENVAHISSEM. PART. MOLLES Non	10	4	0,05
Oui	41	30	
Strontium 85 < 5	18	9	0,01
> 5	24	20	
HISTOLOGIQUES			
Grade nécr. après CT < 50%	5	5	0,001
> 50%	11	4	
CLINIQUES			
SEXE ♂	35	19	0,03
♀	18	16	
DOULEUR Non	20	9	0,04
Oui	33	26	

Les paramètres qui influencent le plus significativement la survie sont les taux sériques initiaux de PAL et de LDH (avec des valeurs de p respectivement de 0,001 et de 0,0001), la taille radiologique de la tumeur en prenant comme limite une taille inférieure à 7cm, comprise entre 7 et 10cm ou supérieure à 10cm ($p = 0,003$), les signes radiologiques de l'envahissement des parties molles ($p = 0,005$) et le taux de nécrose tumorale ($p < 0,01$). Les 5 patients dont la nécrose était mineure inférieure à 50% sont tous décédés alors que dans le groupe des effets objectifs majeurs avec une nécrose supérieure à 50%, 2 patients sur 11 seulement sont décédés. (Figures 1, 2, 3, 4, 5 , 6, 7)

D'autres facteurs, tels que la VS, l'âge, le délai du diagnostic, la présence d'une réaction périostée, le caractère lytique ou condensant, la rapport de captation du Technetium 99 et le sous-groupe histologique, ne semblent pas significatifs ; le sexe féminin apparait comme facteur de mauvais pronostic seulement vis à vis de la survie sans récidive ($p = 0,03$).

Figure 1

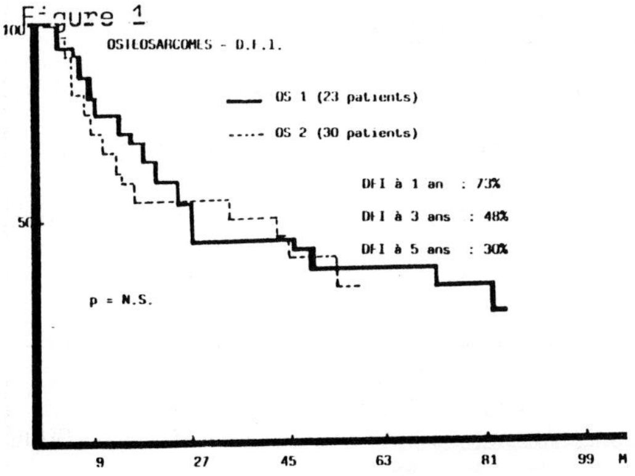

Figure 2

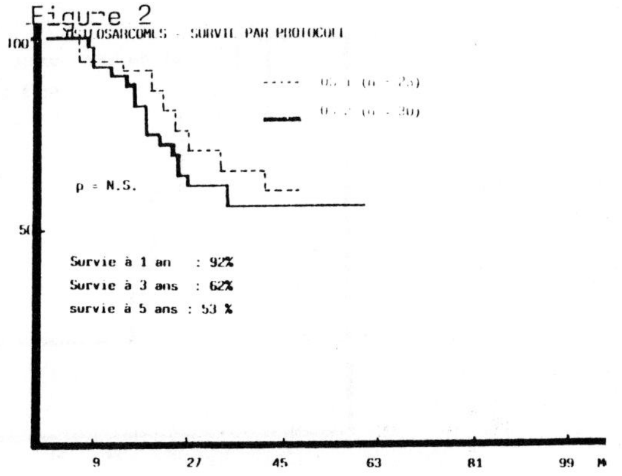

Figure 3

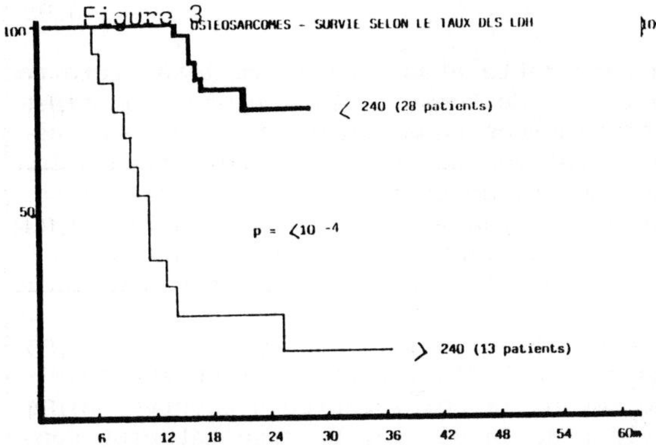

Figure 4

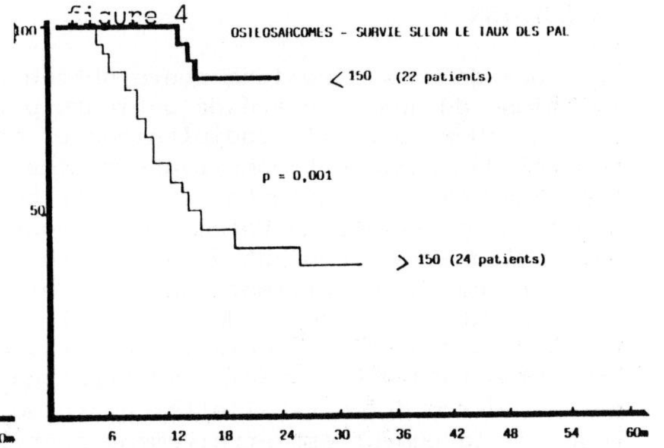

Figure 5

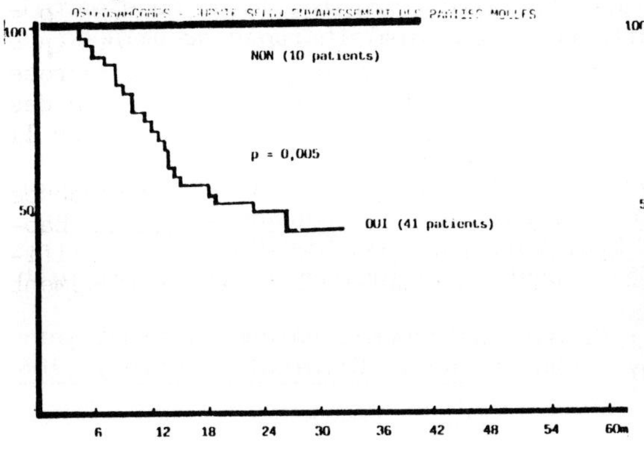

Figure 6

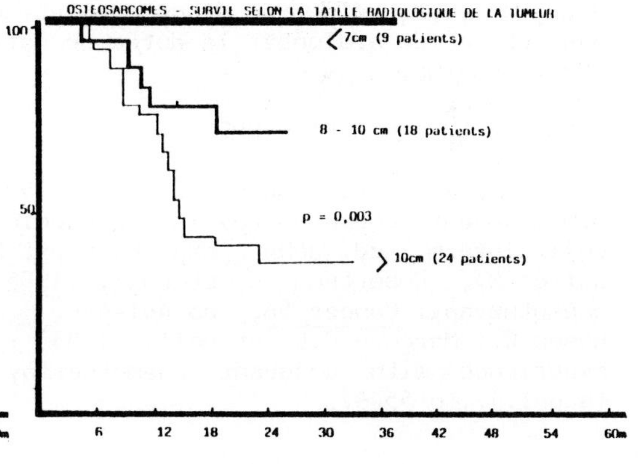

Figure 7

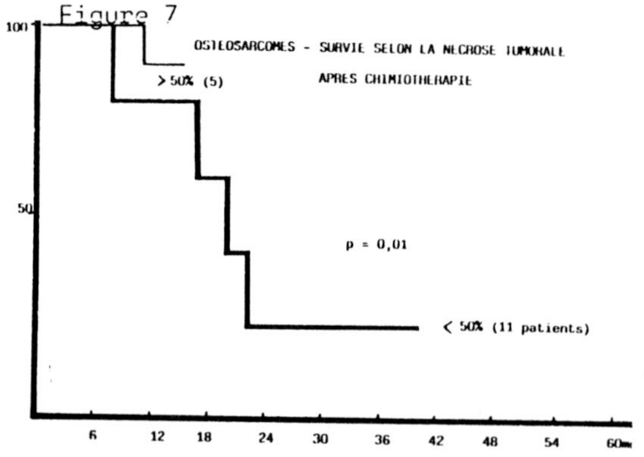

DISCUSSION

Le taux de survie au long cours obtenu dans cette étude doit être interprété en fonction du nombre élevé de patients porteurs de tumeurs volumineuses supérieures à 10cm de taille radiologique et considérées comme au-dessus de toute ressource de traitement conservateur. Les tentatives de traitement par irradiation exclusive dans ce contexte ne donnent que des résultats médiocres au prix de séquelles importantes. Parmi les 39 patients irradiés, nous observons 21 échecs carcinologiques locaux et 9 cas de troubles fonctionnels et trophiques graves.
Il est banal d'affirmer que l'administration d'un programme de chimiothérapie néoadjuvante de courte durée (1 à 2 mois dans cette étude) offre l'avantage de traiter au plus tôt la maladie métastatique infraclinique.
Les résultats obtenus ici démontrent qu'en dépit d'une stérilisation incomplète de la lésion primaire, l'effet histologique de la chimiothérapie observé au niveau de la tumeur est étroitement corrélé avec la survie. Ce résultat brut confirme l'hypothèse et laisse évoquer une efficacité cytotoxique comparable sur les micrométastases et le foyer tumoral organisé. Les études ultérieures ont tenté d'exploiter la signification pronostique de cette réponse initiale : les régimes de chimiothérapie plus intensifs et administrés en intra-artériel sont plus régulièrement actifs sur la tumeur principale. Cependant, avec l'objectif d'éviter toute sélection d'une population cellulaire tumorale, il ne nous parait pas utile de prolonger la durée de cette phase de chimiothérapie au-delà de la 10ème semaine.

REFERENCES BIBLIOGRAPHIQUES

Delepine N., Delepine G. et coll. (1986) : Evaluation of the optimal length of neo-adjuvant chemotherapy in osteogenic sarcoma. In "Neo-adjuvant chemotherapy" coll. Inserm., ed. John Libbey Eurotext Ltd, Vol. 137, pp 581-586.
Jaffe N., Robertson R. et coll. (1985) : Control of primary osteosarcoma with chemotherapy. Cancer 56, pp 461-466.
Rosen G., Marcove R.C. et coll. (1983) : Primary ostéogenic sarcoma : eight year experience with adjuvant chemotherapy. Cancer Res. Clinical Oncology 106 (suppl.), pp 55-67.

Résumé

53 young adult patients with osteogenic bone sarcomas were treated according 2 programs of treatment.
In the 1st assay, 23 patients were given 1 to 2 courses of Vincristine, High dose Methotrexate (HD MTX) (7,5g/m2) and folinic acid as rescue, at 10 days of interval. Local treatment included only radiotherapy (65 to 72 gy in 7 weeks)

and then the patients returned to chemotherapy for 6 to 8 monthly courses combinng VCR, HD MTX, Fol. acid rescue and Adriamycin (ADM) (60mg/m2). In the 2nd assay, 30 patients were given 1 to 2 courses of ADM (60mg/m2) and Cis-platinum (Cis-DDP) (100mg/m2) either by intra-veinous (10 cases) or intra-arterial (20 cases). The local treatment included exclusive radiotherapy in 16 patients, radical surgery in 6 cases, association of radiotherapy at 30gy and surgery in 8 cases. After local treatment, 6 to 8 monthly courses were given including ADM, Cis-DDP and Cyclophosphamide (CPM) (700mg/m2).
The overall survival at 5 years iss 53% and the disease free survival is 30% and related to an high percentage of local relapse in patients whom local treatment was only radiotherapy ((21/39).
Among the parameters of prognosis of significant value, appear :
- the radiological size of the tumor ($p = 0,003$),
- the radiological signs of softt tisssue involvement ($p = 0,005$),
- the initial seric level of alkaline phosphatase ($p = 0,001$)
  and LDH ($p = 0,0001$),
- the histological grading of response to cytotoxic drugs ($p = 0,01$).

Neo-Adjuvant Chemotherapy. Ed. Cl. Jacquillat, M. Weil, D. Khayat. Colloque INSERM/John Libbey Eurotext Ltd. © 1988. Vol. 169, pp. 529-534.

Pre-operative chemotherapy in patients with osteosarcoma. A follow up

H.P. Honegger, M.D. Cserhati, A. Von Hochstetter, P. Grosscurth and G.U. Exner

University Hospital Zürich, Section of Oncology, Institut of Pathology, Section of Cell biology and Clinic for Orthopedics and Triemli Hospital Zürich, Switzerland

SUMMARY

30 patients with osteosarcoma (OSA) underwent preoperative chemotherapy (CT) with the T7, T10, T12 regimen of Rosen or the German COSS protocol. Preoperative CT was well tolerated. Histologic examination of resected specimens after preoperative CT revealed extensive necrosis in 57 % of our patients. Extensive necrosis was associated with a longer relapse free (DFS) and over all survival (OS)compared to patients with tumors with lesser or no histologic changes (p=0,002; p=0,08 resp.). 8 of 27 patients with extremity OSA were amputated (29 %), 19 (71 %) underwent a limb salvage procedure (LSP). OS and DFS was longer for limb salvage procedures than for amputations (p=0,02; p=0,01 resp.). Local recurrences were seen in 26 % after LSP. The incidence of lung metastases after amputations was 88 % and 21 % after LSP.

KEY WORDS

Osteosarcomas, preoperative chemotherapy, limb sparing surgery.

INTRODUCTION

Preoperative chemotherapy was introduced into the management of osteosarcomas in order to destroy micrometastases as early as possible, it allowed an evaluation of the tumor under therapy and histologic examination as an assessment of the effect of therapy (Benjamin 1984, Rosen 1984). Additional CT is later given in an adjuvant fashion.
In Zürich preoperative CT for osteosarcoma OSA was started in 1979, in 1981 we embarked on a multidisciplinary program for these tumors, some data have been published earlier (Cserhati 1984; Honegger 1983, 1986), the actual report provides a longer follow up and includes new patients up to november 1987.

MATERIAL AND METHODS

From 1979 to 1987, 30 patients with histologically confirmed OSA were consecutively admitted to the study, regardless of age and location of the primary tumor. 27 were located at extremities as shown in table 1, one was found in the pelvic area, 2 patients were treated preoperatively for lung metastases, their primaries had been treated with surgery only. As usual, the initial work up consisted of bone scans, CT's of lungs and primary, abdominal ultrasound and hematologic and blood chemistry studies. There were 20 males and 10 females, median age 18 years.

Table 1: Characteristics of patient population

	Total	group A	group B
Patients	30	13	17
median age	18	20	17
male:female	20:10	7:6	13:4
Site of primary			
femur	15	5	10
tibia/fibula	7	2	5
humerus	5	3	2
pelvis	1	1	--
lung (mets)	2	2	--
Therapy			
T7	9	6	3
T10	6	1	5
T12	12	4	8
COSS	3	2	1

Intravenous preoperative CT was applied according the T7, T10 or T12 protocols of Rosen, (Rosen 1976, 1979, 1982), the CT proposed by COSS followed those guidelines (Winkler 1984). High dose methotrexate was given with hydration, alcalinisation of the urine and citrovorum factor rescue. Serum levels of methotrexate were measured at 24 and 48 houres. Ifosfamide (Holoxan) was followed by mesna in usual dosage.
Morphologic assessment of necrosis was performed as described earlier (Honegger 1984). Our patient population was divided into 2 groups, depending on the amount of necrosis after CT in the resected specimen. Group A consisted of cases where predominantly viable tumor covered more than 50 % of the cross-sectional surface area. In group B, on the other hand, the devitalised areas made up more than 50 % of the surface area. CT was completed after surgery and patients were followed in out patient clinics.

Disease free (DFS) and over all survival (OS) were calculated from the date of resection after preoperative CT until november 1987. Survival curves are plotted according the Kaplan and Meier (Kaplan 1952). Statistical analysis was carried out by the log rank test (Peto 1977).

RESULTS

1. Findings after intravenous preoperative chemotherapy

2/3 of our patients experienced shrinking of the primary tumor, in 3/4 the intensity of bone pain decreased. Metastases did not develop during preoperative CT. Preoperative CT was generally well tolerated, significant hematologic or renal toxicities did not occur. 1 of 30 patients (3,3 %) died early in the postopera-tive phase, he was tumorfree at autopsy, his death could not be attributed to his earlier chemotherapy. 17 of the OSA population (17/30=57 %) or 17 of 27 patients with extremity OSA (= 63 %) showed over 50 % necrotic areas in the resected specimens. A high amount of necrosis was noted more often after T10 (5 of 6) and T12 (8 of 12) than after T7 (3 of 9). 10 of 15 patients (66 %) with OSA of the femur, 5 of 7 (71 %) with OSA of tibia/fibula and 2 of 5 (40 %) of humerus OSA belonged to group B.

2. Surgical technique

In 2 patients lung metastases were removed, the patient with a pelvic OSA underwent an attempt to resect the primary. Of 27 patients with extremity OSA, 8 (29 %) had an amputation; the 19 limb sparing procedures (LSP) consisted of 5 rotation osteo-plasties (26 %), 7 tumor bone prostheses (37 %), 4 resections plus arthrodeses (21 %) and 3 tumor resections (16 %).
Of group A with OSA of the extremities, 4 of 10 patients (40 %) were amputated, wereas only 4 of 17 of group B (24 %). LSP were carried out in 60 % of group A patients and in 76 % of group B patients. Reasons for amputations were on one hand locally advanced tumors (with extensions into the soft tissue parts); on the other hand, several tumors in the knee area had to be amputated, for anatomical circumstances precluded a LSP.

Figure 1:

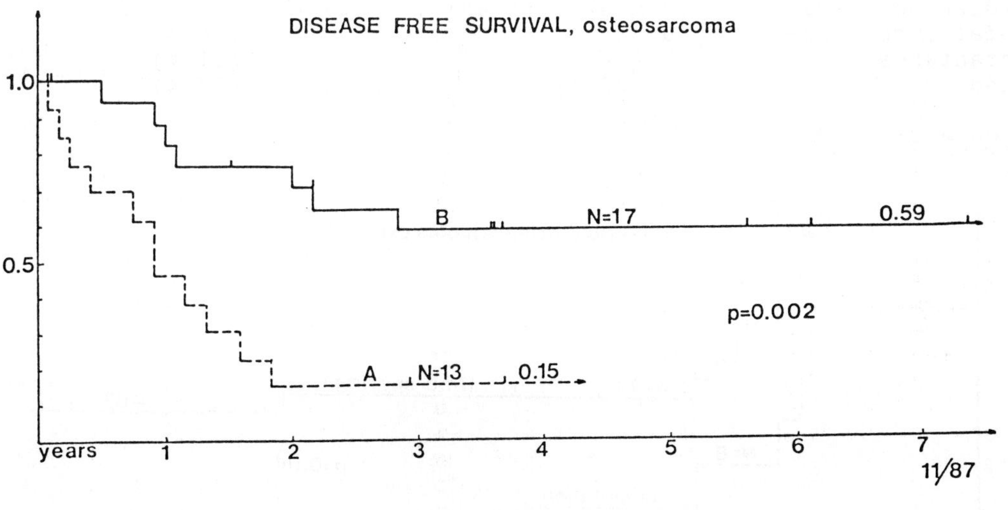

3. Follow up

Median observation time for 30 patients with OSA is 28 months (range 1-89 months) and 27 months for patients with extremity OSA. Analysis for DFS and OS of the total group gave significant differences between patients of group A and B. DFS and OS was longer for group B patients than for group A (p=0,002 and 0,08 resp.) (Fig. 1). If the case of the patient that died early after the operation without tumor is withdrawn, the difference in survival between the 2 groups is significant at the p=0.045 level. Age below 20 years was associated with a significantly better survival than older (p=0,003); male do worse than female patients regarding OS (p=0,12).

4. Course of patients with extremity osteosarcomas

DFS and OS was better for group B than for group A (p=0,01; p=0,29 resp.). Again, if the early postoperative death is discarded, OS is significantly better at the p=0,045 level. If patients with amputations are compared to those with LSP, DFS and OS favor the limb sparing procedures significantly (p=0,015, p=0,04 resp.) (Fig. 2). 8 patients after amputations were observed for a median time of 23 months (range 5-48 months), no local recurrences were noted, but 7 of 8 (88 %) developped lung metastases and 6 of 8 (75 %) are dead. 19 patients with LSP had a median observation time of 27 months (range 1 to 89 months), in this group 5 (26 %) local recurrences were discovered, as well as lung metastases in 4 patients (21 %). 7 of these 19 patients (37 %) have. It is interesting, that local recurrences were observed in 3 of 6 patients (50 %) of group A and only in 2 of 13 (16 %) of group B patients after LSP, (p=0,10, Chi square test) (table 2).

Table 2: Course of extremity OSA

	amputation	limb salv. procedures
number	8	19
median obs.time	23 months (5-48)	27 months (1-89)
local recurrence	0	5 (26 %)
metastases	7 (88 %)	4 (21 %)
died	6 (75 %)	7 (37 %)

Figure 2:

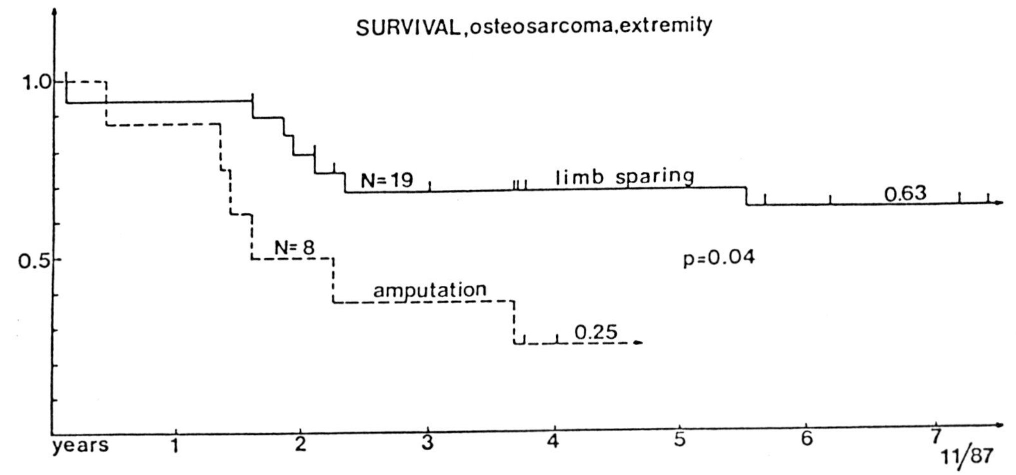

DISCUSSION

Our follow up analysis of 30 patients with OSA confirmes that assessment of necrosis in tumors after preoperative CT represents a reliable prognostic factor. DFS and OS are significantly longer for group B patients (defined as over 50 % necrosis in the primary tumor) in the whole patient group as well as for extremity OSA. In our hands, a limb salvage procedure in extremity OSA is not associated with an adverse risk despite the fact, that 26 % had local recurrences. On the contrary, patients who underwent limb salvage procedures have a significantly better DFS and OS than those after amputations. This is certainly due to a selection bias, since amputees had in our series locally more advanced tumors and less favorable response to preoperative CT. Our series illustrates, that a more radical procedure (amputation) is not able to improve the result, despite maximal resection, these patients develop lung metastases and die earlier and more often than those with a more favorable response after CT and lesser surgery. Our series is small it can not judge the value of adjuvant CT, which is now recommended for extremity OSA (Link, 1986). The impact of the preoperative chemotherapy remains an open question, it will hopefuly be answered after completion and analysis of the ongoing randomised study in the USA addressing that problem (Link 1987).

REFERENCES

Benjamin RS, Chawla SP, Murray JA: Preoperative Chemotherapy for osteosarcoma. A treatment approach facilitating limb salvage with major prognostic implications. In: Adjuvant Therapy of Cancer IV (Jones S, Salomon S eds) p. 601 (1984) (Grune and Stratton)

Cserhati M, Honegger HP, von Hochstetter A: Zürich bone sarcoma study. Concepts of the clinical, morphological and functional study. Verlag Dtsch. Krebs Gesellschaft, Band 4, (1984), Beitrag 4/27, Verlag Karger, Basel

Honegger HP, Cserhati M, von Hochstetter A: Zürcher Erfahrungen mit präoperativem, hochdosiertem Methotrexat bei Osteosarkomen, Schweiz. med. Wschr. 113, 663, 1983.

Honegger HP, Cserhati MC, von Hochstetter A, Grosscurth P, Exner GU. Experience with preoperative high dose methotrexate containing chemotherapy in patients with osteosarcoma. In Neo-adjuvant chemotherapy, Collegue, INSERM/John Libbey Eurotext, Ltd. Vol 137, 573, 1986.

Kaplan EL, Meier P: Nonparametric estimation from incomplete observations. J. Amer. statist. Ass. 53, 457 (1958)

Link M, Goorin A, Miser A et al. The effect of adjuvant chemotherapy on relapse free survival in patients with osteosarcoma of the extremity. N. Engl. J. Med. 314, 1600, 1986.

Link M, personal communication, october 1987 at Sarcoma Meeting in Florida, USA

Peto R, Pike M, Armitage P: Design and analysis of randomized clinical trials requiring prolonged observation of each patient. Analysis and examples. Brit. J. Cancer 35, 1 (1977)

Rosen G, Murphy ML, Huvos AG: Chemotherapy, en bloc resection and prosthetic bone replacement in the treatment of osteogenic sarcoma. Cancer (Philad) 37, 1, (1976)

Rosen G, Marcove R, Caparros B: Primary osteogenic sarcoma. The rational for preoperative chemotherapy and delayed surgery. Cancer (Philad) 43, 2163 (1979)

Rosen G, Caparros B, Huvos AG: Preoperative chemotherapy for osteogenic sarcoma. Cancer (Philad) 49, 1221 (1982)

Rosen G, Nirenberg A: Chemotherapy for primary osteogenic sarcoma. Ten year evolution, and current status of preoperative chemotherapy. In: Adjuvant Therapy of Cancer IV (Jares S, Salomon S eds) p. 593, (1984) (Grune and Stratton)

Winkler K, Beron G, Kotz R: Neoadjuvant chemotherapy for osteogenic sarcoma. Results of a cooperative German/Austrian study. J. clin. onc. 2, 617, (1984)

Address of first author: PD Dr. med. HP. Honegger, Leiter Med. Onkolog. Dienst, Stadtspital Triemli, 8063 Zürich

Neo-Adjuvant Chemotherapy. Ed. Cl. Jacquillat, M. Weil, D. Khayat. Colloque INSERM/John Libbey Eurotext Ltd. © 1988. Vol. 169, pp. 535-539.

Osteosarcoma. Why is T10's Rosen protocol reproducible or not ? High values of short length of neo-adjuvant chemotherapy, of methotrexate pharmacokinetics, of salvage chemotherapy by ifosfamide-platine-pirarubicine for bad responders

N. Delepine[1,2], G. Delepine[2,3], J.C. Desbois[1], H. Cornille[1,2], C. Jasmin[2], A. Astier[4] and G. Mathé[2]

[1] *Unité d'Oncologie Pédiatrique-Service de Pédiatrie Générale (Pr. Desbois). Hôpital Hérold-Robert Debré, 49 Bld Sérurier, 75019 Paris, France*
[2] *ICIG-SMST, Hôpital Paul Brousse, 14 avenue Paul-Vaillant-Couturier, 94800 Villejuif, France*
[3] *Unité d'Orthopédie Oncologique, Clinique du Pré-Gentil, 93110 Rosny, France*
[4] *Service de Toxicologie, Hôpital Henri Mondor, 94010 Créteil, France*

ABSTRACT

In order to reproduct T10's results, we started in 1984 a pilot study. On 27 evaluable patients, DFS is 91 % at 15 months and actuarial event free survival 83 % at 33 months. The major factors of good results seem us to be :
- 1° individual adaptation of HDMTX dosage to obtain the minimal effective serum level : 1000 micromol/l ;
- 2° short lenght of neoadjuvant chemotherapy (inferior to one month) ;
- 3° early rescue of bad responders by IFOSFAMIDE-PLATINE-PIRARUBICINE;
- 4° adequacy of surgery avoiding local relapses ;

KEYWORDS

Osteogenic osteosarcoma, neoadjuvant chemotherapy.
Methotrexate pharmacokinetics, ifosfamide, platine, pirarubicine.
Limb-salvage surgery.

INTRODUCTION

Till 1979, Rosen's results in the treatment of high grade osteosarcomas are promising. His long term results confirm the first datas : 65 % (17/26) for the T4, 91 % (30/33) for the T7, 84 % (71/85) for the T10, 84 % (37/44) for the T12, of the patients are alive with no evidence of disease (ANED). The median follow up of the entire group of 208 patients is 70 months. Excluding 20 documented local recurrences 155/188 patients (82 %) are alive and free of disease at over a 6-1/2 year median time.
Despite these encouraging results, doubtness about them data always plane and many authors think that T10 is not reproductible and EORTC osteosarcoma group wrote in Madrid in November 1987 in ECCO4 : "HD methotrexate : useful or not ? is the remaining question !
In 1984, we decided to treat our patients by a modified T10. We present here our preliminary results and the considerations about them.

PATIENTS

From 1984 to 1987, 27 non previously treated non metastatic patients with high grade limb osteosarcomas received modified T10. There were 18 males, 9 girls aged from 6 to 27 (average 16,5). Locations were 3 fibulas, 1 humerus, 7 tibias, 15 inferior femurs, 1 upper femur.

METHODS

Biopsy was performed as soon as possible after CT scan or NMR and histologic result obtained in less than 24 hours in most cases.
Neoadjuvant chemotherapy began immediately after biopsy and diagnosis, by 3 (or 4) weekly high dose methotrexate.
First course was adapted to age. Teenagers received 12 g/m2 (as children) because growth was not yet totally terminated, even only on plate bones, and hormonal changes are probably still important at this period of life.
In any case, methotrexate dose was adapted to individual pharmacokinetics after the first course and this study confirmed the necessity to consider teenagers as children on this plane, because we have had to increase MTX dose, but never to decrease.
Methotrexate was infused in six hours after a six hours prehydratation infusion (half 14 % sodium bicarbonate, half 5 % dextrose with K+ Cl-, with a total of 750 cc fluid sqm in 6 hours). Perfusion was stopped immediately after end of MTX, and hydratation was performed per os to obtain a minimal diuresis of 1,6 l/sqm at the first day and 2 l/sqm the next 3 days. Alcalinisation was performed as usually to maintain urine pH > 8 and folinic acid rescue began at the 20th hour following the beginning of the MTX infusion, at the habitual dose of 15 mg/m2 every six hours, at least ten times.

MTX pharmacokinetics permitted to study the toxicity of MTX and relation between efficacy at maximum level at the end of the infusion. We choose, as Rosen suggests it, to require a pic level of 1000 micromol minimum at the end of the sixth hour (end of infusion). When this level was not obtained at the first course (with 12 g/sqm in young < 21, and 8 g/sqm > 21) we increased at the second course, the dose of MTX from 2 g/sqm and so one, at the following course if necessary. In fact, we obtain fast always the choosed level, early from the second course.
We performed three courses of HDMTX, and if possible the fourth : in the absence of important headaches (frequent in young children), of hepatic renal or hematologic disturbances.
Surgery was performed the fourth or fifth day following the last course of HDMTX to avoid dead time and possibilities of multiplication of residual tumors cells. In this serie, limb salvage surgery was always performed. Secondary amputation was necessary in two cases of infection prosthesis (by skin infection in two tibia locations). No local recurrence was observed till now.

Perioperative chemotherapy began the next day following surgery as the state of the patient permitted it. Nevertheless, all patients received BCD (Bleomycin 15 mg/sqm J1-J2, Cyclophosphamide 600 mg/sqm J1-J2, Actinomycin D 600 microg/sqm J1-J2) in the three days following operation. Vomiting and nausea were a little more important than usually but chemotherapy was feasible and seems us important pointing out the "dormant cells" which could be in in cycle only a few days after surgery.

Post operative chemotherapy began fifteen days after BCD, by two weekly HDMTX followed by THP-ADR 30 mg/m2 x 3, and fifteen days later (or three weeks function of hematologic normalisation) by two weekly HD-MTX + BCD.
At the fifteenth week of chemotherapy, we distinguished good and bad respondors. Good respondors (more than 95 % of dead or very altered cells and efficacy estimated on digital angiography, NMR, and/or CT scan received four cycles of chemotherapy (each two HD-MTX + BCD or THP-ADR (alternated).
Bad responders received four cycles of two HD-MTX + IPA a week later (IFOSFAMIDE 3 g/sqm J1-J2, CDDP 120 mg/sqm - J3, THP-ADR 35 mg/sqm - J3) three weeks rest between two cycles.

RESULTS

Among 27 patients, we noted 9 bad responders and 16 good responders. In February 1988, overall survival in remission is 25/27 (91 %), 24 in first CR (89 %), 1 in 2nd CR 1 year after thoracotomy, 2 died inmetastatic disease at 24 and 30 months. They were two of the first patients of this serie and they only received initially 8 g/m2 because age > 17.
Furthermore pharmacokinetics and her application was no so good established before June of 1986.
Actuarial event free survival (EFS) is 89 % at 15 months, 83 % at 33 Months.

DISCUSSION

Are Rosen's results reproductible or not ? The answer is of most importance. If not, multicentric randomized studies with and without HD-MTX are useful. If Rosen's results can be confirmed, such studies are non ethical.
Our data supports Rosen's results. Other studies don't We will now try to explain why, about some examples :

Edmondson and Green (1984) didn't find any efficacy of HD-MTX on their 19 patients compared to 19 others without HD-MTX. But this study used too low dose (7,5 g/m2), without reference to age or seric level, and with a too large intervall (3 weeks).

The scandinavian Sarcoma group (1987) tried to reproduce T10. But MTX dosage was only 8 grammes/sqm up 8 years, dosage that doesn't give in our experience an effective MTX serum level. That explains that good responders were only 18 % and continuously disease free survival 66 %.

A large cooperative study was started in France in Lyon and Villejuif. Results confirm the good prognosis of good responders but fail in rescuing bad responders.
But in these 2 studies, HD-MTX ignore individual pharmacokinetics (so that minimal efficacy pic should not be always obtained in young patient and adolescent) and preoperative chemotherapy was fast always too long (12 weeks).
We demonstrated in earlier study with ADR-CDDP that long neoadjuvant chemotherapy is dangerous in bad responders.Another bad prognostic factor in Lyon's study seems to be the high rate of local reccurence (10 %) after conservative surgery.
Up to date, we didn't find any example of study with weekly HD-MTX with pharmacokinetics monitoring of efficacy plasma level > 1000 micromol/l in a short <1 month) neoadjuvant chemotherapy and early rescue for bad responders, that fails.

CONCLUSION

Our data supports Rosen's results. The most important factors in reproducing T10 sems to be :

1° Appropriate serum level of MTX controlled by pharmacokinetics.

2° Short lenght of neoadjuvant chemotherapy ;

3° Early rescue of bad responders by I.P.A. ;

4° Adequacy of limb salvage surgery obtained by enough experimented surgeon (at least one en bloc resection per month).

REFERENCES BIBLIOGRAPHIQUES

Blondet R, Brunat-Mentigny M, Rebattu P., Moyen B. (1987) : Results of combined chemo-surgical therapy in 46 osteosarcomas without metastasis in Consensus Meeting on Osteosarcoma, istituto orthopedico Rizzoli. Bologno - April 9th - 10th.

Delepine N., Trifaud A., Jasmin C., Favre R., Brun B., Delepine G., Tubiano-Hulin M., Kerbrot P., Dionet C., Lucas P. (1986) Chimiotherapie de l'ostéosarcome par l'association Adriamycine-Cisplatinum. Risques de la chimiothérapie néoadjuvante lorsque insuffisamment efficace. Bulletin du Cancer, 73, 3, 288-293

Delepine N., Delepine G., Trifaud A, Voisin MC, Mazabrand A., Jasmin C (1986) : Evaluation of the optimal length of neoadjuvant chemotherapy in osteogenic osteosarcoma. In Néoadjuvant chemotherapy. Colloque Inserm/John Libbey Eurotext Ltd. Vol. 137, 581-586.

Edmonson JH, Green SJ, Ivins JC, Gilchrist GS, Creagan ET, Pritchard DJ, Smithson WA, Dahlin DC, Taylor WF (1984) : A controlled pilot study of high-dose methotrexate as post surgical adjuvant treatment for primary osteosarcoma. J. Clin. Oncol. 2 (3), 152-6

Kalifa C, Dubousset J, Contesso G, Varuel D, Lumbroso R (1987) : Experience of T10 protocol in the treatment of osteosarcomas April 1981-July 1986. In Consensus Meeting on Osteosarcoma, istituto ortopedico Rizzoli. Bologna April 9th-10th.

Rosen G., Marcove RC, Caparros B and al (1979) : Primary osteogenic sarcoma. The rationale for preoperative chemiotherapy and delayed surgery. Cancer, 43, 2163-2177

The Scandinavian Sarcoma Group by p; solheim (1987) Adjuvant chemotherapy in patients with osteosarcoma preliminary results Proceedings, 899, ECCO4 - Madrid

Résumé

Depuis 1984, les auteurs ont traité 27 malades évaluables atteints d'ostéosarcome ostéogénique des membres non métastatique. En Février 1988, le taux actuariel de rémission complète est de 83 % à 33 mois, confirmant les résultats de Rosen T10.

L'analyse comparative d'autres séries récentes de résultats moins satisfaisants souligne la valeur pronostique majeure des facteurs suivants :

1° Individualisation des doses de méthotrexate afin d'obtenir le pic minimal d'efficacité (> 1000 micromol/l)

2° Chimiothérapie preopératoire courte (< 1 mois), strictement hebdomadaire

3° Introduction précoce del'association Ifosfamide-Platine-Pirarubicine dans le traitement des répondeurs insuffisants

4° En cas de chirurgie conservatrice, expérience suffisante du chirurgien afin d'éviter, au maximum, les récidives locales.

Neo-Adjuvant Chemotherapy. Ed. Cl. Jacquillat, M. Weil, D. Khayat. Colloque INSERM/John Libbey Eurotext Ltd. © 1988. Vol. 169, pp. 541-544.

Surgical implications of neo-adjuvant chemotherapy : the experience at the Istituto ortopedico Rizzoli in osteosarcoma (OS) and malignant fibrous histiocytoma (MFH)

F. Gherlinzoni, M. Mercuri, M. Avella, R. Casadei, R. de Cristofaro, A. Ferruzzi, A. Ferraro, R. Capanna and M. Campanacci

Bone Tumor Center, Istituto ortopedico Rizzoli, Via Pupilli 1, 40136 Bologna, Italy

ABSTRACT

215 cases of OS and 12 cases of MFH of bone treated between 1983 and 1987 are described. All patients (pts) were given preoperative chemotherapy with methotrexate (MTX) and cisplatinum (CDP) and postoperative chemotherapy with MTX, adriamycin (ADM), CDP and bleomycin (BCD).

The results are compared with a group of pts who were treated only with postoperative adjuvant chemotherapy or who were treated only with surgery.

Infection was the most frequent complication.

KEYWORDS: Neoadjuvant chemotherapy, osteosarcoma, malignant fibrous histiocytoma, complications.

INTRODUCTION

In the beginning of the eighties, after the introduction of neoadjuvant chemotherapy (NAC) the tendency to perform limb salvage procedures instead of amputations has dramatically increased. The vast indications to perform conservative surgery represent a major progress in the treatment of malignant bone tumors, but increase the complication rate.

In this paper surgical advantages and complications of NAC in pts with OS and MFH are considered. Amputations were required in 21% of the cases and conservative surgery was feasible in 79%. This high rate of limb salvage procedures is due not only to NAC, but also to a different approach surgeons have regarding the feasibility of performing conservative surgery. This has also become possible using the new imaging techniques such as CT scan and NMR.

SUBJECTS AND METHODS

From 1983 to July 1987 at the Bone Tumor Center of the Istituto Ortopedico Rizzoli in Bologna 227 pts previously treated by NAC were operated: in 215 of these pts the histological diagnosis was OS and in 12 was MFH; all tumors were located in the extremities. 122 pts were males and 105 females ranging in age from 3 to 56 years.

Preoperative chemotherapy was given with two different protocols: the first, used from 1983 to 1985 comprised of two cycles of MTX i.v. randomized for high and low doses (750 mg/m^2 in 45-60 minutes versus 7.500 mg/m^2 in 6 hrs). The rescue with Citrovorum factor was performed in both cases 24 hours after the beginning of MTX infusion. Six days after each MTX infusion 120-150 mg/m^2 of CDP i.a. were given in 72 hours. Surgery was performed 6 to 7 weeks after biopsy. The second protocol activated from 1986 comprised of two cycles of MTX high doses (7.500 mg/m^2 in 6 hrs) and ADM (45 mg/m^2 for 2 days) i.v. and 2 cycles of CDP (120-150 mg/m^2 in 72 hrs) i.a. Surgery was performed 8 to 9 weeks after biopsy. Amongst the 227 pts., 178 (79%) had limb salvage surgery while only 49 (21%) had demolitive surgery. Following surgery, necrosis induced by preop chemotherapy was rated: "good" for necrosis > or = 90%, "fair" for necrosis between 60 and 90% and "poor" for necrosis <60%.

RESULTS

The postop complications observed in the 227 pts treated with NAC were analyzed. The surgical complications in our series were divided into minor and major. Moreover, 15 mechanical failures of prosthetic devices were observed, but these complications will not be considered as they are not directly related to NAC. 18% of our pts had one or more minor complication, such as transient nerve palsy, delayed wound healing not requiring plastic surgery or haematomas treated by suction. These complications did not compromise the biological and mechanical outcome of surgery. 14% of our pts had one or more major complication: 1 pt died due to postoperative pulmonary embolism and 3 permanent nerve palsies were observed. These complications were probably not related to NAC. Severe delayed wound healing and infections may be considered directly related to immunosuppression induced by chemotherapy. Infection was observed in 26 (11%) pts: 3 cases (6%) following amputations and 23 (13%) following limb salvage procedures. In this last group the infection was treated by surgical debridement and drainage in 9 cases and removal of implants in 6 cases, whereas 8 pts required a secondary amputation to be cured. Therefore, infection represents the most important and frequent complication in our series.

DISCUSSION

NAC produces many advantages in the treatment of OS not only in terms of disease-free pts but also on the clinical and histological response of the tumors. Regarding clinical symptoms NAC in almost all pts induced a decrease of pain, swelling and edema; in many cases after preop chemotherapy also tumor size decreased. The most surprising impact of NAC is seen in the radiological response of the tumor: following preop chemotherapy, ossification of the mass is sometimes evident, with reduction in size, but especially the periphery of the tumor is better defined with respect of the peritumoral adjacent tissues. The so called "reactive zone" around the tumor often is better demarked and calcified and this allows a better definition of the following surgical margins to be achieved. Angiograms demonstrate a reduced vascularization of the tumor. The better definition of the margins of the tumor is especially useful in planning conservative surgery to exclude neurovascular bundle involvement. NMR is the most recent technique used to define and identify healthy and tumor tissues. Particularly, NMR is useful to define the extension of the tumor in the medullary canal and to precisely assess a possible involvement of nerves and vessels. NMR may also be used to evaluate the necrosis induced in the tumor by preop chemotherapy before surgery, but to this aim MR spectroscopy seems to give better results.

As previously mentioned, infection is the major complication of this treatment. The high rate of infection in limb salvage surgery led us to review our infection rate in the three surgical techniques most frequently used at our Institution for resection and reconstruction in bone tumors. The infection rate in pts treated without chemotherapy, with adjuvant chemotherapy and with NAC was considered. We evaluated the infection rate in three surgical procedures: 1) in distal femur and/or proximal tibia resections and reconstructions with Kotz prosthesis, 2) in proximal humerus resections and reconstructions with modular cemented prosthesis and 3) in pts treated with distal femur or proximal tibia resection and reconstruction with temporary arthrodesis with a Kuntscher rod and a spacer of cement or polyethylene. This difference is present but not statistically significant.

CONCLUSIONS

After the introduction of NAC the use of limb salvage surgery was dramatically increased; NAC allows a better definition of the anatomical margins of the tumor, evident on the pathological specimen analysis and on the radiological studies. The evaluation of necrosis induced by preoperative chemotherapy allows a modification of the postoperative chemotherapy courses according to the rate of necrosis, since it is already proven that the tumor responce to preoperative chemotherapy is statistically correlated to prognosis. We can conclude that NAC presents few local and surgical complications. A higher infection rate seems to be the only major complication enhanced by this treatment.

These results, the number of "good" responders and the continuously disease-free patients convinces us to continue to further improve this treatment.

Table I

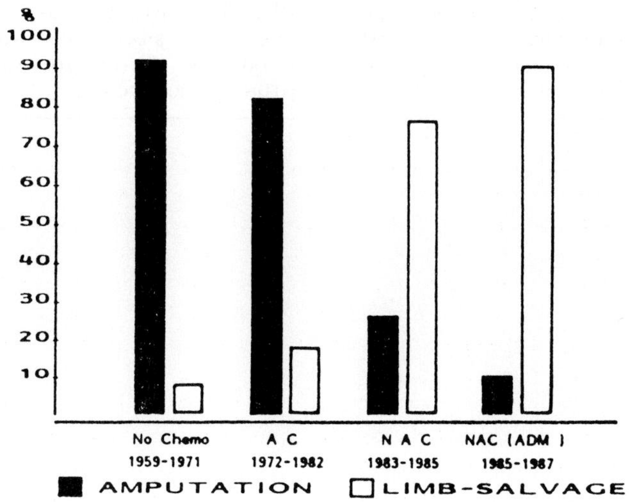

Table II

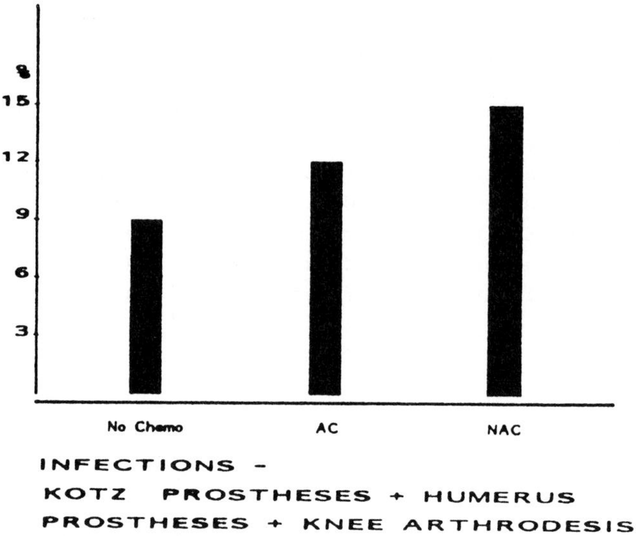

Supported in part by a grant from the Italian National Research Council, Special Project "Oncology" N° 87.02810.44, and by a grant from Regione Emilia-Romagna, law N° 1970 of May 13th, 1986.

Résumé

215 cas d'ostéosarcomes et 12 cas d'histiosarcomes fibreux malins des os ont été traités entre 1983 et 1987. Tous les malades ont reçu une chimiothérapie pré-opératoire avec Méthotrexate et Cis.Platyl. Une chimiothérapie post-opératoire par Méthotrexate-Adriamycine-Cis.Platyl et Bléomycine.
Les résultats obtenus sont comparés avec un groupe de malades traité seulement avec chimiothérapie adjuvante ou par chirurgie exclusive. Les infections ont été les complications les plus fréquentes.

Neo-Adjuvant Chemotherapy. Ed. Cl. Jacquillat, M. Weil, D. Khayat. Colloque INSERM/John Libbey Eurotext Ltd. © 1988. Vol. 169, pp. 545-554.

Comparison of two protocols of treatment of Ewing's sarcoma : the respective roles of monobloc resection, post-operative radiotherapy and of intensification and diversification of post-operative chemotherapy

N. Delepine[1], G. Delepine[2], J.C. Desbois[1], H. Cornille[1], P. Touzet[3], M. Housset[4], N. Tubiana-Hulin[5], M.C. Voisin[6], A. Trifaud[7], G. Mathé[2] and C. Jasmin[2]

[1]*Hôpital Hérold-Robert Debré, 49 Bld Serurier, 75019 Paris, France.*
[2]*Hôpital Paul Brousse, 14 avenue Paul-Vaillant-Couturier, 94800 Villejuif, France.*
[3]*Hôpital Enfants Malades, 149-161 rue de Sèvres, 75730 Paris Cedex 15, France*
[4]*Hôpital Necker, 149-161 rue de Sèvres, 75730 Paris Cedex 15, France*
[5]*Centre René Huguenin, 5 rue Gaston Latouche, 92210 St Cloud, France.*
[6]*Hôpital Henri Mondor, 51 avenue du Maréchal de Lattre de Tassigny, 94010 Créteil, France*
[7]*Hôpital de la Conception, Marseille, France*

Between 1982 and 1987, thirty-five patients with Ewing's sarcoma patients were treated with two consecutive protocols SE_4 and SE_5. In both protocols, preoperative chemotherapy consisted of cycles of 150mg/m^2/day cyclophosphamide for 7 days and 35mg/m^2 THP-adriamycin on day 8 every 15 days (CYTHA) followed by surgical and histological evaluation for tumor necrosis after 6 and 3 cycles of CYTHA respectively.

Post-operative radiotherapy and 6 supplementary cycles of CYTHA were given to all patients. In the SE_5 protocol, monobloc resection of the tumor was performed in all but two pelvic tumors and post-operative radiotherapy omitted for good histological responders defined as having complete tumor necrosis or only a few isolated viable tumor cells. Surgery was followed by peri-operative iphosphamide-Messna (3g/m^2/day on days 2 and 3 post-operatively). In good histological responders, CYTHA was alternated with V/VA = Vincristine/Vincristine-Actinomycin D (2mg/m^2). In bad histological responders, PIA, a combination of 120mg/m^2 cisplatin, 3g/m^2/day x 2days iphosphamide and 45mg/m^2 THP-adriamycin was alternated with CYTHA and V/VA.

Actual disease-free and overall survival at 2 years are 33% and 76% for SE_4 and SE_5 respectively. A comparison of the SE_4 and SE_5 protocols shows that despite the high efficacy, in histologic terms of CYTHA as preoperative chemotherapy, a more intensive and diversified postoperative chemotherapy is necessary to salvage a significant proportion of both good and bad histological responders. Postoperative radiotherapy is probably not required after monobloc resection for good histological responders. Our results confirm that chemotherapy alone can cure some patients and that the final outcome of Ewing's sarcoma mainly depends on the efficacy of post operative adjuvant chemotherapy which should alternate combinations of drugs known to be active on Ewing's sarcoma.

MOTS CLEFS

Sarcome d'Ewing, résection monobloc, radiothérapie, chimiothérapie intensive et diversifiée.

KEY WORDS

Ewing's sarcoma, monobloc resection, radiotherapy, intensive and diversified chemotherapy.

INTRODUCTION

The treatment of Ewing's sarcoma remains controversial. Indeed, there is a lack of consensus concerning indications and treatment modalities of the primary tumor. Although, it is generally stated that Ewing's sarcoma is a radiosensitive tumor which can be sterilized locally in 86% of cases by doses of 45 to 65 Gy applied over large fields (Perez and al, 1977), most authors now agree that only distal lesions have a low rate of local recurrence after radiotherapy. For other tumor localizations (axial skeleton and proximal tumors), rates of local relapse can be as high as 35% after radiotherapy (Pilepich and al, 1981) (Bacci and al, 1985) (Tepper and al, 1980). It is possible that with the increase in the duration of survival observed with adjuvant chemotherapy, local relapses now have a higher chance of being detected, whereas previously rapid death occured due to early metastasis. Indeed, an autopsy study has demonstrated the high incidence (65%) of clinically-undetected local relapses in Ewing's sarcoma patients (Telles and al, 1978).

In 1978, Rosen et al. (1978) recommended the use of conservative surgery followed by radiotherapy to increase local control. Pritchard et al. (1981) have also underlined the interest of surgical treatment in Ewing's sarcoma.

Adjuvant chemotherapy remains the major factor in curing Ewing's sarcoma. However, there are many schemes of treatment which differ in the types of drugs and their modality of use, i.e. sequential or semi-continuous chemotherapy, sequential use of single drugs or combination chemotherapy and the length of treatment (Rosen and al, 1981) (Nesbit and al, 1981).

We report here the results of two consecutive trials - SE_4 and SE_5-that we have conducted since 1982 in patients with Ewing's sarcoma. The SE_4 protocol was based on the results of Hayes et al (1983). These authors reported the high efficacy (assessed by surgical and histological evaluation of tumor necrosis) of a simple chemotherapeutic scheme based on tumor cell recruitment with moderate doses of cyclophosphamide and adriamycine, administered sequentially every two weeks.

In the SE_4 protocol, the effectiveness of chemotherapy was also evaluated surgically but since postoperative radiotherapy was used as the main locoregional treatment, monobloc resection of the tumor was not mandatory. Furthermore, the same chemotherapeutic regimen was used post-operatively in order to study the correlation between the respective chemosensitivity of the primary tumor and of the micrometastatic disease, a crucial point for the design of adjuvant chemotherapy for Ewing's sarcoma and one which has not been yet elucidated.

The early occurrence of a high rate of local and systemic relapses despite the high histologically-proven great efficacy of the preoperative chemotherapy prompted us to change our protocol of treatment.

In the SE_5 protocol, we used the same preoperative chemotherapy but introduced a systematic monobloc resection of the primary tumor followed by a more intensive and diversified peri- and post-operative chemotherapy. Since we also postulate that both the local control and the final outcome of the disease depend mainly on the efficacy of the chemotherapy, locoregional radiotherapy was limited to bad histological responders.

The comparison of SE_4 and SE_5 indeed suggests that intensive and diversified chemotherapy can salvage a significant proportion of Ewing's sarcoma patients. Monobloc resection of the primary tumor can be performed in most if not all patients and provides satisfactory functional results and local control.

PATIENTS AND METHODS

From 1982 to 1987, 35 consecutive untreated patients with histological diagnosis of Ewing's sarcoma were registered and included in our protocols. Sixteen patients were included in protocol SE_4 between 1982 and 1984 and nineteen patients in protocol SE_5 between 1985 and 1987. Table 1 shows the characteristics of patients included in each protocol : age and tumor site were comparable in both groups. Three patients presented with distant metastases in the SE_5 protocol group against 1 in the SE_4 group. There were more male patients in the SE_5 group.

Table 1 : Patient characteristics

Characteristics	Group 1 (SE_4)	Group 2 (SE_5)
Number of patients	16	19
Metastatic	1	3
Male/Female	11/5	10/9
Median age (range)	17 (6-27)	17 (6-27)
Localization of tumors :		
Pelvis	2	3
Sacrum	1	1
Vertebra	1	2
Rib	1	2
Femur	7	9
Tibia	2	0
Fibula	1	2
Humerus	1	0

Table 2 gives the schemes of protocols SE_4 and SE_5. In the SE_4 protocol, 150 mg/m^2/day cyclophosphamide was administered IV or orally within 2 days after biopsy for 7 consecutive days, followed on day 8 by 35 mg/m^2 THP-Adriamycin (IV), a less cardiotoxic anthracycline as efficient as adriamycin (Mathé and al, 1988). This sequence (CYTHA) was repeated six times every 15 days. In order to obtain a histological evaluation of tumor necrosis after the initial chemotherapy, the tumor was surgically removed (simple exeresis or complete resection). Tumor regression was considered as good (GHR) when there were only a few isolated viable tumor cells in the specimen or none at all. All other cases (small islands or larger zones of viable tumor cells) were classified as bad histological regressions (BHR).

Table 2 : Schemes of SE_4 and SE_5 protocols

	SE_4	SE_5
Preoperative treatment	Biopsy → CγTHA x 6 → Surgery	Biopsy → CγTHA x3 → Surgery + perioperative IPM.
Post-operative treatment		
Good histological response	CγTHA x 6 + Radiotherapy 35 Gy	CγTHA x 3 V/VA x 6 CγTHA x 6
Incomplete histological response	CγTHA x 6 + Radiotherapy 45-50 Gy for central lesions, 60 Gy on distal lesions	IPA x 3 V/VA x 6 IPA/CγTHA x 3 + Radiotherapy 35gy.

CγTHA Days 1 to 7 Cyclophosphamide 150 mg/m^2/day
Day 8 THP-adriamycin 35 mg/m^2

V/VA : Weekly alternance of vincristine (VCR) 2 mg/m^2 ($\leqslant$2mg) and of VCR 2 mg/m^2 ($\leqslant$2 mg) + Actinomycin D 2 mg/m^2

IPM Iphosphamide 3 g/m^2 x 2 days on days 2 and 3 after surgery + Messna 3 g/m^2 in three injections

IPA IPA 3 g/m^2 + Messna 3 g/m^2 days 1 and 2.
Cisplatin 120 mg/m^2 with forced diuresis. THP-ADM 45 mg/m^2 every 4 weeks.

Every 3 weeks after surgery, the patients received 6 cycles of CYTHA. The loco-regional treatment was completed by an irradiation of the site of the primary tumor and a large field encompassing the entire affected bone, followed in the case of extremity lesions by an additional 10-15 Gy to a radiation field limited to the initial tumor area. Thirty Gy was given in case of good histological regression and 60 Gy for distal lesions or 45-50 Gy on central lesions if the necrosis was histologically incomplete (BHR).

In protocol SE_5, only 3 cycles of CYTHA were given before surgery which consisted a monobloc resection whenever possible. Perioperative IV iphosphamide (IPM) was used : ($3g/m^2$/day for 2 days with an equivalent IV dose of Messna ($1g/m^2$ every 8 hours).

In the case of GHR, CYTHA was alternated with V/VA : a weekly alternance for 6 weeks of vincristine 2 mg/m^2 (maximum dose 2 mg) and a combination of 2 mg/m^2 vincristine with 2 mg/m^2 actinomycin D (maximum dose 2 mg) given IV on the same day.

In the case of BHR, a third combination of drugs (IPA) consisting of 3 g/m^2 IPM on days 1 and 2 with messna 3 g/m^2 on the same days followed on day 3 by 120 mg/m^2 Cisplatin with hydratation and forced diuresis and 45 mg/m^2 THP-adriamycin. IPA was repeated every 4 weeks. The whole chemotherapeutic scheme for BHR was : IPA x 3 followed by 6 cycles of V/VA and 3 alternated cycles of IPA and CYTHA. There was no dose adaptation : when there were less than 1500 polys/mm^3 and/or less than 100,000 platelets/mm^3, the treatment was delayed until recovery. A 35-45 Gy irradiation was always given at the end of chemotherapy in the case of BHR and was used in some early SE_5 patients even in the case of GHR.

C.T. scans of the primary tumor and the lungs, bone scintigraphy, blood counts, creatininemia, were mandatory for the inclusion of the patients as well as a confirmed diagnosis of Ewing's sarcoma. All radiologic investigations and bone scintigraphy examinations were repeated every three months. Blood counts, creatininemia, ECG and, if required, echocardiography and/or cardiac scintigraphy were repeated before each cycle of chemotherapy.

RESULTS.

Figure 1 shows that the overall survival (OS) and disease-free survival (DFS) at 2 years in the SE_4 protocol (33%) was highly inferior to the SE_5 protocol (76%). Although the mean follow up of SE_5 patients is still too short to give an exact evaluation of the curative potential of this protocol, it is clear that we can expect a very significant improvement in DFS with SE_5 compared to SE_4.

Table 3 shows the high rates (over 50%) of good histological responses obtained with both protocols. There is no difference between SE_4 and SE_5 although preoperative chemotherapy consisted of 6 cycles of CYTHA in SE_4 and only 3 cycles in SE_5 and despite the fact that more monobloc resections were performed in SE_5 patients. It should be mentioned that CYTHA has a remarkable immediate clinical effect with a rapid disappearance of local pain, and a noticeable and often complete regression of the palpable soft tissue tumor in the case of distal lesions.

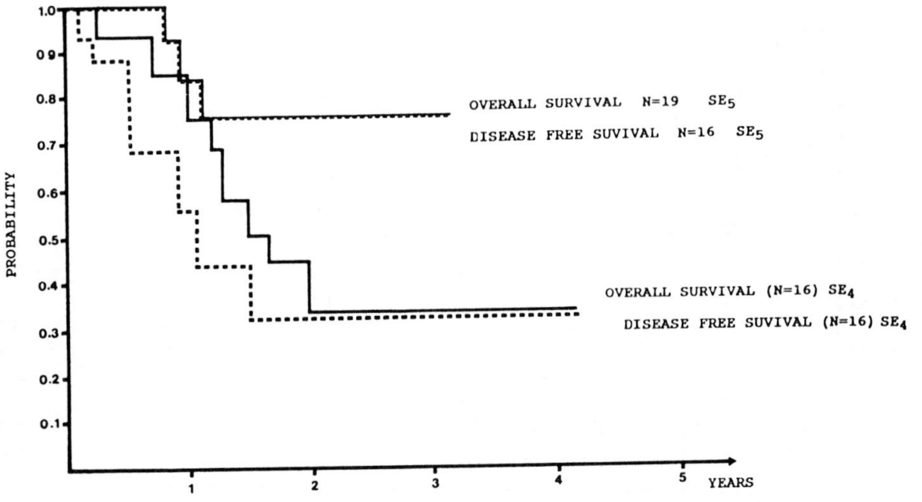

Figure 1 : Overall survival (OS) and disease-free survival (DFS) of Ewing's sarcoma patients treated with protocols SE_4 and SE_5.

Table 3 : Treatment failures of SE_4 and SE_5 protocols

	SE_4	SE_5
Initial local relapses	4/16	2/19
Distant metastases	6/16	3/19

As shown in Figure 2, the histological response was highly predictive of the overall and disease-free survival. It is worthy of note that all the bad responders in protocol SE_4 relapsed within 2 years. The comparison of the results of SE_4 and SE_5 suggests that the diversification and intensification of the chemotherapy (mainly for bad responders but also for good responders) is responsible for this improvement. Monobloc resection also seems to have played a role (Figure 3).

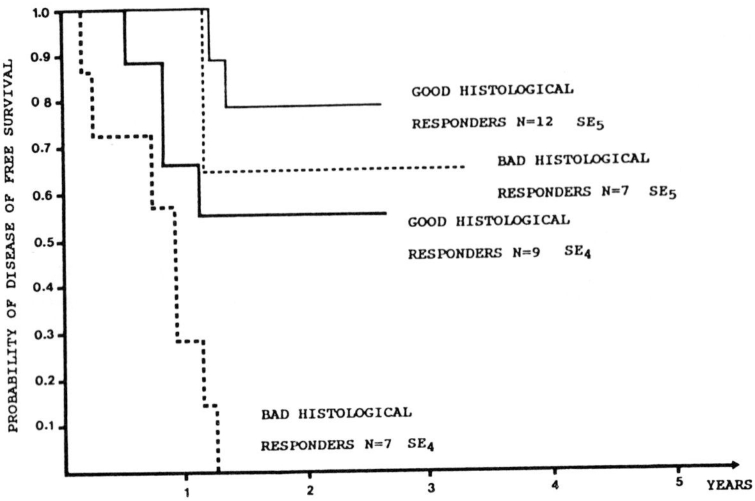

Figure 2 : Probability of disease-free survival of Ewing's sarcoma patients according to the histological response.

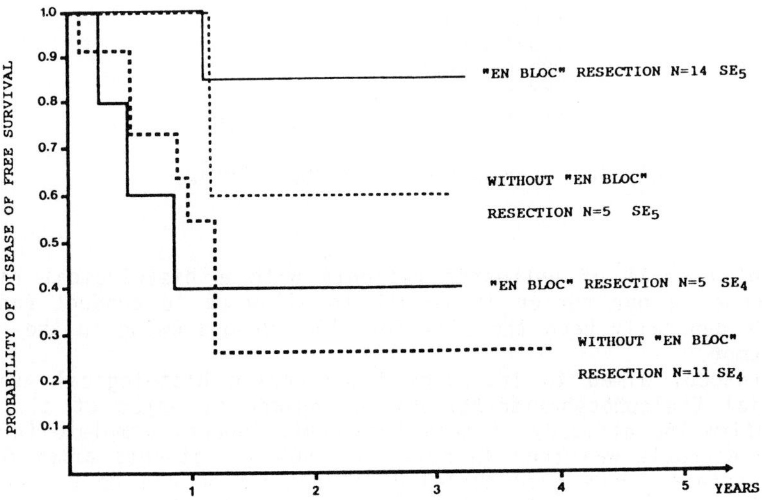

Figure 3 : Probability of disease-free survival of Ewing's sarcoma patients according to the type of surgical treatment.

The sites of relapse are given in Table 3 which shows the low incidence of isolated loco-regional recurrence ; it is noteworthy that of the three local recurrences observed with the SE_5 protocol, one occurred in a fibula lesion after a monobloc resection followed by a 45 Gy local irradiation ; the two others were seen in two pelvic lesions which were treated with a marginal resection followed by a 45 Gy irradiation. The third pelvic lesion in which a monobloc resection was performed has not recurred after 2 years.

Finally, as shown in Table 4, the overall tolerance of the chemotherapy was acceptable. The toxicity of protocol SE_4 was minimal (only grade 1 and 2) with no delay in chemotherapy. Preoperative toxicity was almost absent from protocol SE_5. SE_5 patients experienced 30% grade 3 hematological toxicity during the post-operative chemotherapy, mainly observed after PIA, causing a mean delay of one week for the subsequent cycle of chemotherapy. Alopecia was universal. Severe nausea and vomiting was attributable to IPA in 90% of SE_5 patients. One SE_5 patient experienced a grade 4 cardiotoxicity.

Table 4 : Main toxic effects of SE_5 protocol

	SE_5*
Hematological toxicity	30% Grade 3
Alopecia	100% Grade 3
Cardiotoxicity	1 patient Grade 4
Hemorragic cystitis	20% Grade 2
Nausea-Vomiting	90% Grade 2 and 3
Gastralgia	30% Grade 2

* Only during post-operative chemotherapy.

DISCUSSION.

The rate of accrual of untreated patients with a histological diagnosis of Ewing's sarcoma in our center is to low to allow us to conduct randomized trials. This has generally been the case for other groups owing to the relative rarity of the tumor.

The SE_4 protocol aimed to introduce a systematic histological evaluation of the sequential Cyclophosphamide-Adriamycin regimen of Hayes et al. (1983). Our results confirm the efficacy of this treatment. Indeed, complete (or almost complete) tumor necrosis was seen in more than 50% of patients after 6 cycles of CYTHA. This rate of very good histological regression can be compared with the best published results of other chemotherapy regimens. The results of protocol SE_5 showed that 3 cycles could induce the same rate of tumor necrosis, indicating that prolonging preoperative chemotherapy is not necessary (and may be harmful) as we have previously shown in the case of osteosarcoma (Delepine and al, 1986).

The disappointing results of protocol SE_4, suggesting that a good histological response indicates neither a complete local cure nor efficacy on micrometastases, prompted us to change our strategy. As shown in Table 3, we performed significantly more "en bloc" tumor resections in the SE_5 protocol. Although we cannot state that "en bloc" resection offers a therapeutic advantage over a simple resection followed by radiotherapy, from our preliminary results in patients treated by "en bloc" resection, supplementary radiotherapy does not appear necessary for good histological responders. In fact, the only local recurrence of a distal lesion in SE_5 patients was seen after a monobloc resection followed by a 45 Gy irradiation.

Radiotherapy was added for in SE_5 patients with incomplete histological regression ; in effect, Bacci et al (1985) have suggested that even incomplete surgical resection followed by radiotherapy is more effective than radiotherapy alone. In our opinion, only "en bloc" resection, not incomplete or marginal resection, is able to improve significantly the rate of local cure but this hypothesis remains to be proven.

Finally, the large difference in disease survival and survival between SE_4 and SE_5 patients shows the necessity of agressive post-operative chemotherapy combining several active drugs in alternating combinations.

Indeed, the comparison of SE_4 and SE_5 disease-free and overall survival at two years for bad histological responders also suggests that intensive chemotherapy with various drug combinations such as PIA can salvage these patients as is the case for other chemo-curable cancers (e.g. testicular cancer). Even in GHR, the addition of V/VA and, possibly, perioperative IPM improved the DFS and OS.

Our preliminary SE_5 results are comparable with the best published results. The 76% actuarial DFS and OS obtained at 2 years is clearly superior to SE_4 and to our previous results (Lemevel and al, 1980). A longer follow-up is required to determine whether perioperative chemotherapy can reduce the rate of late metastases, a phenomenon more frequently seen in patients with Ewing's sarcoma, since the introduction of intensive chemotherapy and the subsequent significant decrease in early deaths due to early metastases. The persisting complete remission of the three primary metastatic patients may indicate that chemotherapy alone can cure some patients with complete tumor necrosis ; "en bloc" resection or, if this is not feasible, intensive radiotherapy are necessary for good (but not complete) and bad histological responders although it is not proven that they have additive beneficial effects. Most probably, local control and disease-free survival both depend on the efficacy of adjuvant chemotherapy. Further progress in the treatment of Ewing's sarcoma can therefore only stem from the early recognition of chemoresistant tumor stem cells and the use of therapy capable of overcoming this resistance.

REFERENCES.

Bacci, G. and coll. (1985) : Localized Ewing's sarcoma of bone : Ten years experience at the istituto ortopedico Rizzoli in 124 cases treated with multimodal therapy. Eur. J. Clin. Oncol. 23, 165-175.

Delepine, N. and coll. (1986) : Evaluation of the optimal lenght of neo-adjuvant chemotherapy in osteogenic osteosarcoma in neo-adjuvant chemotherapy, first international Congress, edited by Jacquillat C, Weil M and Khayat D, published by Editions INSERM and John Libbey Eurotext. 581-586.

Hayes, F.A. and coll. (1983) : The response of Ewing's sarcoma to sequential Cyclophosphamid and Adriamycin induction therapy. Cancer. 27, 1051-1054.

Lemevel, V. and coll. (1980) : Treatment of Ewing's sarcoma by radiotherapy and adjuvant chemotherapy : results at 3 and 5 years. La Nouvelle Presse Med. 9, 359-362.

Mathé, G. and coll. (1988) : Minimal cardiotoxicity of THP-Adriamycin (Pirarubicin) in hamster and in cancer patients. Its greater cardiac tolerance than that of other anthracyclins. In press.

Nesbit, M.E. and coll. (1981) : Multimodal therapy for the management of primary non-metastatic Ewing's sarcoma of bone : an intergroup study. Natl. Cancer Inst. Monogr. 56, 255-262.

Perez, C.A. and coll. (1977) : Analysis of local tumor control in Ewing's sarcoma : preliminary results of a cooperative intergroup study. Cancer. 40, 2864-2873.

Pilepich, M.V. and coll. (1981) : Radiotherapy and combination chemotherapy in advanced Ewing's sarcoma. Intergroup study, Cancer. 47, 1930-1936.

Pritchard, D.J. (1981) : Surgical experience in the management of Ewing's sarcoma of bone. Natl. Cancer Inst. Monogr. 56, 169-171.

Rosen, G. and coll. (1978) : Curability of Ewing's sarcoma and consideration for future therapeutic trials. Cancer. 41, 888-899.

Rosen, G. and coll. (1981) : Ewing's sarcoma. Ten years experience with adjuvant chemotherapy. Cancer. 47, 2204-2213.

Telles, N.C. and coll. (1978) : Ewing's sarcoma. Autopsy study cancer. 41, 2321-2329.

Tepper, J. and coll. (1980) : Local control of Ewing's sarcoma of the bone with radiotherapy and combination chemotherapy. Cancer. 46, 1969-1973.

Acknowledgments : We wish to acknowledge the excellent secretarial assistance of Mrs N. Balliet and J. Couvrat-Desvergnes. This work was supported by the Fondation Daher.

Résumé

Trente cinq patients atteints de sarcome d'Ewing ont été traités entre 1982 et 1986 par deux protocoles consécutifs SE_4 et SE_5. La chimiothérapie préopératoire associant cyclophosphamide (150 mg/m^2/jour x 7 jours) et THP adriamycine 35 mg/m^2 au jour 8 (CYTHA) tous les 15 jours pendant 3 (SE_5) ou 6 (SE_4) cycles. L'intervention - résection simple ou monobloc - permettait l'évaluation histologique de la réponse tumorale.

Dans le protocole SE_4, l'intervention étant suivie de 6 cycles de CYTHA associés à une radiothérapie loco-régionale de 35 Gy chez les bons répondeurs (quelques cellules tumorales résiduelles isolées ou plus de cellules viables) ou 60 Gy chez les mauvais répondeurs (autres cas). Dans le protocole SE_5 tous les patients recevant de l'Iphosphamide (3g/m^2/j x 2 jours) péri-opératoire et CYTHA + Vincristine/Vincristine-Actinomycine D (V/VA) pour les bons répondeurs ou une alternance de CYTHA, V/VA et PIA (Cisplatine, Iphosphamide et THP-adriamycine). La radiothérapie complémentaire était réservée aux mauvais répondeurs.

La survie sans récidive et la survie globale à 2 ans sont de 33% pour SE_4 et 76% pour SE_5. Nos résultats confirment l'efficacité de CYTHA et l'inutilité de prolonger la chimiothérapie préopératoire plus de 3 cycles (ou 6 semaines) 2) la place réduite de la radiothérapie réservée à la résection non-monobloc 3) le rôle majeur d'une chimiothérapie postopératoire intensive et diversifiée.

Neo-Adjuvant Chemotherapy. Ed. Cl. Jacquillat, M. Weil, D. Khayat. Colloque INSERM/John Libbey Eurotext Ltd. © 1988. Vol. 169, pp. 555-560.

Neo-adjuvant chemotherapy for Ewing's sarcoma

J. Graham-Pole, R. Marcus, D. Springfield, W. Donnelly, G. Elfenbein, W. Enneking, J. Fort, T. Gillespy, S. Gross, N. Mendenhall, S. Spanier and R. Vander Griend

University of Florida, Departments of Pediatrics, Therapeutic and Diagnostic Radiology, Orthopedics, Pathology and Medicine, Box J-296, JHMHC, 1600 SW Archer Road, Gainesville, Florida, 32610, USA

ABSTRACT

Adjuvant chemotherapy (ACT) has significantly increased disease-free survival (DFS) in patients with Ewing's sarcoma. Recent trials of neoadjuvant chemotherapy (NCT) have tried to further improve this outcome, and also to modify treatment of the primary lesion. We have shown retrospectively that primary tumor size is the single most important prognostic factor, and designed three protocols incorporating NCT, with delayed and modified local irradiation (LRT), intensifying treatment for patients with higher risk of relapse. The latter have received shorter-course, more intensive NCT/ACT, with 'end-intensification' using myelo-ablative therapy supported by autologous marrow infusions.

Our results indicate that short very intensive treatment is effective in high-risk patients, with a projected 70% DFS in 19 patients on our most intensive regimen. This compares with 73% projected DFS in 14 'standard-risk' patients receiving less intensive NCT plus ACT and delayed LRT or surgery. Our other high-risk regimen produced poor (10%) DFS in 10 patients, attributable either to inadequate intensity of NCT/ACT, or to excessive delay of LRT, or to the wrong choice of end-intensification. Large-scale randomized studies will resolve these questions.

KEY WORDS

Ewing's sarcoma, Neoadjuvant, Adjuvant, Chemotherapy, Irradiation

INTRODUCTION

The introduction of adjuvant chemotherapy (ACT) 20 years ago produced gratifying improvements in outcome for patients with Ewing's sarcoma (ES) (Hustu, 1968; Rosen, 1974). Most reported 40%-50% DFS, compared with historical data of 10%-20% DFS with surgery or LRT alone. In the last decade, however, progress has slowed, and major questions remain about optimal therapy, both for the primary lesion and for micrometastases. What is the best way to achieve local eradication with acceptable morbidity? Can LRT be modified, and is there a major role for surgery? What options are available for intensifying systemic therapy? Is the increased risk justifiable? Can a staging system be developed that will help in individual treatment planning?

In 1982, we analyzed a retrospective in the outcome of patients with biopsy-proven ES treated at the University of Florida (UF), since 1966, to give us baseline data for prospective studies to address the above questions. Our plans were: (1) to institute NCT, and delay LRT, with the aim of attacking micrometastases as soon as possible; (2) to reduce local morbidity from concurrent LRT and intensive chemotherapy; (3) to define those patients at highest risk of relapse, on whom to test more intensive NCT plus. This is a preliminary report of our progress to date.

PATIENTS AND METHODS

The patients in our retrospective survey (Marcus, 1984) had all received LRT immediately after diagnosis plus ACT, using combinations of vincristine and cyclophosphamide, with or without dactinomycin, and/or doxorubicin. We correlated DFS with multiple factors, including age, sex, primary site, primary size, presence of metastases, and intensity of ACT.

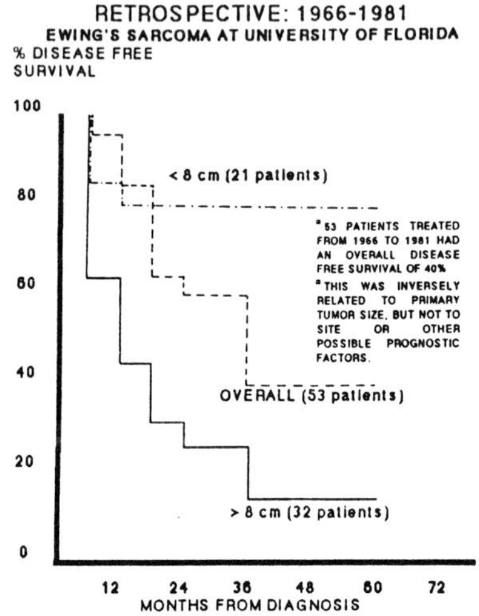

Fig. 1. Effect of Tumor Size on DFS: Retrospective Survey

Figure 1 shows that the only factor correlating significantly with DFS is size of the primary lesion. This held up for both pelvic and non-pelvic lesions, showing that site was not an independent prognostic factor. Since others have made similar observations of the prognostic importance of tumor size (Jurgens, 1988), we adopted a clinical staging system for our prospective studies of NCT, delayed LRT, and standard or intensified ACT, patients with a maximal diameter $\leq$ 8 cm pms, patients with metastases being placed in a 'standard-risk' (SR) group and those with larger primaries in a 'high-risk' (HR) group.

Figure 2 and Table 1 show the treatment regimens for patients with ES since Feb. 1982. The SR and first HR regimen (HR-1) consisted of NCT for 12 weeks, followed by LRT week 12-18. LRT was identical in all three protocols. The initial field was the primary lesion plus a 4 cm margin, which received 3600 cGy at 120 cGy twice a day, usually including the whole bone in HR patients. A 1440-2400 cGy boost was given to the residual mass at the start of LRT plus a 2 cm margin also at 120 cGy twice daily, to a total of 5040-6000 cGy. Metastases were treated with 1000-1500 cGy. Patients with expendable bones and those under 10 years were considered for surgery. ACT was continued until week 54 in the SR and week 40 in the HR-1 group. The latter underwent 'end-intensification' therapy, in the form of a myelo-ablative dose of melphalan (Graham-Pole, 1984), with reinfusion of cryopreserved marrow (ABMT). Because the results in HR patients remained unfavorable, we adopted HR-2 in Jan. 1985, making 3 modifications to HR-1, based on a recently developed NCI Pediatric Oncology Branch protocol (Miser, 1987). (a) We shortened and intensified the NCT phase, starting LRT at 6 weeks; (b) we shortened and intensified the ACT phase, finishing at about 18 weeks post-diagnosis; (c) we changed the end-intensification to total body irradiation (TBI) plus further intensive chemotherapy.

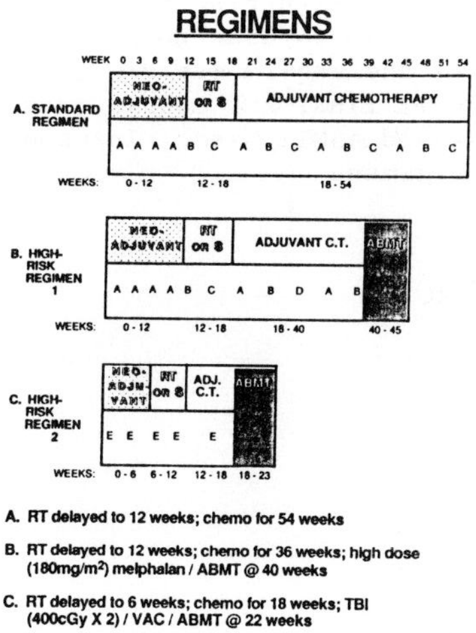

Fig. 2. Standard & High-risk Treatment Regimens

Table 1. Code to Treatment Regimens

CODE TO REGIMENS

A. Cyclophosphamide 150mg/m ^{2} po days 1-7.
Doxorubicin 35 mg/m ^{2} I.v. day 8.

B. Cyclophosphamide 150mg/m ^{2} po days 1-7.
Dactinomycin 1.5mg/m ^{2} I.v. day 8.

C. Vincristine 1.5mg/m ^{2} I.v. (max 2.0mg) days 1, 8, 15.
Doxorubicin 50mg/m ^{2} I.v. day 2.
Cyclophosphamide 1000mg/m ^{2} I.v. day 2.

D. Vincristine 1.5mg/m ^{2} I.v. (max 2.0mg) days 1, 8, 15.
Doxorubicin 75mg/m ^{2} I.v. day 2.
Cyclophosphamide 1000mg/m ^{2} I.v. day 2.

E. (cycle 1-2) Vincristine 2.0mg/m ^{2} I.v. (max 2.0mg) day 1
Doxorubicin 45mg/m ^{2} I.v. days 1 & 2.
Cyclophosphamide 900mg/m ^{2} days 1 & 2.

(cycle 3-5) Vincristine 2.0mg/m ^{2} I.v. (max 2.0mg) day 1.
Doxorubicin 30mg/m ^{2} I.v. days 1 & 2.
Cyclophosphamide 900mg/m ^{2} days 1 & 2.

RT 3600 cGy (4cm margin) original lesion
1440 - 2400 cGy (2cm margin) residual lesion
5040 - 6000 cGy @ 120 cGy BID total dose

S Resection of lesions in 'expendable bones' (ankle, rib, scapula) or in children < 10 years old.

All patients were evaluated and monitored with plain radiographs, computer tomography and/or magnetic resonance imaging, radionuclide bone scans, full blood counts, renal, hepatic, cardiac and pulmonary function studies. These protocols were approved by our Institutional Review Board, and informed written consent was obtained from all patients and/or their legal guardians.

Table 2. UF Patients with ES: Feb. 1982 - Nov. 1987

PATIENTS

	LOWER RISK	HIGHER RISK	
		REGIMEN 1	REGIMEN 2
NUMBER	14	10	19
MALE	9	8	10
FEMALE	5	2	9
AGE			
<10	5	0	3
10 - 20	7	9	13
>20	2	1	3
AXIAL	4	8	8
EXTREMITY	10	2	11
MAX DIAMETER (mean cm)	6	13	14
METASTASES AT DIAGNOSIS	0	4	6
SOFT TISSUE EXTENSION	7	10	19

Table 2 shows details of the 43 subjects entered on these protocols between Feb. 1982 and Nov. 1987. There is a 2:1 ratio of HR to SR patients, and ten (34%) HR patients had metastases at diagnosis. There was a clearcut division between HR and LR patients in terms of primary tumor size. There were more skeletal than axial lesions in the SR and HR-2 than the HR-1 group.

Treatment-related complications were predictably commoner in HR patients. The latter all had temporary episodes of grade 3-4 hematological and gastrointestinal toxicity. Recovery was slowest during the ABMT phase, with a median hospital time of 28 days. Patients on the HR-2 regimen were also often hospitalized with fever and neutropenia for several days during the NCT/ACT phases. 5 HR-2 patients (26%) had major reductions in cardiac contractility. In two, this followed TBI and ABMT, proving fatal in one and reversible in the other. It affected the other three following their final ACT course, and although temporary it caused us to abort the planned ABMT phase. Instead, they received further ACT to week 54, as per the SR regimen.

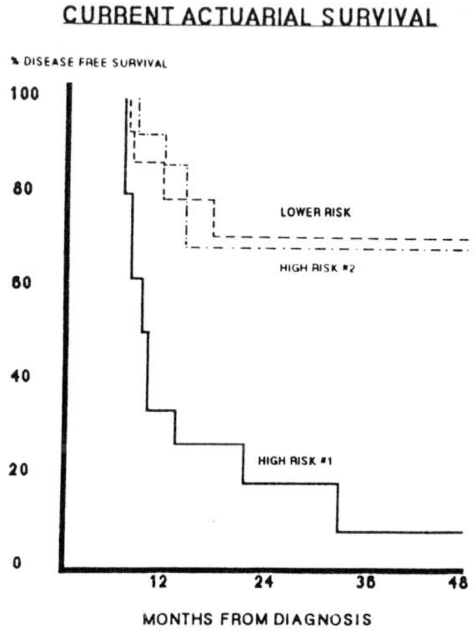

Fig. 3. Predicted DFS of Standard and High-Risk Patients

Figure 3 shows the current DFS in these 43 patients. With a 2+ year median follow-up, Kaplan-Meier analysis indicates a probability of 73% and 70% DFS in the SR and HR-2 groups respectively. Included in the latter are the 3 not undergoing ABMT. Primary control has been excellent in the SR patients, with three having surgical resections and one of the other 11 having a local recurrence. Only one HR-2 patient has had a local recurrence. 9 of the 10 HR-1 patients had complete or partial local responses to NCT, but 3 developed local recurrences. Four HR-1 patients developed metastases during ACT before reaching the ABMT phase. Of the 6 completing all treatment, 5 relapsed at 1,1,2,9 and 23 months post-treatment. All survivors are apparently well, with to date no evidence of chronic disability.

DISCUSSION

Several recent studies have evaluated NCT for patients with ES (Rosen, 1981; Hayes, 1984; Jurgens, 1988). NCT serves the dual purpose of launching an earlier attack on micrometastases and achieving rapid shrinkage of the primary tumor, with the aim of either tapering the subsequent LRT field, or rendering more primaries resectable. Although Jurgens (1988) reported an encouraging actuarial DFS with this approach, it was countered by a high (23%) local failure rate. This group also noted the highly significant influence of tumor size on outcome (80% and 31% DFS for patients with small and large primaries respectively). Our own experience suggests that eradicating the primary tumor correlates closely with systemic disease control. Even though we reduced the LRT booster fields following NCT, we have seen only 2 of 33 (6%) local relapses plus a total of 6 (18%) systemic relapses in SR and HR-2 patients. This compares with 3 (30%) local and 6 (60%) systemic relapses in HR-1 patients.

Our principle finding is the improved systemic control achievable with intensive treatment given immediately after diagnosis. The differences between HR-1 and HR-2 are the intensity and duration of both NCT and ACT, the timing of LRT, and the nature of the end-intensification. Althjough we cannot say which factor contributes most to the better outcome in HR-2 than HR-1, intensive short-duration therapy seems more effective than more protracted less intensive treatment even though the short-term morbidity is greater. Hospitalization for fever and neutropenia was almost the rule after each course in HR-2 patients, and gastrointestinal toxicity was also severe. A major concern is the frequency of cardiac toxicity induced by doxorubicin and/or TBI. The one death was in a 15 year old girl with a cardiac ejection fraction of 55% at week 18, who developed intractable low-output failure 1 week post ABMT. At autopsy her heart showed no pathognomonic changes implicating anthracycline irradiation but we were unable to document an infectious or other cause. We have withheld the ABMT phase in 3 other patients whose ejection fractions fell below 50%.

Whether such aggressive treatment is justifiable in HR patients can only be resolved by large-scale randomized trials with appropriate stratifications.

While the principle of more intensive shorter-course treatment seems sound, it may be optimal to include newer agents such as ifosphamide and etoposide that may prevent the emergence of resistant clones while not adding synergistic toxicity.

REFERENCES

Graham-Pole, J.(1984): High-dose melphalan therapy for children with refractory neuroblastoma and Ewing's sarcoma. Am. J. Ped. Hem. Onc. 6, 17-26.

Hayes, F.A.(1983): The response of Ewing's sarcoma to sequential cyclophosphamide and adriamycin induction therapy. J. Clin. Oncol. 1, 45-51.

Hustu, H.O.(1968): Treatment of Ewing's sarcoma with concurrent radiotherapy and chemotherapy. J. Pediatr. 73, 249-251.

Jurgens, H.(1988): Multidisciplinary treatment of primary Ewing's sarcoma of bone. Cancer 61, 23-32.

Marcus, R.B.(1984): The effect of primary tumor size on the prognosis of Ewing's sarcoma. Rad. Oncol. Biol. Phys. 10, (Suppl 2), 88.

Miser, J.(1987): Treatment of high-risk sarcomas with an intensive consolidation followed by autologous bone marrow transplantation. Proc. ASCO 6, 218.

Rosen, G.(1974): Disease-free survival in children with Ewing's sarcoma treated with radiation therapy and adjuvant four-day sequential chemotherapy. Cancer 33, 384-393.

Rosen, G.(1981): Combination chemotherapy in the multidisciplinary treatment of Ewing's sarcoma. Natl. Cancer Inst. Monogr. 56, 289-299.

Résumé

La chimiothérapie adjuvante a significativement augmenté la survie sans rechute des patients porteurs de sarcome d'Ewing. Les essais récents de chimiothérapie néoadjuvante ont tenté d'améliorer encore le pronostic et de modifier le traitement de la lésion primaire.

Nous avons montré rétrospectivement que la taille de la tumeur primaire était le facteur pronostic le plus important et nous avons prévu trois protocoles de chimiothérapie néoadjuvante pour les malades avec un risque important de rechute, avec un traitement plus intensif, une irradiation plus ou moins retardée et une intensification finale par chimiothérapie aplasiante et greffe de moelle autologue. Nos résultats montrent que des cures intensives et courtes sont efficaces chez des malades à haut risque avec une survie sans rechute projetée de 70 % chez 19 malades dans notre protocole le plus intensif, ceci se compare avec une survie sans rechute de 73 %, pour 14 malades standart recevant une chimiothérapie néoadjuvante moins intensive plus une chimiothérapie adjuvante plus une radiothérapie ou une chirurgie retardée. Notre autre protocole de traitement de haut risque n'a apporté qu'une survie sans rechute de 10 % chez 10 malades, attribuable soit à une intensité insuffisante de chimiothérapie néoadjuvante ou adjuvante ou un retard excessif de la radiothérapie ou à un mauvais choix du traitement d'intensification finale.
Des études randomisées sur une grande échelle, résoudront ces questions.

Neo-Adjuvant Chemotherapy. Ed. Cl. Jacquillat, M. Weil, D. Khayat. Colloque INSERM/John Libbey Eurotext Ltd. © 1988. Vol. 169, pp. 561-563.

Sarcome d'Ewing : combien existe-t-il de formes de la maladie ?

C. Jasmin[1], N. Delepine[2] et G. Delepine[1]

[1]*Hôpital Paul Brousse, BP 200, 94800 Villejuif, France.*
[2]*Hôpital Hérold, 7, place Rhin et Danube, 75019 Paris, France*

RESUME

Le sarcome d'Ewing fait partie de la liste limitée des affections malignes chimiocurables. En effet, la chimiothérapie adjuvante a permis d'obtenir des taux de guérison de 40 à 60% dans les sarcomes d'Ewing localisés contre moins de 10%, il y a quelques décades.

Les différences de chimiocurabilité des sarcomes d'Ewing selon la localisation de la tumeur primitive indépendemment de sa taille et l'existence de métastases tardives observées essentiellement dans les tumeurs pelviennes suggèrent l'existence de formes chimio-incurables de sarcomes d'Ewing liées à la présence de cellules souches tumorales protégées par leur micro-environnement qui ne peuvent être éradiquées par la chimiothérapie adjuvante classique ou néoadjuvante.

Ces formes localement résistantes devraient faire l'objet d'essais de chimiothérapie adjuvante à très fortes doses suivie de greffe de moelle compatible et/ou de nouvelles approches thérapeutiques telles que l'utilisation de modificateurs des réponses biologiques.

MOTS CLEFS

Sarcome d'Ewing, contrôle local, cellules souches tumorales, chimiocurabilité, radiorésistance.

KEY WORDS

Ewing's sarcoma, local control, tumor stem cell, chemo-curability, radio-resistance.

With modern chemotherapy, the long-term survival rate of patients with localized Ewing's sarcoma has been raised from less than ten percent with surgery alone to forty-sixty percent (Gehan 1981, Glaubiger 1981, Rosen 1981). This success has allowed to put in evidence an heterogeneity of the local and systemic evolution of the disease which was not clearly seen when the prognosis was almost uniformly fatal.

Indeed, despite an overall prognostic improvement, local recurrence rates remain elevated ; more than 20% of large tumors will display local recurrence even after intensive radio-chemotherapy (Telles 1978, Evans 1984, Kinsella 1984).

The radiosensitivity of Ewing's sarcoma does not clearly show a dose-effect relation-ship ; indeed, some tumors have been sterilized with low dose radiotherapy (40 gy or less) whereas some tumors have recurred after doses superior to 60 gy. It is worthy to note that radio-resistant forms have most often a metastatic evolution. Furthermore, chemo- and radio-resistance are also correlated.

The major prognostic influence of local sterilization has been demonstrated by Oberlin et al (1985) and in our serie (Delepine, 1987) : local recurrence and systemic relapse have been observed in tumors in which a pathological examination of the whole tumor resected after neoadjuvant therapy has demonstrated the presence of residual tumor cells. In one case from our serie, residual malignant tumor stem cells was revealed only after an in vitro culture of the resected and microscopically sterilized surgical specimen.

In the case of pelvic tumors, the size and localization of the primary tumor are independant prognostic factors : the local control rate of small or medium size pelvic tumors is lower than for distal tumors of compatible or even large size. Conversely, even large extrasquelettal tumors display an excellent cure rate with radiochemotherapy.

Finally, these results underline the importance of local factors controlling the chemocurability and the radiosensitivity of Ewing's sarcoma. These local factors may play a role in the long-term cure rate of the disease independently form the size of the primary tumor.

In view of these considerations, we are currently using preoperative chemotherapy followed by "en bloc" resection of the primary tumor in order to determine by histopathological examination and, if possible, by in vitro cell-cultures the presence of residual tumor stem cells in the resected tumor. We believe that most chemo-resistant Ewing's sarcomas can be detected at this stage of the treatment and may deserve new therapeutic approaches such as intensive marrow-ablative chemotherapy rescued with histocompatible bone marrow transplantation and/or the use of biological response modifiers (i.e. adoptive immunotherapy).

REFERENCES

Delepine, N. (1987) : Response of Ewing's sarcoma to sequential cyclosphosphamide and adriamycin induction therapy (I.T.) in 30 patients. 4th European Conference on Clinical Oncology and Cancer Nursing, 1-4 Novembre, Madrid.

Evans, R. (1984) : Local recurrence, rate and sites of metastases, and time to relapse as a function of treatment regimen, size of primary and surgical history in 62 patients presenting with non-metastatic Ewing's sarcoma of the pelvic bones. Int. J. Radiation Oncology Biol. Phys. 11, 129-136.

Ewing, J. (1921) : Diffuse endothelioma of bone. Proc. NY Pathol. Soc. 21, 17-24.

Gehan, E.A. (1981) : Prognostic factors in Ewing's sarcoma. Natl. Cancer Inst Monogr 56, 273-278.

Glaubiger, D.L. (1981) : Influence of prognostic factors on survival in Ewing's sarcoma. Natl. Cancer Inst. Monogr. 56, 285-288.

Kinsella, T.J. (1983) : Extraskeletal Ewing's sarcoma : Results of combined modality treatment. J. of Clin. Oncol. 1, 489-495.

Kinsella, T.J. (1984) : Local treatment of Ewing's Sarcoma : Radiation therapy versus surgery. Cancer Treat. Rep. 68, 695-701.
Oberlin, O. (1985) : The response to initial chemotherapy as a prognostic factor in localized Ewing's sarcoma. Europ. J. Cancer Clin. Oncol. 21, 463-467.
Rosen, G. (1981) : Ewing's sarcoma : ten-year experience with adjuvant chemotherapy. Cancer 47, 2204-2213.
Telles, N.C. (1978) : Ewing's sarcoma : an autopsy study. Cancer 41, 2321-2329.
Thomas P.R.M. (1984) : The management of Ewings' sarcoma : Role of radiotherapy in local tumor control. Cancer Treatments reports 68, 703-710.

REMERCIEMENTS

This work was supported by Fondation Daher.

Résumé

Ewing's sarcoma belongs to the limited list of chemocurable malignancies. Indeed adjuvant chemotherapy currently produces 5 yr survival rates of 40-60% in localized Ewing sarcoma as compared to less than 10% only a few decades ago.
The differences of chemocurability according to the localization of the primary tumor independently from its size and the existence of late metastases occuring mostly in pelvic tumors suggest the existence of some forms of chemo-incurable Ewing's sarcomas due to the presence of primitive tumor stem cells which cannot be eradicated by classical or neoadjuvant chemotherapy. These forms may deserve trials of adjuvant high dose chemotherapy with bone marrow transplantation and/or new approaches such as the use of biological responses modifiers.

Gynecology

Gynécologie

Neo-Adjuvant Chemotherapy. Ed. Cl. Jacquillat, M. Weil, D. Khayat. Colloque INSERM/John Libbey Eurotext Ltd. © 1988. Vol. 169, pp. 567-572.

Locally advanced cervical carcinoma: an open non-randomized trial on neo-adjuvant PBM chemotherapy followed by radical surgery

S. Mancuso, P. Benedetti-Panici, G. Scambia, S. Greggi, G. Baiocchi and A. Gallo

Department of Gynecology and Obstetrics, Catholic University, 8, largo A. Gemelli, 00168 Rome, Italy

Abstract

Thirty-six previously untreated patients with locally advanced cervical carcinoma (FIGO Stages IB-III, tumor volume >4cm) received three courses of preoperative cisplatin (P), bleomycin (B) and methotrexate (M) chemotherapy. Eighty-nine per cent patients received 100% of programmed doses. Nausea and vomiting (100%), and grades II-III myelotoxicity (22%) represented the major toxic effects. Clinical evaluation of response after chemotherapy revealed 77.8% overall response (CR: 11.1%, 4/36; PR:66.7%, 24/36). All 28 responders underwent Piver types :II-IV radical hysterectomy plus systematic para-aortic and pelvic lymphadenectomy. The overall pathological response rate was 58.3% (CR: 11.1%, 4/36; PR: 47.2%, 17/36). Vaginal lesions showed the highest response rate (82%) and surgical resection margins were tumor-free in 96.4% (27/28) of cases. Eighteen per cent (5/28) lymph node metastases was lower than the expected in such a group of patients. To date, two local recurrences have been detected (median follow-up for the 28 operated patients: 10 months).

Introduction

It has recently been suggested that neoadjuvant chemotherapy may play an important role in the treatment of advanced solid tumors (1, 2). The activity of cisplatin-containing regimens has been reported in both previously untreated cervical carcinoma (3, 4) and non-irradiated recurrent disease (3-6). We report the results of an open non-randomized phase II trial on 36 consecutive patients with locally advanced cervical carcinoma treated with preoperative cisplatin (P), bleomycin (B) and methrotrexate (M) followed by radical surgery. The aim of the study was to evaluate the toxicity, clinical response, operability and pathologic response induced by this treatment.

Material and Methods

From January to December 1986, 38 consecutive patients suffering from primary cervical carcinoma entered the study. Eligibility criteria included: tumor volume >4cm; F.I.G.O. stages IB-III; no previous treatment; age <70 years; performance status (WHO) 0-2; no renal, pulmonary, hepatic or cardiac impairment; normal blood count; no severe non-malignant systemic disease or active infection; no second malignancy (except for adequately treated basal cell carcinoma of the skin); life expectancy >3 months; informed written consent and expected cooperation of patient in treatment and follow-up. The following pre-treatment procedures were considered mandatory: cervical Pap-smear and colposcopy; cervical and vaginal biopsies; pelvic and hepatic ultrasonography; gynecologic examination under general anesthesia; endocervical and endocavitary curettage; chest x-ray; i.v. pyelography; sigmoidoscopy and cystoscopy. All these procedures (except for curettage, sigmoidoscopy and cystoscopy, if previously negative) were repeated two to three weeks after the end of chemotherapy in order to evaluate clinical response. ECG, pulmonary, renal and hepatic function tests, complete blood count, audiometry and neurologic examination were performed before and after each course to monitore toxic side-effects. PBM was administered according to the following schedule: cisplatin (P) 100mg/m2 i.v., day 1; bleomycin (B) 15 mg i.v., days 1,8; methotrexate (M) 300mg/m2 i.v. + leucovorin rescue, day 8, for three courses, every 21 days. Clinical responders were eligible for surgical treatment only if tumor volume reduction to <4 cm had been achieved and extra-cervical disease was judged radically resectable. Surgery consisted of Piver type III-IV radical hysterectomy and systematic para-aortic and pelvic lymphadenectomy. WHO response evaluation criteria were adopted. Patient characteristics are listed in Table 1.

Table 1. Patient Characteristics

Median age: 53 (range: 37-6)		
Patients entered		38 (100%)
Patients evaluable		36 (94,7%)
FIGO Stage:	IB-IIA	6 (16,7%)
	IIB	15 (41,7%)
	III	15 (41,7%)
Histotype:	Squamous cell	28 (77,8)
	Adenocarcinoma	8 (22,2)
Grade:	Well diff.	4 (11,1%)
	Mod. well diff.	19 (52,8%)
	Poorly diff.	13 (36,1%)
Patients undergoing surgery:		28 (77,8%)
Radical Hysterectomy:	Type III	17 (60,7%)
	Type IV	11 (39,3%)
Mean No.lymph nodes removed: 60 (range: 37-128)		
para-aortic: 22 (range: 12-41)		
pelvic : 39 (range: 19-76)		

After surgery, complete responders and patients with negative nodes and negative surgical resection margins received no further treatment. Adjuvant chemotherapy (further two PBM cycles) and/or radiotherapy were given to patients with positive nodes and/or positive surgical resection margins, respectively.

Results

Thirty-six of the 38 patients admitted completed all three cycles of chemotherapy (two refused treatment after the first course and one progressed after the second). Eighty-nine percent (32/36) received 100% of programmed doses: in one patient M was discontinued after the first dose because of grade III allergic skin reaction and in a further two reduced by 50% in the third cycle because of mylosuppression. Nausea and vomiting were experienced by all patients. Grades II and III myelotoxicity occurred in 12% and 10% of cases, respectively, and no pulmonary and renal toxicity was observed. Clinical response to PBM regimen is shown in Table 2.

Table 2. Clinical Response to Chemotherapy in Relation to Stage

FIGO Stage	No. of Patients	Response			
		CR	PR	NC	P
IB-IIA	6	1	5	0	0
IIB	15	1	11	2	1
III	15	2	8	3	2
Total	36	4(11.1%)	24(66.7%)	5(13.9%)	3(8.3%)

CR: Complete Response; PR: Partial Response; NC: No Change; P: Progression.

All 28 responding patients underwent radical surgery. Of the 8 non-responders, six were submitted to external pelvic radiotherapy. The other two patients died in the first two months after chemotherapy. Intraoperative complications arose in two cases (one hemorrage due to a vascular lesion and one ureteral lesion) both having a good outcome. Postoperative moderate-degree complications occurred in 46% (13/28) of the patients and were mainly represented by lymphocysts, pulmonary microembolisms and deep venous thromboses. Pathologic response to treatment is described in Table 3. The overall histologically confirmed response rate was 58.3% (21/36) with 11.1% (4/36) complete responses. A clinical overestimation of response occurred in 25% (7/28) of cases. Vaginal lesions showed the highest overall response rate (82%) followed by cervical lesions (81%) and parametrial lesions (77%). Surgical resection margins were free of tumor in 96.4% (27/28) of cases. Lymph node metastases were detected in 5/28 patients (17.8%), three of these having shown only pelvic positive nodes and the remaining two both para-aortic and pelvic. The median follow-up is now 10 months for the 28 patients who underwent surgery. To date, two local recurrences, four and seven months after surgery, have been observed.

Table 3. Pathologic Response in Relation to Stage

FIGO Stage	No. of patients	Response			Lymph Node Status	
		CR	PR	NC	N-	N+
IB-IIA	6	1	5	0	6	0
IIB	12	1	8	3	9	3
III	10	2	4	4	8	2
Total:	28	4(11.1%)	17(47.2%)	7(19.5%)	23(82.1%)	5(17.8%)

CR: Complete Response; PR: Partial Response; NC:No Change; N-: Negative Lymph Nodes; N+: Positive Lymph Nodes;

Discussion

Preoperative PBM regimen and radical surgery resulted a feasible combined treatment in our series. The clinical and pathological overall response rates achieved (77.8% and 58.3%, respectively) indicate that cervical carcinoma is a chemosensitive tumor. Furthermore, PBM chemotherapy rendered operable 77.8% patients despite their advanced stage and initial bulky tumor. According to the data of Sardi et al. (7) vaginal lesions showed the highest regression rate (82%). The 17.8% incidence of lymph node metastases seems to be lower than the expected in these patients with unfavourable prognostic factors. This data suggests a therapeutic role of preoperative chemotherapy on lymphatic metastases. Thus, considering the well recognized prognostic importance of lymph node status in cervical carcinoma, it seems reasonable to suppose a substantial benefit from this neoadjuvant treatment in disease cure. This hypothesis must, however, be confirmed in the light of a longer follow-up and calls for phase III randomized trials.

References

1) Rosen G, Marcove RC, Huvos AG, et al: Primary osteogenic sarcoma: Eight-years experience with adjuvant chemotherapy. J Cancer Res Clin Oncol 106(suppl):55, 1983

2) Kish J, Drelichman A, Jacobs J, et al: Clinical trial of cis-platin and 5-FU infusion as initial treatment for advanced squamous cell carcinoma of the head and neck. Cancer Treat Rep 66: 471, 1982

3) Kim DS, Moon H, Kang KJ: Primary chemotherapy and post-operative adjuvant chemotherapy in the treatment of squamous cell carcinoma of the uterine cervix. Gynecol Oncol 22:59, 1985

4) Belinson JL, Stewart JA, et al: Bleomycin, vincristine, mitomycin-C and cisplatin in the management of gynaecological squamous cell carcinomas. Gynecol Oncol 20:387, 1985

5) Friedlander ML, Atkinson K, Coppleson JMV, et al: The integration of chemotherapy into the management of local advanced cervical cancer: A pilot study. Gynecol Oncol 19:1, 1984

6) Alberts DS, Martinbeau PW, Surwit EA, et al: Mitomycin-C, bleomycin, vincristine and cis-platinum in the treatment of advanced, recurrent squamous cell carcinoma of the cervix. Cancer Clin Trials 4:313, 1981

7) Sardi JE, Di Paola GR, Cahan A, et al: A possible new trend in the management of the carcinoma of the cervix uteri. Gynecol Oncol 25: 139, 1986

Résumé

36 malades atteintes de cancer avancé du col (FIGO Stade IB-III, volume tumoral supérieur à 4 cm) ont reçu 3 cures de Cisplatyl-Bléomycine et Méthotrexate en pré-opératoire. 89 % des malades ont reçu 100 % de la dose programmée. Des nausées et vomissements, une myélotoxicité de grade 2-3 chez 22 % des malades ont représenté les effets toxiques. L'évaluation clinique de la réponse après la chimiothérapie a révélé 77,8 % de réponse globale, dont 11,1 % réponse complète et 66,7 % réponse partielle. Les 28 répondeurs ont subi une hystérectomie radicale type III-IV, de plus une lymphadénectomie para-aortique et pelvienne systématique. Le taux de réponse pathologique global a été de 58,3 %. Les lésions vaginales ont montré le plus haut taux de réponse (82 %) et la résection chirurgicale des marges était stérilisée dans 96,4 %. 18 % des métastases ganglionnaires ont été moins importantes que prévues. A ce jour, deux rechutes locales ont été dépistées (suivi médian pour les 28 malades opérées 10 mois).

Neo-Adjuvant Chemotherapy. Ed. Cl. Jacquillat, M. Weil, D. Khayat. Colloque INSERM/John Libbey Eurotext Ltd. © 1988. Vol. 169, pp. 573-577.

Concurrent radiation therapy, cisplatinum and mitomycin-C in patients with poor prognosis carcinoma of the cervix

Vinay K. Malviya***, Y. Kim**, Norman Gove* and Gunter Deppe*

*Division of gynecologic oncology, Hutzel Hospital**
*** Gershenson radiation center, Wayne state university*
*Hutzel hospital*** Wayne State University 4707 St. Antoine, Detroit, Michigan 48201 USA*

ABSTRACT

Fifteen patients with poor prognosis squamous cell cancer of the cervix were treated with concurrent radiation therapy (RT) and chemotherapy between February, 1986 and July, 1987. Treatment consisted of intravenous Mitomycin-C 10 mg/m^2 on days 1 and 43 and Cisplatinum 50 mg/m^2 on days 1, 22 and 43. All patients received external RT - 5,000 rads in 28 fractions and brachytherapy - 4,000 rads to point A. Additionally, patients with paraaortic lymph node involvement received 4,000 rads paraaortic RT. The toxicity of this regimen was assessed using SWOG criteria. Toxicity was acceptable and did not delay RT. In addition, local control (complete response) was noted in all patients within one month of completion of therapy and maintained despite distant metastases. At the time of this report, ten of the fifteen patients are alive, 9-22 months after initiation of treatment. Chemotherapy with cisplatinum and Mitomycin-C concurrent with radiation is an effective and well tolerated regimen for advanced cervical cancer and merits further study.

KEYWORDS

Concurrent radiation and chemotherapy, cisplatinum, Mitomycin-C, poor prognosis cancer of cervix.

Early cancer of the cervix (Ca Cx) is curable by surgery or radiation therapy (RT) but cure rates fall sharply with advanced disease (Jampolis, 1975; Hanks, 1983; Perez, 1983). Strategies to improve the results of primary treatment in patients with advanced cancer of the cervix are directed towards improved local control of tumor, effective management of lymph nodes, and presumed microscopic distant metastases. The incidence of pelvic recurrence after RT ranges from 7% (Stage I) to 75% (Stage IV)(Brady, 1986). Doses of radiation cannot be increased indefinitely due to risk of complications, treatment techniques must be directed to enhance biologic effects of irradiation on tumor cells by the use of hypoxic tumor sensitizers, hyperbaric oxygen, hyperthermia and high LET particle radiation (Thomas, 1982; Maruyama, 1985). "Poor prognosis" cervical cancer patients include patients with Stage III and IVA disease and patients with any FIGO stage of the disease with biopsy proven and/or paraaortic lymph node involvement.

Chemotherapy has a limited role in the management of primary cervical cancer. Although several cytotoxic drugs have been shown to induce tumor regression, the highest response rates are seen with cisplatinum (DDP)(Thigpen, 1981) and Mitomycin-C (MMC)(Muscate, 1982)(38% and 22% respectively). When used singly, both may act as radiosensitizers and MMC has been effective in bulky tumors with hypoxic cancer cells. We have previously demonstrated that MMC is selectively concentrated in the uterine cervix of the mouse model after intravenous administration (Malviya, 1986).

Seventy-five percent of patients with poor prognosis squamous cell cancer of the cervix recur with RT alone, and do so with some component of pelvic failure. The five-year survival rates are 30-40% for Stage III and 14-19% for Stage IV (Marcial, 1977). The majority of patients who fail have disease in the pelvis, in addition to distant metastases.

In this pilot study, we investigated the concurrent use of cisplatinum and Mitomycin-C with RT in poor risk patients with squamous cell cancer of the cervix. The goals of our study were to determine the toxicity of this regimen and to investigate whether the concurrent use of cisplatinum and MMC would delay completion of standard radiation therapy protocols.

METHODS

Between February, 1986 and July, 1987, fifteen patients (mean age: 51.4 years) with poor prognosis squamous cell Ca Cx were treated as outpatients concurrently with DDP, MMC and RT (Fig. 1).

FIG. 1 PROTOCOL: CONCURRENT RT, MMC & CISPLATINUM

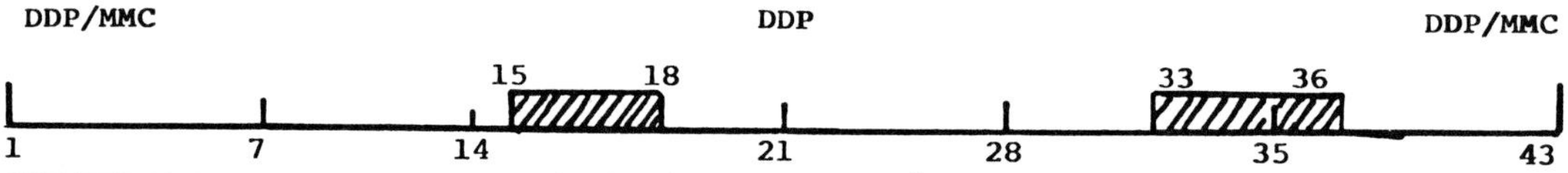

CHEMOTHERAPY:	**Cisplatinum 50 mg/m² - days 1, 22, 43**
	MMC 10 mg/m² - days 1, 43
EXTERNAL RT:	**180 cGy/day, 5 days/week - 5400 cGy**
PARAAORTIC RT:	**150 cGy/day, 5 days/week - 4500 cGy**
INTRACAVITARY CS-137:	**3000 cGy to Pt A, days 15 - 18 and days 33 - 36**

Eight of these patients had FIGO Stage IIIB disease with extension to both pelvic side walls and one patient had Stage IIB disease with pelvic lymph node involvement. Three patients with Stage IB cancer of the cervix had positive paraaortic lymph nodes at the time of radical hysterectomy, while three patients had metastatic involvement of pelvic lymph nodes, but negative paraaortic lymph nodes. NO clinical or radiologic evidence of distant metastases was present. None of our patients had received prior chemotherapy or radiation therapy.

MMC was given intravenously 10 mg/m² on days 1 and 43 (Fig. 1) Following adequate hydration with two liters of normal saline, DDP was administered as an intravenous infusion, (50 mg/m² with 50 grams of mannitol in one liter of normal saline) on days 1, 22 and 43.

Radiation was given to the pelvis, unless the paraortic node contained metastatic disease. In the later cases, the paraaortic area was irradiated along with the pelvis (Table 1).

POOR PROGNOSIS CANCER OF THE CERVIX
RADIATION PORTALS

STAGE	PELVIS	PARAAORTIC & PELVIS
IB	3	3
IIB	1	---
IIIB	8	---

If the paraaortic region was involved, a total dose of 4,500 cGy to the paraaortic and 5,400 cGy to the pelvis was given before the Cesium implant. Otherwise, pelvic irradiation was given in 5 steps; External beam irradiation to 2,980 cGy using 4 fields box technique; a Cesium implant; parametrial boost to 1,200 - 2,000 cGy using opposing an anterior and a posterior fields with custom fabricated stepwedges; a Cesium implant, and a parametrial boost with stepwedges. Cesium implantation was done with a Fletcher-Suite applicator and 3,000 cGy was delivered to the Point A on each application. External beam therapy was performed with a linear accelerator using 15 MEV x-rays. Daily dose to the pelvis was 180 cGy and to the paraaortic 150 cGy.

Pelvic radiation was given with 4 fields; opposing anterior and posterior, and opposing right and left lateral fields. Each field was shaped with custom-made Cerrobend blocks to exclude as much normal tissue was possible from radiation. Physical examination and CT scan findings were used in shaping of the radiation ports. Radiation therapy was postponed if the granulocyte count was less than $1000/mm^3$ and platelet count was less than $100,000/mm^3$.

All patients completed three courses of chemotherapy according to protocol and were considered evaluable for toxicity and response. Toxicity was graded according to the Southwestern Oncology Group (SWOG) criteria. The response was evaluated by pelvic computerized tomography (CT) and by examination under anesthesia. Complete response was defined as the absence of measurable disease and complete resolution of all symptoms.

RESULTS

All patients completed the study protocl and were evaluable for response. The results of this study are presented in Table II.

RESULTS

STAGE	ALIVE & WELL (MONTHS)	ALIVE WITH DISEASE (MONTHS)	DEAD OF DISEASE (MONTHS)
IIIB Ca Cx	4/8 (9,9,14,22)	1/8 (14)	3/8 (5, 5, 14)
IIB w/PLN*	1/1 (14)	---	---
IB w/PALN**	2/3 (9, 15)	---	1/3 (15)
IB w/PLN	2/3 (11, 19)	---	1/3 (9)

* PLN - Pelvic Lymph Node ** PALN - Paraaortic Lymph Node

Of eight patients with Stage IIIB disease, four are alive with no evidence of disease and one is alive with a single lung metastasis that has been resected. Three patients have died of widespread metastases to the lungs, skull, ribs, pericardium, supraclavicular and inguinal lymph nodes. All patients have been followed for 5 to 22 months (median: 11 1/2 months). The patient with Stage IIB cancer of the cervix and positive pelvic lymph nodes is alive with no evidence of disease at 14 months. Two of the patients with Stage IB disease and paraaortic lymph node involvement are alive with no evidence of disease. One patient died of widespread distant metastases at 15 months (median follow-up: 15 months; range: 9-15 months). Of the three with Stage IB disease and positive pelvic lymph nodes, two are alive without disease, while the third died of extensive metastatic disease to the lung, brain and bones (median follow-up: 11 months; range: 9-19 months). We noted complete local response one month after completion of the treatment protocol in all patients and this was maintained despite appearance of distant metastases in some patients.

Chemotherapeutic toxicity was moderate and consisted of grade II nausea and vomiting in all patients. One patient required multiple hospitalizations during extended radiation therapy for recurrent partial small bowel obstruction. Grade I diarrhea occurred in 3/15 patients and was related to radiation therapy and metoclopromide. It was easily controlled with Lomotil. At no time during the course of the study was it necessary to interrupt radiation therapy due to myelosuppresion. The nadir granulocyte count was $1800/mm^3$.

Major complications occurred in three patients including MMC extravasation with necrosis of the dorsum of the hand in one patient. Another patient developed a rectovaginal fistula ten months after completion of RT and one patient developed a sigmoid stricture. Both these patients required terminal sigmoid end colostomy, while the patient with a sigmoid stricture required entero-enteral bypass for persistent small bowel obstruction.

DISCUSSION

This pilot study confirms the efficacy and acceptable toxicity of concurrent chemotherapy and radiation therapy in patients with advanced, poor prognosis, squamous cell cancer of the cervix. A complete local response was noted within one month after completion of therapy in our patients which was maintained despite appearance of distant metastases. In contrast, after RT alone, local response is usually seen within three months.

The pelvic control rate at one year in patients with Stage IIIB disease with bilateral parametrial involvement after RT alone is 43% (Thomas, 1984). In our patients, pelvic control was 100% - much better than expected from radiation alone for this extent of disease. The appearance of distant metastases in 6 of 15 patients (40%) is not surprising in these patients with a poor prognosis. The median follow-up of all patients was 14 months (range: 5-22 months).

The toxicity of chemotherapy with concurrent radical RT was unknown to us at the inception of this study, as was the feasibility of combining chemotherapeutic drugs with RT. One possible cause for the failure to achieve local control with RT is the existence of hypoxic cells within large tumors which tend to be more resistant to ionizing radiation than well oxygenated cells (Kennedy, 1980). Mitomycin-C is effective against hypoxic cells in vivo and in vitro and may be important in its role as a radiopotentiator as well as a chemotherapeutic agent (Thigpen, 1981; Rockwell, 1983).

DDP, in addition to being a radiosensitizer, appears to be the most active drug in squamous cell cancer of the cervix (Douple, 1978; Douple, 1979). Conceptually, the synchronous administration of chemotherapy with RT is logical because radiation enhancement induces increased tumor cell kill at the tumor site. Enhanced local response and tumor regression prevents reseeding of the circulation from the primary tumor, thereby preventing distant metastasis.
We have demonstrated a shorter response time by combining chemotherapy and radiation therapy in patients with poor prognosis cervical cancer; however, longer follow-up of our ten surviving patients is required to determine its impact in improving cure rates. Randomized multi-institutional trials are needed to determine the role of adjuvant chemotherapy in the treatment of patients with advanced, but localized, primary disease.

REFERENCES

Jampolis, S.(1975): Analysis of sites and causes of failure of irradiation in invasive squamous cell carcinoma of intact cervix. Radiology, 115:681-685.

Hanks, GE.(1983): Pattern of care outcome studies. Cancer, 51:959-967.

Perez, CA.(1983): Radiation therapy alone in the treatment of carcinoma of uterine cervix. Cancer, 51:1393-1402.

Brady, L.(1986): Failure patterns in gynecologic cancer. Radiat Oncol Biol Phys, 12:549-557.

Thomas, GM.(1982): A Phase I study of misonidazole and pelvic irradiation in patients with carcinoma of the cervix. Br J Of Cancer, 45:860.
Piver, MS.(1979): Hydroxyurea combined with radiation to beat Stage IIIB and IV cervical cancer confined to the pelvis. Int J Radiat Oncol Biol Phys, 5:317.
Piver, MS.(1983): Hydroxyurea: A radiation potentiator in carcinoma of the uterine cervix. A randomized double blind study. Amer J Obstet Gynecol, 147:803.
Dische, S.(1983): Carcinoma of the cervix: Anemia radiotherapy and hyperbaric oxygen. Br J Radiol, 56:251.
Shingleton, HM.(1987): Cancer of the cervix: Diagnosis and treatment. Radiat Therapy, Pp. 188, Churchill Livingston (edn).
Maruyama, Y.(1985): Clinical trial of ^{252}CF neutron brachytherapy vs conventional radiotherapy for advanced cervical cancer. Int J Radiat Oncol Biol Phys, 11: 1475-1482.
Thigpen, T.(1981): Cisplatinum in treatment of advanced or recurrent squamous cell carcinoma of the cervix. A phase II study of the gynecologic oncology group. Cancer, 48:899.
Thigpen, T.(1981): Chemotherapy in the management of advanced or recurrent cervical and endometrial carcinoma. Cancer, 48:658.
Muscate, MS.(1982): Chemotherapy of cervical carcinoma. Sem Oncol, 9:373.
Malviya, VK.(1986): Pharacokinetics of Mitomycin-C in plasma and tumor tissue of cervical cancer patients and in selected tissues of female rats. Gynecol Oncol, 25:160-170.
Marcial, VA.(1977): Carcinoma of the cervix: present status and future. Cancer, 39:945-958.
Thomas, G.(1984): Concurrent radiation, Mitomycin-C and 5-fluorouracil in poor prognosis carcinoma of the cervix: Preliminary results of a phase I-II study. Int J Rad Oncol Biol Phys, 10:1785.
Kennedy, KA.(1980): Preferential activation of Mitomycin-C to cytotoxic metabolites by hypoxic tumor cells. Cancer Res, 40:2356.
Rockwell, S.(1983): Effects of Mitomycin-C alone and in combination with x-rays on EMT 6 mouse mammary tumors in vivo. J.N.C.I., 71:765.
Douple, EB.(1978): Platinum complexes as radiosensitizers of hypoxic mammalian cells. Brit J Cancer, 37:98-102.
Douple, EB.(1979): Radiosensitization of hypoxic tumor cells by cis and trans dischlorodiammine dichloroplatinum (II). Int J Rad Oncol Biol Phys, 5: 1369-1372.

Résumé

15 malades atteintes de cancer épidermoïde du col de mauvais pronostic ont été traités par irradiation et chimiothérapie entre février 1986 et juillet 1987. Le traitement a consisté en Mitomycine C 10 mg/m2 aux jours 1 et 43, Cis.platyl 50 mg/m2 aux jours 1, 22, 43. Ces malades ont reçu une radiothérapie externe de 4000 rads en 28 fractions et une curiethérapie de 4000 rads. De plus, les malades ayant un envahissement des ganglions para-aortiques ont reçu une radiothérapie par voie aortique de 4000 rads. La toxicité de ce traitement d'après les critères du SVOG était acceptable et n'a pas retardé la chimiothérapie. De plus le contrôle local a été noté chez toutes les malades à un mois du traitement et a été maintenus en dépit de métastases à distance.

Actuellement 10 des 15 malades sont vivantes de 9 à 22 mois après le début du traitement. La chimiothérapie par Cis.Platyl et Mitomycine C associé à une irradiation est un traitement efficace et bien toléré pour les cancers du col avancé et mérite d'autres études.

Neo-Adjuvant Chemotherapy. Ed. Cl. Jacquillat, M. Weil, D. Khayat. Colloque INSERM/John Libbey Eurotext Ltd. © 1988. Vol. 169, pp. 579-583.

Cisplatine-adriamycine séquentielle (PA3), cytoréduction chirurgicale précoce et chimiothérapie intrapéritonéale (IP) dans le cancer avancé de l'ovaire

A. de Gramont, G. Gonzalez-Canali, M. Krulik, C. Louvet, B. Demuynck, L. Marpeau, A. Pigné, J. Barrat, D. Gallot, M. Malafosse, B. Lagadec, J. Cady et J. Debray

Groupe d'étude et de Recherche sur les cancers de l'Ovaire et Digestifs (GERCOD) Paris, France

RESUME

Quarante patientes de moins de 70 ans atteintes de cancer épithélial de l'ovaire stade III stade IV ont reçu respectivement : 1) 3 patientes sans maladie résiduelle après la laparotomie initiale et 10 patientes avec une maladie résiduelle inférieure à 2 cm, 6 cycles de Cisplatine 80 mg/m2 J1 et Adriamycine 50 mg/m2 J3 (PA3) toutes les 4 semaines suivis d'un second-look et de 3 cycles de Cisplatine intrapéritonéal 200 mg/m2 en cas de réponse complète ou de 6 en cas de maladie résiduelle, le Cisplatine étant remplacé par la Mitoxantrone 25 mg/m2 si les cytologies étaient positives; 2) 22 patientes avec une masse résiduelle de plus de 2 cm de diamètre ont reçu 3 cycles de PA3 suivis par une chirurgie de cytoréduction précoce et 6 autres cycles de PA3 avant le second-look et l'IP si les masses résiduelles au second look avaient moins de 2 cm. 5 stades IV ont reçu 6 cycles de PA3, un second look et l'IP en cas de rémission complète extra-abdominale. 33 patientes étaient évaluables, il y a eu 13 réponses complètes (38%), 50% en cas de masse inférieure à 2 cm et 38% en cas de masse de plus de 2 cm. Le taux de réponse partielle était de 35%, stable de 9% et progressif de 18%.
La chirurgie de cytoréduction a été réalisée chez 21 patientes, 14 (66.7%) n'avaient plus de masse supérieure à 2 cm à l'issue de cette seconde cytoréduction. 27 patientes ont reçu une chimiothérapie intrapéritonéale.
La toxicité du PA3 a été neutropénie fébrile 4 cas, paresthésie : 3 cas, insuffisance rénale : 1 cas, insuffisance cardiaque : 1 cas. Avec le Cisplatine IP, 2 patientes ont fait une insuffisance rénale.
La probabilité de survie à 2 ans est de 63%, 87,5% en cas de masse inférieure à 2 cm, 64% en cas de masse supérieure à 2 cm. La survie à long terme après chimiothérapie IP ne peut encore être évaluée.
En conclusion, un taux de réponse élevé est observé avec le PA3, la chirurgie cytoréduction seconde est efficace pour deux tiers des patients, l'impact de l'IP sur la survie demande plus de recul pour être évalué.

INTRODUCTION

Dans le but d'améliorer la survie des cancers avancés de l'ovaire, un protocole thérapeutique (084) a été institué, comportant :

1) Une chimiothérapie systémique comportant l'association séquentielle Cisplatine-Adriamycine, dérivée du CHAP II (1)
2) Une chirurgie de cytoréduction précoce après 3 cycles de chimiothérapie pour les patientes ayant des masses résiduelles de plus de 2 cm de diamètre à la première laparotomie (3)
3) Une chimiothérapie intrapéritonéale de consolidation après second-look (4).

MATERIELS ET METHODES

Les patientes éligibles devaient avoir un cancer épithélial de l'ovaire stade III et IV de la FIGO, pas d'antécédent de cancer, de radiothérapie ou de chimiothérapie, être âgées de moins de 70 ans et avoir un indice de performance compris entre 0 et 3 selon l'OMS.
Le traitement comportait :
1) laparotomie et cytoréduction,
2) si la plus grosse masse résiduelle avait moins de 2 cm de diamètre, 6 cycles de chimiothérapie systémique type PA3
3) si la plus grosse masse avait plus de 2 cm de diamètre, 3 cycles de PA3 étaient suivis d'une chirurgie de cytoréduction précoce, puis de 6 autres cycles de PA3
3) Un second-look avec nouvelle cytoréduction si nécessaire,
4) Une chimiothérapie intrapéritonéale si la plus grosse masse résiduelle avait 2 cm ou moins de diamètre.

CARACTERISTIQUES DES PATIENTES

Quarante patientes sont entrées dans l'étude âgées en moyenne de 54,1 ans, 82,5% avaient un indice de performance de 0 à 1 et 17,5% de 2 à 3.
La classification FIGO était de IIIA pour une patiente, IIIB pour 5, IIIC pour 29 (72,5%) et IV pour 5.
L'histologie était séreuse pour 27 (67,5%), mucineuse pour 1, endométrioïde pour 3, mixte pour 1, Cellules claires pour 1, indifférenciée pour 7.
La maladie résiduelle macroscopique après la laparotomie initiale dans les stades III était nulle dans 3 cas (7,5%), de moins de 2 cm dans 10 cas (25%) et de plus de 2 cm dans 22 cas (55%).
La chimiothérapie systémique (PA3) comportait Jour 1 Cisplatine 80 mg/m2 en perfusion avec les règles habituelles d'hydratation.
Jour 3 Adriamycine à 50 mg/m2, cycle administré tous les 28 jours si les globules blancs étaient supérieurs à 4000/mm3, les plaquettes à 120 000/mm3 et la créatininémie inférieure à 15 mg/l

RESULTATS

Réponses
34 patientes sont évaluables. Les 6 non-évaluables avaient dans 3 cas plus de maladie résiduelle macroscopique après la première laparotomie, dans un cas il s'agissait d'un décès précoce par embolie pulmonaire chez une patiente stade IV, et dans les 2 derniers cas, le second look n'a pas été réalisé en raison de la toxicité de la chimiothérapie systémique, une des patientes était répondeuse complète clinique et l'autre répondeuse partielle.
Le PA3 a permis d'obtenir 38% de réponse complète, soit 50% en cas de résidu tumoral inférieur à 2 cm de diamètre, 38% en cas de résidu tumoral supérieur à 2 cm et 0 dans les stades IV. Le taux de réponse partielle était de 35%, de maladie stable 9% et de maladie progressive 18%.

Résultats de la chirurgie de cytoréduction précoce.
Celle-ci a été réalisée chez 21 patientes ayant des tumeurs résiduelles de plus de 2 cm de diamètre, après 3 cycles de PA3.
Les 3 cycles de PA3 ont pu être évalués, il y avait 1 réponse complète, 16 réponses partielles, 2 maladies stables et 2 maladies progressives.
Après cytoréduction, 3 patientes n'avaient plus de maladie résiduelle macroscopique, et 11 n'avaient pas de masse résiduelle supérieure à 2 cm de diamètre. 66,7% des malades avaient ainsi des tumeurs résiduelles de moins de 2 cm. Pour 4 patientes le résidu tumoral a été supérieur à 2 cm et pour 3 malades, la cytoréduction précoce a été impossible du fait de l'extension des lésions.
Entre la chirurgie de cytoréduction et le second-look, chez les patientes ayant des résidus de plus de 2 cm de diamètre, les 6 cycles complémentaires de PA3 ont permis d'observer des réponses complètes, mais aucune patiente ayant une masse supérieure à 2 cm de diamètre à l'issue de la chirurgie de cytoréduction ne s'est retrouvée dans cette situation au moment du second look.

La chimiothérapie intrapéritonéale
Celle-ci a été réalisée chez 27 patientes ayant une masse résiduelle de moins de 2 cm au second-look. Elle a été réalisée par un système totalement implantable (Infuse-a-port) chez 13 patientes en rémission complète et 14 patientes avec un résidu inférieur à 2 cm de diamètre. Chez 4 patientes le protocole n'a pu être conduit jusqu'à son terme en raison d'une perforation rectale dans un cas et une obstruction du cathéter par de la fibrose dans 3 cas.

Survie
Avec un recul moyen de 25 mois en février 1988, la probabilité de survie pour l'ensemble des patientes est de 92,5% à 1 an (écart-type 4.2 ans) et à 2 ans de 63% (écart-type 9.3%). Pour les patientes ayant une maladie résiduelle initiale inférieure à 2 cm de diamètre, la probabilité de survie à 1 an est de 100% et à 2 ans de 87,5%. Pour celles ayant une masse résiduelle de plus de 2 cm, la probabilité de survie à 1 an est de 95,5% et à 2 ans de 64%. La survie des stades IV est de 60% à 1 an et de 0 à 2 ans (5 patientes seulement). L'impact à long terme de la consolidation intrapéritonéale ne peut encore être évaluée.

Toxicité
En dehors de l'alopécie à l'Adriamycine et des vomissements au Cisplatine dont la fréquence augmente avec le nombre de cycles, les accidents les plus sévères ont été pour le PA3 une neutropénie fébrile dans 10% des cas, une paresthésie dans 7,5% des cas, une insuffisance rénale dans 1 cas et une insuffisance cardiaque dans 1 cas. Pour la chimiothérapie intrapéritonéale, en dehors des incidents liés au cathéter, une insuffisance rénale liée au Cisplatine a été observée dans 2 cas (7,4%). Il n'y a pas eu de décès directement lié à la toxicité du traitement.

DISCUSSION

L'association Cisplatine-Adriamycine séquentielle est particulièrement active dans les cancers avancés de l'ovaire avec un taux de réponse complète de 38% auquel s'ajoute 35% de réponse partielle. Ceci se compare favorablement avec l'administration simultanée de ces 2 drogues qui donnait dans notre expérience 26% de réponse complète et 18% de réponse partielle

(3). La chirurgie de cytoréduction seconde apparait également utile aux patientes avec grosse masse résiduelle, puisque après 3 cycles de PA3 les 2/3 de ces patientes se retrouvent avec une maladie résiduelle de moins de 2 cm de diamètre. L'utilité de la poursuite du PA3 après la chirurgie de cytoréduction précoce apparait par contre contestable puisque en dehors de l'augmentation du nombre de réponses complètes pathologiques, aucune des patientes restant avec une maladie résiduelle importante n'a bénéficié de la poursuite des cycles.
La chimiothérapie intrapéritonéale est prometteuse, réalisable avec cathéter implantable chez plus de 80% des patientes. Il est cependant trop tôt pour évaluer son bénéfice sur la survie.

CONCLUSION

Avec un recul encore faible, on peut conclure à une amélioration probable de la survie avec ce traitement combinant l'administration séquentielle de Cisplatine et d'Adriamycine, la chirurgie de cytoréduction précoce et la chimiothérapie intrapéritonéale surtout pour les patientes ayant initialement des masses résiduelles après la première laparotomie de plus de 2 cm de diamètre.

REFERENCES

1 Brûckner HW, COHEN CJ, FEUER E et al : Long-term follow-up of stage III & IV ovarian cancer : controlled clinical trials utilizing cisplatin (P), doxorubicin (A), cyclophosphamide (C) and hexamethylmelamine (H). Proc Am Soc Clin Oncol, 1987, 6, 121.

2 de Gramont A, Drolet Y, Louvet C, Dray C, Krulik M, Pigne A, Lavoie A, Painchaud M, Blouin R, Tessier C, Ouellet P, Brissaud P, Debray J, Barrat J : la chimiothérapie dans 143 cancers épithéliaux avancés de l'ovaire : Expérience de l'Hôtel Dieu de Quebec et de l'Hôpital Saint-Antoine (Paris). J Gynecol Obstet Biol Reprod, 1986, 15, 105-109.

3 Howell SB, Zimm S, Markman M, Abramson IS, Cleary S, Lucas WE, Weiss RJ : Long-term survival of advanced refractory ovarian carcinoma patients with small-volume disease treated with intraperitoneal chemotherapy. J Clin Oncol, 1987, 5, 1607-1612.

4 Parker LM, Griffiths CT, Janis D : advanced ovarian carcinoma : integration of surgical treatment and chemotherapy with cyclophosphamide (C) Adriamycin (A) and cis-diamminodichloroplatinum (P). Proc Am Soc Clin Oncol, 1983, abstract C-599, 153.

Résumé

40 patients under 70 year-old with stage III-IV epithelial ovarian cancer from Jan 84 to Mar 87 received : stage III, 3 pts without residual mass and IIIB, 10 pts with residual mass <2cm, 6 courses of DDP 80mg/m2 Day 1 and Adriamycine 50mg/m2 Day 3 every 4 weeks followed by second-look laparotomy (SL) and 3 courses of DDP 200mg/m2 IP if pathological CR and 6 if residual disease. 22 pts Stage III with mass >2cm had 3 courses of PA3 followed by debulking surgery and 6 other courses of PA3 before SL and IP when residual masses at SL were <2cm. Stage IV (5 pts) received 6 PA3, SL and IP if complete extra-abdominal remission.

6 patients were not evaluable: 3 Stage III remaining disease-free, 1 early non-therapy related death and 2 who wrer not eligible for second-look. Debulking surgery was effective in 66.7% of pts and resulted in 14 pts with residual disease <2cm and 7 pts with residual masses >2cm. CR was achieved in 38% (III with residual mass < 2 cm : 50%, III with residual mass > 2 cm : 38%), PR in 35%, Stable in 9% and Progressive Disease in 18%. 27 patients received IP, technical failure due to totally implantable system occured in 4 patients.

2-year survival was 63% (SD 9%) in all pts (III < 2 cm 87.5%, III > 2 cm 64%, IV 0%). Toxicities were febrile neutropenia 10%, paresthesia 7.5%, renal failure 2.5%, arythmia 2.5% for PA3 and renal failure 2 pts for IP.

This procedure shows an improvement in treatment of advanced ovarian cancer, specially on patients with bulky disease.

Pharmacokinetics

Pharmacocinétique

Neo-Adjuvant Chemotherapy. Ed. Cl. Jacquillat, M. Weil, D. Khayat. Colloque INSERM/John Libbey Eurotext Ltd. © 1988. Vol. 169, pp. 587-593.

Pharmacocinétique et pharmacologie cellulaire de l'idarubicine et de la pirarubicine, comparées à la daunorubicine et à la doxorubicine

J. Robert, B. Schott et S. Huet

Fondation Bergonié et Université de Bordeaux II, 180, rue de Saint-Genès, 33076 Bordeaux Cedex, France

RESUME

Nous avons étudié la pharmacologie cellulaire de deux nouvelles anthracyclines, la pirarubicine et l'idarubicine, analogues respectifs de la doxorubicine et de la daunorubicine, sur un modèle de cellules en culture sensibles et résistantes à la doxorubicine. Nous avons montré que les nouvelles molécules sont plus actives que les molécules parentales et que leur résistance croisée n'est que partielle. Elles s'incorporent dans les cellules plus rapidement, et à des taux plus élevés. La pharmacocinétique de ces deux nouvelles anthracyclines a été étudiée dans deux séries de malades traités par injections quotidiennes répétées pendant 3 ou 5 jours. Nous avons observé qu'elles ont toutes deux une demi-vie plus brève et un volume total de distribution plus élevé que les molécules de référence. Leur métabolisme est toutefois très différent : l'idarubicine est transformée majoritairement en idarubicinol et la pirarubicine compte parmi ses métabolites la doxorubicine elle-même, qui ne devient importante qu'au décours de la troisième injection du médicament.

MOTS CLEFS

Anthracyclines, pharmacocinétique, pharmacologie cellulaire.

INTRODUCTION

Plusieurs nouvelles anthracyclines sont actuellement en cours de développement dans des essais de phase I et II. Parmi elles, l'idarubicine (4-déméthoxy-daunorubicine) et la pirarubicine (4'-O-tétrahydropyranyldoxorubicine) sont apparues comme des agents prometteurs à l'issue de l'expérimentation préclinique _in vitro_ et _in vivo_ ; les essais cliniques en cours semblent confirmer l'intérêt de ces molécules et justifient un approfondissement des recherches expérimentales tout autant qu'une évaluation des paramètres pharmacocinétiques caractérisant ces molécules chez l'homme. En particulier, il est nécessaire d'explorer un plus grand nombre de modèles cellulaires afin d'étendre et de généraliser les constatations initiales. La comparaison systématique, sur une série de modèles bien définis, des propriétés pharmacologiques des nouvelles molécules avec celles des anthracyclines de référence est nécessaire à ce stade, car elle permet de guider rationnellement la conduite du clinicien dans le choix des schémas thérapeutiques et des protocoles des essais ultérieurs. Quant aux études pharmacocinétiques précoces, elles apportent des informations complémentaires indispensables et indissociables des études expérimentales, qui ne peuvent appréhender des phénomènes tels que la distribution et l'élimination des médicaments ou leur métabolisme hépatique.

Nous présentons ici les données que nous avons obtenues sur l'idarubicine et sur la pirarubicine, d'une part à l'aide d'un modèle cellulaire sensible ou résistant à la doxorubicine, d'autre part après administration intraveineuse chez un petit nombre de malades inclus dans les protocoles d'essais thérapeutiques. Nous essaierons de montrer que ces anthracyclines nouvelles possèdent des caractères communs qui les différencient des molécules de référence, mais qu'elles conservent aussi des caractères propres confirmant l'originalité de chaque structure dans la série des anthracyclines.

MATERIELS, MALADES ET METHODES

Culture cellulaire

La lignée étudiée est originaire du glioblastome C6 du rat, sensible ou résistante à la doxorubicine. La lignée résistante a été obtenue dans notre laboratoire (Vrignaud et coll., 1986) par exposition à des quantités progressivement croissantes de doxorubicine. Cette lignée pousse normalement en présence de 0,5 µg de doxorubicine par ml de milieu. Elle présente l'ensemble des caractères de la résistance pléiotropique (multidrug resistance) ; le rapport des doses de doxorubicine entraînant la même cytotoxicité dans les lignées sensible et résistante est d'environ 400 ; l'incorporation de doxorubicine dans la lignée résistante est réduite d'un facteur 10 dans nos conditions habituelles de mesure (cf. infra). Les cellules sont cultivées en routine dans du DMEM additionné de 10 % de sérum foetal de veau, à 37° dans un incubateur avec 5 % de gaz carbonique et 80 % d'humidité ; ces cellules poussent en monocouches dans des boîtes de Pétri et sont repiquées une fois par semaine environ.

Evaluation de la cytotoxicité

Les cellules sont transplantées dans des boîtes de Pétri de 10 ou 20 cm² de telle sorte que, trois jours plus tard, les incubations puissent être réalisées lorsque 5.10^5 cellules tapissent le fond de la boîte. Ces incubations sont réalisées pendant 2 h à 37° avec des concentrations de médicament pouvant aller de 0,0032 à 100 µg/ml. La croissance cellulaire est alors reprise après lavage, et les cellules sont comptées deux générations cellulaires plus tard. Le comptage est réalisé dans un hémocytomètre après remise en suspension des cellules. La cytotoxicité est évaluée comme étant la concentration de médicament inhibant de 50 % la croissance cellulaire (IC_{50}).

Mesure de l'incorporation des anthracyclines

Les cellules sont transplantées comme précédemment, mais de telle sorte que les incubations puissent être réalisées sur 2.10^6 cellules. Ces incubations ont été réalisées pendant des temps variables (15 min à 24 heures) avec une concentration fixe de 1 µg de médicament par ml de milieu. Les cellules sont récupérées à la fin de l'incubation, rapidement, afin d'éviter toute évolution ultérieure des concentrations intracellulaires. Les anthracyclines sont extraites après précipitation des protéines par le TCA (Noel et coll., 1978) et dosées par spectrofluorométrie à l'aide d'un appareil Jobin Yvon JY3 (470 mm pour l'excitation et 550 mm pour l'émission). Les protéines sont dosées dans le culot acido-insoluble.

Malades inclus dans les études pharmacocinétiques

Huit malades atteints d'une rechute de leucémie aiguë myéloblastique ont été traités par idarubicine intraveineuse à la dose de 7 à 9 mg/m² par jour pendant 5 jours consécutifs. Pour 4 d'entre eux, des prélèvements sanguins répétés ont été réalisés dans les 24 heures suivant la première injection ; pour les quatre autres, ces prélèvements ont été réalisés dans les 24 heures suivant la dernière injection, puis à intervalles de 24 h pendant 5 jours.

Six malades souffrant d'une tumeur solide au stade métastatique ont été traités par pirarubicine à la dose de 20 mg/m² par jour pendant 3 jours consécutifs. Des prélèvements sanguins répétés ont été réalisés au décours de chacune des injections, puis à intervalles de 24 h pendant 3 jours.

Dans tous les cas, le sang a été recueilli sur EDTA, centrifugé immédiatement, et le plasma congelé jusqu'au dosage.

Dosage des médicaments et de leurs métabolites

L'extraction a été réalisée sur des petites colonnes de silice greffée C18 (Sep-pak, Waters) selon une technique mise au point pour la doxorubicine (Robert, 1980). Le dosage a été réalisé par chromatographie liquide à haute performance avec détection fluorométrique selon une technique classique (Israel et coll., 1978). L'analyse mathématique a été réalisée selon une méthode non-lin permettant d'obtenir la décomposition de la courbe concentration = f (temps) en plusieurs exponentielles. Les métabolites ont été étudiés par une approche non modélisée permettant de calculer seulement la demi-vie d'élimination par régression linéaire et l'aire sous la courbe par la règle du trapèze.

RESULTATS ET DISCUSSION

Pharmacologie cellulaire

La cytotoxicité des deux nouvelles anthracyclines peut être comparée à celle des molécules de référence. Le tableau I montre que, dans les cellules sensibles, la pirarubicine est trois fois plus active que la doxorubicine, et l'idarubicine trois fois plus active que la daunorubicine. La résistance croisée des nouvelles anthracyclines avec les anciennes n'est que partielle, alors que la résistance croisée entre daunorubicine et doxorubicine est complète. Des résultats analogues avaient été obtenus séparément sur d'autres modèles, ce qui permet de généraliser l'observation (Arcamone et coll., 1976 ; Kunimoto et coll., 1983).

L'incorporation des nouvelles anthracyclines est plus importante que celle des molécules de référence dans les conditions usuelles d'incubation que nous avons choisies (2 h d'incubation avec une concentration de 1 µg/ml de milieu) ; cela est plus marqué pour les cellules résistantes que pour les cellules sensibles (Tableau I). Il est à noter que le rapport des incorporations dans les cellules sensibles et résistantes est très étroitement corrélé avec le rapport des IC50 : c'est un argument en faveur du rôle déterminant de la réduction de l'incorporation du médicament dans le mécanisme de la résistance.

La cinétique d'incorporation des nouvelles anthracyclines a été étudiée. Elle permet de déterminer par exemple le temps au bout duquel un plateau est atteint, ou, de façon plus précise, le pourcentage de ce plateau atteint au bout d'un temps déterminé, par exemple 30 minutes (Tableau I). Il apparaît que les nouvelles anthracyclines s'incorporent plus rapidement que les molécules de référence : pour la pirarubicine comme pour l'idarubicine, plus de 80 % de la valeur du plateau sont atteints en 30 min, contre 20 % pour la doxorubicine et 50 % pour la daunorubicine, qui sont donc d'incorporation plus lente. Cette incorporation plus rapide des nouvelles molécules a déjà été signalée sur des modèles différents (Kunimoto et coll., 1983 ; Munck et coll., 1985).

Tableau I. Principales caractéristiques de la pharmacologie cellulaire de la pirarubicine et de l'idarubicine comparées à celles de la doxorubicine et de la daunorubicine.

	doxorubicine	pirarubicine	daunorubicine	idarubicine
Cytotoxicité : IC50 (µg/ml)				
. cellules sensibles	0.076	0.025	0.028	0.010
. cellules résistantes	30	3.6	22	0.78
. facteur de résistance	400	140	800	80
Incorporation (2h, 1 µg/ml)				
. cellules sensibles	1.64	5.23	4.07	5.03
. cellules résistantes	0.15	1.12	0.24	3.05
. rapport d'incorporation	10.9	4.67	17.0	1.65
. cinétique d'incorporation (pourcentage de l'incorporation totale atteint en 30 min)	19	84	57	82

Pharmacocinétique

Les deux médicaments suivent une cinétique plasmatique obéissant à un modèle à deux compartiments, alors que la pharmacocinétique de la doxorubicine est plutôt décrite par un modèle à trois compartiments. La répétition des injections ne semble pas influencer de façon appréciable les paramètres cinétiques des médicaments inchangés. Le tableau II rassemble les principaux paramètres que nous avons calculés dans cette étude, ainsi que ceux obtenus pour la doxorubicine dans une étude antérieure (Robert et coll., 1987). Nous ne disposons pas de données personnelles sur la daunorubicine, et la littérature ne nous a fourni que peu de renseignements (Rahmann, 1984). Ce qui caractérise les nouvelles anthracyclines, c'est la disparition du pic de concentration très élevé que l'on observe après une injection en flash de doxorubicine, ainsi qu'un raccourcissement de la demi-vie d'élimination (12 à 18 heures au lieu de 30 à 40 heures). On observe également que les volumes de distribution de la pirarubicine et de l'idarubicine sont très élevés, ce qui suggère une fixation tissulaire importante. Il résulte de tout cela une clairance plasmatique totale double ou triple de celle de la doxorubicine prise comme référence.

Le métabolisme des deux anthracyclines étudiées est différent. L'idarubicine est à l'origine de l'idarubicinol, métabolite 13-dihydrogéné dont la concentration dépasse rapidement celle de l'idarubicine inchangée. Ce métabolite est actif dans les modèles *in vitro* (Casazza et coll., 1983) et il contribue certainement à l'activité clinique de l'idarubicine. Sa demi-vie prolongée entraîne son accumulation progressive dans le plasma, et sa concentration circulante est deux fois plus élevée après la cinquième injection d'idarubicine qu'après la première (Tableau III). La pirarubicine présente, elle aussi, un métabolite 13-dihydrogéné (pirarubicinol), mais tout à fait mineur. Elle est aussi capable de se transformer en doxorubicine, et ensuite en doxorubicinol. En raison de la demi-vie prolongée de ces derniers par rapport à celle de la pirarubicine, ils vont s'accumuler progressivement dans le plasma et, au décours de la troisième injection, c'est la doxorubicine qui est la principale espèce moléculaire circulante.

Tableau II. Principaux paramètres pharmacocinétiques des nouvelles anthracyclines

		doxorubicine (Robert et coll.,1987)	pirarubicine	daunorubicine (Rahmann et coll.,1984)	idarubicine
$A \times 10^3$	(L^{-1})	83.6 ± 6.2	3.24 ± 0.53	-	1.65 ± 0.26
$B \times 10^3$	(L^{-1})	0.873 ± 0.131	-	-	-
$C \times 10^4$	(L^{-1})	2.80 ± 0.28	3.71 ± 0.27	-	3.10 ± 0.23
α	(h^{-1})	9.76 ± 0.27	2.19 ± 0.20	7.70	2.62 ± 0.50
β	(h^{-1})	0.660 ± 0.109	-	0.20	-
$\gamma \times 10^2$	(h^{-1})	2.45 ± 0.22	5.78 ± 0.32	0.05	3.80 ± 0.54
P.Cl	$(L.h^{-1}/m^2)$	29.5 ± 1.8	90.4 ± 4.9	95	68.0 ± 9.2
Vd(ss)	(L/m^2)	801 ± 87	1449 ± 138	1297	1672 ± 114
MRT	(h)	28.2 ± 3.1	15.2 ± 1.1	-	28.5 ± 4.1

Tableau III. Métabolisme chez l'homme de la pirarubicine et de l'idarubicine

	Rapport des AUC métabolite/médicament	
	Première injection	Dernière injection
Métabolites de la pirarubicine		
pirarubicinol	0.223 ± 0.104	0.270 ± 0.118
doxorubicine	0.428 ± 0.052	0.780 ± 0.092
doxorubicinol	0.359 ± 0.055	0.633 ± 0.085
Métabolites de l'idarubicine		
idarubicinol	1.31 ± 0.22	3.50 ± 0.72
Métabolites de la doxorubicine		
doxorubicinol	0.327 ± 0.020	-
Métabolites de la daunorubicine		
daunorubicinol	3.9	-

CONCLUSION

Les deux nouvelles anthracyclines que nous avons étudiées, la pirarubicine et l'idarubicine, analogues respectivement de la doxorubicine et de la daunorubicine, présentent des analogies intéressantes sur le plan cellulaire : cytotoxicité élevée, résistance croisée faible, incorporation rapide et importante. Sur le plan pharmacocinétique, leur demi-vie brève et leur volume de distribution élevé les rapprochent mais la nature des métabolites formés les oppose.

REFERENCES BIBLIOGRAPHIQUES

Arcamone, F., Bernardi, L., Giardino, P., Di Marco, A., Casazza, A.M., Pratesi, G., Reggiani, P. (1976) : Synthesis and antitumor activity of 4-demethoxydaunorubicin, 4-demethoxy-7, α-diepidaunorubicin, and their βanswers. Cancer Treat. Rep. 60, 829-832.

Casazza, A.M., Barbieri, B., Fumagalli, A., Geroni, M.C. (1983) : Biologic activity of 4-demethoxy-13-dihydrodaunorubicin. Proc. Am. Assoc. Cancer Res. 24, 251.

Israel, M., Pegg, W.J., Wilkinson, P.M., Garnick, M.B. (1978) : Liquid chromatographic analysis of adriamycin and metabolites in biological fluids. J. Liquid Chromatogr. 1, 795-809.

Kunimoto, S., Miura, K., Takahashi, Y., Takeuchi, T., Umezawa, H. (1983) : Rapid uptake by cultured tumor cells and intracellular behavior of 4'-O-tetrahydropyranyladriamycin. J. Antibiot. 36, 312-317.

Munck, J.N., Fourcade, A., Bennoun, M., Tapiero, H. (1985) : Relationship between the intracellular level and growth inhibition of a new anthracycline, 4'-O-tetrahydropyranyladriamycin in Friend leukemia cells variants. Leuk. Res. 9, 289-296.

Noel, G., Peterson, C., Trouet, A., Tulkeres, P. (1978) : Uptake and subcellular localization of daunorubicin and adriamycin in cultured fibroblasts. Eur. J. Cancer 14, 363-368.

Rahman, A., Goodman, A., Foo, W., Harvey, J., Smith, F.P., Schein, P.S. (1984) : Clinical pharmacology of daunorubicin in phase I patients with solid tumors : development of an analytical methodology for daunorubicin and its metabolites. Semin. Oncol. 11, 36-44.

Robert, J. (1980) : Extraction of anthracyclines from biological fluids for HPLC evaluation. J. Liquid Chromatogr. 3, 1561-1572.

Robert, J., Bui, N.B., Vrignaud, P. (1987) : Pharmacokinetics of doxorubicin in sarcoma patients. Eur. J. Clin. Pharmacol. 31, 695-699.

Vrignaud, P., Londos-Gagliardi, D., Robert, J. (1986) : Cellular pharmacology of doxorubicin in sensitive and resistant rat glioblastoma cells in culture. Oncology 43, 60-66.

Résumé

Several new anthracyclines are currently developped in preclinical and clinical phase I and II studies. Among them, idarubicin (4-demethoxydaunorubicin) and pirarubicin (4'-O-tetrahydropyranyldoxorubicin) appear as very promising agents. We have studied the cellular pharmacology of these two drugs in a model of doxorubicin-sensitive and -resistant rat glioblastoma cells in culture. Both drugs were more efficient than the parent compounds in doxorubicin-sensitive cell killing and their cross-resistance with doxorubicin was only partial. Drug incorporation in the sensitive or resistant cells was higher for the new anthracyclines than for the original ones when exposed to the same drug extracellular concentrations, and the plateau concentrations were obtained earlier with the new compounds. As usual, resistant cells incorporated much less drug than sensitive ones. We have also studied the pharmacokinetics of both drugs in humans after daily repetitive i.v. administrations. Idarubicin was characterized by an important metabolism to an active 13-dihydroderivative, idarubicinol, similarly to the conversion of daunorubicin to daunorubicinol. Idarubicinol had a much longer elimination half-life than idarubicin (50 h vs 20 h) and progressively accumulated in plasma. Pirarubicin could be converted to doxorubicin. Due to the long elimination half-life of doxorubicin as compared to that of unchanged pirarubicin (30-40 h vs 16 h), doxorubicin progressively accumulated in plasma after the repetitive administrations of pirarubicin. Both new compounds were characterized by a high volume of distribution as compared to those of doxorubicin and daunorubicin, and by a rapid total plasmatic clearance. Similarly to all anthracyclines, they were mainly excreted through bile. In conclusion, these two new anthracyclines present several interesting features and share some pharmacologic characteristics which may be responsible for their clinical properties. Attention must be paid to the metabolism of these compounds, which is very different.

Neo-Adjuvant Chemotherapy. Ed. Cl. Jacquillat, M. Weil, D. Khayat. Colloque INSERM/John Libbey Eurotext Ltd. © 1988. Vol. 169, pp. 595-598.

Clinical application of the pharmacokinetic study of the nitrosourea fotemustine (S 10036)

F. Lokiec*, J. Santoni*, D. Khayat**, K. Beerblock*, J.P. Bizzari**, Cl. Jacquillat** and J. Rouëssé*

** Centre René Huguenin, 92211 Saint-Cloud; ** Hôpital Pitié Salpétrière, 75013 Paris, France*

MOTS CLEF

FOTEMUSTINE - PHARMACOKINETIC STUDIES - CLINICAL APPLICATION

INTRODUCTION

Diethyl 1- [3- (2 chloroethyl) -3-Nitrosoureïdo] ethyl phosphonate (Fotemustine, S 10036) is a nitrosourea entered into clinical trials due to its rationale in chemical design, optimal log P value and activity in the NCI panel screen (1). Despite intensive use of the nitrosourea compounds in clinical situations (2), pharmacokinetics of these drugs have not been extensively studied in regard to technical problems related to this class of compounds, especially their high instability in aqueous solutions, and plasma with a short half - life and difficulties in finding an appropriate and accurate assay method (3). Clinical development of Fotemustine was based on pharmacokinetic considerations. During the pharmacokinetic phase I study, we used the pharmacokinetic parameters to choose the optimal dose and the therapeutic regimen and during the phase II study, we tried to correlate the pharmacokinetic behaviour of Fotemustine with clinical response.

MATERIALS AND METHODS

Treatment plan. Fotemustine chemotherapy was administered over a one hour period by IV infusion in 5 % glucose. A weekly schedule of administration was selected with one administration every week for 3 to 4 consecutive weeks followed by a 4 to 5 weeks rest period. For the pharmacokinetic phase I study, on the basis of the clinical phase I trial (4), the starting dose was 100 mg/sqm.

Sampling Schedule. Pharmacokinetics were monitored for 3 hours following Fotemustine infusion. In all cases, at least 12 samples were collected : before infusion immediately afterwards and at 10, 20, 30 minutes post-infusion, and at 1, 1.5, 2, 3 hours afterwards. Blood samples (5 ml) were obtained through a indewelling cannula and collected into EDTA tubes. The tubes were immediately cooled and protected from light after collecting and plasma was separated by cold centrifugation (+ 4°C) at 3 000 rpm for 3 minutes.

Analytical method. Fotemustine was assayed by a HPLC method using Millipore, Waters apparatus. The drug was twice extracted from the plasma with 5 ml of cold diethyl ether, the organic phase was separated and evaporated to dryness. The residue was then dissolved in 200 µl of the mobile phase (methanol : perchloric acid 0.01 M 40 : 60 v/v). The mobile phase flow rate was 1 ml / minute and Fotemustine was UV detected at 254 nm. All the analytical steps were carried out at a low temperature (+ 4°C) and protected from light.

Calculation of Pharmacokinetic Parameters. The pharmacokinetic curves were constructed by the least square method. The analytical pharmacokinetic program had been written for a IBM 4341 computer, and we used a classic one or two open compartment model for Fotemustine.

Pharmacokinetic phase I study. During the pharmacokinetic phase I study, 8 patients suffering from various malignancies (colon : 2, head and neck : 1, breast : 1, lung : 1, brain tumor : 1, melanoma : 1, and unknown origin : 1 patient) were included. According to the treatment plan, 4 patients received 100 mg/sqm, 2 patients 125 mg/sqm and 2 patients 150 mg/sqm. A total of 9 courses were analyzed at a dose level of 100 mg/sqm, 8 courses at 125 mg/sqm and 4 courses at 150 mg/sqm.

Phase II study. Based on recommandations of the phase I study, 22 patients with various tumors (head and neck, renal carcinoma and melanoma) entered the study and a total of 83 pharmacokinetics were performed.

RESULTS

Main pharmacokinetic parameters of Fotemustine are characterized by short half life and by inter and intra individual variations.

Pharmacokinetic phase I study. During the pharmacokinetic phase I study, doses were escalated from 100 mg/sqm to 125 and 150 mg/sqm. Analysis of results of the first course are presented in table 1 and statistical analysis by Student's t test do not show any statistical significant effect on plasmatic clearance (p = 0.374), or AUC (p = 0.275), when increasing the doses.

Table 1.

STATISTICAL ANALYSIS ON AUC AND PLASMATIC CLEARANCE
AT DIFFERENT DOSE LEVEL (PHARMACOKINETIC PHASE I STUDY)

DOSE (mg/sqm)	Mean ± s.e.m.			STUDENT t TEST
	100	125	150	
Courses -	4	3	3	
AUC (µg/l × h)	5.1 ± 1.1	7.7 ± 0.01	4.5 ± 1.38	p = 0,275 NS
Plasmatic clearance (l/h)	36.7 ± 10.6	33.9 ± 2.4	62.9 ± 21.7	p = 0,374 NS

Phase II study. Using the 100 mg/sqm dosage and the weekly schedule of administration, 22 patients with various tumors (and especially head and neck, melanoma and kidney) were analyzed. Similar patient to patient variations were observed and especially concerning the systemic clearance as shown for example in table 2 (patient n°1) and 3 (patient n°2).

Table 2.

PHARMACOKINETIC PARAMETERS IN PATIENT NUMBER 1 (MELANOMA)

Course	C_0 (µg/ml)	$T_{1/2}$ (h)	AUC (µg/l x h)	Cl (l/h)	V_C (l)	V_{dss} (l)
1	3.14	0.30	1.36	110.12	47.74	18.64
2	5.10	0.23	1.74	86.27	29.36	9.46

Course	C_0 (µg/ml)	$T_{1/2}\,\alpha$ (h)	$T_{1/2}\,\beta$ (h)	AUC (µg/l x h)	Cl (l/h)	V_C (l)	V_{dss} (l)
3	6.13	0.16	2.66	6.88	21.77	24.46	62.37

Table 3.

PHARMACOKINETIC PARAMETERS IN PATIENT NUMBER 2 (HEAD AND NECK CARCINOMA)

Course	C_0 (µg/ml)	$T_{1/2}\,\alpha$ (h)	$T_{1/2}\,\beta$ (h)	AUC (µg/l x h)	Cl (l/h)	V_C (l)	V_{dss} (l)
1	19.9	0.16	1.45	6.52	24.83	8.14	13.39

Course	C_0 (µg/ml)	$T_{1/2}$ (h)	AUC (µg/l x h)	Cl (l/h)	V_C (l)	V_{dss} (l)
2	17.52	0.19	4.85	33.38	9.24	2.49
3	3.5	1.21	6.17	26.25	46.16	35.21

DISCUSSION

Even if great individual difference may be expected in patient with a disease causing metabolic alteration (even in the organs not directly involved), studies on nitrosourea compounds have always pointed out a large (greater than 10 fold sometimes) patient to patient variations.

Data reported in this study with Fotemustine show the same patient to patient variations and especially in regard to the clearance that in our study may vary from 110 l/h to 1 l/h, indicating substantial different patient to patient drug exposure.

The pharmacokinetic phase I study with a dose escalation of 1 to 1.5 ratio from the starting dose (150 mg/sqm compared to 100 mg/sqm) do not show any statistical change in AUC values despite the accuracy of statistical analysis due to the small number of patient. Moreover, since the patients treated with the same dose (100 mg/sqm) during the phase II study, present the same huge variations in AUC, its meaning has to be investigated.

Some explainations could involved "in vivo" serum breakdown of nitrosourea, body fat content and changes in the pattern of blood flow to body organs (5).

Our preliminary results need to be confirmed on larger series but point out a special attention in characteristics of the patient and of the tumor in analysing pharmacokinetic parameters, when intending to correlate these parameters with activity and/or toxicity.

REFERENCES

1 - Cudennec C.A., Lavielle G., Deloffre P., Bizzari J.P. (1987) : Pre-clinical antitumor activity of the new nitrosourea, Servier 10036. Proceeding 15th International Congress of Chemotherapy, pp 243

2 - Serrou B., Schein P.S., Imbach J.L. (1981) : Nitrosoureas in cancer treatment, Inserm symposium 19th

3 - Ames M.M., Powts G. (1983) : Pharmacokinetics of nitrosoureas, Pharmacokinetics of antitumor agents in humans

4 - Khayat D., Lokiec F., Bizzari J.P., Weil M., Meeus L., Sellami M., Rouesse J., Banzet P., Jacquillat C. (1987) : Phase I clinical study of the new amino acid-linked nitrosourea, S 10036, ministered on a weekly schedule. Cancer Research. 47, pp 6782-6785

5 - Levin V.A., Hoffman W., Weinkam R.J. (1978) : Pharmacokinetics of BCNU in man : a preliminary study of 20 patients. Cancer Treat. Rep. 62, pp 1305-1312

Résumé

Application clinique des études de pharmacocinétique de la nitrosourée Fotemustine (S 10036).
La Fotemustine (S 10036) est une nouvelle nitrosourée actuellement en essai clinique de Phase II dont le développement clinique a été axé sur l'approche pharmacocinétique. La Fotemustine est administrée en perfusion intraveineuse lente d'une durée d'une heure dans du glucosé à 5 %. La méthode de dosage utilisée est une méthode CLHP avec détection UV.
Au cours de la Phase I, les paramètres de pharmacocinétique ont été analysés afin de déterminer la dose et le meilleur schéma thérapeutique à adopter pour les études de Phase II. L'étude de Phase I pharmacocinétique a porté sur 8 patients et a permis d'apprécier les variations de ces paramètres en fonction des doses croissantes administrées, soit 100, 125 et 150 mg/m^2.
Les caractéristiques principales de la Fotemustine se traduisent par une demi-vie courte ainsi que par une grande variabilité inter et intra-indivuelle du C_0, de l'aire sous la courbe et de la clairance plasmatique.
En fonction des résultats obtenus au cours des essais cliniques de Phase I et de pharmacocinétique, le choix de 100 mg/m^2 a été retenu et les essais de Phase II ont été initiés dans différentes indications (cancer du rein, mélanome malin, cancer ORL). Les mêmes variations inter et intra-individuelles sont observées et plus particulièrement en ce qui concerne la clairance plasmatique.
La corrélation entre réponse clinique et paramètres pharmacocinétiques a été recherchée.

Neo-Adjuvant Chemotherapy. Ed. Cl. Jacquillat, M. Weil, D. Khayat. Colloque INSERM/John Libbey Eurotext Ltd. © 1988. Vol. 169, pp. 599-603.

Active 5-FU pharmacokinetics : evidence for improvement of the therapeutic index

G. Milano, A. Thyss, J. Santini, J. Vallicioni, M. Schneider and F. Demard

Centre Antoine-Lacassagne, 06054 Nice Cedex, France

ABSTRACT

This study describes the pharmacoclinical correlates for the widely used regimen of cisplatin plus continuous 5-day 5-FU as first-line chemotherapy of head and neck cancer, and the benefit of such data for real-time therapy management. Pharmacokinetic analysis of 177 cycles for 72 patients (group G1) revealed that both the time-concentration product (AUC) for the entire cycle and the half-cycle AUC (AUC D1-D3) were predictive of cycle toxicity. Real-time analysis of individual AUC D1-D3 values was used to decide whether to reduce the dose during the second half of the cycle for a total of 210 cycles (69 pts, group G2); the dose in the second half of the course was reduced in 40% of the G2 courses. There was no statistical difference in response rates between G1 and G2, but a statistically significant reduction was observed in the incidence of toxic cycles (≥ grade2) between G1 and G2 (G1 = 32% vs G2 = 13.5%; $p < 0.01$).

KEYWORDS

5-fluorouracil, pharmacokinetics, head and neck carcinoma, therapeutic index

INTRODUCTION

Chemotherapy by 5-fluorouracil (5-FU) tends to be used for disease sites other than the digestive tract, where its efficacy remains limited (Buroker, 1985). This is the case for head and neck carcinomas, where very high response rates have been observed when the drug is combined with cisplatinum (CDDP) (Thyss, 1986a; Amrein, 1985; Kish, 1982). This combination protocol is accompanied by a non-negligible percentage of toxic manifestations (Amrein, 1985) that are often acceptable but sometimes severe, depending on the dose (Merlano, 1987) or the specific site (Kies, 1987). One of the major objectives of clinical pharmacokinetics is to improve the therapeutic index on an individual basis. On a limited population of head and neck carcinoma patients treated by CDDP-5-FU, we previously showed that digestive and/or hematologic tolerance was linked to the degree of total body exposure to the drug during the cycle (C x T, area under curve, AUC) (Thyss, 1986b).

The present study extends and confirms this concept of a pharmacoclinical association on a larger population; in a second step, data obtained were used for a prospective study in an attempt to improve the therapeutic index.

SUBJECTS AND METHODS

The Subjects

The study population is described in Table I. These 146 patients with head and neck carcinoma treated at our institution between 1983 and 1987 were divided into two groups, G1 and G2. Group G1 corresponds to a retrospective pharmacoclinical study during which 5-FU blood concentrations were systematically measured for individual courses. Establishment of Group G1 allowed us to compare the distribution of pharmacokinetic parameters as a function of response and tolerance to treatment. Group G2 corresponds to patients entered in a prospective study based on the pharmacoclinical conclusions of the initial analyses of group G1data.

Chemotherapy Regimen

Treatment consisted of: Day 0: 6 hr hydration with 2 liters of 5% dextrose, NaCl 6 g/l, and KCl 3 g/l, followed by CDDP 100 mg/m2 1 mg/min iv in 0.5 liter normal saline with 0.25 liter 1.6% mannitol, and then 1 liter of 5% dextrose, NaCl 6 g/l and KCl 3 g/l. Days 1-5: 5-FU 1000 mg/m2/24 hr by continuous iv infusion with a controlled flow pump. The protocol called for three courses per patient every three weeks (D0 = D20).

Evaluation of Response and Toxicity

Before treatment, lesions were evaluated and biopsied during endoscopy under general anesthesia for all patients. Response was evaluated by the same physician by multiple biopsies obtained under identical conditions, 10 days after completion of the last chemotherapy course. Clinical response was defined using the product of two perpendicular lesion diameters. Complete response (CR) corresponded to disappearance of all clinically visible or palpable lesions; partial response (PR) was defined as tumor regression over 50%; no response (NR) corresponded to tumor regression of 50% or less, stable disease or progressive disease. For patients who underwent surgery after chemotherapy, the histologic response was evaluated by examination of the surgical specimen. Hematologic and digestive tract toxicities were evaluated using WHO criteria.

Pharmacokinetic analysis

Two blood samples were collected every day (8 am, 5 pm) during each 5-FU course. 5 ml of venous blood were obtained on EDTA tubes, and samples were immediately brought to the laboratory and centrifuged (10 min., 2500 rpm). Plasma was stored at -20°C until analyzed (within 1-3 days). For Group G2, the tubes corresponding to the first two days of 5-FU administration and the tube obtained at 8 am on the third day (first half of the 5-FU cycle) were grouped and immediately analyzed the same day to determine the half-cycle AUC (AUC D1-D3) and thus modify or not the second half-cycle 5-FU dose. A previously described HPLC technique (Christophidis, 1979) was used for 5-FU measurements. The limit of sensitivity was 5 ng/ml. AUC (product of concentration per time, area under curve) was calculated by the trapezoidal rule.

Statistics

Comparisons of distribution were made using Student's t-test. Threshold values were tested using the chi-square test.

TABLE I - STUDY POPULATION

	N° subjects	Mean age (yr) (range)	Males/females	Stage T1-T2	T3-T4	N° courses administered
TOTAL	146	61 (36-82)	124/22	40%	60%	387
G1	77	61 (36-82)	67/10	28%	73%	177
G2	69	61 (42-79)	57/12	52%	48%	210

RESULTS

Figure 1 shows the respective distribution of individual 5-FU AUC values for all Group G1 courses with respect to toxic and nontoxic courses. Comparisons were made for total course AUC (AUC D1-D5) and first half-course AUC (AUC D1-D3). In both cases, the distributions were significantly different between toxic and nontoxic courses.We identified a threshold AUC D1-D3 value of 15,000 ng/ml/hr that predicted cycle toxicity (chi-square = 39.8, $p < 0.001$). Over 30,000 ng/ml/hr, 13 of 14 courses were toxic. It was decided to used these AUC data to establish a nomograph (Fig. 2) for treatment monitoring in a prospective study group, G2.

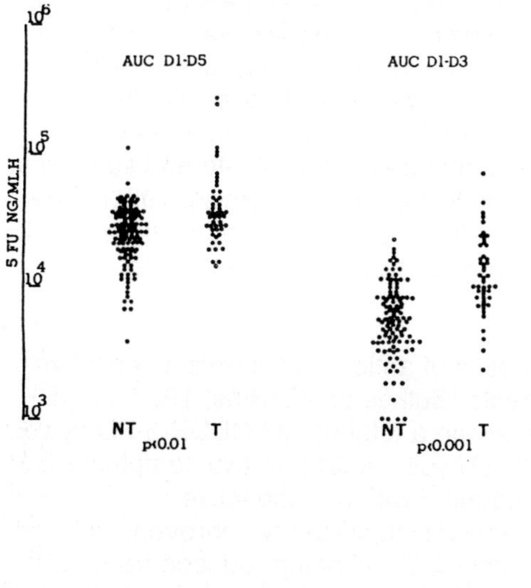

Figure 1: 5-FU AUC distribution in group G1 for toxic (T) and nontoxic courses (NT)

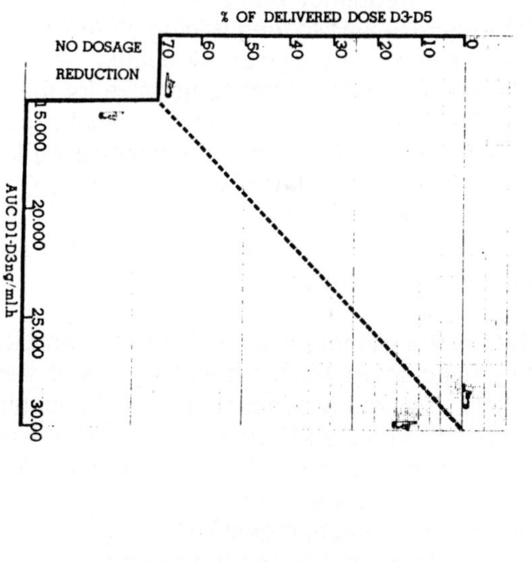

Figure 2: Nomogram for 5-FU dose adjustment during the 2nd half of the course as a function of 5-FU AUC D1-D3

Table II shows the respective treatment responses and toxicity rates in groups G1 and G2. Moderate and severe toxicity (≥ grade 2) were reduced from 32% (G1) to 13.5% (group G2), $p < 0.01$. These results were significant for grade 2 but not for grades 3 and 4 because of the small size of this second set of patients. The dose in the second half of the course was reduced in 40% of cycles; most 5-FU reductions were between 30% and 50% of the scheduled dose for days 3-5. Responses were comparable between the two groups, with even a higher response rate for G2 than for G1.

TABLE II - COMPARISON OF TOXICITY AND RESPONSE IN G1 AND G2

	% toxic cycles			% response to therapy			
	Grade 2	Grades 3,4	Grades 2,3,4	NR	PR	CR	PR + CR
G1	23	9	32	19	50	31	81
G2	7	6.5	13.5	13	39	45	84
Comparison	p<0.01	NS	p<0.01	NS	NS	NS	NS

DISCUSSION

Multiple-drug chemotherapy using CDDP and 5-FU is one of the most efficient first-line therapeutic approaches for advanced head and neck carcinomas. While treatment tolerance is usually acceptable, a non-negligible incidence of toxicity has been reported (Merlano, 1987; Amrein, 1985). In this combination regimen, continuous 5-FU administration (Amrein, 1985) has improved hematologic tolerance in comparison to bolus injections (Merlano, 1987). Stomatitis remains the major toxicity with continuous 5-FU; the frequency was 21% in 131 treatment cycles reported by Amrein et al. (1985). Toxicity may lead to lengthening of the interval between cycles as well as reduction of the total number of cycles scheduled. In both cases, the dose intensity is reduced; theoreticall, this might be pejorative for the optimal cytotoxic activity of a phase-specific drug such as 5-FU. Effectively, clinical experience has shown that the number of CDDP-5-FU cycles is of prime importance for the complete response rate and survival in advanced head and neck cancer (Rooney, 1984). In these patients (Thyss, 1986a), we previously found that the clinical response to CDDP-5-FU is a major prognostic factor. It is thus important not to shorten the chemotherapy program because of excessive unanticipated toxicity.

One of the ultimate goals of clinical pharmacokinetics of anticancer agents is effective improvement of the therapeutic index of treatments (Sulkes and Collins, 1987; Allen, 1983). This study conducted on 146 patients receiving a total of 387 CDDP-5-FU cycles attains this goal and confirms our previous results (Thyss, 1986b). In two complementary steps, a retrospective pharmacokinetic analysis coupled with a prospective pharmacoclinical application, tolerance to treatment was significantly improved, with hematologic and/or digestive tract toxicity attributable to 5-FU being reduced from 32% to 13.5%. This emphasizes the value of drug AUC as one of the best pharmacokinetic parameters for predicting pharmacodynamic events (Powis, 1985). HPLC is now widely used in most clinical biochemistry laboratories, and 5-FU analysis can thus easily be performed on a routine basis to monitor treatment.

Although dose reduction was possible in 40% of G2 cycles, response rates were comparable to those in G1, with an even higher response in G2 (64%) than in G1 (21%). Although this may be due to the lower percentage of elevated tumoral stages in G2, this could also be due to better acceptability of treatment in G2 owing to less toxicity.

REFERENCES

Allen L.M. (1983)): Pharmacokinetic principles of antineoplastic drug therapy. J. Clin. Pharmacol. 23, 71-81.

Amrein P.C., Weitzman S.A. (1985): Treatment of squamous-cell carcinoma of the head and neck with cisplatin and 5-fluorouracil. J. Clin. Oncol. 12: 1632-1639

Buroker T.R., Moertel G.G., Fleming T.R. et al. (1985): A controlled evaluation of recent approaches to biochemical modulation or enhancement of 5-fluorouracil therapy in colorectal carcinoma. J. Clin. Oncol. 12: 1624-2631.

Christophidis N., Mihaly G., Vajda F., Louis W. (1979): Comparison of liquid- and gas-liquid chromatographic assays of 5-fluorouracil in plasma. Clin. Chem. 25: 83-87.

Kies M, Rosen S.T., Tsang T.K., Shetty R. et al. (1987): Cisplatin and 5-fluorouracil in the primary management of squamous esophageal cancer. Cancer 60: 2156-2160

Kish J., Drelichman A., Jacobs J., Hoschner J. et al. (1982): Clinical trial of cisplatin and 5-FU infusion as initial treatment for advanced squamous cell carcinoma of the head and neck. Cancer Treat. Rep. 66: 471-474.

Merlano M., Grimaldi A., Brunetti I, Modenesi M. et al. (1987): Simultaneous cisplatin and 5-fluorouracil as second-line treatment of head and neck cancer. Cancer Treat. Rep. 71: 485-488.

Powis G. (1985): Anticancer drug pharmacodynamics. Cancer Chemother. Pharmacol. 14: 177-183.

Rooney M., Kish J., Jacobs J., Kinzie J. et al. (1984): Improved complete response rate and survival in advanced head and neck cancer after three-course induction therapy with 120-hour 5-FU infusion and cisplatin. Cancer 55: 1123-1128.

Sulkes A. and Collins J.M. (1987): Reappraisal of some dosage adjustment guidelines. Cancer Treat. Rep. 71: 229-233

Thyss A., Schneider M., Santini J., Caldani C., Vallicioni J., Chauvel P. and Demard F. (1986,a): Induction chemotherapoy with cisplatinum and 5-fluorouracil for squamous cell carcinoma of the head and neck. Brit. J. Cancer 54: 755-760.

Thyss A., Milano G., Renée N., Vallicioni J., Schneider M. and Demard F. (1986,b): Clinical pharmacokinetic study of 5-FU in continuous 5-day infusions for head and neck cancer. Cancer Chemother. Pharmacol. 16: 64-66.

Résumé

Cette étude décrit les corrélations pharmacocliniques observées lors de l'administration du protocole cisplatin-5-FU continu sur 5 jours en première ligne thérapeutique à des cancers ORL et l'utilisation de ces données pour l'optimisation du traitement en temps réel. L'analyse pharmacocinétique de 177 cycles (72 patients, groupe G1) a montré qu'à la fois le produit de la concentration par le temps (AUC) pour tout le cycle et pour la moitié du cycle (AUC J1-J3) étaient prédictifs de la toxicité liée au cycle. Les valeurs individuelles de l'AUC J1-J3 ont été utilisés en temps réel pour décider ou non d'une réduction de dose dans la deuxième moitié du cycle. Ceci a été appliqué à 210 cycles (69 patients, groupe G2). La dose de la deuxième moitié de cycle a été réduite dans 40% des cas. Il n'y avait pas de différence significative dans la réponse entre G1 et G2. Par contre, on a observé une réduction significative dans l'incidence des cycles toxiques ($\geq$ grade 2) entre G1 et G2 (G1 = 32% vs G2 = 13.5%, $p < 0.01$).

Neo-Adjuvant Chemotherapy. Ed. Cl. Jacquillat, M. Weil, D. Khayat. Colloque INSERM/John Libbey Eurotext Ltd. © 1988. Vol. 169, pp. 605-609.

Pharmacokinetic and resistance to anthracyclines in living cells studied by microspectrofluorometry

Michel Manfait[1], Teddy Rasoanaivo[1], Jean-Marc Millot[1], Jean-François Angiboust[1] and Mauro Gigli[2]

[1] *Laboratoire de Spectroscopie Biomoléculaire, UER de Pharmacie, 51096 Reims Cedex, France.*
[2] *Farmitalia Carlo Erba S.p.A., R. and S., Chimica Analitica, Milano, Italia*

ABSTRACT

The anthracycline (adriamycin ADM and/or aclacinomycin ACM) - DNA association has been studied by quantitative microspectrofluorometry. This non destructive analysis technique expanded within one living cell, owing to spatial localization from micro-volume (10 μm^3), enables us to obtain fluorescence emission spectra from an anticancer drug localized in the nucleus. Fluorescence spectra have been analysed in terms of difference in spectral shape and fluorescence yield between free, DNA-bound drugs and metabolites. The contribution of each spectral component to the total signal was calculated by least squares linear regression with an error of less than 10 %.

Kinetic studies of drug accumulation in the nucleus were performed as a function of time and of drug concentration into the culture medium. When, sensitive and resistant cells were exposed to several corresponding growth inhibitive doses, the nuclear drug concentration witch resulted was pratically the same, indicating a direct correlation between the biological effect and the drug amount actually present in the nucleus. On the other hand, resistant cells incubated with the ADM-ACM association show an ADM nucleic concentration equivalent to the one measured in sensitive cells.

This new method presents interesting advantages over other current techniques of uptake determination. Information is directly obtained in a non destructive way, avoiding expensive and, not always available, 14 C - labelled drugs.

INTRODUCTION

It is obvious that in a cancer chemotherapy and more specifically the one concerning the use of anthracycline antitumor agents, there is no systematic connection between the plasma concentration or even the drug incorporation into the tumor cell nor its therapeutic efficiency. Then in this case only a study of subcellular pharmacokinetic and quantitative ditribution of the drug, performed on the living cell, will be representative of any incorporation of drugs as well as the performance to pharmacological target. The knowledge of the nucleus-cytoplasm distribution and drug-target interactions will allow a better understanding of the anthracycline effectiveness and the cellular resistance to these drugs. Compared to the usual techniques (HPLC (Fourcade, 1982), flow cytophotometry (Tapiero, 1982), and radio labelling compounds), the microspectrofluorometry, a non destructive methodology (Ginot, 1984 ; Manfait, 1988), allows the quantitative analysis from an isolated living cell of drug incorporation within the nucleus and/or cytoplasm, and the formation of metabolites. Then, it also defines the nature of the interaction between the drug and its pharmacological target leading to the required therapeutic efficiency.

MATERIELS AND METHODS

Instrumentation

A microspectrofluorometer was composed from a conventional optical microscope coupled to a spectrograph with a multichannel detector. Fluorescence data acquisition as well as their mathematical treatments were performed by a computer. The microscope objective focused the laser beam on a subcellular fraction and collected the fluorescence emission which was analyzed by the spectrograph. Cells were observed in physiological buffer through a 100 X water immersion objective, in conditions not altering the cell viability (laser power 4 µW, acquisition time ca. 0.1 sec). The diameter laser spot (2 µm) and the deep field (5 to 10 µm) allowed the analysis of a constant (20 μm^3) volume of the sample.

Drugs and cells

Adriamycin hydrochloride (ADM) and aclacinomycin (ACM) were kindly supplied by Farmitalia Carlo-Erba S.p.a., Milan, Italy and Roger Bellon Laboratoires, Paris, France respectively. Drug concentration in PBS solution was determined spectrophotometrically at 480 and 435 nm.

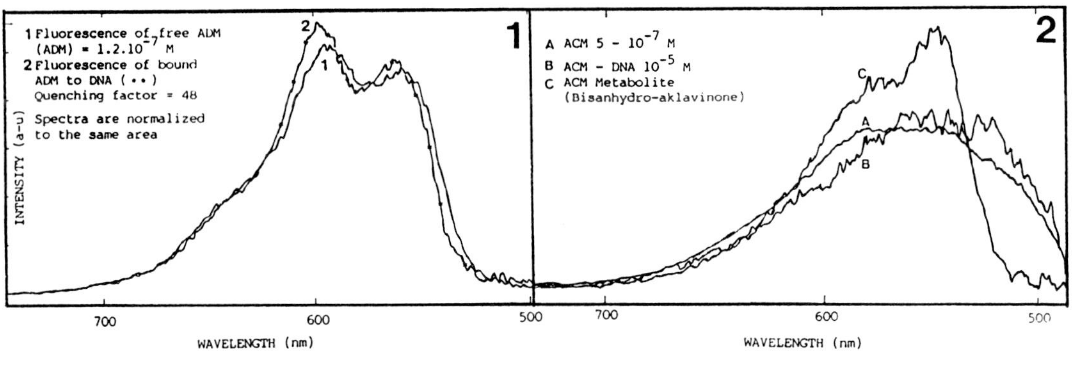

Figure 1 : Fluorescence emission spectra of free (1) and DNA-bound ADM (2) in PBS solution.
Figure 2 : Fluorescence emission spectra of free (A), DNA-bound ACM (B) and ACM metabolite (C) in PBS solution.

RESULTS AND DISCUSSION

Fluorescence emission spectra of free and DNA - bound drug in solution

Figure 1 gives the fluorescence emission spectra of both free ADM and bound ADM to calf thymus DNA after normalization to the same integrated area. The ratio I(free)/I(bound) corresponding to the quenching factor is found to be 48. In figure 2 are given three experimental spectra which will be used in the quantitative analysis of an intranuclear ACM spectrum. These profiles correspond to those of free ACM, DNA-bound ACM (quenching factor = 200), (Du Vernay, 1978) and the major fluorescent metabolite (bisanhydro-aklavinone).

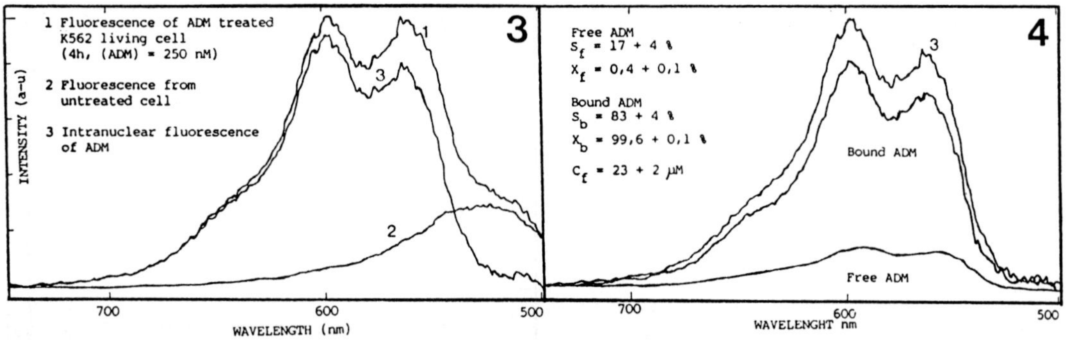

Figure 3 : Fluorescence emission spectrum from ADM-treated cell nucleus (1) from untreated nucleus (2) ; subtracted ADM spectrum (3).
Figure 4 : Quantitative analysis of ADM emission spectrum from a K562 cell nucleus in terms of free and DNA-bound ADM contributions.

Quantitative analysis of the adriamycin uptake in K562 living cell nuclei

A quantitative study (Gigli, 1988) allows to determine the ADM concentration in the nucleus of a living K562 tumor cell isolated from a human erythroleukaemia (figures 3 and 4). Figure 3-1 shows the fluorescence spectrum in the nucleus of a cell treated for 4 hours with ADM (250 nM). The intrinsic fluorescence of an untreated cell is given by figure 3-2. By least squares linear regression, a procedure on a computer evaluates this spectral contribution to the total fluorescence of a treated cell nucleus and gives by subtraction the intranuclear ADM fluorescence emission spectrum (figure 3-3). Simultaneously, this spectrum (figure 4) is analyzed according to free and bound drug components (taking into account their fluorescence quantum yield). From the area fractions (intensity according to a given concentration) and fluorescence yields of free and bound drug contributions, one can determine the drug molar fractions (free and bound) and the whole ADM concentration in the nucleus with an error less than 10 %. Here, nuclei of treated cells (4 hours, 250 nM ADM) point out an ADM concentration of too higher magnitude of order, than the extracellular medium. Moreover, the drug appears mainly bound to DNA (99.6%).

As an example, a kinetic study of ADM intranuclear as a fonction of time, or extracellular ADM concentration in sensitive and resistant cells, is reported in figure 5. Sizeable difference between drug uptake in nuclei of sensitive cells and resistant cells is apparent at any incubation conditions. After a 4 hour incubation, the ADM concentration in sensitive cell nuclei is 6 times higher than the one measured in resistant cell nuclei.

Relationship between cell growth inhibition and ADM nuclear concentration

Figure 6 shows the inhibition curves for sensitive and resistant K562 cell strains versus the extracellular ADM concentration. A quantitative analysis points out that to a given growth inhibition (90, 70, 50, 20%), the sensitive and resistant cells reveal the same nuclear ADM concentration . This important result shows that in a given growth inhibition, sensitive and resistant cells require the same ADM nuclear concentration (figure 7). This relationship confirms DNA as a potential target of this anthracycline.

Adriamycin-aclacinomycin association

ADM intranuclear incorporation in K562 sensitive and resistant cells incubated in the presence of ADM-ACM association has been determined as a fonction of ACM in various concentrations (figure 8). Whatever the extracellular concentration of ACM, sensitive cells exhibit the same ADM intranuclear incorporation. In similar conditions, K562 resistant cells show an increase of ADM intranuclear concentration correlated with ACM doses in the culture medium.

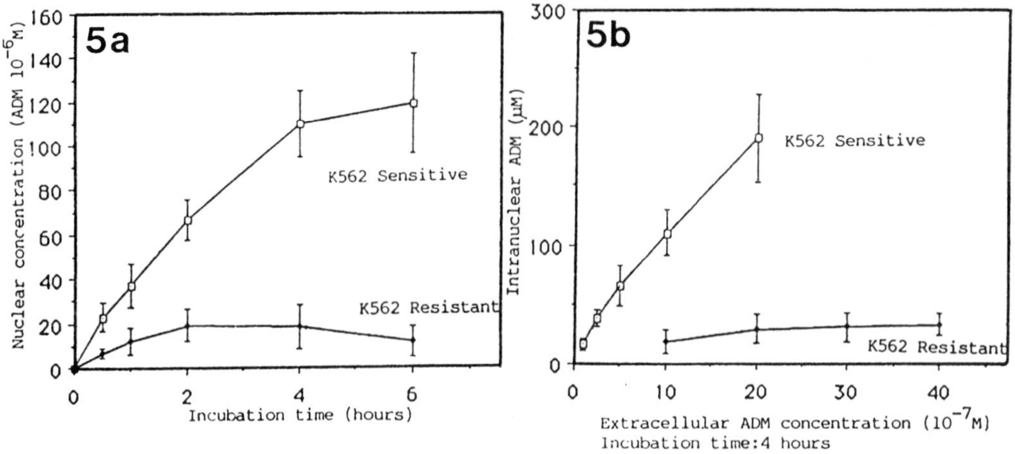

Figure 5 : Kinetic of ADM uptake into the cell nucleus as a function of incubation time, initial drug conc. in the medium 1 µM (A) or as a function of ADM conc. (B).

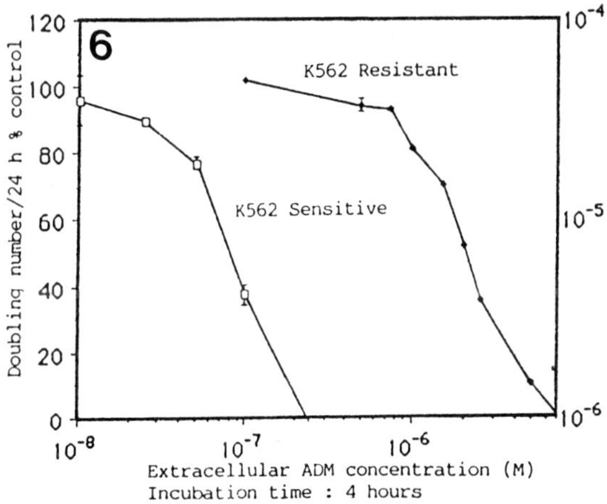

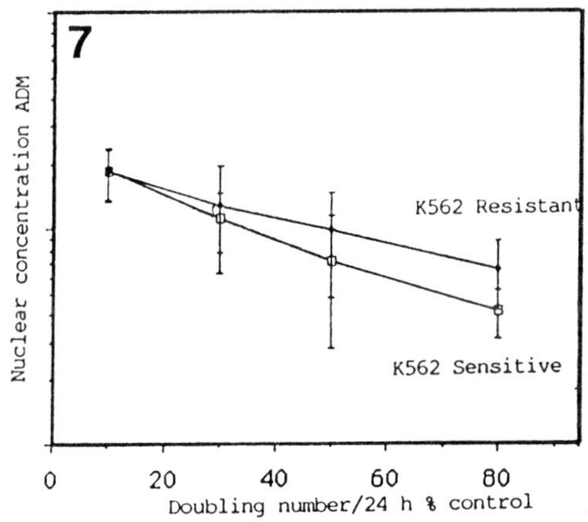

Figure 6 : Growth inhibition by ADM in sensitive and resistant K562 cells.
Figure 7 : Relationship : ADM uptake in the nucleus and growth inhibition.

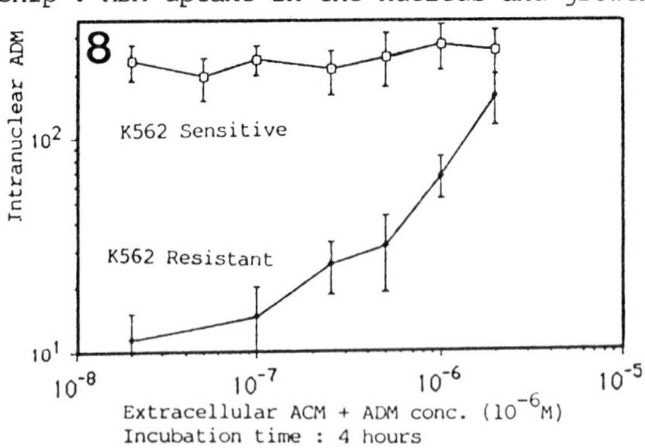

Figure 8 : Intranuclear ADM uptake in sensitive and resistant K562 cells as a function of ACM conc. in the medium in presence of a constant ADM conc.

CONCLUSION

The laser microspectrofluorometry is a noticeable experimental technique suited for the recording within cellular micro-volumes of fluorescent molecules of emission spectra.
This technique offers many other advantages over destructive methods based on the study of anthracycline incorporation in cells.

REFERENCES

Du Vernay V.H., Patcher J.A., Crooke S.T. (1978) : Deoxyribonucleic acid binding studies on several new anthracycline antitumor antibiotics. Sequence preference and structure-activity relationships of Marcellomycin and its analogues as compared to Adriamycin. Biochimestry, 18, 4024-4030.

Fourcade A., Fahri J.J., Bennoum M., Goldschmidt E., Tapiero H. (1982) : Rate of Aclacinomycin A and its metabolites effect on cell growth and macromolecular synthesis. Biochem. Pharmac., 1819-1824.

Gigli M., Doglia S.M., Millot J.-M., Valentini L., Manfait M. (1988) : Quantitative study of doxorubicin in living cell nuclei by microspectrofluorometry. Biochim. Biophys. Acta. in press.

Ginot L., Jeannesson P., Angiboust J.-F., Jardillier J.-C., Manfait M. (1984) : Interaction of Adriamycin in sensitive and resistant leucemic cells : a comparative study by microspectrofluorometry. Studia Biophysica, 104, 145-153.

Manfait M., Gigli M., Millot J.-M., Rasoanaivo T., Amirand C., Nocentini S., Turpin P.-Y., Vigny P., Doglia S.M. (1988) : New perspectives of microspectrofluorometry on living cells. In Spectroscopy of Biological Molecules Vol. 2, ed E.D. Schmid, Chichester : John Wiley & Sons.

Tapiero H., Fourcade A., Vaigot P., Farhi J.J. (1982) : Comparative uptake of adriamycin and daunorubicin in sensitive and resistant friend leukemia cells measured by flow cytometry. Cytometry 2, 298-302.

Résumé

La microspectrofluorimétrie laser développée à l'échelle de la cellule vivante isolée, grâce à la localisation spatiale du microvolume analysé, permet de déterminer, dans des conditions non léthales, les concentrations subcellulaires absolues d'anticancéreux du groupe des anthracyclines. Un spectre de fluorescence obtenu dans un noyau cellulaire est analysé en termes de contributions spectrales du médicament sous la forme libre et liée à la cible nucléaire . la pharmacologie de l'incorporation d'ADM dans les noyaux de cellules K562 sensibles et résistantes met en évidence des concentrations 6 fois supérieures dans le noyau des cellules sensibles. Pour une inhibition de croissance identique ces concentrations sont sensiblement les mêmes pour les deux types de cellules. Dans le cas d'une association ADM-ACM les cellules résistantes présentent une incorporation intranucléaire en ADM proche de celle observée dans les cellules sensibles.

Statistics

Statistiques

Neo-Adjuvant Chemotherapy. Ed. Cl. Jacquillat, M. Weil, D. Khayat. Colloque INSERM/John Libbey Eurotext Ltd. © 1988. Vol. 169, pp. 613-620.

Applications of predictions of prognosis in a clinical trial in acute leukemia

E.A. Gehan, M.J. Keating and E.J. Freireich

University of Texas, System Cancer Center, Houston, Texas, USA

ABSTRACT

A Bayesian analysis was performed of a clinical trial of AMSA-OAP in previously untreated patients with acute leukemia reported by Keating et al (1987). The trial was conducted in three stages and posterior probabilities were calculated at each stage that the treatments (AMSA-OAP versus AD-OAP) are equally preferred or that AD-OAP was preferred. Retrospective justification was provided for the changes in the design of the trial that were made based on frequentist analyses. The Bayesian approach is contrasted with the frequentist approach to the analysis of the results from this study and the implications discussed for the conduct of clinical trials.

KEY WORDS

Predictions of prognosis; clinical trial in acute leukemia; Bayesian analysis

INTRODUCTION

A clinical trial of AMSA-OAP in previously untreated patients with acute leukemia was reported by Keating, Freireich, et al (1987). This clinical trial involved an innovative strategy for the assignment of patients to treatment. Patients were assigned to treatment based upon predicted probabilities of complete remission (PPR values) derived using six prognostic factors. Patients with unfavorable prognosis received AMSA-OAP for remission induction and patients with favorable prognosis received AD-OAP. A further aspect of the study was that as the new treatment was found to be promising in patients with unfavorable prognosis, it was administered to patients with a more favorable prognosis.

The clinical trial of AMSA-OAP proceeded in three stages, each with expanded criteria for administration of AMSA-OAP so that ultimately all patients in the third stage received AMSA-OAP.

A historical control group of 325 patients was available who received AD-OAP from 1973 to 1977 and the complete remission rate in these patients was 61%. A logistic regression model was derived from an analysis of these patients which enabled predictions to be made of the probability of complete remission based on age, antecedent hematologic disorder, temperature status, BUN value, hemoglobin, and liver size. In the analysis, patients in the current study were paired with those from the historical control group for the evaluation of a possible improvement in complete remission rate. So the primary analysis was based on the differences between pairmates in the AMSA-OAP study and those receiving AD-OAP in the historical control group.

In this paper, our objective is to describe a Bayesian approach to the analysis of the results from this study, to contrast it with the frequentist (P-value) approach and to discuss briefly the implications of the Bayesian approach for the conduct of clinical trials.

CONTRAST BETWEEN CLASSICAL (FREQUENTIST) APPROACH AND BAYESIAN APPROACH

Table 1 summarizes the main points in comparing the frequentist and Bayesian approaches. The classical approach uses P-values which give the probability of the observed data or more discrepant data, assuming a null hypothesis is true. If P is less than .05, one ordinarily doubts the null hypothesis and concludes that there is some real difference between the treatments. The calculation of P-values depends upon the data observed and also data not observed, (i.e. the more discrepant data) and also on experiments done or not done.

In contrast, the Bayesian approach uses posterior probabilities of hypotheses (such as the posterior probability that Treatment A is better than B), given the observed data and prior information. In the Bayesian approach, results depend only on data observed and experiments done.

The classical approach uses prior information generally in the planning of studies. In the Bayesian approach, prior information is used explicitly in the calculation of posterior probabilities.

In the classical approach, analyses are tied very closely to the actual design of the study, so that account must be taken of interim analyses performed while the study is in progress. For example, it has been demonstrated that if interim analyses of studies are performed at a significance level of P=.05, the overall significance level at the end of the study is much greater than P=.05. In contrast, a Bayesian can carry out an analysis and calculate posterior probabilities at any time during conduct of the study.

Finally, the Bayesian approach is conditional based upon the likelihood of the current data and the prior information. The classical approach is unconditional involving averaging over data that might have been obtained but was not or experiments that might have been performed but were not.

CLINICAL TRIAL OF AMSA-OAP

Treatment was determined in the clinical trial of patients with acute leukemia based upon the predicted probabilities of response from the historical control data; a patient received either AMSA-OAP or AD-OAP in the current study. For example, if the predicted probability of remission was less than .4, it was considered ethical to administer a new treatment (AMSA-OAP). In the initial stage of the trial, 21 patients received this treatment and the complete remission rate was 43%. This may be compared with the 18% expected complete remission rate, if these patients had been treated with AD-OAP.

Favorable patients, that is those with PPR values $\geq$.4, received AD-OAP. In the initial stage of the trial, 63 patients received AD-OAP, the CR rate was 70% and this may be contrasted with the 75% CR rate to be expected if treatment was given with AD-OAP.

A clinical evaluation was made of these data and a decision taken to expand the criteria for administration of AMSA-OAP. There were three stages in the conduct of the clinical trial of AMSA-OAP. As the CR rate with AMSA-OAP continued favorable in the second stage of the trial, ultimately all patients received AMSA-OAP in the third stage of the study.

ANALYSIS OF THE STUDY

The analyses of the study reported by Keating et al (1987) were based upon the frequentist approach and certain criticisms of this analysis can be made. Table 2 shows that basically the analyses involved paired data by subgroup into AMSA-OAP unfavorable, AMSA-OAP favorable, and AD-OAP favorable subgroups. All together, there were 242 pairs of patients entered into study, 108 receiving AD-OAP and 133 receiving AMSA-OAP. The historical control group consisted of 325 patients who received AD-OAP.

The criticisms are as follows: the P-values calculated and reported assumed that it was a fixed sample size study, rather than one which was conducted in three stages with changing criteria for administration of AMSA-OAP. No account was taken of the sequential conduct of the study. Finally, the decisions about expanding criteria were based mostly on the clinical evidence accumulating in each stage of study and were not based upon rigid statistical criteria.

BAYESIAN ANALYSIS OF CLINICAL TRIAL

I would like now to describe a Bayesian approach to the analysis of these data, which may be used in the calculation of posterior probabilities relating to the relative effectiveness of the treatments and these probabilities may be calculated at each stage of the trial.

The setup is given in Table 3: let θ be the proportion of pairs of patients in which AMSA-OAP is preferred to AD-OAP. This would occur if the patient receiving AMSA-OAP had a response and the paired patient from the historical control group did not respond. A preference would be recorded for AD-OAP if that patient had a complete remission, while the patient receiving AMSA-OAP was a non-responder. There would be no preference between the treatments if either both patients responded or did not respond.

Next, p is the prior probability that the two treatments are equal in effectiveness. Cornfield (1966) utilized this approach in a Bayesian analysis of sequential clinical trials.

At any point during the conduct of the study, n_A and n_B are the number of preferences available for A and B respectively. In this Bayesian analysis, two probabilities will be calculated that have been used by Berry (1987) in of clinical trials. The first is the current probability that the treatments are equally preferred, which may be characterized as the probability that $\theta = 1/2$, given the current data concerning the number of preferences. An expression for this is given in Table 3.

Secondly, assuming a uniform prior information on θ in the interval 0 to 1, one can calculate the probability that $\theta < 1/2$, which gives the current probability that AD-OAP is preferred. Clearly, if this probability becomes very small, say less than .05, this provides strong evidence that there is only a very low probability that AD-OAP is preferred and that therefore there would be a preference for AMSA-OAP.

At the end of the first stage of the trial, the results are given in Table 4. For the AMSA-OAP patients, there were 21 pairs of patients and 12 in which a preference could be recorded. There were 9 preferences for AMSA-OAP and 3 for AD-OAP. The current probability that $\theta = 1/2$ is .41, a relatively low value and the current probability that AD-OAP would be preferred is .07. If one calculated a standard P-value at this point, one would obtain P=.15. Consequently, based upon nearly statistically significant evidence that AMSA-OAP was better than AD-OAP, there was some rationale for expanding the criteria for administering AMSA-OAP from PPR $>$.40 up to PPR$<$.60.

At the bottom of Table 4, results are given in the favorable group of patients who received AD-OAP. In the 63 pairs of patients, preferences could be reported among 28, 13 for AD-OAP and 15 for AD-OAP in the historical control study. Note that the complete remission rates were nearly identical for the two groups of patients, being 70 and 71%.

A Bayesian calculation of the current probability that $\theta = 1/2$ was equal to .81 and there was little evidence that AD-OAP was the preferred treatment, the posterior probability being .57. The standard frequentist P-value at this point was .85, again suggesting no real difference between the two treatments.

A summary of the data from the three stages of the trial is given in Table 5. At the top, the data for the AMSA-OAP unfavorable patients are given. Note that at the end of the third stage of the trial, 50 patients had been entered and preferences could be determined in 24 pairs of patients. Complete remission rates were 43% in the first stage of the trial and ended at 38% after Stage III. Complete remission rate in the paired patients receiving AD-OAP was only 14% in Stage I, but had increased to 22% at the end of Stage III. The Bayesian posterior probability that Treatment B or AD-OAP was better was .07 at the end of Stage I, .05 at the end of Stage II, and remained at .05 at the end of Stage III. Consequently, the probability that AD-OAP was the preferred treatment was relatively low and a Bayesian statistician could support the conclusion for preferring AMSA-OAP based upon these data. Note that the standard P-value was only .15 at the end of the third stage of the study, a non-significant difference between the treatments.

In the patients with intermediate prognosis, that is between PPR of .40 and .60, a total of 41 pairs of patients were entered and preferences could be recorded in 19 pairs. The complete remission rate from AMSA-OAP was 56% at the end of Stage III compared to 44% in the paired patients receiving AD-OAP. The Bayesian probability of no preference between the treatments was .66 and the probability that AD-OAP was preferred was .12. The P-value of .36 at the end of Stage III suggested no significant difference between treatments. Consequently, data for patients with intermediate prognosis provides no strong of a preference for AMSA-OAP relative to AD-OAP; in fact there is moderate evidence of the approximate equivalence of the therapies in this group of patients.

Among patients receiving AD-OAP, ultimately there were 108 patients who received AD-OAP, preferences could be recorded in 45 pairs of patients and the complete remission rate was 73% for AD-OAP compared with 71% in the patients in the historical control group. Note from Table 5 that at the end of Stage II, the probability that $\theta = 1/2$ was equal to .84, quite strong evidence of the equivalence in response rates between these two treatments.

A key point is that the Bayesian probabilities can be calculated after each successive pair of patients or at each stage of the trial, without any consideration that these were interim analyses. On the other hand, the P-values should take into account that they were being performed on an interim basis. Of course, in the planning stage of the trial, one should have some idea of what types of Bayesian probabilities would lead one to change the design of the study, should they be observed. In this particular study, in the AMSA-OAP administered to unfavorable patients, there was moderately strong evidence even at the end of Stage II that AMSA-OAP was the preferred treatment, while the data in the intermediate prognosis patients was not conclusive.

DISCUSSION

The Bayesian approach used prior information explicitly. In the calculation of the current probability that treatments are equally preferred, a p-value of 1/2 was assumed, quite strong evidence of the equivalence of the two treatments. As data accumulated during the trial, the current probability of treatment equivalence was modified.

In the calculation of the Bayesian probability that AD-OAP was preferred, it was assumed that the preference rate for either treatment could have been anywhere in the interval 0 to 1, which is complete ignorance about the preference rate. Generally, one could incorporate prior information concerning the relative merits of the treatments or arrange for the estimated response rate to AMSA-OAP to be any particular value.

In the actual trial analyzed, calculating the current probabilities provided retrospective justification for the changes in the design that actually were made.

Finally, it should be noted that other types of probability calculations could have been made in this trial. For example, the probability that the preference rate was between .45 and .55 could have been calculated, which would mean that the response rates for the two treatments were effectively equivalent. Another type of calculation that could be made is: what is the current probability that the new treatment has a higher response rate by 20% or more than the standard treatment.

At the University of Texas Cancer Center, it is planned to utilize the Bayesian approach in the analysis of clinical trials, so that interim analyses can be performed at any time during the conduct of studies.

Table 1 Contrast Between Classical (Frequentist) Approach and Bayesian Approach to Inferences

Classical	Bayesian
Uses P-values	Uses posterior probabilities of hypotheses, given observed data and prior information
Depends on data observed and not observed, experiments done and not done	Depends on data observed and experiment done
Uses prior information generally	Uses prior information explicitly
Analysis tied to design (e.g. number of interim analyses)	Analyze at any time
Unconditional	Conditional

Table 2 Analyses of Study Reported in Keating et al (1987) Jour. of Cl. Oncology 5, 5, 710-721

Paired data analyses by sub-group

AMSA-OAP	unfavorable	(PPR<.60)	91 pairs
AMSA-OAP	favorable	(PPR≥.60)	43 pairs
AD-OAP	favorable	(PPR≥.40)	108 pairs

Historical control group

- 325 patients who received AD-OAP
- logistic regression equation for predicting CR

Criticisms

- P-values assumed fixed sample size study
- No account taken of sequential conduct of study
- Decisions in 3 stages of study taken on clinical evidence and not statistical tests

Table 3 — Bayesian Analysis of Clinical Trial of AMSA-OAP in Acute Leukemia

Set-Up: Paired Data: 134 AMSA-OAP, 108 AD-OAP
θ = parameter giving proportion of pairs in which AMSA-OAP is preferred

p is prior probability
n_A, n_B are number of preferences of A, B

1. Non-Zero prior prob. p that $\theta = 1/2$ (Cornfield {1966}) and 1 - p distributed uniformly over $\theta \neq 1/2$
then, under conditions of binomial sampling,

$$Pr(\theta = 1/2 \mid n_A, n_B) = \left[1 + \left(\frac{1-p}{p}\right) 2^{n_A+n_B} \int_0^1 \theta^{n_A}(1-\theta)^{n_B} d\theta\right]^{-1}$$

gives current prob. that treatments are equally preferred

2. Assume uniform prior on θ in (0,1)

$$Pr(\theta < 1/2 \mid n_A, n_B) = \frac{(n_A+n_B+1)!}{n_A!\, n_B!} \int_0^{1/2} \theta^{n_A}(1-\theta)^{n_B} d\theta$$

gives current prob. that AD-OAP is preferred

Table 4 — Changes in Study Design at End of Stage I

A. AMSA-OAP Unfav. (A) vs AD-OAP Unfav. (B)
PPR < .40

Data: No. pairs = 21 — CR rate (A) = 43%
$n_A = 9$, $n_B = 3$ — CR rate (B) = 14%

Current prob. $\theta = 1/2$ is .41
Current prob. B better is .07
Paired data P is .15

Decision: Expand criteria for administration of AMSA-OAP from PPR<.40 to PPR<.60

b. AD-OAP Fav. (A) vs AD-OAP Fav. (B)
PPR> .40

Data: No. pairs = 63 — CR rate (A) = 70%
$n_A = 13$, $n_B = 15$ — CR rate (B) = 71%

Current prob. $\theta = 1/2$ is .81
Current prob. B is better is .57
Paired data P = .85

Decision: Restrict criteria for administration of AD-OAP from PPR $\geq$ .40 to PPR $\geq$ .60

Table 5 Summary of DT7995 Data by Stage

Treatment Group		Stage 1	Stage 2	Stage 3
	No. pts.	21	38	50
	No. pref.	12	19	24
AMSA-OAP	CR% (AMSA-OAP)	43%	39%	38%
	CR% (AD-OAP)	14%	21%	22%
	PR (θ = 1/2|data)	.41	.51	.52
	PR (B better|data)	.07	.05	.05
	P	.15	.17	.15
	No. pts.	-	22	41
AMSA-OAP	No. pref.	-	11	19
.40≤PPR≤.60)	CR%(AMSA-OAP)	-	50%	56%
	CR%(AD-OAP)	-	36%	44%
	PR(θ = 1/2|data)	-	.66	.66
	PR(B better|data)	-	.17	.12
	P	-	.55	.36
	No. pts.	63	108	-
	No. pref.	28	45	-
AD-OAP	CR%(AD-OAP)	70%	73%	-
PPR>.40	CR%(AD-OAP) (Hist.Control)	71%	71%	-
	PR(θ = 1/2|data)	.81	.84	-
	PR(B better|data)	.71	.38	-
	P	.85	.88	-

REFERENCES

Berry, D.A. (1987): Interim Analyses in Clinical Trials - The Role of the Likelihood Principle. The Amer. Statistician, 41, 2, 117-122.

Cornfield, J. (1966): A Bayesian Test of Some Classical Hypotheses - with Applications to Sequential Clinical Trials. Jour. of Amer. Stat. Assoc., 61, 315, 577-594.

Keating, M.J., Gehan, E.A., Smith, T.L. et al (1987): A Strategy for Evaluation of New Treatments in Untreated Patients: Application to a Clinical Trial of AMSA for Acute Leukemia. J. Clin. Oncology, 5, 5, 710-721.

Neo-Adjuvant Chemotherapy. Ed. Cl. Jacquillat, M. Weil, D. Khayat. Colloque INSERM/John Libbey Eurotext Ltd. © 1988. Vol. 169, pp. 621-625.

The prognostic value of patient age in initial diagnosis of operable breast cancer : implications for neo-adjuvant chemotherapy

Bernard Chevallier*, Véronique Mosseri**, Yvon Graic*, Jean-Paul Dauce*, Philippe Bastit* and Bernard Asselain**

* *Centre H. Becquerel, rue d'Amiens, 76038 Rouen, France*
** *Clinical Research Department, Institut Curie, 26, rue d'Ulm, 75231 Paris, France*

ABSTRACT

This study is based on 645 female patients (ptes) who had undergone immediate surgical removal of an invasive mammary adenocarcinoma without distant metastasis. With unifactorial analysis (Log-rank test), 5 years relative actuarial overall survival of patients 35-70 and >70 was very similar (87% and 89,6% respectively) and significantly better than that of patients ≤ 35 (76,4%). Considering disease-free survival, patients ≤ 35 had the worse prognosis, followed by age group > 70 and by age group 35-70, the difference between the 3 age group being significant (p<0.0001). Multifactorial analysis (COX) revealed subsequently that age ≤ 35 was an independant prognostic factor affecting both disease-free and overall survival.This multivariate analysis also revealed that disease-free survival was strongly related with tumour size,lymph node invasion, capsular rupture, SBR grade and PR. Multifactorial analysis of overall survival showed that it was strongly associated with the same prognostic factors than disease-free survival,plus menopausal status and ER. A prognostic score taking into account these factors was calculated for disease-free survival and for overall survival and enabled us to categorize the study sample into four groups having a good, intermediate or poor prognosis. We have confirmed the validity of these two models on a separate group of subjects using a test sample procedure and good score reproducibility was observed. These results show that patient age of ≤ 35 is an autonomous prognostic factor in operable breast cancer and could indicate more aggressive treatment for this particular age group.
KEY WORDS : BREAST CANCER, AGE AT DIAGNOSIS, PROGNOSTIC FACTORS, MULTIFACTORIAL ANALYSIS.

Among the factors influencing overall survival and the length of disease-free survival of operable breast cancer, lymph node invasion (9, 14), tumor size (4) and histoprognostic grade (5) are the best established. The prognostic value of patient age at time of first diagnosis is still the subject of some controversy (1, 3, 6, 10, 11, 12). In this retrospective study we have examined the importance in prognosis of age at diagnosis and compared it to the weighting of other prognostic factors.

PATIENTS AND METHODOLOY

Between october 1977 and december 1983, 651 consecutive female patients underwent surgical treatment for cancer in one breast, in the Cancer Center H. Becquerel in Rouen. All the cases were invasive adenocarcinomas with one or more tumour foci. Six patients diagnosed as having one or more fixed homolateral axillary lymph node were not considered in the study since they were too small in number to provide a basis for viable statistical analysis. The remaining 645 female patients were free of any metastasis. The first step in treatment was invariably surgical: modified radical mastectomy (n=310), tumorectomy or quadrantectomy (n=335), axillary lymph node dissection (n=615). Adjuvant radiotherapy was given to 507 patients, adjuvant chemotherapy to 43 and adjuvant hormonotherapy to 94. None of the adjuvant treatments were randomized. Further, the adjuvant therapies used were employed in a number of combinations. In all cases the procedure adopted for measurement of estrogen (ER)and progesterone (PR) receptor levels was the following : biopsy of tumour tissue prior to mammectomy, single saturation dosage according to the

Charbon-Dextran technique. For ER and PR, a level >5 femtomoles per milligramme of cytosolic protein (fmoles/mg) was taken as positive (ER + or PR+) and one of ≤ 5 fmoles/mg as negative (ER- or PR-). Quality control tests were carried out twice yearly on ER and PR dosage by the European Organisation for Cancer Research and Treatment and by the National Federation of Anti-Cancer Centres. Histoprognostic grading was established by use of the SCARFF BLOOM/RICHARDSON technique. TNM (UICC 1978) classification was employed in the categorization of tumor size in clinical terms as well as clinical axillary lymph node invasion. Menopause was defined as cessation of menstruation for one year or more. Clinical follow-up was bi-annual for the first five years and annual thereafter. Last updating of the data took place in july 1986, and the study period was therefore 106 months maximum and 30 months minimum (Mean period = 59 months). Unifactorial analysis was applied to eleven parameters likely to influence recurrence of tumour growth (see left column table I). Disease-free survival and overall survival were calculated using the actuarial technique of KAPLAN and MEIER (7). The level of statistical significance of the difference between the curves obtained (p) was evaluated with the Log-Rank test (8). Percentage differentials were tested by application of the Chi-2 test. Factors showing prognostic value in the unifactorial analysis were subsequently subjected to multifactorial analysis using COX's proportional hazard survival regression models (2). In this way, it was possible to determine a prognostic score. The higher the score, the poorer the patient's prognosis. We then chosed to divide the score range into 4 groups.

The 645 subjects included in the study were grouped by random selection into two independent samples with the aim of checking the validity of our model.

- a base group of 323 patients to which the COX model was again applied in order to establish a new prognostic score SC'.

- a test sample of 322 patients on which the prognostic value of the SC' score was verified. The intention of this was to confirm that the score remained of value when applied to an independent sample.

RESULTS

The average age of the patients at the time of the initial diagnosis was 57, the extremes of the age-range falling at 28 and 86. There was 22 patients aged ≤ 35, 531 between 35 and 70 years old and 92 which age was > 70. Fifty-one local recurrences, 7 homolateral lymph node recurrences and 6 homolateral recurrences within the same general area were observed. Twenty-one of the patients showed progression in the controlateral breast. Metastatic spread occured in 144 patients. Out of 104 deaths, 91 were associated with the progression of cancer growth. Two patients succumbed to endometrial cancer diagnosed during the follow-up period.

Unifactorial analysis

Table I shows the influence of the eleven parameters considered on disease free survival and on overall survival. Overall survival and disease free survival were examined for 3 age-groups : ≤ 35, 35 to 70, > 70 years. Examination of the sensitivity of this grouping showed that for the series of cases included here, these thresholds were close to optimal. The effect of these 3 age groupings does not disappear over time. Those patients aged between 35 and 70 at first diagnosis have the best chance of survival and the longest period free of any relapse. Patients aged under 35 at initial diganosis have the poorest prognosis. Finally, those aged over 70 show in actuarial terms a poor overall survival rate but a disease-free survival intermediate between the two groups already mentioned. The overall survival rate has been corrected by means of the mortality statistics for the French population as a whole over the period 1973 to 1977 as published by INSEE. The poor outcome associated with ages over 70 disappears when such correction is applied. In so far as statistically different prognoses are concerned, there remain only two age groups : ≤ 35 and > 35.

Multifactorial analysis

Such analysis was applied only to the 9 factors found to be significant in univariate analysis. The influence of menopausal status was examined independently, as was the interaction between menopause and ER>5. The results given by the model for survival and disease free survival are detailed in table II. Seven prognostic factors are of importance in predicting patient survival, plus the interaction between menopause and oestrogen receptor already mentioned above. Six parameters are influential in predicting the length of the disease-free survival. The pronostic scores (PS) obtained are derived directly from table II :

- For overall survival : PS = 0.971. Age + 0.872. Menopause -0.92.(Ménopause + RO>5) + 0.46.Tumour size + 0.472. Histological lymph node invasion + 0.606. Capsular rupture + 0.669.histopathological grade - 0.561. PR.

- For disease free survival : PS = 0.932. Age + 0.406. Tumour size + 0.369. Lymph node invasion + 0.401. Capsular rupture + 0.556. histopathological grade - 0.561. PR.

The scores range respectively between - 1.89 and + 2.1 (disease-free survival) and - 1.8 to + 4.7 (overall survival). The curves for overall survival and disease-free survival as functions of the prognostic score have been bracketed in four ranges of increasing seriousness. For both survival and disease-free survival the differences between the groups are of a high level of significance (p < 0.0001).

Confirmation of the prognostic score

Score SC' is very close to score SC as derived from the study of the whole group of 645 subjects. Thus the survival rates after 5 years for groups 1, 2, 3,4 (formed by division of whole range of score SC') are respectively, 93, 89, 75 and 57 % in the base sample and 90, 84, 75 and 40 % in the test sample. The trust-worthiness of SC' is thereby confirmed in the test sample. The differences between groups 1, 2, 3 and 4 are highly significant ($p < 0.0001$). The same process was successfully applied to the disease-free survival.

DISCUSSION

The aim of the present study was, on the one hand, to evaluate the importance of different age brackets at the time of first diagnosis of breast cancer on disease-free survival and on overall survival and, on the other, to compare the prognostic value of age to the other prognostic factors already recognized in the context of operable breast cancer. Certainly, the isolation of factors indicating a high risk of relapse after surgical treatment of breast cancer is of the greatest interest. Used alone or in combination such factors allow identification of high risk of recurrence groups of patients for which adjuvant therapies are prescribed in order to lenghten disease-free survival and overall survival (9). Besides the existence of metastatic or inflammatory conditions, the usual criterias considered in breast cancer prognosis are the following : number of axillary lymph nodes involved (9), size of tumor (4, 3) and histoprognostic grade (5). Prescription of adjuvant treatment is currently made on the basis of these factors. Traditionnaly, age at diagnosis has not been taken into account when considering adjuvant therapies. This can no doubt be explained by the disagreements evident in the relevant literature where the importance of age group on disease-free survival and survival are concerned.

The univariate analysis which we have applied to disease-free survival and overall survival confirms the value of traditional prognostic criterias : tumour size, clinical or histological axillary lymph node invasion, lymph node capsule rupture and histopathological grade. Our study brings out a negative effect for a patient age ≤ 35 at time of initial diagnosis in so far as disease free survival and overall survival are concerned. This negative effect does not fade over time. The results given in the literature for the prognostic value of age at diagnosis are contradictory. Some studies (12,13) associate youth and poor outcome. Others (10) find the youngest patients to have the better prognosis. Finally, there are studies which fail to demonstrate any correlation between age at diagnosis and prognosis of operable breast cancer. These differences can be partly accounted for by the small numbers of patients often involved, as well as by the length of the periods devoted to patient observation and to their follow up, which are short in some cases. Other studies use age ranges which are too wide (10, 11), no attempt having been made to confirm the possible increase in analytical discrimination through a decrease in the number of years in each bracket. The results recorded in the national registers of cancer occurrence for France (14), Norway (6) and Sweden (1) are of especial interest. These three records cover 113,000 patients with a minimum follow-up of 13 years. In all three cases there is an association between poor outcome and the youngest of the women involved. Only the Norwegian and Swedish registers give a corrected actuarial suvival rate which is shorter for women aged over 74. Some weight can be attached to these three publications given the large number of subjects involved, the lengthy follow-up period and the non-controversial nature of the methodology used.

To date, no multifactorial study have isolated age as an independant prognostic factor. Our results show that age is a specific prognostic criterion possessing its own importance and which must be considered independently of the other factors traditionnally taken into account in breast cancer prognosis. In view of the results still published, the reasons for the concept of a poorer outcome in young than in old breast carcinoma patients seems unclear. Adami et al.(1) demonstrated that the difference in prognosis between young and old women can not be explained by hormonal factors such as menopause. Host (6) suggested that women aged 70 or more have generally more advanced disease at diagnosis. It is also our findings. These older women may also be treated less intensively. An other explanation is that breast tumors in younger women is *per se* biologically more malignant than in older age groups. These findings might indicate a more aggressive initial treatment for women ≤ 35.

The validity of our prognostic scoring has been confirmed by test sample. There is no evidence to our knowledge of any similar confirmatory procedure in the available literature. Further confirmation of our scoring would be provided by its testing by another research team.

ACKNOWLEDGMENTS

This study has been made possible with the financial assistance of the anti-cancer Committee for the department of Seine-Maritime.

FACTOR STUDIED	DISEASE-FREE SURVIVAL (p)	OVERALL SURVIVAL (p)
Age (years) (-35; 35 to 70; +70)	< 0.0001 (-35 < +70 < 35 to 70)	< 0.005 (-35 = +70 < 35 to 70)
Familial history of breast cancer (Yes; no)	NS (p = 0.51)	NS (p = 0.57)
Menopausal status (Pre;post)	NS (p = 0.39)	NS (p = 0.06)
Clinical size of the tumor (T0, T1, T2, T3)	< 0.0001 (T3 < T2 < T1-T0)	< 0.0001 (T3 < T2 < T1-T0)
Clinical lymph node involvement (N0, N1a, N1b)	< 0.001 (N1b < N0-N1a)	<0.0001 (N1b < N1a-N0)
Histological lymph node involvement (0; 1 to 3; +3)	< 0.0001 (+3 < 1 to 3 < 0)	< 0.0001 (+3 < 1 to 3 < 0)
Lymph node capsular rupture (Yes; no)	< 0.0001 (Yes < no)	< 0.0001 (Yes < no)
Number of tumor foci (1; +1)	NS (p = 0.68)	NS (p = 0.70)
Histopathological grading [(1, 2, 3, non gradable (NG)]	< 0.0001 (3 < 2, NG < 1)	< 0.0001 (3 < 1, 2, NG)
ER (fmoles/mg. : -5; +5)	< 0.01) (-5 < +5)	< 0.0001 (-5 < +5)
PR (fmoles/mg. : -5; +5)	< 0.001 (-5 < +5)	< 0.0001 (-5 < +5)

Table I : Univariate analysis of prognostic factors : influence on disease-free survival and on overall survival.
Legend : NS = not significant.
p = degree of statistical significance.

FACTOR STUDIED	DISEASE-FREE SURVIVAL (p)	DISEASE-FREE SURVIVAL ß coefficient	OVERALL SURVIVAL (p)	OVERALL SURVIVAL ß coefficient	Prognosis better if
Age	< 0.001	+0.932	< 0.02	+0.971	> 35
Menopausal status	NS	-	< 0.002	+0.872	pre
Post menopause + ER>5	NS	-	< 0.0003	-0.92	
Clinical size of the tumor	< 0.005	+0.406	< 0.01	+0.46	T1
Clinical axillary lymph node involvement	NS	-	NS	-	
Histological axillary lymph node involvement	< 0.003	+0.369	< 0.005	+0.472	N < 3
Lymph node capsular rupture	< 0.05	+0.401	< 0.03	+0.606	Absent
Histopathological grading (SBR)	< 0.0003	+0.556	< 0.005	+0.669	SBR = 1
ER	NS	-	NS	-	
PR	< 0.0004	-0.561	< 0.004	-0.622	≥ 5 fmoles/mg.

Table II : Multivariate analysis of prognostic factors.
Results on disease-free survival and overall survival.
Legend : NS = not significant.

REFERENCES

1- ADAMI H. O.; MALKER B.; HOLMBERG L.; PERSSON I.; STONE B. (1986) : The relation between survival and age at diagnosis in breast cancer.
New Engl. J. Med., 315, 559-563.
2- COX D. R. (1972) : Regression models and life table.
J. Roy. Statis. Soc. B., 34, 187-220.
3- CUTLER S.J., AXTELL L.M. (1969) : Adjustment of long term survival rates for deaths due to intercurent disease.
J. Chron. Dis., 2, 485-491.
4- FISHER B.; SLACK N. H.; BROSS I. D. (1969) : Cancer of the breast : size of neoplasm and prognosis.
Cancer, 24, 1071-1080.
5- FREEDMAN L. S.; EDWARDS D. S.; McCONNELL E. M.; DOWHNHAM D. Y.(1979) : Histological grade and other prognostic factors in relation to survival of patients with breast cancer.
Br. J. Cancer, 40, 44-55.
6- HOST H.; LUND E. (1986) : Age as a prognostic factor in breast cancer.
Cancer, 57, 2217-2221.
7- KAPLAN E. L.; MEIER P. (1957) : Non parametric estimation from incomplete observation.
J. Am. Statis. Ass., 53, 457-471.
8- MANTEL N. (1966) : Evaluation of survival data and two new rank order statistic arising in its consideration.
Cancer Chemother. Rep., 50, 163-191.
9- MOURIDSEN H.T.; PALSHOF T. (1983) : Adjuvant systemic therapy in breast cancer : a review.
Eur. J. Cancer Clin. Oncol., 19, 1753-1770.
10- MUELLER C.B., AMES F., ANDERSON G.D. (1978) : Breast cancer in 3558 women : age as a significant determinant in the rate of dying and causes of death.
Surgery, 83, 123-132.
11- NOYES R. D., SPANOS W.J., MONTAGUE E. D.(1982) : Breast cancer in women aged 30 and under.
Cancer, 49, 1302-1307.
12- RIBEIRO G., SWINDELL R. (1981) : The prognosis of breast carcinoma in women aged less than 40 years.
Clin. Radiol., 32, 231-236.
13- STOLL B.A (1976) : Does the malignancy of breast cancer vary with age?
Clin. Oncol., 2, 73-80.
14- Enquête Permanente Cancer (1982) : Fédération Nationale des Centres de Lutte Contre le Cancer. 1975-1981. DOIN Ed., 82-87.

Résumé

Cette étude porte sur 645 patientes (ptes) opérées d'emblée d'un adénocarcinome mammaire invasif non métastasé L'analyse unifactorielle (Test du Log-rank) a mis en évidence une liaison statistiquement significative entre la survie globale et plusieurs facteurs: l'âge, la taille de la tumeur, le grade histopronostique SBR, l'envahissement ganglionnaire axillaire clinique et histologique, la rupture capsulaire, le taux de récepteurs d'oestrogènes (RO) et de progestérone (RP). La liaison avec le statut hormonal pré ou post ménopausique est à la limite de la signification. L'uni ou la multifocalité tumorale est sans liaison. De la même façon, l'intervalle libre sans récidive est lié significativement aux mêmes facteurs que la survie globale. Une analyse multifactorielle (COX) a montré dans un deuxième temps que la survie globale était très liée à l'âge, à la taille de la tumeur, à l'envahissement ganglionnaire, à la rupture capsulaire, au grade SBR, au statut ménopausique, à RO et à RP. L' analyse multifactorielle de l'intervalle libre sans récidive a révélé qu'elle était très liée à l'âge, à la taille tumorale, à l'envahissement ganglionnaire, à la rupture capsulaire, au grade SBR et à RP. Un score pronostic prenant en compte ces facteurs a été calculé pour l'intervalle libre sans récidive et pour la survie globale, et a permis de séparer la population étudiée en trois groupes depronostic bon,intermédiaire ou mauvais. Ces résultats montrent qu'un âge $\leq$ 35 ans est un facteur autonome de mauvais pronostic qui suggère un traitement plus aggressif pour ce groupe particulier.
MOTS CLES : CANCER DU SEIN, AGE AU DIAGNOSTIC INITIAL, FACTEURS PRONOSTIQUES, ANALYSE MULTIFACTORIELLE.

Neo-Adjuvant Chemotherapy. Ed. Cl. Jacquillat, M. Weil, D. Khayat. Colloque INSERM/John Libbey Eurotext Ltd. © 1988. Vol. 169, pp. 627-629.

Impact of treatment starting time, dose-related factors and induced amenorrhoea on survival of breast cancer patients treated with adjuvant CMF

P. Pronzato, E. Campora, D. Amoroso, G. Bertelli, M.P. Cusimano, I. Brunetti, E. Baldini, F. Botto, C. Midolo, P.F. Conte, M.R. Sertoli and R. Rosso

Istituto Nazionale per la Ricerca sul Cancro, Viale Benedetto XV, 10, Genova, 16132, Italy

SUMMARY

In this study a series of factors potentially influencing the outcome of adjuvant chemotherapy have been taken into account. 229 patients with histologically node positive breast cancer have been treated with 12 cycles of intravenous CMF. The interval between mastectomy and start of chemotherapy, the individual dose intensity and the number administered cycles were able to influence survival, while induced amenorrhoea had no impact. Results of univariate analysis have been confirmed in a multivariate model.

KEY WORDS

breast cancer, adjuvant chemotherapy, dose intensity, multivariate analysis

INTRODUCTION

In the seventies a series of trials carried out in Europe and U.S.A.has shown that adjuvant chemotherapy is able to prolong disease free survival and overall survival of node positive breast cancer patients, mainly in premenopause.
The most largely employed regimen is the combination of Cyclophosphamide, Methotrexate and 5-Fluorouracil. In the present trial a consecutive series of 229 patients entered a program of adjuvant chemotherapy consisting of 12 cycles of CMF administered intravenously every 21 days.
Since factors like the interval between the surgical removal and the first cycle, the level of administered dose, the interval between cycles and the induction of amenorrhoea in premenopausal patients are theretically able to influence the results of the treatment, we have studied all the possible and available factors in univariate and multivariate models.

SUBJECTS AND METHODS.

229 patients entered the trial. Characteristic of patients were : median age 51 years (range 27-70); premenopause: 118 patients, postmenopause: 111 patients; pathological tumor size: pT1 in 71, pT2 in 113, pT3 in 17, pT4 in 28 patients; median number of axillary lymphnodes involved 3 (range 1-28).
Patients were treated with Cyclophosphamide 600 mg/sm, Methotrexate 40 mg/sm and 5-Fluorouracil 600 mg/sm intravenously every 21 days, provided bone marrow recovery had occurred.
The dose intensity of drugs administered was calculated on the basis of a modification of the methods of Hryniuk and Coppin (2-4).
Survival analysis was performed by Kaplan Meier method. Results were compared by log-rank test and Cox multivariate model.

RESULTS.

4-year overall survival (S) and relapse free survival (RFS) were 78% and 56.8%, respectively.
Patients who experience chemotherapy induced amenorrhoea had S and RFS comparable to other patients.
Median value of individual received dose intensity was 90%. We found that a cut-off of 80% divided patients in two groups with different prognosis: patients with dose intensity >80% had better S and RFS ($p = 0.02$).
S of patients was positively affected by a short time (<35 days) from mastectomy to the first cycle and by administration of all the 12 planned cycles ($p = 0.01$ in both cases).
Cox multivariate model has shown the indipendent prognostic value of the considered factors.

CONCLUSION.

Adjuvant chemotheapy has shown a certain effectiveness in prolonging survival of node positive breast cancer patients (1-3).
Our study suggest that optimal results can be obtained by paying attention to time and dose of drugs administered: infact, dose reductions and treatment delays decrease the chemotherapy dose intensity with possible negative effects on outcome.

REFERENCES.

Bonadonna G, Valagussa P, Zambetti M, Buzzoni R, Moliterni A.(1987): Milan adjuvant trials for stage I-II breast cancer. in Adjuvant Therapy of Cancer V, ed.Salmon SE, pp. 211-221. Orlando,Florida: Grune-Stratton.

Coppin CML (1987): The description of chemotherapy delivery: options and pitfalls. Sem Oncol 14,34-42.

Fisher B, Redmond C, Fisher ER, Wolmark N (1986): Systemic adjuvant therapy in treatment of primary operable breast cancer : National Surgical Adjuvant Breast and Bowel Project Experience.
NCI Monogr 1, 35-43.

Hryniuk W, Levine MN (1986): Analysis of dose intensity for adjuvant chemotherapy trials in stage II breast cancer.
J Clin Oncol 4,1162-1170.

Résumé

Dans cette étude, une série de facteurs pouvant eventuellement influencer le résultat de la chimiothérapie adjuvante ont été considérés. 229 malades atteints de cancer du sein avec des ganglions positifs ont été traités par 12 cycles de CMF I.V.. L'intervalle entre la mastectomie et le début de la chimiothérapie l'intensité individuelle de la dose, le nombre de cycle administré ont tous influencé la survie alors que l'aménorrhée n'a eu aucun impact. Les résultats d'une analyse monofactorielle ont été confirmés par un modèle multifactoriel.

Neo-Adjuvant Chemotherapy. Ed. Cl. Jacquillat, M. Weil, D. Khayat. Colloque INSERM/John Libbey Eurotext Ltd. © 1988. Vol. 169, pp. 631-637.

Application d'une technique d'agrégation de similarité pour la classification pronostique d'une population de mélanomes malins primitifs

J. Maral*, P. Parisot, F. Marcotorchino, G. Forget*, P. Banzet** et Cl. Jacquillat*

Centre Scientifique IBM France, 13 place Vendôme, 75001 Paris, France
** Service d'Oncologie Médicale Pitié Salpêtrière, Hôpital de la Salpêtrière, 47 bd de l'Hôpital, 75013 Paris, France*
*** Groupe Mélanome Malin Laboissière-Saint Louis, Hôpital Saint-Louis, 2 place du Dr. Fournier, 75010 Paris, France*

ABSTRACT

The "old" principle of "paired comparaisons" allows the use of classical criteria of association as tools for classification. This is due to the possibility offered to linearize two dimensional as well as multi-dimensional cross-association criteria on multiway contingency tables. Thses statistical cross association measures expressed in contingency tables environement give rise to quadratic mathematical formulations, in scientific papers dealing with categorical data. This possibility to linearize some of these criteria allows :

. Generalization of cross association measures to multidimensional contingency tables.

. Generalization of the "Association analysis" of Williams-Lambert and Mac Naughton-Smith (research of the parameter the "most correlated" with the other among a set of variables to a virtual parameter maximizing the association within a set of variables). This problem generalizes the methodology of "similarity aggregation" associated to the Condorcet's criterion developed by P. Michaud and F. Marcotorchino to other types of cross-association measures.

The Maximal Association Theory was used as a tool to classify in prognostic classes a population of 982 malignant melanoma patients. A first partition was made on data censored in 1982. Actualisation of the method whose results were compared to classical multiregression model.

INTRODUCTION

En médecine et en particulier en cancérologie les méthodes de classifications basées sur les facteurs pronostiques permettent :

1) de valider la valeur des paramètres choisis
2) de définir les populations à haut risque
3) d'adapter l'attitude thérapeutiques à la gravité de la maladie

Les méthodes de classifications usuelles ne sont adaptées qu'à des variables quantitatives et à des variables homogènes. Les données manquantes sont difficiles à prendre en compte.

Nous avons choisi une méthodologie basée sur le principe de la comparaison par paires.
Le critère de Condorcet est un critère logique datant du 18ème siècle. On travaille sur un tableau qui croise les individus 2 par 2. Chaque variable est considérée comme une opinion comparant les individus 2 à 2 en terme de similarité.
On cherche à optimiser une opinion globale tenant en compte l'ensemble des opinions particulières.
La règle de majorité par paire ne permet d'optimiser ce critère que localement et l'opinion globale peut être paradoxale (non transitive).
La solution à ce problème de paradoxe est une règle de majorité globale sous contrainte, le résultat doit être une partition répondant aux règles de transitivité et de symétrie.
Cette formulation se ramène à un problème linéaire donc résolvable exactement par programmation. Cette technique a été mise au point au Centre de Recherche d'IBM France par F. Marcotorchino et P. Michaud (4, 5).

Les intérêts de cette méthode sont en particulier :

. La possibilité de traiter des données hétérogènes et manquantes

. Une classification sans à priori sur le nombre de classes et sans interprétation des résultats comme dans les méthodes graphiques car la solution est une partition (6).

POPULATION ETUDIEE

Nous avons appliqué cette technique aux patients suivis dans le Groupe de Recherche sur les Mélanomes Malins St Louis-Lariboisière.
Les dossiers des patients sont informatisés depuis 1973.
Ils ont été traités par chirurgie large + greffe et inclus dans 3 protocoles successifs randomisés de chimiothérapie ou d'immunothérapie adjuvante (sans qu'il soit obervé d'influence sur la survie des patients) (1 , 2 , 3).

Parmi ces malades, nous avons selectionné 561 patients inclus entre 1976 et 1986. Les facteurs pronostiques que nous avons pris en compte pour la classification sont :

- le sexe
- l'épaisseur de la lésion mesurée selon Breslow en 4 classes
- le niveau d'invasion histologique (niveau III, IV, ou V)
- la topographie de la lésion que nous avons regroupée en 3 classes :
    - * tête et cou
    - * tronc
    - * membres
- le type histologique (SSM, nodulaire)
- l'existence ou non d'une ulcération

Les différents facteurs pronostiques sont intercorrélés (tableau 1).
Parmi les corrélations les plus importantes l'épaisseur est liée avec la plupart des autres facteurs. Cette lésion est bien sur très étroite avec le niveau.
Nous retrouvons aussi les notions classiques : le sexe et la topographie sont liés, etc...

Classe 2 — 58 pts
: Epaisseur 2-3 mm
: Membres
: Femme
: Ulcération
: Nodulaire

Classe 3 — 73 pts
: Epaisseur 1-2 mm
: Ulcération
: Membres
: SSM
: Femme

Classe 4 — 48 pts
: Epaisseur 1 mm
: Niveau II-III
: Femme
: Membres

Autres (3 classes) : Tête et cou
13 pts

Les classes 3 et 4 sont en fait la classe 3 de la 1ère population éclatée en 2 selon l'épaisseur.
Il s'agit de femmes SSM, membres :

classe 3 : 1 à 2 mm
classe 4 : moins de 1 mm

Les autres classes regroupent les sujets présentant un mélanome de la tête et du cou.

Cette classification elle aussi correspond à une hiérarchie pronostique comme le montrent les courbes de survie sans rechute (Fig. 2).

Figure 2 : AVANT 1/1/1980 - BILAN 82 - DFI

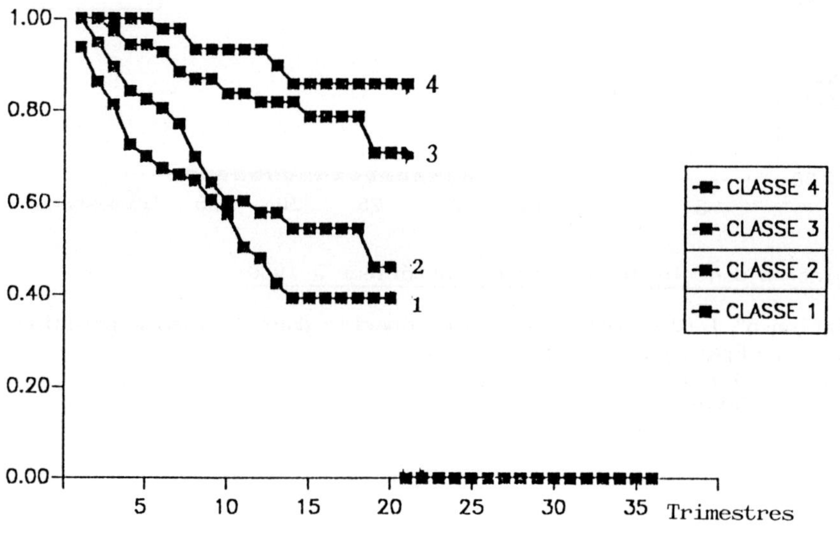

Tableau 2

Classe 1 73 pts	Epaisseur 3 mm Niveau V Homme
Classe 2 63 pts	Epaisseur 2-3 mm Mélanome nodulaire Localisation : membres Ulcération Femme
Classe 3 129 pts	Epaisseur 1 et 1 à 2 mm Pas d'ulcération Tronc

La partition obtenue avec les facteurs est bien une classification pronostique. Les courbes de survie (dans la figure 1) sans rechute montrent bien que la classe 1 regroupe les individus de mauvais pronostic, la classe 3 les individus de bon pronostic et la classe 2 les individus de pronostic intermédiaire.

Figure 1 : APRES 1/1/1980 - BILAN 87 - DFI

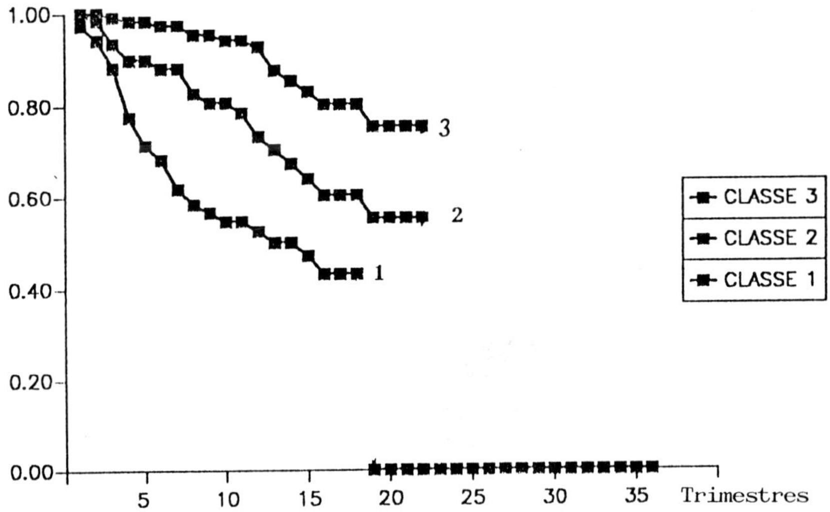

2 - Population dont le diagnostic est antérieur à 1980

La population n° 1 (277 patients) a été répartie dans 4 classes principales

Classe 1 82 pts	Epaisseur 3 mm niveau V Homme

Tableau 1 (Matrice des CHI-2)

	S	E	N	L	H	V
Sexe (S)		XXX		XXX		
Epaisseur (E)	XXX		XXX	X	XXX	XXX
Niveau (N)		XXX		XX	XX	XXX
Localis.(L)	XXX	X	XX		XX	X
Histology (H)		XXX	XX	XX		XXX
Ulcération (U)		XXX	XXX	X	XXX	

X $p < 0.05$
XX $p < 0.01$
XXX $p < 0.001$

Nous avons isolé 2 sous-populations, distinctes dans le temps, d'effectif semblable :

Une première population de patients dont le diagnostic a eu lieu avant 1980.
La deuxième population regroupe des patients inclus entre 1980 et 1986.
De manière à étudier les 2 populations avec le même recul, dans une analyse, la date de suivi de la population 1 a été artificiellement ramenée au 1.1.1982. Cela nous a permis :

- de comparer les partitions obtenues pour les 2 populations et
- de valider ainsi les classifications.

Le suivi des patients de la population n°1 après 1982 confirme la valeur pronostique de la classification obtenue.

ANALYSE

1 - <u>Population des patients diagnostiqués après 1980</u>

Pour la population 2 trois classes principales ont été obtenues. Les caractéristiques présentées tableau sont celles de la majorité des patients de la classe.

3 - Suivi de la population 1

Le suivi des patients de cette population jusqu'à aujourd'hui confirme la partition réalisée avec une date d'observation en 1982

Tableau 2 : Rechute en fonction des classes

Classe	1	2	3	4
N. Sujets	82	58	73	48
Rec. avant 82	49 (59,8 %)	30 (51,8 %)	21 (28,8 %)	12 (25 %)
Rec. depuis 82	8 (24,2 %)	6 (21,4 %)	4 (7,7 %)	5 (13,9 %)

La courbe de DFI prolongée en 1987 confirme ces résultats (figure 3).

Figure 3 : AVANT 1/1/1980 - BILAN 87 - DFI

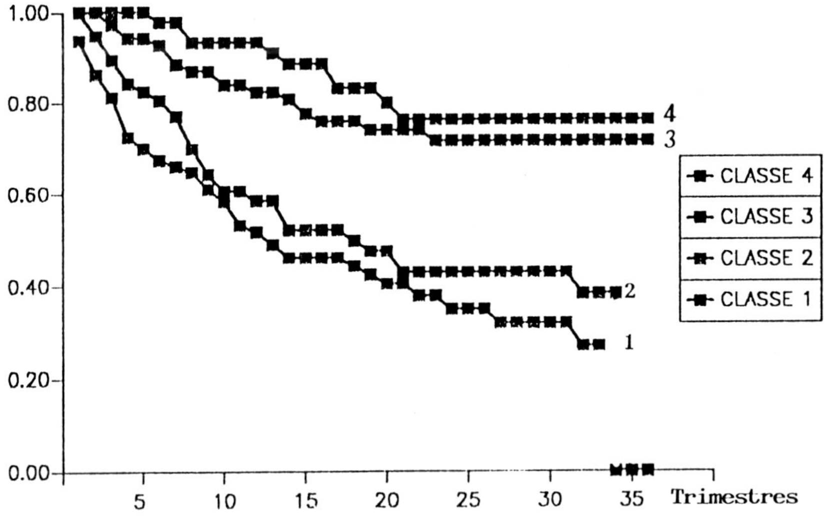

Cette technique de classification permet donc selon les caractéristiques d'un nouveau patient de l'affecter à la classe pronostique dont il est le plus proche.

CONCLUSION

Cette étude montre que la technique d'aggrégation par similarité nous a permis de réaliser une partition des patients atteints de mélanomes malins primitifs selon leur caractéristique pronostique, sans à priori sur le nombre de classes désirées.
La partition obtenue a bien une valeur pronostique et prédictive, ce qui a été vérifié par la mise à jour à 5 ans des données tronquées.

L'affectation d'un nouveau patient s'effectue selon des règles simples. Cette technique pouvant être étendue à la classification pronostique des maladies malignes. Elle présente l'avantage de ne pas nécessiter d'à priori sur le nombre de classes, de pouvoir traiter des données quantitatives ainsi que des données tronquées.

BIBLIOGRAPHIE

1 - P. BANZET, J. MARAL, J. BONVALET et coll
Pronostic factors of primary malignant melanoma. Observations in two randomized trials
Proc. ASCO, 1982, 183 - Abst. C713

2 - A. BRESLOW
Thickness, cross-sectional aeras and depths of invasion in the prognosis of cutaneous melanoma
Ann. Surg. 1970, 172, 902-903

3 - Cl. JACQUILLAT, P. BANZET, J. MARAL
Clinical trials of chemotherapy and chemo-immunotherapy in primary malignant melanoma
Recent Results in Cancer Research, 1982, 80, 254-258

4 - F. MARCOTORCHINO
Association maximale et aggrégation relationnelle (un thème général de la classification)
Neo-Adjuvant Chemotherapy - Colloque INSERM/John Libbey Vol 137, 1986, 835-842

5 - F. MARCOTORCHINO, P. MICHAUD
Optimisation en analyse ordinale des données
Masson Paris 1979

6 - P. PARISOT
Application of similarity aggregation techniques to a population of paraplegic patients
J. of Applied Stochastic Models and Data Analysis
J. Wiley London 1985

Neo-Adjuvant Chemotherapy. Ed. Cl. Jacquillat, M. Weil, D. Khayat. Colloque INSERM/John Libbey Eurotext Ltd. © 1988. Vol. 169, pp. 639-643.

The « Nouvelle Informatique » and the future of clinical trials

A.J. Valleron* and C. Chastang**

** Unité de Recherches Biomathématiques et Biostatiques de l'INSERM U. 263 et Université Paris 7, 2 place Jussieu, 75251 Paris Cedex 05, France*
*** Département Biostatistique et Informatique Médicale, Hôpital Saint-Louis, et Université Paris 7, 1, avenue C. Villefois, 75475 Paris Cedex 10, France*

ABSTRACT

This paper describes the changes expected in the fields of clinical trials following the new dramatic changes in computer technologies, namely the increased power of local -and cheap- microcomputers and the facility of communication between computers, therefore between users, through networks. Positive aspects of these changes are emphasized and possible risks concerning the confidentiality and the safety of data banks are described.

The aim of this paper is to show that the dramatic technological changes in informatics which have occured during the last 5-10 years will unavoidably lead to major modifications in the design, conduct, analysis and diffusion of results of clinical trials, and specially of multicenter cooperative clinical trials.

What can be called the "nouvelle informatique" has three main characteristics of importance.

First, the power of most micro computers expressed in terms of size of the central memory, amount of information that can be locally stored or speed of computations have so greatly increased that they exceed the computing needs of most clinical trials. For example, the file corresponding to a large clinical trial (two groups of one thousand sujects, each of them with 200 items, (400 000 values) can be stored on a single diskette of most microcomputers.

Previously computer facilities had to be centralized because those which possessed as much memory were rare and expansive. Now any clinic will be able to store the data concerning a whole cooperative clinical trial and analyse them.

The second charateristic is that most of the software necessary to handle a clinical trial is now available on personal computers. Data entry, file creation and editing is provided by specialised programs. Software previously implemented on large computers are now available to PC users (for example the popular SAS or BMDP). In future, interfacing with users will be improved and even expert systems will be developed to help the non-biostatistician use such facilities . Again this will help clinicians to participate to the analyses of the clinical trials they have in charge, by contrast with the past where analyses were done distantly.

The third -and main- characteristic of the "nouvelle informatique" is that it is distributed. The borders between micro, supermicro, mini, supermini and main frames are difficult to define and depend upon the criteria which are used ; size of the memory, number of MIPS (Millions of Instructions per second), I/O capacity, etc, cost. Teleinformatics brought an actual revolution : all categories of machines can now communicate, through standard or specialized telephone lines. Therefore the microcomputer(s) of a clinic can now be considered as the gate toward the exterior. Such microcomputers can communicate with any distant computer centre through TRANSPAC in France,TELENET in USA or similar systems in other countries. The future choice of this center will just rely on the quality of this center, not on his proximity with the clinic where the trial is done . Such connexions with distant centers do not actually exist in practice because there are numerous practical problems to be solved. However scientists of life sciences are now in the position of taking advantage of more than 10 years experience of their colleagues in "hard sciences" (physics, informatics, electronics) who now currently use for example in Europe the European Academic Research Network (EARN) or in USA networks such ARPANET or CSNET, where many problems of standardisation have been solved. In the next few years (2, 5, 10 ?) any user of a microcomputer will be able to take advantage of the possibility that exists now, namely to access any other computer in the world by typing a few commands and paying a small fee. We will soon arrive at the time of "distributed informatics" when everybody will use its three main functions :

- access to distant computers whose characteristics exceed the local possibilities
- access to software that is not locally available and to factual or bibliographic databases.
- communication with other individuals or groups, via computer mail. The experience accumulated over several years in "Hard Sciences" by network users demonstrates that this third function is quite important.

These characteristics of the "Nouvelle Informatique" will inevitably lead to important changes in the field of clinical trials. We shall first consider, step by step, which changes -most of them very positive- will result from the "Nouvelle Informatique" and review some of the negative effects of these changes that have to be taken into account in advance.

The "Nouvelle Informatique" and the five steps of a clinical trial :

- FORMULATING THE QUESTION

At this essential step, the facility to communicate between potential partners of the clinical trial will be used to interact more deeply, through computer mail, than in the past where basic discussion was concentrated in a few late afternoon meetings. Participants will be able to contribute without consideration of distance using the computer mail as a permanent forum. Facilitation of access to bibliographic data bases and to updated registries of ongoing clinical trials will also be of importance at this step.

- WRITING THE PROTOCOL

Current research using artificial intelligence technologies are providing tools ("protocol writers") which embody the various rules underlying the writing of a portocol. All the classical steps (case definition, randomisation procedure, ...) are included and alternatives are proposed. Software for critical evaluation of the necessary number of subjects is also available. Questionnaires are automatically generated and editing is facilitated.

- CARRYING OUT THE TRIAL

All components of this stage will be facilitated : first of all, data entry will be done once and once only, without the various past intermediaries between the form filled at the bed of the patient to the storage of the data in a distant computer. The local program will incorporate functions for verification of data coherence and correction and editing will occur immediately. More important, programs will automatically check the clinical profile of any new patient acceptable for inclusion into a trial. Information on these clinical trials, including computer mail addresses of the coordinators of the trial will be on line. Thus more patients than before will be recruited into clinical trials just because the trials will be more widely known and open to new clinicians. This is of importance when one considers that in France only 3% of the 20000 new cases of lung cancer per year are recruited into clinical trials.

The conduct of many clinical trials requires an adjustment of the doses that a patient receives, and perhaps also changes in treatment during the course of the study according to a priori well defined - but sometimes quite complex - criteria. These procedures, e.g. the automatic adjustment of doses according to body weight, will be facilitated by the computer.

- ANALYSING THE RESULTS

The principles of the statistical analysis of clinical trials will not obviously be changed by the new informatical technologies. The major change induced by the concept of distributed informatics is that the analysis will not be centralized on the computer of the biostatistician in charge of the clinical trial but will be available to all users who can analyse their own local data concerning their own patients and will be able to analyse the total data base provided by all participants (inasmuch as they are authorized to do so). Indeed the computational power of local microcomputers will be sufficient for this purpose and, inaddition, the statistical libraries available on microcomputers contain all the necessary software including ; multivariate analysis, Cox analysis, etc... which were previously "restricted" to biostatisticians working on mainframes. In addition, there is a trend toward building expert systems that facilitate the use of software by non statistician scientists. These systems will provide on line HELP procedures and allow the user to question the "expert" about the various underlying hypotheses. Exactly what the clinician wanted to do before. Therefore, the data center will be in the future only in charge of "specialised" analyses, such as those requiring the writing of special procedures (e.g. Monte Carlo simulation of trials to estimate consequences of various models of loss of follow up, ...).

- PUBLISHING THE RESULTS

The last step of a clinical trial concerns the diffusion of the results. The usual manner of communication is in medical journals. The use of computer networks will cause an explosion of the diffusion of results. Indeed the results will constitute data banks that will be accessible world wide. The data sets themselves will be made available in order that any distant user may reanalyse with his own views the clinical trial. Results will be accessible from every where. They will also be accessible by new readers, such as general practitioners who, at present, do not read that much the specialized journals where clinical trials are published. The possibility to constitute databases opened to general practitioners will greatly enhance the practical diffusion of medical knowledge linked to clinical trials. We can note, for instance, that in France in May 1988, 22000 out of 50000 general practitioners have a potential access by terminal to such facilities.

NEXT PREDICTIBLE RISKS

We have just seen that the "Nouvelle Informatique" will induce major changes in the conduct of clinical trials and in the relationship between clinicians and between clinicians and biostatisticians.

Some risks, however should be mentioned : first, the risk of undue interim analyses will increase just because they will be easy to perform by any participant at any time and, in the absence of good statistical training of

these new "statisticians", will increase to risk of unjustified termination of the trial. The solution will besound biostatistical knowledge of all participants (and not just a superficial training in the use of statistical packages). We can also predict a development of sequential analysis.
A second major risk concerns the security of the informatic system. For example, the dose adjustment during the trial will be automatised. There is a first technological risk that some data may be accidentally modified during the transmission through networks. Softwares exist that use redundancies systems to avoid that risk. There is even a risk that a "pirate" modifies from a distant terminal the doses and the schedules of a subject and this risk is very important where double blind trials make surveillance difficult. Such security problems are well known and solutions exist including data crypting, connexion security, isolation of mass memories containing the data from the networks, use of cards of access. Anyway this is, together with the obvious need for confidentiality, one of the major present limitations to a completely positive judgment of the impact of informatics on clinical trials.

Résumé

Cet article décrit les changements profonds qui devraient survenir dans la conduite, l'analyse et la diffusion des résultats des essais thérapeutiques suite aux modifications importantes de la technologie informatique en termes de puissance de calcul (désormais disponible à faible coût pour des utilisateurs qui devaient autrefois recourir à des centres de calculs extérieurs) et en termes de communication (facilitée par la téléinformatique permettant la mise en place de réseaux d'ordinateurs et, plus important, de réseaux d'utilisateurs).

Si les aspects positifs de cette évolution inévitable sont soulignés, quelques dangers prévisibles sont également indiqués : le risque d'analyse statistique intérimaire "sauvage" menant à des interprétations non rationnelles des essais, le danger en ce qui concerne la confidentialité et la sécurité des informations transmises au moyen des réseaux informatiques.

Progress in biology of metastasis and of chemoresistance

Progrès dans la biologie des métastases et de la chimiorésistance

Neo-Adjuvant Chemotherapy. Ed. Cl. Jacquillat, M. Weil, D. Khayat. Colloque INSERM/John Libbey Eurotext Ltd. © 1988. Vol. 169, pp. 647-650.

The basis of multidrug resistance to anticancer drugs

Victor Ling

The Ontario Cancer Institute, 500 Sherbourne Street, Toronto, Ontario, M4X 1K9, Canada

Successful chemotherapeutic management of patients with disseminated malignant disease may be severely limited by the development of resistant tumor cells. Multidrug resistance (MDR) frequently develops in cultured cell lines and in transplantable tumors. MDR is complex, but its predominant feature is resistance to a wide range of structurally unrelated cytotoxic drugs, many of which are anticancer drugs (1,2). Reduced drugs accumulation appears to be the basis of the resistance. A wide variety of biochemical changes have been detected in MDR cell lines (2) but the most consistent change is the increased expression of P-glycoprotein, a plasma membrane glycoprotein of approximately 170,000 daltons. Monoclonal antibodies developed against P-glycoprotein detect the presence of this membrane component in different MDR human and animal tumor cell lines (3). Moreover, the level of P-glycoprotein expression correlates with the degree of drug resistance.

Insights into the role of P-glycoprotein in drug resistance come from genetic and structural studies. Structural analysis of P-glycoprotein cDNAs from mouse, human and hamster indicates that P-glycoprotein is highly conserved (4-6). Striking homology between P-glycoprotein and a number of bacterial proteins, particularly hemolysin transport protein (HlyB protein), is observed (6). P-glycoprotein can be viewed as an ancient protein resulting from a tandem duplication of a primitive HlyB-like gene. The hydropathy profiles of the two proteins are similar and reveal an extensive transmembrane region, resembling those found in pore-forming plasma membrane proteins. A model is proposed for multidrug resistance in which P-glycoprotein functions as an energy-dependent export pump to reduce intracellular levels of anticancer drugs. It is envisioned that the cytoplasmic domain couple energy from ATP to export drugs through a channel formed by the transmembrane segments of P-glycoprotein.

P-glycoprotein appears to be encoded by a small family of closely related genes (7). In many MDR lines, increased P-glycoprotein expression is accompanied by gene amplification. Thus it is possible that co-amplified flanking genes contributes to the plethora of changes observed in different MDR lines (8). However, gene transfection studies indicate that transfer of a single member of the P-glycoprotein genes is sufficient to mediate multidrug resistance (9-11) and that this protein is causative of multidrug resistance.

Initial studies to determine if multidrug-resistant tumor cells involving increased P-glycoprotein expression occur in cancer patients have been undertaken by various groups (12-14). Increased expression of P-glycoprotein, or its mRNA has been reported in a variety of solid tumors, leukemias, and myelomas. Further studies will be required to determine if there is a prognostic correlation between P-glycoprotein level and response to chemotherapy. Nevertheless these studies do show, that multidrug resistance involving P-glycoprotein expression can occur in a variety of malignancies.

REFERENCES

1. V. Ling, J. Gerlach, and N. Kartner (1984). Multidrug resistance. Breast Cancer Research and Treatment 4: 89-94.

2. J. Gerlach, N. Kartner, D. Bell and V. Ling (1986). Multidrug resistance. Cancer Surveys 5: 25-46.

3. N. Kartner, D. Evernden-Porelle, G. Bradley and V. Ling (1985). Monoclonal antibodies detecting P-glycoprotein in multidrug-resistant cell lines. Nature 316: 820-823.

4. P. Gros, J. Croop and D. Housman (1986). Mammalian multidrug resistance gene: Complete cDNA sequence indicates strong homology to bacterial transport proteins. Cell 47: 371-380.

5. C. Chen, J.E. Chin, K. Veda, D.P. Clarke, I. Pastan, M.M. Grohesman and I.B. Roninson (1986). Internal duplication and homology with bacterial transport proteins in the mdr-1 (P-glycoprotein) gene from multidrug resistant human cells. Cells 47: 381-389.

6. J.H. Gerlach, J.A. Endicott, P.F. Juranka, G. Henderson, F. Sarangi, K.L. Deuchars, and V. Ling (1986). Homology between P-glycoprotein and a bacterial hemolysin transport protein suggests a model for multidrug resistance. Nature 324: 485-489.

7. J. Riordan, K. Deuchars, N. Kartner, N. Alon, J. Trent and V. Ling (1985). Amplification of P-glycoprotein gene in multidrug-resistant mammalian cell lines. Nature 316: 817-819.

8. A.M. Van der Bliek, T. Van der Velde-Koerts, V. Ling and P. Borst (1986). Overexpression and amplification of five genes in a multidrug-resistant Chinese hamster ovary cell line. Mol. Cell. Biol. 6: 1671-1678.

9. P. Gros, Y.B. Nericeh, J.M. Croop, and D.E. Houseman (1986). Isolation and expression of a complementary DNA that confers multidrug resistance. Nature 323: 728-731.

10. K.L. Deuchars, R-P. Du, M. Naik, D. Evernden-Porelle, N. Kartner, A.M. Van der Bliek, and V. Ling (1987). Expression of hamster P-glycoprotein and multidrug resistance in DNA-mediated transformants of mouse LTA cells. Mol. Cell. Biol. 7: 718-724.

11. K. Veda, C. Cadarelli, M.M. Gottesman, and I. Pastan (1987). Expression of a full-length cDNA for human MDR1 gene confers resistance to colchicine, doxorubicin, and vinblastine. Proc. Natl. Acad. Sci. USA. 84: 3004-3008.

12. D. Bell, J. Gerlach, N. Kartner, R. Buick and V. Ling (1985). Detection of P-glycoprotein in ovarian cancer: a molecular marker associated with multidrug resistance. J. Clinc. Oncology 3: 311-315.

13. D.D.F. Ma, R.A. Davey, D.H. Harmon, J.P. Isbister, R.D. Scurr, S.M. Mackertich, G. Dowden, and D.R. Bell (1987). Detection of a multidrug resistant phenotype in acute non-lymphoblastic leukemia. The Lancet Jan. 17, 135-137.

14. J.H. Gerlach, D.R. Bell, C. Karakousis, H.K. Slocum, N. Kartner, Y.M. Rustum, V. Ling and R.M. Baker (1987). P-glycoprotein in human sarcoma: Evidence for multidrug resistance. J. Clinical Oncology. 5:1452-1460.

Neo-Adjuvant Chemotherapy. Ed. Cl. Jacquillat, M. Weil, D. Khayat. Colloque INSERM/John Libbey Eurotext Ltd. © 1988. Vol. 169, pp. 651-654.

Acquired and natural resistance to folate antagonists : implications for adjuvant chemotherapy

J.R. Bertino, G. Pizzorno and E. Mini

Memorial Sloan-Kettering Cancer Center, Yale U. Sch. of Med., USA and U. of Florence, Italy

MTX is usually employed in the clinic for the treatment of breast and head and neck cancer as a weekly or bi-weekly pulse injection, especially when used in combination with other agents. For certain tumors capable of efficiently transporting and polyglutamylating this drug may provide a therapeutic benefit, since MTX a consequence, is retained in cells for long periods of time, thus resulting in prolonged inhibition of DNA synthesis. We have found that in human squamous cell cancer lines, polyglutamylation of MTX varies considerably. For example, a cell line not able to polyglutamate MTX significantly was refractory to a high pulse dose of MTX given over 4h; in contrast, another cell line capable of extensive polyglutamylation of MTX after a 4h exposure was sensitive to this drug. Both cell lines were equally sensitive to long term (72h) exposures to drug. Recently we reported that acquired resistance high dose (3,30 uM) 24h pulses of MTX in the human T lymphoblast cell line CCRF-CEM is also associated with impaired polyglutamylation of MTX. In this circumstance as well, resistance is scheduled dependent, and the "resistant" cell line remains sensitive to long term (72h) exposures to this drug. These data underscore the importance of polyglutamylation as determinant of MTX sensitivity to low dose continuous exposure may still be present in tumor cell populations unable to polyglutamate this drug. The clinical message that may be derived from these studies is that natural or acquired resistance to MTX may be a function of the dose schedule employed in that low dose continuous MTX maybe useful in "MTX resistant" patients.

Key Words

Squamous cell carcinoma
Methotrexate
Drug resistance
Polyglutamylation

INTRODUCTION

A persuasive argument can be made for NEO-Adjuvant chemotherapy: irradiation treatment with cytotoxic drugs may shrink the primary tumor, thus improving operability or local control with x-rays; and this information re tumor responsiveness may be used to determine post definitive treatment use. A more important rationale for the use of chemotherapy in conjunction with surgery or irradiation (either pre or post) is the possibility that this modality will eliminate micro-metasasis that if left untreated, eventually will result in relapse. There is firm experimental evidence that supports the value of adjuvant chemotherapy for this purpose; micrometastasis may be more susceptible to chemotherapy than are larger primary tumors because they may be growing more rapidly, and perhaps more importantly have less of a probability of having drug resistant cells, if the number of drug resistant cells is proportional to the tumor size.

The limited success of this approach in the treatment of breast cancer, colon cancer, and in epidermoid cancer of the head and neck is likely due to the presence of a more significant drug resistant population than believed. For example, if micrometastasis contain less that 10^8 cells, and the mutation frequency is one in 10^6 cells, combinations of drugs with different mechanisms of action and resistance mechanisms, i.e. CAF for breast cancer, cisplatin and 5 FU for cancer of the head and neck, would be more effective than current results indicate.

Therefore, an important avenue to explore is the possibility that these epithelial tumors are more heterogenous than believed, and that large proportions of the tumor cell population may be inherently resistant to individual drugs. It follows then that if we are to improve the results of adjuvant therapy, an assessment of sensitivity to the drugs to be used should be made, and that treatment programs will have to be more flexible, taking this information into account. In this report we describe the disparate sensitivity of well known squamous cell carcinoma cell lines to high dose pulses of methotrexate (MTX) as well as the basis for this result, as an example of the problem that may be encountered clinically.

RESULTS

Three human cell lines, obtained from patients with epidermoid cell carcinoma were studied (TABLE I). The cell lines were maintained as monolayers, in

RPMI media containing 10% dialysed fetal bovin serum. We determined the ED^{50} of each of these cell lines to both a 24 and 72 hr exposure of varying concentrations of MTX (TABLE 1). Although these cell lines were derived from patients with squamous cell carcinoma who had not been previously treated with chemotherapy, the A253 cell line was markedly insensitive to a 24 hr exposure to MTX; there was less of a difference in the ED^{50} for a 72 hr exposure between the three cell lines. We studied the factors known to be important in tumor cell sensitivity to MTX in these cell lines. The level of the target enzyme dihydrofolate reductase (DHFR), uptake of MTX in the three cell lines, and the affinity of MTX for DHFR from each of the cell lines were all similar. Since we had previously demonstrated that acquired resistance to high dose pulses of MTX was due to impaired polyglutamylation of this drug, we tested the cell lines for this activity. As shown in TABLE II, the A253 cell line is markedly impaired in its ability to polyglutamate MTX, while the FaDu cell line is comparable to the results we have obtained in the CCRF-CEM parent strain, also highly sensitive to MTX administered as a 24h pulse (Pizzorno et al, 1988). The SQCC/YI cell line was slightly less efficient than the FaDu cell line in its ability to polyglutamate MTX, and its sensitivity to this drug was also slightly less than the FaDu cell line.

As was also observed for the MTX resistant CCRF-CEM cell line that is resistant on the basis of impaired polyglutamylation, when a longer exposure of MTX was used (72h) there was almost no difference in the ED_{50} values for cytotoxicity between the parent cell line and the MTX resistant line. This observation strongly supports our conclusion that impaired polyglutamylation is responsible for resistance to "pulse" (24h) MTX; since in this circumstance cytotoxicity would depend to a great extent on the ability of the cell to polyglutamate and thus retain this drug. Other studies have also emphasized the importance of this event to MTX cytotoxicity and selectivity. Normal tissues (G.I. mucosa, bone marrow cells) have limited ability to polyglutamate MTX (Koizumi et al, 1985; Poser et al, 1981; Fry et al, 1983).

These results provide an additional example of how mechanisms of natural and acquired resistance to a drug may be identical when a tumor cell population contains a substantial number of drug resistant cells. When there is no decrease in the tumor cell volume, we conclude that the tumor is inherently resistant to the drug. Acquired resistance results when the tumor population is decimated by the drug, but eventually (months to years) drug resistant cells accumulate and result in relapse. These and other studies show that at least for one drug, we now have the ability to assess sensitivity to a tumor cell population (Rodenhuis et al, 1986), and encourages further efforts to test the usefulness if these observations in adjuvant trials. Whether inherent resistance is due to gene damage caused by the carcinogen, is also worthy of further study (Srimatkandada et al, 2988). Finally, this work indicates that in some circumstances drug resistance may be only relative, and that other dose schedules may still be effective.

TABLE I Cytotoxicity to MTX after exposure to 24h or 72h in three human squamous cell lines.

CELL LINE	ED_{50} (uM)		RATIO
	24h	72h	24/72h
A253	5000	40	125
$ScCC/Y_1$	500	30	15
FaDu	300	20	15

TABLE II MTX polyglutamate formation in three human squamous cell carcinoma lines.

CELL LINE	MTX	glu_1	glu_2	glu_3	glu_4	glu_5	glu_6	TOTAL
A_{253}	51.3	7.4	11.8	3.6	5.9	0.3	15.8	81.6
SQ CC/Y_1	64.5	26.0	44.0	44.8	29.3	0.9	75.0	209.5
FaDu	70.8	65.5	103.1	56.2	22.2	1.9	80.3	319.7

Cells were incubated with [3H -MTX (10uM) for 24h in complete medium. MTX polyglutamates were determined as described (Pizzorno et al, 1988).

REFERENCES

Pizzorno, G., Mini, E., Coronello M., McGuire, J.J., Moroson, B.A., Cashmore, A.R. Lin, J.T., Mazzei, T., Periti, P., and Bertino, J.R. (1988) Resistance to methotrexate in CCRF-CEM cells after short-term, high dose treatment is associated with impaired polyglutamylation. Cancer Res. in Press.

Koizumi, S.G. Curt, R.L. Fine, J.D. Griffin, J., and Chabner, B.A.(1985) Formation of methotrexate polyglutamates in purified myeloid precusor cells from normal human bone marrow. J. Clin. Invest 74: 1008-1014.

Poser, R.C., Sirotnak, F.M. and Chello, P.L. (1981).Differential synthesis of methotrexate polyglutamates in normal proliferative and neoplastic mouse tissues in vivo Cancer Res.,41: 4441-4446.

Fry, D.N., Anderson, L.A., Borst, M., and Goldman, I.D. (1983). Analysis of the role of membrane transport and polyglutamylation of methotrexate in gut and the Ehrlich tumor in vivo as factors in drug sensitivity and selectivity. Cancer Res. 43: 1087-1092.

Rodenhuis, S. McGuire, J.J., Narayanan, R., and Bertino, J.R. (1986). Development of an assay system for the detection and classification of methotrexate resistance in resistance in fresh leukemia cells. (1986) Cancer Res. 46: 6513-6519.

Srimatkandada, S., Schweitzer, B.I., Moroson, B.A., Dube, S., and Bertino, J.R. Selective amplification of a polymorphic dihydrofolate reductase gene in a methotrexate resistant human colon carcinoma cell line, HCT-8. Submitted for publication.

Résumé

Le Méthotrexate est généralement utilisé dans le cancer du sein, de la tête et du cou par injection mensuelle ou bi-mensuelle en particulier en association avec d'autres agents. Dans certaines tumeurs capables de transport et de polyglutamation, le médicament peut être bénéfique au plan thérapeutique puisque le Méthotrexate est retenu dans les cellules pendant longtemps ceci provoquant une inhibition prolongée de la synthèse de l'ADN. Nous avons trouvé que dans les lignées de cellules épidermoïdes humaines, la polyglutamation du Méthotrexate varie considérablement ainsi une lignée incapable de polyglutamation est résistante à des doses rapides de Méthotrexate en 4 heures. Au contraire, une autre lignée capable de polyglutamation extensive du Méthotrexate est sensible à une exposition de 4 heures au Méthotrexate. Mais les deux lignées sont également sensibles à l'exposition à long terme (72 heures). Récemment nous avons montré que la résistance acquise à de hautes doses de Méthotrexate de 24 heures, sur les lignées lymphoblastiques humaines CCRFCEM est également associée avec une altération de la polyglutamation du Méthotrexate. Dans ces circonstances également, la résistance dépend de la durée du traitement et les lignées résistantes demeurent sensibles à des expositions prolongées (72 heures). Ces données soulignent l'importance de la polyglutamation comme déterminant de la sensibilité à de faibles doses d'exposition continue. Ainsi la résistance naturelle ou acquise peut être fonction de la durée d'administration et de faibles doses continues peuvent être utiles chez des malades résistants au Méthotrexate.

Neo-Adjuvant Chemotherapy. Ed. Cl. Jacquillat, M. Weil, D. Khayat. Colloque INSERM/John Libbey Eurotext Ltd. © 1988. Vol. 169, pp. 655-660.

Relationship of membrane potential to acquired and intrinsic multiple drug resistance

Theodore J. Lampidis, Alain Fourcade and Haim Tapiero

Institut de Cancérologie et d'Immunogénétique, Département de Pharmacologie Cellulaire, Moléculaire et de Pharmacocinétique (CNRS UA 1163), Hôpital Paul Brousse, 94800 Villejuif, France (A.F., H.T.)Papanicolaou Comprehensive Cancer Center, Department of Oncology, University of Miami, School of Medicine, Miami, Florida 33136, (TJL) USA

ABSTRACT

We review data here which demonstrate that cells with acquired multiple drug resistance (MDR) share a number of biochemical changes with cells that have intrinsic MDR. Among the changes that may directly affect lowered drug accumulation and therefore have relevance for a mechanism of MDR are lowered transmembrane potentials that have been found in both these cell types. This data is supported by the observation that the drugs which the MDR cell types studied here are resistant to, are positively-charged. The results overall are consistent with the interpretation that electrically negative membrane potentials influence the cellular accumulation of certain lipophilic positively-charged compounds. Since active efflux has been widely reported in tumor cells with acquired resistance, and in the cell types considered here, it appears that two separate processes affect the transport and accumulation of these positively charge compounds, acive efflux and transmembrane potentials. If and how these two processes are related remain to be investigated.

INTRODUCTION

In a number of in vitro studies it has been shown that by exposing tumor cells to a single drug they can acquire resistance to a variety of seemingly unrelated compounds (1-3). Cells which acquire this kind of multiple drug resistance (MDR) have been shown to have an increased ability to efflux these agents as compared to their sensitive parental cell counterparts (4-7). Moreover, drug efflux has been demonstrated to be effectively blocked by the calcium channel blocker, verapamil (8, 9) and a number of other agents (9-12). By blocking drug efflux and consequently increasing intracellular drug levels, resistant cells can be rendered sensitive. A relationship between the ability to efflux these compounds and the appearance of certain high molecular weight glycoproteins has also been widely reported (13-15). More recently, the isolation and transferance of a gene which confers multiple drug resistance and the appearance of the high molecular weight glycoprotein in the recipient cell has been demonstrated (16, 17).

Thus a number of studies have shown that MDR is directly linked to lowered drug accumulaion which is associated with increased efflux and the appearance of specific glycoproteins.

It is the intend here to review data which link a new parameter, membrane potentials, to drug resistance, lowered drug accumulation and MDR mRNA expression in cell types which have acquired and those that have intrinsic MDR. These data will emphasize that cellular changes associated with acquired MDR parallel those with intrinsic MDR.

RESULTS AND DISCUSSION

MEMBRANE POTENTIALS AND INTRINSIC MULTIPLE DRUG RESISTANCE

Recently, we have shown that a number of positively-charged anti-cancer agents such as adriamycin (ADM), daunorubicin (DNR), THP-ADM, and vincristine preferentially accumulate in, and are more cytotoxic to (10), a human breast carcinoma cell line, MCF-7, as compared to an epithelial cell line derived from normal tissue, CV-1. Similar results were obtained in these cells with a number of fluorescent dyes which are also positively-charged i.e. Rhodamine 123 (Rho 123), Rhodamine 6G, an Safranin O (19). Using microelectrodes we found that these increases in drug accumulation and preferential cytotoxicity correlate with increased transmembrane potentials in MCF-7 vs CV-1 cells (19). These results are consistent with the interpretation that electrically negative membrane potentials influence the cellular accumulation of certain lypophilic positively-charged compounds.

Since mitochondria have highly negative membrane potentials and the latter group of compounds have been shown to localize specifically in mitochondrial, Davis et al. (20) used high K+ medium and specific inhibitors of mitochondrial membrane potential to demonstrate that both plasma and mitochondrial membrane potentials were contributing to the accumulation of Rhodamine 123. More recently, it has been shown that mitochondria isolated from MCF-7 cells had a higher membrane potential than those isolated from CV-1 (21). Thus for these cell lines data has emerged which suggests that membrane potentials play a key role in the differential accumulation of certain positively-charged compounds and consequently to their relative resistance to them.

On the other hand, we have reported (10, 22) that decreased accumulation of Rho 123, ADM and their respective positively-charged analogs are also related to the ability of normal epithelial cells to efflux these compounds. Efflux of these drugs from CV-1 cells was shown to be blocked by the calcium channel antagonist, verapamil (22). This implies that either the efflux pump and/or membrane potentials are involved with differtial accumulation of positively-charged compounds in cells which display intrinsic MDR.

MEMBRANE POTENTIALS AND ACQUIRED MULTIPLE DRUG RESISTANCE

Increased efflux and its inhibition by verapamil in these intrinsically resistant normal epithelial cells parallels results reported for a number of different tumor cell types which have acquired MDR (8, 9, 10).

Dano (4), Skovsgaard (5) and other investigators (6) have shown that by lowering glucose and using metabolic inhibitors, drug efflux from tumor cells with acquired MDR could be blocked, suggesting that drug efflux is an active process and thus proposing the existence of an "efflux pump". Working with Friend leukemia cells that have acquired MDR by stepwise exposure to increasing levels of ADM we found that these cells also have increased efflux and reduced accumulation of ADM and Rho 123. Moreover, we find that the drugs these cells are resistant to are also positively-charged (10).

We therefore investigated whether differential membrane potentials could be playing a role in drug accumulation of tumor cells with acquired MDR. With flow cytometry we have found significantly higher levels of the membrane potential probe 3,3-dihexyl-oxacarbocyanine (DiOC6(3)) in sensitive vs resistant FLC (23, 24). This data agrees with the preliminary report by Gupta et al. (25) in which they showed lower membrane potentials in two MDR tumor cell types as compared to their parental sensitive cell counterparts. Thus it appears that for anti-cancer agents as well as other compounds that are positively-charged two separate processes also affect their transport and accumulation in tumor cells with acquired MDR, plasma membrane potentials and active efflux if and how these two processes are related remains to be investigated.

MDR mRNA EXPRESSION IN INTRINSIC AND ACQUIRED MDR

A class of MDR genes have been isolated from cells with acquired resistance which are also responsible for the expression of these high molecular weight glycoproteins (16-18). However, the normal function of these genes remains unknown. A clue that they do have a role in normal tissue function comes from the work of Fojo et al. (26) and Thiebaut (27), in which it is shown that MDR mRNA expression is found in widely-varying amounts in different normal tissues i.e. adrenal gland, kidney, lung, etc. Ames (28) suggests that the homology between the expression of these MDR genes found in eukaryotic cell and those previously found for the influx of certain amino acids in prokaryotic cells implies a conservation of normal function for these genes. Recently, we have reported (29) that the above mentioned CV-1 cell line isolated from normal tissue is poitive for MDR mRNA expression. Thus this provides clear evidence that a cell line not previously exposed to chemotherapeutic agents which therefore did not acquire MDR, displays intrinsic resistance and expresses MDR mRNA.

CONCLUSIONS

Although several biochemical changes have been reported to be associated with acquired MDR in different tumor cell types it is unclear whether any of them are directly responsible for this process. It is clear however, that reduced drug accumulation is fundamental to this kind of resistance. Thus changes which are related to reduced intracellular drug levels in MDR cells are pertinent to the mechanism of resistance. Here we describe data which shows that lowered membrane potentials in cells with either intrinsic or acquired MDR correlates with reduced drug accumulation in these cell types relative to their sensitive cell counterparts (19, 23, 24). The fact that the drugs which these cell types are resistant to carry an overall positive-charge indicates that differences in membrane potentials may play a key role in the mechanism(s) responsible for MDR.

Acknowledgements

This work was supported by NIH CA 37109, Eastman Kodak, ARC, INSERM CRE 85.2024 and Roger Bellon Laboratories.

REFERENCES

1. BECK W.T. The Cell biology of multiple drug resistance. Biochem. Pharmacol. 36 : 2879-2887, 1987.

2. RONINSON I.B. Molecular mechanism of multidrug resistance in tumor cells. Clin. Physiol. Biochem. 5 : 140-151, 1987.

3. MYERS C., COWAN K., SINHA B., and CHABNER B. The phenomenon of pleiotropic drug resistance in Important Advances in Oncology, J.B. Lippincott Company 1987, pp. 27-38.

4. DANO K. Active outward transport of daunomycin in resistant Ehrlich ascites tumor cells. Biochem. Biophys. Acta 323 : 466-483, 1973.

5. SKOUSSGAARD T. Mechanism of cross-resistance between vincristine and daunorubicin in Ehrlich ascites tumor cells. Cancer Res. 38 : 4722-4727, 1978.

6. INABA M. and JOHNSON R. Uptake and retention of adriamycin and daunorubicin by sensitive and anthracycline-resistant sublines of P388 leukemia. Biochem. Pharmacol. 27 : 2123-2130, 1978.

7. TAPIERO H., FOURCADE A., VAIGOT P. and FARHI J.J. Comparative uptake of adriamycin and daunorubicin in sensitive and resistant Friend leukemia cells measured by flow cytometry. Cytometry 2 : 298-302, 1982.

8. TSURUO T., IIDA H., TSUKAGOSHI S. and SAKURAI Y. Overcoming of vincristine resistance in P388 leukemia in vivo and in vitro through enhanced cytotoxicity of vincristine and vinblastine by verapamil. Cancer Res. 41 : 1967-1972, 1981.

9. TSURUO T., IIDA H., TSUKAGOSHI S. and SAKURAI Y. Increased accumulation of vincristine and adriamycin in drug-resistant P388 tumor cells following incubation with calcium antagonists and calmodulin inhibitors. Cancer Res. 42 : 4730-4733, 1983.

10. TAPIERO H., BOULE D., ITTAH-CORCOS N., FOURCADE A. and LAMPIDIS T.J. Manipulation of drug accumulation : mechanisms to overcome resistance in Mechanisms of Drug Resistance in Neoplastic Cells (Eds Wooley P. and Tew K.) pp. 329-345. Academic Press, New-York 1987.

11. RAMU A., FUCHS Z., GATT S. and GLAUBIGER D. Reversal of acquired resistance to doxorubicin in P388 murine leukemia cells by perhexiline maleate. Cancer Res. 44 : 144-148, 1984.

12. GANAPATHI R., GRABOWSKI D., ROUSE W. and RIEGLER F. Differential effect of the calmodulin inhibition trifluoperazine on cellular accumulation, retention and cytotoxicity of anthracyclines in doxorubicin-resistant P388 mouse leukemia. Cancer Res. 44 : 5056-5061, 1984.

13. JULIANO R.L. and LING V. A surface glycoprotein modulating drug permeability in chinese hamster ovary cell mutants. Biochem. Biophys. Acta 455 : 152-162, 1976.

14. HAMADA H. and TSURUO T. Functional role for the 170 to 180 kDa glycoprotein specific to drug-resistant tumor cells as revealed by monoclonal antibodies. Proc. Natl. Acad. Sci. USA 83 : 7785-7789, 1986.

15. KARTNER N., RIORDAN J.R. and LING V. Cell surface glycoprotein associated with multidrug resistance in mammalian cell lines. Science 221 : 1285-1288, 1983.

16. RONINSON I.B., ABELSON H.T., HOUSMAN D.E., HOWELL N. and VARSHAUSKY A. Amplification of specific DNA sequences correlates with multidrug resistance in chinese hamster cells. Nature 309 : 626-628, 1984.

17. FOJO A., LEBO R., SHIMIZU N., CHIN J.E., RONINSON I.B., MERLINO G.T., GOTTESMAN M.M. and PASTAN I. Localization of multidrug resistance associated DNA sequences to human chromosome 7. Somatic Cell Mol. Genet. 12 : 415-420, 1986.

18. SHEN D.W., FOJO A., RONINSON I.B., CHIN J.E., SAFFIR R., PASTAN I. and GOTTESMAN M.M. Multidrug resistance of DNA-mediated transformants is linked to transfer of the human mdR 1 gene. Mol. Cell. Biol. 6 : 4039-4044, 1986.

19. LAMPIDIS T.J., HASSAN J., WEISS M. and CHEN L.B. Selective killing of carcinoma cells in vitro by several different cationic lipophilic compounds : a cellular basis. Biomed. Pharm. 39 : 220-226, 1985.

20. DAVIS S., WEISS M.J., WONG J., LAMPIDIS T.J. and CHEN L.B. Mitochondrial and plasma membrane potentials cause unusual accumulation and retention of rhodamine 123 by human breast adenocarcinoma-derived MCF-7 cells. J. Biol. Chem. 260 : 13844-13850, 1985.

21. MODICA-NAPOLITANO J.S. and APRILLE J.R. Basis for the selective cytotoxicity of rhodamine 123. Cancer Res. 47 : 4361-4365, 1987.

22. LAMPIDIS T.J., KRISHAN A., PLANAS L. and TAPIERO H. Reversal of intrinsic resistance to adriamycin in normal cells by verapamil. Cancer Drug Deliv. 3 : 251-259, 1986.

23. HASMANN M., VALET G., TAPIERO H. and LAMPIDIS T.J. Plasma and mitochondrial transmembrane potentials in adriamycin resistant and positive Friend leukemia cells as determined by flow cytometry. Proc. Amer. Assoc. Cancer Res. 28 : 1120, 1987.

24. HASMANN M., VALET G.K., TAPIERO H., TREVORROW K. and LAMPIDIS T.J. Membrane potential differences between adriamycin sensitive and resistant cells as measured by flow cytometry. Submitted, 1987.

25. GUPTA S., VAYUVEGULA B., SWEET P., STEPECKEY M., MURRAY S., JACOBS R. and SLATER L. Membrane potential changes associated with pleiotropic drug resistance. Abstract AFCR Clinical Res. 34 : 881A, 1986.

26. FOJO A.T., VEDA K., SLAMON P.J., POPLACK D.G., GOTTESMAN M.M. and PASTAN I. Expression of a multidrug-resistance gene in human tumors and tissues. Proc. Natl. Acad. Sci. USA 84 : 265-269, 1987.

27. THIEBAUT F., TSURUO T., HAMADA H., GOTTESMAN M.M., PASTAN I. and WILLINGHAM M.C. Cellular localization of the multidrug-resistance gene product P-glycoprotein in normal human tissues. Proc. Natl. Acad. Sci. USA 84 : 7735-7738, 1987.

28. AMES G.F.L. The basis of multidrug resistance in mammalian cells : homology with bacterial transport. Cell 47 : 323-324, 1986.

29. SAVARAJ N., LU K., KUO T., CASTELLO C., TAPIERO H. and LAMPIDIS T.J. Reduced drug accumulation and increased P-glyprotein expression in a normal cell line. Proc. Amer. Assoc. Cancer Res. 29 : 1988, in press.

Digestive cancers

Cancers digestifs

Neo-Adjuvant Chemotherapy. Ed. Cl. Jacquillat, M. Weil, D. Khayat. Colloque INSERM/John Libbey Eurotext Ltd. © 1988. Vol. 169, pp. 663-666.

Best timing of adjuvant chemotherapy for gastric cancer

Toshifusa Nakajima and Mitsumasa Nishi

Division of Surgery, Cancer Institute Hospital, Kamiikebukuro 1-37-1, Toshimaku, Tokyo 170, Japan

ABSTRACT

A retrospective analysis of five independent randomized studies of adjuvant chemotherapy for gastric cancer was made to know the best timing when to initiate chemotherapy in relation to the surgery. The total number of the patients involved were 1012. Early use of chemotherapy revealed to be effective on the advanced stage diseases rather than early disease. Delay in initiation resulted in taking a longer time for the clinical benefit to be manifest. These findings suggest that an adjuvant chemotherapy should be initiated immediately or within a few days after surgery.

KEY WORDS

Adjuvant chemotherapy, gastric cancer, timing of initiation

INTRODUCTION

The gastric cancer is still the leading cause of death in Japan. To improve the treatment results of gastric cancer, we have performed various adjuvant chemotherapies since 1960. Except for some trials in the United States conducted as early as in 1960s, most adjuvant chemotherapies were initiated one or two months after major surgery(Douglass,1988). Most Japanese trials of adjuvant chemotherapy for gastric cancer(Nakajima,1988) are also initiated after surgery, though not so late as one month. Recent trend in adjuvant chemotherapy(Frei,1982) namely, the neoadjuvant chemotherapy recommends the perioperative (preferably preoperative) initiation of treatment. However, experimental chemotherapy(Skiper, 1986,Goldie,1986) indicates that the best results could be obtained at the least tumor burden. In this regards, the present report deals with the retrospective review of our past five independent controlled studies related to the timing of chemotherapy and its clinical benefit.

PATIENTS AND METHOD OF STUDY

From 1961 to 1977 at The Cancer Institute Hospital,Tokyo, patients with gastric cancer who had curative gastrectomy entered the five consecutive studies by random allocation. Total number of the patients were 1012, 24.9% of whole cases (4070) treated in our hospital during the same period. Treatment results were evaluated by postoperative survivals related to the timing of adjuvant chemotherapy to the surgery.

RESULTS

From 1969 to 1970, a trial was carried out with intraoperative i.a, and i.p administration of mitomycin C(MMC), followed by intermittent oral administration of cyclophosphamide(CPM) for three years after surgery. MMC was injected into the hepatic and splenic arteries and spread into the peritoneal cavity. These multichemotherapy regimen was compared with surgery plus intraoperative chemotherapy, and surgery alone. This trial was abandoned because of frequent liver dysfunction caused by intrahepatic MMC, which seemed to be related to the later development of liver metastasis. A trial initiated immediately after surgery was carried out from 1966 to 1968 with large dose(0.4mg/kg on day 1 and 0.2mg/kg on day 2) of MMC. This regimen was effective exclusively on stage III disease:5 year survival rate was 45% for chemotherapy group and 32% for the control group(surgery alone). From 1961 to 1966, a study was done, where 0.08mg/kg of Mitomycin C was given a few days after surgery, one shot i.v. twice a week for five weeks. Five year survival rate of whole case was 45.9% for treated group and 35.9% for the control group(surgery alone). The effect was prominent in stage III disease(37.3% vs 18.6%). A chemotherapy trial (1971 to 1973), which compared single MMC with multi-drug regimen, was initiated a few days after surgery. The regimen of single MMC was identical with the previous trial. This combination chemotherapy was known as MFC therapy and consisted of MMC,5-FU and cytosine arabinoside, given ten times after surgery. MFC therapy was superior to MMC group, and to the control(surgery alone). Five year survival rate was 66.9% for MFC, 64.3% for MMC, and 50.0% for surgery alone.
The next trial(1974 to 1977) was composed of MFC therapy followed by oral 5-FU for two years after surgery, an alternate combination therapy(MF'C), where 5-FU in MFC plus 5-FU was substituted by futraful(FT), a kind of masked compound of 5-FU, and surgery alone. The chemotherapies were initiated two weeks after surgery. MFC + 5-FU and MF'C + FT therapies were superior to surgery alone. Five year survival rate was 69.6% for MFC + 5-FU, 62.7% for MF'C + FT, and 48.0% for surgery alone. It took three years for the clinical benefit to be manifest.

Table 1. Timing of Adjuvant Chemotherapy in Terms of the Effect

Pre-op	Intra-op	Post-op	Post-op maintenance	Effect
	i.a ⇩		p.o	Abandoned due to liver dysfunction
		i.v ⇩		Stage III
		i.v ⇩		Stage II and III
		i.v ⇩		Stage II and III
		i.v ⇩	p.o	Stage II (and III)

Table 1 shows the summarized results of adjuvant chemotherapy in regard to the timing of initiating chemotherapy.

DISCUSSION

Table 2. Gastric Cancer treated at Cancer Institute Hospital

	Curative gastrectomy (5yr. surv.)	Non-curative gastrectomy (5yr. surv.)	No resection (5yr. surv.)	Total (5yr. surv.)
1946~49	123 (41.5%)	75 (1.3%)	57 (0%)	255 (20.4%)
1950~59	1,057 (47.7%)	531 (3.4%)	383 (0%)	1,971 (26.5%)
1960~69	1,383 (60.9%)	583 (6.7%)	237 (0%)	2,203 (40.0%)
1970~79	1,631 (72.9%)	453 (6.7%)	138 (0%)	2,222 (53.9%)
1980~86	1,778 ( )	284 ( )	47 ( )	2,109 ( )
Total	5,972 (59.4%)	1,926 (5.0%)	862 (0%)	8,760 (37.4%)

Table 2 shows the treatment result of gastric cancer in our hospital from 1946 to 1986. Five year survival rate is 37.4% for all cases, and 59.4% for patients with curative surgery. A steady improvement in the survival rate was observed in the group of curative surgery, and there is a large difference in the survival rate between 1950s and 60s. The improvement in the survival rate seems to be attributable to the increase in the early stage cancer, and also to the incorporation of adjuvant chemotherapy to the routine treatment modalities.

Since 1961, we have carried out 8 adjuvant chemotherapy trials for gastric cancer. The timing of initiating chemotherapy varies from intraoperative administration to two weeks after surgery. According to the experimental chemotherapy, the best results could be expected when the chemotherapy is initiated at the least tumor burden, namely immediately after surgery. This idea has lead the concept of neoadjuvant chemotherapy. Our present analysis does not allow a definitive conclusion in term of the best timing when to initiate an adjuvant chemotherapy, because the regimens of our adjuvant chemotherapy are different from each other. However, some common findings through 5 trials suggest that early use of adjuvant chemotherapy is more effective on the advanced stage diseases than the late use, regardless of the dose intensity. Intraoperative administration of MMC into the hepatic artery should be avoided because of frequent postoperative liver dysfunction, which might have been enhanced by the anesthetic influence.

Neoadjuvant chemotherapy seems, in general, to be accepted as identical with preoperative chemotherapy(Frei,1986) but experimental data provide no evidence for the superiority of preoperative to the postoperative chemotherapy. When the curative surgery can be expected, it seems reasonable to assume that the control of micrometastasis by adjuvant chemotherapy is easier after eradication of the primary tumor than before, because the impact of curative surgery on the prognosis is much stronger than that of chemotherapy. Then, neoadjuvant chemotherapy should include postoperatives.

Prolonged oral administration of 5-FU, or its derivatives is generally used in Japan as a maintenance therapy. The significance of such maintenance therapy should be re-evaluated from the standpoint of biological cell kinetics(Hill, 1986).

CONCLUSION

Adjuvant chemotherapy should be initiated as early as possible after surgery. However, surgical and anesthetic interventions should be taken into account when the intraoperative i.a. chemotherapy is given.

REFERENCES

Douglass,H.O.,Jr(1988): Western surgical adjuvant trials in gastric cancers: Lessons from current trials to be applied to the future. In "Gastric Cancer (Contemporary Issues in Clinical Oncology, Vol.8)" ed. Douglass,H.O.Jr. pp 145-172. Churchill Livingstone, New York

Nakajima,T. and Nishi,M. (1988): Adjuvant chemotherapy, immunochemotherapy, and neoadjuvant therapy for gastric cancer in Japan. In "Gastric Cancer (Contemporary Issues in Clinical Oncology, Vol.8)" ed. H.O.Douglass,Jr. pp 125-143, Churchill Livingston, New York, 1988

Frei,E.,III (1982): Clinical cancer research: an embattled species. Cancer 50: 1979-1992

Skipper,H.E. (1986): Experimental adjuvant chemotherapy: An overview. Recent Results Cancer Res.103:6-29

Goldie, J.H. and Coldman,A.J. (1986): Theoretical considerations regarding the early use of adjuvant chemotherapy. Recent Results Cancer Res.103:30-35

Frei,E.III, Miller,D., Clark,J.R., Fallon,B.G. and Ervin,T.J. (1986): Clinical and Scientific considerations in preoperative (neoadjuvant) chemotherapy. Recent Results Cancer Res.103:1-5 Hill,B.T.(1986): Implications of certain cell kinetics and biological parameters for preoperative chemotherapy. Recent Results Cancer Res.103:40-53

Neo-Adjuvant Chemotherapy. Ed. Cl. Jacquillat, M. Weil, D. Khayat. Colloque INSERM/John Libbey Eurotext Ltd. © 1988. Vol. 169, pp. 667-671.

Results of a randomized neo-adjuvant program of chemotherapy before surgery and/or radiotherapy in the treatment of 156 esophageal carcinoma

Michel Resbeut*, Christian Chenal, Jacques Vignoud, Jean-Paul Malhaire, Elisabeth Leprise, Sylvain Bourdin, Dominique Barral and Marie H. Pejovick

** Institut J. Paoli-I. Calmettes, BP 156, 13273 Marseille Cedex 9, France*

SUMMARY

Based on the chemotherapy (CH) response rate in a previous pilot study, this trial between 01/83 and 06/86 was designed to test if survival and recurrences would differ in CH treated group (80 pts) from control group (76 pts). The two groups include locally advanced disease. Neoadjuvant program is Methotrexate 100 mg/m2 I.V. + 200 mg/m2 12 hours infusion and folinic acid rescue days 1 and 21, Cisplatin 120 mg/m2 + Vindesine 3 mg/m2 days 2 and 22. Then locoregional treatment is surgery if possible and post-operative radiotherapy (RT) in 35 pts, or only RT with a split course regimen (30 Gy/10F-2 weeks rest-28 Gy/14F). We note CH toxicity WHO > grade 3 in 5 pts with 4 deaths (2 renal damage and 2 infections) and 14% (5/35) surgery deaths related. CH response rate (including pts with only 1 course) : 43.9% (42.5% PR + 1.4% CR). RT response rate (including partial treatment : 42.8% (22.4% PR + 20.4% CR). Response rates of CH and RT are 67.5% (42.5% PR + 25% CR). Resectability rate : 80% (16/20) in CH group vs 60% (9/15) in control group. The 3 year survival is 7.2% vs 10.6% and after surgery, 22% in the both groups but for much less advanced disease. Bad prognostic factors are : weight loss > 10% and non operable tumors. In conclusion, this neoadjuvant program is not of benefit on survival or recurrence rate in the treatment of esophageal squamous cell carcinoma.

INTRODUCTION

The prognosis of squamous celle carcinoma of esophagus remains extremely poor. Despite technical advances in both surgery (S) and radiation therapy (RT), overall 5-year survival rates are in the 5-20% range (9). It is important to emphasize that only 30% and sometime less (11) of patients (pts) are in operable condition when the diagnosis is established because of poor general condition, advanced locally disease or distant mestastases. Long term results of S or RT are similar. It is difficult to obtain locoregional (LR) control which has a major impact for patient palliation as well as cure. Since 10-15 years, several chemotherapy (CH) attempts have been undertook and approximately major objective regressions are seen in 50% of the pts (3). Based on a previous pilot study (12) a randomized trial with or without neoadjuvant CH before LR treatment was begun at Cancer Centers of Lorient, Nantes, Rennes and Brest to validate the impact of such a program on LR control and survival.

METHODS AND MATERIRALS

Between january 1983 and june 1986, 156 pts with SCC of esophagus were entered into a clinical trial in which the planned course of treatment was randomized CH before S and/or RT. To be eligible for this trial, all patients had to have biopsy-proven SCC of the thoracic esophagus without distant mestastase except supraclavicular node. The pretreatment workup included physical examination and endoscopic examination of the esophagus, trachea and bronchial tree with a systematic search of a head and neck cancer. Esophagogram, chest X-ray, liver echography, bone scan, routine blood studies including screening of liver and renal function were perfomed on all pts. Serum creatinine $<$ 133 umol/L, a WBC count of 4,000/uL and a platelet count of 100,000/uL were required. Pts with previous cancer treated for cure were eligible but not those with concomittant malignancy.

80 pts were included in the CH group. CH was given as follows : on day 1, Methotrexate 100 mg/m2 in I.V. bolus followed by Methotrexate 200 mg/m2 12 hours infusion and folinic acid as rescue 50 mg x 2. Vindesine 3 mg/m2 was given on day 2 just before Cisplatin 120 mg/m2 with prehydratation and mannitol induced diuresis. A second course started on day 21. 76 pts were included in the control group. In both groups S was performed when possible followed by post-operative RT. Otherwise a split-course RT was performed (RT protocols are detailed in table 1). In the CH group RT or S starded on day 45. Response was assessed after CH on day 42. In pts without S response was also assessed 1 month after RT (including CH group and control group pts). Standard criteria of complete and partial response (CR and PR) were used and are detailed elsewhere (3,4). Pts characteristics are noted in table 2.

Table 1 - Radiation therapy protocols

Split-course	30 Gy/10F/13 days and 2 weeks rest
	28 Gy/14F/18 days : middle or lower third
	or 32 Gy/16F/22 days : upper third
Post operative RT	50 Gy/25F/33 $\pm$ boost (10 Gy)

Biologic equivalent dose : supra clavicular node : 50 Gy $\pm$ boost and spinal cord : 40 Gy

Table 2 - Patient Characteristics

	CH Group	Control Group
Pts entered	80	76
Male	95%	99%
Median age	57	59
Median karnofsky (range)	80 (40-100)	80 (50-100)
Median weight loss	6.2% (-25% ; 3.5%)	5.9% (-48.5% ; 3.9%)
Size (standard deviation)	6.1 cm (2.7 cm)	7.2 cm (3.3 cm)
Supra clavicular node	10%	7.8%

RESULTS

In the CH group response assessment is avalaible on 73 of 80 pts (tumor progression before starting CH : 4 and denials : 3). 10 pts had only one course of CH (tumor progression : 0 and renal damage after the first course of CH : 1). After CH, among the pts without S, 13 did not receive the planned split-course RT (deaths : 11 and tumor progression : 2). 20 pts were operated without the planned post-operative RT in 6 cases (death : 5 and tumor progression : 1). Pts dead prior day 42 are assumed as no responders. 73 pts received at least one course of CH ; among them response rates are PR : 42.5% (31/73) and CR : 1.4% (11/73). In pts treated with 2 courses of CH, response rates are respectively PR : 54.2% and CH : 2.1%. The median duration of response is identical for CR or PR : 12 months (1-32). After CH, 40 pts without S received the planned split-course RT ; 1 month after this RT with prior CH response rates are PR : 42.5% and CR : 25%. 20 pts underwent S after CH with a 80% resectability rate. In the whole CH group, the actuarial 3-year survival rate in 80 pts is 7.2% (standard deciation 3.6%), this rate is 8.8% for pts treated with 2 courses of CH and 22% for operated pts.

In the control group, 3 pts did not receive RT (tumor progression : 2 and denial : 1). 7 pts had only the first part of the split-course RT (deaths : 3, tumor progression : 3 and denial : 1). 15 pts underwent S and among them, 3 pts did not receive the planned post operative RT (death : 1, denial : 1 and "in-situ carcinoma" : 1).
Responses rates in the 55 pts treated with RT without S are : PR 22.4% and CR 20.4%. The median durations of responses are respectively 6 months (1-40) and 11 months (1-46). 15 pts underwent a S prior any other treatment with a 60% resectability rate. In the whole control group, the actuarial 3-year survival rate in 73 pts is 10.6% (standard deviation 3.9%). This rate is 22% for operated pts.

TOXICITY

CH related toxicity : 2 pts died from renal failure and 2 others from infections (only one during a leukopenic episode). We noted also 2 renal toxicity (serum creatinine $>$ 266 umol/L without death and in one of these 2 cases, second course of CH was not given. 3 pts had leukopania with WBC counts $<$ 1,000 cells/m3 and sepsis requiring antibiotic therapy. Thrombocytopenia was less frequent and a patient had platelet count $<$ 20,000. Almost all pts experencied vomiting and needed anti-emetic treament.

S related toxicity : 4 pts died after S in the CH group (liver cirrhosis decompensation : 1 and respiratory distress : 3) and 1 pts died after S in the control group (hemothorax) but this difference between CH and control group is not significant.

RT related toxicity : we did not seen major complication related to RT. In particular, even after CH, no one pulmonary complication was noted. All the esophagobronchial fistulae are related to tumor progression.

DISCUSSION

CH response rates are similar to those reported in the previous pilot study (12) and in the litterature (3, 4, 13). However, it is well known that the evaluation of the response is very difficult as well as initial staging. Theoretical advantages of a first line CH on the primary tumor and on the micro-metastases were not confirmed in this study. This neo-adjuvant program of CH did not improve survival or LR control and did not protect against metastatic evolution. We noted a simular number of distant metastases in the two groups (15 vs 22 in the control group). At time of death LR control is uncommun with 57 failures in 71 pts in the CH group vs 53 failures in 65 pts in the control group. Even when S is performed at time of death this LR control is not obtained in 10 of 17 pts dead in the CH group and 4 of 11 pts dead in the control group. We can note that the overall response rate to RT with prior CH was 67.5% (PR : 42.5% and CR : 25%) which is better than response rates to RT alone especially for CR and it is important for the comfort of the pts.

We found only two factors of prognosis : weight loss $>$ 10% and operability ($p < 0.01$).

Two courses of CH are perharps not enough especially for responders pts but, with a similar approach ; DESAI (2) in a randomized study obtains 30% 3-year survival rate in the CH group vs 4% with S alone and 5% with RT alone.

Concurrent RT and CH allows to combine cytotoxic and radiosensitizing effects of drugs (7). This approach seems able to improve results in particular when RT is combined with Cisplatin and 5 FU (8, 10) and POPLIN (10) obtains 18 CR in 71 pts, but median durations of response remain 12 months in the whole group and 32 months after CR. Results are similar without S (8).

As KELSEN (5), we think that CH in the treatment of SCC at the esophagus is "still an experimental approach" but it is a very interesting way of research and new attempts must be done with CH regimen allowing to obtain more aften CR without intolerable toxicity. More recent combinations of drugs than the regimen of this study give an higher CR response rate before the LR treatment. In particular, CH regimens including 5 FU and Cisplatin (1, 6) seem attractive and able to widely shrink the tumor before or during the LR treatment.

However the goal is survival and not response rates even if the lR control is an important point for patient palliation.New randomized studies are needed to evaluate the impact of more recent CH regimens on survival.

REFERENCES

1 - Adjani J., Mc Murtrey M., Rich T., Blackburn R., Chang-Tung E., Faintuch J., Lenin B. and Mountain C. (1987) : Combined modality therapy with effective prolonged systemic compnent for the locally advanded squamous cell carcinoma of the esophagus. In ASCO Proceedings, n°320

2 - Desai P.B.,Aduani S.H., Sharma S., Saikia T. and Gopal R. (1987) : A comparison of surgery, radiotherapy and combination chemotherapy in the treatment of locally advanced esophageal carcinoma. In ASCO Proceedings, n°289

3 - Kelsen D. (1984) : Chemotherapy of esophageal cancer. Seminars In Oncology vol.11, n°2, pp 159-168

4 - Kelsen D., Hilaris B., Counley C., Chapman R., Lesser M., Dukeman M., Heelan R. and Bains M. (1983) : Cisplatin, Vindesine and Bleomycin chemotherapy of loco-regional and advanced esophageal carcinoma. The American J. of Med. vol.75, pp 645-652

5 - Kelsen D. (1987) : Multimodality therapy of esophageal carcinoma : Still an experimental approach. Journal of Clin. Oncol. vol.5, n°4, pp 530-531

6 - Kies M.S., Rosen S.T., Chmiel J.S. and Shields T.W. (1987) : Cisplatin and infusion 5 FU in primary management of squamous esophageal cancer. In ASCO Proceedings, n°327

7 - Kolaric K., Maricic Z., Roth A. and Dujmovic I. (1980) : Chemotherapy versus chemoradiotherapy in inoperable esophageal cancer. Oncology, suppl. 1 pp 77-82

8 - Leichman L., Herskovic A., Leichman C.G., Lattin P.B., Steiger Z., Tapazoglou E., Rosenberg J.C., Arbulu A., Asfaw I. and Kinzie J. (1987) : Nonoperative therapy for squamous cell of esophagus. Journal of Clin. Oncol. vol.5, n°3, pp 365-370

9 - Moertel C. (1973) : The esophagus. In Holland J., Frei E. eds. Cancer Medecine Philadelphia Lea and Febiger. pp 1526-1579

10 - Poplin E., Fleming Th., Leichman L., Seydel H., Steiger Z., Taylor S., Vance R., Stuckey W. and Rivkin S. (1987) : Combined therapies for squamous cell carcinoma of the esophagus, a southwest oncology group study. Journal of Clin. Oncol. vol.5, n°4, pp 622-628

11 - Resbeut M., Leprise-Fleury E;, Roussel A. (1987) : Le cancer de l'oesophage en Normandie-Bretagne. Description de la population de malades traitée à Caen-Rennes-Lorient de 1980 à 1984. In Journées de Radiologie Paris 4-5 novembre 1986 J. Eur. Radiother. vol.7, n°3, pp 139-147

12 - Resbeut M., Leprise-Fleury E., Ben-Hassel M., Goudier M.J., Morice-Rouxel M.F., Douillard J.Y and Chenal Ch. (1985) : Squamous cell carcinoma of the esophagus. Treatment by combined Vincristine-Methotrexate plus Folinic acid rescue before radiotherapy. Cancer 56, pp 1246-1250

13 - Spielmann R., Kac J., Rougier P., Le Chevalier T. and Rouesse J. (1987) : Phase II study of 5 FU infusion, Cisplatin and Vindesine in squamous carcinoma of esophageal. in ASCO Proceedings n°368

Résumé

Sur la base d'une étude pilote antérieure, cet essai a inclus 156 patients (pts) porteurs d'un cancer épidermoïde de l'oesophage. La chimiothérapie (CH) première a été randomisée (2 cures à J1 et J21 de Méthotrexate-Vindesine-Cisplatine) et a été administrée à 80 pts. A partir de jour 45, ou d'emblée pour les 76 autres pts, le traitement loco-régional comprenait une chirurgie chaque fois que possible (35 cas), suivie d'une radiothérapie (RT) post-opératoire ou bien, une RT en split-course. Le taux de réponse à la CH est : 43,9% (RP : 42,5% et RC : 1,4%) sur 73 pts évaluables. 4 décès son reliés à la CH. Cette CH n'améliore pas le contrôle loco-régional ni la survie à 3 ans (7,2% vs 10,6% dans le groupe controle).

Neo-Adjuvant Chemotherapy. Ed. Cl. Jacquillat, M. Weil, D. Khayat. Colloque INSERM/John Libbey Eurotext Ltd. © 1988. Vol. 169, pp. 673-682.

Disease oriented phase II study with cisplatin/5FU/etoposide in patients with advanced squamous cell carcinoma of the esophagus

P. Preusser*, H. Wilke*, W. Achterrath**, L. Lenaz**, W. Pircher*, J. Meyer*, M. Blum* and H. Bünte*

** University Hospitals Münster, Hannover, ** Clin. Research Anticancer, Bristol Myers, New-York, USA*

INTRODUCTION

Retrospective analysis of several disease oriented phase II studies in advanced inoperable esophageal cancer shows the following overall response rates:

	Pat. n	CR n (%)	CR + PR n (%)	Lit.
Cisplatin/5Fu	37	3(8%)	13(35%)	7
Cisplatin/5Fu/ADM	21	2(10%)	7(33%)	9
Cisplatin/5Fu/ADM/Etoposide	18	4(22%)	12(67%)	3

Comparing the studies with Cisplatin/5Fu versus Cisplatin/5Fu/ADM shows no differences in CR and overall response rates.

Adding Etoposide to Cisplatin/ADM/5Fu doubled CR and overall response rates, suggesting that Etoposide is active in esophageal cancer.

Therefore, Cisplatin/5Fu/Etoposide was of interest from the clinical point of view.

Furthermore, the combination was of interest because of the following experimental data:

- synergism between Cisplatin/Etoposide (14) and Cisplatin/5Fu (1,14), and 5Fu/Etoposide in vitro (6) and in vivo (13)
- lack of cross resistance between Cisplatin and Etoposide (16, 17), Cisplatin and 5Fu (10), and Etoposide and 5Fu (10)

- different molecular mode of action of Cisplatin, 5Fu, and Etoposide with complementary inhibition of cell metabolism (4,14,15).

Considering these clinical and experimental data, a disease oriented phase II study with Cisplatin/5FU/Etoposide seemed well justified.

Patients and Methods

A total of 23 patients (22 with extensive disease, one with loco-regional disease acc. to MSKCC-staging criteria) have been entered into the study since June 1986.

Patients' characteristics are shown in table 1.

Inclusion and exclusion criteria, and criteria for premature withdrawal from treatment are shown in tables 2 - 4.

Tables 5 and 6 show staging and control examinations, laboratory screen and response evaluation.

TABLE 1

Patients' characteristics

No of pts	23
No of pts evaluable	20
age	42-65 years (mean 57 yrs)
males / females	20 / 0
performance status	WHO-grade I: 4 pts
	WHO-grade II: 16 pts

Extent of disease

Classification acc. to TNM	No of evaluable pts
T_2 N_1 M_0	1
T_3 N_0 M_0	2
T_3 N_1 M_0	3
T_3 N_1 M_1	3
T_4 N_0 M_0	1
T_4 N_1 M_0	3
T_4 N_1 M_1	7

Classification acc. to MSKCC	No of evaluable pts
loco-regional disease	1
extensive disease	19

TABLE 2

Inclusion criteria

- histologically confirmed advanced squamous cell carcinoma of the esophagus
- measurable or evaluable disease
- no prior chemotherapy or radiotherapy
- no brain metastases
- age ≤ 65 years
- performance status ≤ II WHO-scale
- life expectancy of at least 3 months
- white blood cell count (WBC) ≥ 4000/mm3, platelet count ≥ 100.000/mm3
- adequate renal function defined as serum creatinine, BUN within the normal range creatinine clearance ≥ 60 ml/min/1,72 m2 (≥ 1,0 ml/sec)
- liver function parameters (SGOT, SGPT, S-bilirubin) within the normal range
- serum electrolytes within the normal range
- normal auditory function
- no acute disease with fever
- informed consent

TABLE 3

Exclusion criteria

- inadequate bone marrow and/or renal function (see inclusion criteria)
- chronic disease requiring long term corticoid therapy
- any active neurological disorder
- pregnancy

TABLE 4

Premature withdrawal from treatment

Patients were taken off study early for any of the following reasons:

- adverse reactions
- progressive disease after the first course of chemotherapy
- no CR or PR after the second course and third course
- progressive disease after initial response
- intolerable toxicity
- if a treatment interval of 35 days had been exceeded
- patient's decision to withdraw
- administrative reasons
- any event which in the investigator's opinion justified treatment discontinuation

---

TABLE 5

Staging and control examinations

Before entering the study, patients underwent the following examinations:

- assessment of measurable tumor parameters by appropriate procedures
- barium esophagram
- esophagoscopy
- tracheabronchoscopy if indicated
- CT: chest / abdomen
  brain if indicated
- sonography: abdomen
- bone scan if indicated
- histology

TABLE 6

Laboratory screen and response evaluation

Hematology, liver and renal function (including creatinine clearance) and serum electrolytes were done before each course of chemotherapy and 4 weeks after the last course. Hematology (WBC, differential count, platelets, Hb) and renal function were controlled weekly.

Audiometry was done before the first and after the last course of chemotherapy.

Electrocardiogram was done before each course.

Tumor response was evaluated by the same procedures as used before start of treatment before each course until maximum response. Subsequently, after every second course and 4 weeks after the last course of chemotherapy.

Criteria for response and toxicity

All patients who had received one course of chemotherapy were considered evaluable for response and toxicity in case of progressive disease.

Patients without progressive disease after the first course were considered evaluable for response and toxicity after they had received at least two courses.

Response, response duration, and toxicity in patients without surgery were assessed acc. WHO-classification.

Treatment

Patients received the following chemotherapy:

Cisplatin 50 mg/m^2 i.v., on days 1 + 7

Etoposide 120 mg/m^2 i.v., on days 3 - 5

5Fu 500 mg/m^2 i.v., on days 3 - 5

Courses were given at 4-weekly intervals provided that patients had recovered from hematologic toxicity.

Treatment consisted of a fixed dose of Cisplatin and 5Fu. After the first course, the dose of Etoposide was modified. If the WBC nadir had been < 1500/mm^3 and/or nadir of platelets < 75.000/mm^3 during the preceding course, the next dose of Etoposide was decreased by 20%.

Results

20 out of the 23 patients entered into the study were evaluable for response and toxicity. Three patients had only one course of chemotherapy and are, therefore, too early for evaluation.

20 patients received 81 (mean 4) courses of chemotherapy and were evaluable for response and toxicity.

5 patients have NC and two have progressive disease.

One patient with NC and one patient with progressive disease underwent radiation and were, therefore, excluded from survival calculation.

Results achieved with Cisplatin/5Fu/Etoposide are summarized in table 7.

TABLE 7

No of pts.	CR n (%)	CR + PR n (%)	mPFI* in months	mS
20	3 (15%)	13 (65%) (44-86%)**	not yet reached	12

** 95% confidence limits * for NED pts.

The overall response rate in 20 evaluable patients was 65% (95% confidence limits 44-86%). It consisted of 3 (15%) CR and of 10 (50%) PR.

After a mean of 3,5 courses (average 2-5), maximum of responses was achieved. Two of three patients with CR after induction chemotherapy received two further courses. Surgery was not performed because the primary tumor was located in the upper third of the esophagus. These clinical CRs were confirmed as pathological CRs by multiple biopsies. The other CR was confirmed as pathological CR by surgery and multiple biopsies.

7 of 10 patients underwent surgery with multiple biopsies after clinical evaluation of stable PR during chemotherapy. All of these PRs were confirmed as pathological PRs.

All patients were disease free after surgery and they received two further courses with Cisplatin/5Fu/Etoposide postoperatively. The remaining three patients responded with PR after two courses. They will receive further chemotherapy till stable PR or CR. After that, they will undergo surgery. Two of three patients with CR are disease free at 2^+ months and at 4^+ months.

One patient died of progressive disease 9 months after induction of a CR. Median progress free interval for patients with PR and NED after surgery has not yet been reached (5^+ - 15^+ months). Median survival of all patients is 12 months (3^+ - 15^+ months). Patients with CR or partial response and NED have a median survival time of 15 months Patients with NC have a median survival of 9 months.

The worst toxicities observed after all courses per patient acc. to WHO-criteria are listed in table 8.

TABLE 8

Toxicity

Toxicity	WHO-grade n (%) 0	1	2	3	4
Leucocytes	2 (10%)	3 (10%)	7 (35%)	7 (35%)	2 (10%)
Thrombocytes	5 (25%)	4 (20%)	7 (35%)	2 (10%)	2 (10%)
Nephrotoxicity	20 (100%)	0	0	0	0
Neurotoxicity	20 (100%)	0	0	0	0
Nausea, vomiting	2 (10%)	1 (5%)	17 (85%)	0	0
Mucositis	19 (95%)	1 (5%)	0	0	0
Diarrhea	12 (60%)	6 (30%)	2 (10%)	0	0
Alopecia	0	0	9 (45%)	11 (55%)	0

Leucocytopenia and thrombocytopenia were observed in 90% and 75% of patients, respectively.
Leucocytopenia and thrombocytopenia of WHO-grade III were observed in 35% and 10%, respectively; of WHO-grade IV in two patients. The nadir of leucocytes and thrombocytes occurred on days 14-18, recovery was on days 20-24.

Nausea and vomiting of different grades was noted in 90% of patients. Severe mucositis and/or diarrhea were not seen. Alopecia of grade II and III occured in all patients. No other toxicities were observed.

Discussion

The concept of chemotherapy ± surgery in patients with squamous cell carcinoma of the esophagus has been explored since 1970 (12).

The combinations Cisplatin/Bleomycin and Cisplatin/Bleomycin/Vindesin produced 15% and 45% objective responses (5,11) in patients with loco-regional and extensive disease (8,11). The objective response rates of Cisplatin/Bleomycin and Cisplatin/Bleomycin/Vindesin were in loco-regional disease 17% and 64% (5,11), and 14% and 29% in extensive disease (5,8,11). Objective response rates of 68% including 16% CR were achieved with Cisplatin/5Fu/Etoposide in 19 patients with extensive disease.

7 of 10 patients with PR after chemotherapy were operable and disease free after surgery.

Comparison of these preliminary data with the results obtained with the more frequently used combination Cisplatin/ Bleomycin/Vindesin (8,11) indicates that Cisplatin/5Fu/Etoposide achieves higher overall response and lower toxicity in extensive disease.

Furthermore, activity of Cisplatin/5Fu/Etoposide in extensive disease is comparable to that of Cisplatin/5Fu/Etoposide/Adriamycin in loco-regional disease (2) and efficiency is higher than that of Cisplatin/5Fu (7) and of Cisplatin/5Fu/Adriamycin (9).

The results with Cisplatin/5Fu/Etoposide show that Etoposide is an important drug in combination chemotherapy of esophageal cancer.

The conclusion from this phase II study is that Cisplatin/5Fu/ Etoposide is an active and safe regimen for treatment of esophageal cancer. It increases operability in patients with extensive disease.

1 Atassi, G., Kenis, Y., Dumont, P., Rozencweig, M.,:
Animal Screening of New Platinum Derivates - Studies with Single Agents and Combinations
Fourth NCI-EORTC Symposium on New Drugs in Cancer Therapy Dec. 14-17, Brussels, Belgium Abstr. 27 (1983)

2 Bedikian, A.Y., Deniord, R., El-Akkad, S.:
Value of Pre-Op Chemotherapy for Esophageal Carcinoma
Proc of ASCO 6, 96, Abstr. 375 (1987)

3 Bedikian, A.Y.:
Phase II Evaluation of 5-Fluorouracil (F), Adriamycin (A), Cis-Platinum (P), and Vepesid (VP-16), FAP-VP-16 Multi-Drug Regimen in Patients (PTs) with Esophageal Carcinoma
Proc of ASCO 146, abstr. C-571 (1984)

4 Chabner, B.A.:
Pyrimidine Antagonists
In: Pharmacologic Principles of Cancer Treatment
Ed: Chabner, B.
Publ: W.B. Saunders Company Philadelphia, London, Toronto, Mexico City, Rio de Janeiro, Sydney, Tokyo 183-212 (1982)

5 Coonley, C.J., Bains, M., Hilaris, B., Chapman, R., Kelsen, D.P.:
Cisplatin and Bleomycin in the Treatment of Esophageal Carcinoma
Cancer 54, 2351-2355 (1984)

6 Damon, L.E., Cadman, E.C.:
Enhanced Cytotoxicity of Fluoropyrimidines by Etoposide in L1210 Cells
Proc of AACR 27, 372, abstr. 1477 (1986)

7 De Besi, P., Sileni, V.C., Salvagno, L., Tremolada, C., Cartei, G., Fosser, V., Paccagnella, A., Peracchia, A., Fiorentino, M.:
Phase II Study of Cisplatin, 5-Fu, and Allopurinol in Advanced Esophageal Cancer
Cancer Treat Rep 70, 909-910 (1986)

8 Dinwoodie, W.R., Bartolucci, A.A., Lyman, G.H., Valez-Garcia, E., Martelo, O.J., Sarma, P.R.:
Phase II Evaluation of Cisplatin, Bleomycin, and Vindesine in Advanced Squamous Cell Carcinoma of the Esophagus: A Southwestern Cancer Study Group Trial
Cancer Treat. Rep. 70, 267-270 (1986)

9 Gisselbrecht, C., Calvo, F., Mignot, L., Pujade, E., Bouvry, M., Danne, O., Belpomme, D., Marty, M.:
Fluorouracil (F), Adriamycin (A), and Cisplatin (P) (FAP): Combination Chemotherapy of Advanced Esophageal Carcinoma
Cancer 52, 974-977 (1983)

10 Hill, B.T.:
Potential of Continuous Tumor Cell Lines for Establishing Patterns of Cross-Resistance and Collateral Sensitivity in Vitro
Drugs Exptl. Clin. Res. XII(1/2/3), 293-298 (1986)

11 Kelsen, D., Hilaris, B., Coonley, C., Chapman, R., Lesser, M., Dukeman, M., Heelan, R., Bains, M.:
Cisplatin, Vindesine, and Bleomycin Chemotherapy of Local-Regional and Advanced Esophageal Carcinoma
Am. J. Med. 75, 645-652 (1983)

12 Kelsen, D.:
Chemotherapy of Esophageal Cancer
Eur. J. Cancer Clin. Oncol. 21, 5-7 (1985)

13 Osswald, H., Kunz, W.:
Therapeutic Synergism of Etoposide and 5-Fluorouracil Combined Sequentially in Advanced Leukemia 1210
J. Cancer Res. Clin. Oncol. 113, suppl, 53, D-Ther 39 (1987)

14 Preusser, P., Achterrath, W., Niederle, N., Seeber, S.:
Cisplatin
Arzneimitteltherapie 2, 50-65 (1985)

15 Ross, W., Wozniak, A., Smallwoood, S., Yalowich, J.C.:
DNA Damage by VP-16: Mechanism and Relationship to Cytotoxicity
In: Etoposide (VP-16) - Current Status and New Developments
Eds: Issell, B.F., Muggia, F.M., Carter, S.K.
Publ: Academic Press Inc. Orlando, San Diego, San Francisco, New York, London, Toronto, Montreal, Sydney, Tokyo, Sao Paulo 49-51 (1984)

16 Seeber, S., Osieka, R., Schmidt, C.G., Achterrath, W., Crooke, S.T.:
In Vivo Resistance towards Anthracyclines, Etoposide, and Cis-Diamminedichloroplatinum (II)
Cancer Research 42, 4719-4725 (1982)

17 Seeber. S.:
Model Studies of Etoposide Resistance
Cancer Treat. Rev. 9, suppl. A, 15-20 (1982)

Neo-Adjuvant Chemotherapy. Ed. Cl. Jacquillat, M. Weil, D. Khayat. Colloque INSERM/John Libbey Eurotext Ltd. © 1988. Vol. 169, pp. 683-686.

Pre-operative simultaneous radio-chemotherapy in squamous cell carcinoma of the thoracic esophagus

Françoise Izar*, Serge Roos**, Adnan Naja*, Gilles Fourtanier** and Roland Bugat*

* *Centre Claudius Regaud, 20-24 Rue du Pont Saint-Pierre 31052 Toulouse, France*
** *Service de Chirurgie générale et digestive, C.H.U. Rangueil, Chemin du Vallon, 31054 Toulouse, France*

ABSTRACT

Ten patients with locally advanced squamous cell carcinoma of the esophagus were preoperativelly treated by synchronous chemotherapy (two courses of 5 Fluorouracil and cisplatinum) and radiation (40 Grays). The toxicity of the treatment was mild. Seven patients were resected for cure. Four of seven had no histologic evidence of cancer in the resected esophagus but with residual positive celiac nodes for one of them. This radio-chemotherapy program achieved increased local tumor control ; however the presumed benefit of this therapeutic approach might be dimmed by initial tumoral extension outside the radiation portals.

KEYWORDS

Esophageal cancer, pilot study, synchronous radio-chemotherapy, toxicity, local control.

INTRODUCTION

This pilot study was designed to evaluate the feasibility and potential effectiveness of synchronous radio-chemotherapy in squamous cell carcinoma of the thoracic esophagus secondarily operated on. In the aim to increase local tumor control, we decided to administer two courses of chemotherapy simultaneously to radiation therapy. Pathologic findings were designed as the short term criteria of evaluation.

PATIENTS AND METHODS

From January to October 1987, ten patients were entered into this clinical trial. All of them were male, the mean age was 66 years (range 50 to 71). The weight loss was superior to 10% for four patients. Three patients had upper third lesions, four had middle third lesions and three lower third lesions.
The pretreatment work-up included esophagogram and esophagoscopy, chest roentgenogram, CT scan of the thorax and abdomen, bronchoscopy and routine blood studies.

The size of the tumor as measured by barium swallow was inferior or equal to 5cm for three patients, superior to 5cm for seven patients.
The treatment plan called for initiating preoperative radiation therapy, cisplatinum and 5 fluorouracil (5-FU) on day 1. Radiation was delivered for five days per week, for 4 weeks at 2 grays per day, for a total of 40 grays. We used X ray beams of 10 Mev energy (Neptune CGR). All the patients were treated with parallel opposed anterior and posterior fields. Both fields were treated on each day of treatment. The mean dimensions of the fields were 15 by 8cm.
Cisplatinum was given at 100 mg/m^2, intravenous, on day 1 and 22. 5-FU was given at 1000 mg/m^2 per day as a 24-hour infusion on days 2-5 and 23-26.

RESULTS

Nine patients completed the pre-operative part of the treatment plan, the remaining patient received only one course of chemotherapy because of transient renal failure related to intercurrent pathology. Bone marrow toxicity was relatively mild, one patient only had a grade 3 toxicity (WHO scale). Nausea and vomiting were noted in the majority of patients, no case of toxicity higher than grade 2 was noticed.

The mean delay to surgery was 34 days. No patients died postoperatively. The morbidity was mild since only one patient had postoperative complications (cervical anastomosis leakage). Two patients had simple exploratory laparotomy : the tumor was still bulky and unresectable for one, the second had liver metastases. One patient had palliative surgery with incomplete resection. Seven patients have been operated on with curative intent. The esophagus was resected through a right thoracotomy after laparotomy for three patients. Four patients had total esophagectomy without thoracotomy for 3 of them.
Four patients had no histologic evidence of cancer in the resected esophagus but one had positive celiac nodes. Three patients had residual local tumor with positive peri-esophageal nodes for two of them.

ESOPHAGEAL TUMOR	NODES	NUMBER OF PATIENTS
-	-	2
-	?	1
-	+	1 *
+	?	1
+	+	2
		7

* (positive celiac nodes)

TABLE I : PATHOLOGIC FINDINGS.

The seven patients with curative surgery are alive, free of disease with a mean follow-up of eight months.

DISCUSSION

According to a mild toxicity which did not delay the surgery, this radio-chemotherapy association led to curative resection in 7 of 10 patients ; four of them were free of residuel primary tumor.
This preoperative treatment is clearly able to enhance local tumor control. However overall survival is still relatively little affected by this therapeutic approach probably because of primary tumoral extension outside of the radiation fields.
For SEYDEL and coll. (1988) some patients treated by combined modality treatment experienced prolonged survival. The patients who could take benefit of this new therapeutic approach, remain to be defined.

REFERENCES

1 - COIA L.R., ENGSTROM P.R., PAUL A., GALLAGHER M., STOLL D., CATALANO R., RICHTER M.R. (1984) :
A pilot study of combined radiotherapy and chemotherapy for esophageal carcinoma.
Am. J. Clin. Oncol., 7, pp. 653-659.

2 - KELSEN D.P., BAINS M., HILARIS B., CHAPMAN R., ALEXANDER J., HOPFAN S., MARTINI N. (1982) :
Combination chemotherapy of esophageal carcinoma using Cisplatin, Vindesine and Bleomycin.
Cancer, 49, pp. 1174-1177.

3 - POPLIN E., FLEMING T., LEICHMAN L., SEYDEL G., STEIGER Z., TAYLOR S., VANCE R., STUCKEY J., RIVKIN S. (1987) :
Combined therapies for squamous cell carcinoma of the esophagus, a southwest oncology group study.
J. Clin. Oncol.,5, pp. 622-628.

4 - SEYDEL G., LEICHMAN L., BYHARDT R., COOPER J., HERSKOVIC A., LIBNOCK J., PAZDUR R., SPEYER J., TSCHAN J. (1988) :
Preoperative radiation and chemotherapy for localized squamous cell carcinoma of the esophagus.
Int. J. Rad. Oncol. Biol. Phys., 14, pp. 33-35.

Résumé

10 malades porteurs d'un épithélioma épidermoïde de l'oesophage thoracique ont été traités par 2 cycles de chimiothérapie associant 5 FLUORO-URACILE (5-FU) et PLATINE, simultanés à une irradiation médiastinale (40 grays).
Cette association thérapeutique s'est accompagnée d'une toxicité modérée.
Sur les 10 malades opérés, 7 avaient une tumeur résécable. A l'examen anatomo-pathologique, la tumeur oesophagienne était stérilisée dans 4 cas mais avec envahissement ganglionnaire sous-diaphragmatique dans un cas.
Au total, cette association thérapeutique permet d'augmenter le taux de contrôle local, toutefois le bénéfice en terme de survie risque d'être masqué par l'extension tumorale initiale en dehors du volume d'irradiation.

Neo-Adjuvant Chemotherapy. Ed. Cl. Jacquillat, M. Weil, D. Khayat. Colloque INSERM/John Libbey Eurotext Ltd. © 1988. Vol. 169, pp. 687-694.

A comparison of surgery, radiotherapy and combination chemotherapy (followed by radiotherapy or surgery) in the treatment of locally advanced esophageal carcinoma. An analysis of 300 treated patients at Tata Memorial Hospital, Bombay, India

P.B. Desai, S.H. Advani, S. Sharma, T. Saikia and R. Gopal

Tata Memorial Hospital, Dr. Ernest Borges Marg, Parel, Bombay 400 012, India

SUMMARY

Esophageal cancer remains one of the most distressing Cancers to treat and manage. Results, the world over, for unselected group of patients range between 5 and 8% salvage at 5 years. The main reasons for such dismal results is a late diagnosis, limitation of treatment due to anatomic restraints and the usually rapid biologic behaviour of the tumour.

It is natural, therefore, that significant attempts have been made by workers in the field to use different treatment methods (surgery, radiotherapy, chemotherapy) either singly or in combination to improve salvage rates in esophageal cancer.

This presentation is a retrospective non randomised and uncontrolled analysis of locally advanced esophageal cancer (>7 cms. on esophagogram) treated by surgery alone, radiotherapy alone and a combination of anterior chemotherapy (Cisplatinum-Methotrexate) followed by either radiotherapy or surgery depending on the site of the lesion; - those in the upper reaches receiving radiotherapy and those in the lower and mid 1/3rd having surgical resections. Hundred patients have been studied in each group with a 5-year follow up in the surgery and radiotherapy group and a 3-year follow up in the group receiving anterior chemotherapy followed by surgery or radiotherapy. Responses to anterior chemotherapy (2 cycles of Cisplatinum 20 mgm/m^2 on day 1 through 5 and day 15 through 20 and Methotrexate 200 mgm/m^2 on day 1 and 15) have been noted in 75% with nearly 10% showing complete responses. The 3 and 5 year survival rates in the surgical and radiotherapy group are 11% and 4% and 10% and 5% respectively. The group of patients with anterior chemotherapy followed by either surgery (lower and mid 1/3rd) or radiotherapy (upper 1/3rd) is 30% at 2 years and 23% at 3 years. It has not been possible to exhibit maintenance chemotherapy after the definitive treatment is over. Addition of effective chemotherapy drugs (Cisplatinum, VPlb, MTX, Bleomycin) and its appropriate interpolation with surgery and radiotherapy appears to be the only method at the present by which one can expect to increase salvage and cures for advanced esophageal cancer.

Cancer of the esophagus continues to exercise the skill and ingenuity of the Surgeon, the Radiotherapist and the Medical Oncologist in an effort to improve its long term control or cure. The disease is usually diagnosed late; The rapid spread of cancer within the rich submucosal lymphatic plexus along the lengths of the esophagus and the therapeutic restraints imposed due to its confines within the mediastinum surrounded by vital structures results in poor overall results. Conventionally, esophageal cancer has been treated either by surgery or radiotherapy with results varying from 4% to 35% (Bains, 1982; Desai, 1979; Earlam, 1980; Pinto, 1975; Rosenberg, 1982; Shiverberg, 1983) depending on the stage of the disease. Numerous recent reports in the literature (Advani, 1985; Kelsen, 1983; Kelsen, 1984; Lad, 1980; Ravry, 1979) now indiate that esophageal cancer responds to cytotoxic drugs frequently enough to merit appropriate and continuing studies to improve results.

The Tata Memorial Hospital, Bombay is a large referral Centre for malignant diseases in India. The centre records over 11,000 new cancer patients per year. Cancer of the esophagus forms 8% of the total load (nearly 900 patients annually) and is the 4th commonest cancer seen in the setting of the Hospital Registry.

SELECTION OF PATIENTS:

This report is a retrospective, non randomised and uncontrolled study involving 300 patients (100 in each group) treated by Radiotherapy, Surgery and Combination therapy (2 cycles of anterior chemotherapy followed by either radiotherapy or surgery) during 1979 -1982. The objective of this study was not only to see the efficacy of local control and relief of dysphagia by either surgery or radiotherapy but also to asses the impact on overall survival at 3 and 5 years. Patients selected were in fair or good general health so as to be able to withstand and complete prescribed therapy (Karnofsky score 70). A complete assessment of the extent of the disease was achieved by a barium swallow esophagogram, a bronchoscopy, a chest skiagram and an isotope liver scan if indicated by an abnormal liver chemistry or a suspected palpable liver. For the last 4 years evaluation by CT scan is used when indicated. Only lesions with long vertical lengths on esophagogram were included in the study, for essentially one is trying to study and decide the optimal method of palliation in an average case of advanced esophageal cancer. Patients with metastatic disease in the neck, abdomen, liver, lungs or a fixed vocal cord and those with poor general condition were excluded from the study.

Radiotherapy:

One hundred patients between 1980 - 1982 with lesions in the mid 1/3rd and upper 1/3rd were treated by radiotherapy alone - by cobalt 60 teletherapy or a linear accelerator and a dose of 60 Gy to the tumour delivered by an anterior and a posterior port.

Responses mainly depended upon the type of lesion (proliferative or infiltrating and ulcerative) and the tumour burden. Most proliferative lesions responded well with rapid restoration of swallowing and resolution of the growth. Patients with ulcerative and infiltrative lesions often responded with more fibrosis and poor control of the primary lesion. Despite a good local control initially, a large initial tumour burden is an important factor in local recurrences and dissemination to distant site (Figs. 1 a.b.c.). A few patients, though controlled of the main tumour were left with fibrosed and narrow esophagus which constantly required dilatation at varying intervals. The 3 and 5 year survivals of patients undergoing full radiotherapy are 10% and 5% respectively (Fig. 2).

Surgery:

A group of 100 patients with lesions in the lower and mid 1/3rd underwent one stage esophageal resection with esophagogastrostomy (left sided intra thoracic anastomosis in case of lower 1/3rd and high right sided intra thoracic anastomosis in case of mid 1/3rd lesions). The overall post-operative mortality was 11%. Fig. 2 shows the survival curves of patients undergoing surgical resections. Majority had palliative resections and the 3 and 5 year survivals were 11% and 4% respectively showing results almost similar to those obtained after radiotherapy. Ability to swallow normally was an important advantage in patients who have had surgery, though a few do require dilatation to overcome anastomotic stenosis (10%).

The overall results with radiotherapy and with surgery alone therefore, leave much to be desired for an average case of advanced esophageal cancer

Anterior Chemotherapy with Definitive Treatment (Radiotherapy or Surgery):

The advent of effective chemotherapeutic drugs (Bleomycin, Methotrexate, Mitomycin etc.) and more particularly after the arrival of Cisplatinum, locally advanced esophageal cancers are now being treated with the addition of chemotherapy prior to definitive radiotherapy or surgery to improve results.

Combination Treatment Protocol:

Logically, therefore, in order to improve the depressing salvage rates obtained by surgery or radiotherapy alone, anterior (front loading) chemotherapy was then incorporated in such lesions. After 2 cycles of chemotherapy, definitive treatment was then offered in the form of radiotherapy (upper 1/3rd lesions) or surgical resection (in lower and mid 1/3rd lesions).

Responses to chemotherapy were significant. A previous publication from our Centre (Advani, 1985) shows a 75% response rate (CR + PR) with Cisplatinum and Methotrexate combination.

The dose schedules employed are:

Cisplatinum - (2 cycles) 20 mgm/m^2 on day 1 through day 5 and day 15 through 20.

Methotrexate - 200 mgm./m^2 on day 1 and 15.

Figs.3 a-f show the type of response achieved. In 10% total responses were achieved and subsequently the resected specimen did not show any evidence of tumour; over all responses were 77%. Radiation as a definitive treatment was given after complete responses in patients with almost normal looking esophagograms with -ve endoscopic findings; nonetheless, it is important to always follow anterior chemotherapy with definitive surgery or radiotherapy - as almost every patient who did not receive conventional radiotherapy or surgery after anterior chemotherapy recurred in 9 months to 1 year locally except two patients who refused definitive treatment after a complete response to chemotherapy remained disease free at 3 and 3 1/2 years.

Table 1 shows the data on 42 evaluable patients who have undergone such combined treatment programme at 3 years. Majority has had radiotherapy after chemotherapy and a few had surgical resections. A 3 year survival rate of 23% is significantly better than 10% and 11% achieved with surgery or radiotherapy alone (Fig.4).

While this study is non randomised and uncontrolled, this retrospective analysis, gives vital information based on historical controls, vis-a-vis the behaviour and overall survivals in esophageal cancer with conventional treatment and/or combination treatment methods. Combination of pre-operative radiotherapy and surgery have not significantly improved results and the current approach of utilising cytotoxic drugs before definitive therapy is one other avenue which needs to be explored. The initial response rates and the results obtained in this study merits further collation of data from other Centres and other studies to mount intensive clinical trials in a controlled and randomised fashion to increase long term control of esophageal cancer worldwide.

Table 1 Locally advanced esophageal cancer

Responses to combination therapy (Cisplat. + MTX)

Total number treated	78	(MTX + Cisplat)
Good response*	60	(77%)
No response	18	
Complete response	7	(10%)

* Tumour reduction > 50%

REFERENCES

Advani, S.H., Saikia, T., Swaroop S. et al (1985):Anterior chemotherapy in esophageal cancer. Cancer 56, 1502-1506.

Bains, M.S., Vagaiwala, M.R., Hilaris, B., Beattie, E.J. (1982):Management of esophageal cancer. In Principles of Cancer Treatment, eds. S.K. Carter, E.Glatstein, R.B. Livingston, Chapter 48, pp 444-455. U.S.A.:McGraw-Hill Inc.

Desai, P.B. (1979):Combination treatment methods in esophageal cancer. In Advances in Medical Oncology, Research and Education. ed. N.Thatcher, vol. 9 pp 389-397. Oxford:Pergamon Press.

Earlam, R., Cunha-Melo, J.R. (1980):Esophageal squamous cell carcinoma - A critical review of surgery. Brit. Journal of Surgery, 67, 381-390.

Kelsen, D., Hilaris, B., Coonley C. et al (1983): Cisplatin, Vindesin and Bleomycin therapy of locoregional and advanced esophageal carcinoma. Am. Jr. Med. 75, 645-652.

Kelsen, D., Bains, M., Hilaris, B., Martini, N.(1984):Combined modality therapy of esophageal cancer. Semin. Onc. 11, 169-177.

Lad, T.E.(1980):Platinum, Mitomycin-C and Bleomycin chemotherapy of esophageal carcinoma. Proc. Am.Soc. Clin. Onc. 21, 419.

Pinto, J.M., Bhalavat, R.L., Nagaraj Rao, D. (1975):Radiotherapy in carcinoma of the esophagus. Indian Cancer 12, 380-388.

Ravry, M.J.R., Moore, M.(1979):The South Eastern cancer study group, A phase I study. Cancer Treatment Reports, 63, 2019-2021.

Rosenberg, J.C., Schwade J.G., Vaikevicius V.K.(1982):Cancer of the Esophagus In Cancer- Principles and Practise of Oncology, eds. V.T. DeVita, S.Helman, .A. Rosenberg. pp 499-533. Philadelphia/Toronto:J.B.Lippincott Co.

Shiverberg, E(1983): Cancer Statistics. CA 33, 9-25.

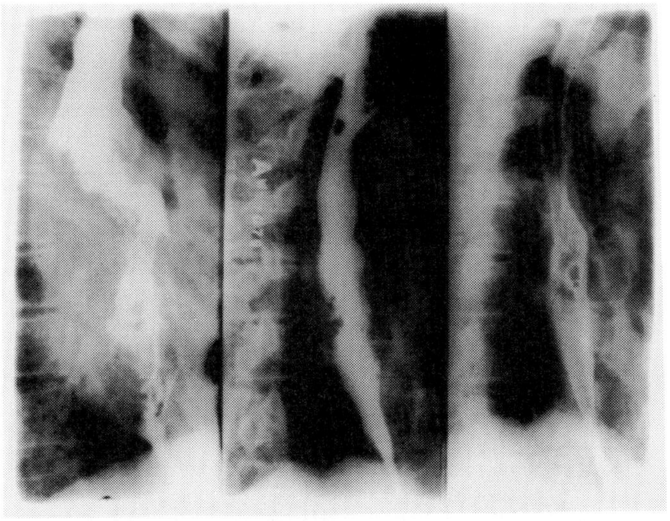

Figs. 1 a.b.c.

Extensive local disease - proliferative - in almost the whole of the esophagus. Excellent local response with 2 courses of chemotherapy and radiotherapy. Locally controlled. Extensive bilateral pulmonary metastasis in 4 months due to large tumour bulk.

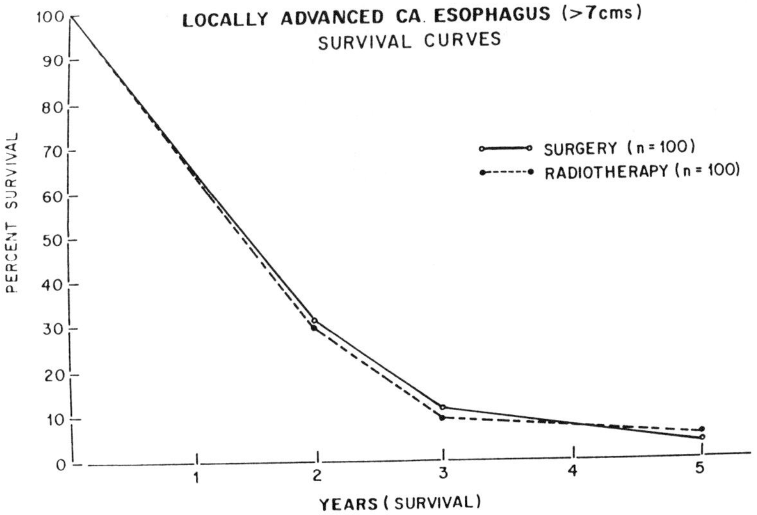

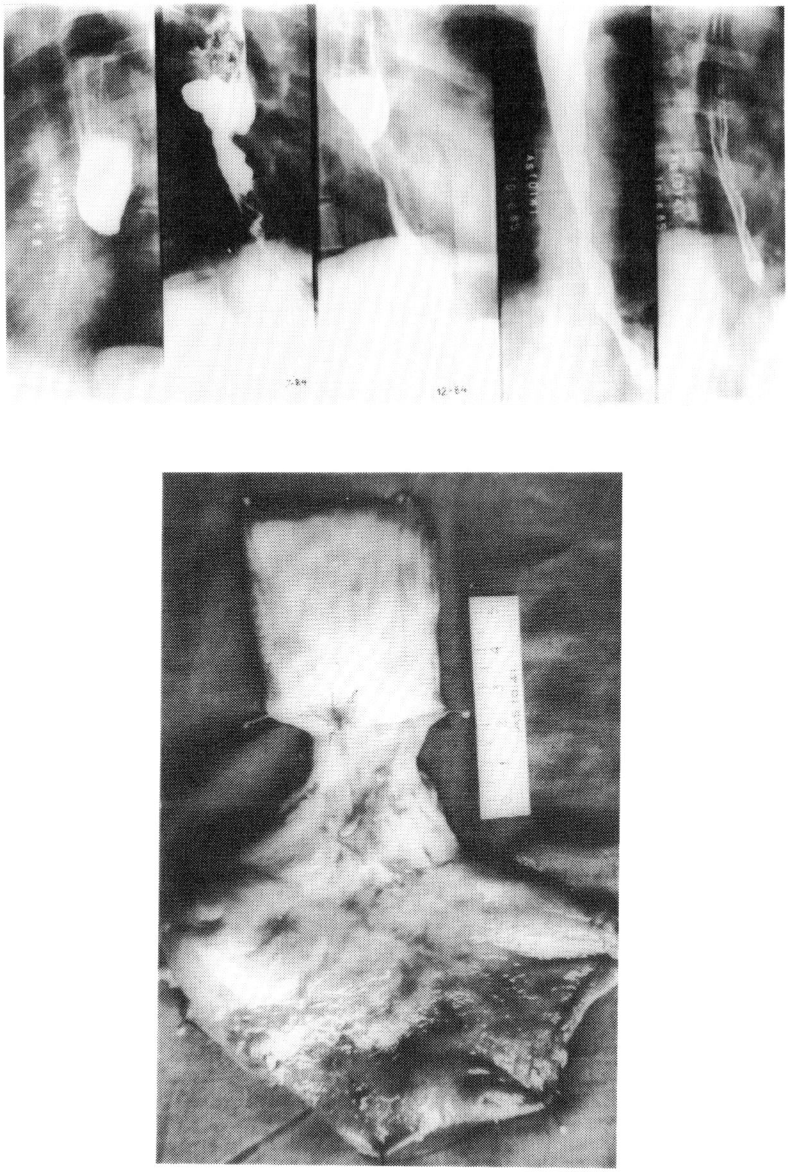

Fig. 3 a - f

Serial x-rays showing an advanced obstructed cancer middle esophagus treated by combination of anterior chemotherapy (4.84), radiotherapy (10.84) and subsequent surgical resection (6.85) because of positive cytology at esophagoscopy(e). Resected specimen shows no evidence of tumour (f). Patient surviving free of disease 4 years after combined therapy during 1984-85.

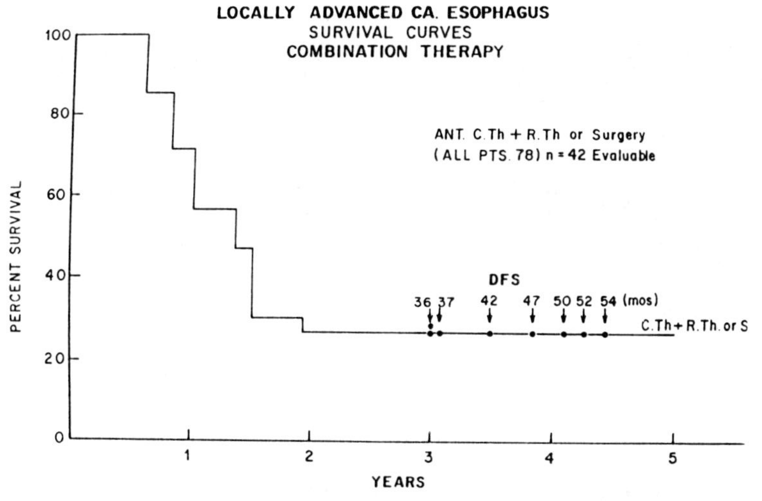

Fig. 4

The dots represent 8 patients surviving free of disease (DFS) from 36 months to 54 months. 23% surviving at 3 years of those evaluable who have completed combination treatment.

Résumé

Le cancer de l'oesophage demeure un des pires pour un groupe non sélectioné de malades, le taux de guérison à travers le monde s'établit entre 5 % et 8 %. Les principales raisons pour un résultat aussi mauvais sont le diagnostic tardif, la limitation du traitement dûe aux conditions anatomiques, et l'évolution rapide de la tumeur. Il est naturel pour cette raison que des essais aient été faits pour utiliser les différentes méthodes de traitement : chirurgie, radiothérapie, chimiothérapie, soit isolément, soit en association pour augmenter les taux de survie. Cette présentation est une analyse rétrospective non randomisée et non contrôlée de cancers de l'oesophage avancés supérieurs à 7 cm sur l'oesophagogramme, traités par chirurgie seule, radiothérapie seule, et une association de chimiothérapie première (Méthotrexate-Cisplatinum) suivie soit par la radiothérapie soit par la chirurgie selon le siège de la lésion. Les malades dont la lésion siège au 1/3 supérieur recevant la radiothérapie et ceux dont la lésion se situe au niveau du tiers inférieur ou moyen ayant des résections chirurgicales. 100 malades ont été étudiés dans chaque groupe, avec un recul de 5 ans pour la chirurgie et la radiothérapie et un recul de 3 ans pour la chimiothérapie suivie de chirurgie ou de radiothérapie. Les réponses à la chimiothérapie première 2 cycles de Cisplatinum 200 mg/m2 du jour 1 au jour 5, du jour 15 au jour 20 et Méthotrexate 200 mg/m2 aux jours 1 et 15, ont été observés dans 75 % des cas, près de 10 % montrant une rémission complète. Les survies à 3 ans et à 5 ans pour le groupe chirurgie ont été 11 % et 4 % et pour le groupe radiothérapie 10 % et 5 %. Le groupe de malades avec chimiothérapie antérieure suivie soit par chirurgie du tiers moyen ou inférieur ou radiothérapie pour le tiers supérieur, 30 % à 2 ans et 23 % à 3 ans. Il n'a pas été possible de reprendre la chimiothérapie àprès le traitement local. L'association de chimiothérapie effective Cis.platinum VP.16-Méthotrexate-Bléomycine et son intercalation appropriée avec chirurgie ou radiothérapie parait la seule méthode actuellement qui puisse augmenter le taux de guérison des cancers avancés de l'oesophage.

Neo-Adjuvant Chemotherapy. Ed. Cl. Jacquillat, M. Weil, D. Khayat. Colloque INSERM/John Libbey Eurotext Ltd. © 1988. Vol. 169, pp. 695-701.

Combined treatment with chemotherapy and hyperfractionation radiotherapy in inoperable esophageal carcinoma

Ph. Martin, D. Martin, D. Serin and F. Reboul

Clinique Sainte-Catherine, Avignon, France

ABSTRACT

Between 12/81 and 5.86, 17 pts with inoperable carcinoma of the oesophagus were treated by combined sequential chemotherapy and multifraction radiotherapy. UICC classification showed 8T2 and 9 T3. During the time of the study, two consecutive chemotherapy protocols were used : VCP (Vindesine, Cyclophosphamide, Cis-Platinum) and VBP (Vindesine, Bleomycine, Cis-Platinum).
Radiation therapy consisted of 3 daily fractions of 1,4 Gy delivred at 4 hours interval during 7 days (29,4 Gy in 21 fractions and 9 days). This schedule was repeated after a 3 week rest and followed by a boost. The total dose was 71,4 Gy. 13 patients completed the whole course of scheduled chemoradiotherapy. One course of chemotherapy was administered during each course of radiotherapy for a total of 2 courses.
Complete endoscopic regression of the tumor was observed in 9 patients out of 17 for a CR rate of 53 %. The determinate CR rate is 69 % (9/13).
Despite this high immediate local control rate, crude survival rates remained poor with 42 % at 12 months, 17 % at 18 months and 6 % at 60 months. There were 11 tumor related deaths. Late adverse effects were significant with 4 cases of oesophageal stenosis.
Thus we failed to demonstrate any survival benefit of this highly aggresive treatment compared to more classical schedules.
Innovative schedules of synchronous radiochemotherapy should be considered in the treatment of this dismal disease.

INTRODUCTION

Due to poor medical status as well as locally advanced disease, inoperable oesophageal carcinoma still carries a very poor prognosis. Conventional fractionation radiotherapy may at best cure only a few patients, with survival figures around 25 % at one year and 5 % at 5 years in most series. Treatment failure is related to persistent or reccurent local disease as well as metastatic disease (1,2).

With single agent chemotherapy, objective responses are always scarce and of brief duration. Aggressive multi-drug regimens seem to be more promising. Advani and al. (3) treated 47 pts. with MTX + DDP, resulting in a 76 % objective response in 42 evaluable patients, without prolongation of survival. Vogl and al. (4) treated 10 pts. with a combination of DDP + MTX + BLM and reported 5 major responses. Le chevalier and al. (5) using a combination of VDS + CTX + DDP + CCNU obtained preliminary encouraging results. Finally, Kelsen and al. with a combination of VDS + DDP + BLM (6) observed 55 % major responses in 53 evaluable patients with an impressive resection rate of 82 % among 28 pts. treated pre-operatively. The combination of DDP + 5FU by continuous infusion is actually being studied by several groups.

During the same period, there has been a renewal of interest for altered fractionation radiotherapy on the basis that reduction of overall treatment time would reduce tumor cell proliferation and repair of sublethal damage and that multiple dialy fractions would increase the differential effect between tumor and normal tissues. The EORTC Radiation Therapy Group (7) reported a pilot study of 3 daily fractions of 1.6 Gy in head and neck tumor to a total dose of 70 Gy. with impressive results and acceptable toxicity. With a somewhat similar protocol, J.C. Horiot (8) treated 179 pts. with an impressive 86 % tumor regression rate and a 48 % local control rate and an actuarial survival of 31 % at 20 months.

Concomittant chemotherapy and radiation therapy has been studied by Steiger (9) using 2 courses of 5FU-MMC and radiation in 25 inoperable patients with 44 % achieving good local palliation. Among 40 pts. treated pre-operatively with 30 Gy. over 3 weeks and 2 courses of 5FU-MMC or 5FU-DDP, 35 pts. went to surgery with 13 (37 %) having non residual microscopic disease and a 2-year survival rate of 30 %. Kolaric (10) treated 15 pts. with ADM + BLM and radiation, resulting in a 60 % response rate with a median duration of response of 5.2 months. According to Byfield, 5FU by continuous infusion is a powerful radiosensitizer with 5 out of 6 pts. treated with concomittant radiotherapy achieving complete response (11).

On the basis of these previous studies, we initiated a pilot study with the objective of testing the therapeutic potential of combined chemotherapy and accelerated radiotherapy with multiple fractions per day.

MATERIAL AND METHODS

Between 12/81 and 5/86, 17 pts. with inoperable biopsy proven carcinoma of the oesophagus were treated by combined sequential chemotherapy and multifractionation radiotherapy. UICC classification showed 8 T2 (N0=6, N2=1, NX=1) and 9 T3 (N0=6, N3=3). Anatomical site was cervical oesophagus in 5, upper thoracic in 2, mid-thoracic in 8 pts (multiple sites : 2 pts). During the time of study, two consecutive chemotherapy protocols were used :

1) VCP (10 pts)	VDS	3 mg/m^2	J1
	CTX	300 mg/m^2	J2-3
	DDP	30 mg/m^2	J2-3-4
2) VBP (7 pts)	VDS	3 mg/m^2	J1
	BLM	10 mg/m^2	J2-3-4
	DDP	30 mg/m^2	J2-3-4

One course of chemotherapy was administered during each course of radiotherapy for a total of 2 courses.

Radiation therapy consisted of 3 daily fractions of 1.4 Gy. delivered at 4 hours interval during 7 days (29,4 Gy in 21 fractions and 9 days). This schedule was repeated after a 3 week rest and followed by a boost of 12.6 GY. in 9 fractions and 3 days. The total dose was 71.4 Gy. in 51 f. and 40 days. The first course was delivered through A-P portals, covering the oesophagus and mediastinal structures, and supra-clavicular or coeliac nodes depending on the anatomical location of the tumor. The second course was delivered through the same fields until a total dose of 46.2 Gy, subsequently through oblique and reduced fields to avoid spinal cord. Total dose was comparable to that of conventionnal treatment. 13 patients completed the whole course of scheduled chemo-radiotherapy (76,5 %).

After completion of treatment every patient was reevaluated at one month by physical examination, baryum study and repeated fibreroptic control with or without biopsy then followed up at regular intervals.

RESULTS

Complete endoscopic regression of the tumor was observed in 9 patients out of 17 for a CR rate of 53 %.
Among the patients that completed the whole treatment programm (13) the determinate CR rate is 69 % (9/13). Of the 9 pts. achieving complete response, 3 developped subsequent local recurrence and 3 had distant metastasis.

All patients with partial or no response died from local persistant disease.

Four patients did not complete the full course of treatment and died respectively from massive bleeding, hepatic cirrhosis, superior vena cava syndrome and hyponatremia. On the other hand, considering the poor medical status of these patients, treatment-related toxicity was acceptable, with only one case of severe myelotoxicity. The most common and disabling side effect was oesophagitis. Serious mucosal reactions with occasional candidosis were maximum by the second week of treatment, leading to cancel the final boost in many cases.

Late adverse effects of this combined treatment were significant with oesophageal stenosis and mediastinal fibrosis, leading to cachexia in one patient despite nutritionnal support. Finally, there was no case of radiation myelopathy.

Despite this high local control rate, crude survival rates remain poor with 42 % at 12 months, 17 % at 18 months and 6 % at 60 months. There are 11 tumor-related deaths, 3 treatment related deaths and 2 deaths related to intercurrent disease (cirrhosis, myocardial infarction).

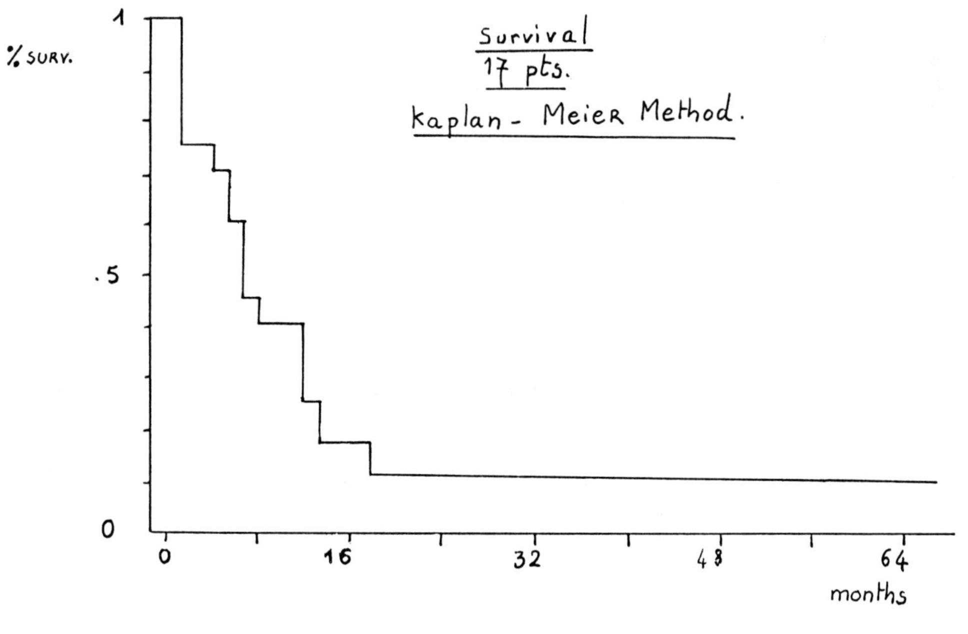

DISCUSSION

In this study, we failed to demonstrate any survival benefit of this particular treatment compared to more classical schedules. However, a high local determinate response rate of 69 % is encouraging considering the far advanced loco-regional disease of these patients. Nonetheless, the local failure rate as well as the distant dissemination remains unacceptably high.

This experience suggests that innovative schedules of aggressive synchronous radio-chemotherapy should be considered in the treatment of this dismal disease.

Using multifractionation radiation therapy, therapeutic gain may be achieved through inhibition of sublethal cellular damage in the tumor cells which affect to a lesser extent the normal cells. In the EORTC study (7), comparing classical fractionation to MFRT, local control was achieved in 35 % of patients with no statistical difference between the two arms. There was no difference in late effects but more pronounced early mucosal reactions with MFRT.

In the experience reported by Roussel (12) from the CFB in Caen, local control was identical with classical fractionation, hyperfractionation and split course radiotherapy. According to Wang (13), the optimum fraction size, total daily dose, overall treatment time and interval between fractions deserve further investigation.

At present, fractions of 1.6 and 1.2 Gy bid with a minimum of 4 hours interval for a total dose of 65-75 Gy. seem to improve control rates with acceptable morbidity in head and neck cancer.

Our two chemotherapy protocols were well tolerated and gave similar results in term of local regression and control. However, we had many local failures and nodal relapses as well as distant metastasis in the few long term survivors, accounting for a modest efficacy of these particular drug combinations. Noteworthy is the difficulty in assessing final complete response after chemotherapy, requiring in all cases histological confirmation.

Among the several drugs with demonstrated activity in oesophageal carcinoma, cis-DDP is included in almost every combination protocols at this time with response rates varying from 15 % to 80 %. The most widely used regimens are PVB and DDP-5FU with response rates of 50 % and 80 % respectively. Remission duration are brief with median survivals around 7 months.

Chemotherapy may be used in a neo-adjuvant setting or simultaneaously with radiation therapy. In the study of Kolaric (10), the response rate was 60 % with a median duration of response of 11 months in complete responders.
In the study of Abitbol (15), with only 9 pts. treated with 5FU-MTX-DDP and radiation, response rate was 89 % with a median survival of 7 months. In the study of Martial (16), there was no complete response after chemotherapy alone but a complete response after subsequent radiotherapy was observed in 60 % with a median survival of 11 months.

Leichman (17) studied two pre-operative adjuvant regimens with MMC-5FU DDP-5FU plus radiation then surgery 3 weeks later. In the patients that were amenable to surgery, 25 % and 47 % respectively had no residual tumor in the resected specimen. The mean survival rate in these patients was 24 months. Finally, Resbeut and al. (18) treated 28 pts. with chemotherapy (DDP-MTX-VCR) and split course radiotherapy with a 43 % response rate (32 % CR) and a median survival of responders of 13 months.

CONCLUSION

The litterature results as well as ours remain unsatisfactory but should lead to persistant evaluation of close combinations of chemotherapy and radiation in a sequential or simultaneous manner in order to improve if possible the prognosis of this dismal disease.

REFERENCES

1 - MARTIAL V.A,GARCIA EV,CINTRON J, YDRACH A.A
Radiotherapy preceded by multidrug chemotherapy in carcinoma of the oesophagus. A pilot study of the Radiation Therapy Oncology Group.
Cancer Clin. Trials 3 : 127-130, 1980

2 - HANCOCK S, GLATSTEIN E
Radiation therapy of oesophageal cancer.
Seminars in oncology, 11 : 144-158, 1984

3 - ADVANI S, SAIKIA T, SWAROOP S, RAMAKRISHNAN G, NA R C, DINSCHAW K, SHARMA S, VYAS J, DESAI P
Anterior chemotherapy in oesophageal cancer.
Cancer, 56 : 1502-1506, 1985.

4 - VOGL S, GREENWALD E, KAPLAN B
Effective chemotherapy for oesophageal cancer.
Methotrexate, Bleomycine, et Cis Diamine-Dichloro -platinum II
Cancer, 48 : 2555-2558, 1981

5 - LE CHEVALIER T, ROUESSE J, CAILLE P, ARRIAGADA R, BALDEYROU P
Vindesine, CCNU, Cis-platinum et Cyclophosphamide dans les carcinomes bronchiques métastatiques.
IGR Actualités carcinologiques, Paris, Masson , 162-166, 1983

6 - KELSEN D, BAINS M, HILARIS B, CUAPMAM R, Mc CORMACK P, ALEXANDER J, HOPFAN S, MARTINI N
Combination chemotherapy of oesophageal carcinoma using Cis-platine, Vindesine et Bleomycine.
Cancer, 49 : 1174-1177, 1982

7 - VAN DEN BOGAERT W, VAN DER SCHUEREN E, HORIOT J.C et al.
The feasibility of high dose multiple daily fractionation and its combination with anoxie cell sensitizers in the treatment of head and neck cancers.
Int. J. Radiat. Oncol. Biol. Phys., 8 : 1649-1655, 1982

8 - HORIOT JC
Clinical experience with multiple fraction per day in the radiotherapy of head and neck carcinoma.
J. Eur. Radiother., 2 : 79-89, 1982

9 - STEIGER Z, FRANKLIN R, WILSON R, LEICHMAN L, ASFAW I, VAISHANPAYAN G, ROSENBERG JC et al.
Complete eradication of squamous cell carcinoma of the esophagus with combined chemotherapy and radiotherapy.
Am. Surg., 47 : 95-98, 1981

10 - KOLARIC K, MARICIC Z, ROTH A, DUJMOVIC I
Combination of Bleomycine and Adriamycine with and without radiation in the treatment of inoperable oesophageal cancer.
A randomized study.
Cancer, 45 : 2265-2273, 1980

11 - BYFIELD J, BARONE R, MENDELSOHN J, FRANKEL S, QUINOL L, SHARP T, SEAGREN S
Infusion 5 Fluorouracil and X ray therapy for non-resectable esophageal cancer.
cancer, 45 : 703-708, 1980

12 - ROUSSEL A, JACOB JH, OLLIVIER JM
Assessment of a short radiotherapy protocol for the treatment of esophageal carcinomas.
In Proceedings ECCO 4, n° 127, 1987

13 - WANG C
The enigma of accelerated hyperfractionated radiation therapy for head and neck cancer.
Int. J. Radiation Oncology Biol. Phys., 14 : 209-210, 1988

14 - KELSEN D
Chemotherapy of esophageal cancer.
Seminars in Oncology, 11 : 159-167, 1984

15 - ABITBOL A, STRAUS M, FRANKLIN G
Infusional chemotherapy and cyclic radiation therapy in inoperable esophageal and gastric cardia carcinoma.
Am. J. Clin. Oncol., 6 : 195-201, 1983

16 - LEICHMAN L, STEIGER Z, SEYDEL H, DINDOGRU A, KINSIE J, TOBEN S, MACKENSIE G, SHELL J
Preoperative chemotherapy and radiation therapy for patients with cancer of esophagus : a potentially curative approach.
Am. J. Oncol., 2 : 75-79, 1984

17 - RESBEUT M, LE PRISE-FLEURY L, BEN-HASSEL M, GOUDIER MJ, MORICE-ROUXEL MF, DOUILLARD JY, CHENAL C
Squamous cell carcinoma of the esophagus treatment by combined Vincristine-Methotrexate plus folinic acid rescue and Cisplatine before radiotherapy.
Cancer, 56 : 1246-1250, 1985

Résumé

Entre Décembre 1981 et Mai 1986, nous avons traité 17 patients porteurs d'un cancer de l'oesophage inopérable (8 T2, 9 T3) par une association séquentielle de polychimiothérapie (2 cures VCP ou VBP) et de radiothérapie multifractionnée. Nous avons délivré une dose élevée, 71, 4 Gy en 51 fractions et 40 jours à raison de 3 fractions par jour espacées de 4 heures en 2 séries de 7 et 10 jours espacées de 3 semaines.
13 patients ont pu arriver au terme du traitement. Le taux de réponses complètes endoscopiques est de 53 % (9/17) pour l'ensemble du groupe et de 69 % (9/13) pour les 13 patients traités à doses pleines.
Malgré ce taux de controle local immédiat intéressant, la survie à long terme reste décevante : 42 % à 1 an, 6 % à 5 ans.
Les complications sont notables dominées par les sténoses oesophagiennes (4/17).
Malgre son aggressivité maximale ce protocole de chimiothérapie séquentielle + irradiation multifractionnée ne semble apporter aucun bénéfice par rapport aux traitements conventionnels.

Neo-Adjuvant Chemotherapy. Ed. Cl. Jacquillat, M. Weil, D. Khayat. Colloque INSERM/John Libbey Eurotext Ltd. © 1988. Vol. 169, pp. 703-706.

Pre-operative chemotherapy in squamous cell carcinoma of the esophagus. 35 cases

J. Vignoud, S. Bourdin, J. Leborgne and J. Paineau

Centre René Gauducheau, Nantes, France

RESUME

From March to December 1986, we treated 48 patients with squamous cell carcinoma of the esophagus by an induction chemotherapy combining CISPLATINUM and 5 FLUOROURACILE. All these patients presented advanced stages :
- 16 synchronous Head and Neck and esophageal carcinoma
- 7 metastatic osophageal carcinoma
- 4 locoregional recurrences after esophageal carcinoma irradiated
- 16 locally advanced esophageal carcinoma

The response rate at the esophageal site appeared particulary high : 64 % and the quality of the responses was impressive.
In regard with these results, we now deliver induction chemotherapy before locoregional treatment, and we treated 35 patients before surgery.

PATIENTS AND METHODS

35 patients with squamous cell carcinoma of the esophagus were juged potentially operable by our surgical team, in regard with general status and locoregional extend of disease.
Medium age was 55 years (33 to 73 years) and the sex ratio was 34 men for 1 woman.
All lesions were locally advanced and staged T2 NX. We noted :
- 6 upper third and cervical localisations
- 24 middle third localisations
- 5 lower third localisations

Induction chemotherapy combined
- CISPLATINUM 100 mg/m2 on day 1
- 5 FLUOROURACILE 1000/m2/day delivered as continuous infusion on days 2, 3, 4 and 5.

3 courses were delivered on days 1, 15 and 30.

Surgery was accomplished on day 50, after evaluation of the response and esophagectomy was performed after thoracotomy.

TOXICITY

Toxicity of this protocol was tolerable :
For **chemotherapy**, we noted 12 toxicities
- 11 low grade toxicities, especially hematologic, grades 1 or 2
- 1 grade 4 hematologic toxicity

And 30 patients received the whole induction treatment, chemotherapy had to be stopped after the 2nd course, once for toxicity, 4 times for progressive disease or no response.

Surgery was always possible in regard of general conditions, had to be post-dated 4 times for hematologic reasons, and the complication rate does not seem to be enhanced by induction chemotherapy : we observed
- 2 deaths, 1 after fistula, 1 by respiratory decompensation
- 1 chylothorax
- 1 cervical abscess

CRITERIA OF RESPONSE

Response was evaluated
- clinically on pain and dysphagia
- radiologically on stenosis and sub-stenosis dilatation
- endoscopically on stenosis and intra-luminal tumor

For these criteria, we where very strict and we considered as responders only patients presenting a very important improvment of the symptoms or an almost return to the normal of radiologic or endoscopic initial constatations, in order to correlated this "clinical" response with surgical and histologic constatations.

Response was also evaluated
- on surgical constatations at thoracotomy : persistent palpable tumor or pathologic nodes in the mediastinum
- on histologic examination of the surgical exeresis in regard with 2 parameters :
  * the initial tumor site where epithelioma persists in certain cases, or is found as microscopical residual disease, or is not found.
  * the epithelium at the tumor site which was found tumoral or totaly repared.

RESULTS

Based on these criteria, the response rate is high :
- 20 responses out 35 patients clinically
- 19 responses out 35 patients on radiologic examination
- 18 responses out 35 patients at endoscopy

Esophagectomy was performed 34 times, one of the patient being discovered as metastatic at laparotomy. Thoracotomy was used 30 times, esophageal stripping 4 times for upper localisations. Esophageal exeresis was realised 34 times, and macroscopic extirpation was radical in 31 out 35 patients.

- 17 patients were considered as surgical responders :
  * no palpable tumor in the mediastinum
  * 17 radical extirpations

Histologic examination of exeresis :
* 17 normal epithelium
* 5 persistent tumors in the sub-mucosa
* 4 sterilised tumors
* 8 microscopic residual tumors
* 2 microscopic residual carcinoma in the nodes

- 17 patients were considered as non-responders, radical resection was performed in 14 cases, histologic examination of the exeresis showed in all cases persistent epithelioma, tumoral epithelium, and node metastasis in 10 cases.

CONCLUSIONS

Induction chemotherapy combining CISPLATINUM and 5 FLUOROURACILE appears as a safe protocole in squamous cell carcinoma of the esophagus.
Toxicity is tolerable, toxicity of surgery is not enhanced by pre-operative chemotherapy.

Clinical response rate is about 50 %.
In responders, improvment is dramatic and confirmed by surgical and histologic constatations.
By reduction of the tumor, chemotherapy improves the rate of radical surgical resections, especially in upper third localisations.

No data about survival is avalaible, but induction chemotherapy appears as a great help for locoregional treatment of squamous cell carcinoma of the esophagus, and should be used for locally advanced disease, especially in upper third localisations.

Résumé

De mars à décembre 1986 nous avons traité 48 malades atteints de cancer épidermoïde de l'oesophage par une chimiothérapie d'induction associant Cis.Platyl et 5 Fluorouracile. Ces malades présentaient des stades avancés. 16 malades avaient de façon synchrone un cancer de la tête et du cou et un cancer de l'oesophage, 7 malades avait des cancers de l'oesophage métastasés. Dans 4 cas il s'agissait de rechutes loco-régionales après irradiation d'un cancer de l'oesophage, dans 16 cas de cancer localement avancé de l'oesophage. Le taux de réponse au niveau de l'oesophage parait particulièrement élevé 64 % et la qualité de la réponse a été impressionnante.

Eu égard à ces résultats, nous administrons maintenant la chimiothérapie d'induction avant le traitement loco-régional. Nous avons traité 35 malades avant la chirurgie.

Locoregional therapy I

Traitements locorégionaux I

Neo-Adjuvant Chemotherapy. Ed. Cl. Jacquillat, M. Weil, D. Khayat. Colloque INSERM/John Libbey Eurotext Ltd. © 1988. Vol. 169, pp. 709-712.

Drug levels in isolated extremity perfusion

H. Walther

Department of General and Oncologic Surgery, Trostberg Hospital (Head : PD Dr. med. K.R. Aigner), FRG

Chemotherapy by isolated regional perfusion was initiated and developed thirty years ago at Tulane University, New Orleans by E.T. KREMENTZ and co-worker (1). Another major parameter was added to regional perfusion with the introduction of hyperthermia in the perfused area in the late 60th from CAVALIERE et all (2).

Meanwhile this method became the treatment of choice in malignant melanoma with intransit metastases.

Techniques have been developed for perfusion for all areas of the body (3), a variety of chemotherapeutic agent have been tested and new agents that are currently becoming available are also under investigation by this technique.

Perfusion technique itself, however, has been unchanged during the last thirty years. For example isolation of the lower extremity is performed by canulation of the iliac vessels and seccured by a tourniquet around the upper tigh. In usual techniques the oxygenated and preheated blood perfused through the limb at a physiological flow rate. Tissue temperature, measured with thermistor probes is increased up to 42° C.

With our modification of common perfusion technique we intend to increase the tissue uptake of cytostatic drugs.

Tissue uptake of cytostatic drugs (MMC, CDDP, L-Pam) is directly related to serum concentration in the perfused area. Increase of response can be achieved by increase of the concentration x time product (Area Under the Curve) at the tumorsite.

Increase of the total dose for AUC enlargement is limited by tissue release of the drugs post treatment, causing bone marrow depression.

Another possibility to increase the AUC in isolated perfusion without the risk of an overdose is time limited intraarterial infusion into the arterial perfusion line under arterial flow rate reduction. The femoral access is performed with a special arterial double canulation system (B. Braun) that guarantees homogenuous heat distribution in the upper and lower limb. In order to achieve permanently high arterial drug levels for enlargement of AUC the drug is infused directly into the arterial line over a 15 to 30 minute period, while at high oxygen tension the roller pump flow rate is decreased to 80 - 120 ml/minute.

Venous return is kept at the same rate in order to maintain blood volume and venous pressure in the extremity stable. At the end of drug infusion blood flow is increased to a maximum. Venous return is heated up to 42° C in the oxygenator. This blood temperature, cooling down to 41 - 41,5° C in the arterial line maintain the tissue temperature of 39,5 - 40° C. Neovascularisation of metastases is thus dilated (K. STORM). In the use of CDDP tissue temperature over 40° C would cause nerve damage.

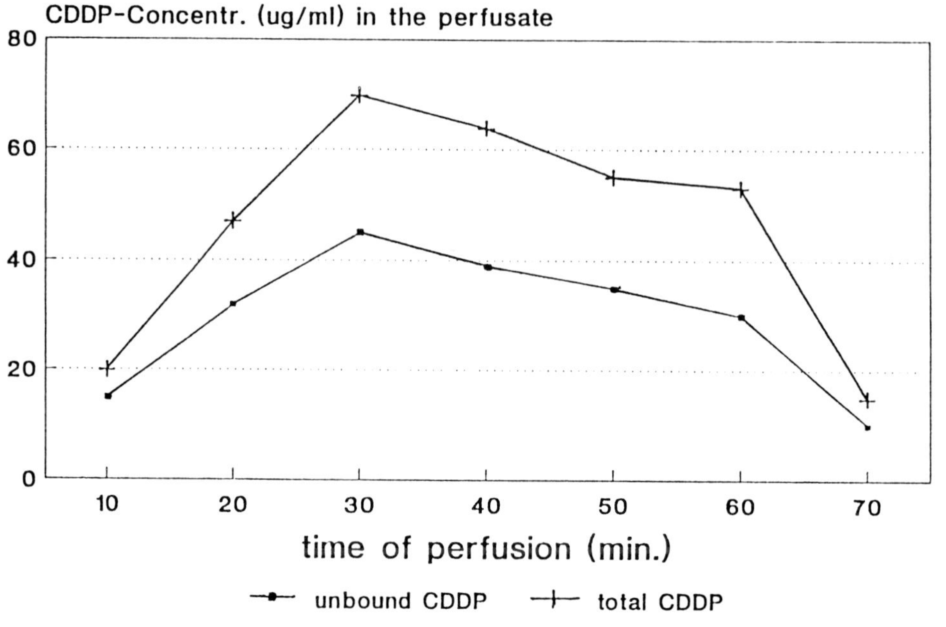

Fig. 1: CDDP plasma levels 100 mg in isolated extremity perfusion

Total amount of CDDP (15 - 20 mg/l limb volume) is given in the oxygenator. After 30 minutes of perfusion time the total amount of CDDP has reached 80 ug/ml, while the unbound CDDP is 40 ug/ml in the perfusate (Fig. 1). These concentration ranges are nearly constant until the end of perfusion.

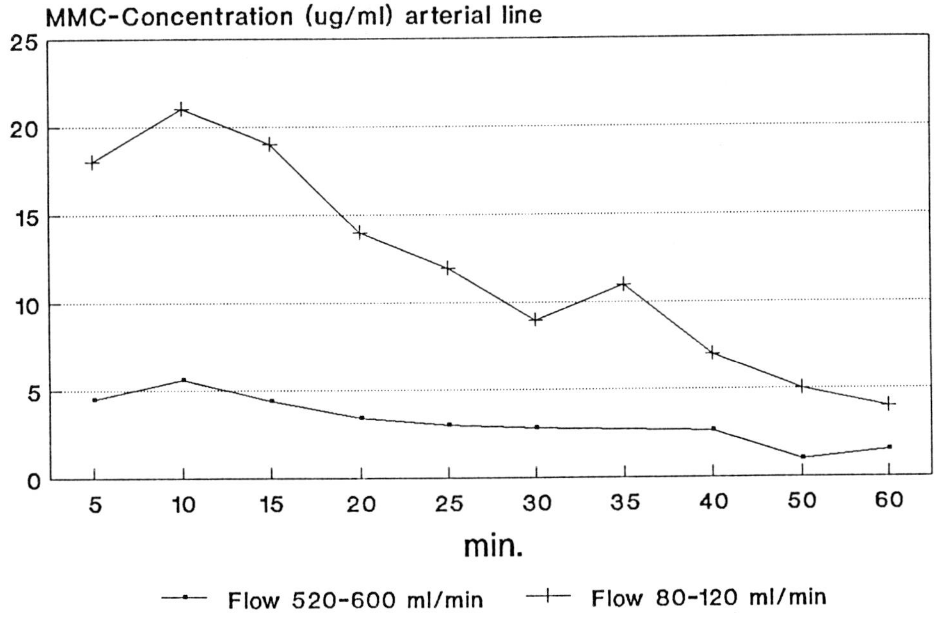

Fig. 2: Mitomycin C - concentration 20 mg in isolated extremity perfusion

Mitomycin C is infused directly into the arterial line over a 20 minute period. With a nearly physiological blood flow of 520 - 600 ml/minute the MMC concentration in the arterial line is about 5 ug/ml (Fig. 2). The same amount of drug (20 mg MMC) and a flow reduction to 80 - 120 ml/minute increase the MMC concentration up to 20 ug/ml. Concentration x time product and tissue uptake are increased.

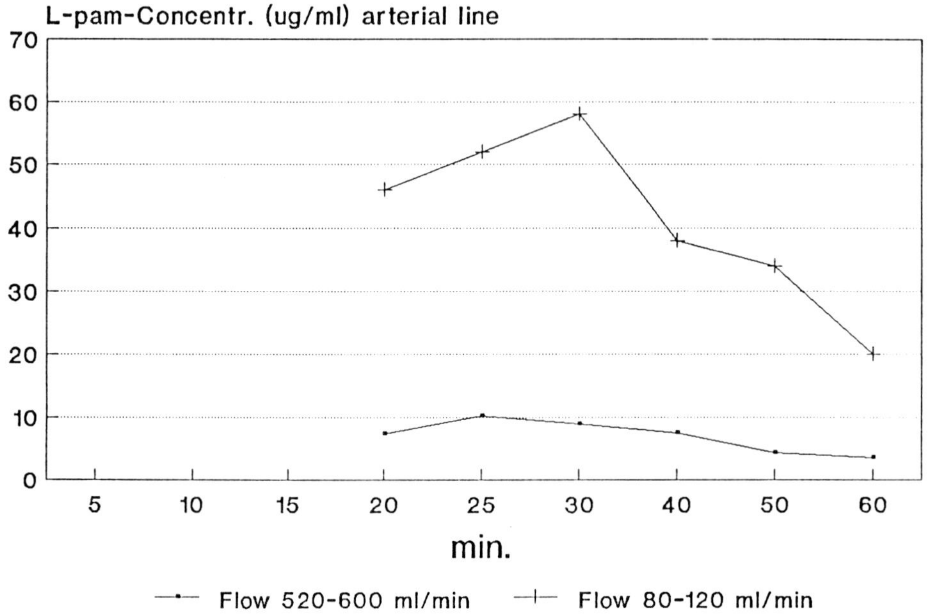

Fig. 3: L-Pam - concentration 70 mg in isolated extremity perfusion

Measurements of L-Pam concentration, infused directly into the arterial line a 20 minutes period too, show the following results (Fig. 3): at high blood flow rates, (520 - 600 ml/minute) only 10 ug/ml can be achieved. Up to 60 ug/ml L-Pam concentration is measured, when the blood flow is decreased down to 80 - 120 ml/minute. Arterial serum levels of L-Pam are six fold higher at the low flow rate.

Conclusions:

A number of advantages have occured from the use of chemotherapy by regional perfusion. With our technical variation (canulation of the deep and superficial femoral artery, infusion of the drug in the arterial perfusion line under arterial flow rate reduction) the effect of the isolated hyperthermic perfusion for treatment of malignant tumors of the extremities can be increased.

References:

1. Ryan RF, Krementz ET, Creech O, Winblad JW, Chamblee W, Cheek H: Selected perfusion of isolated viscera with chemotherapeutic agents using extracorporeal circuit. Surg. Forum 8: 158 - 161, 1957.

2. Cavaliere R, Ciocatto EC, Giovanella BC, Heidelberger C, Johnson RO, Margottini M, Mondori B, Monicca G, Rossi-Fanelli A: Selective heat sensitivity of cancer cells: Biochemical and clinical studies. Cancer 20: 1351 - 1381, 1967.

3. Aigner KR, Walther H, Tonn J, Wenzl A, Hechtel R, Merker G, Schwemmle K: First experimental and clinical results of isolated liverperfusion with cytotoxis in metastases from colorectal primary. Recent Results in Cancer Research 86. Springer-Verlag, pp. 99 - 102, 1983.

Neo-Adjuvant Chemotherapy. Ed. Cl. Jacquillat, M. Weil, D. Khayat. Colloque INSERM/John Libbey Eurotext Ltd. © 1988. Vol. 169, pp. 713-715.

Neo-adjuvant versus adjuvant chemotherapy by means of isolated extremity perfusion in recurrent malignant melanoma

Martin Manner, Peter Schlag, Thomas Hupp and Werner Tilgen*

Departments of Surgery and Dermatology, University of Heidelberg, Im Neuenheimer Feld 110, 6900 Heidelberg, FRG*

Abstract: For recurrent malignant melanoma isolated extremity perfusion with cystostatics can be performed as adjuvant or neo-adjuvant chemotherapy in combination with local excision. The aim of this study was to compare pre- and posterative isolated limb perfusion in regard to local and distant tumor control. Fifteen patients with recurrent malignant melanoma of the extremities were treated with isolated limb perfusion before (n=7) and after (n=8) local excision. Hyperthermic extremity perfusion (39°C) with Alkeran (Melphalan[R]) (1mg/kg BW) and Cisplatinum (Platinex[R]) (1mg/kg BW) was performed for 60 minutes in each case. During a median follow-up time of 21 months, a local recurrence was found in four out of eight patients with adjuvant perfusion chemotherapy as compared to two out of seven with neo-adjuvant treatment. The median local disease free survival time of patients was 13 vs. 17 months but overall recurrence free survival time was 13 vs. 6 monts for adjuvant and neo-adjuvant treatment, respectively. It is therefore concluded, that a neo-adjuvant perfusion chemotherapy allows a better control of local tumor disease in recurrent malignant melanoma.

Key words: malignant melanoma, tumor recurrence, isolated extremity perfusion.

Introduction: The prognosis of patients with locally recurrent malignant melanoma with or without regional satellitosis or lymphnode metastases is poor despite wide surgical excision. Since the introduction of the extremity perfusion by CREECH et al (1958), this method has been increasingly used for the treatment of local recurrence of malignant melanoma of the extremity. A five year survival rate of 40% of patients with recurrent malignant melanoma was found bei KREMENTZ et al (1979). The rational of isolated chemotherapy perfusion is to achieve high concentration of the cytostatics at the site of the tumor recurrence without systemic side effects. The tumor-toxic effect may be further increased with high oxygen tension, mild acidosis and hyperthermia of the perfusate. For locally recurrent melanoma, perfusion chemotherapy can be performed either before (neo-adjuvant) or after (adjuvant) surgical excision. This study was designed to compare the results of adjuvant and neo-adjuvant perfusion chemotherapy regarding local and distant tumor control of already metastasized malignant melanoma.

Material and Method: Between 1982 and 1987 31 patients with locally recurrent malignant melanoma were treated with isolated extremity perfusion. 16 patients were treated with perfusion chemotherapy only. In 15 patients, perfusion chemotherapy was combined with surgical excision. 8 patients had adjuvant chemotherapy 2-6 weeks after the operation. Neo-adjuvant chemotherapy was performed at the time of operation or 2 weeks before surgery. For limb perfusion, the iliac vessels were surgically exposed and cannulated. The extremity was perfused with a pump oxygenator containing a heat exchanger in the circuit. Perfusion was performed at a temperature of 39°C for 60 minutes using Alkeran (1mg/kg BW) and Cisplatinum (1mg/kg BW).
The tumor staging was according to M.D.Anderson classification (STEHLIN et al 1975).

Tab. I: STAGING OF LOCAL RECURRENCE OF MALIGNANT MELANOMA (M.D.Anderson)

Stage II: Local recurrence with or without regional satellitosis $<$2cm

Stage III: Local recurrence with satellitosis $>$2cm or intransit or regional lymphnode metastases

Stage IV: Local recurrence and distant metastases

Tab. II: STAGING OF PATIENTS WITH COMBINATION OF SURGERY AND PERFUSION CHEMOTHERAPY

	Stage II	Stage III	Stage IV
adjuvant	3	5	0
neo-adjuvant	2	3	2

Results: Median follow-up time was 16 months for the adjuvant chemotherapy group and 26 months for the neo-adjuvant chemotherapy group. Local recurrence was observed in 4 of 8 patients with adjuvant chemotherapy and 2 of 7 patients with neo-adjuvant chemotherapy. Distant metastases were found in 2 of 8 patients with adjuvant chemotherapy and 3 of 7 patients with neo-adjuvant chemotherapy. No patient died in the adjuvant therapy group, whereas 3 of 7 patients with neo-adjuvant therapy died, all of them due to tumor progression. The median local disease free survival time was 13 months in the adjuvant group and 17 months in the neo-adjuvant group. The median overall recurrence free survival time was 13 and 6 months, respectively.

Comment: The reduced survival following neo-adjuvant compared to adjuvant chemotherapy may be partially due to more advanced tumor disease in the neo-adjuvant group. The occurence of distant metastases is similar in both groups, whereas a local recurrence was more frequent in the adjuvant (4/8) than in the neo-adjuvant (2/7) group. Although the number of patients is small, this difference becomes even more pronounced for the ratio of local recurrence free survival time and overall tumor free survival time. This ratio was 1 (13 month/13 months) in the adjuvant and 2,8 (17 months/6 months) in the neo-adjuvant therapy group, however, this difference was statistically not significant.

Conclusions: The overall recurrence free time is similar following adjuvant and neo-adjuvant chemotherapy. However, neo-adjuvant perfusion therapy seems to allow better control of local tumor disease than adjuvant perfusion therapy. Further studies including a larger number of patients comparing adjuvant and neo-adjuvant perfusion chemotherapy have to demonstrate, whether this difference in results is significant or not.

References:

1. Creech O Jr., Krementz ET, Ryan RF, Winthed JN (1958): Chemotherapy of cancer: Regional perfusion utilizing an extracorpeal circuit. Human Surg. 148: 616
2. Krementz ET, Carter D, Sutherland CM, Campbell M (1979): The use of regional chemotherapy in the management of malignant melanoma. World J Surg 3: 289-304
3. Stehlin JS, Giovanella BC, De Ipoly PD; Muenz LR, Anderson RF (1975): Results of hyperthermic perfusion for melanoma of the extremities. Surg. Gynecol. Obstet 104 (3): 339-349

Résumé

Pour les rechutes de mélanomes malins, des perfusions isolées des extrémités avec des cytostatiques peuvent être faites en adjuvant ou en néoadjuvant en association avec une excision locale. Le but de cette étude a été de comparer les perfusions de membres isolés en pré et post-opératoires eu égard au contrôle local et à distance, chez 15 malades avec des rechutes de mélanomes malins des extrémités. Les perfusions isolées de membres avant (7 malades) et après (8 malades) excision locale. Les perfusions ont été faites en hyperthermie à 39°C avec de l'Alkéran (Melphalan[R]) 1 mg/kg deux fois par semaine, CIS.PLATYL 1 mg/kg deux fois par semaine. pendant 60 minutes dans chaque cas. Après un suivi médian de 21 mois, une rechute locale a été observée chez 4 des 8 malades traités par chimiothérapie adjuvante et 2 des 7 malades traités par chimiothérapie néoadjuvante. La survie sans rechute locale a été de 13 contre 17 mois (CNA), mais la survie sans rechute de façon plus générale a été de 13 mois pour la chimiothérapie adjuvante contre 6 mois pour la chimiothérapie néoadjuvante mais au départ les malades avec chimiothérapie néoadjuvante étaient plus graves. Il semble que les perfusions locales de chimiothérapie néoadjuvante assurent un meilleur contrôle local de la tumeur dans les rechutes de mélanomes malins.

Neo-Adjuvant Chemotherapy. Ed. Cl. Jacquillat, M. Weil, D. Khayat. Colloque INSERM/John Libbey Eurotext Ltd. © 1988. Vol. 169, pp. 717-721.

Neo-adjuvant intra-arterial doxorubicin and its regional concentration during complex treatment of uterine tumors

János Stumpf, György Németh and Apostolos Georgopoulos*

Oncoradiology of the 'Weil Emil' Hospital, Budapest, Hungary, Uzsoki utca 29, H-1145.
**1st Chemotherapy Clinic of the Medical University, Vienna, 1100 Lazarettgasse 14, Austria*

ABSTRACT

Multimodality treatment /neoadjuvant intraarterial (i.a.) cytostatics, irradiation and surgery if possible/ was carried out in 23 patients with advanced tumor of the uterine cervix. Long term i.a. cannulation of the visceral branch of the hypogastric artery was made by puncture of the femoral artery and a totally implantable catheter system was used. Cytostatics /Doxorubicin and CDDP/ were administered with 5 mg/hour dose rate, total dose of CDDP about 250 mg in four weeks, Doxocubicin each 60 mg at the start and at the end of cannulation. /4 weeks interval./

Early results are promising, nearly all patients responded. This effect may be attributed to the neodajuvant strategy and to the locoregional administration. Response rate is dose-dependent and i.a. administration is connected with high local cytostatic 'offer'.

Local cytostatic concentration was monitored with intravaginal diffusion chamber method. Two diffusion chambers were fixed in the vagina during i.a. infusion and samples were taken regularly.

In case of unilateral Doxorubicin infusion /because of unilateral tumor invasion/ up to tenfold drug-concentration was measured on the cannulated side. This considerable difference may be responsible for tumor control-effect.

KEYWORDS

Locoregional tumor treatment, drug distribution monitoring, uterine tumors

INTRODUCTION

Regional administration of cytostatics f.i. intraarterial infusion has been widely used during the last decade to control advanced solid tumors. (Schwemmle, Aigner, 1983). Usually this method of treatment was carried out as a last chance therapy, but lately more and more often as a part of complex treatment. On the basis of promising results, regional chemotherapy was suggested as basal treatment of cancer (Stephens, 1980). In our institution complex treatment protocol has been elaborated for advanced uterine malignancies in the early 80th (Stumpf, 1986). The protocol consists of: neo-adjuvant intraarterial cytostatic treatment, irradiation and surgery if possible.

Early results are promising. 12 of 23 patients have shown complete remission (CR) and 4 of the 23 partial remission (PR). Overall response rate 16/23. About half of the patients responded well to regional cytostatic treatment, and surgery could have been carried out after the first step of therapy. This unusually good local response rate can be attributed partly to the neo-adjuvant strategy and partly to the high regional drug 'offer' due to long term character of drug administration (Stumpf, 1987).

THEORETICAL BASIS AND PRACTISED DRUG DELIVERY

Pharmacokinetics of intraarterial chemotherapy has been matter of discussion for many years (Stephens, 1983; Bier et al., 1983; and Aigner, 1987).

In all kind of regional treatment /intraarterial infusion, haemofiltration and even in perfusion therapy/ administered amount of cytostatics is usually indicated in mg/m^2. However this terminology may be useful to determine general toxicity in intraarterial administration but it is less or not relevant in the latter mentioned two methods /both regarding tumor control and general toxicity/. It must be pointed out that tumor control depends on regional drug 'offer' thus depending prevalently of both, infused dose of cytostatic and blood flow in the cannulated artery. This widely differs and may be rather low f.i. in head and neck tumors (Kreidler et al., 1983). Blood flow in the cannulated artery can be detected, the given dose of cytostatics in mgs/passing blood volume during the time period of infusion in mls may be a more relevant terminology for dosage (mg/ml).

DIFFUSION CHAMBER METHOD TO MONITOR DRUG DISTRIBUTION IN THE PELVIC REGION

Diffusion chamber method to detect intercellular fluid concentration was used in animal experiments (Georgopoulos, 1983; and Porpaczy, 1983). The method was adapted for clinical use (Stumpf, 1985).

Diffusion chambers (Fig. 1.) were placed into the vagina and fixed on it's lateral walls (Fig. 2.). In case of unilateral tumorous infiltration of the small pelvis only one side cannulation and intraarterial infusion was carried out. (Doxorubicin.) The catheter was placed into the visceral branch of the hypogastric artery, therefore homolateral half of the pelvis can be taken as 'infused area' (Fig. 3b.). Tumor 'target area' (Fig. 3a.) should be within the infused one. Homolateral half of the vagina and of the paracolpium should be within the infused area as well.

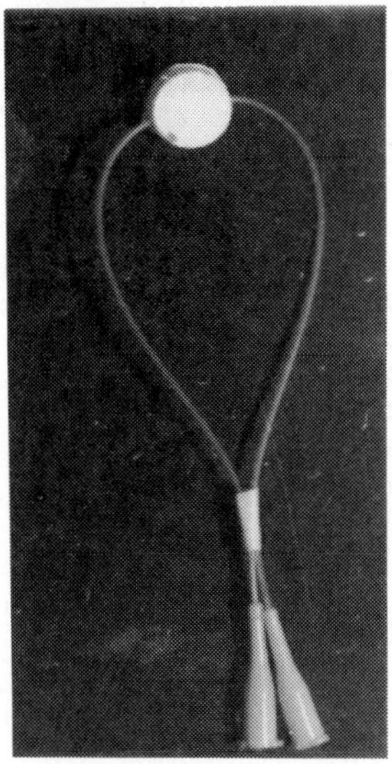

Fig. 1. Diffusion chamber with pipes

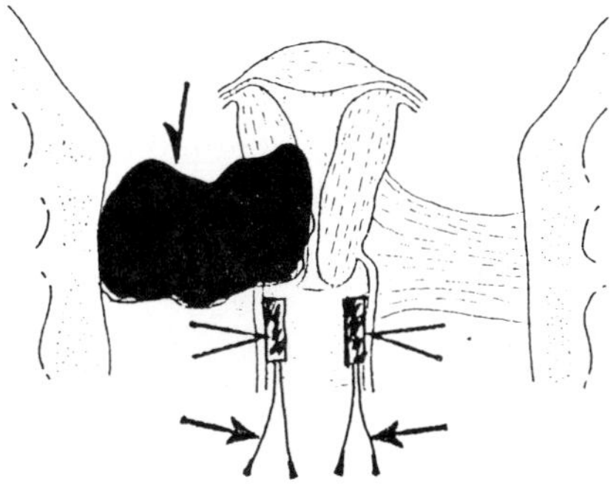

Fig. 2. Measurement in a Stage-III/A cervical tumor (pelvic infiltration, diffusion chamber, pipes leading out of the vagina for sample taking).

Fig. 3. Unilateral regional cytostatic treatment of pelvic tumor

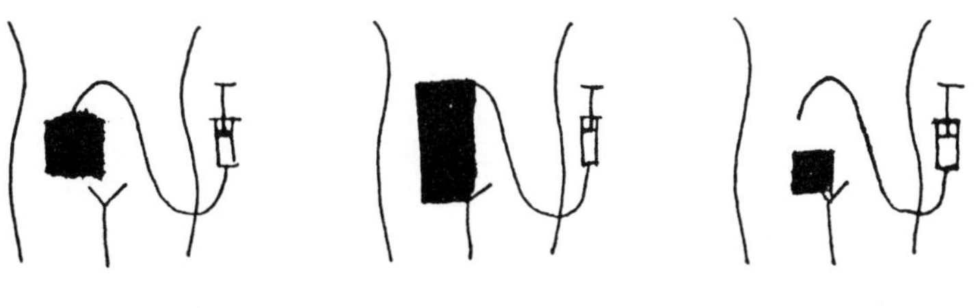

a/ target area b/ infused area c/ monitored area

This can be taken as 'monitored area' (Fig. 3c.) in case target- and monitored area are really within the infused one, Doxorubicin concentration measured in the diffusion chamber's fluid will reflect to the target area while drug concentration in the other side diffusion chamber will reflect to the non-target areas. Intraarterially administered cytostatics will reach non-infused regions only after having passed inferior caval vein, lung and heart and will distribute in the non-infused areas like administered intravenously. Difference in the two chambers cytostatic concentration is a function of regional /i.a./ administration versus i.v. application. In this in vivo study up to a tenfold difference was detected.

SUMMARY

Individual pharmacokinetic patterns of different cytostatic drugs and blood vessel anatomy in the infused region may considerably influence local cytostatic 'offer'. Suitable small amount of cytostatics can be measured by different methods f.i. HPLC. Intravaginal diffusion chamber method gives the possibility to monitor drug distribution in vivo therefore to carry out regional cytostatic treatment individually.

REFERENCES

Schwemmle, K., Aigner, K. (1983): Vascular perfusion in cancer therapy. Springer, Berlin-Heidelberg-New York,Tokyo.

Stephens, F.O., Harker, G.J., Crea, P. (1980): The intra-arterial infusion of chemotherapeutic agents as basal treatment of cancer: evidence of increased drug activity in regionally infused tissues. Aust. NZ J. Surg. 50. 597-602.

Stumpf, J., G, Vadon, Gy. Németh, (1987): Intervention Radiology and Previous Arteriography in the Management of Uterine Malignancies. 14th Int. Cancer Congress Budapest, 1986. Vol. 6. 195-212, Karger, Basel/Akadémia Kiadó.

Stumpf, J., Vadon, G., Németh, Gy. (1985): Radiotherapy Combined with Intraarterial Chemotherapy in Advanced Tumours of the Uterine. Progress in Radio-Oncology III, Ed. K.H. Karcher, H.D. Kogelnik, T. Szepesi, Vienna.

Stephens, F.O. (1983): Pharmacokinetics of Intra-Arterial Chemotherapy. In: Vascular perfusion in cancer therapy. Springer, Berlin-Heidelberg-New York, Tokyo.

Bier, J., Loer, E., Franke, J. (1983): Kinetics of 57-Co Bleomycin in sheep after intraarterial injection in the head and neck region. In: Vascular perfusion in cancer therapy. ed. K. Schwemmle, K. Aigner, Springer, Berlin-Heidelberg, New York, Tokyo.

Aigner, K. (1987): Personnal communication

Kreidler, J.F., Petzel, J.R. (1983): Combined treatment of maxillofacial carcinoma by intraarterial proliferation block and irradiation. Recent Results in Cancer Research, 86. 152-161.

Georgopoulos, A., Porpaczy, P., Schmidbauer, C.P., Rameis, H., Schramek, P., Schütze, E.: The diffusion chamber technique for quantitative determination of antibiotics and cytostatics in interstitial fluids. In: Tissue levels of antimicrobial and antineoplastic agents. ed. Eickenberg, H.U., Georgopoulos, A., Rameis, H., Vienna, 1983. 13rd ICC Proceedings.

Porpaczy, P., Schmidbauer, P., Georgopoulos, A., Endler, A.T.(1983) Pharmacokinetics of high-dose methotrexate in dogs. An experimental model with diffusion chambers. Cancer Chemother. Pharmacol. 11., 172-176.

Stumpf, J., A. Georgopoulos, Gy. Németh (1985): Intraarterial Chemotherapy of Collum Tumors, Measurement of Intercellular Drug Level in vivo (Chamber Diffusion Technique) In: Recent Advances in Chemotherapy. ed. Joji Ishigami, University of Tokyo Press, 1298-1299.

Résumé

La chimiothérapie régionale fut réalisée dans le cas de 23 malades comme une partie de la thérapie complexe dans le cancer du col utérin. Les résultats préliminaires sont encourageux. La tumeur devint opérable dans 12 cas sur 23 (Stage III-IV).

La chimiothérapie régionale avait été la premiere étape de la thérapie complexe et elle fut suivie par la radiothérapie /curiethérapie et téléthérapie/.

La distribution de la cytostatique (Doxorubicin) fut mesurée avec la méthode de la chambre de diffusion intravaginale. Au cours de l'examen 2 chambres furent fixées aux 2 cotés latéraux du vagin. Dans la cas ou la chimiothérapie régionale /infusion intraartérielle/ était unilatérale, des différences considérables furent détectables dans la concentration de la cytostatique dans les deux chambres /la concentration du coté infusé est plus grand au maximum d'un ordre de grandeur, plus exactement de 1,5 a 11 fois/.

La concentration du coté non-infusé est comme si la cytostatique était donnée intraveineusement. Il semble logique que c'est cette différence de la concentration qui est la cause des résultats thérapeutiques plus avantageux.

La méthode de la chambre de diffusion intravaginale n'est pas dangereuse pour les malades et elle rend possible le mesurage 'in vivo' de la distribution locale de la cytostatique. Cette monitorisation de la chimiothérapie régionale facilite l'individualisation de la thérapie.

Neo-Adjuvant Chemotherapy. Ed. Cl. Jacquillat, M. Weil, D. Khayat. Colloque INSERM/John Libbey Eurotext Ltd. © 1988. Vol. 169, pp. 723-728.

Intra-arterial infusion chemotherapy as a primary treatment in cancer of uterine cervix limited to the pelvis

J. Iglesias*, J.A. Lejarcegui*, X. Cot**, J.M. Lailla*, A. Tarrats*, E. Davi*, J. Ausin*, M. Marquez***, P. Jou***, B. Guix**** and J. Gonzalez-Merlo*

School of Medicine-University of Barcelona, Spain
* *Department of Gynaecology*
** *Angio-radiology Service*
*** *Department of Pathology*
**** *Department of Radiotherapy*

SUMMARY:

Percutaneous intraarterial infusion chemotherapy via the internal iliac arteries was performed in 19 patients with invasive cancer of the uterine cervix as a primary treatment. The drugs used were Mytomycin-C, Bleomycin and Cis-Platinum in cycles of 52 hours which were repeated, in some cases, 21 days apart. Complete responses were observed in 4 patients. Partial responses were seen in 12 patients and no response in 3 patients. 8 patients were treated surgically and 9 patients received radiotherapy after the infusion. The effect of chemotherapy was more evident in exophytic tumors with less effect on the parametria. Tumor masses can be reduced and patients can then be treated by surgery or radiotherapy.

KEY WORDS:

Intraarterial chemotherapy, cancer uterine cervix.

INTRODUCTION:

Chemotherapy has been traditionally reserved as a last resort for those patients where sugery and radiation therapy have been unsuccessful, with poor results (1,8,11).

At present, chemotherapy drugs such as Cis-platinum, in combination with other anti-neoplastic medications, are available and are associated with a high tumour response in patients suffering from advanced carcinoma of the cervix (3,9).

The failure of radiation therapy to control large pelvic tumours could be related to radio resistance of the hipoxic cells in the tumoural mass (5,6)

It is possible to reduce the volume of the tumour and thus control the disease (7) using a cytostatic intraarterial infusion as a primary treatment. The idea is to place the patient in a more favorable position for sugery, or, if this is not possible, for radio-therapy.

Chemotherapy could be used as a primary treatment in patients with stage II-B and III cervical cancer, which cannot be successfully treated with traditional local therapy methods (2,9).

Chemotherapy delivered intraarterially increases retention of the medication in the tumour and the surrounding area as the drugs are perfused directly to the artery irrigating this region. In secondary, systemic circulation, the chemotherapy drugs have much less harmful side effects (10).

MATERIAL AND METHODS

19 patients with invasive carcinoma of the uterine cervix were given intraarterial chemotherapy.

A conditioning factor was that the tumour be confined to the pelvis and irrigated by the internal iliac artery system. This was checked by selective angiography. Possible node metastases were determined by lymphangiography.

The chemotherapeutic medication was administered with catheters placed percutaneously in each internal iliac artery using the Seldinger technique. The drugs were delivered using an arterial infusion pump (Eckli-PE-300 BL, Neuchatel, Switzerland). The technique was performed using a local anaesthetic and was well tolerated by the patients. The patients rested during the hours the infusion was given.

The chemotherapy agents and doses used were: Mytomycin-C 10 mg/m^2 over four hours of infusion; Bleomycin 25 mg/m^2 over 24 hours, and Cis-platinum 100 mg/m^2 over 24 hours. Before commencing treatment hyperhydration and heparinization were carried out.

The intravenous hydration was begun the night before the angiography. It was necessary to obtain not less than 2 litres of urine over the duration of the chemoterapy treatment. For the heparinization we used 5000 U prophylactic calcic heparin applied subcutaneosly every eight hours. The last dose was administered eight hours before withdrawing the catheters.

The medications were administered in 1 or 2 cycles, 21 days apart, depending on the tumour response.

Toxicity parameters to be assessed were: stomatitis, nausea, vomiting, diarrhea, pulmonary, cardiac, cutaneous, nervous and renal complications. Thorough checks on platelets, granulocytes and creatinine were carried out. Required laboratory values were: platelets in excess of 110,000; granulocytes in excess of 1800; creatinine less than 2 mg/100 ml and bilirrubin lower than 5 mg/10 ml. The stage of the disease was catalogued in accordance with the classification of the International Federation of Obstetrics and Gynaecology and is shown in table 1.

Table 1. Distribution by stages

Stage	I B	2 patients
Stage	II A	1 patient
Stage	II B	6 patients
Stage	III B	10 patients

The diagnosis was confirmed histologically in all cases and the pathology is shown in table 2.

Table 2. Pathology

Non queratinizing squamous carcinoma	6 patients
Keratinizing squamous carcinoma	4 patients
Basal cell carcinoma	4 patients
Glassy cell carcinoma	2 patients
Adenosquamous carcinoma	1 patient
Mucoid carcinoma	1 patient
Undifferenciated carcinoma	1 patient

The pre-treatment clinical study included: Clinical history; the physical examination of the patient; measuring the size of the tumor; complete blood tests; radiography of the thorax; ultrasound; bone and liver gammagraphy and lymphangiography. Computerized axial tomography was used in some selected cases.

To sum up, the patients local and generalized disease was assessed along with the toxic effects of the treatment.

These evaluations, especially the laboratory and clinical test, were carried out after each cycle of treatment. The number of cycles depended on the local tumor evolution. Which was determined by pelvic examination.

As soon as a favorable surgical situation was reached, the patients were operated. We never carried out more than two cycles of treatment. If after the second cycle of treatment, pelvic examination showed no favorable change for surgical treatment the patients were then treated by radiotherapy.

RESULTS

Nineteen patients, aged 34 to 74 were given intraarterial chemoterapy as a primary treatment, using the methods described above.

12 patients received two cycles of chemotherapy while the remaining received only one.

Table 3 shows the patients who received chemotherapy prior to surgery.

In the patient, Case I, stage III-B, with right parametrial infiltration two cycles of chemotherapy were given. The mass regressed completely, with full mobility of both parametria, thus permitting a Wertheim-Meigs operation. The pathological examination revealed no neoplastic tissue, except for the cytotoxic effects which will be explained later. This patient had a positive right iliac node. The patient is now free from disease thirty nine months after commencement of treatment.

Four patients had only one cycle of treatment before radical hysterectomy was performed and three of them are free from disease 9, 15 and 35 months respectively; the other patient had an unsatisfactory surgery and she has persistent disease 26 months after treatment. Four other patients had two cycles with complete response in all of them. Two are well, 7 and 39 months respectively, one has persitent disease 13 months and one died 10 months after treatment from renal failure and sepsis.

Table 3. Surgical Group

Case nº	Stage	Cycles and response	Oper.	Survival months	Present Status
1	III B	+ PR + CR	WM	39	NED
2	I B	+ PR + CR	WM	10	✠ Renal failure Sepsis
3	I B	+ PR	WM	35	NED
4	II B	+ PR	Unsat.	26	PD
5	II A	+ PR	WM	15	NED
6	II B	+ PR	WM	9	NED
7	II B	+ PR + CR	WM	7	NED
8	III B	+ PR + CR	WM	13	PD

PR= Partial response CR= Complete response WM=Wertheim-Meigs
PD= Persistence Disease NED= No Evidence of Disease

Table 4. Radiotherapy Group

Case nº	Stage	Cycles and response	R.X.	Survival months	Present Status	Cause Death
9	III B	+ PR + PR	Co-60	12	✠	Renal failure Sepsis
10	III B	+ PR + PR	6 Mev	37	NED	
11	III B	+ No + No	-	19	✠	Sepsis
12	III B	+ PR + PR	Co-60	22	✠	Sepsis
13	III B	+ PR + PR	Co-60	9	✠	Renal failure.Sepsis
14	III B	+ PR + PR	6 Mev CS	32	P.D.	
15	II B	+ PR + PR	Co-60 CS	30	P.D.	
16	II B	+ PR + PR	6 Mev	14	✠	Fecaloid perit.
17	II B	+ No	6.Mev	24	P.D.	
18	III B	+ No	-	1	✠	Cardio-Renal failure
19	III B	+ PR	6 Mev	9	NED	

CS = Cesium

Table 4 shows the results obtained with patients where reduction of the tumor was not so evident. These patients were later treated by radiotherapy except cases 11 and 18; both died from persistent disease and sepsis and cardio-renal failure respectively. Case number 11 had a mucoid adenocarcinoma.

Case 10 had a favorable response to 6 Mev. linear accelerator radiotherapy and she is free from disease 37 months after treatment with a dose of 46 Gy.

Although partial reduction of the tumoral mass was obtained in cases 9, 12, 13 and 16, the patients died 12,22,9 and 14 months after treatment. The cause of death was sepsis in three and a fecaloid peritonitis in the fourth.

Cases 14 and 15 were treated with Radiotherapy and Caesium and they have persistent disease 30 and 32 months respectively.

Case 17 showed no response, she was treated with Radiotherapy and has a persistent disease 24 months after treatment.

Finaly Case 19, stage III B had a partial response after infusion, she was then treated with Radiotherapy and she is free from disease 9 months after treatment.

Side effects consisted of two echimosis in the punction site and nausea and vomiting in eleven patients.

Post chemotherapy pathology varies from case to case. In some cases there is little evidence of the effect of the cytotoxic drugs on neoplasic cells and only some cytoplasmic vacuolation is seen with the presence of nuclei with irregularly distributed chromatin and some signs of karyorrhexis.

In other cases, however, the cytotoxic and tumor reducing effects were extremely evident and wide areas of necrosis were observed, with accumulation of foaming type histiocytic elements and giant multinucleate cells, that phatogocytate cholesterol crystals.

To conclude, tumor response to chemotherapy was complete in four cases and partial in twelve. No response was obtained in three cases. As far as side effects were concerned, most patients tolerated the treatment well. No patient had reduction of leucocytes or platelets, or renal or pulmonary complications which prevented or delayed a second cycle of chemotherapy. Only case 16 presented a neurological disorder, of a paraplegic type in both lower extremities. This patient recovered slowly but, even after computerized axial tomography and nuclear magnetic resonance, it did not become clear whether the complication was due to the chemotherapy or to a possible metastasis in the spinal cord. This patient also presented ulceration of the vulva as a result of chemotherapy.

DISCUSION

Intraarterial chemotherapy increases the concentration of chemotherapy drugs in the tumor and the surrounding area, thus, reducing the amount of the drugs in systemic circulation, producing less harmful secondary effects (10).

Cis-platinum in combination with other chemotherapy drugs showed high tumor response in advanced stages of carcinoma of the uterine cervix (3,4,9) and this was the reason for choosing this particular combination.

In our study we observed that the effect of chemotherapy is more evident in primary tumours, specially in exophytic forms, than in the parametrium.

The high incidence of distant metastasis in stages II-B and III of cancer of the cervix, explains the failure of the traditional methods of local application of treatment (9). Therefore, new techniques should be sought and new guidelines for treatment established. What we are trying to do with the technique of intraarterial infusion chemotherapy is to reduce the tumour mass and make it possible for later surgery or radiotherapy.

REFERENCES

1. Carlson, J.A. Jr., Freedman, R.S., Wallace, S. et al. (1981): Intraarterial Cis-platinum in the management of squamous-cell carcinoma of the uterine cervix. Gynecol. Oncol. 12:92-93.
2. Carlson, V.; Delclos, L.; Fletcher, G.H. (1967): Distant metastases in squamous-cell carcinoma of the uterine cervix. Radiology, 88: 961-966.
3. Friedlander, M.L.; Kate, S.B.; Sullivan, A. et al. (1983): Cervical carcinoma: A drug responsive tumor. Experience with combined Cis-platin, Vinblastine, Bleomycin. Gynecol. Oncol. 16, 257-281.
4. Friedlander, M.L.; Atkinson, K.; Coppleson, J.M.V. et al. (1984): The Integration of Chemotherapy into the Management of Locally Advanced Cervical Cancer. A pilot study. Gynecol. Oncology 19, 1-7.
5. Fletcher, G.H. (1983): Clinical dose response curves of human malignant tumors. Brit. J. Radiol. 46, 1-12.
6. Hall, E.J. (1972): Radiation dose rate: A factor of importance in radiobiology and radiotherapy. Brit. J. Radiol. 45, 81-87.
7. Jones, T.K., Levitt, S.H. (1979): Combination chemotherapy and radiation therapy. Int. J. Radiat. Oncol. Biol. Phys. 5, 2147-2149.
8. Morrow, C.P.; Di Saia, P.J.; Maugan, C.P. et al. (1977): Continuous pelvic arterial infusion with Bleomycin for squamous carcinoma of the cervix recurrent after irradiation therapy. Cancer Treat. Rep. 61, 1403-1405.
9. Perez, C.A.; Breaux, S.; Madox-Jones, H. et al (1983): Radiation therapy alone in the treatment of carcinoma of uterine cervix. Cancer 51, 1393-1402.
10. Stephens, F.O. (1983): Selective embolization and organ perfusion with cytostatics. In "Recent results in Cancer Research", edited by K. Schwemmle and K. Aigner. Vol. 86, pag. 1-12. Springer-Verlang. Berlin-Heidelberg.
11. Swenerton , K.D.; Evers, J.A.; White, G.W. et al. (1979): Intermittent pelvic infusion with Vincristine, Bleomycin and Mytomycin-C for advanced recurrent carcinoma of the cervix. Cancer Treat. Rep. 63; 1379-1381.

Résumé

Des perfusions intra-artérielles percutanées de chimiothérapie par les artères iliaques internes ont été effectuées chez 19 malades atteintes de cancer invasif du col utérin, comme premier traitement. Les médicaments ont été Mitomycine-C, Bléomycine et Cis.Platyl en cycle de 52 heures qui ont été répété dans certains cas après 21 jours. Une réponse complète a été observée chez 4 malades, des réponses partielles ont été observées chez 12 patients et 3 malades n'ont eu aucune réponse. 6 malades ont été traitées chirurgicalement, 9 malades ont reçu une radiothérapie après la perfusion. L'effet de la chimiothérapie est plus évident dans les tumeurs exophytiques avec moins d'effets sur les paramètres. Les masses tumorales peuvent être réduites, les patientes peuvent alors être traitées par chirurgie ou radiothérapie.

Neo-Adjuvant Chemotherapy. Ed. Cl. Jacquillat, M. Weil, D. Khayat. Colloque INSERM/John Libbey Eurotext Ltd. © 1988. Vol. 169, pp. 729-732.

Intra-aortic infusion of methotrexate in squamous cell carcinoma of penis

Maw-Chang Sheen and Chun-Hsiung Huang*

Department of Surgery, Department of Urology, Kaohsiung Medical College, Kaohsiung, Taiwan, Republic of China*

ABSTRACT

From 1985 to 1987 five patients with advanced squamous cell carcinoma of penis were treated with continuous intra-aortic infusion chemotherapy. The catheter was inserted retrogradely through lateral circumflex artery into abdominal aorta. The catheter tip was located below the branching of inferior mesenteric artery and above the bifurcation of abdominal aorta. Intra-aortic infusion with methotrexate 50 mg/24hr and simultaneous intramuscular injection of leukovorin 6 mg/6hr were given for a mean of 9 days. Then they were followed with long term intermittent intra-aortic infusion with mitomycin C 2 mg pluse 5 FU 250 mg or methotrexate 25 mg every week. Two patients obtained complete response and one had partial response. The side effects were mild and tolerable. This therapeutic modality is a simple and effective method for palliation of advanced penile carcinoma with its unique advantage in functional and anatomical preservation of organ.

KEY WORDS

Intra-aortic infusion, penile carcinoma

INTRODUCTION

Penile carcinoma is extremely uncommon in our country. The treatment most commonly used is partial penectomy with or without inguinal lymphadenectomy. Amputation of the penis in most cases is followed by loss of sexual function. Therefore there are still a lot of patients refuse penectomy because they would rather die than living without a penis. These patients are always seeking for some folk measures to preserve their penis.

As result, the disease became advnaced when they were first seen in our clinic. Radiotherapy has been used in the treatment of penile carcinoma to preserve sexual function, but urethral stricuture, skin change and even penile atrophy may follow radiotherapy. Systemic chemotherapy has had a very limited used in penile carcinoma. In order to avoid anatomical and functional deficits, regional chemotherapy was tried to those patients who refuse or are unsuitable for penectomy.

SUBJECTS AND METHODS

From November 1985 to February 1988, 5 cases of advanced penile carcinoma (Table 1) were referred for regional chemotherapy. The age ranged from 42 to 68 years old with an average of 53 years old. Four cases received no prior therapy except herb drugs. The fifth case is a recurrent case after penectomy and inguinal lymphadenectomy.

Table 1. Results of Intra-aortic Methotrexate (MTX)

Case No.	Age (y/o)	Stage	Total Dose (MTX)	Results
1	51	$T_3N_2M_0$	700 mg	CR
2	42	$T_4N_2M_0$	450 mg	CR
3	56	$T_3N_2M_0$	350 mg	NR
4	51	$T_3N_2M_0$	500 mg	NR
5	68	$T_0N_3M_0$	350 mg	PR

The Catheterization Method (Sheen, 1984)

One minimeter inner diameter and 2 minimeter outer diameter teflon tube were used for catheterization. A 5 cm incision was made on inguinal area. The teflon catheter was inserted through the larteral circumflex branch of the profound femoral artery retrogradely into the abdominal aorta. The catheter tip was located between the branching of inferior mesenteric artery and the bifurcation of abdominal aorta. After the catheter was properly placed, the distal portion of the catheter was inserted subcutaneously along the anterolateral trunk using a specially designed 70 cm in length introducer and brought out to the skin surface through a stab wound near the infraclavicular region and fixed. The catheter can be kept in place for long term treatment.

The Treatment Regimens

Initially, the patient was infused continuously with methotrexate 50 mg every 24 hours using a portable pump until the development of side effect. Simultaneously, citrovorum factor 6 mg was given intramuscularly every 6 hours. The average total dose of methotrexate given is 450 mg. Then the patients were followed in outpatient department with long term intermittent one shot of methotrexate 25 mg or Mitomycin C 2 cm pluse 5 FU 250 mg weekly until the occurrence of intolerable side effect.

RESULTS (Table 1)

Of those 4 patients without previous treatment, 2 patients had complete remission and the other 2 with response of shot duration were classified as nonresponder. The fifth patient with penectomy showed partial response. The most common side effects seen are skin rash, leukopenia and anorexia, etc.

Case Reports

Case No. 1, a 52-year-old patient had noted a slow growing tumor of penis for 3 years. On physical examination, the tumor was 6 x 4 cm in size. Bilateral inguinal lymph nodes were palpable. No evidence of distant metastasis was found. The pathological diagnosis by Broader's classification is grade II keratiznizing squamous cell carcinoma.

Continuous infusion of methotrexate was given for 11 days and was stopped due to skin rash and malaise. Total dose of methotrexate given was 550 mg. The tumor regressed considerably and leaving only erosion of the glans of penis. Later, the patient was follow-up on outpatient department with intermittent one shot of methotrexate for about 3 months until slight elevation of GOT and GPT. These enzymes decline to normal level soon after the switch of methotrexate to 5 FU and mitomycin C. The penis had healed with normal sexual function 6 months after therapy.

One year after initiation of infusion therapy, the catheter ruptured while infusing with 5 FU and mitomycin C. Extravasation of the drug occurred and necrosis of the overlying skin on left side inguinal area was found. Infusion therapy was stopped and no further anticancer durg was given. No evidence of recurrence is noted so far, that is one year and six months after therapy.

Case No. 2, a 42 years old patient had suffered from ulcerating penile tumor for 2 years. On physical examination, the mass was 14 x 13 cm in diameter. All the penis became neorotic except urethra. Bilateral inguinal nodes were palpable. No distant metastasis was found. Pathologic diagnosis is grade II keratinizing squamous cell carcinoma.

Continuous infusion of methotrexate was given for 11 days with a total dose of 450 mg and was stopped because of stomatitis, ginginval bleeding and skin rash. The mass regressed considerably leaving only a skin defect, 8 x 6 cm in diameter. The patient was followed at OPD and received maintainous therapy. The wound healed completely 3 months after therapy. He was relatnctant to receive any further treatment after 4 months' intermittent therapy.

Eighteen months after discontinue of therapy that is 22 months after initiation of therapy, the tumor recurred. Another catheter was inserted from left circumflex artery. Second course of continuous methotrexate infusion was given for 16 days. The total methotrexate given is 700 mg. The tumor regressed remarkedly again and leaving only a 2 cm diameter ulceration at the time of follow-up (1988, Feb).

DISCUSSION

Two of 4 previous untreated penile carcinoma revealed complete remission to intra-aortic methotrexate. The side effect is mild and tolerable. The functional and anatomical preservation is good. Intra-aortic infusion chemotherapy seems to be a simple and effective treatment for palliation of advanced penile carcinoma. More cases and longer follow-up are indicated to make a conclusion.

REFERENCES

Sheen, M.C. (1984): Chemotherapy for metastatic liver cancer by intra-aortic infusion. J. Formosan Med. Assoc. 83, 576-584.

Résumé

De 1985 à 1987, 5 malades avec des cancers avancés du pénis ont été traités par chimiothérapie continue intra-aortique. Le cathéter était inséré par voie rétrograde à travers l'artère circonflexe dans l'aorte abdominale. L'extrêmité du cathéter était placée au-dessous de l'embranchement de la mésentérique inférieure et au-dessus de la bifurcation de l'aorte abdominale. Une infusion intra-artérielle avec du Méthotrexate 50 mg/24 h. et simultanément une injection de Leucovorine 6 mg toutes les 6 heures, a été donnée sur une moyenne de 9 jours, puis elles étaient suivies par des infusions intra-aortiques intermittentes de Mitomycine 2 mg et de 5.Fu 250 mg, Méthotrexate 25 mg toutes les semaines. Chez deux malades une rémission complète a été observée, chez un malade, une réponse partielle. Les effets secondaires ont été modérés et tolérables. Cette modalité thérapeutique est simplet et efficace dans la paliation des cancers avancés du pénis avec l'avantage unique de préserver la fonction et l'anatomie de cet organe.

Neo-Adjuvant Chemotherapy. Ed. Cl. Jacquillat, M. Weil, D. Khayat. Colloque INSERM/John Libbey Eurotext Ltd. © 1988. Vol. 169, pp. 733-737.

Chimiothérapie intra-artérielle hépatique pour métastases hépatiques d'origine colo-rectale

Ph. Rougier, M. Ducreux, D. Elias, J. Lumbroso, J.P. Droz et Ph. Lasser

Institut Gustave Roussy, 94800 Villejuif, France

La chimiothérapie intra-artérielle hépatique (CIAH) permet d'augmenter l'exposition tumorale aux cytostatiques en augmentant à la fois la concentration locale en antinéoplasique et le temps de contact (ROUGIER). Son utilisation dans les métastases des adénocarcinomes colo-rectaux est justifiée par la chimio-résistance habituelle de ces tumeurs aux doses habituellement utilisées (MOERTEL).

Entre 1983 et 1987, nous avons traité par CIAH 58 patients ayant des métastases hépatiques (MH) d'origine colorectale selon deux techniques différentes :

- La CIAH discontinue par le 5 FU (groupe 1) et,
- La CIAH continue par le FUDR (groupe 2)

METHODES :

- La CIAH discontinue par le 5 FU (groupe 1) a été réalisée au moyen d'un cathéter artériel, placé chirurgicalement dans l'artère gastro-duodénale et reliée à un accès sous-cutané. Les perfusions de 5 FU ont été réalisées en utilisant une pompe ou un pousse-seringue portable, à la dose de 1 g/m2 par perfusion de 6 heures. Le rythme des CIAH a été journalier pendant 7 jours à partir du 4 ème jour post-opératoire puis hebdomadaire après la sortie des patients. Les perfusions ont été poursuivies jusqu'à la progression tumorale ou la thrombose artérielle. Les doses ont été adaptées à la tolérance.

- La CIAH continue par le FUDR (groupe 2) a été réalisée au moyen d'une pompe implantable (Infusaid 400) placée au niveau de la fosse iliaque droite. La dose de FUDR était de 0,3 mg/kg/jour pendant 14 jours alternant avec 14 jours de repos pendant lesquels la pompe était remplie avec du sérum physiologique et de l'héparine (10 000 ui).

POPULATION

58 Patients ont été traités, 42 dans le groupe 1 et 16 dans le groupe 2. L'importance des métastases était similaire dans les 2 groupes les patients avaient plus de 4 métastases dans 75 % des cas et un envahissement hépatique inférieur à 25 % chez 26 % des patients, compris entre 25 et 75 % chez 63 % des patients, et supérieur à 75 % chez 11 %.

RESULTATS

Le taux de réponse, selon les critères de l'OMS ont été identique dans les 2 groupes (52 et 53 %), de même que la survie à un an (79 + ou - 12 %) et la médiane de survie (14 et 18 mois). Des métastases extra-hépatiques se sont développées dans les 2 groupes chez 81 et 75 % des patients. Les patients qui avaient des métastases bien perfusées au contrôle angioscintigraphique ont eu une survie supérieur aux autres (P<0,02).

<u>LES COMPLICATIONS</u> : ont été différentes selon les techniques : avec la CIAH discontinue les thromboses artérielles ont été observées dans 66 % des cas au bout d'un délai moyen de 3 mois ; des ulcérations ou une inflammation gastroduodénale dans 12 % des cas ; et une (leucopénie grade II a été observée chez 19 % des patients. Avec la CIAH continue (groupe 1) aucune thrombose n'a été observée mais une hépatite clinique a été notée dans 50 % des cas, une cholangite sclérosante dans 25 % des cas et une inflammation, ou ulcération gastro-duodénale dans 50 % des cas.

<u>LE CONFORT</u> des patients est bon avec les deux méthodes aussi longtemps que la maladie tumorale est contrôlée et que n'apparaissent pas de complications. Le nombre de venues à l'hôpital de jour ont été deux fois plus nombreuses pour les patients du groupe 1.

<u>DISCUSSION</u> : La CIAH dans notre expérience permet de contrôler l'évolution des métastases d'origine colo-rectale dans la majorité des cas, mais les patients développent dans 80 % des cas des métastases extra-hépatiques qui sont souvent responsables de leur décès ce qui limite l'efficacité de ces CIAH sur la survie. Celle-ci semble cependant augmentée (Balch, Nieder Ruse, Kemeny) et un essai randomisé est actuellement en cours en FRANCE pour mieux définir ce bénéfice.

Les deux méthodes de CIAH : discontinue et continue semblent également efficaces sur les métastases. Cependant le confort, tout au moins au début est supérieur avec les pompes implantables. Ultérieurement il faut prendre en compte la toxicité hépatique et biliaire importante du FUDR administré en continu et qui gêne le traitement. Il est probable que la dose et le rythme d'administration du FUDR joue un rôle et actuellement il semble plus prudent de commencer le traitement à la dose de 0,2 mg/kg/jour. Il est également important de surveiller très étroitement la fonction hépatique car l'interuption précoce de la CIAH et sa reprise à dose très diminuée après retour à la normale des transaminases est l'attitude qui semble le mieux éviter l'apparition d'une cholangite sclérosante.

Sur le plan du coût, malgré le coût élevé des pompes implantables, du fait de la réduction de moitié du nombre des visites à l'hôpital, celui-ci est identique pour les 2 techniques dès lors que la CIAH dure un an ou plus.

CONCLUSION

Quelle que soit la technique, la chimiothérapie intra-artérielle hépatique permet d'obtenir, dans les métastases de cancers colo-rectaux, une régression tumorale objective dans 50 % des cas environ, surtout si les métastases sont bien perfusées par voie artérielle. Son efficacité est limitée par l'apparition de métastases extra-hépatiques et les complications locales. Les études randomisées sont indispensables pour déterminer clairement son avantage en terme de survie et ses indications.

BIBLIOGRAPHIE

BALCH, C.M. ; CRIST, M.M. ; SOONG, S.J. :
A prospective phase II clinical trial of continuous FUDR regional chemotherapy for colorectal metastases to the liver using a totally implantation dru infusion pump.
Ann. Surgo 198: 567-573 (1983).

KEMENY, N. ; DALY, J. ; REICHMAN, B. ; GELLER, N. ; BOTET, J. ; ODERMAN, P. :
Intrahepatic or systemic infusion of lurorodeoxyuridine in patients with liver memtastases from colorectal carcinoma. A randomized trial.
Ann. Int. Med. 107: 459-465 (1987).

MOERTEL, C.G. :
Chemotherapy of gastrointestinal cancer.
N. Engl. J. Med. 299: 1049-1052 (1978).

NIEDERHUBER, J.E. ; ENSLUBGER, W. ; GYVES, J. :
Regional chemotherapy of colorectal cancer metastasis to the liver.
Cancer 53: 1336-1343 (1984).

ROUGIER, Ph. :
Chimiothérapie intra-artérielle hépatique des métastases isolées des adénocarcinomes colo-rectaux.
Gastroenterol. Clin. Biol. 10: 120-122 (1986).

Résumé

IAHC in non resectable LMCR is an active treatment in terms of response rate. In order to determine whether the modalities and drugs influence the clinical results of IAHC we retrospectively compared our results according to two different techniques : discontinuous (DIAHC) and continuous IAHC (CIAHC). A total of 59 pts were treated : - DIAHC was administered to 42 pts with an 8-hour weekly perfusion of 5FU (1 g/m2) via an arterial subcutaneous access. - CIAHC was administered to 16 pts with a 14-day infusion of FUDR every 28 d. (0.3 mg/kg/d) by an implantable pump (INFUSAID 400). Liver involvement was similar in the two groups. The results were similar for DIAHC and CIAHC in terms of response rate : 52 % vs 53 %, for median survival : 14 months vs 18 months, and for overall survival : one year survival (79 ± 12 %). We must underline that survival was better for pts with well vascularized metastasis ($P < 0.02$). Toxicity and tolerance were different : 1) For pts with DIAHC arterial thrombosis was observed in 66 %, 19 % had leucopeny grade II ; 12 % gastrointestinal toxicity, and only one pt (2 %) hepatic toxicity. 2) With CIAHC chemical hepatitis was observed in 50 % of pts, biliary sclerosis in 25 % and gastroduodenitis in 50 %. Patient comfort was better with the implanted pump which requires fewer hospital visits. However the initial cost was more expensive.
Conclusion : IAHC is efficient whatever the technique employed and better in well vascularized metastases. A randomized trial is currently in progress to demonstrate its efficiency on survival.

Locoregional therapy II

Traitements locorégionaux II

Neo-Adjuvant Chemotherapy. Ed. Cl. Jacquillat, M. Weil, D. Khayat. Colloque INSERM/John Libbey Eurotext Ltd. © 1988. Vol. 169, pp. 741-745.

The possible role of adjuvant hepatic artery 5-fluorouracil and hepatic radiation in the management of pancreatic carcinoma

A.L. Wiley Jr., G.W. Wirtanen, M.P. Mehta and G. Ramirez*

*Sections of Radiation Oncology and Medical Oncology, *Department of Human Oncology, University of Wisconsin Medical School, Madison, Wisconsin, USA*

ABSTRACT

Since subclinical hepatic metastases are frequently present at time of diagnosis of pancreatic carcinoma, any meaningful effort to improve survival must include "effective prophylactic" liver therapy, in addition to concurrent "effective" treatment of the pancreatic primary. We report the results of a prospective, unrandomized clinical trial of a two week liver and pancreas infusion (by hepatic artery) of 5-Fluorouracil (5-FU) and pancreatic irradiation to 50-60 Gy, combined with prophylactic irradiation of the liver with approximately 20 Gy. Of 21 evaluable patients, 17 completed therapy without excessive toxicity and had a median survival of 50 weeks. Contrary to historical controls, the liver in our series was not a common first site of failure, suggesting that the combination of hepatic artery 5-Fluorouracil and 20 Gy liver radiation may suppress subclinical (microscopic) liver metastases without significant hepatotoxicity. Recurrent tumor in the pancreatic bed, however, remained a common site of failure. Future clinical investigation of this form of combined therapy as an attempt to eradicate micro-metastasis in the liver (combined with more aggressive local pancreatic therapy) seems appropriate.

KEY WORDS: Pancreatic carcinoma; subclinical liver metastases; hepatic artery 5-FU.

INTRODUCTION

Cancer of the pancreas first described by Bigsby (1835)[3] remains one of the most lethal of all malignancies with more than a 99% fatality rate.[4]

The incidence of pancreatic cancer in the United States is increasing, the rate of which is second only to lung cancer. The more than 25,000 cases recorded in 1985 represent the second most common gastrointestinal tumor, the seventh most common malignancy and the fifth most common cause of cancer death.[1]

Only 8% of lesions are localized sufficiently to permit radical resection[14] and the five year survival of these patients is less than 4%.[21] For the unresectable lesions, median survival without treatment is 3-4 months.[17] Early nonsurgical approaches included both external beam irradiation as well as implantation techniques,[6,10] but results were poor due to the low doses (35-40 Gy) and, as we have previously reported, inadequate tumor localization procedures has caused frequent "geographic miss".[22]

More recent reports employing more than 40 Gy photon dose, fast neutrons, and intra-operative radiation[20] have resulted in a doubling of the median survival to 6-8 months.[8,7] Higher doses of 160-200 Gy with interstitial implants[11] into the pancreatic tumor bed unfortunately have not improved survival. Liver and other locoregional failures too frequently are the cause of death even with local control of the primary pancreatic mass. Single agent chemotherapy has resulted in a 6-27% objective response rate and multi-agent chemotherapy in 13-43%[11,5] but the median survival is only 4-6 months. Combined intravenous 5-FU and radiation therapy[18,19,13] to the pancreatic bed gives only minimally improved survival. These studies clearly indicate that surgery and/or high dose radiation therapy to the pancreatic bed alone does not significantly improve survival, and some effective form of prophylactic treatment of subclinical liver metastases is necessary. Achieving an "effective" therapy for eradicating subclinical liver metastases is not a trivial problem as the 50 Gy/5 weeks of whole liver radiation alone required for 90% control of subclinical disease is not possible, since this whole liver radiation dose produces lethal radiation hepatitis.[9,12] Our previous extensive experience with both hepatic artery 5-FU and liver radiation prompted us to design a protocol to combine hepatic artery 5-FU and x-ray therapy as a therapy which would not damage the liver and yet offer some hope of controlling the almost certain hepatic micro-metastases.

In summary, we designed and carried out this study to address the challenge of obtaining both local pancreatic cancer control and control of subclinical hepatic metastasis, with a combination of hepatic artery 5-FU and radiation to the liver and pancreas.

SUBJECTS AND METHODS

Therapy

This pilot study was designed to evaluate the toxicity and effectiveness of combined radiation therapy and hepatic artery 5-FU infusion for biopsy-proven, unresectable, adenocarcinoma of the pancreas.

Exclusion criteria included tumor extending beyond a 20x20 cm radiation field, distant metastases, including hepatic angiographic evidence of metastases, ascites and previous chemotherapy or radiotherapy as well as ECOG performance status less than 3. Regional node involvement was not considered as distant. Informed consent was required of all patients.

The majority of patients underwent exploratory laparotomy and some form of surgical by-pass. Tumor debulking was not attempted in any patient. Metastatic work-up including chest x-ray, liver scans and/or liver functions, CEA, selective hepatic arteriography, and CT scans, generally including intra-arterially contrast enhanced computerized tomography, as well as ultrasound evaluation in some patients. We evaluated and staged[22,23,24,25,2] the liver for gross metastases from pancreatic cancer, by the sensitivity of hepatic angiography and often intra-arterially contrast enhanced computerized tomographic scanning, prior to the initiation of therapy - so that the question of possible suppression of subclinical hepatic disease by this therapy could be evaluated.

The treatment regimen consisted of a two-week continuous selective hepatic artery infusion of 5-FU (15 mg/kg/day), utilizing the percutaneous transbrachial artery technique of catheter insertion and placement.[24,25] Common hepatic artery infusion, proximal to the gastroduodenal artery was used for tumor arising in the head of the pancreas, while splenic artery and proper or common hepatic artery catheters may be used for tumor in the body or tail.

Angiography and fluoroscopy with the injection of radio-opaque contrast assured that the 5-FU infusion was directed to the liver and pancreas. For quality control and to insure precision delivery of the 5-FU infusion, the infusion catheter position was checked fluoroscopically at least twice a week. These studies also gave us useful appreciation of tumor boundaries for radiation portal definition. Our development and use of percutaneously placed transbrachial artery catheters, we believe, is an important improvement in the quality control of continuous intra-arterial delivered chemotherapy - and is preferred over the surgical placement - since it allows for outpatient catheterization and importantly for relatively simple readjustment of the catheter should catheter position change during the 2-week infusion period (such readjustment is not possible with surgically placed catheters).

Two weeks following the completion of infusion, patients were re-evaluated for disease progression, and radiotherapy was initiated. This consisted of a maximum dose of 20 Gy (1.5 Gy/fractions) to the liver, pancreas and parapancreatic and celiac nodes, using 10 MV photons. Opposed anterior and posterior fields were generally used. After a further two-week break and repeat CT evaluation for disease progression, the entire pancreas was treated (1.7 Gy/fraction) to a total dose of approximately 40 Gy. Rotational and/or lateral tumor boost fields then brought the total dose to the gross tumor-bearing region to 50-60 Gy. Either 10 MV or 4 MV x-rays or Cobalt-60 were used for the boost fields.

Six weeks following completion of radiation therapy, repeat liver scans were generally obtained and patients without evidence of progression were often given systemic 5-FU at 15 mg/kg/wk. Patients were followed until death with serial liver scans, abdominal CT scans, ultrasound, chest x-rays, serum chemistry, CBC and CEA levels as indicated.

Patients

A total of 27 patients were entered on the protocol.

Abdominal and/or back pain, weight loss and jaundice were the most common symptoms, present in about two-thirds of patients. An abdominal mass was very uncommon, present in only three patients.

The American Joint Committee on Cancer (AJCC) staging system was employed. Five patients had T_1 disease while twenty-one were T_3. One patient was not laparotomized and hence staging data is not available. Fourteen patients had positive regional lymph nodes and twelve were N_0. Tumor grade was inadequately defined in eight patients. (One patient was diagnosed by needle biopsy and the grade was therefore not available.)

Tumor location analysis revealed that the head was involved in the vast majority of patients (88%) while the tail was the most infrequently involved region (12%). The body was involved in 24% of patients.

RESULTS

Survival

Six of the 27 patients should not have been entered on the protocol - 2 because of problems with the histologic diagnosis, i.e., one had no histologic diagnosis of cancer and one had a diagnosis of adenocarcinoma of the stomach. There were also four who, on retrospective review, had distant metastases prior to commencing therapy. For these reasons we report the survival of all the 27 patients entered, as well as that of the 21 who were actually eligible for the protocol. The median survival of the total 27 patients entered on the protocol was 29 weeks; but the overall survival curve of the 21 patients who were eligible for the protocol was 40 weeks. Of these 21 patients, four were unable to complete the first phase of their treatment (3 out of 4 completed the initial infusion, but received only a small fraction of the planned radiation). The median survival for the 17 patients who completed the initial intra-arterial 5-FU and the radiation therapy was 50 weeks.

Toxicity

One patient developed multiple subdiaphragmatic and intrahepatic abscesses secondary to his primary surgery and died as a result of this. Another patient developed large bowel obstruction approximately nine months after completion of therapy and at surgery was found to be free of tumor, but had much fibrosis around the inferior mesenteric artery, and devitalized large bowel was responsible for the patient's demise.

One patient required embolectomy from a catheter-related embolus.

5-FU-related GI toxicity occured in 5 patients. One required celiac nerve block for pain and another developed a severe chronic gastric ulcer, requiring surgery. 5-Fluorouracil-related transient neutropenia resulted in discontinuation or interruption of chemotherapy occured in 3 patients.

Two patients experienced myelosuppression requiring interruption of therapy while undergoing radiation therapy.

Failure Patterns

The 17 patients who completed radiation therapy were analyzed for failure patterns. The local tumor bed was the first site of failure in 12 patients (70%). As far as we can determine the liver was the first site of failure in only one patient. Two patients presented with metastatic supraclavicular nodes as the first clinical site of failure. One patient died of pneumonia unrelated to therapy and another from fibrosis of the inferior mesenteric artery.

The mean time to disease progression in this subgroup of 17 patients who completed therapy was 41 weeks. The mean time to death following disease progression was 13 weeks.

REFERENCES

American Cancer Society (1985): Cancer Facts and Figures.

Bell, E.T. (1957): Carcinoma of the pancreas, I. A clinical and pathological study of 609 necropsied cases. Am. J. Path. 33(3), 449-523.

Bigsby, J. (1835): Observations, pathological and therapeutic, on diseases of the pancreas. Edinb. Med. Surg. J. 44, 85-102.

Buncher, C. (1980): Epidemiology of pancreatic cancer. In: Tumors of the Pancreas, ed. A. Moosa, pp 415-427, Baltimore: Williams and Wilkins.

Carter, S. (1975): The integration of chemotherapy into a combined modality approach for cancer treatment. VI. Pancreatic adenocarcinoma. Cancer Treat. Rev. 2, 193-214.

Cavanaugh, P., Haslam, J. (1973): Radiation therapy in the treatment of irresectable adenocarcinoma of the pancreas. Cancer 32, 1341-1345.

Cohen, L., Woodruff, K., Hendrickson, F., et al (1985): Response of pancreatic cancer to local irradiation with high energy neutrons. Cancer 56, 1235-1241.

Dobelbower, R. (1979): The radiotherapy of pancreatic cancer. Semin Oncol. 6, 378-389.

Fletcher, G.H. (1980): Textbook of Radiotherapy, 3rd edn, pp 192-196, Philadelphia: Lea & Febiger.

Handley, W. (1934): Pancreatic cancer and its treatment by implanted radium. Ann.

Surg. 100, 215-223.

Hilaris, B., Henschke, U., Holt, J. (1968): Clinical experience with long half-life and low energy encapsulated sources in cancer radiation therapy. Radiology 91, 1163-1167.

Ingold, J.A., Reed, G.B., Kaplan, H.S., et al (1965): Radiation hepatitis. Am. J. Roentgenol. 93, 200-208.

Klassen, D., MacIntyre, J., Catton, G., et al (1985): Treatment of locally unresectable cancer of the stomach and pancreas: A randomized comparison of 5-fluorouracil alone with radiation plus concurrent and maintenance 5-fluorouracil - An Eastern Cooperative Oncology Group Study. J. Clin. Oncol. 3, 373-378.

Mange, J., Gage, R. (1964): Radical pancreato-duodenectomy: 22 years experience with the complications, morbidity rate and survival rate. Ann. Surg. 160, 711-722.

Mikhailichenko, V.A. (1977): On pancreatic cancer spread in the adjacent organs. Vopr. Onkol. 23(1), 32-36 (Translation).

Mohiuddin, M., Cantor, R.J., et al (1988): Combined modality treatment of localized unresectable adenocarcinoma of the pancreas. Int. J. Radiat. Oncol. Biol. Phys. 14, 79-84.

Moertel, C., Reitemeier, R. (1969): Advanced Gastrointestinal Cancer, Clinical Management and Chemotherapy, p 218, New York: Harper and Row.

Moertel, C. (1976): Chemotherapy of gastrointestinal cancer. Clin. Gastroenterol. 5, 777-793.

Moertel, C., Childs, D., Reitmeir, R., et al (1968): Combined 5-FU and supervoltage radiation therapy of locally unresectable gastrointestinal cancer. Lancet 3, 865-867.

Nishimura, A., Nakano, M., Otsu, H., et al (1984): Intraoperative radiotherapy for advanced carcinoma of the pancreas. Cancer 54, 2375-2384.

Tepper, J., Mardi, G., Suit, H. (1976): Carcinoma of the pancreas: Review of MGH experience from 1963 to 1973. Cancer 37, 1519-1524.

Wiley, A.L., Wirtanen, G.W. (1977): Radiotherapy of carcinoma of the pancreas - Does the local control probability relate to "geographic miss" and suboptimal effective dose to tumor volume? XIV International Congress of Radiology, Rio de Janeiro, Brazil, Book of Abstracts.

Wiley, A.L., Jr., Wirtanen, G.W. (1981): The role of computerized tomography in staging and radiotherapy treatment planning for gastrointestinal malignancies. Brit. J. Radiol. Suppl. 15, 44-47.

Wiley, A.L., Jr., Wirtanen, G.W., Chien, I.C. (1983): Utilization of special computerized tomography and nuclear medicine techniques for quality control and for optimization of combined precision chemotherapy and precision radiation therapy. In: Diagnostic Imaging in Medicine, ed. E. Reba, pp 574-589, NATO-ASI Series, Martinus Nijhoff Publishers.

Wiley, A., Wirtanen, G., Holden, J., et al (1977): Utilization of a selective tumor artery catheterization technique for the intra-arterial delivery of chemotherapeutic agents and radiopharmaceuticals in a combined chemotherapy-radiotherapy clinical research program. In: Radiobiological Research and Radiotherapy, pp 389-412, Vienna: IAEA Pub. No. ISBN 92-0-010377-4, Vol. 1.

Wiley, A.L., Jr., Wirtanen, G.W., et al (1981): Preliminary results on the treatment of unresectable pancreatic carcinoma with a combination of precision chemotherapy and precision radiotherapy. In: New Directions in Therapy, pp 97-106, New York: Masson Publ. Co.

Neo-Adjuvant Chemotherapy. Ed. Cl. Jacquillat, M. Weil, D. Khayat. Colloque INSERM/John Libbey Eurotext Ltd. © 1988. Vol. 169, pp. 747-751.

Exclusive or combined intra-arterial treatment of hepatic metastasis using fluoro-uracile, adriamycin and mitomycin C (FAM) chemotherapeutic regimen

D. Khayat, A. Le Cesne, M. Weil, N. Azar, V. Cour, C. Vu Thi Myle, G. Auclerc, L. Thill, X. Vallantin and Cl. Jacquillat

SOMPS, Hôpital de la Salpêtrière, 47 boulevard de l'Hôpital, 75013 Paris, France

Since 1983, 34 evaluable patients (pts) were treated using exclusive intra-arterial (IA) or combinet IA and intra-veinous (IV) chemotherapy for hepatic metastases. Metastasis were from breast, colorectal, lung cancer (33 cases) or from unknown origin (1 case). Pts aged from 24 to 77 years (mean : 55), received the FAM protocol including IA Fluoro.uracil (1gr/sqm/day for 3 days) with Adriamycin (40 mg/sqm, day 1) and Mitomycin (10 mg/sqm, day 1) administrated either by IA (12 pts) or by simultaneous IV route (22 pts).

The intra-arterial access consisted in a percutaneous radiologically placed catheter in most of the cases, in a surgically implanted port or in a combination or both (2 to 3 cycles using a percutaneous catheter followed by a surgically implanted port). A total of 170 cycles were evaluable. Toxicity was very mild : 8 leukepenia, 3 thrombocytopenia, 1 liver enzymes raise and 11 cases of local pain. Amont the 34 pts, 4 complete and 10 partial responses were observed (36 %) with a median response duration of 9 months and a median actuarial survival of 18 months. The exclusive IA or combined IA and IV infusion of FAM chemotherapy seems to be an effective and safe therapeutic approach of hepatic metastasis.

Mots clés / key words :
Chimiothérapie loco-régionale, intra-artérielle, métastases hépatiques.

Loco-regional chemotherapy, intra-arterial, hepatic metastases.

Hepatic involvement represents a frequent aspect of the metastatic process of cancer with a frequency as high as 70 % in case in intra-abdominal primary tumors (1).

Median survival, from the time of hepatic metastases occurrence, is usually very short, ranging from 2 to 6 months, because of their rare operability and their lack of chemosensitivity using intra-veinous anti-cancer drugs.

However, this chemo-resistance seems to be more relative than absolute (2) and can be, at least in *in vitro* models, circumvinted by the increase of drug concentration in the tumor blood supply. Both, this increase in the hepatic tumors drug exposure and the decrease of systemic drug concentration due to the hepatic extraction define the pharmacokinetic advantage of hepatic intra-arterial chemotherapy (3).

We therefore started in 1983 a prospective trial aimed at studying the feasability and the efficacy of a 3 drugs combination regimen (Fluoro-Uracil, Adriamycin and Mitomycin C) in the intra-arterial or combined intra-arterial and intra-veinous treatment of hepatic metastasis.

MATERIAL & METHODS

Thirty nine consecutive patients carrying hepatic metastasis 24 females (62 %) and 15 men (38 %), aged from 24 to 77 years (mean : 55 years), have been prospectively included in the study from 1983 till 1985.

Hepatic metastases were from breast cancer (22 cases : 56 %), colorectal cancer (15 cases : 38 %), lung cancer (1 case : 3 %) or from unknown primary tumor (1 case : 3 %). Nine of these patients (23 %) had synchronous hepatic metastases (8 colorectal and 1 breast) and and 31 (77 %) had metachronous (mean time between primary and metastatic tumors : 19 months) hepatic metastases.

Three patients (8 %) had simultaneous extra-hepatic metastasis (2 lung, 1 spleen) at the time of their entry in the present study.
The extend of the liver involvement was as followed : 26 patients had a greater than 50 % involvement (67 %), 9 had a limited involvement with 2 to 3 nodules (23 %) and 4 patients (10 %) had a single hepatic metastasis that was considered as non operable.

These patients were treated using the FAM chemotherapeutic regimen including 5.Fluoro-Uracil (1gr/sqm/day, continuous infusion from day 1 to day 3), Adriamycin (40 mg/sqm, day 1) and Mitomycin C (10 mg/ sqm, day 1) repeated every 3 to 4 weeks according to hematologic status.
Concerning chemotherapy, two distinct periods can be distinguished in the study : during the first period, the 3 drugs were infused directly into the hepatic artery (12 patients : 31 %). However, because of the high extra-hepatic progression rate, we then started to combined intra-arterial (5 FU) and simultaneous intra-veinous (Adriamycin and Mitomycin C) routes of infusion (27 patients : 69 %).

Two methods were used for hepatic artery infusion : 36 pts had a percutaneous (Seldinger) placement of their catheter which was then withdrawn after each cycle and 26 pts had a surgical implantation of an intra-arterial port connected to a subcutaneous access chamber either at entry (3 pts) or after 2 to 3 cycles using Seldinger technic (23 pts).

A total of 170 cycles were performed : 116 using Seldinger technic and 54 using a surgically implanted arterial port.

RESULTS

Among the 39 pts included in the study, 34 pts were evaluable for response. Five pts were considered non evaluable (13 %) beacause of early death (before the 3rd week (1pt), lost of follow-up (2 pts) or protocol violation (2 pts)).

Four complete responses (RC = 10 %) and 10 partial responses (PR = 26 %), as considered on CT-scans with a parallele decrease in blood tumor marquers when initially elevated, were observed (36 %). The overall response rate was higher in hepatic metastases from breast origin (4 CR and 6 PR = 56 %) than in hepatic metastases from colorectal origin (3 PR = 21 %)(Table I).

TABLE I

Primary Tumor	CR	PR	MR	ST	PD
Colorectal (14 pts)	-	3	4	3	4
Breast (18 pts)	4	6	2	2	4
Lung (1 pt)	4	6	2	2	4
Unknown (1 pt)	-	1	-	-	-
TOTAL (34 pts)	4 (12 %)	10 (29 %)	7 (21 %)	5 (15 %)	8 (24 %)

The median duration of response, calculated from the time of entry into the study till disease progression was 9 months with a median actuarial survival of 18 months.

As mentioned, the outcome of patients treated using a unique intra-arterial route (12 pts) or using a combined simultaneous intra-arterial and intra-veineous infusion (22 pts) was totaly different. Patients treated using only intra-arterial chemotherapy had a higher response rate (50 % : 1 CR and 5 PR) when compared with the results obtained in the combined IA/IV chemotherapeutic group (33 % : 3 CR and 5 PR) but had also a higher extra-hepatic pregression rate : 4 extra-hepatic progression (66 %) among the 6 responders in the IA group compared to no extra-hepatic progression among the 8 responders of the IA/IV combined group.

Hematologic toxicity was very mild with 8 leucopenia (1 grade III : 1 % and 7 grade II : 4 %) and 3 thrombocytopenia (3 grade II : 2 %). A significant increased in serum liver enzymes was only observed in 1 case (1 %) but abdominal pain or hepatalgia were relatively frequent occuring in 11 pts (6 %).

A high rate of accidents was observed in the group of patient (36 pts) receiving chemotherapy through a percutaneous placed catheter. Indeed, among the 116 cycles of chemotherapy given in that group, 28 accidents occured. There was 9 technical failures to selectively catheterise the hepatic artery, 6 sub-acute ischemias of the upper limb, 1 compressive axillary hematoma, 3 hepatic artery dissections, 3 prolonged arterial spasms, 1 right hemiparesia related to a cerebral emboly, and 5 hepatic artery narrowring occuring after the second or the third catheterism. At opposite, only one accident (infection) was observed when surgically implanted ports were used. However, these ports were thrombosed in 10 cases with a mean duration time of 6 months.

DISCUSSION

We report here the result of hepatic intra-arterial (IA) alone or combinet with intra-veinous (IV) chemotherapy in the treatment of hepatic metastases. Thirty four evaluable patients were treated by a combination of IA Fluoro.5.Uracil and Adriamycin and Mitomycin C which were administrad either by IA route (12 pts) or by simultaneous IV route (24 pts). The shift between exclusive IA treatment (group I) and combined IA and IV (group II) treatments was aimed at preventing the high extra-hepatic metastasis progression rate which was initially observed in group I. Indeed, although the response rate on hepatic metastases appeared slightly higher when the 3 drugs were infused directely in the hepatic artery (6 pts/12 = 50 %), this was associated with a concommittent high frequency of disease progression on extra-hepatic metastases (4 extra-hepatic progression amoung the 6 responders). As expected, the use of the combined IA/IV routes lead us to a better control of the extra-hepatic component of the metastatic process (8 hepatic responders (33 %) without any extra-hepatic progression).

Systemic or hepatic toxicity was very mild and no toxic related death is reported; however, a very high vascular accidents frequency were noted when chemotherapy was given through a percutaneous radiologically (Seldinger) placed catheter (26 accidents among 116 cycles : 24 %). At opposite, no major toxicity was reported with the use of surgically implanted ports. However, surgically implanted ports were related to a high frequency (38 %) of vascular or catheter thrombosis which occured after a mean time of 6 months. More recently, the use of low dose aspirin seems to be able to better prevent such artery and/or catheter thrombosis.

The large spread of implanted ports the lack of local toxicity, the improvement in the systemic tolerance, and the high response rate with a prolonged control of hepatic metastases seem to indicate that intra-arterial or combined intra-veinous and intraarterial chemotherapy is an effective and safe therapeutic approach of hepatic metastases.

REFERENCES

1 - Cancer Facts and Figures. (1982) New York American Cancer Society, 8.
2 - Link K.H. and Beger H.G.(1988) : Chemosensitivity of solid tumors at high drug concentrations. Proceeding of 2nd International Congress on Neo-Adjuvant Chemotherapy, John Libbey Ed. London.
3 - Chen H.S.G. and Gross J.F. (1980) : Intraarterial infusion of anticancer drugs. Theoretic aspects of drug delivery and review of responser. Cancer Treat. Rep., 64, 31-40.

Acknowledgment :

We are gratefull to Miss Brigitte Cédreau for her help. This work was supported by a Grant from the Centre de Recherches Appliquées à la Chimiothérapie (C.R.A.C.) - Paris, and from the Comité de Paris de la Ligue Nationale Française Contre le Cancer.

Résumé

Au cours des trois dernières années, 34 patients évaluables ont été traités pour métastases hépatiques par administration par voie intra-artérielle (IA) d'une polychimiothérapie associant 5.FU 1gr/m2/jour pendant 3 jours, Adriamycine (ADR) 40 mg/m2/J1, et Mitomycine C (MMC) 10 mg/m2/J1. Parmi ces patients 12 ont reçu la totalité des trois drogues par voie IA et 20 l'ont reçue simultanément par voir IA (5FU) et IV (ADR-MMC). Ces pts âgés de 24 et 77 ans (médiane : 55 ans) présentaient des métastases hépatiques d'origine mammaire, colique, pulmonaire ou inconnue. Sur le plan thérapeutique, cette chimiothérapie IA a été administrée par l'intermédiaire d'un cathéter artériel hépatique par voie transcutanée dans la majorité des cas, par la pose d'emblée d'un cathéter totalement implanté avec chambre d'accès sous-cutanée ou par conjonction de deux thérapeutiques dans certains cas (pose d'un réservoir après 2 ou 3 cures de chimiothérapie par voie per-cutanée). Au total 170 cures de protocole FAM ont été analysées. Sur 34 pts évaluables sur le plan de la réponse tumorale, nous avons observé sur notre série, 10 réponses partielles supérieures à 50 %, et 4 réponses complètes soit un total de 36 %. Le taux de réponse varie peu en fonction de l'origine de la tumeur. La médiane de réponse est de 9 mois après le début de l'IA hépatique. La tolérance hématologique a été satisfaisante ($\lesssim$ 10% grade IV). Aucune toxicité hépatique ou autre n'a été observée. Seul l'abord transcutané (radiologique) a entrainé un certain nombre de complications locales. Au total, ce protocole de chimiothérapie combinée IA/IV associant 5FU-ADR-MMC semble très intéressant au plan de la tolérance ($\lesssim$ 10% de toxicité hématologique grave) et de l'efficacité thérapeutique (41% de réponse ; médiane =9 mois).

Neo-Adjuvant Chemotherapy. Ed. Cl. Jacquillat, M. Weil, D. Khayat. Colloque INSERM/John Libbey Eurotext Ltd. © 1988. Vol. 169, pp. 753-760.

Pre-operative regional chemotherapy in management of gastric cancer. 5-year survival results

F.O. Stephens

Department of Surgery, University of Sydney, Sydney, Australia

Gastric cancer has been amongst the more common internal neoplasms affecting mankind. Although decreasing in incidence in Europe, North America and Australasia it is still amongst the 10 most common causes of cancer death in both sexes (1).

At the time of diagnosis approximately 40% of patients are considered incurable by surgical resection and of the remainder treated by gastrectomy with some prospect of cure 5-year survival has been in the order of 15% (2-7).

The situation is quite different in Japan where gastric cancer in males is the most common internal cancer. There mass screening and routine more intensive diagnostic techniques have allowed a high incidence of detection of the disease in its early stages. This together with extended radical surgical resection has resulted in much improved 5-year survival statistics.

Encouraging results of the use of "neo-adjuvant" chemotherapy given regionally by intra-arterial infusion prior to subsequent standard treatment with radiotherapy and/or surgical resection in treating advanced localized cancers in head and neck, breast and cancers and sarcomas in limbs provided the stimulus for a pilot study of the use of a similar technique in management of gastric cancer (8).

MATERIALS AND METHODS

Thirty-five successive patients referred to the Sydney Hospital Surgical Oncology Service with a diagnosis of gastric cancer were managed initially with intra-arterial chemotherapy prior to consideration of gastrectomy.

Prior to treatment routine examinations included gastroscopy with biopsy, liver/spleen scans, and CT abdominal examination.

Chemotherapy was given into the coeliac axis after cannulation by a transfemoral approach by the radiologist using a Seldinger catheter. The catheter was securely tied into position by suture in the groin allowing the patient some freedom of movement in the hospital ward.

Correct position of the catheter was confirmed by injection of blue dye (Disulphine Blue or Patent Blue) into the catheter during gastroscopic examination. The catheter position was adjusted if necessary until the blue dye flowed into the gastric mucosa containing the region of the carcinoma. Confirmation of correct catheter position was made at gastroscopy at weekly intervals.

In some patients laparoscopy was also carried out to look for evidence of tumour spread. At laparoscopy blue dye was again injected into the catheter to confirm the flow of dye into the gastric wall surrounding the region of the neoplasm.

The regimen of chemotherapy used was BCNU 150mgm/m^2 (as a once only dose) followed by:

Day 1 - 5FU 500 mgm/m^2

Day 2 - Adriamycin 15mgm/m^2

Day 3 - Mitomycin C 4mgm/m^2

Each drug was given over a 24-hour period in 1 litre of normal saline.

Then two rest days were allowed infusing 1 litre of saline only with a further cycle repeated every 5 days for a total period of 4 to 6 weeks. Treatment was deferred if there was depression of bone marrow (white cell count less than 2,000 or platelet count lessthan 100,000). Treatment was stopped if the patient became severely anorexic or uncomfortable which was usually between 4 to 6 weeks.

Sixteen of the 35 patients presented with advanced cancers considered quite incurable by gastrectomy. In these patients the cancers presented with a fixed mass, or involved the whole stomach, or involved other organs i.e. pancreas or liver. These patients were considered incurable by standard means and were referred to as the "palliative group".

In 19 patients the cancers were all confirmed to be invasive carcinoma but appeared to be confined to the stomach and possible adjacent lymph nodes only with no evidence of involvement of other tissues or viscera. These patients were designated the "potentially curable" group.

After 4 to 6 weeks of intra-arterial chemotherapy the patients were allowed to go home for 3 to 4 weeks before being readmitted for consideration of gastrectomy.

RESULTS

TOXICITY

As is usually the case with regional chemotherapy, regional toxicity was more apparent in most patients than systemic toxicity.

Regional Toxicity

Most patients with gastric pain initially had some pain relief soon after commencing treatment. However, virtually all patients subsequently developed epigastric discomfort, anorexia and in some cases epigastric pain. All patients tolerated treatment for a minimum of 4 weeks but between 4 and 6 weeks severe anorexia and discomfort necessitated cessation of chemotherapy in most patients. Only one patient claimed not to have had any epigastric discomfort or anorexia.

In 3 cases there was some blood stained vomiting which in one patient necessitated urgent gastrectomy. That patient subsequently survived for more than 5 years tumour free.

Systemic Toxicity

Reduced white cell count necessitated deferment of treatment on one or more occasions in 12 patients but in no patient was it necessary to stop chemotherapy due to bone marrow depression.

No patient suffered significant alopecia.

SURVIVAL

The Palliative Group

Although patients in this group who had been referred with abdominal pain usually had some temporary pain relief, in fact there were no cures in this group of patients. The longest survivor was in fact 6 years but 14 of these 16 patients succumbed within a period of 5 to 16 months. In 7 of these patients gastrectomy was not carried out.

The "Potentially Curable" Group

Of the 19 patients in the "potentially curable" group all completed between 4 and 6 weeks chemotherapy and subsequently underwent gastrectomy. Eleven survived for 5 years without evidence of tumour recurrence. One of those 11 patients has subsequently died of other causes.

On gastroscopic examination after completion of chemotherapy in the 19 patients there was apparent complete tumour regression in 4, a partial tumour regression in 11 and no evidence of tumour regression in 4. Following gastrectomy 6 of the 19 patients were found to still contain some metastatic neoplasm in the adjacent lymph nodes, 2 of these 6 patients have subsequently died but the other 4 remain well more than 5 years later.

DISCUSSION

Fortunately in Australia as in other western societies gastric carcinoma has become less common in recent years. However, it remains one of the top 10 causes of cancer death in both sexes.

The standard treatment by gastrectomy has been unsatisfactory as even in those patients designated as having "potentially curable" and resectable carcinoma 5-year survival has been in the order of 15%.

Possibilities of improving upon this poor survival rate have rested with:

a) Cancer prevention.

b) Early detection and early treatment.

c) More radical surgical resection.

d) A new approach in management.

Change in dietary habits and better food storage methods may have played a part in the reduced incidence of gastric cancers in western societies. In Japan early detection of minimal disease has resulted in significantly increased survival results after standard gastrectomy. Some improvement of survival results in Japan may also be due to more radical surgery for more established cancers.

The possibility of improving results by the use of neo-adjuvant chemotherapy delivered on a regional basis was explored after apparently improved survival with similar treatment for other types of neoplasms supplied by a regional artery. The coeliac axis is a single artery which supplies the stomach and surrounding lymph nodes as well as the liver via the hepatic artery and portal vein. The liver could be the site of microscopic metastatic disease so that the flow of agents directly into the liver may well be advantageous possibly eradicating microscopic potential metastatic foci. The chemotherapeutic agents BCNU, 5FU, Adriamycin and Mitomycin C are all known to be effective against gastric cancer so their combination was considered to be appropriate for use in this trial.

The achievement of 63% 5-year survival in successive patients who would otherwise have been considered to have a likelihood of 5-year survival in the order of 15% by gastrectomy alone has been encouraging. This suggests that further trials of neo-adjuvant chemotherapy in treatment of gastric cancer are indicated possibly comparing results of chemotherapy given by intra-arterial infusion as compared to the more simply delivered preoperative systemic administration of the same agents.

REFERENCES

1. Silverberg, E.: Cancer statistics. Ca 1985;35:19-35.

2. Cories, R.L. and Carter, S.K.: A review of chemotherapy in gastric cancer. Cancer 1974;34:1576-1578.

3. Editorial: Management of advanced gastric cancer; a more promising future. Med. J. Aust. 1980;1:402-403.

4. Franz, J.L. and Cruz, A.B.: The treatment of gastric cancer with combined surgical resection and chemotherapy. J. Surg. Oncol. 1977; 9:131-137.

5. Nelson, P.G. and Collier, N.: Carcinoma of the stomach: the need for a new approach. Aust. N.Z. J. Surg. 1982;52:358-362.

6. Sinha, V.N. Shorter, E.A. and Katz, B.: Carcinoma of the stomach in a large community hospital. Am. J. Surg. 1970;119:256-260.

7. Goffin, J.C. and Machin, D.: Treatment of patients with gastric cancer by surgery, radiotherapy and chemotherapy. Recent Results of Cancer Res. 1978;68:208-211.

8. Stephens, F.O.: Clincial experience in the use of intra-arterial infusion chemotherapy in the treatment of cancers in the head and neck, the extremities, the breast and the stomach. Recent Results of Cancer Res. 1983;86:122-127.

Résumé

PRE-OPERATIVE REGIONAL CHEMOTHERAPY IN MANAGEMENT OF GASTRIC CANCER - 5 YEAR SURVIVAL RESULTS

F. Stephens, Dept. Surg., Sydney University, AUSTRALIA

Between 1976 and 1983,35 successive patients referred to the Sydney Hospital surgical oncology service with a diagnosis of gastric cancer were managed initially with intra-arterial chemotherapy given by coeliac axis infusion for a period of 4-6 weeks before consideration of gastrectomy.

In 16 patients (designated the "palliative" group) the cancer was considered to be incurable when referred. There was either total involvement of the stomach, a fixed mass or spread of tumour into pancreas, liver or other adjacent viscera. In none of these patients has cure been achieved.

In 19 patients (designated the "potentially curable" group) the cancer was considered treatable by gastrectomy alone but standard expectation of results would have been in the order of 15% 5 year survival. Following regional chemotherapy in these 19 patients there was an apparent complete tumour regression in 4, a partial tumour regression in 10 and no evidence of significant regression in 5. After chemotherapy all 19 patients in this group then underwent a gastrectomy. Twelve of these 19 patients (63%) survived 5 years with no evidence of residual gastric cancer.

Neo-Adjuvant Chemotherapy. Ed. Cl. Jacquillat, M. Weil, D. Khayat. Colloque INSERM/John Libbey Eurotext Ltd. © 1988. Vol. 169, pp. 761-768.

Supra-selective intra-arterial infusion chemotherapy of breast cancer : BCPLSC protocol and phase I study

P. Michel, A. Hulet, C. Chastel*, J. Bacq, J. Bernier, M.A. Millet, D. Marchal*, J. Lardinois, P.E. Vancutsem and J.C. Legrand***

* *Service de Chirurgie, Hôpital Civil de Charleroi, Belgique*
** *Service de Radiothérapie-Oncologie, Hôpital Civil de Charleroi, Belgique*
*** *Service d'Oncologie Médicale, Hôpital Civil de Charleroi, Belgique*

Following previous qualitative and quantitative studies, in which we demonstrated the interest of a selective intra-arterial route, combined with co-injected starch microspheres, in the therapeutical approach of breast cancer, an experimental protocol was started and called "BREAST CANCER PRIMARY LOCAL-SYSTEMIC CHEMOTHERAPY".
The Phase 1 Study, the aim of which is principally to estimate and control local toxicity, is limited to T3-T4 patients, and is now on course.
The first results seem to evidence a fast and important local response, though vascular toxicity of cytostatic drugs is essential matter. So, ideal regimen, drugs and doses, are to be specified.

INTRODUCTION : (1,2,3,4,7,10,11,12,14,15,16,17,18,19,21)

La notion de perfusion intra-artérielle "supra-sélective" dans le cancer du sein découle de travaux effectués par différents auteurs au cours des 8 dernières années.
En 1980, STEPHENS décrivait 4 cas de stade III et IV, perfusés par voie trans-humérale au niveau de l'artère sous-clavière; KOYAMA, en 1985, et AIGNER, en 1987, firent de même.
STEPHENS (1985) perfectionna sa technique par un abord direct de l'artère mammaire interne; TIMMERMANN (1987) y ajouta celui de l'artère mammaire externe; et SUGITACHI (1986), celui de l'artère scapulaire inférieure, ces voies devant être considérées comme sélectives.

De notre côté, nous réalisons des investigations qualitatives (1985) et quantitatives (1987), relatives à une perfusion du sein par l'artère dite principale interne (API) du sein; ces investigations, complétées par une étude pré-clinique poursuivie encore actuellement, mettaient en évidence un accroissement de la dose tumorale de la drogue injectée, de l'ordre de 16 fois; cet accroissement est dû à l'utilisation conjuguée de cette voie supra-sélective et de microsphères dégradables d'amidon (DSM).
Il faut remarquer que KOYAMA et SUGITACHI avaient eux-mêmes tenté d'augmenter la diffusion locale de la drogue injectée, en utilisant respectivement de l'angiotensine et un procédé de chémo-embolisation.

Dès 1986, nous jugions donc opportun de mettre en application un protocole de phase 1, dans le but principal d'évaluer la pra ticabilité clinique de cette technique; ce protocole mettait en oeuvre un traitement combiné systémique et intra-artériel, et fut baptisé BCPLSC : Breast Cancer Primary Local-Systemic Chemotherapy.

DESCRIPTION :

La sélection des patientes repose principalement sur les 3 critères suivants : âge inférieur à 65 ans, tumeur classée T3, T4 ou PEV, et disposition d'un examen cytologique positif formel.
Sous anesthésie locale, l'API est alors cathétérisée.

Le traitement chimiothérapique local est au départ basé sur le schéma utilisé par STEPHENS (1980), et est constitué de l'association de 4 droques : Fluoro-Uracile, Adriamycine, Vincristine et Metotrexate, utilisées à des doses de 10 ou 20 % des doses systémiques usuelles; la dose de DSM utilisée est de 120 mg (Spherex° 2 ml à 60 mg/ml).
Simultanément, une perfusion intra-veineuse de type FAC est administrée; un maximum de 3 cycles à 3 semaines d'intervalle est prévu, en fonction de la réponse et/ou de la toxicité locale éventuelle.
Ce traitement néo-adjuvant est alors suivi d'une chirurgie et des traitements adjuvants habituels, en fonction du TNM initial et de la réponse clinique.

DONNEES TECHNIQUES : (5,6,8,9,13,22)

La cathétérisation de l'API est précédée d'une artériographie numérisée mammaire interne, de manière à définir l'espace intercostal d'émergence de l'API, qui est ensuite repérée de manière précise par un examen ultra-sonique (Doppler).
Le dispositif de perfusion intra-artérielle utilisé comprend un système Port-A-Cath épidural et une pompe portable à perfusion continue de sérum physiologique; ce dispositif est rincé quotidiennement par 2 ml de sérum hépariné à 2 %.
Avant la mise en route du traitement local, une évaluation isotopique comparative est réalisée, afin de préciser le gain obtenu par rapport à la voie intra-veineuse.
Enfin, l'administration des drogues cytostatiques et des DSM est synchrone, réalisant une chémo-embolisation transitoire.
Les différentes drogues sont injectées successivement à 24 h d'intervalle.

PREMIERS RESULTATS : (20)

Deux patientes, respectivement de stade IV et III, entrèrent dans ce protocole en avril 86; par la suite, et pour des raisons diverses dont surtout l'âge avancé de ces cas de stade évolué, aucune patiente ne s'est révélée éligible.
Toutefois, ces 2 cas n'ont certes pas manqué d'être instructifs à de multiples égards.

En tout premier lieu, la praticabilité de cette perfusion continue intra-artérielle supra-sélective devait être prouvée : elle est en effet réalisable, moyennant un soin et une précision technique comme requis en microchirurgie, de même qu'une maintenance particulièrement attentive; la première patiente a pu ainsi être perfusée durant 7 semaines.
Cette perfusion intra-artérielle ne représente pas un traitement lourd : les doses utilisées sont faibles et déduites des doses systémiques, l'ensemble du dispositif

est peu encombrant et suffisamment fiable pour permettre un traitement ambulatoire.
La toxicité locale semble surtout se manifester au niveau vasculaire, ce qui peut amener une thrombose progressive de l'artère cathétérisée; cette observation nous a conduit à expérimenter, dans le 3ème volet de notre étude pré-clinique, une drogue peu aggressive de ce point de vue : la Mitoxantrone.

Le faible diamètre (0,8 à 1,5 mm) de l'artère cathétérisée ainsi que le caractère très anastomotique du réseau artériel du sein pourrait faire craindre une perfusion assez parcellaire de la glande mammaire; ce serait le cas si la perfusion était réalisée sans microsphères; l'embolisation artériolaire transitoire qu'elles provoquent entraîne en réalité un remplissage de proche en proche de tout le réseau mammaire, débordant même vers les régions voisines, axillaires, sus- et sous-mammaires, déterminant ainsi pratiquement la perfusion d'un hémithorax antérieur.
L'efficacité locale de cette perfusion est probable, mais il est difficile de l'évaluer dans le cadre de ce traitement combiné. Nous avons toutefois assisté à une importante fonte de la masse néoplasique dans les 2 cas, et, par ailleurs, ces 2 patientes sont suivies depuis 22 mois et ne présentent aucun signe de récidive locale; il s'agissait de T4 ulcérés dans les 2 cas; elles ont été mastectomisées, mais n'ont pas reçu de radiothérapie post-opératoire.

Enfin, la disparition de métastases sus-claviculaires homolatérales dans le premier cas laisse espérer une certaine efficacité "régionale" de ce traitement; cette observation est corroborée par la mise en évidence d'une reprise lymphatique de la Mitoxantrone injectée lors de certains tests pré-cliniques (dosages ganglionnaires, coloration de collecteurs lymphatiques).

EVOLUTION :

Nous pensons actuellement que les enseignements exposés ci-dessus, étayés par les résultats très encourageants des derniers tests pré-cliniques quantitatifs, nous permettent de poursuivre l'application d'un protocole du même type, utilisant cette fois la Mitoxantrone en monothérapie intra-artérielle, combinée à un CAF systémique, et ce, dans les cancers du sein inflammatoires ou localement avancés (BCPLSC Phase 2).
D'autre part, un traitement intra-artériel pur néo-adjuvant pourrait être envisagé dans les cas intermédiaires (T2-T3), afin de pouvoir les traiter de manière conservatrice; un tel protocole est actuellement à l'étude et sera dénommé : Breast Cancer Primary Loco-Regional Chemotherapy (BCPLRC Phase 1-2).

BIBLIOGRAPHIE :

1. AIGNER K.R., MULLER H., WALTHER H.
STRAUBE H.
Arterial Infusion of Primary and Metastatic Breast Cancer
ICRCT 87, Ulm/Donau, 1987, 82

2. CALVO D.B., PATT Y.Z., WALLACE S., CHUANG V.P., BENJAMIN R.S., PRITCHARD J.D., HERSCH E.M., BODEY G.P., MAVLIGIT G.M.
Phase 1-2 Trial of Percutaneous Intra-Arterial Cio-Diamminedichloro platinum for Regionally Confined Malignancy
Cancer, 1980, 45, 1278-1283.

3. DAKHIL S., ENSMINGER W.D., KYUNG CHO, NIEDERHUBER J.E., DOAN K., WHEELER R.
Improved regional selectivity of hepatic arterial BCNU with degradable microspheres
Cancer, 1982, 50, 631-635

4. ENSMINGER W.D., GYVES J.W., STETSON P., WALKER S.
Phase 1 Study of hepatic arterial degradable starch microspheres and mitomycin
Cancer Research, 1985, 45, 4464-4467

5. GRISOLI J.
Recherches anatomiques sur les artères de la glande mammaire
Thèse Médicale, Marseille, 1943, 40

6. HAKANSSON L., STARKHAMMER H., MORALES O., SJODHAL R., EKBERGS., SVEDBERG J.
Effect of degradable starch microspheres on the passage of intra-arterially co-injected molecular weight substances through the liver
ICRCT 85, Giessen, 1985, 63

7. KOYAMA H., NISHIZAWA Y., WADA T., KABUTO T., SHIBA E., IWANAGA T., TERASAWA T., WADA A.
Intra-arterial infusion chemotherapy as an induction therapy in multidisciplinary treatment for locally advanced breast cancer
Cancer, 1985, 56, 725-729

8. LALARDRIE J.P., JOUGLARD J.P., MITZ V., CARLIN G.
La vascularisation artérielle du sein
Chirurgie Plastique du Sein, Masson, Paris, 1974, 19-22

9. LEVIN D.C.
Augmented arterial flow and pressure resulting from selective injections through catheters : clinical implications
Radiology, 1978, 127, 1, 103-108

10. MICHEL P., HULET A., CHASTEL C., VERHELST G.
Microvascularisation du sein cancéreux : perspective thérapeutique ?
Acta Chirurgica Belgica, 1985, 85, 374-377

11. MICHEL P., BERNIER J., BACQ J., HULET A., CHASTEL C., VERHELST G.
Perfusion intra-artérielle sélective du sein cancéreux : étude quantitative
Acta Chirurgica Belgica, 1987, 87, 92-95

12. MONTAQUE E.D., GUTIERREZ A.E., BARKER J.L., TAPLEY N.V., FLETCHER G.H.
Conservation surgery and irradiation for the treatment of favourable breast cancer
Cancer, 1979, 43, 1058-1061

13. SALMON M.
Les artères de la glande mammaire
Annales d'anatomie pathologique, 1939, 16, 4, 477-500

14. SHAH P., BAKER L.H., VAITKEVICIUS V.K.
Preliminary experiences with intra-arterial Adriamycin
Cancer treatment reports, 1977, 61, 8, 1565-1567

15. STEPHENS F.O., CREA P., HARKER G.J.S., ROBERTS B.A., HAMBLY C.K.
Intra-arterial chemotherapy as basal treatment in advanced and fungating primary breast cancer
The Lancet, 1980, 2, 435-438

16. STEPHENS F.O.
Clinical experience in the use of intra-arterial infusion chemotherapy
Recent results in cancer research, 1983, 86, 122-127

17. STEPHENS F.O.
The use of intra-arterial chemotherapy in the treatment of locally advanced breast cancer
ICRCT 85, Giessen, 1985, 52-53

18. SUGITACHI A., TAKATSUKA Y.
TACE enhances adriamycin action against breast cancer
Oncology News, Nov-Dec 1986, 3

19. TIMMERMANN J.
Regionale Tumortherapei des Stad.IV eines Mammacarcinoms
ICRCT 87, Ulm/Donau, 1987, 81

20. VAN BELLE S.J.P., DE PLANQUE M.M., SMITH I.E., VAN OOSTEROM A.T., SCHOEMAKER T.J., DENEVE W., McVIE J.G.
Pharmacokinetics of mitoxantrone in humans following single-agent infusion or intra-arterial injection therapy or combined-agent infusion therapy
Cancer chemotherapy and pharmacology, 1986, 18, 27-32

21. VILCOQ J.R., CALLE R., STACEY P., GHOSSEIN N.A.
The outcome of treatment by tumorectomy and radiotherapy of patients with operable breast cancer
International Journal Radiations, Oncology, Biology, Physics, 1981, 7, 1327-1332

22. ZIESSMAN H.A., THRALL J.H., GYVES J.W., ENSMINGER W.D., NIEDERHUBER J.E., TUSCAN M., WALKER S.
Quantitative hepatic arterial perfusion scintigraphy and starch microspheres in cancer chemotherapy
Journal of nuclear medicine, 1983, 24, 871-875

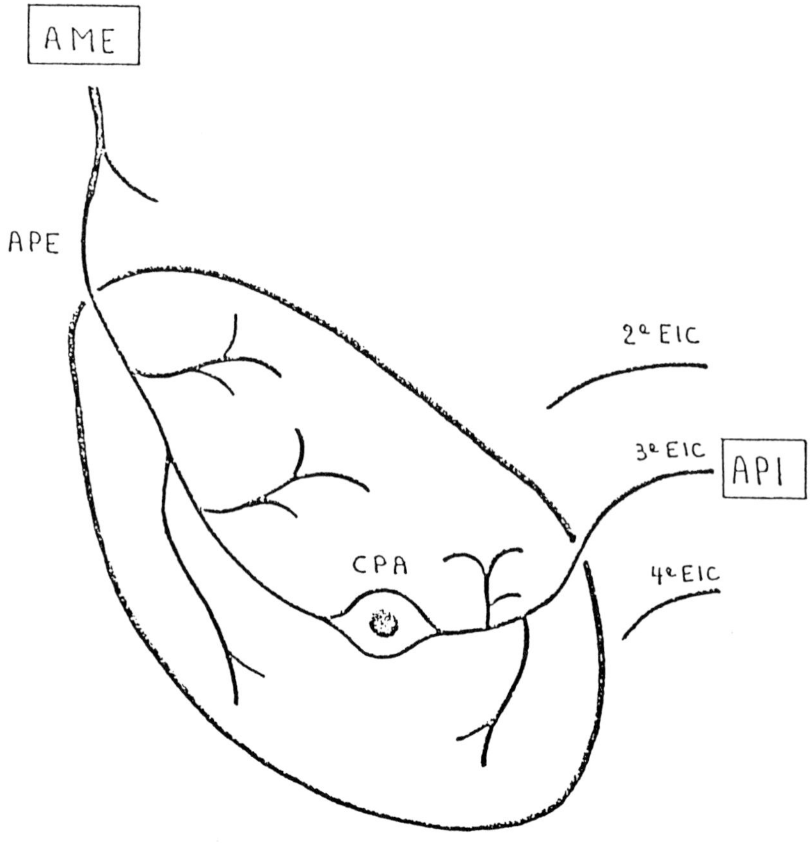

(D'après LALARDRIE)

FIG.1: VASCULARISATION ARTERIELLE DU SEIN

AME = Artère Mammaire Externe
APE = Artère Principale Externe
API = Artère Principale Interne
EIC = Espace Intercostal
CPA = Cercle Péri-Aréolaire

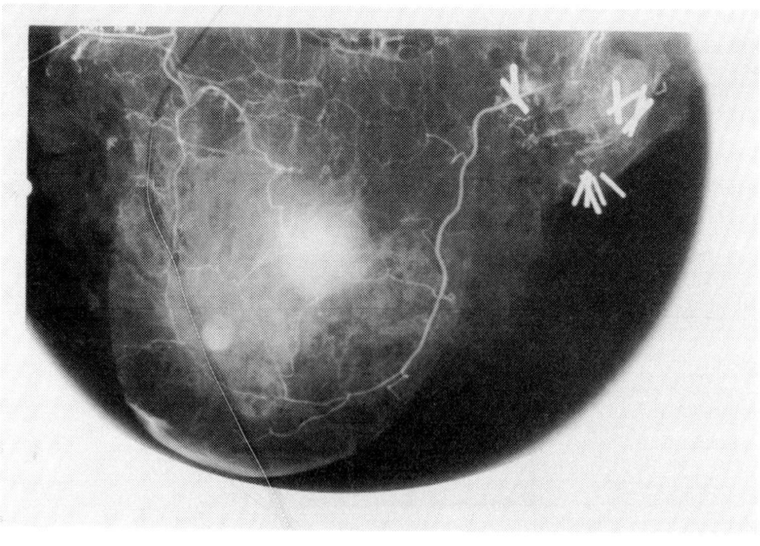

(Fig.2)

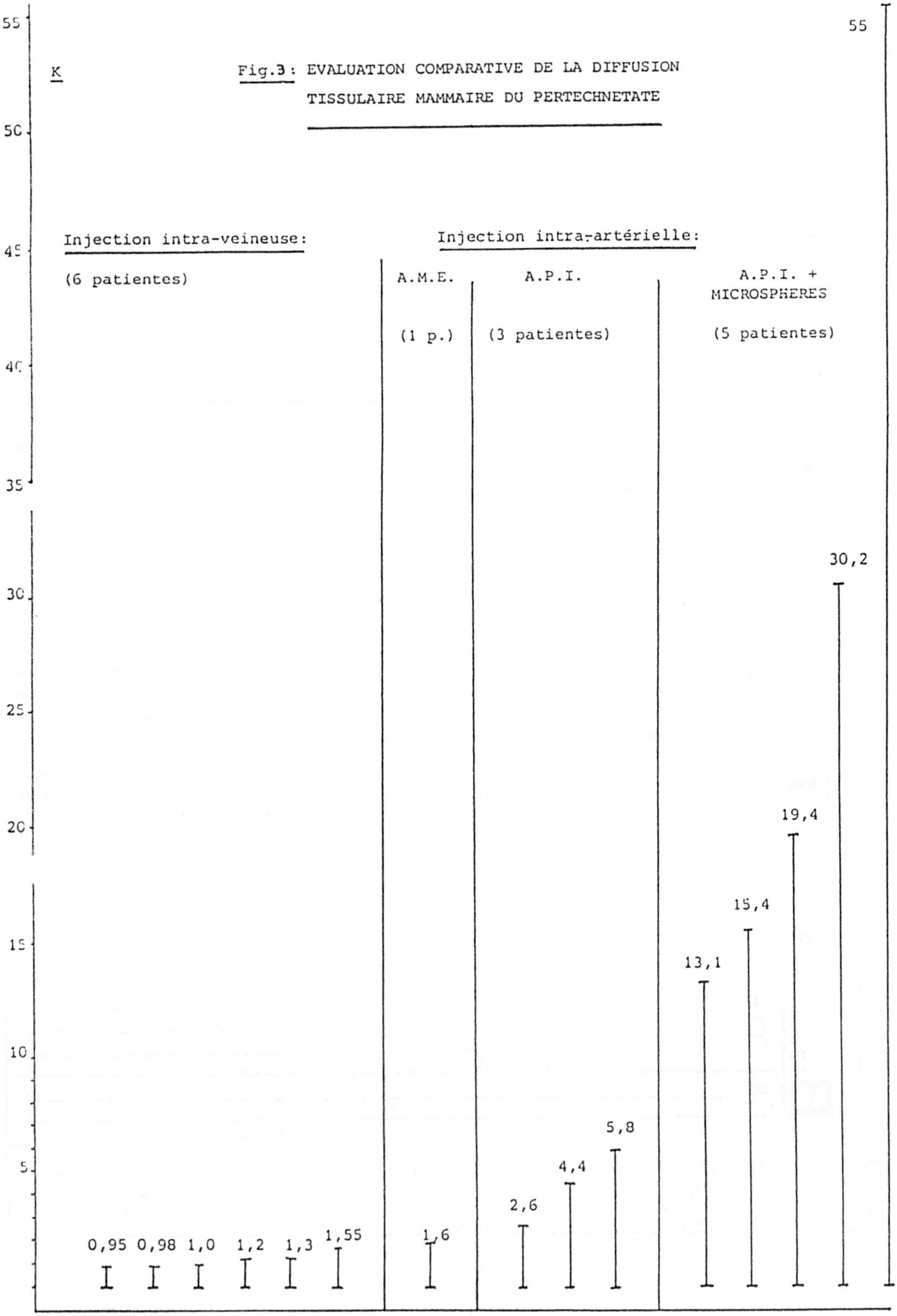

Fig.3 : EVALUATION COMPARATIVE DE LA DIFFUSION TISSULAIRE MAMMAIRE DU PERTECHNETATE

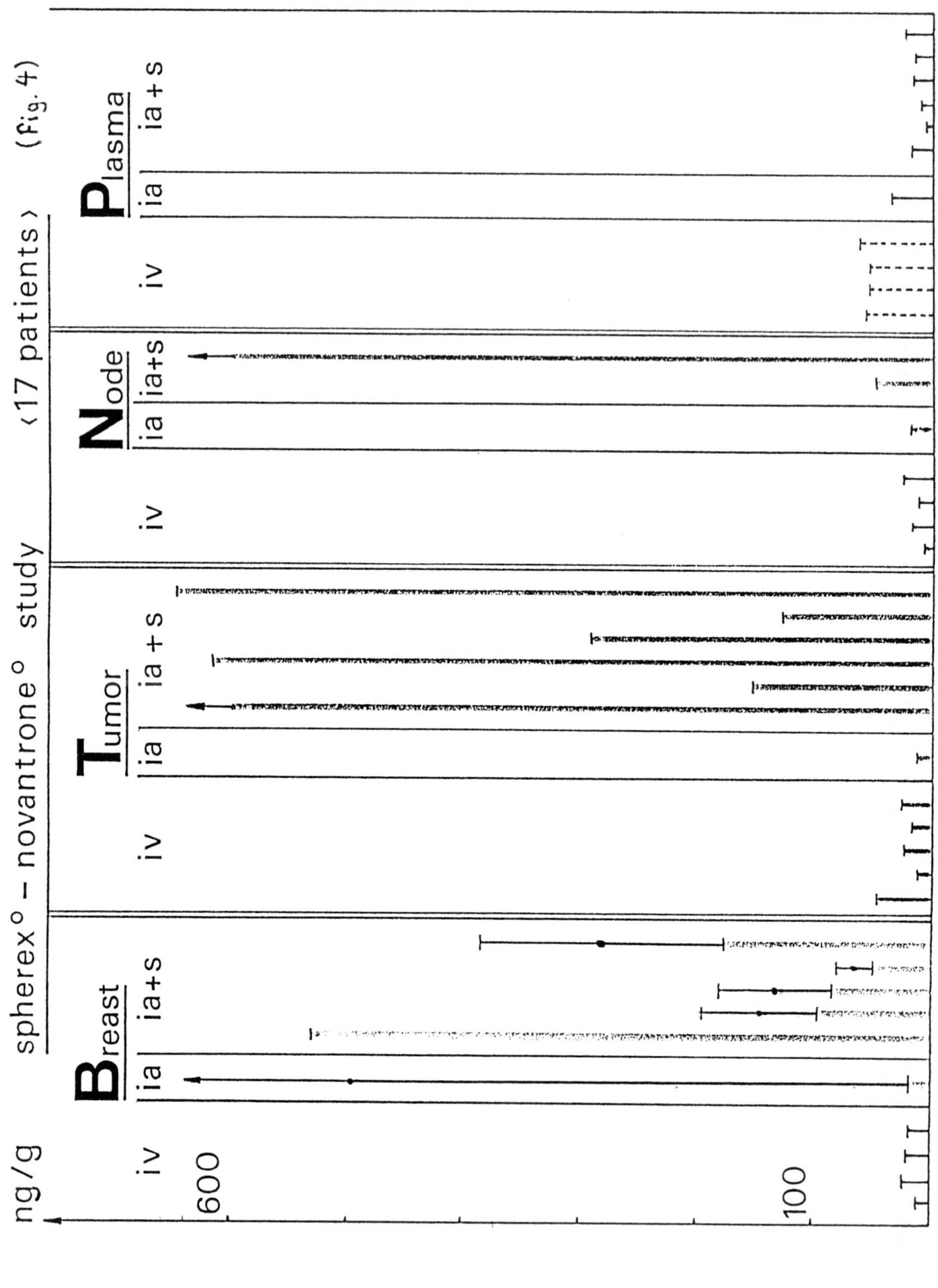

spherex° - novantrone° study
‹17 patients›
(fig. 4)
ng/g
Breast
Tumor
Node
Plasma
iv
ia
ia+s
600
100

Neo-Adjuvant Chemotherapy. Ed. Cl. Jacquillat, M. Weil, D. Khayat. Colloque INSERM/John Libbey Eurotext Ltd. © 1988. Vol. 169, pp. 769-773.

Chimiothérapie intra-artérielle d'induction. Essai cavité buccale 2 du groupe tête et cou EORTC

J.M. Richard*, J.L. Lefèbre**, R. Molinari***, F. Blanchet****, P. Dor***** et H. Sancho-Garnier*

* *Institut Gustave Roussy. 94805 Villejuif, France*
** *Centre Oscar Lambert, 59020 Lille, France*
*** *NCI Milan, Italie*
**** *Centre François Baclesse, 14021 Caen, France*
***** *Institut J. Bordet, Bruxelles, Belgique*

RESUME

Résultats à 5 ans d'un essai thérapeutique randomisé comparant chirugie +- radiothérapie versus chimiothérapie intraartérielle + chirurgie +- radiothérapie dans le traitement des carcinomes du plancher buccal. Une différence significative sur la survie a été mise en évidence en faveur du groupe comportant une chimiothérapie.

MOTS CLEFS

Chimiothérapie intraartérielle, essai thérapeutique randomisé, tête et cou, plancher buccal.

INTRODUCTION

La chimiothérapie néoadjuvante permet elle d'améliorer la survie dfes malades: telle est la question à laquelle nous nous efforçons de répondre à l'Institut Gustave Roussy depuis 1970. Notre premier essai thérapeutique s'était adressé à ,des tumeurs T4 et avait permis de constater un gain minime sur la survie de trois mois environ, donc sans conséquence pratique.(1) Cependant, nous avions pu constater deux faits importants:

- l'association chimiothérapie intraartérielle-chirurgie paraissait la plus performante.
- la localisation qui répondait le mieux à la chimiothérapie au niveau de la cavité buccale était le plancher de la bouche.

Nous avons alors proposé un essai thérapeutique randomisé au groupe tête et cou de l'EORTC. Ce groupe connaissait bien la technique intraartérielle grâce à un premier essai comparant l'action de la Bleomycine à celle du méthotrexate. (2)

MATERIEL ET METHODE:

Dans cet essai étaient inclus les patients présentant un carcinome épidermoïde du plancher buccal histologiquement confirmé et justiciables d'une chirurgie d'éxérèse.Les causes d'exclusion étaient les petites lésions T1, les adénopathies fixées bilatérales, les métastases à distance, les patients agés de plus de 70 ans, les malades traités antérieurs et les localisations multiples. Enfin les patients avec pathologie artérielle ou respiratoire contr'indiquant la chimiothérapie étaient également exclus.

Les patients étaient randomisés par centre coopérateur.

La chimiothérapie était administrée par voie artérielle (voie de la temporale superficielle) en infusion continue, mais en cas d'échec initial ou secondaire de la voie artérielle il était prévu d'administrer la même chimiothérapie par voie veineuse. Les drogues utilisées étaient la vincristine (1mgr au jours 1, 5 et 9) et la Bleomycine (15 mgr de J1 à J12).

La chirurgie consistait pour la lésion primitive en une pelvimandibulectomie interruptrice ou non. Pour les adénopathies un évidement radical était prévu en cas d'adénopathie palpable. Pour les N0, un évidement sousmento-maxillaire, sous digastrique et sus omohyoïdien était réalisé avec examen extemporané peropératoire; si les ganglions étaient envahis l'évidement était complèté.

Il faut préciser que 3 patients ne purent avoir de chirurgie en raison de la progression rapide des lésions: 2 dans le bras chirurgie seule, 1 dans le bras chimiochirurgie.

La radiothérapie postopératoire n'était effectuée qu'en cas d'envahissement ganglionnaire sur les aires ganglionnaires cervicales (50 Gy + surdosage de 15 Gy sur les zônes en rupture capsulaire) et sur le lit tumoral en cas de résection insuffisante (65 Gy).

RESULTATS:

Centres coopérateurs		Randomisation	
IGR: France	50 cas	Chirurgie:	63 cas
Lille: France	38 cas		
Milan: Italie	24 cas	Chimio-chirurgie:	64 cas
Caen: France	10 cas		
J.Bordet: Belgique	5 cas	Un T1 exclus	

Les facteurs pronostiques cliniques ne montrent pas de différence significative.

	chirurgie (63)	chimio-chirurgie (64)
Age	52,9	53,3
Sexe (F)	2 (3%)	0
T2	29 (47%)	26 (41%)
T3	30 (48%)	27 (42%)
T4	4 (6%)	11 (17%)
N0	42 (67%)	37 (58%)
N1 N2	16 (25%)	23 (36%)
N3	5 (8%)	4 (4%)

La radiothérapie a été effectuée de la même façon en ce qui concerne les doses et les étalements dans les deux groupes.

	chirurgie (63)	chimio-chirurgie (64)
RX L.Prim.	43 (68%)	35 (55%)
Durée	41 jours	42 jours
Dose L.P.	54,8 GY	55,9 Gy
RX Gang.	43 (68%)	37 (58%)
Dose	55,3 Gy	57,8 Gy

Au point de vue anatomopathologique, les résections insuffisantes ont été un peu plus fréquentes dans le groupe chirurgie seule.

		chirurgie (63)	chimio-chirurgie (64)
Résect.suff.		50 (79%)	57 (89%)
Envahiss.	N+	33 (55%)	34 (58%)
Gg.	R+	19 (30%)	23 (36%)
Embolies		2 (3%)	5 (8%)

Sur le plan de la chimiothérapie 73% des patients ont reçu la chimiothérapie intraartérielle comme prévu, 18% ont eu une voie d'administration mixte en raison d'incident de cathéter et 9% ont reçu uniquement une chimiothérapie systémique.
La toxicité résumée dans le tableau suivant a été faible. La chimiothérapie n'a été interrompue que dans 3 cas.

	FAIBLE*	MODEREE**	SEVERE***
Neurologique	6 (3mixt.)	1	
Cutanées	1		1 (sys)
Asthenie	3	1	
Allergie			1
Temperature	2 (1sys)		1 (SYS)
Alopecie	2		

*: sans modification du traitement
**: avec " "
***: avec interruption du traitement

L'étude de la régression tumorale clinique a permis de constater peu de régressions complètes (6%) avec 48% de régressions objectives au niveau de la lésion primitive. Les adénopathies ont régressé de façon moins importante que la lésion primitive.

REGRESSION CLINIQUE

	LESION PRIMITIVE (64)	ADENOPATHIES (26)
RC	4 (6%)	3 (11%)
RP	27 (42%)	1 (4%)
< 50%	16 (25%)	8 (30%)
NR	15 (23%)	14 (52%)

L'étude histologique des pièces opératoires fait apparaitre une discordance avec l'appréciation clinique de la régression: l'anatomopathologiste constate en effet 15% de régressions complètes, phénomène qui s'explique par la nécrose et la sclérose résiduelle postchimiothérapique que le clinicien ne peut distinguer d'un reliquat tumoral.
En ce qui concerne les adénopathies, la régression histologique est en gros parallèle à la régression clinique mais constate par contre même en cas de régression très importante la persistance de cellules tumorales dans le tissu periganglionnaire traduisant la rupture capsulaire.

La survie
La courbe de survie en Kaplan Meier montre une différence de survie globale en faveur du groupe chimiothérapie et si l'on ajuste les résultats sur le T et le N cette différence est significative (p=0,04). Autrement dit, l'espérance de survie des malades ayant bénéficié de la chimiothérapie passe de 3 à 7 ans.

COURBE DE SURVIE PAR TRAITEMENT

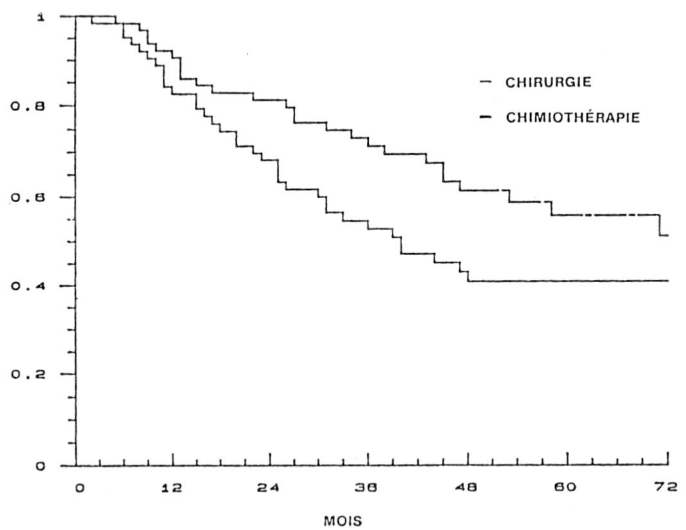

Par contre le desease free calculé de la date de randomisation à la date du premier échec ne montre pas de différence. Cette apparente contradiction peut être expliquée par l'étude des causes d'échec.

TYPE DE PREMIER ECHEC

	CHIRURGIE (63)	CHIMIO-CHIRURGIE (64)
Rec.Loc.	18	10
Rec.Gg.	3	8 (4 N-)
Rec.L.Reg.	1	1
Metastases	7	5
2ème Loc.	14	15

On peut en effet constater que:
- les récidives locales sont moins nombreuses dans le groupe chimiothérapie avec un nombre d'évènements très voisin.
L'analyse définitive qui est presqu'achevée permettra de préciser les autres facteurs qui sont intervenus pour expliquer cette différence de survie et fera l'objet d'une prochaine publication.

CONCLUSION

Grace à la chimiothérapie intraartérielle cet essai a pu démontrer qu'une chimiothérapie d'induction pouvait améliorer la survie des patients atteints de carcinomes épidermoïdes du plancher buccal. Ce résultat a pu être obtenu malgré une chimiothérapie actuellement dépassée sur le plan des drogues utilisées.
Ceci nous pousse d'une part a poursuivre la voie d'administration intraartérielle, d'autre part a continuer des études structurées portant sur des localisations dont les éléments pronostiques et l'histoire naturelle sont identiques.

REFERENCES BIBLIOGRAPHIQUES

Richard J.M., Sancho H., Lepintre Y., Rodary J., Pierquin B. (1974).Intra-arterial methotrexate chemotherapy and telecobalt therapy in cancer of the oral cavity and oropharynx. Cancer 34:491-496.

Molinari R.(1982). A randomised EORTC trial comparing intra-arterial infusion with Methotrexate versus Bleomycine as initialtherapy in carcinoma of the oral cavity. Eur. J. of Cancer clinic. oncol. 807-812.

Résumé

Intraarterial neoadjuvant chemotherapy: oral cavity 2 trial of the head and neck cooperative group (EORTC).
RICHARD J.M., LEFEVRE J.L., MOLINARI R., BLANCHET F., DOR P.,SANCHO-GARNIER H.
The results, at 5 years of a randomised therapeutic trial comparing surgery +- radiotherapy with intraarterial chemotherapt and surgery +- radiotherapy in the treatment of carcinoma of the floor of the mouth are reported. A significant improvement in survival was noted in those patients receving intraarterial chemotherapy as part of their treatment.

Neo-Adjuvant Chemotherapy. Ed. Cl. Jacquillat, M. Weil, D. Khayat. Colloque INSERM/John Libbey Eurotext Ltd. © 1988. Vol. 169, pp. 775-778.

Chimiothérapie intra-artérielle d'induction : essai thérapeutique cavité buccale postérieure du groupe tête et cou EORTC

B. Luboinski*, R. Molinari**, F. Blanchet***, A. Kramar*, M. Luboinski* et J.M. Richard*

* *Institut Gustave-Roussy, 94805 Villejuif, France*
** *N.C.I. Milan, Italie*
*** *Centre François Baclesse, 14021, Caen, France*

RESUME

Résultats à 5 ans d'un essai thérapeutique randomisé comparant chirurgie versus chimiothérapie-chirurgie associés à une radiothérapie post-opératoire dans le traitement des carcinomes de la cavité buccale postérieure et de l'oropharynx. Aucune différence significative sur la survie n'a été mise en évidence entre les deux groupes.

MOTS CLEFS

Chimiothérapie intra artérielle, essai thérapeutique randomisé, tête et cou, cavité buccale postérieure et oropharynx.

INTRODUCTION

Cet essai thérapeutique résulte de la stratification d'un essai thérapeutique plus vaste englobant également les carcinomes du plancher buccal. Il a paru intéressant de séparer ces deux groupes de localisation en raison de leur pronostic différent.

MATERIEL ET METHODE

Dans cet essai étaient inclus les patients présentant un carcinome épidermoïde de la cavité buccale postérieure ou de l'oropharynx : trigone rétro-molaire, zone de jonction linguale, sillon glosso-amygdalien, pilier antérieur de la loge amygdalienne, confirmés histologiquement et justiciables de chirurgie. Les causes d'exclusion étaient les lésions classées T_1, les adénopathies fixées, bilatérales, les métastases à distance, les patients âgés de plus de 70 ans, les malades traités antérieurs et les localisations multiples. Etaient également exclus les patients avec pathologie artérielle ou respiratoire contr'indiquant la chimiothérapie.

La randomisation était effectuée par centre coopérateur :

Centres coopérateurs	Randomisation	
I.G.R, France : 67 cas	Chirurgie	47*
Milan, Italie : 24 cas	Chimio-chirurgie	48
Caen, France : 4 cas		

* Deux patients ont refusé la chirurgie.

La chimiothérapie était adminstrée par la voie de l'artère temporale superficielle en infusion continue. En cas d'échec de cette voie la chimiothérapie était administrée par voie veineuse aux mêmes doses. Les drogues utilisées étaient la vincristine (1 mg jours 1,5 et 9) et la bléomycine (15 mg de J_1 à J_{12}).
La chirurgie consistait pour la lésion primitive en une buccopharyngectomie transmaxillaire et pour les adénopathies un évidement cervical radical était prévu pour les adénopathies palpables. Pour les N_0, un évidement sous-mento-maxillaire, sous digastrique et sus-omo-hyoïdien était réalisé avec examen histologique per opératoire. Si les ganglions étaient métastatiques, l'évidement était complété.

La radiothérapie post-opératoire était systématique sur les aires ganglionnaires et le lit tumoral à la dose de 50 Gy en cas de N- et de résection suffisante. Un surdosage de 15 Gy était délivré en cas de N+ ou de résection insuffisante.

RESULTATS

Les facteurs pronostiques ne montrent pas de différences significatives : l'âge est le même dans les deux groupes (M= 53 ans),il y a 3 femmes (6%) dans le groupe chirurgie, 4 (8%) dans le groupe chimiothérapie.

La répartition TNM montre une légère prédominance des T_3 et des N_1b-N_2ab.

	Chirurgie (47)	Chimio-chirurgie (48)
T_2	24 (51%)	17 (36%)
T_3	22 (47%)	29 (60%)
T_4	1 (2%)	2 (4%)
N_0-N_{1a}	31 (66%)	26 (54%)
N_{1b}-N_{2ab}	11(23%)	17 (35%)
N_3	5 (11%)	5 (10%)

La radiothérapie a été effectuée de la même façon en ce qui concerne les doses et les étalements dans les deux groupes.

Il n'existait pas de différence entre les deux groupes pour la qualité de la résection chirurgicale et l'envahissement ganglionnaire

	Chirurgie (47)	Chimio-chirurgie (48)
Résection suffisante	36 (77%)	38 (79%)
Envahissement gangl.		
N+	31 (68%)	30 (65%)
R+	16 (34%)	20 (42%)
Embolies	7 (15%)	8 (17%)

La chimiothérapie a été délivrée par voie intra artérielle dans 37 cas, par voie mixte (intra artérielle et intra veineuse) dans 4 cas, par voie veineuse dans 7 cas. 1 patient est décédé à la suite d'une erreur de protocole, pour le reste la toxicité a été considérée comme légère dans 9 cas et sévère dans un cas (hématologique) avec interruption du traitement.

L'étude de la régression clinique montre peu de réponses complètes.

Régréssion clinique

	Lésion primitive (48)	Adénopathies (22)
RC	3 (6%)	3 (14%)
RP	17 (35%)	2 (9%)
<50%	18 (38%)	4 (18%)
NR	7 (15%)	11 (50%)
Inconnu		2 (9%)

SURVIE

La courbe de survie de KAPLAN MEIER ne montre aucune différence entre les deux groupes. La médiane de recul est de 55 mois. Au moment de l'analyse 56 patients sont décédés, la médiane de survie est de 3 ans dans les deux groupes.

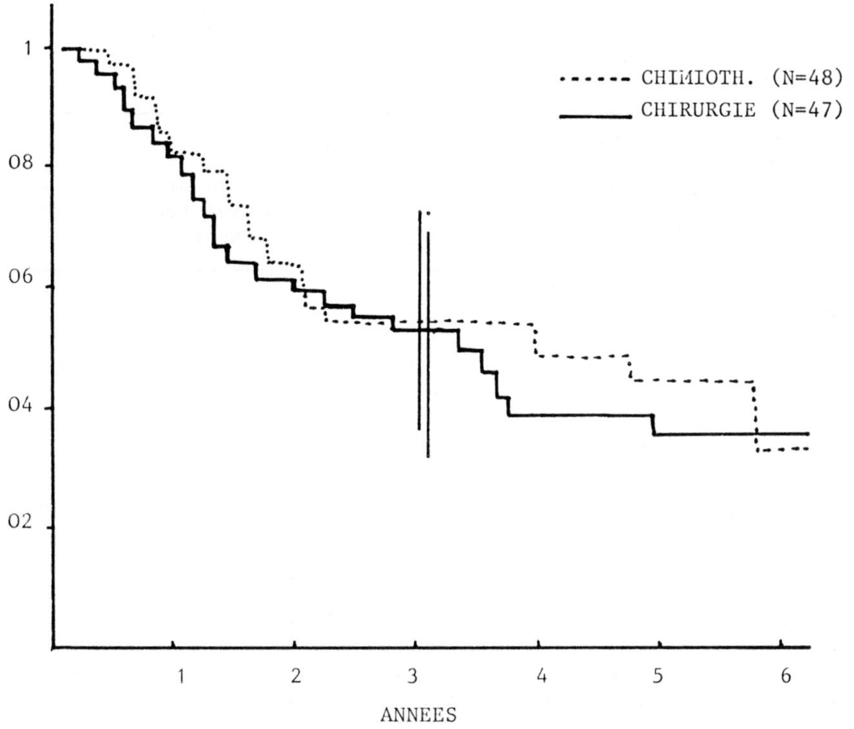

La récidive locorégionale constitue le mode le plus fréquent du premier échec.

Type de premier échec

	Chirurgie (47)	Chimio-chirurgie (48)
Récidive locale	8	7
Récidive ganglionnaire	2	3
Récidive loco-régionale	0	4
Métastases	8	6
2ème localisation	5	6

CONCLUSION

Contrairement aux résultats obtenus pour le plancher buccal, la chimiothérapie d'induction intra artérielle n'a apporté aucune amélioration de la survie des carcinomes de la cavité buccale postérieure et de l'oropharynx. Toutefois les drogues utilisées sont actuellement dépassées. Il nous parait intéressant actuellement de poursuivre ce type d'étude avec des associations de drogues plus efficaces, en conservant une stratification qui permet d'étudier des localisations de même pronostique.

REFERENCES BIBLIOGRAPHIQUES

Richard, J.M, Sancho, H, Lepintre, Y, Rodary, J, Pierquin, B, (1974): Intra Arterial methotrexate chemotherapy and telecobalterapy in cancer of the oral cavity and oropharynx. Cancer 34, 491-496

Molinari, R, (1982):A randomised EORTC trial comparing intra arterial infusion with methotrexate versus bleomycine as initial therapy in carcinoma of the oral cavity. Eur. J. of Cancer Clinic.oncol. 807-812

Résumé

The results at 5 year of randomised therapeutic trial comparing surgery versus chemotherapy and surgery, both followed by post operative radiotherapy are reported no difference was noted in survival between the two groups.

Neo-Adjuvant Chemotherapy. Ed. Cl. Jacquillat, M. Weil, D. Khayat. Colloque INSERM/John Libbey Eurotext Ltd. © 1988. Vol. 169, pp. 779-783.

Combined intra-arterial and systemic chemotherapy for paranasal sinus carcinoma

I.W. Dimery, Y.Y. Lee, P. van Tassel, H. Goepfert, K. McCarthy, R. Byers, O. Gullamendegui and W.K. Hong

University of Texas, M.D. Anderson Hospital and Tumor Institute, Houston, Texas 77030, USA

ABSTRACT

In our experience, recurrent or advanced, previously untreated paranasal sinus carcinoma (PNSC) has demonstrated a low response rate to intravenous systemic combination chemotherapy continuous as compared to other primary head and neck tumor sites. Because of the usual aggressive biologic behavior of these tumors, a prospective analysis of intra-arterial chemotherapy by super-selective internal maxillary artery catheterization and infusion of cisplatin + bleomycin combined with intravenous infusion of 5-fluorouracil (5-FU) x 5 days was undertaken to evaluate its efficacy in the overall treatment of advanced (AJC Stage IV) or recurrent PNSC.

INTRODUCTION

Carcinoma of the paranasal sinuses (maxillary, ethmoid, and nasal cavity), upon presentation, is usually locoregionally confined; however, because of its proximity to surrounding vital structures (i.e., orbital contents and cavernous sinus) craniofacial resection may be required for treatment. Despite aggressive combined treatment including postoperative radiotherapy, the overall 2 to 5 year determinant survival is 59% and 42%, respectively for all patients (1).

Those patients with tumors originating in the suprastructure may extend intracranially or into the pterygoid or sphenopalatine fossa and may only be candidates for palliative therapy. Therefore, an alternative approach to therapy is indicated in cases of advanced disease.

Intra-arterial chemotherapy has been employed as a treatment modality for head and neck carcinoma for the past 20 years with a variety of agents, especially cisplatin and bleomycin, with a reported increase in tissue levels and in response rates of from 2 to 4 times greater as compared to the intravenous route (2-4). Systemic toxicity may also be milder (5). A report from Lee et al reviewed our experience in the treatment of both recurrent and untreated sinus carcinoma by super-selective arterial catheterization resulting in an improved therapeutic index (6).

The I.V. continuous infusion of 5-FU in combination with cisplatin has resulted in excellent clinical response in previously untreated cancers (7). In some cases surgery has been entirely circumvented (8). Therefore, we have combined intra-arterial cisplatin and bleomycin with 5-FU continuous infusion x 5 days for 3 cycles of treatment followed by surgery and/or radiotherapy. The outcome of treatment was examined in regards to 1) the initial response to chemotherapy, 2) the histologic findings at surgical resection, and 3) induction chemotherapy and radiotherapy as a substitute for radical craniofacial surgery.

METHODOLOGY AND PATIENTS

Using standard techniques, a femoral artery puncture is performed and a 5-French catheter is introduced and the external carotid is selectively catheterized under fluoroscopic guidance and positioned just distal to the facial artery. A 2-French catheter is then introduced through the 5-French catheter and advanced to the desired position and connected to the pulsatile pump for administration of the chemotherapy.

Chemotherapy

Cisplatin (100 mg/m^2) with mannitol diuresis and bleomycin (30 u) are infused intra-arterially over a period of 1 to 1-1/2 hours in the radiology suite. All catheters are then removed. 5-FU (1000 mg/m^2/day) is then administered by intravenous infusion for 5 days. The entire procedure is repeated every 3 to 4 weeks for 3 to 4 courses. Re-evaluation is then performed by physical examinations and computerized tomography (CT scan) or magnetic resonance imaging (MRI scan). Surgery and radiotherapy are then planned according to the initial results obtained with chemotherapy.

Patients

Patients eligible for this study were those with Stage IV or recurrent PNSC not amenable to curative surgery and/or radiotherapy, normal renal ($Cr \leq 1.5$ mg/dL), and hematologic function (granulocytes $\geq 2,000$ cells/mm^3 and platelets $\geq 100 \times 10^3$/mm^3).

RESULTS

Patient characteristics (Table 1)	
Entered into study	17
Evaluable for toxicity	17
Evaluable for response	13
Unable to infuse	2
Early death	2
Male/Female	12/5
Median age in years (range)	61 (25-72)
Previous treatment	
None	12
Radiotherapy	2
Surgery and radiotherapy	3
Site of disease	
Maxillary sinus	11
Ethmoid sinus	2
Nasal cavity	2

Stage of disease	
T4	14
(6/14 with intracranial extension)	
T3	1
N0	11
N1	2
N2b	2

Histology	
Squamous cell carcinoma	9
Lymphoepithelioma	2
Adenoid cystic	2
Neuroendocrine	1
Adenocarcinoma	1

Seventeen patients were entered into this treatment program. Fifteen patients were catheterized and infused. Two patients were unable to be infused secondary to arterial spasms (1) and prior surgical ligation of the maxillary artery (1). Most patients were previously untreated, with T4 intracranially extending maxillary sinus carcinoma. Histologically, 60% of patients treated had squamous cell carcinoma.

Treatment response (Table 2)		
Median courses (range)	3 (1-4)	
Total number of courses administered	40	
Response to chemotherapy (n = 13)		
Complete response	3 (23%)	10 (77%)
Partial response	7 (54%)	
Minor response	2 (15%)	
Progression	1 (8%)	
Response to radiotherapy only (n = 7)		
Complete response	4 (57%)	5 (71%)
Stable residual disease	1 (14%)	
Progression and death	2 (28%)	
(Too early)	1	
Response to surgery +/- radiotherapy (n = 4)		
Complete response	4 (100%)	
(Too early)	1	
Overall response (n = 11)		
Complete response	8 (73%)	
Stable residual (> 12 months)	1 (9%)	
Dead of disease	2 (18%)	

Fifteen patients received 40 courses of chemotherapy. Two patients died within 2 weeks of infusion and were not evaluable for response. Seventy-seven percent responded to chemotherapy with 23% (3/13) attaining a complete response and 54% (7/13) with residual disease. Seven (53%) patients received radiotherapy only with 4 (57%) of those attaining complete response. Four others underwent surgical resection followed by surgical resection and were rendered disease-free. Five patients underwent surgical resection. Two patients had minimal residual disease, one had carcinoma *in situ* and two had gross disease (1- positive margins, 1 - negative margins post-operatively). Overall, of 13 patients (2 - too early to evaluate), 8 were disease-free, and 1 had minimal residual disease at 150+ weeks. Of those who achieved final complete response, 1 patient relapsed in the cervical nodes at 82 weeks and was treated with radiotherapy.

Toxicity

Seventeen patients were evaluable for toxicity. The predominant side effect of the treatment was gastrointestinal with nausea and vomiting occurring in 10 (59%) and mucositis in 5 (29%). Six (35%) developed myelosuppression with granulocytes < 1,500 cells/mm^3 in 6 (35%) without infections and platelets < 1 z 10^5/mm^3 in 1 (6%). Transient elevations of creatinine (1.7 - 2.0 mg/dL) occurred in 2 (11%) but subsequently returned to < 1.5 mg/dL.

DISCUSSION AND CONCLUSIONS

Successful treatment was accomplished in 13 patients with advanced PNSC. Initial induction treatment and radiotherapy resulted in the circumvention of surgery in 4 patient. In 3/5 patients undergoing surgery, minimal residual disease was removed underscoring the effectiveness of this approach. The two patients dying after infusion both had post-mortem examinations which did not disclose any unusual findings and cause of death was deemed secondary to either a cardiovascular event and advanced disease, respectively. Toxicity was relatively mild and reversible and in only one patient was a catheter-related (spasm) event observed necessitating discontinuance of the procedure.

Whether this early experience with our approach of super-selective arterial catheterization and infusion of cisplatin/bleomycin and peripheral 5-FU is superior to that of others is to be determined. This method allows a very distal catheter placement resulting in higher local drug concentration. The addition of intra-arterial chemotherapy with a variety of drugs has been utilized by others in an effort to improve the local control rate and prolong the disease-free survival in previously untreated or palliate those with recurrent disease (9-11). Small series or case reports indicate the optimum responses which can be obtained by this method (12-14). Knegt et al described the anatomy-sparing approach of typical 5-FU and low-dose radiotherapy plus surgical necrotomy (15); whereas, Shibuya et al did not observe benefit in those he treated with multi-modality therapy consisting of intra-arterial 5-FU concurrent with radiotherapy (16). The selective entry of patients who are of an ideal performance status and who are initially resectable would ultimately gain long-term benefit over a population with more advanced disease. In a similar fashion for other head and neck tumors in which partial response is attained (residual disease remains), overall survival only favors complete responders. This approach may facilitate achieving such a result more consistently in advanced PNSC.

We conclude that: 1) Superselective internal maxillary artery catheterization and intra-arterial infusion of cisplatin and bleomycin + systemic 5-FU is an effective mode of therapy for a selective population of good-risk patients with advanced paranasal sinus carcinoma; 2) Toxicity was tolerable in most patients with very few catheter-related problems; 3) Overall response rate appears to result in a higher response rate than systemic chemotherapy alone; 4) The definitive treatment following the chemotherapy (surgery and/or radiotherapy) seems to be effectively delivered despite the advanced stage at presentation resulting in an acceptable overall and disease-free survival; and 5) additionally and importantly, four patients with advanced PNSC who would have required craniofacial surgery attained CR after combined chemotherapy and radiotherapy.

REFERENCES

1. Goepfert, H.(1983): Cancer of the paranasal sinuses and nasal cavity. In Surgical Oncology, ed E.M. Copeland, III, pp 77-91. John Wiley and Sons, Inc.

2. LeHane, D.E.(1980): Intra-arterial cisplatinum administration for advanced squamous cell carcinoma of the head and neck region. Int. Head and Neck Oncol. Res. Conf., (Abstract).

3. Sessions, R.B.(1982): Intra-arterial cisplatin treatment of adenoid cystic carcinoma. Arch Otolaryngol 108, 221-224.

4. Bitter, K.J.(1976): Pharmacokinetics behavior of bleomycin-cobalt 57 with special regard to intra-arterial perfusion of the maxillo-facial region. Maxillofac Surg 4, 226-231.

5. Stewart, D.J.(1983): Clinical pharmacology of intra-arterial cis-diamminedichloroplatinum (II). Cancer Res 43, 917-920.

6. Lee, Y.Y.(1986): Intra-arterial chemotherapy of head and neck tumors. Am J Neurorad 7, 343-348.

7. Jacobs, J.(1986): Combined modality therapy utilizing cisplatinum combinations: Development of effective chemotherapy in patients with previously untreated head and neck cancer. Am J Surg 152, 451-455.

8. Jacobs, C.(1987): Chemotherapy as a substitute for surgery in the treatment of advanced resectable head and neck cancer. A report from the Northern California Oncology Group. Cancer 60, 1178-1183.

9. Zielke-Temme, B.C.(1980): Combined intra-arterial chemotherapy, radiation therapy, and surgery for advanced squamous cell carcinoma of the head and neck. Cancer 45, 1527-1532.

10. Moseley, H.S.(1981): Advanced squamous cell carcinoma of the maxillary sinus, results of combined regional infusion chemotherapy radiation therapy and surgery. Am J Surg 141, 522-525.

11. Sakai, S.(1983): Multidisciplinary treatment of maxillary sinus carcinoma. Cancer 52, 1360-1364.

12. Sessions, R.B.(1982): Intra-arterial cisplatin treatment of adenoid cystic carcinoma. Arch Otolaryngeal 108, 221-224.

13. Horu, Y.(1981): Long term remission of an advanced head and neck tumor following intra-arterial infusion with cis-dichlorodiammine platinum. J Surg Oncol 18, 189-192.

14. Arbit, E.(1979): Craniofacial resection following chemotherapy. Indian J Cancer 16, 74-79.

15. Knegt, P.P.(1985):Carcinoma of the paranasal sinuses: Results of a prospective pilot study. Cancer 56, 57-62.

16. Shibuya, H.(1982): Reappraisal of trimodal combination therapy for maxillary sinus carcinoma. Cancer 50, 2790-2794.

New developments in melanoma

Nouveaux développements dans le mélanome

Neo-Adjuvant Chemotherapy. Ed. Cl. Jacquillat, M. Weil, D. Khayat. Colloque INSERM/John Libbey Eurotext Ltd. © 1988. Vol. 169, pp. 787-790.

Multicentric study of the nitrosourea fotemustine (S 10036) in advanced malignant melanoma (AMM) including patients with cerebral metastases

Cl. Jacquillat[1], D. Khayat[1], P. Banzet[2], M. Weil[1], P. Fumoleau[3], M. Namer[4], M.F. Avril[5], R. Lauvin[6], P. Kerbrat[7], C. Vilmer[8] and J.P. Bizzari[1]

From Hôpital La Pitié-Salpétrière, Paris[1], Hôpital St Louis, Paris[2], Centre René Gauducheau, Nantes[3], Centre A. Lacassagne, Nice[4], Institut Gustave Roussy, Villejuif[5], Hôpital Sud, Rennes[6], Centre E. Marquis, Rennes[7], Centre René Huguenin, Saint-Cloud[8], France

MOTS CLEF

NITROSOUREA FOTEMUSTINE, MALIGNANT MELANOMA, CEREBRAL METASTASES, MULTICENTRIC STUDY

INTRODUCTION

Fotemustine (S 10036) - diethyl 1 - [3 - (2chloroéthyl) - 3 - nitrosoureïdo] - ethylphosphonate - is a nitrosourea of third generation characterized by the grafting of a phosphono alanine carrier group to a nitrosourea radical in order to increase the passage through the cell membrane and the blood brain barrier.

Initial concept of this new molecule leads to pharmacodynamic considerations i.e. difference in membrane permeabilities to amino acids between healthy and cancer cells (1), and increase of intracellular penetration using the amino acids transport system (2,3).

Due to the pharmacological toxicity on the NCI tumor panel screen, the rationale of the chemical design - defined by an optimal partition coefficient octanol/water (log P) within the range of optimal activity (4,5) and the decreased mutagenic activity compared to BCNU (Carmustine), Fotemustine was tested in phase I clinical trial (6).

During this phase I study, 3 clinical responses have been observed and especially in CLL and in melanoma.

Based on these data, a multicentric phase II study was then initiated in various tumors. Preliminary results of the phase II study in disseminated malignant melanoma have been already reported (7). We report here the results of the french multicentric phase II study which confirms these preliminary results.

PATIENTS AND METHODS

One hundred and five patients from 14 differents institutions suffering from disseminated malignant melanoma were entered in this French multicentric study.

Informed consent was obtained in all patients. Patients had to fulfill all the following criteria : histologically confirmed diagnosis of melanoma, mesurable or evaluable lesions with documented progression within 2 months prior to entry in the study, life expectancy of at least 12 weeks, age between 18 and 80 years, Karnofsky greater than 50 %, correct hematological status, normal hepatic and renal functions unless abnormalities were clearly due to metastatic disease, no chemotherapy for the previous 28 days (or 42 days if prior treatment with nitrosourea).

Among the 105 patients, 95 patients were evaluable for antitumor activity and 10 patients (9,5 %) were not evaluable (non eligible : 1 patient, protocol violation : 7 patients, early death : 2 patients).

Median age was 51 years (range 20 - 79), sex ratio 1.15 (51 men and 44 women), median Karnofsky was 80 % (range 50 - 100 %).

Before entering the trial, 1 patient never received any treatment, 26 patients were treated by surgery and 62 patients (65.3 %) had received prior chemotherapy (40 with 1 regimen and 22 patients with 2 or more regimen).

Site of metastases was : cerebral (23 patients = 24.2 %), ocular (2 patients = 2.1 %), visceral (41 patients = 43.2 %) and non visceral (29 patients = 30.5 %).

According to the recommandations of the phase I study, therapeutic regimen consisted in an induction therapy of 100 mg/sqm every week during 3 to 4 consecutive weeks in 1 hour IV infusion, followed by a 4 to 5 weeks rest period. On patients with clinical response and/or stabilisation, maintenance therapy was initiated consisting of 100 mg/sqm every 3 weeks.

Toxicity was evaluated every week. Clinical and/or radiological evaluation of mesurable and/or evaluable lesion was appreciated at week 4 and 8.

Responses were scored according to WHO criteria and classified into : complete response (CR), partial response (PR), minor response (MR), stabilisation (ST) and progressive disease (PD).

RESULTS

Clinical efficacy

Among the 105 entered patients, 95 patients are evaluable for activity. One complete response, 24 partial responses, 4 minor responses and 17 stabilisations were observed, with an overall response rate of 26.3 %.

According to metastatic sites, responses have been observed in cerebral (5/23 = 21.7 %), visceral (11/43 = 26.6 %) and non visceral (9/29 = 31 %) metastases.

Based on prior chemotherapy, we observed a response rate of 36.4 % (12/33) in patients with no prior chemotherapy versus 21 % (13/62) in patients with one or more previous chemotherapeutic regimen.

Median duration of response was 16 weeks (7 - 76 weeks).

Toxicity

As expected, toxicity was mainly hematological characterized by delayed thrombocytopenia (7.2 % grade IV, nadir at day 36) and leucopenia (11.2 % grade IV, nadir at day 42). Gastro intestinal toxicity analysed during the 279 administrations was very mild (72.3 % grade 0 and I).

Increase in hepatic enzyme value was also observed but was transient and always reversible.
No death related toxicity has been reported.

DISCUSSION

Chemotherapy has been generally of limited clinical benefit in disseminated malignant melanoma (6) and DTIC is being reported as the most active single agent treatment with a response rate of 20 - 22 % (8,9).

The results observed during the phase I and the preliminary phase II study (7) have focused on the antitumor activity of this molecule in disseminated malignant melanoma, primary brain tumor and hematological malignancies.

Based on these data, the multicentric phase II study was initiated and the results presented here on 95 evaluable patients confirm the clinical activity of this molecule on disseminated malignant melanoma overall with a response rate of 26.3 % (95 % confidence interval : 17.5 - 35.2) and so whatever the involved metastatic site (especially the cerebral metastases) and/or the previously therapeutic status of the patients.

As expected (10), limiting toxicity was hematological and well controled. Given the high response rate and responses obtained in cerebral metastases, Fotemustine appears to be a good candidate for chemotherapeutic combination study and especially with Deticene is order to increase the response rate and duration of response of disseminated malignant melanoma.

REFERENCES

1 - Foster D.O. and Pardee A.B. (1969) : Transport of amino acids by confluent and nonconfluent 3T3 and polyoma virus-transformed 3T3 cells growing on glass cover slips. J. Biol. Chem., 244, pp 2675-2681,

2 - Christensen H.N. (1969) : Some special kinetic problems of transport. Adv. Ensymol, 32, pp 1-20,

3 - Vistica D.T. (1979) : Cytotoxicity as an indicator for transport mechanism. Evidence that melphalan is transported by two leucine-preferring carrier systems in the L 1210 murine leukemia cells. Biochim. Biophys. Acta, 550, pp 309-317,

4 - Montgomery J.A. (1976) : Chemistry and structure-activity studies of the nitrosoureas. Cancer Treat. Rep., 60, pp 651-664,

5 - Hansch C., Smith N., Engle R. and Wood H. (1972) : Quantitative structure-activity relationships of antineoplastic drugs : nitrosoureas and triazeneimidazoles. Cancer Chemother. Rep., 56, pp 443-456,

6 - Khayat D., Lokiec F., Bizzari J.P., Weil M., Meeus L., Sellami M., Rouesse J., Banzet P. and Jacquillat C. (1987) : Phase I clinical study of the new amino acid-linked nitrosourea, S 10036, ministered on a weekly schedule. Cancer Res., 47, pp 6782-6785,

7 - Khayat D., Bizzari J.P., Weil M., Frenay M., Naman H., Namer M., Banzet P., Jacquillat CL. (1987) : Phase II study of the new nitrosourea S 10036 in advanced malignant melanoma. AACR, Atlanta

8 - Hill G.J., Moss S.E., Golomb F.M., and al. (1981) : DTIC and combination therapy for melanoma : III, DTIC post-operative adjuvant study Central Oncology Group Protocol 7040. Cancer ; 47, pp 2256-62

9 - Carter R.D., Krementz E.T., Hill G.J. and al. (1976) : DTIC (NSC 45388) and combination therapy for melanoma : I -Studies with DTIC, BCNU (NSC 409962), CCNU (NSC 78037), Vincristine (NSC 67574) and Hydroyyurea (NSC 32065). Cancer Treat Rep., 60, pp 601-3

10 - Carter S.K. (1973) : An overview of the status of the nitrosoureas in other tumors. Cancer Chemother. Rep. 4, pp 35-46

Résumé

Au cours d'une étude multicentrique de phase II, l'activité antitumorale et la toxicité d'une nouvelle nitrosourée, la Fotemustine (S 10036) ont été recherchées dans l'indication mélanome malin (y compris chez des patients porteurs de métastases cérébrales) sur 95 patients. Les caractéristiques de ces patients sont les suivantes : 51 hommes, 44 femmes, âge médian 51 ans (extrêmes : 20 - 79), pas de chimiothérapie antérieure (33 patients), sites métastatiques : cérébral (23 patients = 24,2 %), oculaire (2 patients = 2,1 %), viscéral (41 patients = 43,2 %) et non viscéral (29 patients = 30,5 %).

Le schéma thérapeutique utilisé comprenait un traitement d'attaque de 100 mg/m²/semaine pendant 3 à 4 semaines consécutives suivi d'une période de repos de 4 à 5 semaines. En cas de réponse clinique et/ou stabilisation, le traitement était poursuivi à raison d'une administration de 100 mg/m² toutes les 3 semaines (traitement d'entretien).

La toxicité est essentiellement hématologique caractérisée par une thrombopénie (7,2 % grade IV) et une leucopénie (11,2 % grande IV) retardées (nadir respectivement à Jour 36 et Jour 42). La toxicité digestive est faible (72,3 % grade 0 et I).

En fonction des critères de réponse WHO, le taux de réponse global est de 26,3 % (1 réponse complète et 24 réponses partielles) avec une durée médiane de la réponse de 16 semaines (extrêmes 7 - 76). Ces réponses ont été observées aussi bien sur des sites métastatiques cérébraux (21,7 %) que viscéraux (25,6 %) ou non viscéraux (31 %).

Enfin, 36,4 % des patients n'ayant jamais reçu de chimiothérapie antérieure ont présenté une réponse clinique (versus 21 % traités auparavant par chimiothérapie).

En conclusion, l'efficacité thérapeutique de la Fotemustine est maintenant confirmée dans cette étude multicentrique de phase II et l'intérêt de cette molécule souligné par les réponses obtenues sur les sites viscéraux et cérébraux de la maladie.

Neo-Adjuvant Chemotherapy. Ed. Cl. Jacquillat, M. Weil, D. Khayat. Colloque INSERM/John Libbey Eurotext Ltd. © 1988. Vol. 169, pp. 791-794.

Biological therapy of malignant melanoma

G.N. Hortobagyi

From the Department of Medical Oncology, The University of Texas, Anderson Hospital and Tumor Institute at Houston, Houston, Texas 77030 USA

Much has been learned about the natural history of malignant melanoma, but developments in therapy have lagged behind our knowledge of prognostic factors. Once distant metastases develop, the disease is incurable with current therapies. Dacarbazine, the nitrosoureas, cisplatin, the vinca alkaloids, and a few other cytotoxic agents produce response rates of 20% in patients with metastatic melanoma. Most responses are partial and transient. Some combinations of cytotoxic agents produce higher response rates, but survival rates have not been improved (1).

A number of biological agents have been evaluated in patients with melanoma (2). Bacillus Calmette-Guerin (BCG), its derivatives (methanol extracted residue, Ribi vaccine, etc.), and Corynebacterium parvum have been employed by intralesional administration, intradermal scarification or injection, and intravenous injection. Levamisole, transfer factor, Poly-IC, immune RNA, mixed bacterial vaccine, OK-432, pseudomonas vaccine, thymosin, and a host of other biological agents have been studied in phase I-II and III trials (3). Intralesional administration of bacterial substances results in objective regression of injected tumors in many instances, but not improved survival rates. The systemic administration of these biologicals has not been consistently associated with either improved response or survival rates. The toxicity of many was severe, and this, coupled with doubts about their efficacy, has led to their abandonment.

However, the identification of lymphokines, and their availability in large quantities for appropriate clinical trials have had a favorable effect on the development of biological therapy against malignant melanoma.

Interferons:

Occasional antitumor effects were observed with the use of partially purified interferon preparations; when recombinant interferon molecules became available in larger quantities the systemic evaluation of their efficacy and toxicity in the treatment of patients with malignant melanoma became a reality. As shown in Table 1, several types of interferon have shown definite antitumor activity, resulting in partial, and sometimes complete responses in patients with metastatic malignant melanoma. Although most responses are transient, this is the first time that the systemic administration of a biological agent has resulted in a reproducible and consistent response rate. However, interferon administered as a single therapeutic agent will not result in a major modification of the natural history of melanoma. Additional clinical trials combining interferons with other antitumor sub-

Table 1. Activity of Recombinant Interferon Against Melanoma

Investigator (Reference)	Type of Interferon	No. of Patients	No. of CR	No. of PR	Response Rate
Creagan et al[4]	IFN α-2a	31	3	4	23
Creagan et al[5]	IFN α-2a	30	1	5	20
Creagan et al[6]	IFN α-2a	35	0	8	23
Slater et al[7]	IFN-α (Le)	23	0	3	13
Ernstoff et al[8]	IFN α-2b	16	2	0	12
Kirkwood et al[9]	IFN α-2b	17	0	2	12
Hawkins et al[10]	IFN α-2b	30	0	1	3
Robinson et al[11]	IFN α-2b	63	2	5	11
International trial[12]	IFN α-2b	64	3	7	16
Hersey et al[13]	IFN α-2a	23	3	2	22
Flodgren et al[14]	IFN α	20	0	0	0
Kirkwood et al[15]	IFN α-2	23	2	3	22
Dorval et al[16]	IFN α-2	24	2	4	25
Legha et al[17]	IFN α-2a	31	0	3	10
		31	0	2	6
Goldberg et al[18]	Lymphoblastoid (α-N1)	33	2	1	9
Retsas et al[19]	Lymphoblastoid (α-N1)	15	0	1	7
Ernstoff et al[20]	IFN- γ	30	0	0	0
Creagan et al[21]	IFN- γ	28	0	3	11
Schiller et al[22]	IFN β + γ	15	0	0	0

IFN = Interferon; CR = Complete response; PR = Partial response

stances will be necessary to determine the full effectiveness of these agents.

Interleukin-2:

Interleukin-2 (IL-2) is a glycoprotein produced by circulating T cells activated by exposure to antigens or mitogens. IL-2 induces T helper cells, cytotoxic cells and the production of autoantibodies. IL-2 induces the expression of specific IL-2 receptors. Limited clinical trials of high doses of IL-2 in patients with malignant melanoma have shown that major antitumor responses are possible (23,24)(Table 2). Because of small sample size and variations in dose and schedule of administration, however, it is uncertain how effective IL-2 therapy really is.

Interleukin-2 and Lymphokine-Activated Killer (LAK) Cells:

LAK cells are activated by IL-2 and have the phenotypic characteristics of OKT-3 and OKT-8 positive cells. They are cytolytic for fresh autologous and allogeneic tumor cells but not for normal cells (25). LAK cells can be induced in vivo and in vitro, and their reinfusion into the host, with the administration of additional IL-2, results in antitumor effects. Several investigators have reported the results of using the combination of IL-2 and LAK cells in the treatment of patients with metastatic malignant melanoma (Table 2). Both partial and complete responses have been obtained (23-25). Although most responses are transient, a few have exceeded one year.

The toxic effects of treatment with IL-2 are considerable. Nausea, vomiting, and diarrhea occur in almost all patients, and chills, pre-renal azotemia, hypotension, and cardiopulmonary abnormalities occur frequently. Several fatalities

Table 2. Activity of Interleukin-2 With and Without LAK Cells Against Malignant Melanoma

Investigator (Reference)	No. of Patients	No. of CR	No. of PR	Response Rate
Interleukin-2				
West et al[23]	8	0	5	62
Rosenberg et al[24]	16	0	5	31
Interleukin-2 with LAK Cells				
Rosenberg et al[24]	26	2	4	23
West et al[23]	10	0	5	50
Dutcher et al[25]	32	0	6	19

LAK = Lymphokine activated killer; CR = Complete response; PR = Partial response

have been reported. The toxic effects mentioned are dose- and schedule-dependent (23). Therefore, additional clinical studies are needed to define the most effective and least toxic, treatment regimens.

Other Biological Agents:

Several anti-melanoma monoclonal antibodies are being evaluated as single agents or as part of immunoconjugates with toxins or cytotoxic agents. The results of these early clinical trials are not available.

Tumor necrosis factor (TNF) has been evaluated in phase I trials and is currently being incorporated in phase II studies. The antitumor efficacy of this agent has not been demonstrated.

Conclusions:

Lymphokines have definite antitumor efficacy, although the toxic effects during the initial clinical trials have been severe. Additional trials with different doses and schedules of administration are warranted, and lymphokine therapy in combination with other antineoplastic treatments must be explored.

References:

1. Nathanson L, Kaufman SD, Carey RW: Vinblastine infusion, bleomycin, and cis-dichlorodiammine-platinum chemotherapy in metastatic melanoma. Cancer 48:1290-1294, 1981.
2. Mastrangelo M, Hersh E, Chirigos M: Agumenting agents in cancer therapy: Summary. IN Augmenting Agents in Cancer Therapy, EM Hersh (ed), Raven Press, New York, 1981, pp. 553-564.
3. Terry WD, Hodes RJ: Newer methods of cancer treatment (Chapter 48, Section 1, Immunotherapy). IN Cancer: Principles & Practice of Oncology, VT DeVita, S Hellman and SA Rosenbert (eds), J.B. Lippincott Company, Philadelphia, 1982, pp. 1788-1877.
4. Creagan ET, Ahmann DL, Green SL, et al: Phase II study of low-dose recombinant leukocyte A interferon in disseminated malignant melanoma. J Clin Oncol 2:1002-1005, 1984.
5. Creagan ET, Ahmann DL, Green SJ, et al: Phase II study of recombinant leukocyte A interferon (rIFN-α A) in disseminated malignant melanoma. Cancer 54: 2844-2849, 1984.

6. Creagan ET, Ahmann DL, Green SJ, et al: Recombinant leukocyte interferon (IFN-αA) plus cimetidine in disseminated malignant melanoma (DMM). Proc Am Soc Clin Oncol 4:126 (abstract C-491), 1985.
7. Slater DE, Krown SE, Pinsky CM, et al: Human leukocyte (lapha) interferon (Le) and cimetidine in malignant melanoma. Proc Am Soc Clin Oncol 3:54 (abstract C-210), 1984.
8. Ernstoff MS, Reiss M, Davis CA, et al: Intravenous (IV) recombinant alpha-2 interferon (IFN α-2) in metastatic melanoma. Proc Am Soc Clin Oncol 2:57 (abstract C-222), 1983.
9. Kirkwood JM, Ernstoff MS: Interferons in the treatment of human cancer. J Clin Oncol 2:336-352, 1984.
10. Hawkins MJ, McCune CS, Speyer JL, Sorell M: Recombinant alpha 2 interferon (IFN α-2)(SCH 30500) in patients with metastatic malignant melanoma (MMM): An ECOG pilot study. Proc Am Soc Clin Oncol 3:51 (abstract C-195), 1984.
11. Robinson WA, Kirkwood J, Harvey H, et al: Effective use of recombinant human α2) in metastatic malignant melanoma (MMM): A comparison of two regimens. Proc Am Soc Clin Oncol 3:60 (abstract C-234), 1984.
12. Data reported in Interferon Letter, Volume 1, No. 3, 1985, Schering-Plough Corportation.
13. Hersey P, MacDonald M, Hall C, et al: Immunological effects of recombinant interferon alfa-2a in patients with disseminated melanoma. Cancer 57:1666-1674, 1986.
14. Flodgren R, Borgstrom S, Jonsson PE, et al: Metastatic malignant melanoma: Regression induced by combined treatment with interferon [HuIFN-α(Le)] and cimetidine. Int J Cancer 32:657-665, 1983.
15. Kirkwood JM, Ernstoff MS, Davis CA, et al: Comparison of intramuscular and intravenous recombinant alpha-2 interferon in melanoma and other cancers. Ann Intern Med 103:32-36, 1985.
16. Dorval T, Palangie T, Jouve M, et al: Clinical phase II trial of recombinant DNA interferon (interferon alfa 2b) in patients with metastatic malignant melanoma. Cancer 58:215-218, 1986.
17. Legha SS, Papadopoulos NEJ, Plager C, et al: Clinical evaluation of recombinant interferon alfa-2a (roferon-A) in metastatic melanoma using two different schedules. J Clin Oncol 5:1240-1246, 1987.
18. Goldberg RM, Ayoob M, Silgals R, et al: Phase II trial of lymphoblastoid interferon in metastatic melanoma. Cancer Treat Rep 69:813-816, 1985.
19. Retsas S, Pristman TJ, Newton KA, Westbury G: Evaluation of human lymphoblastoid interferon in advanced malignant melanoma. Cancer 51:273-276, 1983.
20. Ernstoff MS, Trautman T, Davis CA, et al: A randomized phase I/II study of continuous versus intermittent intravenous interferon gamma in patients with metastatic melanoma. J Clin Oncol 5:1804-1810, 1987.
21. Creagan ET, Ahmann DL, Long JH, et al: Phase II study of recombinant interferon-gamma in patients with disseminated malignant melanoma. Cancer Treat Rep 71:843-844, 1987.
22. Schiller JH, Storer B, Willson JKV, Borden EC: Phase II trial of combined recombinant beta and gamma interferons in patients with advanced malignant melanoma. Proc Am Soc Clin Oncol 6:244 (abstract 961), 1987.
23. West WH, Tauer KW, Yannelli JR, et al: Constant-infusion recombinant interleukin-2 in adoptive immunotherapy of advanced cancer. N Engl J Med 316:898-905, 1987.
24. Rosenberg SA, Lotze MT, Muul LM, et al: A progress report on the treatment of 157 patients with advanced cancer using lymphokine-activated killer cells and interleukin-2 or high-dose interleukin-2 alone. N Engl J Med 316:889-897, 1987.
25. Dutcher JP, Creekmore S, Weiss GR, et al: Phase II study of high dose interleukin-2 (IL-2) and lymphokine activated killer (LAK) cells in patients (PTS) with melanoma. Proc Am Soc Clin Oncol 6:246 (abstract 970), 1987.

Symposium THP-adriamycin (pirarubicine)

THP-adriamycine (pirarubicine)

Neo-Adjuvant Chemotherapy. Ed. Cl. Jacquillat, M. Weil, D. Khayat. Colloque INSERM/John Libbey Eurotext Ltd. © 1988. Vol. 169, p.797.

Introduction

Claude Jacquillat

Groupe hospitalier Pitié-Salpétrière, Paris, France

La découverte des anthracyclines marque une date capitale dans l'histoire de la chimiothérapie anticancéreuse.
Il n'est pas excessif de parler du pronostic des leucémies aiguës, des sarcomes ou des cancers du sein avant ou après la découverte des anthracyclines.
Pour ceux qui, comme moi, ont vécu cette histoire, le scepticisme dans la thérapeutique des cancers est devenu impossible : nous sommes devenus des "croyants" en chimiothérapie.
Toutefois, notre expérience nous a très vite enseigné que ces médicaments puissants étaient de maniement difficile, que l'intensité thérapeutique était nécessaire, que la toxicité hématologique était inévitable mais que le savoir-faire devait permettre de la surmonter : il n'y a pas d'ordre contemplatif pour les croyants en chimiothérapie anticancéreuse.

Enfin, l'histoire des anthracyclines nous enseigne que des modifications mineures modifient l'activité de ces médicaments (Adriamycine), qu'elles élargissent leur spectre d'activité ou qu'elles modifient leur cinétique d'action (Rubidazone).

L'intérêt clinique qui s'attache aux divers dérivés de première génération dont les indications thérapeutiques sont précises et diverses, justifie la poursuite de la recherche de dérivés nouveaux, d'où l'importance de la réunion qui va se dérouler.

Neo-Adjuvant Chemotherapy. Ed. Cl. Jacquillat, M. Weil, D. Khayat. Colloque INSERM/John Libbey Eurotext Ltd. © 1988. Vol. 169, pp. 799-802.

Historique des anthracyclines

Marise Weil

Groupe hospitalier Pitié-Salpétrière, Paris, France

C'est en 1962 que DUBOST isole un nouvel antibiotique d'une culture de streptomycine coeruleorubidus, la Rubidomycine. De leur côté, DI MARCO et ses collaborateurs isolent un antibiotique d'une culture de streptomyces peucitius la Daunomycine. L'étude de la structure de ces deux composés montre qu'ils sont identiques. Comme le disait Jean BERNARD, la Rubidomycine partage avec Homère et Shakespeare l'honneur d'une parternité disputée. Pour tenir compte de cette double paternité, le produit allait être appelé DAUNORUBICINE.

Son étude expérimentale a été assurée par René MARAL dont le souvenir doit être rappelé chaque fois qu'il est question des premières anthracyclines.
Dès cette époque, le mécanisme d'intercalation est décrit avec la fragmentation de l'ADN, la génération des radicaux libres, l'action membranaire.

L'étude clinique a été conduite à Saint Louis par Claude JACQUILLAT. En 1967, le Premier Colloque International sur la Daunorubicine mettait en évidence l'exceptionnelle activité de la Daunorubicine dans les leucémies aigues myéloblastiques où, pour la première fois, des taux de rémission complète supérieurs à 50 % étaient observés. Très vite on observe que les leucémies à promyélocytes constituaient en particulier une indication privilégiée.
A l'époque, la pharmacocinétique n'était guère à la mode et la posologie et le rythme d'administration furent empiriques. Il s'agissait d'obtenir le plus rapidement possible la rémission complète qui mettrait le malade à l'abri des infections et des hémorragies.
La dose unitaire avait été de 2 mg/kg, l'administration était quotidienne et la dose moyenne nécessaire avait été en moyenne de 11 mg/kg

Dans une étude avec l'A.L.G.B., 3 posologies avaient été étudiées :
- 60 mg/m^2 x 3 jours consécutifs,
- 60 mg/m^2 x 5 jours consécutifs,
- 60 mg/m^2 1 fois par semaine.

Les résultats du traitement hebdomadaire avaient été défavorables. Ceci n'étant pas lié sans doute à des propriéts pharmacocinétiques particulières du médicament mais à la cinétique des blastes et des cellules souches normales. D'ailleurs, en association avec Endoxan et Vincristine, ce rythme hebdomadaire avait donné des résultats convenables dans les lymphomes non-hodgkiniens.

Chez les 11 premiers enfants traités pour des rechutes, le traitement avait été poursuivi pendant la rémission et la dose totale avait été de plus de 40 mg/kg en 5 mois soit des doses supérieures à 1.500 mg/m². Chez 6 de ces enfants, une toxicité cardiaque a été observée après un intervalle libre de quelques mois. Chez un patient, l'intervalle a été particulièrement long puisque les signes cliniques de l'insuffisance cardiaque sont apparus en 1979 alors que la Daunorubicine avait été arrêtée en 1969. Il a bénéficié, il y a quelques mois, d'une greffe cardiaque et va très bien !

Comme vous le savez tous, cette insuffisance cardiaque est liée à une fibrose myocardique.
Dès cette époque, deux laboratoires, Rhône Poulenc en France, Farmitalia en Italie consacraient une activité importante à la recherche de nouveaux dérivés.

En 1969, Farmitalia produit l'Adriamycine par hydrolyse acide de la Daunorubicine.
Cette modification chimique, somme toute mineure, a des conséquences cliniques importantes : le spectre d'activité de l'Adriamycine est nettement plus large que celui de la Daunorubicine.

Si l'Adriamycine est moins efficace que la Daunorubicine dans le traitement des leucémies aigues, elle est en revanche plus active dans le traitement des lymphosarcomes non hodgkiniens et des tumeurs solides. A quoi attribuer des différences ?

Expérimentalement la demi-vie plasmatique et la rétention cellulaire sont plus longues pour l'Adriamycine que pour la Daunorubicine.
Au niveau de la cellule, l'incorporation est plus faible pour l'Adriamycine mais en raison d'une concentration lysosomiale moindre, la fixation au niveau de l'A.D.N. est plus importante.

L'Adriamycine a été utilisée selon plusieurs schémas :

Quotidien : 30 mg/m², 3 jours de suite (ostéosarcomes)
Intermittent : 75 mg/m², toutes les 3 semaines (CHOP)
Hebdomadaire : 35 mg/m², toutes les semaines (VTMFAP)

Eu égard à la toxicité locale des anthracyclines, les prescriptions d'administration avant l'avénement des réservoirs implantables visaient à réduire le plus possible la durée de contact entre le médicament et la paroi veineuse et nous recommandions que le produit soit injecté dans la tubulure et qu'ensuite la veine soit rincée.

Il existe des arguments valables en faveur de l'administration prolongée d'un certain nombre de produits : c'est le cas du 5 FU, de la Bléomycine, de la Cytosine Arabinoside et les réservoirs implantables, complétés par les pompes ambulatoires permettent d'avoir recours à ces traitements prolongés sans inconvénient pratique et psychologique pour nos patients.

Y-a-t-il des arguments en faveur des perfusions prolongées d'Adriamycine ?
Les données pharmacocinétiques chez l'homme n'apportent aucun arguement en faveur des perfusions I.V. prolongées. Par contre, deux études signalent une toxicité cardiaque réduite.

La notion de la perfusion intra-veineuse prolongée est d'ailleurs très variable, allant de 2 à 30 jours. Cette dernière posologie n'a fait l'objet d'aucune étude comparative.

Il est probable que nous ne pourrons pas répondre à cette question puisque de nouveaux dérivés sont actuellement en cours d'étude.
Avant que vous les abordiez, je voudrais vous parler de deux dérivés synthétisés par Rhône Poulenc tandis que Farmitalia développait l'Adriamycine.

La RUBIDAZONE ou Benzoyl Hydrazone DNR a été étudiée sur le plan expériemntal en 1972 par René MARAL. Il montra que ce dérivé semi-synthétique était moins toxique que la DNR chez la Souris, le Chien et le Lapin.

Une toxicité cardiaque était observée chez le Rat et le Hamster mais à des doses équitoxiques plus élevées que pour la DNR. L'index thérapeutique était double de celui de la DNR.

Chez la Souris, DEPREZ De CAMPANEERE, BAURAIN et TROUET ont montré que la demi-vie de la Rubidazone et sa répartition tissulaire suggèrent qu'elle est une pro-drogue de la DNR avec ses caractéristiques pharmacocinétiques propres.
Chez l'homme BENJAMIN et ses collègues ont montré que la disparition de la Rubidazone était plus lente que celle de la DNR avec une excrétion relativement diminuée de Daunorubicinol.

En 1972, nous avons entrepris les phases I et II et avons démontré l'activité importante de la Rubidazone dans les leucémies avec une moins grande brutalité d'action que pour la DNR. Nous préconisons des doses de l'ordre de 3 à 5 mg/kg, 5 jours de suite. Une ou deux doses additionnelles était(ent) donnée(s) si nécessaire. La dose nécessaire pour obtenir la rémission étant de l'ordre de 750 mg/m^2. BENJAMIN proposait lui, des doses voisines de 450 mg/m^2.

Dans deux circonstances, la Rubidazone nous paraissait nettement supérieure à la DNR en raison de sa cinétique d'action différente :
- les leucémies aiguës de l'adulte en particulier les leucémies aiguës lymphoblastiques ;
- et les leucémies monoblastiques où la libération brutale d'une grande quantité de lysozyme résultant d'une lyse cellulaire trop brutale peut entraîner des accidents rénaux irréversibles.

Si la Rubidazone a eu la carrière honorable qu'elle méritait, il n'en est pas de même pour la Diethoxyacétoxy DNR ou Détorubicine également étudiée expérimentalement par René MARAL.

L'étude pharmacocinétique que nous avons conduite chez l'homme avec Claude BONNET et J. KHAYAT a montré que la Détorubicine se transformait très rapidement en Doxorubicine mais que celle-ci avait une répartition tissulaire différente de la Doxorubicine originaire. Toujours est-il que la Détorubicine est un médicament actif dans les lymphomes et dans les sarcomes des tissus mous. L'étude de ce produit pourtant intéressant mais dont le spectre d'activité était voisin de celui de l'Adriamycine a été interrompu par arrêt de sa synthèse.

Avoir participé de très près aux premières études des anthracyclines est un privilège qui convainc de l'intérêt de la chimiothérapie.
Il est intéressant de noter qu'au-delà de leurs propriétés communes, ces dérivés de première génération, peut-être en raison de leur cinétique d'activité propre, ont une spécificité relative : à telle variété de leucémies tel dérivé ; aux tumeurs solides, la Doxorubicine ou l'un de ses dérivés.
Des faits semblables doivent sans doute être recherchés pour les anthracyclines de 2ème génération, la 4'épirubicine et la Pirarubicine en particulier.

Neo-Adjuvant Chemotherapy. Ed. Cl. Jacquillat, M. Weil, D. Khayat. Colloque INSERM/John Libbey Eurotext Ltd. © 1988. Vol. 169, pp. 803-806.

Activité expérimentale de la THP-doxorubicine

F. Lavelle

Département de Cancérologie, Centre de Recherches de Vitry, Rhône-Poulenc Santé, BP 14, 94403 Vitry-sur-Seine Cedex, France

La daunorubicine (DNR) et la doxorubicine (DOX) ont suscité de nombreux travaux de microbiologie et de chimie visant à obtenir de nouvelles anthracyclines d'efficacité antitumorale et/ou d'indice thérapeutique améliorés. Plus d'une centaine d'anthracyclines d'origine naturelle et plus d'un millier d'analogues obtenus par hémisynthèse et par synthèse totale sont actuellement connus (1).

Des modifications portant sur la fonction OH présente en 4' sur le sucre permettent de moduler l'activité et la toxicité de la doxorubicine (2). C'est ainsi qu'a été obtenue par hémisynthèse la 4'-O-tétrahydropyranyldoxorubicine (THP-DOX) dans le groupe d'H. UMEZAWA au Japon (3).

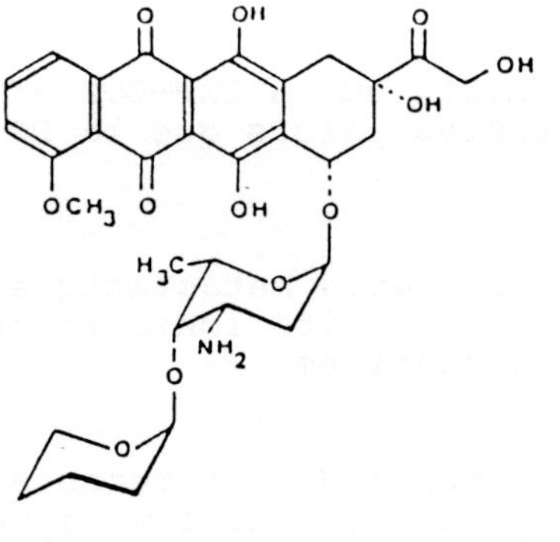

Activité antitumorale expérimentale

La THP-DOX a fait l'objet d'études comparatives avec la DOX dans plusieurs laboratoires (3, 4, 5, 6).

Les résultats sont résumés dans le tableau ci-dessous.

Tumeurs	THP-DOX	DOX
L1210 (ip/ip)	++	++
L1210 (ip/iv)	++	+
3LL	++	+
3LL métastatique	++	-
C26	+	++
C38	++	++
M5076	++	-
B16	+	-
L1210 (+ cis DDP)	++	-

Les différences d'activité les plus significatives ont été obtenues :

1/ Sur la leucémie L1210 où la THP-DOX administrée i.v. exerce une activité curative, alors que la DOX ne conduit qu'à des rémissions.

2/ Sur le carcinome de Lewis métastatique (3LL) où seule la THP-DOX exerce une activité inhibitrice sur la croissance des métastases pulmonaires.

3/ Sur l'histiocytosarcome M 5076 métastatique où là encore seule la THP-DOX, administrée i.v. après exérèse de la tumeur primaire, réduit le nombre des métastases hépatiques.

4/ Sur le carcinome du colon C26 où cette fois la DOX présente une efficacité supérieure à celle de la THP-DOX.

5/ Sur la leucémie L1210 où la THP-DOX exerce une activité synergique avec le cis DDP.

Toxicologie

La cardiotoxicité expérimentale comparative de la THP-DOX et de la DOX a été tout particulièrement étudiée par DANTCHEV et coll. (7).

La THP-DOX et la DOX sont administrées, à doses équithérapeutiques chez la souris, 3 fois/semaine pendant 4 semaines consécutives chez des hamsters dorés (dose unitaire 3 mg/kg).

La cardiotoxicité est évaluée après étude histologique du muscle cardiaque (8) :

Score de cardiotoxicité

Produit	1 sem.	2 sem.	3 sem.	4 sem.
THP-DOX	0-1	1	1-2	1-2
DOX	1-2	2-3	2-3	

Il s'avère donc qu'administrée à doses équithérapeutiques chez la souris, la THP-DOX apparaît moins cardiotoxique que la DOX dans un modèle d'administration chronique chez le hamster.

La THP-DOX administrée par voie i.v. en traitement unique est plus myelotoxique que la DOX chez le chien et le singe.

La THP-DOX a fait l'objet d'une étude de toxicité chronique chez le rat (i.p.; doses : 0,005 - 0,6 mg/kg/semaine pendant 6 mois). Le profil de toxicité générale et les impacts sont identiques à ceux que l'on note avec la DOX. Ni nouvelle toxicité, ni toxicité retardée n'ont été observées.

CONCLUSION

La THP-DOX répond aux critères expérimentaux requis pour l'étude clinique d'un nouvel analogue d'anthracyclines :

- activité antitumorale expérimentale supérieure à celle de la DOX, à doses équitoxiques sur le plan général
- diminution de la cardiotoxicité, à doses équithérapeutiques avec la DOX
- absence de nouvelle toxicité et de toxicité retardée.

(1) Progress in Medicinal Chemistry, 21, 1984, 169-236

(2) Cancer Res., 45, 1985, 5995-5999

(3) J. Antibiotics, 32, 1979, 1082-1085

(4) Cancer Res., 42, 1982, 1462-1467

(5) Anthracyclines : Current status and future developments MASSON Edit., 30, 183-188

(6) Proceedings 15th International Congress of Chemotherapy, 1987, 606

(7) Biomedicine and Pharmacotherapy, 38, 1984, 322-328

(8) Cancer Treat. Rep., 62, 1978, 865-879

Neo-Adjuvant Chemotherapy. Ed. Cl. Jacquillat, M. Weil, D. Khayat. Colloque INSERM/John Libbey Eurotext Ltd. © 1988. Vol. 169, pp. 807-810.

Pharmacocinétique de la THP-adriamycine

J. Robert

Fondation Bergonié, Bordeaux, France

INTRODUCTION

De nombreux analogues d'anthracyclines ont été synthétisés, mais peu d'entre eux sont entrés en pratique clinique. Un nouveau composé, la pirarubicine (4'-O-tétrahydropyranyldoxorubicine, figure 1) provient du laboratoire d'Umezawa (1). Il est entré en phase II en Europe, en particulier dans un essai ouvert organisé par l'EORTC. Dans notre Centre de Lutte contre le Cancer, douze malades ont été inclus, dont six ont fait l'objet d'une analyse pharmacocinétique détaillée. Une étude sur la pharmacocinétique de la pirarubicine a été publiée en 1987 (2) et des présentations préliminaires ont été faites (3, 4). Toutes sont basées sur des injections en flash réalisées toutes les trois semaines. Nous présentons ici nos résultats obtenus après des injections fractionnées sur trois jours consécutifs.

Figure 1
Structure de la pirarubicine

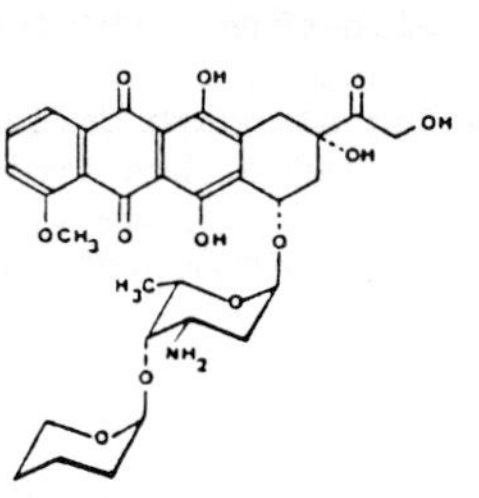

MALADES ET METHODES

Six malades (cinq femmes et un homme) sont entrés dans l'étude pharmacocinétique. Leur âge médian était de 55 ans (limites : 33 et 68) et tous avaient un cancer progressif, prouvé par l'histologie. Ils avaient tous été lourdement prétraités et quatre avaient reçu auparavant de la doxorubicine. Ils n'avaient aucun signe d'insuffisance hépatique ou rénale et avaient une qualité de vie de grade OMS 1 ou 2.

Les injections de pirarubicine ont duré de 3 à 5 minutes et des échantillons de sang ont été obtenus après chaque injection quotidienne aux temps suivants : 5, 10, 20, 40 min ; 1, 2, 4, 8, 12 et 24 heures ; un prélèvement a été également réalisé 48 et 72 heures après la dernière injection. Le sang était recueilli sur des tubes à EDTA et centrifugé immédiatement. Le plasma a été conservé à - 30° jusqu'à l'analyse. Les urines ont été recueillies par fractions de 12 heures pendant les trois jours de traitement et par fractions de 24 heures pendant les deux jours suivants. Elles ont été filtrées si nécessaire et congelées jusqu'à l'analyse.

Une quantité connue de daunorubicine a été ajoutée aux échantillons comme standard interne ; l'extraction de la pirarubicine et de ses métabolites a été réalisée sur des colonnes de silice greffée C18 (Sep-pak, Waters), comme nous l'avons déjà publié pour la doxorubicine (5). Nous avons vérifié que cette technique permettait d'obtenir un rendement quantitatif. Une chromatographie liquide à haute performance a été réalisée sur colonne de microbondapak C-18 (Waters) avec un mélange tampon formiate d'ammonium/acétonitrile (66/34) comme phase mobile, avec un flux de 3 ml/min. La détection était faite grâce à un spectrophotomètre Perkin-Elmer modèle LS1, avec une longueur d'onde d'excitation de 480 nm et une longueur d'onde d'émission de 592 nm. Dans ces conditions, une séparation complète de tous les pics fluorescents présents dans le plasma est réalisée en environ sept minutes. L'identification des pics a été faite par comparaison des temps de rétention avec ceux de standards connus.

Les données concernant la pirarubicine ont été traitées selon un modèle non-linéaire déjà utilisé (6), basé sur l'équation donnant la concentration plasmatique C(t) en fonction du temps t :

$$C(t) = \frac{D}{T} \sum_{i=1}^{i=n} A_i \left(e^{\alpha_i T} - 1\right) e^{-\alpha_i t}$$

dans laquelle D est la dose injectée, T la durée de l'injection, Ai et αi les paramètres de chaque courbe exponentielle et n le nombre de compartiments. Les données concernant les métabolites ont été traitées sans modélisation ; les demi-vies d'élimination ont été calculées par régression linéaire et les aires sous la courbe (AUC) selon la règle du trapèze.

RESULTATS

Un maximum de quatre pics ont été observés dans les extraits plasmatiques et urinaires après injection de pirarubicine. Ce sont, par ordre de polarité croissante, la pirarubicine elle-même, la 13-dihydropirarubicine (pirarubicinol), la doxorubicine et le doxorubicinol.

Pour la pirarubicine elle-même, un modèle à deux compartiments rendait mieux compte des résultats expérimentaux qu'un modèle à trois compartiments ; avec ce dernier, la déviation standard de la valeur estimée était généralement plus grande que l'estimée elle-même. Les trois courbes plasmatiques successives étaient tout à fait semblables (figure 2) et aucune différence significative n'a pu être détectée entre les paramètres pharmacocinétiques obtenus les jours 1, 2, et 3. Les valeurs de ces paramètres (± SEM) sont présentées ci-dessous :

$A = 3{,}24 \pm 0{,}53 \times 10^{-3}\ L^{-1}$
$B = 3{,}71 \pm 0{,}27 \times 10^{-4}\ L^{-1}$
$\alpha = 2{,}19 \pm 0{,}20\ h^{-1}$ (demi-vie de distribution = 22 min)
$\beta = 0{,}0578 \pm 0{,}0032\ h^{-1}$ (demi-vie d'élimination = 13 h)
Clairance plasmatique totale = $90{,}4 \pm 4{,}9\ L \cdot h^{-1} \cdot m^{-2}$
Volume total de distribution = $1\,449 \pm 138\ L \cdot m^{-2}$

Le principal métabolite de la pirarubicine est la doxorubicine ; sa concentration est très faible après la première injection mais augmente progressivement de jour en jour (figure 2) ; elle devient même supérieure à celle de la pirarubicine à partir du troisième jour de traitement. Le rapport des aires sous la courbe doxorubicine/pirarubicine, mesurées pendant les 24 heures qui suivaient chaque injection, ont été les suivants :
jour 1 : 0,428 ; jour 2 : 0,607 ; jour 3 : 0,780.

Les autres métabolites identifiés de la pirarubicine sont le pirarubicinol et le doxorubicinol ; tous les deux ne sont présents dans le plasma qu'à faible concentration ; alors que le pirarubicinol est resté pratiquement inchangé pendant les trois jours de traitement, le doxorubicinol augmente progressivement en suivant une courbe analogue à celle de la doxorubicine.

L'excrétion urinaire totale cumulée de la pirarubicine et de ses métabolites n'a jamais excédé 5 % de la dose injectée. Les quantités absolues de pirarubicine et de pirarubicinol dans l'urine sont constantes dans les fractions 0-12 h et 12-24 h respectivement ; les quantités absolues de doxorubicine et doxorubicinol dans l'urine augmentent en revanche progressivement de jour en jour pendant et après le traitement. Par conséquent, la proportion de doxorubicine parmi les produits fluorescents excrétés dans l'urine, qui n'était que de 20 % le premier jour, s'élève à 60 % deux jours après la fin du traitement.

Figure 2

Evolution des concentrations plasmatiques de pirarubicine (trait plein) et de son principal métabolite, la doxorubicine (pointillés) au cours d'un traitement de 3 jours par pirarubicine

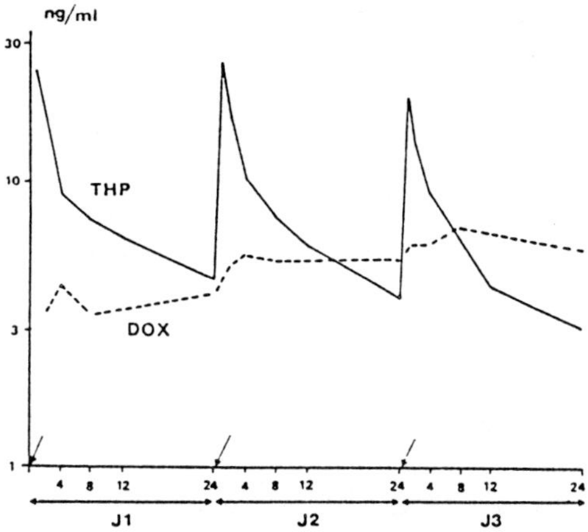

DISCUSSION

Le comportement pharmacocinétique de la pirarubicine inchangée dans le plasma est similaire à celui décrit par Miller et Schmidt (2). Ces auteurs ont observé cependant une phase de distribution très rapide, de demi-vie 1 à 4 minutes, avant les deux phases que nous avons étudiées. Ils ont également trouvé, dès la première injection, des taux de doxorubicine circulante beaucoup plus élevés que les nôtres. Raber et al. (4) ont posé la question de savoir si la présence de doxorubicine dans les échantillons était réelle ou artefactuelle. Nous pensons que la doxorubicine est un métabolite réel de la pirarubicine puisqu'il est possible d'en observer l'accumulation ; une production artefactuelle ou une contamination pré-existante aurait donné des résultats identiques les trois jours de traitement. Cependant, les taux très élevés observés par Miller et Schmidt (2) peuvent être en partie dus à une dégradation de la pirarubicine avant l'analyse.

L'accumulation progressive de doxorubicine et de doxorubicinol dans le plasma et l'urine après une injection de pirarubicine est probablement liée à la demi-vie prolongée de ces composés, qui est de 30 à 40 heures, alors que la demi-vie de la pirarubicine n'est que de 13 à 14 heures. La doxorubicine est la principale espèce moléculaire circulante dans le plasma à partir du troisième jour de traitement. Si la pirarubicine a des propriétés spécifiques intéressantes en termes de spectre antitumoral ou de cardiotoxicité, comme on peut le penser à la suite des études précliniques (7), cette originalité peut être perdue par un schéma d'administration inapproprié qui aboutit à la formation de quantités appréciables de doxorubicine. Le retour à des intervalles classiques de trois semaines doit donc être suggéré à la suite de notre travail.

REFERENCES

(1) Umezawa H, Takahashi Y, Kinoshita M et al. J Antibiot 1979 ; 32 : 1082-4.
(2) Miller AA, Schmidt GG. Cancer Res 1987 ; 47 : 1461-5.
(3) Majima H, Iguchi H, Tone H. Jap J Cancer Chemother 1986 ; 13 : 542-8.
(4) Raber M, Legha S, Gorski C, Krakoff I. Proc Am Assoc Cancer Res 1987 ; 28 : 223.
(5) Robert J. J Liq Chromatogr 1980 ; 3 : 1561-72.
(6) Robert J, Bui NB, Vrignaud P. Eur J Clin Pharmacol 1987 ; 31 : 695-9.
(7) Dantchev D, Paintrand M, Hayat M, Bourut C, Mathé G. J Antibiot 1979 ; 32 : 1085-6.

Neo-Adjuvant Chemotherapy. Ed. Cl. Jacquillat, M. Weil, D. Khayat. Colloque INSERM/John Libbey Eurotext Ltd. © 1988. Vol. 169, pp. 811-812.

Cellular response to pirarubicin

Haim Tapiero

Département de Pharmacologie Cellulaire, Moléculaire et de Pharmacocinétique, I.C.I.G. (CNRS UA 1163), Hôpital Paul Brousse, 14, avenue Paul Vaillant Couturier, 94800 Villejuif, France

The majority of malignancies occuring in the adult population are refractory to presently available chemotherapy. This raised the perplexing questions about the reasons for failure of drugs. One of the most probable reason is the low concentration of drug at the site(s) of action.

It is function of dose given which recognizes the magnitude of the response by optimally balancing the desirable and the undesirable effects. How aften and how long recognizes the importance of time. It will depend upon the pharmacokinetics phase and thus relates the dose frequency and the route of administration to drug concentration. Our aim here is to study the relationship between accumulation, retention and cytotoxicity of anthracyclines which belong to doxorubicin derivatives. The cellular uptake of the new anthracycline pirarubicin is 50 times faster than that of doxorubicin. The subcellular distribution analysis shows that more than 95 % of either doxorubicin or pirarubicin is accumulated and retained in the nuclear fraction. Since the cytotoxic effect of anthracyclines is related to the amount accumulated, we assumed that following short cell exposure to the same drug concentration, pirarubicine will be more cytotoxic than the less rapidly incorporated doxorubicin. This assumption was supported by our results in which ID50 was observed after 100 minutes exposure to 0.1 ug/ml doxorubicin whereas the same effect was reached after only 2 minutes exposure to pirarubicin. Moreover, uptake is a passive process and since the rate of incorporation varies between pirarubicin and doxorubicin one can expect that cell density is an important parameter in the modulation of the intracellular concentration. Here we show that in contrast to doxorubicin the intracellular amount of pirarubicin decrease with the cell density. Because the uptake of pirarubicin occurs differently, it is postulated that the administration modalities have to be modulated according to the characteristics of this drug, the size and the localization of the tumor.

Another parameter related to treatment failure is the relative development of resistance in tumors initially responsive to treatement.

How patients with malignancies usually sensitive to various drugs rapidly develop broad based resistance during relapse is still unknown. Despite the appearance of a form of multidrug resistance (MDR) in these patients, little is known about its biochemical expressions in contrast to the clinical situation. The relationship and function of the biochemical and pharmacological features to experimental and especially clinical MDR are presently unknown. Here we show that the level of resistance to pirarubicin is significantly lower than doxorubicin or daunorubicin in cells with high level of resistance to these latter drugs. This low level of resistance is associated with higher accumulation of drug in these resistant cells.

Recently, we have shown that intracellular accumulation of doxorubicin or daunorubicin was found to be increased in human breast carcinoma cell line (MDF-7) or colon carcinoma (HT-29) as compared to an epithelial cell line derived from monkey kidney (CV-1).

This increase correlates with greater sensitivity of the carcinoma cell line to doxorubicin. Here, we demonstrate that normal epithelial CV-1 cells are 20 to 40 times more sensitive to pirarubicin than to doxorubicin. Human breast carcinoma cells are significantly more sensitive to pirarubicin than CV-1 cells. These data demonstrate selectivity for doxorubicin and pirarubicin in human breast and colon carcinoma cell lines. Moreover, in the cell types with acquired or intrinsic resistance considered here, it appears that transport, accumulation and consequently cytotoxicity differs between pirarubicin and doxorubicin. It is therefore suggested that pirarubicin may be a relative good alternative compound in tumour cells resistant to doxorubicin or daunorubicin.

Neo-Adjuvant Chemotherapy. Ed. Cl. Jacquillat, M. Weil, D. Khayat. Colloque INSERM/John Libbey Eurotext Ltd. © 1988. Vol. 169, pp. 813-819.

A phase II trial of tetrahydropyranyl-doxorubicin in patients with advanced breast cancer

J.M. Extra[1], S. Leandri[1], M. Espie[1], F. Morvan[2], L. Mignot[3], C. Ferme[1] and M. Marty[1]

[1] *Dpt of Medical Oncology, Hôpital Saint-Louis, Paris, France*
[2] *Dpt of Medical Oncology, Centre Hospitalier, Pontoise, France*
[3] *Dpt of Medical Oncology, C.M.C. Foch, Suresnes, France*
[4] *Dpt of Medical Oncology, CMS Bligny, Bligny, France*

INTRODUCTION

Tetrahydropyrannyl doxorubicin is a new class 2 anthracycline with experimental antitumor activity similar to that of doxorubicin and very reduced, if any, cardiotoxicity. Phase I trials have shown that leucopenia was the dose limiting toxicity and that dose levels of 60 mg/m² in good risk patients (pts) and 45 mg/m² in poor risk patients every 3 weeks could be recommanded.

We therefore initiated a phase II study in women with advanced breast cancer to evaluate potential antitumor activity of THPA.

MATERIALS AND METHODS

Eligibility criteria

Women with pathological confirmation of adenocarcinoma of the breast were eligible if they had :

- demonstrated metastatic progression except for isolated CNS metastasis ;
- failed conventionnal chemo/or hormonotherapy,
- life-expectancy > 8 weeks.

Patients with evidence of bone-marrow failure (leucocytes < 3 G/l and/or platelets < 100 G/l) except when due to bone-marrow involvement, of severe liver dysfunction (>WHO grade 2), or renal failure (>WHO grade 2) or cardiac dysfunction were not eligible.

On the other hand previous anthracyclin therapy whatever the doses used or previous aminoanthraquinone therapy nor heart irradiation were criteria for ineligibility.

Drug administration

THPA -provided by R. Bellon laboratories- was administered as a short (10 minutes) IV infusion.
Starting dose was 45 mg/m² in patients at risk for neutropenia (abnormal counts prior THPA, extended field radiation therapy, prior severe neutropenia, prior ametycine therapy >45mg/m².

Other patients received a dose of 60 mg/m².

THPA was administered IV every three weeks or at longer intervals in case of toxicity.

Patients monitoring
Prior THPA physical examination and adequate ultra-sound radiologic or nuclear imaging to measure at least 1 metastatic site were performed. Complete blood cell counts, electrolytes renal and liver function tests as well as EKG and measure of left-ventricular function were done.

During therapy physical examination, complete blood cell counts, electrolytes, renal and liver function tests as well as EKG were performed weekly for the first 6 weeks. Thereafter, those examinations were conducted every 3 weeks or when clinically indicated.

Evaluation of tumor masses was done every 2 courses or if clinically suggested.

Toxicity was assessed according to WHO grading recommandations.

RESULTS

Patients characteristics
From September 1986 to December 1987, 32 patients were enrolled in this study.Two patients were not eligible (bone marrow and liver failure) or had major protocole violation (1 pt). Twenty nine patients are evaluable for toxicity and 26 for antitumor activity ; one is too early.

Main characteristics of these patients are shown in table 1. 24/31 pts had previously received antineoplastic chemotherapy either as adjuvant chemotherapy and/or as treatment of metastatic progression. Details on main cytotoxic agents previously received are shown in table 2. Patients had a median number of 3 measurable/evaluable distinct metastatic sites. The most significant are described in table 3.

Pretherapeutic tolerance parameters are shown in table 4 : 6 pts had leucocytes < 4 G/1 and or platelets < 100 G/1 ; in 3 of them bone marrow involvement was demonstrated. Two patients had pre-existing cardiac abnormalities thought to be compatible with the treatment : in none of them was it attributed to previous anthracycline therapy. Four patients had severe liver dysfunction related to liver metastasis. Finally 2 of them had increased serum creatinine related to hypercalcemia.

In relation to heavy prior therapy and poor condition of most patients in this study starting dose was 60 mg/m2 in 9 pts and 45 mg/m2 in 22.

TOXIC EVENTS
Toxicity was evaluated in 29 pts , as 1 pt had received THPA for less than 3 weeks.

Leucopenia:

Leucopenia has been the major side effect. Grade related to dose level is shown in table 5 depicting the most severe event in each patient. All patients experienced leucopenia during at least one course of therapy. While in most cases leukopenia -even if severe- appeared of short duration (<5 days), it was responsible for 2 toxic deaths in those patients (at day 22 in 1 pt with grade 3 hyperbilirubinemia ; at day 75, after a third course in one patient treated with 60 mg/m2). Leucopenia was not cumulative in those patients who received more than 2 courses. It was somewhat impredictible, as the most severe event occurred between 1st and 3d course without any significant relationship to clinical and biological parameters as determined before each course. Although dose was selected according to "hematolgical risk", no clear relation between dose and grade of toxicity is apparent in that study.

Thrombocytopenia

Thrombocytopenia was a much rarer event. Five patients experienced grade I thrombocytopenia, 3 grade II, 1 grade III and 1 grade IV, for a 34 % overall incidence of thrombocytopenia : the grade III and IV were seen in those 2 pts with reduced pretherapeutic platelet count. In all cases thrombocytopenia was associated with grade III or IV leucopenia.

Nausea and vomiting

Digestive tolerance of THP-dox has been good : 9 pts experienced grade I nausea, 10 grade II although no specific antiemetic therapy was given. Such 65 % incidence of minor nausea and vomiting was almost completely abrogated by subsequent antiemetic therapy.

Alopecia

Alopecia has been minimal with 5 pts experiencing grade 1 alopecia (24 %)

Liver abnormalities

Only those abnormalities which appeared or worsened during THP-Dox therapy were taken into account whatever their cause has been ; they were seen in 6 (20 %) pts.

- 3 pts showed increased serum bilirubin (gr 1 in 2, 2 in 1), without clinical or therapeutic consequences, and associated with increased transaminases.
- 6 pts had grade I increased in transaminases.

Renal dysfunction

No renal dysfunction other than related to hypercalcemia or infectious shock (1 pt) was seen.

Cardiac tolerance

Cardiac events (arythmia) occurred in 2 pts, one of them with anamnesis of supraventricular arythmia. Relationship with THP-Dox appears doubtful. Those 2 patients with prior cardiac abnormalities did tolerate well drug administration. No cumulative cardiac toxicity was observed in those patients, even when they received large cumulative doses after prior anthracyclines/aminoanthraquinone therapy (table 6).

Deaths

Six patients eventually died while on study (table 7) : 2 deaths are clearly due to septicemia in patients with grade IV drug-related neutropenia. A of them had grade 3 hyperbilirubinemia before initiation of THP-Dox. The other patients died of progressive disease.

RESPONSES

Only those patients having received at least two courses of THP-Dox and showing at least a 50 % tumor regression for at least 2 courses (40 days) have been taken into account : 5 partial responses (but no complete response) have been observed in 26 patients evaluable for a response rate of 19 %.

Responses were observed in nodes, skin, bone, lung and liver metastasis. Whenever response was observed, THP-Dox was used as maintenance therapy. Duration of response have been 60 days, 75 days, 120+ days, 180+ days, 365 days.

Two minor responses of 90 days duration were observed.

DISCUSSION

In this phase II study of THP-Dox in advanced breast cancer, a 20 % response rate was observed in heavily pretreated patients. As 3/5 PR were observed at a dose level of 60 mg/m2 while 9 pts were treated at that dose level, there is a suggestion that a dose effect relationship might exist. This dose as well as heavy prior chemo-hormonotherapy may account for a lower response rate as compared to other studies (P. Pouillart, personnal communication). Such a response rate is indeed suggestive of significant activity in such patients. Neutropenia has been the major side effect, encountered in all patients. Although of short duration, it may be associated with life-threatening infections ; severity of neutropenia did not correlate well with the dose used ; liver dysfunction and specifically hyperbilirubinemia could be associated with more severe myelosuppression. Thrombocytopenia was infrequent.

Non hematological toxicities appear very limited with THP-Dox: nausea and vomiting have been mild, alopecia rare ; no liver or renal abnormalities could be unequivocally attributed to THP-Dox. Finally the drug appears to have very little if any cardiotoxicity.
THP-Dox appears to be an active agent in metastatic breast cancer even after anthracycline therapy. Its lack of non hematological toxicity can allow for association with non myelosuppressive agents. On the other hand if THP-Dox was to be used with myelosuppressive agents, dose reduction should be defined.

Other schedules, such as the weekly schedule should be studied in view of the very short duration of neutropenia.

Age (median,range) :	59y (35-75)			
Metastatic progression number	1	2	3	>3
	4 pts	10	15	2

	Number of pts
Previous adjuvant chemotherapy	14
Without anthracyclines	2
With anthracyclines	12
Previous chemotherapy for metastasis	24
1 regimen :	10
2 regimen :	9
3 regimen :	4
>3 regimen:	1
Previous hormone-therapy for mets	19
Previously received anticancer agents	
none	7
4	3
5	9
6	2
7	3
8	7
Distinct metastatic organ sites:	
1	3
2	4
3	10
4	4
5	7
6	3
Status (WHO) 0-2	21
3-4	10

Table 1 : main characteristics of the treated patients.

	Nb of patients	dose (median, range) mg/m2
Cyclophosphamide	24	5400 (1800 - 13000)
Methotrexate	24	2700 (140 - 7500)
Class I anthracyclines	21	225 (90 - 400)
Fluorouracile	20	10000 (700 - 30000)
Vinca	18	12 (6 - 30)
Ametycine	17	30 (10 - 60)
Mitoxantrone	14	60 (25 - 100)
Ellipticinium	9	720 (150 - 1000)

Table 2 : Cytotoxic agents previously received. Doxorubicine and 4'epidoxorubicine have been gathered as class I anthracyclines using a conversion factor of .75 for epirubicin. Vincristine and vindesine have also been grouped using a conversion factor of .5 for vindesine

Metastatic sites	Number of patients with
Lung	21
Bone	20
Liver	20
Soft tissue	19
Lymph nodes	15
Peritoneum	4
Ovary	3
G.I. tract	2

Table 3 : main metastatic sites. No CNS involvement was clinically demonstrated at initiation of THP-doxorubicine.

	Grade 0	GrI	Gr II	Gr III	Gr IV
Leucocytes	23	6	0	0	0
Platelets	27	2	0	0	0
Heart	27	1	1	0	0
Alopecia	24	0	2	5	0
Liver					
Bilirubin	24	3	0	2	0
Transaminases	21	4	4	0	0
Alkaline phosph.	18	3	5	1	1
Serum creat.	26	2	1	0	0
Serum calcium	26	2	1	0	0

Table 4 : pretherapeutic toxicity parametters (29 patients)

Dose level (mg/m²)	number evaluable	Gr I	Gr II	Gr III	Gr IV
45	20	3	3	8	6
60	9	0	1	4	4

Table 5 : leucopenia during phase II study. The most severe event in any single patient has been selected.

n° of patient	Prior AC dose	Prior DHAD dose	THP-DOX dose
1	360	0	225
2	0	0	180
3	150	0	135
4	120	0	135
5	225	0	120
6	0	0	135
7	120	24	270
8	225	30	135
9	0	0	135
10	225	24	225
11	400	60	45
12	0	0	125
13	90	72	60
14	360	0	360
15	260	0	270
16	0	30	180
17	180	72	135
18	250	0	135
19	350	72	225
20	120	100	135
21	0	37	120
22	140	0	60
23	0	68	270
24	180	0	720
25	1200	0	660
26	280	30	225
27	0	0	180
28	180	30	90
29	250	40	60

Table 6 : cumulative doses (mg/sqm) of class I anthracyclines (AC), mitoxantrone (DHAD) and THP-Dox in the study patients. Doxorubicine and 4'epidoxorubicine have been gathered as class I anthracyclines using a conversion factor of .75 for epirubicin.

Initial status	date of death	primary cause for death
3	32	Lung progression
1	112	Lung and liver progression
4	37	Costal metastatic fractures
2	70	Neutropenia/infection
2	22	Neutropenia/infection
3	35	Progression

Table 7 : deaths during study.

Neo-Adjuvant Chemotherapy. Ed. Cl. Jacquillat, M. Weil, D. Khayat. Colloque INSERM/John Libbey Eurotext Ltd. © 1988. Vol. 169, pp. 821-822.

La pirarubicine (THP-adriamycine) dans les cancers du sein avancés en première ligne. Un essai phase II multicentrique avec doses fractionnées (3 jours)

P. Fumoleau*, P. Kerbrat, A. Monnier, M. Spielmann, B. Chevallier, A. Cattan, C. Chevreau, T. Delozier, M. Mousseau, B. Coiffier, M.J. Goudier, M. Namer et P. Herait

* *Centre René Gauducheau, 44035 Nantes, France*

La THP-ADRIAMYCINE est une nouvelle anthracycline obtenue par hémisynthèse à partir de la Doxorubicine par H. UMEZAWA et coll. La découverte représente l'aboutissement de recherches visant à obtenir de nouvelles anthracyclines ayant un index thérapeutique supérieur à la dauno et doxorubicine.

Plusieurs essais cliniques, phase I, ont été réalisés tant au Japon (MAJIMA, OGAWA, OKA et WAKI) qu'en Europe (KLEEBERG et MATHE). A partir de ces résultats, plusieurs schémas thérapeutiques ont été proposés pour les phases II : 20 à 50 mg/m^2 en bolus IV q. 3 semaines, 20-25 mg/m^2 J1, 2, 3 toutes les 3 semaines, 20 mg/m^2 par semaine, 7 mg/m^2 J1 à J5 toutes les 3 semaines.

OKA a publié en 1984 une synthèse des phases II effectuées au Japon. La plupart des différents chémas qu'il proposait à l'issue des résultats de la phase I ont été utilisés. Pour les cancers du sein avancés (2/3 ayant déjà reçu une chimiothérapie et 1/5 une anthracycline), le taux de réponse est de 24 %.

En tenant compte de ces publications, des résultats phases I et II obtenus par MATHE et coll., des données pharmacocinétiques (TAPIERO) et pour harmoniser ce protocole avec l'essai phase II, CLINICAL SCREENING GROUP, la dose initialement retenue a été 25 mg/m^2/jour 3 jours consécutifs toutes les 3 semaines mais, compte tenu de neutropénies sévères lors de la première cure, la dose de départ a été ensuite ramenée à 20 mg/m^2/J.

Le but de cet essai phase II est donc de définir l'efficacité antitumorale et la toxicité de la PIRARUBICINE en première ligne chez des malades atteintes de cancer du sein avancé.

Les critères d'inclusion sont ceux classiquement retenus pour un essai phase II en retenant qu'il s'agit d'une étude de chimiothérapie de première ligne en phase avancée : les patientes antérieurement traitées par chimiothérapie adjuvante avec ou sans anthracycline sont éligibles à condition que le délai entre la fin de la chimiothérapie adjuvante et l'inclusion dans l'étude soit supérieur à un an, que la dose cumulée antérieure d'anthracyclines en mg équivalentes soit inférieure à 300 mg/m^2, d'un bilan cardiologique normal (clinique, ECG, écho). Les cibles "os seul" ont été exclues.

Onze centres ont participé à l'essai. 51 patientes ont été incluses, 49 sont éligibles avec les caractéristiques suivantes :

- âge moyen : 54 ans avec des extrêmes de 36 et 67 ans.
- post-ménopause : 31/49 (63 %), pré-ménopause 18/49 (37 %).

- Trente et une patientes (63 %) n'ont pas reçu de chimiothérapie adjuvante. Dix-huit ont été traitées en adjuvant par CMF dans 5 cas, avec anthracyclines dans 13 cas (dose moyenne : 280 mg/m^2, extrême 95-300 mg/m^2).

- Toutes les patientes ont une ou plusieurs cibles (viscérales, ganglionnaires ou tissu mou) mesurables, répondant aux critères d'éligibilité Les plus souvent rencontrées sont les localisations au niveau des tissus mous (30 %), hépatiques (26 %) et pulmonaires (24 %).

La posologie de départ a été de 3 x 25 mg/m^2 compte tenu de la modification du protocole.

I) L'évaluation de la réponse a été faite selon les critères d'évaluation internationaux. 37 patientes sont actuellement évaluables pour la réponse et 12 non évaluables (9 trop tôt, 2 décès toxiques précoces et 1 décès précoce non lié à la drogue (embolie pulmonaire sur phlébite).

Le taux de réponse est de 43 % avec un intervalle de confiance (27-59) dont 5 réponses complètes, 11 réponses partielles et 1 seule progression. Pour les 27 patientes non précédemment traitées en adjuvant, il est retrouvé 3 réponses complètes et 9 réponses partielles avec un taux de réponse de 44 %. La durée des réponses est de 1 à 9 mois +. Pour les 10 patientes précédemment traitées en adjuvant, il est retrouvé 2 réponses partielles et 2 réponses complètes. La durée des réponses est de 2 à 5 mois +.

L'analyse des réponses en fonction du site tumoral permet de retrouver les taux de réponses suivants : Foie 1/13 (8 %), Poumon 5/12 (42 %), Ganglion 8/11 (73 %), Sein et Tissus sous-cutanés 9/15 (60 %).

II) La toxicité maximale hématologique évaluée par le grade, observée au moment du nadir est la suivante :

1°) neutropénie grade (3+4) 72 % au moment du nadir avec une récupération rapide à J21. A la dose de 20 mg/m^2 x 3, cette toxicité maximale est de 50 % et de 33 % si l'on tient compte de l'ensemble des cycles (n=179) et de l'ajustement des doses prévu dans le protocole (75 mg/m^2 puis 60 mg/m^2 puis 45 mg/m^2).

2°) thrombopénie grade (3+4) 19 %

3°) anémie " (3+4) 29 %

Les autres toxicités, grade > 2 rencontrées, sont les suivantes :

1°) infection : toxicité maximale 15 % (dont 2 décès toxiques par septicémie à la dose de 25 mg/m^2 x 3), évaluée sur 179 cycles 5 %.

2°) vomissements : toxicité maximale 11 % et de 8 % si évaluée sur l'ensemble des cycles.

3°) stomatite : toxicité maximale 12 % et seulement 2 % si évaluée sur l'ensemble des cycles.

4°) alopécie 19 % sans grade 4.

Aucune toxicité cardiaque n'a été rencontrée.

III) Cet essai phase II montre l'intérêt de la Pirarubicine dans les cancers avancés du sein avec un taux de réponse de 43 % en première ligne. La toxicité hématologique rencontrée à 3 x 25 mg/m^2 est le facteur limitant, mais à la dose de 3 x 20 mg/m^2, cette toxicité devient parfaitement acceptable.

Des études de phase III utilisant la PIRARUBICINE se trouvent ainsi justifiées.

Neo-Adjuvant Chemotherapy. Ed. Cl. Jacquillat, M. Weil, D. Khayat. Colloque INSERM/John Libbey Eurotext Ltd. © 1988. Vol. 169, pp. 823-824.

Pirarubicin (04'0 tetra hydro-pyranyl-doxorubicin) in solid tumors

J.P. Armand, N. Guiochet, P. Cappelaere, J. Chauvergne, P. Fumoleau, R. Metz, Ph. Bastit, C. Lhomme, Th. Le Chevalier, P. Herait and M. Schneider

Institut Gustave-Roussy, Villejuif, France

Numerous Anthracyclin analogues have been synthetized but only few of them have entered in clinical use in leukemia and solid tumour.

Pirarubicin-THP-Doxorubicin (4'0 tetra-hydro-pyranyl-doxorubicin) synthetized by UMEZAWA has shown a broad antitumor activity in animal similar to DOXORUBICIN with no significant cardiotoxicity in golden hamster models.

THP is incorporated in cancer cell more rapidly than Doxorubicin, cellular pharmacokinetic studies have suggested the superiority of a 3 days IV bolus schedule over the classical one day schedule. This was the rational for Phase I study which already confirm that myelotoxicity was the limiting toxicity with little hair loss and no cardiotoxicity in patient treated over a 750mg/m^2 dosage. Phase II trials has been conducted in different localisation out of breast cancer, 9 localisations have been explored, 4 are closed to enter (head and neck, lung, melanoma, kidney) 5 localisations are recruting patients (ovary, cervix, endometrium, sarcoma, colo-rectal). The drug was given as a first line chemo in renal, colorectal and lung cancer, as a second line without anthracyclin in melanoma, head and neck, cervix and in anthracyclin pretreated patients with sarcoma, ovary and endometrium.

Because of a serious, reversible and deep leucopenia and thrombopenia seen on day 15, the schedule was changed from 25 mg/m^2/d x 3 every 4 weeks, to 20 mg/m^2/d x 3 every 3 weeks.

189 patients have been entered, 11 are non evaluable, 40 to early, 138 evaluable for response.

* TOXICITY : the reduction from 75 (46 patients) to 60 mg/m^2/3d (46 patients) has considerably improved the hematological toxicity at D15. At the 1st cycle 9 % instead of 39 % of patients had a nadir < 1000 WBC/mm^3, and 48 % instead of 65 % a nadir < 2000 WBC/mm^3.

Same effect was reported for the 2nd cycle (65 patients). A nadir of less than 500 PMN/mm^3 was observed at D15 in 24 % of patients treated at 60 mg/m^2 and in 42 % at 75 mg/m^2 the platelet nadir was observed at D15, severe (< 25 x 10^3 platelets/mm^3) in 14 % at 75 mg/m^2 and 7 % at 60 mg/m^2. Treatment was stopped in 3 patients based on abnormalities observed on ECG, VEF no clinical heart failure was reported. If we consider the reported hematological nadirs we can estimate that dosage of 20 mg/day of THP is an optimal one for the 3 days regimen.

* RESULTS : 20 patients with renal carcinoma, free of any previous chemotherapy have been entered with only 1 partial response (PR), 5 % objective response (OR). 17 melanoma has been entered with no response.
In 47 head and neck patients (one third non pretreated by chemo) 4 PR were observed 11 % OR (0-16 %). Most of them interesting targets non previously irradiated.
Out of 24 non small cell lung cancers (70 % adenocarcinoma) 2 PR were reported out of 17 evaluable patients.
All these localisations are closed to enter. The 3 x 20mg/m^2/d schedule has not shown any significant activity despite the limiting white blood cell toxicity has been reached. Other types of cancer are still in evaluation. Endometrium 2/11 CR, cervix 1/9 CR, colorectal 1/10, sarcoma 0/8, ovarian 0/16.

CONCLUSION : These preliminary results using the 3 days schedule seem to indicate no improvment of the spectrum of activity of this new anthracyclin (melanoma, head and neck, colorectal, cervix). In acquired anthracyclin resistant situation THP has not shown any indication of a non cross resistant activity.
The probable activity expected in anthracyclin sensitive tumor will have to be explored in non anthracyclin pretreated patients to check if THP obtains the remarquable activity reported previously in breast cancer and confirm its better cardiac tolerance.

Neo-Adjuvant Chemotherapy. Ed. Cl. Jacquillat, M. Weil, D. Khayat. Colloque INSERM/John Libbey Eurotext Ltd. © 1988. Vol. 169, pp. 825-826.

Essai phase I-II d'administration intra-artérielle hépatique de la pirarubicine avec étude pharmacocinétique comparant l'administration intra-artérielle et intraveineuse : données préliminaires

J.N. Munck et Ph. Rougier

Institut Gustave Roussy, Villejuif, France

Les etudes pharmacocinetiques comparant l'administration intraarterielle et systemique de l'adriamycine ont montre un faible avantage a l'administration de cette molecule selon cette voie (Garnick M.G., Cancer Research 39: 4105-4110, 1979). Le developpement de la Tetrahydro Pyranyl Adriamycine (THP-ADM) moins cardiotoxique et possedant des proprietes de penetration intracellulaire plus rapide que l'adriamycine (Munck J.N. ,Leukemia Research 44: 5544-5549, 1984) nous a conduit evaluer cette drogue en perfusions courtes par catheter intraarteriel hepatique relie a un acces sous cutane chez des patients atteints de metastases hepatiques ou de tumeur primitive hepatique ou des voies biliaires.Quatres patients ont ete inclus (1 avec des metastases de cancer colique, 1 avec des metastases d' un cancer anal, 1 cancer fibrolamellaire et 1 cancer des voies biliaires).La THP-ADM a ete admistree en une perfusion courte de 45 minutes toutes les 3 semaines quelque soit la dose et la voie d'abord, initialement a la dose de 40 mg/m2 puis par paliers croissants chez le meme malade de 10mg/m2 par cycle en l'absence de toxicite (> grade 2 OMS). Uniquement a l'issue du premier cycle intraarteriel, chez chaque patient a ete intercale un cycle aux doses identiques par voie intraveineuse peripherique. Des dosages pharmacocinetiques ont ete effectues a chaque administration.Deux patients ont atteint le palier de 60mg/m2 dose maximale toleree par voie veineuse debut Janvier 1988.Il n'y a eu aucune toxicite locale, hematologique hepatique ou cardiaque chez les deux patients qui ont atteint le palier de 60mg/m2 intraarteriel ; chez un des deux patients des nausees et vomissements grade 2 sur un jour ont ete constatees a partir de 60mg/m2; il n' a pas eu d'alopecie.Les donnees pharmacocinetiques ont montre a la comparaison des taux systemiques selon la voie d'administration que la voie veineuse exposait a des concentrations bien superieures a celles obtenues par voie arterielle: l'estimation des aires sous la courbe respectives evalue le rapport AUC veineux sur arteriel a environ 7. Les prelevements effectues a 60 mg/ m2 ne montrent pas de differences notables avec les doses des paliers initiaux et ont autorises le passage au palier de 70mg/ m2.

Les cibles tumorales evaluables sont sans changement.

Des donnes supplementaires concernant les autres patients et les paliers superieurs chez les deux premiers seront presentees.

Neo-Adjuvant Chemotherapy. Ed. Cl. Jacquillat, M. Weil, D. Khayat. Colloque INSERM/John Libbey Eurotext Ltd. © 1988. Vol. 169, pp. 827-831.

Essai de chronothérapie avec l'association THP-adriamycine/CDDP

F. Lévi[1,2], M. Bénavidès[1,2], C. Chevelle[3], F. Le Saunier[3], J.L. Misset[1], A. Reinberg[2] et G. Mathé[1]

[1]ICIG (CNRS UA04-1163) et SMST Hôpital Paul-Brousse, 94804-Villejuif, France
[2]Unité de Chronobiologie et Chronopharmacologie (CNRS UA-581), Fondation A. de Rothschild, 75019-Paris, France
[3]Service de Radiothérapie et d'Oncologie, Centre Hospitalier Général, 10003-Troyes, France

La moindre toxicité extrahématologique de la THP-adriamycine conduit à tenter de remplacer l'adriamycine par cette nouvelle anthracycline dans les protocoles de chimiothérapie. La combinaison d'adriamycine et de cisplatine constitue l'un des traitements standards des cancers avancés de l'ovaire. L'efficacité de cette combinaison est semblable à celle des combinaisons à trois drogues ou davantage lorsque les critères d'évaluation sont le taux de réponse ou la survie des patients (1,2). Dans une étude Phase II menée chez 41 patientes souffrant de cancer ovarien, la chimiothérapie par THP-Adriamycine seule a entraîné un taux de réponses objectives de 27 %, ce qui est comparable à celui obtenu avec l'adriamycine (3). Par ailleurs, l'heure d'administration de la combinaison adriamycine-cisplatine influence sa toxicité chez l'Homme (4). Parmi les facteurs responsables de ce rythme circadien (de période = 24 heures) interviennent le rythme circadien des divisions cellulaires dans la moëlle osseuse (5,6) et celui qui affecte la pharmacocinétique des médicaments utilisés (7,8,9).

Un essai Phase II de la combinaison de THP-adriamycine et de cisplatine a donc été mené chez 26 patientes souffrant de cancer avancé de l'ovaire. L'horaire d'administration des 2 médicaments était tiré au sort entre deux schémas (cf méthodologie) afin de préciser l'existence d'un horaire éventuel de tolérance optimale à cette combinaison. Le choix des horaires d'administration était fondé sur les résultats de l'étude clinique menée avec l'association adriamycine-cisplatine (4) et sur ceux de l'expérimentation animale.

En effet, l'heure d'injection de 20 cytostatiques d'utilisation courante influence de façon importante et prévisible sa toxicité chez le Rat ou la Souris (10,11). L'heure de meilleure tolérance à la THP-adriamycine se situe dans la seconde moitié de la phase de repos (lumière) de la Souris (12). La compréhension de ces phénomènes passe par l'étude du devenir du médicament dans l'organisme en fonction du moment de son administration (chronopharmacocinétique), et ceux liés aux variations temporelles de la susceptibilité de systèmes-cibles (chronesthésie).

Afin d'étudier ce dernier aspect, la moëlle fémorale de souris a été prélevée à différents moments du nycthémère, incubée in vitro pendant une heure à différentes concentrations, puis mise en culture en agar selon la technique de la formation de colonies monocytogranulocytaire (GM-CFU). Cette technique permet d'évaluer la capacité proliférative de la moëlle osseuse.

Une variation circadienne caractérise cet index et semble affecter la susceptibilité in vitro de la moëlle osseuse à la THP. Ces résultats s'accordent bien à ceux obtenus in vivo et indiquent que la toxicité hématologique de la THP est moindre dans la seconde moitié de la phase de repos diurne chez la souris (13,14).

METHODOLOGIE

Il s'agit d'une étude de type Phase II destinée à préciser le taux de réponses de patientes atteintes de cancer avancé de l'ovaire (stade III-IV, selon la FIGO) à la combinaison THP-CDDP. La THP était administrée par voie veineuse directe à la dose de 50 mg/m², puis le CDDP à la dose de 100 mg/m² sous forme d'une perfusion de 4 h, débutant 10 h après l'injection de THP.
Un cycle était administré toutes les 3-4 semaines selon des critères stricts de tolérance hématologique et rénale, lesquels guidaient aussi d'éventuelles modifications de doses. En cas de réponse clinique majeure, une laparotomie dite de "énd look" était effectuée avec biopsies multiples systématiques de façon à préciser la qualité de la réponse chirurgicale. Afin de préciser le rôle éventuel joué par l'horaire d'injection de ces agents, les patientes étaient stratifiées selon le stade (IIIA ou IIIb-IV), puis randomisées pour recevoir le protocole A (THP à 6.00 h, puis CDDP de 16.00 à 20.00 h) ou B (THP à 18.00 puis CDDP de 4.00 à 8.00 h). La sévérité de la toxicité était évaluée selon le système de cotation de ROMS.

RESULTATS ET DISCUSSION

26 patientes sont rentrées dans ce protocole, dont 10 antérieurement traitées. 11 ont reçu le protocole A et 15 le protocole B. 80 % présentaient une maladie dont le plus gros nodule excédait 2 cm. 25 sont évaluables pour la réponse.

Efficacité

13/25 patientes ont présenté une réponse clinique complète après 6 cycles et 3/25 une réponse objective > 50 %, soit un taux de réponse clinique de 64 %. La durée médiane de réponse était de 10 mois et la durée médiane de survie de 18 mois. Ces résultats sont comparables à ceux obtenus dans la littérature avec cette population de patientes.
L'intervention de 2nd look a révélé l'absence de maladie microscopique chez 4/14 patientes et a permis l'exérèse apparemment complète des lésions résiduelles chez 6/14 patientes, soit un total de 10/25 (40 %). Le pronostic à long terme de ces deux catégories de patientes paraît semblable (2).

Tolérance

Une patiente est décédée des suites d'une toxicité hématologique et rénale sévère (schéma B).
L'incidence des cycles où apparaît une anémie sévère (grade 3-4) est trois fois supérieure dans le schéma B que le schéma A (28 % vs 9 % ; $p<0.02$). Deux fois plus de toxicité rénale (grade 1-3) sont associés à l'administration du schéma B qu'à celle du schéma A (30 % vs 12 % ; $p<0.05$). En ce qui concerne la neutropénie et la thrombopénie, l'heure d'administration n'en influence la sévérité de façon statistiquement significative que chez les patientes non-antérieurement traitées, et pendant les trois premiers cycles de traitement.
Ceci s'explique par l'ajustement des doses, fonctions de la numération des neutrophiles et des plaquettes dans chaque intercycle.
Il apparaît qu'en moyenne, la dose de THP s'est maintenue à 100 % de la dose initiale chez les patientes recevant le schéma A, alors qu'elle a du être réduite progressivement jusqu'à 75 % de la dose initiale au 6ème cycle dans le schéma B ($p<0.01$).

De même la dose de CDDP a du être réduite dès le 1er cycle chez les patientes recevant le schéma B et seulement après le 3ème cycle chez celles traitées par le schéma A (p 0.07).

CONCLUSIONS

La combinaison THP-CDDP est efficace dans les cancers de l'ovaire. Sa toxicité hématologique et rénale peut être réduite par l'administration de THP tôt le matin et de CDDP en fin d'après-midi ainsi que nous l'avions rapporté de façon préliminaire (15). Aucune cardiotoxicité n'a été observée aux doses utilisées. La prise en compte de l'horaire d'administration de cette combinaison semble permettre d'en augmenter les doses administrées et peut ainsi conduire à en accroître l'efficacité thérapeutique. Cette hypothèse est actuellement éprouvée au sein d'un essai multicentrique. Par ailleurs, l'existence d'un rythme circadien de la prolifération des cellules cancéreuses des tumeurs ovariennes est maintenant acquise (16) et peut contribuer à une différence d'efficacité antitumorale des deux schémas comparés.

REFERENCES

1. UMEZAWA H., TAKAHASHI Y., KINOSHITA M., NAGANAWA H., MASUDA T., ISHIZUKA N., TATSUTA K., TAKEUCHI T. : Tetrahydropyranyl derivatives of daunomycin and adriamycin. J. Antibiotics 1979 ; 32 : 1082-1085.
2. KOMIYAMA T., MATSUZAWA Y., OKI T., INUI T., TAKAHASHI Y., NAGANAWA H., TAKEUCHI T., UMEZAWA H. : Baumycins, new antitumor antibiotics related to daunomycin. J. Antibiotics 1977 : 30 : 619-621.
3. UMEZAWA H., YAMADA K., OKI T. : Comparative experimental studies on 4'-O-tetrahydropyranyl-adriamycin and adriamycin. In MATHE G. el Coll. : Anthracyclines : Current status and future developments, MASSON Edit., 1983 ; Chap. 30 : 183-188.
4. KUNIMOTO S., MIURA K., TAKAHASHI Y., TAKEUCHI T., UMEZAWA H. : Rapid uptake by cultured tumor cells and intracellular behavior of 4'-O-tetrahydropyranyladriamycin. J. Antibiotics 1983 ; 36 : 312-317.
5. TSURUO T. IIDA H., TSUKAGOSHI S., SAKURAI Y. : 4'-O-tetrahydropyranyladriamycin as a potential new antitumor agent. Cancer Research 1982 ; 42 : 1462-1467.
6. Studies on 4'-O-tetrahydropyranyladriamycin (THP-ADM) Dossier d'expertise MEIJI, Juillet 1981.
7. DANTCHEV D., PAINTRAND M., BOURUT C., PIGNOT I., MARAL R., MATHE G. : Comparative experimental study and evaluation of the degree of cardiotoxicity and alopecia of twelve different anthracyclines using the golden hamster model. In "Anthracyclines : curent status and future developments", MATHE G., DE JAGER R. & MARAL R., eds, MASSON Publ., New York, 1983 : Chap. 5 : 25-36
8. DOMAE N., ANDO S., KAGAWA D., UEDA T., KUBO A., UCHIDA M., NAKAMURA T., UCHINO H. : Comparative studies of cardiomyopathy induced in rabbits by various anthracyclines and anthraquinones. J. of Japan Soc. for Cancer Therapy 1984 ; 10 : 304 (Abst. P 14-3).
9. GIOVANNINI L., BERTELLI A.A.E., DELL'OSSO L., ROMANO M.R., MAZZANTI L., BERTELLI A. : Toxicological evaluation of aclacinomycin (ACM) and thepirubicin (THP) in rats. 14th International Congress of Chemotherapy, KYOTO - JAPAN, juin 1985, p. 324 (Abst. P 18-32).
10. MUNCK J.N., FOURCADE A., BENNOUN M., TAPIERO H. : Relationship between the intracellular level and growth inhibition of a new anthracycline 4'-O-tetrahydropyranyladriamycin in Friend leukemia cell variants. Leukemia Research 1985 ; 9 : 289-296.
11. TAPIERO H., OSTRONOFF M., FOURCADE A., BLUM J.P., TRINCAL G. : Comparative accumulation and retention in cells of adriamycin, epi- adriamycin, THP-adriamycin, daunorubicin and demethoxy-daunorubicin. Proceedins of the 14th. International Congress of Chemotherapy, Kyoto, 1985 ; Anticancer Section, 1 : 627-628.

REFERENCES (suite et fin)

12. MILLER A.A., SCHEULEN M.E., SCHMIDT C.G. :
Clinical pharmacology of tetrahydropyranyl-adriamycin
Proceedings of the 14th. International Congress of Chemotherapy, Kyoto, 1985 ; Anticancer Section, 1 : 619-620.

13. MAJIMA H. :
Preliminary phase I study of 4'-0-tetrahydropyranyl-adriamycin hydrochloride (THP).
13th International Cancer Congress , Seattle - USA, September 8-15 1982 ; Abst. 2310 : 405.

14. OGAWA M., MIYAMOTO H., INIGAKI J., HORIKOSHI N., EZAKI K., INOUE K. IKEDA K., USUI N., NAKADA H. :
Phase I clinical trial of a new anthracycline : 4'-0-tetrahydropyranyl adriamycin
Investigational New Drugs 1983 ; 1 : 169-172.

15. OKA S.
Clinical results of aclacinomycin and THP-adriamycin in Japan.
In progress in Cancer Chemo-Immunotherapy, Tokyo 1984 ; 86-102.

16. WAKUI A., YOKOYAMA M., KONNO K., NAKAI Y., SAKANO T., KOYAMA Y., IMAMURA Y., NAKAJIMA O., NIIJIMA T., AKAZA H. :
Phase I trial of 4'-0-tetrahydropyranyl-doxorubicin (THP) : a multi-institutional cooperative study.
Gan to Kagaku Ryoho 1985 ; 12 : 118-124.

17. KLEEBERG U.R., RICHTER VON ARNAUD H.P., MILLER A.A., SEEBER S. :
Phase I study of a new anthracycline-derivative in patients with dissiminated cancer.
Proceedings of the 14th International Congress of Chemotherapy, Kyoto, 1985 ; Anticancer Section, 1 : 623-624.

18. DE VASSAL F., BRIENZA S., MUSSET M., DESPAX R., MACHOVER D., GOLDSCHMIDT E., RIBAUD P., MATHE G. :
THP-ADM Phase II trial in metastatic tumors.
Communication au Symposium "Anthracyclines Roger Bellon", Marrakech Maroc, 29-30 mai 1986 - Poster.

19. MAJIMA H., OHTA K. :
Clinical Studies of (2"R)-4'-0-Tétrahydropyranyl Adriamycin (THP)
Biomedicine Pharmacotherapy, 1987, 41 : 237-243

20. KERBRAT J.P., FUMOLEAU P., MONNIER A. & al :
First line THP-Adriamycin (T) in advanced breast cancer (BC) - A french cooperative Phase II trial with a 3-day schedule;
Submited to publication

21. MARINO J.P., BRIENZA S., DANTCHEV D., MISSET J.L. & al :
Reduced cardiotoxicity of THP-ADRIAMYCIN in cancer patients.
Proceedings ECCO-4/Madrid 1987 : 82 (Abst. 310)

Neo-Adjuvant Chemotherapy. Ed. Cl. Jacquillat, M. Weil, D. Khayat. Colloque INSERM/John Libbey Eurotext Ltd. © 1988. Vol. 169, pp. 833-835.

THP-adriamycine : rapport efficacité/tolérance avec étude clinique de la cardiotoxicité. Conclusion et synthèse

G. Mathé et J.L. Misset

ICIG (CNRS UA-04 1163 et Assoc. Cl. Bernard) et SMST, Hôpital Paul-Brousse, 94804 Villejuif, France

THP-Adriamycin was shown by Hamao Umezawa and coworkers to be as/or more active and less toxic than adriamycin, which is one of the most efficient cytostatics in cancer chemotherapy.

Moreover, we have been very much interested in the results of our experimental study of its cardiac and hair toxicities, which have appeared to be the least among those of all anthracyclins.

Japanese colleagues after a classical phase I trial proposed a starting dose of 30–50 mg/m²/month for phase II trials. We started a phase II trial in breast cancer patients, at the dose of 30–50 mg/m²/month. As we had registered 9 % response only with this schedule in advanced cancer patients, and there after have modified the modality of application.

We have based this change on the results of our pharmacokinetic study, which had shown that THP-adriamycin cell influx and efflux is much more rapid than that or adriamycin, suggesting the possible interest of a longer application duration, and we shifted to an original protocol comprising three day infusion per cycle with escalating doses of 20, 30 and 40 mg/m²/day, each four weeks.

We have already published the results of our first phase II trial of THP-adriamycin in breast carcinoma according to those modalities. We have concluded that this new analog was, in advanced breast cancer patients, a) as efficient as adriamycin (we had registered 32 % responses) and b) excellently tolerated, significantly better than all other anthracyclins.

To this day, we have submitted to THP-adriamycin phase II trials, 88 patients, among which there are 32 breast cancer women. With the three days modality of administration we registered a 28 % per trial response rate but a 44 % response rate if we consider only the 16 patients who had not previously received adriamycin.

In this setting equimyelotoxic doses appeared to us to be 40 mg of adriamycin and 50 mg of THP-adriamycin.

In other solid tumors, phase II studies a still ongoing but we already observed encouraging responses in Kidney and colorectal tumors. Japanese colleagues also observed responses in ovarian and urothelial cancers.

We have studied THP-ADM in combination in wide range of situations.

In advanced breast cancer THP-adriamycin (THP-ADM) was combined with vincristine

(VCR), fluorouracil (FU) or the combination of fluorouracil and folinic acid (FU-Fol) according to a study we have previously published, and cyclophosphamide (CPM) or ThioTEPA (TTP), this regimen was given to 71 patients. The overall response rate was 52 % but in the 20 patients without previous chemotherapy and who received full dose, the response rate was 70 % including 5 (25 %) complete responses.

40 patients were submitted to the same combination as primary (neo-adjuvant) therapy for operable breast cancer. The incidence of clinical complete remission was 32 % and that of partial response (50 % of the tumor volume) was 42 %. The incidence of the histopathologic complete remissions was 18 %, of the partial remission 64 % (>50 % of the tumor volume), comprising 18 % with a minimal local residual disease (5mm diameter). This initial chemotherapy is new part of our strategy protocol including breast conservation after restaging.

THP-ADM has also been applied in combination together with cis-platinum both applied in a chronomodulated regimen in 25 patients with ovarian carcinoma, 80 % of which had bulky disease at initiation of therapy : CR rate was 40 % at surgical restaging and overall response rate was 64 % (F. Lévi).

In Hodgkin disease, combined only with Vinca alcaloids and Bleomycin, 3 patients out of 6 in relapse entered sustained CR as well a 3 out of 5 in first perceptible phase. Encouraging results have also been obtained in high grade non Hodgkin's lymphoma.

In pediatric tumors, THP-ADM has now routinely replaced ADM in most combination protocols. Results are already known to be at least as good as previously in osteosarcoma and Ewing's tumors (G. and N. Delépine).

The most interesting property of THP-ADM appears to be its markedly reduced cardiotoxicity for which we have now entended experience and clinical evidence of much better tolerance. On the experimental model of golden hamster THP-ADM belongs together with aclacinomycin A to the least cardiotoxic group of anthracyclins at electron microscopic studies of the heart.

On the clinical ground, 57 patients treated for various tumors with THP-ADM alone or in combination, have received more than 500 mg/m^2 of anthracyclins (the maximum received dose being 1650 mg/m^2, and the median 800 mg/m^2).

The total dose of THP-adriamycin ranged from 90 mg/m^2 to 1170 mg/m^2, with a median of 605 mg/m^2. It was usually applied for a relapse after a previous course of adriamycin. The total dose of which varied from 0 to 700 mg/m^2, and the median was 309 mg/m^2 for the 37 patients who had effectively received adriamycin prior to THP-adriamycin.

Clinical congestive heart failure was only observed in two patients, at the respective cumulative doses of anthracyclins of 1650 mg/m^2 (adriamycin 525 mg/m^2 ; THP-adriamycin : 1125 mg/m^2 for the first patient and 805 mg/m^2 of THP-adriamycin without adriamycin for the second).

One of these two congestive heart failure completely regressed at discontination of therapy with histological control of myocardium normalisation (this patient had not received Adriamycin previously). The other died with heart failure of progressive tumor. Two other patients had THP-adriamycin discontinued after cumulative doses of anthracyclins of 937 mg/m^2 and 1103 mg/m^2 respectively, because we had noticed a hardly detectable decrease of ventricular function, measured by ultrasound echography or mugascan. None of them developped any clinical congestive heart failure.

Moreover, with the exception of the four above-mentioned patients, none had a decreased ejection fraction among those forty patients who had serial measurements with cumulative doses higher than 890 mg/m^2 of THP-adriamycin, following 320 mg/m^2 of adriamycin.

Using the method of Von Hoff for determining the risk of CHF after anthracyclin therapy, THP-ADM appears far less cardiotoxic not only than ADRIAMYCIN itself but also than other drugs of the anthracyclin and anthraquinone series to day available.

REFERENCES

1. Levin L. & Hryhiuk W. Dose intensity analysis of chemotherapy regimens in ovarian carcinoma. J. Clin. Oncol., 1987, 5, 756–767.

2. Thigpen T. & Blessing J. Current therapy of ovarian carcinoma. An overview. Semin. Oncol., 1985, 12, 47–52.

3. Majima H. & Ohta K. Clinical studies of (2"R)-4'0-tetrahydropyranyladriamycin (THP). Biomed. & Pharmacother., 1987, 41, 237–243.

4. Hrushesky W. Circadian timing of cancer chemotherapy. Science 1985, 228, 73–75.

5. Killman S.A., Cronkite Z.E.P., Fliedner T.M. & Bond V.T. Mitotic indices of human bone marrow cells. I. Number and cytologic distribution of mitoses. Blood 1962, 19, 743–750.

6. Mauer A.M. Diurnal variation of proliferative activity in the human bone marrow. Blood 1965, 26, 1–7.

7. Reinberg A., Lévi F., Smolensky M. Chronopharmacocinétique clinique. J. Pharmacol., 1984, 15 (suppl. 1), 95–124.

8. Hrushesky W., Borch R.F. & Lévi F. Circadian-time dependence of cisplatin urinary kinetics. Clin. Pharm. Ther., 1982, 32, 330–339.

9. Lévi F., Metzger G., Bailleul F., Reinberg A. & Mathé G. Circadian-varying plasma pharmacokinetics of doxorubicin (DOX) despite continuous infusion at constant rate. Proc. Am. Ass. Cancer Res., 1986, 27, 693 (abstract).

10. Lévi F., Boughattas A. & Blazsek I. Comparative chronotoxicity of anticancer agents. Ann. Rev. Chronopharm., 1987, 4, sous presse.

11. Lévi F., Hrushesky W., Blomquist C., Lakatua D., Haus E., Halberg F. & Kennedy B.J. Reduction of cis-diamminedichloroplatinum nephrotoxicity in rats by optimal circadian drug timing. Cancer Res., 1982, 42, 950–955.

12. Lévi F., Mechkouri M., Roulon A., Bailleul F., Lemaigre G., Reinberg A. & Mathé G. Circadian rhythm in tolerance of mice for the new anthracycline analog 4'tetrahydropyranyladriamycin (THP). Eur. J. Cancer Clin. Oncol., 1985, 21, 1245–1251.

13. Ferlé-Vidovic A., Blazsek I. & Lévi F. Circadian time-dependence of murine bone marrow tolerance for the anticancer agent 4'-0-tetrahydropyranyladriamycin (THP). Ann. Rev. Chronopharmacology 1986, 3, 195–197.

14. Lévi F., Blazsek I. & Ferlé-Vidovic A. Circadian and seasonal changes in murine bone marrow colony forming cells affect host tolerance for the anticancer agent 4'-tetrahydropyranyladriamycin (THP). Exp. Hematol., 1988, sous presse.

15. Lévi F., Bailleul F., Misset J.L., Chevelle C., Le Saunier C., Despax R., Vannetzel J.M., Machover D., Reinberg A. & Mathé G. Large improvement of hematologic and renal tolerance for 4'tetrahydropyranyladriamycin (THP) and cisdiamminedichloroplatinum (CDDP) at selected dosing times in patients with ovarian cancer. Proc. Amer. Soc. Clin. Oncol., 1986, 5, 190 (abstract).

16. Klevecz R.R., Shymko R.M., Blumenfeld D. & Braly P.S. Circadian gating of S phase in human ovarian cancer. Cancer Res., 1987, 47, 6267–6271.

Symposium Carboplatinum (Paraplatin)

Carboplatine (Paraplatine)

Neo-Adjuvant Chemotherapy. Ed. Cl. Jacquillat, M. Weil, D. Khayat. Colloque INSERM/John Libbey Eurotext Ltd. © 1988. Vol. 169, pp. 839-843.

Le paraplatine en gynécologie

M. George*, C. Lhomme* et C. Toussaint**

* *Service de gynécologie, Institut Gustave-Roussy, Villejuif, France*
** *Centre Eugène Marquis, Pontchaillou, Rennes, France*

Le Paraplatine (carboplatine, CBDCA, JM8) est un analogue du platine qui, dès les essais de phase I, a montré une activité dans le cancer de l'ovaire. Sa toxicité, principalement médullaire (1), est moindre que celle du cisplatine (CDDP). Le paraplatine a été très rapidement introduit dans le traitement des cancers épithéliaux de l'ovaire. En effet, malgré les progrès réalisés en thérapeutique, le cancer de l'ovaire représente la première cause de mortalité par tumeur gynécologique. L'utilisation du CDDP a permis d'augmenter les taux de réponse tumorale et la durée de survie des malades. Mais le CDDP a d'une part, une toxicité rénale imposant une hyperhydratation, nécessitant l'hospitalisation des malades, et d'autre part, une toxicité digestive (nausées et vomissements) difficile à contrôler. Ces 2 effets secondaires et leurs conséquences rendent la qualité de vie des malades médiocre et incitent à rechercher un traitement mieux toléré.

* LE PARAPLATINE EN MONOTHERAPIE DANS LE CANCER DE L'OVAIRE

. Résultats des études de phase II

- A la dose de 300 mg/m2/mois, Evans et col. ont observé 2 rémissions cliniques complètes et 5 réponses partielles (taux de réponse : 25%) chez 28 malades ayant reçu du CDDP (2). A cette dose, la principale toxicité observée a été une myélotoxicité d'intensité modérée : aucune malade n'a eu moins de 1000 globules blancs/mm3 et une seule a eu un taux de plaquettes inférieur à 20 000/mm3. Deux malades ont eu une aggravation d'une neuropathie secondaire au CDDP, et une autre a majoré une insuffisance rénale évaluée par la diminution de la clairance de la créatinine.
- A la dose de 400 mg/m2/4 semaines, Calvert et col. ont rapporté 8 rémissions complètes et 11 réponses partielles chez 28 malades (taux de réponse : 68%) (3). Parmi ces malades, 13 n'avaient jamais reçu de chimiothérapie, et les 15 autres avaient été traitées antérieurement par une chimiothérapie ne comportant pas de CDDP. Les effets secondaires observés ont été des nausées et des vomissements d'intensité modérée, et une toxicité médullaire modérée (nadir médian des globules blancs 3400/mm3, nadir médian des plaquettes 98000/mm3).
- La comparaison des résultats de ces 2 études à ceux rapportés dans la littérature pour le CDDP, montre que le Paraplatine semble avoir une activité comparable à celle du CDDP, mais que sa toxicité est différente : toxicité digestive et rénale faible, myélotoxicité modérée et absence de neurotoxicité.

. Résultats des études de phase III

En raison des résultats observés dans les essais de phase II, le Paraplatine a été comparé au CDDP dans le traitement de première ligne du cancer de l'ovaire par

Wiltshaw et col. (4). Les traitements, attribués par tirage au sort, ont été, soit le Paraplatine 400 mg/m2 toutes les 4 semaines, soit le CDDP 100 mg/m2 toutes les 4 semaines. En l'absence de progression, les malades ont reçu 5 cycles de traitement. La réponse au traitement a été évaluée de façon chirurgicale (laparatomie ou laparoscopie) au terme de ces 5 cycles. Si la réponse était confirmée, les malades ont poursuivi le traitement, à la même dose pour le Paraplatine et à une dose réduite pour le CDDP (20 mg/m2), pendant 5 autres cycles. Les autres malades ainsi que celles ayant une toxicité inacceptable ont reçu l'autre bras du traitement. Le tirage au sort a permis d'équilibrer dans les 2 groupes les principaux facteurs pronostiques : âge, état général, stade FIGO, type et grade histologiques, taille du résidu tumoral laissé en place après la 1ère chirurgie. Les taux de réponse clinique, de rémission complète histologique, la durée des réponses et la médiane de survie sont identiques pour les 2 traitements (Tableau I). Par contre, les 2 traitements diffèrent quant à leur toxicité (Tableau II). La myélotoxicité a entraîné le retard de 30% des traitements dans le groupe Paraplatine, mais toutes les malades n'ont pas reçu les 10 cycles de CDDP prévus en raison de sa toxicité digestive ou de sa neurotoxicité. cette étude montre que, donné en monochimiothérapie et en traitement de 1ère ligne, le Paraplatine a la même activité antitumorale que le CDDP.

TABLEAU I : Comparaison de l'activité du paraplatine et du cisplatine dans le cancer de l'ovaire

	PARAPLATINE	CISPLATINE
Nombre de malades	58	59
Taux de réponse clinique (%)	55	57
Taux de rémission complète histologique (%)	21	20
Médiane de survie (jours)	600 (61-1104)	517 (61-1097)

TABLEAU II : Comparaison des effets secondaires du paraplatine et du cisplatine

TOXICITE (%)	PARAPLATINE	CISPLATINE
Rénale (clairance de l'EDTA)	18	81
Nausées, vomissements	43	91
Leucopénie	70	44
Thrombopénie	2	0
Transfusion	29	25
Neurotoxicité	2	22
Ototoxicité (clinique)	5	18

* LE PARAPLATINE EN COMBINAISON DANS LE CANCER DE L'OVAIRE

Le groupe coopérateur de gynécologie de l'EORTC a comparé l'efficacité et la tolérance de 2 polychimiothérapies l'une comportant du Paraplatine, l'autre du CDDP, comme traitement de 1ère ligne des cancers de l'ovaire stade IIB, III, IV (5). Trois cent quarante et une malades ont reçu selon le tirage au sort soit la combinaison CHAP 5 (doxorubicine 35 mg/m2 i.v. jour 1, CDDP 20 mg/m2 jour 1 à 5, cyclophosphamide 100 mg/m2 et héxaméthylmélamine 150 mg/m2 per os jour 14 à 28, 1 cycle tous les 35 jours, soit la combinaison CHAC1 dans laquelle le CDDP est remplacé par le paraplatine 350 mg/m2 i.v. jour 1. Le traitement devait être entrepris dans les 4 semaines suivant une chirurgie de réduction tumorale aggressive. En cas de réponse à la chimiothérapie une réintervention chirurgicale était pratiquée après le 6ème cycle de chimiothérapie. L'analyse préliminaire des résultats concerne

236 patientes et montre que le CHAC 1 a été mieux toléré que le CHAP 5 (Tableau III). D'autre part, cette analyse montre qu'il n'y a pas de différence statistiquement significative entre les traitements pour les taux de réponse et les médianes de survie.

Tableau III : principaux effets secondaires des associations CHAP 5 et CHAC 1

	CHAC 1	CHAP 5
Nausées, vomissements*	94 Durée 1 jour	99 Durée 5 jours
Atteinte neurologique*	16	51
Alopécie*	76	88
Nadir globules blancs**	2.0	2.1
Nadir plaquettes **	70	66

* % des malades
** valeur médiane x 10^9/l

La conclusion de cette étude est que le Paraplatine a permis aux malades d'avoir un traitement mieux toléré, donné en ambulatoire, et d'activité antitumorale similaire à celle obtenue avec le CDDP. D'autres associations sont en cours d'étude : cyclophosphamide-Paraplatine ou doxorubicine - cyclophophamide-Paraplatine. Leurs résultats seront bientôt disponibles.

Tableau IV : Comparaison de l'activité des combinaisons CHAC 1 et CHAP 5 dans le cancer de l'ovaire

	CHAC 1 NB de malades	CHAP 5 NB de malades
Malades incluses	167	159
Malades évaluées pour la réponse	107	95
Réponses complètes	30	37
Maladie résiduelle minime	9	11
Réponses partielles	12	7
Progressions	41	30
Stabilité des lésions	12	9
Décès précoces	3	1
Médiane de survie (mois)	21 IC : 18-27	25 IC : 22-28

* LE PARAPLATINE DANS LES AUTRES CANCERS GYNECOLOGIQUES

L'activité du Para platine a été évaluée par des études de phase II dans d'autres localisations gynécologiques.

- Dans le cancer du col de l'utérus, il a été observé 20 réponses partielles et une rémission complète chez 77 malades ayant une forme avancée de la maladie (6,7).
- Dans le cancer de l'endomètre, une étude a rapporté 5 réponses partielles chez 15 malades (8). Une autre étude n'a pas observé de réponse parmi 14 malades ayant échappé à une 1ère chimiothérapie, mais a obtenu une rémission complète chez 8

malades n'ayant reçu de chimiothérapie (9).

CONCLUSION

En gynécologie, le Paraplatine a été étudié principalement dans le cancer de l'ovaire. Dans cette indication, les études cliniques comparatives qui ont été publiées, montrent que le Paraplatine a une activité anti-tumorale équivalente à celle du cisplatine en terme de réponse clinique et de survie à 2 ans.
La faible toxicité digestive et le caractère ambulatoire du traitement font que le Paraplatine doit procurer une amélioration de la qualité de vie des malades.

REFERENCES BIBLIOGRAPHIQUES

1. LENAZ L.
   Paraplatin: compendium of recent data.
   Bristol-Myers Company, New York, 1987.
2. EVANS B.D., RAJU K.S., CALVERT A.H., HARLAND S.J., WILTSHAW E.
   Phase II study of JM-8 : a new platinum analog in advanced ovarian carcinoma.
   Cancer Treat Rep, 67, 997-1000, 1983.
3. CALVERT A., HARLAND S.J., HARAP K.R., WILTSHAW E., SMITH L.E.
   JM-8 development and clinical projects.
   In Platinum Coordination Complexes in Cancer Chemotherapy. Hacker M.P.(ed)
   Martinus Nijhoff Publishing, Boston, 1984, 241-252.
4. WILTSHAW E.
   Ovarian trials at the Royal Marsden.
   Cancer Treat Rev 12 (sup A), 67-71, 1985.
5. VAN DER BURG M.E.L., TEN BOKKEL HUININK W., VAN OOSTEROM A., DALESIO O., ROTMENSZ N., VERMORKEN J., GEORGE M., NEIJT J.P., VEENHOF C.
   Combination chemotherapy with carboplatin replacing cisplatin for ovarian cancer. A randomized phase II trial of the Gynecological Cancer Cooperative Group of the EORTC.
   Satellite symposia proceedings of the ECCO-4, Madrid, 1987, p.84.
6. LIRA PUERTO V., CARUGATTI A., MUGGIA F., COLOMBO N. and PAVLOVSKY S.
   Randomized study of CHIP versus CBDCA in recurrent and metastatic cervix cancer.
   Proc. Am. Soc. Clin. Oncol., 1986, 5 (Abst. 464), p.119.
7. ARSENEAU J.C., HATCH K., STEHMAN F. and BLESSING J. for the Gynecologic Oncology Group (GOG).
   Phase II study of carboplatin in advanced squamous cell carcinoma of cervix.
   Proc. am. Soc. Clin. Oncol., 1985, 4 : p. 120 (Abst. C-468).
8. LONG H.J., PFEIFLE D.M., WIEAND H.S.
   Phase II evaluation of carboplatin (CBDCA) in advanced endometrial cancer: a collaborative trial of the North Centra Cancer Treatment Group and Mayo Clinic.
   Proc. Am. Soc. Clin. Oncol., 1987, 6 : 114, (Abst. 448).
9. GEORGE M., DE OLIVEIRA C.F., LANDONI S., TUMOLO S., VAN OOSTEROM A.T., ZANABONI F., ROTMENSZ N., and VERMORKEN J.B.
   Phase II study of carboplatin (CBDCA) in recurrent or advanced endometrial cancer (EC).
   Proceedings of the ECCO 4, Madrid, 1987, p.209, 795 (Abst. 79).

FOCUS ON PARAPLATIN IN GYNECOLOGY

M. GEORGE*, C. LHOMME*, C.TOUSSAINT**

* Service de gynécologie, Institut Gustave Roussy, Villejuif , France

** Centre Eugène Marquis, Pontchaillou, Rennes, France

Paraplatin is a platinum analog which has proven to be useful in ovarian carcinoma with a toxicity profile different from cisplatin. In monotherapy, in phase II as well as in phase III studies, Paraplatin has given the same response rate and median survival time than cisplatin. In combination therapy also in a randomized comparative study carboplatin and cisplatin had the same activity. Nevertheless carboplatin gave a better quality of life than cisplatin. In phase II studies in cervix and endometrium cancers, Paraplatin has also shown signs of activity in previously untreated patients.

KEY WORDS
Carboplatin, ovarian neoplasms, cervix neoplasms, uterine neoplasms, endometrium.

Neo-Adjuvant Chemotherapy. Ed. Cl. Jacquillat, M. Weil, D. Khayat. Colloque INSERM/John Libbey Eurotext Ltd. © 1988. Vol. 169, pp. 845-849.

Etude de phase II de l'association carboplatine-ifosfamide dans les cancers bronchiques à petites cellules métastatiques

Rosa-Anna Subirana, Thierry Le Chevalier, Pierre Ruffié, Rodrigo Arriagada, Marc Spielmann et Thomas Tursz

Institut Gustave-Roussy, 94805 Villejuif Cedex, France

RESUME

Trente patients porteurs d'un carcinome bronchique à petites cellules, présentant au moins une métastase et non pré-traités ont été inclus dans une étude de phase II visant à tester une association de chimiothérapie comportant : Carboplatine 300 mg/m2 et Ifosfamide 4 gr/m2 administrés une fois tous les 28 jours.

Vingt quatre malades sont actuellement évaluables : 16 (67 %) ont présenté un réponse objective (1 rémission complète et 15 réponses partielles). La survie médiane est de 6+ mois ; elle est de 8+ mois pour les malades ayant présenté une réponse objective et de 5 mois pour les autres.

La NSE était élevée chez 19 patients. Sa normalisation a été obtenue après 1 cycle de chimiothérapie chez 6 malades dont la survie médiane est de 8,5+ mois. Cette normalisation après la première cure de chimiothérapie semble donc être un facteur pronostique.

La toxicité a été acceptable : il n'a été observé que trois cas d'hématotoxicité de grade IV et 1 cas de grade III réversible.

Le taux de réponse chez des malades métastatiques, la très bonne tolérance du traitement et l'absence de résistance croisée avec d'autres combinaisons chimiothérapiques efficaces nous incitent à inclure l'association Carboplatine-Ifosfamide dans des protocoles d'alternance de chimiothérapie.

MOTS-CLEFS

Carboplatine, Ifosfamide, Phase II, Cancers bronchiques à petites cellules métastatiques.

Le Carboplatine est un analogue du Cis-platinum qui a été sélectionné sur la base de son activité anti-tumorale (1-2). Il ne présente pas de néphrotoxicité significative ni d'ototoxicité et s'est révélé moins émétique que le cis-platinum dans les études cliniques de phase I (3). Sa toxicité limitante est hématologique, notamment sur la lignée plaquettaire (3).

Le Cis-platinum utilisé seul, avec 13 % de réponses sur 98 malades, n'est pas une drogue majeure dans le traitement des cancers bronchiques à petites cellules (CPC) bien que la plupart des patients inclus dans cette série aient été pré-traités. Cependant, l'association VP 16-Cis-platinum s'est révélée très active avec 80 à 100 % de taux de réponse chez des malades non pré-traités. Le Carboplatine utilisé seul a donné un taux de réponse de 41 % chez 56 malades (4). L'association VP 16-Carboplatine a donné 86 % de taux de réponse dans une série de 44 malades non pré-traités dont 22/26 avec une maladie limitée et 16/18 avec une maladie disséminée (5).

L'Ifosfamide est la drogue la plus active lorsqu'elle est utilisée seule dans les CPC avec un taux de réponse de 63 % chez 52 patients (6).

Les taux de réponse obtenus avec l'Ifosfamide et le Carboplatine utilisés seuls nous ont conduits à évaluer l'efficacité et la toxicité de leur association dans les CPC métastatiques non prétraités.

MALADES ET METHODES

Les malades inclus dans cette étude avaient tous un diagnostic de CPC prouvé histologiquement avec présence de métastases à distance.

Les critères d'exclusion étaient les suivants : tumeur non mesurable, index de Karnofsky < 40 %, âge > 75 ans, malade antérieurement traité par chimiothérapie ou radiothérapie, créatinine > 150 mmol/l, infection intercurrente, maladie cardiovasculaire sévère ou mal contrôlée incluant les infarctus du myocarde récents (< 6 mois) ou une insuffisance cardiaque congestive, antécédents de tumeurs malignes (en-dehors des épithéliomas basocellulaires ou des cancers stade I du col utérin), espérance de vie < 2 mois, numération formule sanguine anormale (globules blancs < 3500/mm3 et/ou plaquettes < 100.000/mm3).

Etaient indispensables avant inclusion dans le protocole : radiographie de thorax de face et de profil ; fibroscopie bronchique ; scanner thoracique, abdominal et cérébral ; scintigraphie osseuse et biopsie médullaire.

Le schéma du traitement prévoyait une combinaison de chimiothérapie associant Carboplatine 300 mg/m2 et Ifosfamide 4 g/m2 administrés la même jour, une fois toutes les 4 semaines. Le protocole était poursuivi jusqu'à progression mais en cas de stabilisation, le traitement était modifié après 2 cures.

Le Carboplatine était reconstitué avec 9.8 ml d'eau et la préparation diluée dans 250 cc de sérum glucosé isotonique et administrée en perfusion intra-veineuse de 30 minutes. L'Ifosfamide était diluée dans 2,2 l/m2 de sérum isotonique et perfusée sur 24 heures. Une hyperdiurèse était établie en utilisant 0,6 l/m2 de sérum glucosé isotonique donné deux heures avant le traitement et 120 ml/m2 de manitol passés en perfusion en Y en 30 minutes, une heure avant la chimiothérapie. Une dose de mesnum identique à la dose d'Ifosfamide était administrée en trois temps durant les 24 heures de la chimiothérapie.

Trente malades, 27 hommes et 3 femmes, dont l'âge moyen était de 59 ans (allant de 37 à 74 ans) ont été inclus dans cette étude de phase II d'Octobre 86 à Février 88. L'index de Karnofski initial moyen était de 80 % (allant de 60 % à 100 %). 13 patients étaient porteurs d'un seul site métastatique et 17 de plusieurs. Les localisations secondaires les plus fréquentes étaient hépatiques dans 15 cas, osseuses dans 7 cas, cérébrales dans 5 cas, surrénaliennes dans 4 cas, médullaires dans 4 cas et ganglionnaires dans 3 cas.

L'Enolase Neuro-specifique (NSE) et l'Antigène Carcino-embryonnaire

(ACE) étaient élevés simultanément dans 8 cas ; la NSE seule dans 11 cas et l'ACE seul dans 4 cas. Un seul malade avait à la fois un ACE et une NSE normaux.

RESULTATS

La réponse à la chimiothérapie a été appréciée quatre semaines après chaque cycle et les résultats ont été évalués en fonction des critères internationaux usuels (7). Le traitement a été poursuivi jusqu'à progression ou après 2 cures en cas de stabilisation.

Vingt quatre patients sont à ce jour évaluables.

Un malade a présenté une réponse complète (prouvée histologiquement), et 15 ont présenté une réponse supérieure à 50 % (taux de réponses objectives de 67 %), 4 malades ont présenté une stabilisation (16,5 %) et 4 une progression (16,5 %). La durée médiane de la réponse a été de 4 mois, allant de 2 à 11 mois.

La survie médiane est de 6+ mois. Elle est de 8+ mois pour les malades ayant présenté une réponse objective à la chimiothérapie et de 5 mois pour les autres. Douze patients sont décédés, 10 de l'évolution de leur maladie et 2 d'affections intercurrentes.

Dix neuf patients présentaient une NSE élevée initialement. Sa normalisation a été observée après 1 cycle de chimiothérapie chez 6 malades dont la survie médiane est de 8,5+ mois ; après 2 cycles chez un malade (survie 2+ mois) et après 4 cycles chez un malade (survie 12 mois). La NSE ne s'est pas normalisée dans 11 cas et la survie médiane de ce groupe est de 5,5 mois.

La toxicité de cette association a été très acceptable : 3 malades ont présenté une hématotoxicité de grade IV, 1 de grade III et 3 une toxicité digestive de grade III. Une alopécie de grade II a été observée chez 11 patients, de grade III chez 5. Une cystite hémorragique est survenue chez 1 malade et, dans un cas, une insuffisance rénale de grade II s'est développée.

La toxicité hématologique n'a jamais été observée après la première cure mais à partir de la seconde. Le Nadir se situe autour du 15ème jour (entre 10 et 20 jours selon les malades).

DISCUSSION

Le traitement des cancers bronchiques à petites cellules repose sur la chimiothérapie. Ses résultats restent dans l'ensemble décevants, la quasi totalité des malades métastatiques rechutant après une période de quelques mois durant laquelle ils répondent au traitement.

Il est donc indispensable pour progresser de découvrir de nouvelles drogues qui, en association avec d'autres, permettent d'obtenir des taux de réponse intéressants. En l'absence de résistance croisée avec d'autres combinaisons, des schémas d'alternance peuvent ainsi être proposés selon le modèle mathématique de Goldie et Coldman (8).

C'est dans cet esprit que nous avons évalué l'efficacité et la toxicité de l'association Carboplatine-Ifosfamide, deux produits dont les taux de réponse en monochimiothérapie sont parmi les plus élevés dans les CPC non prétraités. Le taux de réponse de 67 % obtenu parmi des malades métastatiques est tout-à-fait intéressant d'autant qu'il n'a pas été observé de résistance croisée avec plusieurs autres combinaisons de drogue dont l'association VP 16 Cisplatinum, avec ou sans Doxorubicine.

La tolérance a été satisfaisante, la seule toxicité limitante étant hématologique.

La combinaison de Carboplatine et d'Ifosfamide peut donc trouver sa place dans des schémas d'alternance de chimiothérapie, en particulier avec le VP 16, la Doxorubicine et éventuellement le Cisplatinum dont la toxicité est différente.

REFERENCES BIBLIOGRAPHIQUES

1.- Harrap, K.R., Jones, M., Wilkinson, C.R. et al. (1980) : Anti-tumour, toxic and biochemical properties of cisplatin and eight other platinum complexes. In Cisplatin : Current Status and New Developments (Prestayko AW, Crooke ST and Carter SK eds). New-York Academic Press, 93-312.

2.- Wilkinson, R., Cox, P.J., Jones, M., et al. (1978) : Selection of potential second generation platinum compounds. Biochimie 60, 851-853.

3.- Calvert, A.H., Harland, S.J., Newell, D.R. et al. (1982) : Early clinical studies with cis-diammine I, I-cyclobutane dicarboxylate platinum II. Cancer Chemother. Pharmacol. 9, 140-147.

4.- Smith, I.E., Harland, S.J., Robinson, B.A. et al. (1985) : Carboplatin : a very active new cisplatin analog in the treatment of small cell lung cancer. Cancer Treatment Report 69, 43-46.

5.- Smith, I.E., Yarnold, J.R., Evans, B.D. (1985) : Carboplatin (JM 8) and Etoposide (VP 16) combination chemotherapy for untreated small cell lung carcinoma (SCLC). Abstracts of the 4th World Conference on Lung Cancer, Toronto, n° 86, p. 95.

6.- Hansen, H.H., RORTH, M. (1980) : Lung Cancer. In Pinedo H.M. ed : The EORTC Cancer Chemotherapy Annual 2. Excerpta Medica. Amsterdam, p. 267-283.

7.- World Health Organisation (1979) : Handbook for reporting results of cancer treatment. WHO Offset Publication n° 48, Geneva.

8.- Goldie, J.H., Coldman, A.J. (1979) : A mathematical model for relating the drug sensitivity of tumors to their spontaneous mutation rate. Cancer Treat. 63, 1727-1733.

PHASE II STUDY OF CARBOPLATIN + IFOSFAMIDE IN METASTATIC SMALL CELL LUNG CARCINOMA.

Rosa-Anna SUBIRANA, Thierry LE CHEVALIER, Pierre RUFFIE, Rodrigo ARRIAGADA, Marc SPIELMANN, Thomas TURSZ.

Institut Gustave-Roussy, 94805 VILLEJUIF Cédex - France.

Carboplatin and Ifosfamide are active agents in small cell lung carcinoma (SCLC) and we are being evaluating the activity of their combination in metastatic SCLC. The chemotherapy (CT) regimen consisted of Carboplatin 300 mg/m2 day 1 and Ifosfamide 4 g/m2 day 1 (+ Mesnum) every 4 weeks.

Thirty patients have been included in this phase II study and 24 are currently evaluable for activity. There are 27 males and 3 females with a median age of 59 y.o. (range 37-74). Thirteen had 1 metastatic site and 17 had > 1 metastatic site. The most frequent metastatic sites were liver (15 cases), bone (7 cases), brain (5 cases), adrenal glands (4 cases), bone marrow (4 cases) and lymph nodes (3 cases). Median performance status (Karnofsky index) was 80 % (range 60-100 %). Among evaluable patients, both CEA and NSE were elevated in 8 patients, CEA alone in 4, NSE alone in 11 and none in 1.

One patient achieved complete remission and a partial response was observed in 15 cases (objective response rate 67 %). Median duration of response was 4 months (range 2-11). Bone marrow toxicity was grade IV in 3 patients, grade III in 1 patient. Alopecia was grade II or less in 18 patients and nausea in 19.

These preliminary results demonstrate the good tolerance and the activity of this combined regimen which can be considered for inclusion in alternating CT schedules.

Neo-Adjuvant Chemotherapy. Ed. Cl. Jacquillat, M. Weil, D. Khayat. Colloque INSERM/John Libbey Eurotext Ltd. © 1988. Vol. 169, pp. 851-854.

Le paraplatine dans les cancers ORL

P. Gehanno

Groupe Hospitalier Bichat-Claude-Bernard, Service ORL, 46, rue Henri Huchard, 75018, Paris, France

Cisplatinum is one of the most active drug used in combination therapy in the treatment of head and neck tumors. Carboplatin, an analog which has been prooved to be less toxic than cisplatin, has been studied in monochemotherapy, in polychemotherapy and in combination with radiotherapy. The published results show that carboplatin has the same level of efficacy than cisplatin.

MOTS CLEFS
Carboplatine, tumeurs, tête et cou.

KEY WORDS
Carboplatin, head and neck, neoplasms.

L'efficacité de la chimiothérapie dans les cancers des voies aérodigestives supérieures est souvent mise en balance par sa toxicité, particulièrement chez des malades dont les problèmes nutritionnels sont souvent au premier plan.
Le carboplatine est un organoplatine dont la tolérance rénale, neurologique et digestive est meilleure que celle du cisplatine.
Il a été étudié dans les cancers ORL en monochimiothérapie, en polychimiothérapie et en association avec la radiothérapie.

1. Monochimiothérapie

Sept études de phase II ont été publiées. Elles ont porté sur 175 malades, tous à un stade avancé de leur maladie et pour la plupart en rechute ou résistants à un premier traitement. Le taux global moyen de réponses de 23% est comparable à celui que donne le cisplatine chez ces malades dont le pronostic est mauvais. L'étude d'Ogawa qui porte sur 28 malades évaluables traités à la dose de 400 mg/m2 toutes les quatre semaines donne un taux de réponse global de 21% (1).

Celle d'Eisenberger qui traite 29 malades à la dose de 60 à 80 mg/m2 par jour pendant cinq jours donne un taux de réponse global de 28%(2).

Avec une dose de 400 mg/m2 répétée toutes les quatre semaines Al-Sarraf et coll. ont obtenu un taux global de réponses de 24% chez 29 malades évaluables (3).

Chez 14 malades recevant une perfusion intra-veineuse continue sur 24 heures de 320 mg/m2, Creekmore obtient un taux de réponse global de 14% (4).

Treize malades évaluables traités par Ohnuma à la dose de 270 à 400 mg/m2 toutes les quatre semaines ont présenté un taux de réponse global de 15% (5).

Calvert et coll. ont traité 33 malades avec une dose de 400 mg/m2 toutes les quatre semaines et ont obtenu un taux de réponse global de 27% (6).

Enfin 29 malades évaluables traités par De Andrès toutes les trois semaines par une dose de 400 mg/m2 ont montré un taux de réponse global de 21% (7).

2. Polychimiothérapie

Les résultats de cinq études portant sur l'association carboplatine + 5-Flurouracile ont été publiés. Cent malades ont été traités par des doses de carboplatine allant de 270 à 440 mg/m2 administrées au J1, et des doses de 5-Fluorouracile de 1 g/m2/j en perfusion continue de J1 à J5 ou de J2 à J6. Les cycles ont été répétés toutes les quatre semaines à l'exception de l'étude de De Andrès où ils ont été répétés toutes les quatre semaines. Chez ces malades pour la plupart déjà traités ou métastatiques d'emblée le taux moyen global de réponses est de 54%.

Chez 27 malades évaluables Forastière et coll. retrouvent un taux de réponse global de 48% (8).

Olver retrouve un taux de 26% chez des malades de mauvais pronostic (9).

L'étude faite par Thorud et coll. retouve 62% de réponses chez 16 malades évaluables (10).

Schröder et coll. observent une réponse chez 12 malades sur 13, soit un taux de réponse global de 92% (11).

Enfin, dans une étude comparative randomisée cisplatine -5-FU versus carboplatine -5-FU, le taux de réponse global est considéré par De Andrès, parmi 18 malades évaluables dans chaque groupe, comme statistiquement non différent. Ce taux de réponse est pour l'association carboplatine-5-FU de 66% (12).

3. Association radiothérapie-chimiothérapie

L'administration de carboplatine associé de façon concomitante à une radiothérapie loco-régionale, étudié par Eisenberger chez 12 malades, donne un taux de réponse global de 75% (13).

En conclusion, l'efficacité du carboplatine tant en monochimiothérapie qu'en polychimiothérapie ou en association à la radiothérapie est identique à celle du cisplatine dans le traitement des cancers de la sphère ORL.

REFERENCES BIBLIOGRAPHIQUES

1. OGAWA M., INUYAMA Y., KATO T., NITANI H., NIIJIMA V., TAZAKI H., KURIHARA M. and KIMURA K.
   Phase II study of carboplatin.
   Proc.Am.Soc.Clin.Oncol., 1987, 6: 20.
2. EISENBERGER M., HORNEDO J., SILVA H., DONEHOWER R., SPAUDING M., VAN ECHO D.
   Carboplatin (NSC-241240) : an active platinum analog for the treatment of squamous cell carcinoma of the head and neck.
   J. Clin. Oncol., 1986, 4 : 1506-1509.
3. AL-SARRAF M., METCH B., KISH J., ENSLEY J., RINEHART J.J., SCHULLER D.E., COLTMAN J.C.A.
   Platinum analogs in recurrent and advanced head and neck cancer: a Southwest Oncology Group and Wayne State University study.
   Cancer Treat Rep., 1987, 71 : 723-726.
4. CREEKMORE S.P., MICETICH K.C., VOGELZANG N., CANZONERI C., CHOUDHURY A., FISHER R.I.
   Low toxicity andsignificant tumor responses in phase II trials of carboplatin (CBDCA) in head and neck, non small cell lung, urothelial and ovarian cancers.
   Proc. Am. Soc. Clin. Oncol., 1985, 4 : 144.
5. OHNUMA T., LEYVRAZ G., COFFEY V., BILLER H., MUGGIA F., HOOLAND J. F.
   Carboplatin : activity in patients with head and neck, renal cell and ovarian carcinomas.
   Proc. Am. Soc. Clin. Oncol., 1984, 6 : 124.
6. CALVERT A.M., GUMBRELL L.A., HENK M.J.
   Paraplatin phase II study in head and neck cancer.
   Proc. Symposium Paraplatin : the British translation, London, 1986, p.25.
7. DE ANDRES BASAURI L., LOPEZ POUSA A., ALBA E., SAMPEDRO F.
   Carboplatin, an active new drug in advanced head and neck cancer.
   Cancer Treat Rep., 1986, 70 : 1173-1176.
8. FORASTIERE A.A., NATALE R.B., TAKASUGI B.J., GOREN M.P., VOGEL W. C., KUDLAHATCH V.
   A phase I-II trial of carboplatin and 5-fluorouracil combination chemotherapy in advanced carcinoma of the head and neck.
   J. Clin. Oncol., 1987, 5 : 190-196.
9. OLVER I.N., BISHOP J.F., WOODS R., ARONEY R., HUGHES P., PAE J., HILLCOAT B.L.
   Carboplatin (CBDCA) and continous infusion 5-fluorouracil (5-FU) in advanced head and neck cancer.
   Proc. Am. Soc. Clin. Oncol., 1987, 6 : 124.
10. THORUD E., TAUSSO J., GUNDERSEN S.
   Phase I study with carboplatin-5-FU to patient with advanced head and neck carcinomas.
   Proc. ECCO, 1987, 4 : 84.

11. SCHRODER M., VOLLING P., ACHTERRATH N., KNEBA M., STENNERT E., NAGEL G.
Phase II trial with carboplatin/5-FU in previously untreated patients with advanced squamous cell carcinoma of the head and neck.
Proc. ECCO, 1987, 4 : 255.
12. DE ANDRES L., LOPEZ POUSA A., BURGUES J., PAREDES M.V., SOLA C., RATTI P.
Randomized trial of neoadjuvant cisplatin and fluorouracil (CF), carboplatin and flurouracil (CBDCA-F) in patients (PTS) with advanced head and neck cancer.
Proc. ECCO, 1987, 4 : 250.
13. EISENBERGER M., BAJAJ K., KENNEDY P., JACOBS M., LAVAGNINO D., ELIAS G., GRAY W.
Phase I-II trial with simultaneous weekly carboplatin (CBDCA) and conventional radiotherapy (RP) for patients with unresectable head and neck cancer.
Proc. Am. Soc. Clin. Oncol., 1987, 6 : 135.

Neo-Adjuvant Chemotherapy. Ed. Cl. Jacquillat, M. Weil, D. Khayat. Colloque INSERM/John Libbey Eurotext Ltd. © 1988. Vol. 169, pp. 855-859.

Focus on paraplatin in pediatrics

L. Brugières*, J.M. Zucker**, M. Chazard***, C. Kalifa*, C. Patte*, F. Flamant* and J. Lemerle*

* *Service de pédiatrie, Institut Gustave-Roussy, Rue Camille Desmoulins, 94805 Villejuif Cedex, France*
** *Institut Curie, 26, rue d'Ulm, 72231 Paris, France*
*** *Laboratoire Bristol, 32, rue de l'Arcade, 75008 Paris, France*

Carboplatin has been developed for clinical trials as a less nephrotoxic, less emetogenic and less ototoxic analogue of cis-platinum. Phase I studies conducted in children have established two schedules of administration : 560 mg/m2 every 28 days in a one-hour infusion (Ettinger 1984 - I.G.R. 1987) and 175 mg/m2 weekly for 4 weeks followed by a 2 weeks' rest (Bacha 1986). Hematotoxicity is dose limiting with thrombopenia more pronounced than leukopenia. Emesis, nephrotoxicity and ototoxicity are mild and rare. Few pediatric Phase II trials have been published to date. In a Phase II study of carboplatin 175 mg/m2/weekx4 in children with recurrent brain tumors, Allen (1987) reports 9/36 responses (CR+PR). In refractory or relapsing neuroblastoma Philip (1987) obtains 5/9 partial responses with VP16 and carboplatin 200 mg/m2/dayx5 every 4 weeks. Many other trials are in progress worldwide. However, as pediatric malignant tumors are rare, large randomized studies comparing the efficacy of carboplatin and cis-platinum are difficult to carry out. The role of carboplatin in the treatment of pediatric malignant tumors has not yet been clearly defined. The lack of non hematological toxicity will allow its use at high doses in intensive chemotherapy regimens followed by bone marrow transplantation. However, replacement of cis-platinum by carboplatin in current multidrug regimens needs further studies.

KEY WORDS
Carboplatin : Carboplatine
Pediatric Oncology :Oncologie Pédiatrique .

INTRODUCTION

Focus on paraplatin in pediatrics

Several studies have established that cis-platinum is a major agent in the treatment of pediatric malignant tumors and in particular neuroblastomas (Hayes et al. 1981), osteosarcomas (Rosen et Nirenberg 1982), brain tumors (Sexauer et al. 1985), germ cell tumors (Flamant et al. 1984). Major dose-limiting side effects such as renal damage, high frequency hearing loss, emesis, have led to the development of platinum analogues.

Carboplatin is a second generation cis-platin analogue which has undergone phase II testing in adults following promising preclinical studies in both hematopoietic and solid tumor animal models. Its greater water solubility, diminished protein binding and rapid renal clearance compared with cis-platinum (Doz et al. 1987) may account for the decreased renal- and ototoxicity seen in preclinical trials. Several schedules have been studied in adult trials : 1 hour bolus and 24-hour infusion every 28 days, bolus doses daily x 5 and weekly bolus doses x 4.

All have shown myelosuppression as the dose limiting toxic effect with thrombopenia more pronounced than leukopenia. Pediatric studies are still rare and partially unpublished. The purpose of this report is to relate the published experience on one hand and the studies conducted by the SFOP (French Society of Pediatric Oncology) in the other hand.

Phase I studies

Only three phase I studies conducted in children have been published as yet. Bacha et al. (1986) reported a phase I study performed in 40 children with advanced cancer.A single course of carboplatin consisted of 4 weekly 1-hour infusions followed by 2 weeks' rest. The carboplatin dose was escalated in five steps from 100 to 210 mg/m2/week. Myelosuppression was dose limiting with thrombopenia more pronounced than leukopenia. The nadir WBC and platelet count occurred 1-2 weeks after the fourth weekly dose with subsequent recovery within 2 ½ weeks. Apart from two heavily pretreated patients, nadir platelet count of under 75.10^3 (grade 2) were limited to the 175 and 210 mg/m2 dose levels. No changes in hemoglobin were observed in any patients. There was no evidence of cumulative hematologic toxicity. Other side effects included transient nausea and vomiting at the higher dose levels and non dose-related reversible changes in creatinine clearance. One patient developed hives. No hepatic toxicity was seen.

Another study from the same group (Allen et al. 1987) was conducted in children with recurrent brain tumors using the same schedule of administration and dose escalation. Twenty-four patients were registered for the phase I study. The major toxicity was hematologic, encountered in 6/12 evaluable patients. Nausea and vomiting were mild and of short duration. No significant renal or auditory toxicity were observed. As in the previous study, the maximal tolerable dose derived from this study was 210 mg/m2/week and the recommended dose 175 mg/m2/week.

Ettinger et al. (1984) published a phase I study conducted in 20 children who received 23 courses of carboplatin in 1-hour infusions every 4 weeks with dose escalation from 350 mg/m2 to 490 mg/m2. Mild neutropenia was seen in 7/16 courses and mild thrombocytopenia in 3/10 courses at doses $\geq$ 420 mg/m2. Mild proteinuria was seen in 11/18 courses. High-frequency hearing loss was noted in one patient at 490 mg/m2 and transient hypomagnesemia in another. The maximum tolerable dose was 670 mg/m^2 and the recommended dose 560 mg/ml (Foster BJ et al. 1985).

Two other phase I studies have been conducted in several centers of the SFOP, in which carboplatin was given as a single 1-hour infusion every 4 weeks, respectively at 400 mg/m2 and 560 mg/m2.

In the first study (400 mg/m2) 14 courses in 9 children are evaluable. Hematologic toxicity was noted in 3 patients : one had medullary involvement with neuroblastoma and presented grade 4 anemia and thrombopenia. Another heavily pretreated patient showed grade 2 thrombopenia occurring between 20 and 25 days after each course. A transient grade 3 neutropenia occurred in the third patient at day 5 after the second course. No other toxicity was noted except mild nausea and emesis.

Thirty-nine courses in 15 patients are evaluable for the second study (560 mg/m2). Severe thrombopenia (> grade 3) was noted after 12 courses in 9 patients, occurring between day 15 and 19 and of short duration. Two patients showed neutropenia (> grade 3) and two others, grade 4 anemia. Nausea and emesis were mild except in 4 patients. High-frequency hearing loss occurred in two patients after a cumulative dose of 960 and 2360 mg/m2 respectively. The other side effects were transient hypomagnesemia in one patient and hives occurring during the infusion of carboplatin in another.

The SFOP studies confirmed the conclusions of Foster et al. (1985). In monochemotherapy and with a 1 hour bolus every 28 days, the recommended dose is 560 mg/m2.

Phase II studies

In children, very few phase II studies have been reported as yet but many trials are in progress.

Allen et al. (1987) reported a phase I-II study conducted in children with recurrent brain tumors. Carboplatin was administered as an intravenous one-hour infusion of 175 mg/m2 every week for four weeks. Fourteen patients were registered on a phase I and 20 on a phase II study. Nine of 36 (25 %) evaluable patients in the combined studies experienced objective response for a median duration of 10 + months. Disease-specific response rates were as follows : medulloblastoma 6/14 (43 %) with 3 RC and 3 PR, pinealoblastoma 1/1 (PR), germinoma 1/2 (CR), brainstem glioma 1/8 (13 %) PR. Response rates were comparable to those obtained with cis-platinum but with less toxicity and easier administration.

Philip et al. (1987) reported a phase II study of carboplatin and VP16 in neuroblastoma. Nine patients with relapsed or refractory neuroblastoma, 6 having previously received cis-platinum (total dose = 120 to 1200 mg/m2), entered the study and received a combination of VP16 100 mg/m2/day over 5 days and carboplatin 200 mg/m2/day over 5 days. 5 partial remissions were observed, 3 patients had a progressive disease and 1 no response. All the patients received an additional therapy after response to this protocol and the duration of the response is therefore difficult to assess clearly. Toxicity was mainly hematologic. All the patients had a WBC count less than 1000 during the post-chemotherapy period. The nadir of WBC was observed at day 15 (10 - 17) and the median duration was 8 days. The nadir of platelets was at day 17 (10 - 35) with a median duration of 9 days at less than 50.000/mm3. The treatment was otherwise well tolerated.

Several phase II studies of carboplatin in monochemotherapy or in combination chemotherapy are in progress worldwide. Three studies are being conducted by the SFOP : a phase II study of carboplatin 200 mg/m2/week x 4 every 6 weeks in the treatment of recurrent brain tumors, a phase II study of carboplatin 600 mg/m2 in 24 h continuous infusion - Vincristine 1,5 mg/m2 and VM26 150 mg/m2 in rhabdomyosarcomas and a phase II study of carboplatin and VP16 in relapsing or refractory neuroblastomas.

CONCLUSION

As pediatric malignant tumors are rare, large randomized studies comparing the efficacy of carboplatin and cis platinum are difficult to carry out. Most information will thus be gained from studies performed in adults. The antitumor spectrum seems to be the same for the two drugs (Von HOFF 1987). High cross-resistance between the two drugs has been shown but might not be total in some cases. The lack of non hematological toxicity will allow the use of high dose carboplatin in intensive chemotherapeutic regimens followed by bone marrow transplantation. However, replacement of cis platinum by carboplatin in current multidrug regimens needs further studies. Hematologic toxicity might lead to incomplete or delayed courses with development of resistant or recurrent disease. Studies in progress have to determine the role that carboplatin will have in pediatric oncology : replacement of cis platinum in current multidrug regimens or as an alternative in patients with pre- existing renal dysfunction.

REFERENCES

Hayes, F.A., Green, A.A., Casper, J., Cornet J., Evans W.E. (1981) : Clinical evaluation of sequentially scheduled cisplatin and VM 26 in neuroblastoma : response and toxicity. Cancer 48, 1715-1718.

Rosen, G. and Nirenberg, A. (1982) : Chemotherapy for osteogenic sarcoma : an investigative method, not a recipe. Cancer Treat. Rep. 66, 1687-1697.

Sexauer, C.L., Khan, A., Burger, P.C., Krischer, J.P., Eys, J.V., Vats, T., Ragab, A.M. (1985) : Cis platin in recurrent pediatric brain tumors : A POG Phase II study. A pediatric Oncology Group Study. Cancer 56, 1497-1501.

Flamant, F., Schwartz, L., Delons, L., (1984) : Non seminomatous malignant germ cell tumors tumors in children. Multidrug therapy in stages III and IV. Cancer 54, 1687-1691.

Doz, F. (1987) : Etude pharmacologique des dérivés du platine dans le traitement des tumeurs solides de l'enfant. DEA de pharmacologie clinique et expérimentale. Université Paris VI.

Bacha, D.M., Caparros-Sison, B., Allen, J.A., Walker, R., Tan, C.T.C. (1986) : Phase I study of carboplatin in children with cancer. Cancer Treat. Rep. 70, 865-869.

Allen, J.C., Walker, R., Luks, E., Jennings, M., Barfoot, S., Tan C. (1987) : Carboplatin and recurrent brain tumors. J. Clin. Oncol. 5, 459-463.

Ettinger, L.S., Siegel, S.E, Baum, E.S., Moel, D.I. and Gaynon, P.S. (1984) : Phase I pediatric trial of cis diammine-1,1- cyclobutane dicarboxylate platinum II. ASCO Abstract C-170.

Foster, B.J., Clagett-Carr, K., Leyland-Jones, B., Hoth, D. (1985) : Results of NCI - sponsored phase I trials with carboplatin. Cancer Treat. Rev. 12, 43-49.

Philip, T., Farge, A., Carrie, C., Bouffet, E., Kremens, B., Brunat-Mentigny, M. (1987) : Phase II studies of combination of drugs with high dose carboplatin in neuroblastoma (800 mg/m2 to 1 g 250/m2) in Fourth symposium on advances in neuroblastoma research. Ewans A.E., d'Angio G.J. and Seeger RC eds, New York Alan liss.

Von Hoff, D.D. (1987) :Wither Carboplatin. A replacement for or on alternative to cis platin ? J. Clin. Oncol. 5, 169-171.

Résumé

Le carboplatine est un organoplatine de 2ème génération intéressant en raison d'une toxicité extrahématologique plus faible que celle du cis-platinum. Les essais de phase II effectués en pédiatrie ont permis de déterminer deux schémas d'administration : 560 mg/m2 en une injection IV toutes les 4 semaines, 175 mg/m^2 et par semaine 4 semaines de suite suivis de 2 semaines de repos. Les publications concernant des essais de phase II en pédiatrie sont encore rares et concernent essentiellement les tumeurs cérébrales et les neurobastomes. De nombreuses études sont en cours pour déterminer la place qu'occupera le carboplatine en oncologie pédiatrique : remplacement du cis platinum dans les protocoles de première ligne ou alternative chez les malades insuffisants rénaux.

Neo-Adjuvant Chemotherapy. Ed. Cl. Jacquillat, M. Weil, D. Khayat. Colloque INSERM/John Libbey Eurotext Ltd. © 1988. Vol. 169, pp. 861-865.

Pharmacologie clinique du paraplatine

L. Lenaz* et M. Chazard**

Bristol Myers
** New-York, USA*
*** Paris, France*

1. INTRODUCTION

Le cisplatine est un des agents anti-tumoraux les plus actifs, avec une efficacité démontrée sur un grand nombre de tumeurs chez l'homme. Cependant des effets indésirables tels que les vomissements, la néphrotoxicité, l'ototoxicité et la neurotoxicité périphérique en limitent la durée d'utilisation, malgré de lourdes modalités d'administration qui imposent une hospitalisation ou un séjour prolongé en hôpital de jour. Pour cette raison la recherche d'analogues du cisplatine possédant un meilleur index thérapeutique a constitué un domaine de recherche extrêmement actif au cours de la dernière décennie. Parmi toutes les molécules ayant faitl'objet d'études cliniques, le Paraplatine (carboplatine, JM-8, CBDCA, cis-diamine-cyclobutane-dicarboxylato platine II) s'est montré le seul dérivé du cisplatine dont l'activité soit équivalente mais qui présente des avantages importants en termes de tolérance.

2. MECANISME D'ACTION ET PHARMACOCINETIQUE

Le cisplatine et le carboplatine partagent le même mécanisme d'action. Leurs dérivés qui sont liés à des molécules d'eau, se fixent sur l'ADN en formant des ponts intra-brins et inter-brins (1). Mais la liaison aux molécules d'eau est beaucoup plus lente avec le cisplatine, et c'est cette particularité qui est supposée être responsable des différences biologiques observées entre les deux molécules. La moindre réactivité physico-chimique du carboplatine se traduit par une fixation plus lente aux protéines plasmatiques et, de ce fait, par une demi-vie plus longue du platine libre ultrafiltrable ainsi que par des phénomènes de clairance rénale différents. Alors que le cisplatine est éliminé par filtration glomérulaire et par sécrétion tubulaire, le carboplatine est éliminé par filtration glomérulaire simple (Tableau 1) (2). La faible concentration du carboplatine dans le tubule rénal expliquerait ainsi la moindre néphrotoxicité du carboplatine. Le fait que le carboplatine soit éliminé principalement par filtration glomérulaire a d'importantes conséquences puisqu'il existe une corrélation entre le taux de filtration glomérulaire, les taux sanguins de carboplatine et la toxicité clinique (3). Ainsi une diminution de la fonction rénale se traduit-elle par une toxicité médullaire accrue. On constate également que cette relation reste linéaire même chez les malades dont la fonction rénale est supérieure à la normale, nécessitant ainsi des posologies plus élevées. Un certain nombre de formules destinées à déterminer la posologie optimale du carboplatine ont été proposées (4-6). L'une d'entre elles a été développée pour s'adapter aussi bien au malade insuffisant rénal qu'à celui dont la fonction rénale est supérieure à la normale (5). Cette formule, proposée par Calvert et coll., est actuellement étudiée de façon prospective mais il est encore trop tôt pour en évaluer les résultats. Aucune relation entre la modalité d'administration (perfusion i.v. simple, ou perfusion continue sur 24 heures voire sur 5 jours) et la tolérance observée n'a été mise en évidence et c'est l'injection unique intermittente qui a pratiquement toujours été utilisée dans les études de phase II et III. La toxicité limitant la posologie du carboplatine est la toxicité médullaire (Tableau 2). Le nadir des plaquettes survient habituellement 2 à 3 semaines après l'administration avec une normalisation à la quatrième semaine. Le nadir des leucocytes survient quelques jours plus tard; il est moins prononcé mais la normalisation est souvent un peu plus longue. Une anémie modérée a été parfois notée, mais elle n'amène pas à diminuer la posologie. Les effets secondaires non-hématologiques sont en général modérés. Une toxicité rénale minime est parfois observée mais elle ne nécessite jamais d'hyperhydratation ni de diurèse forcée. Des signes d'ototoxicité et de neuropathies périphériques sont rarement observés; ils sont généralement légers et se retrouvent essentiellement chez les malades antérieurement traités par le cisplatine. Seule la moitié des malades traités par carboplatine présente des vomissements qui sont en général bien contrôlés par des traitements anti-émétiques standard (Tableau 3).Chose importante pour la qualité de vie des malades, la durée de ces vomissements ainsi que celle de l'anorexie résiduelle sont brèves, contrairement à ce que l'on observe avec le cisplatine. Un nombre limité d'études utilisant de hautes doses de carboplatine a montré que jusqu'à 1.500 mg/m2 /cure la seule toxicité significative était la toxicité médullaire. A des doses plus élevées, une hépatotoxicité réversible a été notée. Egalement à ces doses, l'administration concomitante d'aminosides a été décrite comme ayant pu contribuer à l'apparition d'une ototoxicité (9).

Tableau 1 : Pharmacocinétique du carboplatine et du cisplatine chez l'homme

	Carboplatine	Cisplatine
Demi-vie		
Platine libre	6 h	1,5 h
Produit inchangé	1,5 h	0,3 - 0,5 h
Elimination urinaire		
24 heures	70 %	30 %
3 jours	80 %	-
5 - 6 jours	-	40 - 50 %
Mécanisme d'élimination urinaire	Filtration glomérulaire	Filtration glomérulaire et sécrétion tubulaire
Fixation aux protéines plasmatiques	Limitée	Pratiquement totale

Tableau 2 : Principaux effets secondaires du carboplatine observés chez 710 malades en majorité pré-traités (adapté de la référence 7).

Toxicité Hématologique	%	Toxicité Digestive	%
Anémie	59	Nausées et vomissements	78
Leucopénie	55	Diarrhée	6
Thrombopénie	32	Constipation	3
Saignements	6		
Infection	4		
Modification de la fonction rénale		**Modifications des paramètres hépatiques**	
Clairance de la créatinine	25	Phosphatases alcalines	36
Uricémie	25	SGPT	16
Azotémie	16	SGOT	15
Créatininémie	7	Bilirubine	4

Tableau 2 : Principaux effets secondaires du carboplatine observés chez 710 malades en majorité pré-traités (adapté de la référence 7).

Modifications des électrolytes sériques	%	Toxicité neurologique	%
Magnésium	37	Périphérique	6
Potassium	16	Dysgueusie	1
Calcium	5		
		Ototoxicité	
		Infra-clinique	15
		Clinique	1
Autres			
Alopécie	2		
Réactions allergiques	2		
Syndrome pseudo-grippal	1		
Douleur au point d'injection	1		

Tableau 3 : Tolérance gastro-intestinale. Comparaison carboplatine - cisplatine (monothérapie) (tiré de la référence 8).

	Cisplatine 100 mg/m2	Carboplatine 400 mg/m2
Nombre d'épisodes de vomissements	16 (a) 3 (b)	2 (a) 2 (a)
Durée des nausées (jours)	3 (a) 3 (b)	0 (a) 0 (a)

(a) traitement anti-émétique : Méthylprednisolone, Lorazepam et chlorpromazine
(b) même traitement que (a) avec des doses plus élevées de métoclopramide.

3. EFFICACITE CLINIQUE

Le carboplatine a une efficacité clinique au moins équivalente à celle du cisplatine (tableau 4) (7). Un certain nombre d'études randomisées carboplatine versus cisplatine, tant en mono - qu'en polychimiothérapie ont été menées dans le traitement des cancers de l'ovaire. Si le carboplatine est utilisé à sa posologie optimale, les taux de réponse ainsi que les médianes de survie sont identiques dans les deux bras de traitement. Ainsi, et pour préserver le concept de dose-intensité, dans une association de plusieurs drogues les modifications de posologie à adopter en fonction des toxicités observées doivent porter plutôt sur les produits associés que sur les organoplatines.Bien qu'il n'existe pas d'études randomisées comparatives dans les autres types de tumeurs, l'activité du carboplatine parait équivalente à celle du cisplatine. Des résultats préliminaires suggèrent que le carboplatine possèderait une activité dans les leucémies aiguës réfractaires (9,10). L'utilisation optimale du carboplatine est toujours à l'étude en particulier en association avec la cyclophosphamide (avec ou sans d'autres drogues) dans le cancer des ovaires, avec l'étoposide (avec ou sans d'autres drogues)dans les cancers du poumon à petites cellules et non à petites cellules, et avec le 5-FU dans les cancers ORL. Des associations avec d'autres drogues ou avec la radiothérapie sont en cours. Enfin, il faut noter que des réponses au carboplatine n'ont été notées que de façon occasionnelle chez les malades résistants au cisplatine. Ceci suggère que carboplatine et cisplatine ont une résistance croisée à peu près totale. D'un autre côté les malades qui ont rechuté après la fin d'un traitement par cisplatine ou chez qui ce traitement a été interrompu pour des raisons de toxicité ont montré un excellent taux de réponse au carboplatine.

Tableau 4 : Spectre d'activité du carboplatine en monothérapie dans les études de phase II (tiré de la référence 7).

Type de tumeur	Nombre de malades évaluables	Nombre d'études	Taux de réponse (Valeurs limites) %
- Ovaires	453		
. pas de traitement antérieur par cisplatine	83	3	32 - 68
. traitement antérieur par cisplatine	370	10	14 - 28
- ORL	159	7	14 - 32
- Poumons : non à petites cellules	136	6	0 - 18
- Poumons : à petites cellules			
- 1ère intention	41	2	60 - 82
- 2ème ou 3ème intention	41	2	0 - 19
- Col utérin	73	3	22 - 29
- Estomac	61	3	0 - 13
- Testicules			
. Tératomes	35	3	10 - 33
. Séminomes	17	1	88
- Mélanome	49	2	4 - 19
- Colon	48	2	0
- Sein	33	3	0
- Cérébrales (enfant)	30	1	30
- Oesophage	30	1	7
- Vessie	26	2	14 - 21
- Mésothéliome	25	2	12 - 25
- Lymphome	23	1	9
- Sarcome	17	1	12
- Rein	16	2	0 - 17
- Thyroïde	5	1	20
- Neuroblastome	3	1	0

REFERENCES BIBLIOGRAPHIQUES

1 . MICETICH K.C. et coll.
A comparison of the cytotoxicity and DNA damaging effects of cis-(diammino)(1,1-cyclobutanedicarboxylato)-platinum (II) (CBDCA) and cis-diamminodichloroplatinum (II) (DDP) on L1210 cells.
Proceedings of AACR, vol.26, march 1985, Abst.1037.

2. HARLAND S.J. et coll.
Pharmacokinetics of cis-diammine-1,1-cyclobutane dicarboxylate platinum (II) in patients with normal and impaired renal function.
Cancer Research, 1984, (44), 1693-1697.

3. EGORIN M.J. et coll.
Pharmacokinetics and dosage reduction of cis-diammine (1,1-cyclobutane -dicarboxylato)platinum in patients with impaired renal function.
Cancer Research, 1984, (44), 5432-5438.

4. EGORIN M.J. et coll.
Prospective validation of a pharmacologically based dosing scheme for the cis-diamminecyclobutanedicarboxylatoplatinum.
Cancer Research, 45, 1985, 6502-6506.

5. CALVERT A.H. et coll.
Carboplatin : prospective pharmacokinetically guided dose-escalation in relation to renal function.
Proceedings of ASCO, vol.6, march 1987, Abst.172.

6. HARLAND S.J. et coll.
What dose of carboplatin can be combined with etoposide and bleomycin in patients with testicular cancer?
Proceedings of ASCO, vol.6, march 1987, abst. 184.
7. CANETTA R. et coll.
Oncology 1 : 61, 1987.
8. ADAMS M. et coll.
A comparison of the toxicity and efficacy of cisplatin (CDDP) and carboplatin (JM8) in advanced ovarian cancer.
Proceedings ECCO, 1987, Abstr. 785.
9. LEE E.J. et coll.
Phase I trial of carboplatin (CBDCA) in relapsed/refractory adult leukemia.
Proceedings of ASCO, vol.6, march 1987, Abst. 617.
10. MEYERS F. et coll.
A phase I trial of infusioncarboplatinum (CBDCA) in relapsed acute leukemia - Evidence of efficacy with limited toxicity.
Proceedings of ASCO, vol.6, march 1987, Abst. 575.

Résumé
Carboplatin is a platinum compound which has been proved to have equivalent efficacy but relevant advantages in terms of toxicity over the parent compound. Carboplatin is less emetogenic, nephro-, oto-, and neurotoxic than cisplatin. Its dose limiting toxicity is myelosuppression. In randomized studies in ovarian cancers, carboplatin and cisplatin produced the same response rate and median survival time. In other tumors carboplatin appears to have the same response rate than cisplatin.

Workshop on lymphokines and other immunological tools in medicine

Lymphokines et autres outils immunologiques en médecine

Neo-Adjuvant Chemotherapy. Ed. Cl. Jacquillat, M. Weil, D. Khayat. Colloque INSERM/John Libbey Eurotext Ltd. © 1988. Vol. 169, p.869.

Characterization and uses of a recombinant secreted $FC_{\gamma}R$

Jay C. Unkeless, Zhengxing Qu, Joseph Odin and John D. Glass

Departments of Biochemistry and Physiology and Biophysics, Mount Sinaï School of Medicine, 1 Gustave Levy Place, 10029 New York, NY, USA

With the recent cloning of murine Fc receptors for IgG (Fcγ R), it has become possible to make recombinant Fc γR protein in large amounts for further biochemical study. We have constructed a plasmid encoding a soluble secreted Fc γ R, transfected it along with a dihydrofolate reductase (dhfr) minigene into a dhrf - CHO cell line, and amplified production of the recombinant protein by selection in methotrexate containing medium. The resultant cell line secretes 2-4 μg of truncated Fc γR per ml/day. The secreted Fc γR was purified by affinity chromatography on IgG-Sepharose. The truncated Fc γR has a M_r of 31-33,000, which shifts to M_r 21,000 after removal of the N-linked oligosaccharide by N-glycosidase F. We confirm that the truncated Fcγ R has 2 disulphide bonds, creating loops of 42-45 amino acids. The activity of the receptor is not dependent on glycosylation, since truncated Fcγ R secreted by tunicamycin treated cells preserved both IgG binding and immunologic reactivity with an anti-Fc γR mAb, 2.4G2.

The truncated Fc γR was examined for reactivity with a variety of anti-Fc γR mAbs, and was found to lack the epitope recognized by mAb 6B7C. This mAb binds to LPS-stimulated B cells and mouse macrophage cell lines, but not the BCL_1 cell line or to peritoneal macrophages, although 6B7C will stain Fcγ R in immunoblots from these cells. We show that the epitope for mAb 6B7C is in the 8 amino acids just outside the membrane spanning domain, and it is this section that is deleted in the truncated Fc γR. Studies are proposed to crystallize the truncated FcγR and to examine the appearance of anti-Fc γR antibodies in murine models for autoimmune disease. Supported by Public Health Service grants AI-24322 and HL-38498.

Neo-Adjuvant Chemotherapy. Ed. Cl. Jacquillat, M. Weil, D. Khayat. Colloque INSERM/John Libbey Eurotext Ltd. © 1988. Vol. 169, pp. 871-872.

Interferons and the cytokine network

Edward de Maeyer

Institut Curie-Biologie, Bât. 110, Centre Universitaire, 91405 Orsay, France

Interferons belong to a network of regulatory cytokines that are all involved in the homeostatic control of cellular function and replication under normal conditions, and that become active participants in host defense during infection. The cytokines, which make up this network of intercellular messengers, are called lymphokines when derived from lymphocytes and monokines when made by monocytes and macrophages. However, because the production of some lymphokines and monokines is not restricted to lymphocytes or macrophages, it seems simpler to refer to all these polypeptides as cytokines. A few cytokines are also called interleukins, a name originally coined to designate substances acting as signals between leukocytes. Since this definition has rapidly proved too restrictive, a substance can now be called an interleukin as long as it is produced by leukocytes, either exclusively or in addition to others cells, and also provided it functions during the immune or inflammatory response. According to this definition, interferons are also interleukins.

In several respects the difference between interferons and many other cytokines is becoming blurred, as it is realized that important properties, first described for interferons, are shared with a number of polypeptide effector molcules. A substance should not be called an interferon if, in addition to its many other biological activities, it does not have significant broad spectrum antiviral action. The antiviral effect should result from the interaction of the polypeptide with specific high affinity plasma membrane receptors -resulting in the activation of cellular genes, encoding proteins directly responsible for the antiviral state- and not via another plasma membrane receptor. This is the basic distinction between interferons and some polypeptide interferon inducers, for example, growth factors or interleukins, which can also act as antiviral proteins, but do so indirectly via the induction of interferon.

By some criteria the IFN system is distinct from the immune system, and by other criteria, it is an integral part of the immune system. Any nucleated cell in the body is able to produce IFN- / , and thus is capable of directly influencing the immune system. Although cells of the immune system itself can make IFN- and , some of them can, in addition, produce their "own" IFN, IFN- , which has important effects not only on immune cells, but on many other cells in the organism.

Host response to infection is an integration of humoral and cellular immunity, inflammatory mediators, and other cytokines. Cytokines influence the production and action of IFNs, and IFNs exert effects on the production and activity of other cytokines. The interaction can be either synergistic or antagonistic, and the outlines of a highly complex regulatory network are emerging. Since most of this work has been performed in vitro, we should exert due caution in the interpretation of data concerning the activity of a highly complex system based on analysis of only a small part of its components, frequently in concentrations considerably above physiological levels and usually removed from its natural context.

Neo-Adjuvant Chemotherapy. Ed. Cl. Jacquillat, M. Weil, D. Khayat. Colloque INSERM/John Libbey Eurotext Ltd. © 1988. Vol. 169, pp. 873-876.

Interféron recombinant α dans les tumeurs solides

C. Gisselbrecht

Département d'Hémato-Oncologie, Hôpital Saint Louis, Paris, France

Les Interférons font partie des nouveaux moyens thérapeutiques pour traiter les néoplasies. Ils agissent sur la croissance tumorale et modifient la réponse immunitaire de l'hôte au cancer et en ce sens, ils se distinguent des médicaments chimiothérapiques classiques. Depuis la production industrielle d'Interféron Alpha 2 recombinant, la plupart des tumeurs solides ont été l'objet d'études pilotes, afin de mieux cerner leur spectre d'activité. Indiscutablement, les Interférons sont doués in vivo de propriétés antinéoplasiques, cependant leur activité pour la plupart des tumeurs solides métastasées reste modeste et ne dépasse qu'exceptionnellement celle de la chimiothérapie. Pour les tumeurs où une activité des Interférons a été décrite, les problèmes concernent la sélection des patients et la possibilité d'améliorer les résultats par des associations chimiothérapiques et Interféron. Le champ d'investigation reste ouvert pour d'autres tumeurs non encore explorées, certaines réponses inhabituelles ou spectaculaires, comme dans les cancers du rein ou les lymphomes T périphériques, laissent entrevoir la possibilité de nouvelles indications thérapeutiques. Enfin, il apparaît que les Interférons sont souvent, surtout actifs lorsque la masse tumorale est peu importante, constatation qui doit amener à développer des stratégies de thérapeutiques adjuvantes.

Interféron Alpha dans le Sarcome de Kaposi :

Chez les patients atteints de SIDA, 30 ou 40 % seront atteints au cours de leur évolution par le sarcome de Kaposi. Depuis 1982, de nombreuses études ont confirmé l'activité de l'Interféron Recombinant Alpha. Le taux de réponse objective à des doses supérieures ou égales à 20 MU/m2/jour est de 30 %. Cette posologie recommandée, entraîne une toxicité aiguë nécessitant une réduction des doses dans un tiers des cas environ. L'utilisation de plus faibles doses d'Interféron, semble moins efficace avec des taux de réponse inférieurs à 10 %. Les associations Interféron-chimiothérapie, que ce soit la Vinblastine, le VP 16 ou la Bléomycine, n'ont pas permis d'améliorer les taux de réponse observés avec l'Interféron Alpha seul. De nombreux auteurs ont essayé de définir les caractéristiques des patients susceptibles d'être améliorés par ce traitement.

Il apparaît que beaucoup plus que le degré d'extension du sarcome de Kaposi, c'est le degré de déficit immunitaire qui conditionne la probabilité de réponse. Les patients atteints de SIDA ayant eu des infections opportunistes, associant des signes généraux d'évolutivité et présentant un déficit en T4 majeur sont moins susceptibles de bénéficier de ce traitement. Dans ces conditions, la question est de savoir si le traitement par Interféron améliore la qualité et la durée de survie. La qualité de vie est certainement améliorée sur le plan cosmétique. De plus, il semble que les patients répondeurs au traitement par Interféron, ont une moins grande fréquence d'infections opportunistes et une plus longue survie que ceux qui ne répondent pas à ce traitement. Cependant, puisque ces réponses surviennent chez des patients avec un état immunitaire relativement peu touché, il n'est pas possible de déterminer si cette amélioration du pronostic reflète un effet de l'Interféron ou l'histoire naturelle de la maladie.

Interféron et Mélanome :

Le mélanome métastasé fait partie des tumeurs les plus résistantes à la chimiothérapie et le taux de réponse rapporté avec le meilleur agent isolé jusqu'à présent la Dacarbazine, n'est que de 14 %. Depuis 1982, de multiples études avec l'Interféron Alpha Recombinant ont été entreprises. Les taux de réponse objectifs les plus communément rapportés sont autour de 20 %, bien que certaines équipes ne retrouvent que des taux très marginaux de l'ordre de 5 %. Il n'en demeure pas moins que les Interférons sont actifs dans les mélanomes et ont une efficacité au moins égale à celle de la chimiothérapie. Les doses recommandées sont supérieures à 10 MU/m2. Peu ou pas d'activités ont été décrites à des doses inférieures et l'utilisation de doses plus importantes, si elle se traduit peut-être par une augmentation du taux de réponse, entraîne par contre, une toxicité rendant difficile l'utilisation de l'Interféron. Parmi les facteurs conditionnant la réponse, les métastases viscérales ont un effet négatif, si bien que ce sont principalement les patients atteints de localisations cutanées multiples en bon état général, qui pourront bénéficier de ce traitement. Cependant, la durée de réponse est généralement brève, et ne semble pas avoir un impact majeur sur la survie. L'association chimiothérapie type Dacarbazine et Interféron semble plus prometteuse, puisque dans une étude randomisée, cette association était significativement plus efficace que l'Interféron seul.

Interféron et Cancers du Rein :

Il n'y a pas de traitement satisfaisant pour les patients ayant un cancer du rein métastatique et les traitements hormonaux ou chimiothérapiques ne donnent au maximum que 10 à 15 % de taux de réponse. L'utilisation des Interférons permet de retrouver un taux constant de 12 %, chiffre comparable à ceux obtenus par les associations chimiothérapiques. La plupart des patients répondeurs ont subi une néphrectomie, ont des métastases pulmonaires, n'ont pas reçu de traitement antérieurement et ont un état général conservé. Il semble donc possible de sélectionner une population de patients avec des facteurs pronostiques permettant d'espérer un bénéfice d'un tel traitement. En ce qui concerne les associations chimiothérapie-Interféron, notamment, avec la Vinblastine, elles laissent espérer une amélioration des résultats obtenus par l'Interféron seul ou le Velbé seul.

Interférons et Tumeurs Carcinoïdes du Pancréas :

Dernièrement, l'utilisation d'Interféron Alpha a été développée chez des patients atteints de tumeur carcinoïde ou de tumeur maligne endocrine du pancréas. Les taux de réponse rapportés dans deux séries sont voisins de 50 % avec une régression des masses tumorales concomittentes avec la réduction des marqueurs tumoraux (5 HIAA-NPK). Ces taux de réponse semblent supérieure à ceux obtenus avec les chimiothérapies. Bien qu'il s'agisse de tumeurs rares, il s'agit d'une nouvelle indication potentielle des Interférons.

Interféron et Lymphomes T :

Les lymphomes T représentent un groupe hétérogène parmi lesquels on peut distinguer trois sous-groupes :

- les lymphomes T cutanés de type Mycosis Fungoïde et syndrome de Sézary,
- les lymphomes T périphériques,
- les lymphomes de type lymphoblastique proches des leucémies aiguës lymphoblastiques.

Les lymphomes T cutanés de type Mycosis Fungoïde, ont été traités ces dernières années par Interféron Alpha Recombinant. Les taux de réponse sur des séries limitées de patients étant donné la rareté de la maladie, sont voisins de 50 %, ce qui place l'Interféron, proche des résultats obtenus par les polychimiothérapies. Les régressions complètes ou partielles ont été observées aussi bien avec des doses de 3 MU/m2, qu'avec de fortes doses (50 MU/m2). La plupart des auteurs recommandent une posologie de 10 MU/m2, mais une étude phase II est poursuivie à l'heure actuelle, avec une posologie de 3 millions 3 fois/semaine. En raison de la difficulté de contrôler à long terme les formes tumorales par la chimiothérapie, la poursuite d'études préliminaires dans ce domaine est importante, afin de mieux cerner les indications, les posologies et les durées de traitement.

En ce qui concerne les lymphomes T périphériques, ils s'individualisent dans les lymphomes non hodgkiniens agressifs, par leur redoutable pronostic, la difficulté de mise en rémission complète et surtout leur taux de rechute plus important que pour les lymphomes B. Dernièrement, nous avons traité 11 lymphomes T périphériques résistants à la chimiothérapie initiale ou ayant rechuté. Le taux de réponse a été de 36 % avec des rémissions complètes chez 2 malades, s'étant poursuivies au delà d'un an. Les posologies employées variaient de 3 MU à 10 MU/24 heures. Il s'agit là de résultats préliminaires méritant confirmation sur une plus grande étude et qui placerait les Interférons comme un des médicaments de ce type grave de lymphome.

Interféron et autres tumeurs :

Dans de nombreux modèles tumoraux, l'action des Interférons est d'autant plus prononcés qu'il s'agit d'une situation où les masses tumorales sont peu importantes, et les maladies lentement évolutives. Deux tumeurs illustrent particulièrement les nouvelles indications thérapeutiques. Tout d'abord, dans le cancer de l'ovaire, où l'Interféron n'a qu'une activité très modeste par voie générale dans les formes évoluées Figo III - IV à hautes masses tumorales. L'Interféron utilisé en intrapéritonéal a permis d'obtenir 36 % de rémissions complètes vérifiées chirurgicalement dans une série de 11 malades. Seules les patientes ayant des masses tumorales inférieures à 5 mm avaient pû bénéficier d'un effet thérapeutique des Interférons. Dans le cadre du traitement des carcinomes de l'ovaire, les chimiothérapies complémentaires ont profondément bouleversé le pronostic initial. Il restera donc à évaluer si les Interférons apportent en intra-péritonéal, un bénéfice thérapeutique.

L'activité des Interférons s'exerce également pour prévenir les récidives dans les tumeurs in-situ, telles que le carcinome superficiel de la vessie. Une étude randomisée a permis de montrer une diminution des récidives locales chez les patients traités par l'Interféron intra-vésical. Cet effet semble supérieur à celui obtenu par l'immunothérapie de type BCG. Cependant, en raison de la variabilité de l'évolution de ce type de tumeurs, des études prospectives randomisées sont nécessaires.

En conclusion, les Interférons ont indiscutablement une activité dans de nombreuses tumeurs solides. Pour certaines tumeurs, il s'agit du traitement préférentiel à proposer en première intention, pour d'autres, l'étude d'association chimiothérapie-Interféron semble nécessaire. Enfin, pour les tumeurs pour lesquelles, une activité a été démontrée, il sera important d'évaluer le rôle des Interférons dans les traitements complémentaires.

Neo-Adjuvant Chemotherapy. Ed. Cl. Jacquillat, M. Weil, D. Khayat. Colloque INSERM/John Libbey Eurotext Ltd. © 1988. Vol. 169, pp. 877-878.

Interferon recombinant α in haematologic malignancies

Moshé Talpaz

M.D. Anderson Hospital, 77030 Houston, Texas, USA

Ladies and Gentlemen, I'got the impossible taste of trying to cover the activity of alfa interferon in myeloproliferative disorders.

Let me focus my presentation of Philadelphia positive chronic myelogenous leukemia. This is a pluripotent stem cell neoplasia, which is characterized by excessive expansion of the myeloïd compartiment. This was also the first human malignancy which was associated with a cy togenetic abnormality, the Philadelphia chromosom.

The etiology of the disease is unknown, although a high incidence was described. Overall, the incidence in the U.S.A. is 1,4 cases of every 100.000 people. The disease is associated with a median survival of 3,5 years and therapies such as Busulfan or Hydroxyurea failed to alter the disease course.

Several investigators were able to indentify groups with different prognosis based on several clinical parameters such as blood and bone marrow basophilis, age and race, and the presence or absence of cytogenetic clonal evolution. Based on this model, we identified three groups of patients :

- high risk with a median survival of 2 years
- low risk with a median survival of 54 months
- intermediate risk group.

This model was extremely useful in evaluating response to interferon alfa or leucocyte interferon was initially provided as a partially pure interferon also known as Cantell interferon.

The very first had the following pattern of response. This particular patient is still in remission after 7 years. Some patients had a slow and cycling pattern of response and it is important not to mix this phenomen with resistance to therapy. Between 1981-1984, 51 minimal tested benign phase CML patients were given partially pure alfa interferon at doses ranging from 3 to 9 x 10.6 units daily. We can see an overall haematologic remission of 71 % and the results were better in the low risk group than in the high risk group.

However, the most interesting observation was that 20 of the patients (39 % of total 56 % of treated) had various degrees of a cytogenetic response meaning that in some patients this treatment was able to suppress the Philadelphia positive cells and restore "normal" cell growth. This treatment did not prevent blast crisis at the time we had 13 blast crisis cases and now we have 16.However, the majority of them occured in 4 patients who were either resistant to interferon alfa or when they developed secondary resistance to interferon. That lymphoïd blast crisis (6 myeloïd and 3) are unclassified. The survival was affected by the prognostic groups being the best in the best prognostic group. At the point after a median follow up of 58 months, 28 of 51 patients are alive and the projected median survival is about 60 months.

Upon the availability of the recombinant interferon, we went to study recombinant alfa interferon. A study initiated in 1984 was closed to new patients entry in 1987. The patients were given doses of 5 x 10.6 IU/m2 of recombinant alfa interferon and the response rate was identical to that seen with partially pure interferon, in 40 patients with early disease. However, in patients with long standing disease the response was poor and was around 25 % with rare cytogenetic responses.

Two studies have been carried out with interferon alfa 2b (INTRONA Schering Corp.) and essentially confirm the activity of alfa interferon in C.M.L. The doses administrated in the studies were the same (5 x 10.6 IU). The response rate is similar to that seen in my studies. Thus confirming the overall response rate. However, there is a difference in complete haematologic remission. We have seen more of phase. The difference between our study and Dr. NIEDERLE's study is the type of patients. On the study, even though the dose was similar. He tested some patients with long standing disease and as I have shown before, those have a poor response.

CONCLUSION :

Duration of previous therapy will affect response rate. Both NIEDERLE and MANDELLI have also observed lower cytogenetic responses and again that will be influenced by patients selection, and treatment dose, which is different between our study and the Italian study.

Higher doses might be associated with better cytogenetic responses. Supporting the hypothesis is the fact that we were the only to see consistent complete cytogenetic remissions, and this is perhaps the most important observation, because in several patients they were durable. We have now 8 of 40 patients with complete sustained remission.

Neo-Adjuvant Chemotherapy. Ed. Cl. Jacquillat, M. Weil, D. Khayat. Colloque INSERM/John Libbey Eurotext Ltd. © 1988. Vol. 169, pp. 879-881.

Applications cliniques des anticorps monoclonaux en cancérologie médicale

J.Y. Douillard

UER Médecine, Centre R. Gauducheau, Nantes, France

La production d'anticorps monoclonaux par hybridation cellulaire a permis une nouvelle approche immunologique des tumeurs sur le plan clinique.

Le répertoire immunologique de la souris a révélé de nouvelles structures antigéniques contre lesquelles des anticorps monoclonaux ont été produits et connaissent un développement clinique en matière de diagnostic in vitro ainsi qu'in vivo et à un moindre degré jusqu'à présent en matière thérapeutique.

Utilisation diagnostique in vitro des anticorps monoclonaux

Parmi les nombreuses structures antigéniques reconnues par la souris sur les tumeurs humaines et contres lesquelles des anticorps monoclonaux ont été produits, certaines molécules sont libérées à partir de la membrane des cellules tumorales et passent dans le torrent circulatoire. Ces marqueurs de tumeur peuvent être dosés par des méthodes immunologiques, selon une technique de "sandwich" dite immunoradiométrique qui remplace maintenant dans la plupart des cas le classique radioimmunoessai basé sur un test d'inhibition.

Aux marqueurs classiques (alpha foeto proteîne, beta HCG, ACE) maintenant dosés à l'aide d'anticorps monoclonaux, viennent s'ajouter de nouveaux outils dans l'arsenal du clinicien.

Dans le domaine des tumeurs génitales de la femme, le CA 125 apporte des éléments importants pour évaluer l'efficacité du traitement et permet de mieux poser les indications thérapeutiques, en particulier dans la décision d'une chirurgie de "second look". De même la sensibilité de ce marqueur permet dans la majorité des cas de tumeurs séreuses de l'ovaire de détecter une récidive à un stade infra-clinique.

Deux autres marqueurs sont maintenant proposés en matière d'adénocarcinomes digestifs et s'ajoute à l'ACE. Le CA 19-9 et le CA 50 reconnaissent des structures biochimiquement voisines et de nature onco-foetale. Leur contribution principale se situe essentiellement dans les cancers du pancréas où ils peuvent aider au diagnostic différentiel et ultérieurement dans le suivi chez les rares malades ayant pu bénéficier d'une resection complète. Pour les autres localisations des adénocarcinomes digestifs ces deux nouveaux marqueurs sont complémentaires de l'ACE et ont un intérêt dans le suivi des patients et la détection précoce des récidives.

Le CA 15-3 utilise deux anticorps monoclonaux réagissant préférentiellement avec les cancers du sein. Son élévation est liée au stade de la maladie et son intérêt réside surtout dans le suivi, pour la détection des récidives, et dans l'appréciation de la réponse au traitement.

En matière de cancer de la prostate, on a récemment rapporté les résultats cliniques d'un nouveau marqueur détecté à l'aide d'anticorps monoclonaux : le PSA (prostate specific antigen). Il s'agit d'un marqueur d'une grande sensibilité qui devrait là encore contribuer à la détection précoce des récidives ou d'une maladie résiduelle. Sa faible spécificité cependant rend illusoire son utilisation dans le dépistage de masse.

En conclusion, plusieurs marqueurs de tumeurs détectés à l'aide d'anticorps monoclonaux sont maintenant à la disposition du clinicien. Leur contribution se situera sans doute au niveau du suivi des malades permettant un diagnostic plus précoce des récidives et un meilleur monitoring de la réponse aux traitements.

Utilisation diagnostique in vivo des anticorps monoclonaux

Plusieurs études animales, complétées par des études cliniques ont montré que des anticorps monoclonaux radiomarqués pouvaient se fixer in vivo sur leur cible tumorale confirmant ainsi les résultats initiaux obtenus avec des anticorps polyclonaux anti-ACE.

Cette méthode diagnostique dite immunoscintigraphique consiste à injecter des anticorps radiomarqués avec un émetteur gamma dont le rayonnement est enregistré par une gamma caméra. Plusieurs types de cancers sont l'objet d'investigations cliniques selon cette techniques : cancers digestifs, ovariens, mammaires, testiculaires, mélanomes, lymphomes. Dans l'ensemble, cette méthode diagnostique paraît complémentaire des autres techniques d'imagerie médicale. Elle présente cependant un avantage qui réside dans la spécificité apportée par l'anticorps monoclonal utilisé. Dans le cadre du suivi de malade en rémission, elle vient logiquement compléter le dosage des marqueurs de tumeurs mentionnés ci-dessus, la suspicion d'une récidive sur une élévation isolée d'un marqueur est l'indication typique de l'immunoscintigraphie à l'aide de l'anticorps correspondant radiomarqué. Des études prospectives sont en cours dans ces situations cliniques, il est encore tôt pour en tirer des résultats dépendent de plusieurs paramètres et pourront peut-être s'améliorer par l'utilisation de radioisotopes plus appropriés et de moyens d'enregistrement plus performants permettant de diminuer la taille limite de détection actuellement de 20 mm.

En conclusion, le marquage d'anticorps monoclonaux à l'aide d'un isotope radioactif et leur injection in vivo apporte un outil complémentaire de diagnostic qui semble permettre la visualisation précoce de récidives infra-cliniques suspectées sur une élévation isolée des marqueurs de tumeurs ouvrant la possibilité d'un traitement plus précoce de ces récidives.

Utilisation thérapeutique d'anticorps monoclonaux

La sérothérapie des tumeurs est une idée ancienne qui ne s'était jusqu'alors pas développée faute d'anticorps disponibles en quantité suffisante. Avec les méthodes actuelles de production d'anticorps monoclonaux, ce problème est pratiquement résolu. Comme nous l'avons déjà dit ci-dessus, ces anticorps peuvent être utilisés comme vecteur dans l'organisme d'une molécule radioactive mais aussi bien d'une drogue ou d'une toxine qui ciblée sur la cellule tumorale pourra y jouer son rôle cytotoxique. Ces méthodes de radioimmunothérapie, ces immunodrogues et ces immunotoxines sont actuellement l'objet d'essais cliniques. Si des résultats ponctuels interessants ont été obtenus chez des malades en phase avancée, il est encore trop tôt pour tirer des conclusions formelles dans ce domaine et des études cliniques plus étendues devront les confirmer.

Un anticorps par ailleurs est une molécule pourvue d'une activité fonctionnelle et certains anticorps monoclonaux possèdent des propriétés cytotoxiques vis à vis des cellules tumorales. Ces propriétés ont servies de bases rationnelles à l'élaboration d'essais cliniques essentiellement en matière de cancers digestifs et de mélanomes. Là encore les résultats sont très préliminaires et il serait hasardeux de tirer des conclusions hâtives. Il faut cependant constater que plusieurs réponses cliniques objectives ont été obtenues dans différentes institutions chez des malades en phase avancée et que ces résultats encourageants doivent inciter au développement d'essais cliniques de type phase 2. Par ailleurs, il se pourrait que l'injection d'anticorps monoclonaux de souris agisse comme une immunisation active responsable finalement d'une réponse autologue anti tumorale.

En conclusion, la possibilité d'obtenir des anticorps monoclonaux en grande quantité permet leur utilisation éventuelle en thérapie soit à l'aide d'anticorps seul soit à l'aide d'anticorps vecteur d'une molécule et ouvre peut-être une perspective thérapeutique nouvelle.

Neo-Adjuvant Chemotherapy. Ed. Cl. Jacquillat, M. Weil, D. Khayat. Colloque INSERM/John Libbey Eurotext Ltd. © 1988. Vol. 169, pp. 883-887.

Infusion of a monoclonal anti-FcR III in patients with refractory ITP

J. Bussel*, R. Kimberly, S. Clarkson, R. Nochman, J. Valinsky and J.C. Unkeless

**New York Hospital (Room N 740), 525 East 58th Street, New York, NY 10021, USA*

INTRODUCTION

Patients with Immune Thrombocytopenia Purpura (ITP) who have undergone splenectomy, still maintain a very low platelet count (< 20,000/ul), and have clinical bleeding symptoms, represent a truly difficult group of patients to manage (1.) Recent reports have confirmed a mortality in excess of 10% in this patient group (2,3.) Treatment is difficult because these patients often do not respond to conventional therapy including cyclophosphamide, azathioprin, danazol, vinca alkaloids, and colchicine. In addition, when they do respond, they usually require continuous/repeated treatment in order to maintain their response. With such treatment, the chance of developing significant toxicity requiring discontinuation of the medicine is high and tachyphylaxis often occurs. A pilot study with intravenous gammaglobulin in these patients suggests that it will be effective in many of these patients but it is an expensive and difficult therapy and will not work for all patients (3.) Therefore, a new therapy of refractory ITP is required.

Studies of the mechanism of action of intravenous gammaglobulin have highlighted the importance of Fc receptor blockade in the treatment of patients with ITP. Fc receptor blockade appears to be responsible for the acute dramatic platelet increase seen in patients receiving intravenous gammaglobulin (4,5.) Studies of a monoclonal anti-FcR antibody (3G8) binding to FcR III showed that it inhibited ligand binding as demonstrated by inhibition of antibody-coated red cell rosetting around neutrophils (6.) Therefore we elected to investigate the use of this monoclonal antibody as a therapy of refractory ITP.

METHODS:

1) Animal Studies

3G8 was prepared by Damen Biotec Company in accordance with the Bureau of Biologic Specifications for mouse monoclonal antibody therapy in humans including general safety testing in animals. Since only chimpanzees had an epitope that cross-reacted with FcR III, they were chosen for the animal studies using 3G8. Infusions in chimpanzees revealed that they did not have any evident toxicity from the infusions. Neutropenia developed as expected but was transient lasting between three and ten days. Antibody coated red cell clearance was utilized as a measure of Fc receptor blockade in the chimps and an antibody to the MN blood group was utilized to pursue these studies. Antibody coated red cell clearance was significantly prolonged by both intact 3G8 as well as by 3G8 FAB although not by an irrelevant monoclonal antibody of the same IgG subclass (7.)

2) Patient eligibility criteria

Patients were chosen for therapy if they had failed to respond to splenectomy, steroids, intravenous gammaglobulin, danazol, vinca alkaloids, and at least one of oral cyclophosphamide or azathioprin. In most cases the patients were completely unresponsive to these therapies. In certain cases, barely adequate platelet counts could be maintained by therapy (i.e. IVGG) that was given at too high a dose and/or too frequent intervals to be sustained. In addition, all patients had low platelet counts < 10,000 without therapy, had had significant clinical bleeding with low counts, and had had their disease for at least two years.

3) Protocol for Infusions

3G8 was infused at an initial dose of 25 mg, chosen to be approximately enough to saturate twice the estimated number of FcR III's in the body. Subsequent infusions during the first week were given only as needed to patients whose platelet counts did not respond to the intial infusion. Three responding patients received second infusions after the first week. Studies that were carried out included: circulating peripheral blood counts, mouse monoclonal antibody levels in the blood, cytofluorometry of neutrophils, antibody coated red cell clearances, natural killer activity, and T cell numbers and subsets.

RESULTS:

Clinical Response

Five of seven patients (including one treated in Paris) had significant increases in their platelet counts in response to infusion of 3G8. Peak platelet counts in the five responders were 450K 302k, 150k, 85k and 36k respectively. Four of the 5 responding patients required only a single infusion of 3G8 except for 1 patient with an atypical response who received 2 infusions. The two non responders could be distinguished despite the fact that they both had minor responses to 3G8, (one even had a peak platelet count of 26,000), because the count decreased within a second 24 hour period and further infusions did not further elevate the platelet counts in these patients. In fact, the platelet count continued to decrease despite a second and third infusion of 3G8 in each. Bleeding symptoms ceased promptly in all patients as the platelet count began to rise indicating that the platelets were hemostatically effective.

In all but one of the 5 responders, the platelet count returned rapidly to baseline within two weeks of the initial infusion. The one exception was a woman whose platelet count did not start to increase until the sixth day after therapy. Her platelet count gradually increased further so that her peak count of 85,000/ul occurred two weeks after the initial infusion of 3G8 and remained elevated above baseline for approximately six more weeks.

Among the four evaluable responders, all had evidence of a lasting effect of 3G8 infusion on their refractory ITP in addition to the more dramatic short-term effects. Three of four patients became responsive to intravenous gammaglobulin again following 3G8 infusion, after they had been unresponsive. Three patients were eventually able to become stable without receiving any therapy within months of their initial 3G8 infusions. The fourth patient was able to be maintained for several months with single infusions of intravenous gammaglobulin every five weeks. She has since gradually deteriorated to the point where she is requiring intravenous gammaglobulin weekly in addition to prednisone and/or danazol.

One patient with extensive preexisting lung disease had a good response to the first infusion of 3G8. A second infusion 8 days later resulted in the development of ARDS to which the patient succumbed.

FcR STUDIES:

Studies of the antibody red cell clearance showed the expected prolongation of the red cell clearance comparing before to after 3G8 infusions in three of the five patients. Surprisingly, in the two refractory patients the red cell clearance actually sped up. 3G8 was detectable in the plasma for three days following intial 3G8 infusion and 3G8 could be detected on circulating neutraphils for an equivalent length of time. Immunoglobulin levels were unchanged by these infusions. A marked neutropenia was seen which occurred as early as 10 minutes after the beginning of the 3G8 infusion with an obsolute neutrophil count < 1,000 in all cases at the nadir. The neutrophil count rebounded back to the pre-treatment baseline between 2 hours and 4 days after the end of infusion. There was a delayed monocytopenia and lymphopenia starting approximately four hours after 3G8 infusion and then returning to baseline by the next morning. Natural killer activity was completely ablated by 3G8 infusion; it returned within 1 week. Leu 7 and leu 11 bearing cells simultaneously disappeared from the circulation.

DISCUSSION:

These results indicate that 3G8 therapy is effective in the treatment of refractory cases of ITP unresponsive to all conventional therapy (8.) The average peak platelet count for the seven patients was 152,000/ul; the median peak platelet count for the patients was 85,000/ul. The usefullness of this treatment is exemplified by the fact that these patients were refractory to intravenous gammaglobulin at the time they received 3G8 which may reflect on the relative "completeness" of the Fc receptor blockade seen after the two therapies. As expected, the acute dramatic results were shortlived in all but one patient.

The long-term effects that were seen were surprising and emphasized the fact that interactions with Fc receptors may lead to more than transient effects. The mechanism for this effect did not appear to be a lasting change in Fc receptor clearance per se. Other possibilities include either the development of anti idiotypic antibody to 3G8 which could cause an "endogenous" Fc receptor blockade also could have been a result of the interaction of the Fc receptor with the monoclonal antibody through some biochemical/hormonal immunomodulation. Alternatively, the transient elimination of NK cells from the peripheral circulation and their subsequent repopulation may have resulted in more effective suppression of autoantibody production. Platelet antibody testing was done without demonstrating a clear long-term decrease in platelet antibody, but the methodology of these types of tests has been generally considered to be not very sensitive.

The fact that this therapy was effective emphasizes the importance of Fc receptor blockade interaction as a means of therapy in ITP. This may have wider applicability in other disorders. Areas of interest would include autoimmune hemolytic anemia and patients who are refractory to platelet transfusion.

REFERENCES:

1. McMillan, R. Chronic idiopathic thrombocytopenic purpura. New Engl J of Med 304:1135, 1981.

2. Ahn, Y.S., Harrington, W.J. N Engl J Med 312(4):243, 1985 (letter)

3. Bussel, J., Pham, L.C., Aledort, L., and Nachman, R. Maintenance treatment of adults with chronic refractory immune thrombocytopenic purpura using repeated intravenous infusions of gammaglobulin. In press Blood 1988.

4. Fehr, J., Hofmann, V., Kappeler, U. Transient reversal of thrombocytopenia in idiopathic thrombocytopenic purpura by high-dose intravenous gammaglobulin. N Engl J Med 306:1254, 1982.

5. Bussel, J.B., Kimberly, R.P., Inman, R.D., Schulman, I.,Cunningham -Rundles, C., Cheung, N., Smithwick, F.M., O'Malley, J.,Barandum, S., Hilgartner, M.W. Intravenous gammaglobulin treatment of chronic idiopathic thrombocytopenic purpura. Blood 62:480, 1983.

6. Fleit, H.B., Wright, S.D., Unkeless, J.C. Human neutrophil Fc receptor distribution and function. Proc Natl Acad Sci 79:3275-9, 1982.

7. Clarkson, S.B., Kimberly, R.P., Bussel, J.B.,Valinsky, J.,Nachman, R.L., Unkeless, J.C. Blockade of immune complex clearance by a monoclonal antibody. J Exp Med. 1986

8. Clarkson, S., Bussel, J.B., Kimberly, R., Valinsky, J., Nachman, R., Unkeless, J. Treatment of refractory immune thrombocytopenic purpura with an Anti-Fcy-Receptor antibody. N Engl J Med 314(19): 1236, 1986.

Résumé

Six clientes avec des cas de PTI qui n'ont pas respondu a aucun therapie conventionnelle etaient traite avec un anticorps monoclonal contre le Fc Recepteur III, s'appellant 3G8. On a commence avec des estudes dans les singes ou on a pu demontrer que l'infusion de l'anticorp 3G8 cree un bloquage presque totale de l'elimination des cellules rouge qui ont des antiglobulines anti M,N sur leurs surface. C'est a dire que on voit le development d'un FcR bloquage profonde apres l'infusion de 3G8. Alors on l'a donne aux 6 clientes. 4 sur 6 ont eu des responses aigues avec des comptes du plaquette montant a 36, 85, 150, and 302 mille plaquettes quand ils ont toujours eu des comptes moins de 10 mille avant l'infusion. On a meme vu des responses qui ont dure dans 3 sur 4. Un homme ont developpe ARDS avec le deuxieme infusion; il a eu beaucoup de maladie dans le systeme respiratoire avant les infusions. Ses infusions indiquent que le bloquage des Fc Recepteurs peuvent faire monter des responses impartantes dans les maladies autoimmunes et que le FcR III c'est le recepteur le plus importante dans PTI.

Neo-Adjuvant Chemotherapy. Ed. Cl. Jacquillat, M. Weil, D. Khayat. Colloque INSERM/John Libbey Eurotext Ltd. © 1988. Vol. 169, pp. 889-897

Involvement of the interleukin 2/interleukin 2-receptor system in the pathophysiology of human acute lymphoblastic leukemias of T and B-cell origin

M. Allouche, V. Georgoulias and C. Jasmin

Unité d'Oncogenèse Appliquée (INSERM U.268), Hôpital Paul Brousse, BP 200, 94804 Villejuif, France

I. T-CELL ACUTE LYMPHOBLASTIC LEUKEMIAS

The proliferation of normal T lymphocytes requires : 1) recruitment into the cell cycle of quiescent T-cell precursors (1-3), 2) expression of IL2 receptors (IL2-R) (4-7) which can be induced by antigenic or mitogenic stimulation (8,9) and 3) the presence of IL2 (7,10,11). IL2-R expressed on activated T and B cells have been identified under both high and low affinity forms (10,12). IL2-dependent cellular proliferation is mediated by high affinity, but not low affinity IL2-R. Recently, it has been demonstrated that high affinity IL2-R are composed of, at least, two binding proteins of molecular weight 70Kd (p70) and 55Kd (p55), respectively (13-15). The p55 protein is recognized by the monoclonal antibody anti-Tac (4,5) and its gene has been cloned (16).

The IL2/IL2-R system is also involved in the proliferation of malignant T-cells from patients infected with the human T-cell leukemia/lymphoma virus type I (HTLI 1). HTLV 1-transformed cells can constitutively produce and respond to IL2 without prior mitogenic or/and antigenic activation, and they express a high number of IL2-R (17). However, long term culture of these T-cell lines requires exogenous IL2 early in the culture (18) ; some of these cell lines subsequently become independent of IL2 but do not produce detectable amounts of IL2 (19).

T-cell colony formation from normal peripheral blood T cell colony-forming cells requires mitogenic or antigenic stimulation and/or the presence of a conditioned medium containing IL2 (3,20,21). Recently, we reported that peripheral blood T-cell colony-forming cells (T-CFC) from patients with T-cell malignancies (T-cell acute lymphoblastic leukemias, T-ALL), can proliferate in vitro in the absence of any exogenous growth factors or mitogenic stimulation (20,23). These T-CFC generate spontaneous colonies which are composed of immature cells bearing a phenotype similar to that of leukemic cells and cytogenetic studies revealed that they derive, at least partly, from the leukemic clone (22,24).

Since leukemic cells from these patients did not spontaneously produce IL2 (25), we were interested to investigate whether the IL2/IL2-R system was involved in the proliferation of immature leukemic T cells.

Spontaneous and IL2-induced proliferation of T-CFC from T-ALL patients.

Mononucleated cells (MNC) from peripheral blood or bone marrow of T-ALL patients were separated by density gradient centrifugation (Ficoll). They were used, either unfractionated, or enriched in leukemic T cells by depletion of mature T cells with E-rosetting, and treatment by monoclonal antibodies (moAbs) anti-CD2 and CD3 and complement (25), according to the cell phenotype. Unfractionated MNC, or blast-enriched cell fractions generated spontaneous colonies in 18 out of 22 (82 %), and 8 out of 13 patients (62 %), respectively, in the absence of any exogenous mitogens or growth factors (25). According to the plating efficiency, two groups of patients could be distinguished : the first consisted of 10 patients with a high spontaneous colony formation (140-1473 colonies/10^5 cells) (group A). The second group consisted of 12 patients with a significantly lower plating efficiency (less than 100 colonies/10^5 cells ; p<0.001 ; group B). Recombinant IL2 (rIL2) could not enhance the plating efficiency of group A patients' T-CFC whereas it greatly enhanced the colony growth of T-CFC from all group B patients. This colony-promoting effect of rIL2 was dose-dependent (Figure 1) (26). rIL2-induced colonies were also composed of lymphoblastoid cells bearing an immature phenotype (55-78 % CD1+ cells) as spontaneous colonies. Moreover, 33-39 % of the colony cells expressed the Tac molecule of the IL2-R (26). Thus, rIL2 could enhance T-cell colony formation from immature T-CFC of leukemic patients. This biological effect of rIL2 was specific, since it was inhibited if the cells were pre-incubated with moAbs, either directed against the active site of IL2 (DMS1) (27), or against the IL2-binding site of the Tac molecule of the IL2-R (anti-Tac) (26). Thus, these observations indicate that some T-ALL patients' T-CFC are activated cells, bearing IL2-R, and can respond to rIL2 (26).

Growth factors involved in the proliferation of leukemic T cells.

An important question during our studies was to define the growth factors involved in the proliferation of T-CFC from group A patients, who display a high number of spontaneous colonies. To investigate this question, blast-enriched cells were seeded in the presence of increasing concentrations of anti-IL2 or anti-Tac moAbs without added growth factors or mitogens. Surprisingly, both moAbs inhibited in a dose-dependent manner the spontaneous colony growth, suggesting that the IL2/IL2-R system is also involved in the spontaneous proliferation of T-CFC.

We then investigated whether blast-enriched T-ALL cells express the Tac subunit of the IL2-R. Although direct staining of the leukemic cells revealed less than 10 % Tac+ cells, cell incubation in the absence of growth factors for 48hr allowed an increased expression of the Tac molecule (Table 1) (26). This phenomenon was independent of the presence of fetal calf serum into the growth medium, and the kinetics of Tac expression varied from patient to patient.

In order to investigate the mechanism of Tac expression on leukemic cells, media conditioned by unstimulated T-ALL cells (LCM) were prepared and were tested for induction of Tac expression on normal resting T cells. Table 2 indicates that 8 out of 12 LCM tested could induce a substantial (more than 10 %) Tac expression. In addition, these same LCM induced T-cell colony formation from unstimulated normal T cells in the absence of PHA or IL2 : this activity was called TCPA for T-cell colony-promoting activity (Table 2). One hypothesis would be that leukemic cells produce one or several activities which can both induce IL2-R expression and IL2 secretion by the patients' cells, resulting in IL2-responsiveness in an autocrine fashion. We have shown that these activities are proteins, produced by actively proliferating cells (28), and that they are distinct from IL1, IL2, BCGF and PDGF.

Taken together these findings clearly indicate that the IL2/IL2-R system is involved in the proliferation of immature leukemic T cells, which are not infected by the HTLV-1. They strongly suggest that activation of the leukemic cells is maintained by a constitutive production of an activity which can induce expression of the Tac subunit of the IL2-R. Studies are in progress to biochemically characterize this activity and to define the functional status of the IL2-R expressed on T-ALL cells.

II - PRE-B ACUTE LYMPHOBLASTIC LEUKEMIAS

Recent studies have demonstrated that IL2 is also involved in the proliferation of normal activated B cells, which can express IL2-R upon antigenic stimulation under both high affinity and low affinity forms (29-36). IL2-R expression, as determined by immunofluorescence or immunoprecipitation with anti-Tac moAb, has also been described on leukemic B cells such as B-cell chronic lymphocytic leukemia (B-CLL) (37,38), hairy cell leukemia (39), and can be induced after stimulation with phytohemagglutinin (PHA) or phorbol myristate acetate (PMA) on common or pre-B acute lymphoblastic leukemia (cALL) (40,41). We were interested in the functional role of IL2 on the proliferation of pre-B leukemic cells, and thus we studied the structure, affinity and functional characteristics of IL2-R expressed on such cells.

Characterization of IL2-R expressed on acute leukemic B cells.

First we described a case of morphologically undifferentiated acute leukemia, which expressed surface markers of both the monocyte/myeloid (My7, My9, OKM1) and the B-cell (CD19) lineages, as well as the Tac molecule on 90 % of the cells. This leukemia was committed to the B-cell lineage, since Southern analysis of DNA from leukemic cells revealed monoclonal rearranged heavy and K light chain immunoglobulin genes (42). The presence of the Tac component of IL2-R on the leukemic cells did not mediate IL2-responsiveness, either in an 3H-thymidine incorporation or in a colony assay (42), thus suggesting that the IL2-R were of low affinity. However, leukemic cells pre-incubated with PMA, generated B cell colonies in the presence of rIL2 (Table 3), in spite of a decrease in the proportion of Tac+ cells. PMA also induced an increased expression of the B-cell associated CD19 antigen (up to 100 % positive cells) and decreased the fraction of My9+ cells. Binding experiments with radiolabelled rIL2, used at doses detecting high affinity IL2-R (inferior to 1nM rIL2), did not reveal any specific cell associated radioactivity, either on unstimulated, or on PMA-incubated leukemic cells. Thus, it is probable that the majority, if not all, of the cells express low affinity IL2-R. However, we cannot exclude the presence of a small number of leukemic cells displaying high affinity receptors that could not be detected with binding experiments or 3H-thymidine uptake assay but that could respond to rIL2 in a colony assay, which reveals only a small number of clonogenic cells (42).

PMA induces functional IL2-R on a pre-B leukemic cell line

In another study, we have examined IL2-R expression on a pre-B leukemic cell line, Reh 6. The Reh 6 line is derived from a patient with cALL, has an immature B cell phenotype, and has rearranged heavy and light chain immunoglobulin genes (43). Cell incubation with PMA induced expression of the Tac molecule of IL2-R in a dose-and time-dependent fashion, with a peak of expression (90-95 % of Tac+ cells) after 48hr in the presence of 10-100ng/ml PMA. Binding experiments with radiolabelled rIL2 revealed a few high affinity (approximately 200 sites per cell with a Kd of 260pM) and a large number of low affinity IL2-R (24000 sites per cell with a Kd of 17nM). By cross-linking of radiolabelled rIL2 to its receptor, we showed the presence of 2 polypeptide chains of 55 and 70Kd, as in normal activated T cells (13). PMA-treated Reh6 cells could specifically bind and internalize IL2. Moreover, IL2-R expressed on PMA-treated cells were functional since rIL2 specifically enhanced the in vitro proliferation of cells in semi-solid, but not liquid cultures (44).

Taken together, our data suggest that PMA could induce functional, high affinity IL2-R on immature leukemic B cells. In addition, leukemic pre-B cell lines may provide a convenient model to elucidate the molecular and biochemical mechanisms that regulate IL2-R expression and IL2-induced proliferation and differentiation of immature B cells.

In conclusion, the IL2/IL2-R system is involved in the proliferation of both immature T and B cells, as demonstrated using leukemic cells. Whether IL2 also plays a role in the differentiation of these immature lymphoid cells is still unknown at the present time.

ACKNOWLEDGEMENTS

This work was supported by a grant from the Association de la Recherche contre le Cancer (ARC). We wish to thank Ms. Colette DELTEIL for expert secretarial help.

REFERENCES

1 - CLAESSON M.H., RODGER H.D., JOHNSON G.R. et al. Clin. Exp. Immunol., 28:526, 1977.

2 - BUICK R.N., MESSNER H.A., TILL J.E. et al. J. Nat. Cancer Inst., 62:249, 1979.

3 - GEORGOULIAS V., MARION S., CONSOLINI R. et al. Cell. Immunol. 95:1, 1985.

4 - UCHIYAMA T., BRODERS S. & WALDMANN T.A. J. Immunol. 126:1393, 1981.

5 - UCHIYAMA T., NELSON D.L., FLEISCHER T.A. et al. J. Immunol. 126:1398, 1981.

6 - LEONARD W.J., DEPPER J.M., UCHIYAMA T. et al. Nature 300:267, 1982.

7 - CANTRELL D.A. & SMITH K.A. Science 224:1312, 1984.

8 - MEUER S.C., HUSSEY R.E., CANTRELL D.A. et al. Proc. Nat. Acad. Sci. 81:1509, 1984.

9 - MEUER S.C., HUSSEY R.E., FABBI M. et al. Cell 36:897, 1984.

10- ROBB R.J., MUNCK A. & SMITH K.A. J. Exp. Med. 154:1455, 1981.

11- GILLIS S. J. Clin. Immunol. 3:1, 1983.

12- ROBB R.J., GREENE W.C. & RUSK C.H. J. Exp. Med. 160:1126, 1984.

13- SHARON M., KLAUSNER R.D., CULLEN B.R. et al. Science 234:859, 1986

14- TSUDO M., KOZAK R.W., GOLDMAN C.K. et al. Proc. Nat. Acad. Sci. 83:9694, 1986.

15- TESHIGAWARA K., WANG H.M., KATO K. et al. J. Exp. Med. 165:223, 1987.

16- LEONARD W.J., DEPPER J.M., CRABTREE G.R. et al. Nature 311:626, 1984.

17- GOOTENBERG J.E., RUSCETTI F.N., MIER J.W. et al. J. Exp. Med. 154:1403, 1981.

18- POIESZ B.J., RUSCETTI F.W., MIER J.W. et al. Proc. Nat. Acad. Sci. 77:6815, 1980.

19- POPOVIC M., LANGE-WANTZIN G., SARIN P.S. et al. Proc. Nat. Acad. Sci. 80:5402, 1983.

20- ROZENSZAJN L.A., SIHOHAM D. & KALECHMAN I. Immunology 29:1041, 1975.

21- TRIEBEL F., ROBINSON W.A., HAYWARD A.R. et al. J. Immunol. 126:2020, 1981.

22- GEORGOULIAS V., BOURINBAIAR A., AMESLAND F. et al. Int. J. Cancer 34:471, 1984.

23- GEORGOULIAS V., AUCLAIR H. & JASMIN C. Leuk. Res. 8:1025, 1984.

24- ALLOUCHE M., BOURINBAIAR A., GEORGOULIAS V. et al. Blood 66:1155, 1985.

25- GEORGOULIAS V., TRIEBEL F., KOSMATOPOULOS C. et al. Leuk. Res. 10:419, 1985.

26- GEORGOULIAS V., ALLOUCHE M., SALVATORE A. et al. Cell. Immunol. 105:317, 1987.

27- SMITH K.A., FAVATA M.F. & OROSZLAN S. J. Immunol. 131:1808, 1983.

28- KOSMATOPOULOS C., ALLOUCHE M., TRIEBEL F. et al. Int. J. Cancer 37:247, 1986.

29- TSUDO M., UCHIYAMA T. & UCHINO H. J. Exp. Med. 160:612, 1984.

30- JUNG L., HARA T. & FU S.M. J. Exp. Med. 160:1597, 1984.

31- WALDMANN T.A., GOLDMAN C.K., ROBB R.J. et al. J. Exp. Med. 160:1450, 1984.

32- ZUBLER R.H., LOWENTHAL J.W., ERARD F. et al. J. Exp. Med. 160:1170, 1984.

33- MINGARI M.C., GEROSA G., CARRA G. et al. Nature 312:641, 1984.

34- MURAGUCHI A., KEHRL J.H., LONGO D.L. et al. J. Exp. Med. 161:181, 1985.

35- MITTLER R., RAO P., OLINI G. et al. J. Immunol. 134:2393, 1985.

36- BOYD A.W., FISHER D.C., FOX D.A. et al. J. Immunol. 134:2387, 1985.

37- LANTZ O., GRILLOT-COURVALIN C., SCHMITT C. et al. J. Exp. Med. 161:1225, 1985.

38- TOUW I. & LOWENBERG B. Blood 66:237, 1985.

39- KORSMEYER S.J., GREENE W.C., COSSMAN J. et al. Proc. Natl. Acad. Sci. 80:4522, 1983.

40- TOUW I., DELWEL R., BOLHUIS R. et al Blood 66:556, 1985.

41- MATSUOKA M., HATORI T., KAWANO F. et al. Leuk. Res. 10:597, 1986.

42- BENTABOULET M., ALLOUCHE M., TSAPIS A. et al. Blood 70:954, 1987.

43- KORSMEYER S.J., ARNOLD A., BAKHSHI A. et al. J. Clin. Invest. 71:301, 1983.

44- ALLOUCHE M., GEORGOULIAS V., AUGERY-BOURGET et al. Submitted.

TABLE 1 : EXPRESSION OF IL2-R ON LEUKEMIC CELLS FROM T-ALL PATIENTS

Patient	Fresh cells	After 48hr incubation
2	34[a]	41
4	0	4
5	0	16
7	0	2
11	9	10
12	2	17

Cells were stained by indirect immunofluorescence with anti-Tac moAb either immediately after separation on Ficoll-Hypaque (fresh cells) or after 48hr incubation in growth medium supplemented with FCS, L-glutamine, and antibiotics, at 37°C in 5 % CO2 in air.

[a] Results are expressed as percentages of positive cells.

TABLE 2 : INDUCTION OF IL2-R (Tac Molecule) EXPRESSION AND T-CELL COLONY FORMATION BY NORMAL T LYMPHOCYTES INCUBATED WITH MEDIA CONDITIONED (LCM) BY T-ALL CELLS

Source of LCM	TCPA	% Tac+ cells
1a	294	9
1b	48	12
2a	206	10
2b	43	12
5b	ND	9
8a	ND	18
8b	ND	12
9b	34	9
12b	363	26
13a	ND	17
14a	ND	15
15a	ND	17
Normal MNC	0	2
α-MEM	0	1

10^6 normal T lymphocytes/ml were incubated for 48hr with 10 % (v/v) of LCM from different patients in the absence of other growth factor or mitogenic stimulation. Washed cells were stained with the anti-Tac moAb by indirect immunofluorescence. TCPA was tested by incubating normal T lymphocytes (5.10^5 /ml) with 10 % (v/v) LCM in 0.8 % methylcellulose in growth medium containing 15 % FCS, antibiotics and glutamide. Colonies (containing more than 50 cells) were counted at day 7 of culture and are expressed as mean number of colonies / 5×10^4 cells.

ND : Not determined.

TABLE 3 : COLONY FORMATION FROM BLAST-ENRICHED PRE-B LEUKEMIC CELLS

Preincubation		Culture	Number of colonies / $5x10^4$ cells	3H-thymidine incorporation (cpm/$2x10^5$ cells)
Days	PMA (100ng/ml)	rIL2 (u/ml)		
0	-	0	0	1365 ± 852
0	-	0.1-10	0	1741 ± 356
2	-	0	91 ± 11[a]	ND[b]
2	-	0.5	130 ± 23	ND
2	+	0	334 ± 26	ND
2	+	0.5	794 ± 92	ND

10^6 cells/ml were preincubated or not with 100ng/ml PMA for 48hr. Cells were washed and reseeded in microtiter wells, either in methycellulose at $5x10^5$ cells/ml, or in liquid culture at 10^6 cells/ml, in the absence or presence of 0.5u/ml rIL2 (1 unit = 40 BRMP units). 3H-thymidine incorporation was measured at 3 days, and the number of colonies at 7 days of culture respectively.

[a] Small colonies containing less than 100 cells.
[b] ND = Not determined.
[c] Large and round colonies containing up to 1000 cells.

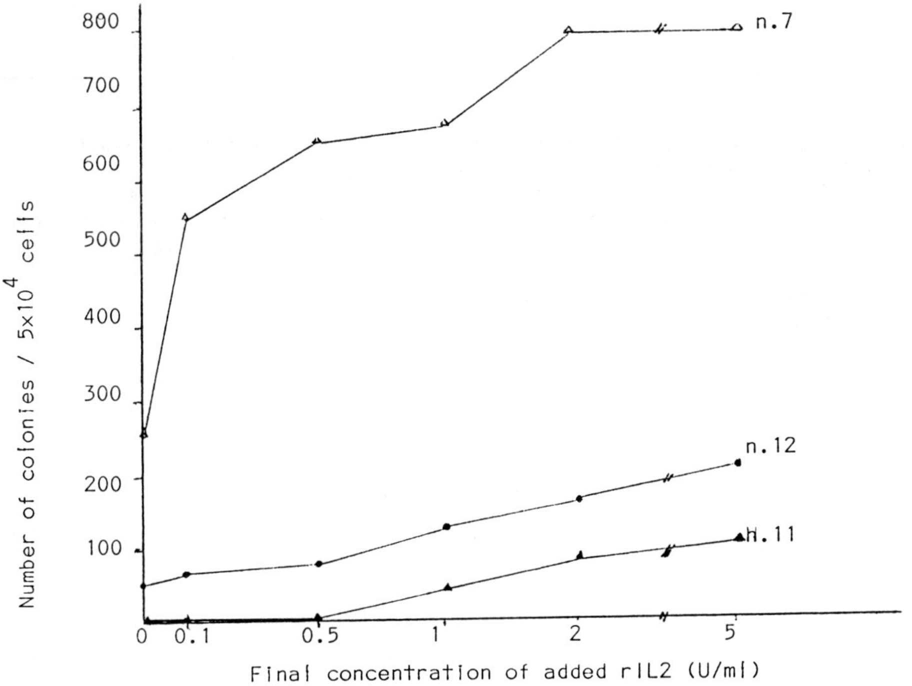

Figure 1

LEGEND

Fig. 1 : Dose-response curves of IL2-induced T-cell colony formation. 5 x 10^5 blast-enriched (E^- $T3^-$) cells/ml were seeded in 0.8 % (v/v) methylcellulose in growth medium supplemented with 15 % FCS, glutamine and antibiotics in the presence of various concentrations of rIL2 and incubated at 37°C, 5 % CO2, for 5-7 days. Aggregates containing more than 50 cells were counted as colonies. One unit of rIL2 = 40 BRMP units.

Neo-Adjuvant Chemotherapy. Ed. Cl. Jacquillat, M. Weil, D. Khayat. Colloque INSERM/John Libbey Eurotext Ltd. © 1988. Vol. 169, pp. 899-901.

Biological activities and potential clinical utility of human recombinant IL-3 and IL-4

Jan E. de Vries, Sem Saeland and Hergen Spits

UNICET, Laboratory for Immunological Research, 69570 Dardilly, France

Recently, we cloned human IL-3 from a cDNA library constructed from an activated T cell line. The immature IL-3 protein consists of 133 aminoacids. This IL-3 differs by one aminoacid at position 27 from the sequence published by Yang et al (Cell, 47, 3, 1986). The deduced molecular weight (M.W) of the mature protein is≃ 14,600. This M.W. of 14,600 does not take into account post translational glycosylation of the polypeptide, which is predicted by the presence of 2 potential N-glycosylation sites, which account for the size heterogeneity ot the protein expressed in Cos-7 cells (20,000, 21,000, 23,000).

IL-3 was used as supernatant from mammalian Cos-7 cells transfected with a pc D-expression vector containing the hIL-3 cDNA sequence. The biological effects of IL-3 were tested on cell fractions from umbilicord and normal bone narrow. Cells were fractionated by "panning" methods according to their expression of the CD34 surface membrane antigen, defined by the monoclonal anti-My-10 antibody. CD34 is expressed on early human hematopoietic progenitors which represent approximately of 1 % of the total bone marrow cell population. This approach was taken in order to characterize direct effects of IL-3 on its target cell thereby minimizing bystander activities mediated by accessory cells. We found that IL-3 added to CD34 enriched cells cultured in semi-solid medium induced the generation of myeloid and erythroid colonies in the presence of human erythropoietin. Based on morphological and cytological criteria, these colonies could be categorized into granulocyte-macrophage (CFU-GM), neutrophilic granulocyte (CFU-G), eosinophil (CFU-EO), monocyte/macrophage (CFU-M), erythroid burst (BFU-e) and mixed erythroid (CFU-mix) consisting of myeloid and erythroid elements. IL-3 did not induce any significant colony formation when tested on CD34-depleted marrow-or cord blood cell fractions. IL-3 also induced proliferation of CD34+ cells in liquid cultures, whereas only minimal cell proliferation was obtained with the CD34 depleted fraction. Culturing of CD34 enriched fractions in the presence of IL-3 resulted in an increase in the numbers of cells of the monocyte/macrophage and granulocyte lineages, as measured by the expression of CD14 and CD15 antigens respectively. In combination with human erythropoietin IL-3 promoted the emergence of erythroid lineage elements, as indicated by a strong induction of cells expressing glycophorin A and of cells of the trombocytic series expressing platelet associated Gp II b-III a complex. In addition, cytological characterization demonstrated that IL-3 induced the differentiation of the eosinophilic lineage.

Collectively, these data indicate that normal hematopoietic progenitor cells enriched for expression of CD34 antigen could be induced to proliferate and differentiate into all myeloid and erythroid lineages both in liquid and semi-solid cultures. In addition, these data indicate that the CD34 enriched cell fraction contained multipotential progenitor cells responding to IL-3.

IL-3 also induced the proliferation in liquid cultures of fresh acute myeloblastic leukemia cells tested. However, no clear correlation between proliferation and FAB classification was noted.

The fact that IL-3 has growth promoting and differentiation inducing activities on early multipotential progenitor cells implies that IL-3 may have important potential clinical utility. IL-3 could be used for the treatment of virally induced cytopenia (AIDS). IL-3 may shorten periods of chemotherapy or irradiation-induced bone marrow hyperplasia and reduce the rate and severity of neutropenia related sepsis. Finally, IL-3 may be of great value to support bone marrow transplantation. GM-CSF also induced proliferation of CD34 enriched cells which however was consistently lower than that obtained with IL-3. Simultaneous addition of IL-3 and GM-CSF to CD34-enriched cells in liquid cultures resulted in an additive growth promoting effect. However, sequential addition of IL-3 and GM-CSF resulted in a strong augmentation of the proliferative response to GM-CSF. In contrast, addition of GM-CSF followed by IL-3 had no enhancing effect. These data indicate that optimal growth promoting effects are obtained when IL-3 and GM-CSF are added sequentially. Although it remains to be tested, it is tempting to speculate that sequential addition of IL-3 and GM-CSF in vivo may also result in enhanced growth of bone marrow cells.

IL-4 inhibits IL-2 induced LAK cell activity

cDNA clones encoding IL-4 have been isolated from a cDNA library constructed from one of our activated cloned T cell lines. The mature IL-4 popypeptide consists of 129 aminoacid residues and the deduced M.W. is ≃ 15,000. The IL-4 molecule has two potential glycosylation sites and naturally produced IL-4 in differentially glycosylated, as determined by it's heterogeneity in M.W. (15,000, 18,000 and 19,000). Recombinant human IL-4 has pleiotropic effects. We have demonstrated that IL-4 acts as a growth factor for activated B cells, T cells and natural killer (NK) cells. In addition, IL-4 induces the expression of CD23 and class MHC antigens on normal and malignant B cells. Finally, IL-4 was shown to induce IgE production by normal B cells.

Here, we report that IL-4 blocks lymphokine activated killer (LAK) cell activity. IL-2 has been shown to induce lymphokine activated killer cell activity against target cells that are not sensitive for fresh natural killer cells. The precursor of these LAK cells have all the characteristics of NK cells. In PBL, the LAK precursor is contained mainly within the CD3- NKH-1+ subset, the majority of which also express CD2. Human IL-4 is unable to induce LAK cell activity against target cells that are not sensitive for fresh NK cell activity. However, IL-4 strongly inhibited the IL-2 mediated induction of LAK cell activity in a dose dependant manner. IL-4 also inhibited the induction of LAK activity induced in CD3- NKH-1+ cells suggesting that the LAK precursor cells is the target of the inhibitory effect of IL-4. IL-4 did not inhibit the activity of LAK cells once they were activated by IL-2, since PBL activated for 24 hrs with IL-2 and subsequently incubated with IL-2 plus IL-4 developed LAK cell activity which was similar to those cells incubated with IL-2 only. Moreover, incubation of T cell clones that have all the phenotypic characteristics of LAK cells (CD3- NKH-1+

or CD3+ CD16+ NKH-1+) with IL-4 did not affect the cytotoxicity of these clones against the NK insensitive target cell Daudi. IL-4 only inhibited the IL-2 mediated LAK activity from PBL, but also from spleen, tonsils and thymocytes. Interestingly, IL-4 inhibited the induction of IL-2 mediated cytotoxic activities of thymocytes against NK insensitive target cells and also against the NK sensitive target cell K562. This latter observation suggest that IL-4 plays a negative regulatory role in the differentiation of NK cells, but that this activity of IL-4 is only restricted to those cytotoxic activities induced by IL-2. Collectively, these data imply that IL-4 may have a potential clinical utility in those situtations where NK cell activity is associated with transplant rejection.

Neo-Adjuvant Chemotherapy. Ed. Cl. Jacquillat, M. Weil, D. Khayat. Colloque INSERM/John Libbey Eurotext Ltd. © 1988. Vol. 169, pp. 903-905.

Facteurs de croissance : de la révolution biologique à la révolution thérapeutique en cancérologie

C. Jasmin

Hôpital Paul Brousse, Laboratoire d'Hématologie, Villejuif, France

Les grands progrès conceptuels et technologiques de la biologie moléculaire dans le domaine du cancer ont marqué la révolution biologique des années 80.

La biologie moléculaire a offert des outils remarquables pour analyser certaines étapes initiales du processus de cancérisation cellulaire et mis en évidence le rôle important de certains gènes appelés oncogènes qui codent pour des facteurs de croissance, des récepteurs de ces facteurs ou des molécules capables de moduler l'expression de notre machinerie génétique combinée à la cytogénétique, elle a permis de localiser ces oncogènes au niveau des chromosomes et de mettre en évidence des remaniements chromosomiques apparemment spécifiques dans la plupart des cancers humains. En particulier, l'étude de cancers héréditaires comme le rétinoblastome a permis d'identifier des gènes anticancer ou anti-oncogènes dont l'altération peut jouer un rôle essentiel dans le développement de la tumeur.

On voit donc se dessiner un modèle de la cancérisation qui résulterait de la perturbation d'une balance subtile de l'expression des gènes essentiels jouant un rôle positif et/ou négatif dans la prolifération et la différentiation des cellules normales.

La biologie moléculaire associée au progrès des méthodes de biochimie et de biologie cellulaire a aussi permis d'identifier, de produire et de purifier des quantités théoriquement illimitées de molécules biologiques qui contrôlent directement ou indirectement la différenciation et la prolifération cellulaire normale et parfois maligne. Ainsi, ont été identifiés des médiateurs des principaux tissus et leurs récepteurs : interleukines et lymphokines pour le système myélo et lymphopoïétique, le facteur de croissance fibroblastique (FGF) pour le tissu conjontif (os, muscles par exemple), le facteur de croissance épidermique (EGF), pour le tissu épithélial (muqueuses par exemple), des facteurs pour le tissu endothélial (PDGF), et même des facteurs associés à la transformation (étape fréquente de la cancérisation) cellulaire (TGF).

Les interleukines et lymphokines permettent aussi de manipuler les réactions immunitaires de l'hôte contre les cellules tumorales et d'autres molécules devraient servir à manipuler l'hôte pour contenir ou détruire sa tumeur, par exemple en agissant sur la vascularisation tumorale ou ce qu'on appelle de manière plus globale (et imprécise) le microenvironnement de la tumeur.

En résumé, l'intervention thérapeutique pourrait s'effectuer à trois niveaux :

a) génotypique : il s'agirait de réparer, de compenser, de stimuler, d'altérer ou de supprimer l'activité et/ou l'activation des oncogènes ou anti-oncogènes.

La biologie moléculaire offre les éventuels outils de telles interventions thérapeutiques : par exemple l'introduction de gènes compensateurs dans des cellules souches normales, modulation de gènes par l'utilisation de séquences dites antisens capables de bloquer spécifiquement l'activation de certains gènes, mutagènese dirigée ... De telles méthodes sont déjà à l'oeuvre dans le cas des maladies génétiques, chez l'animal et même chez l'homme, et pourraient s'appliquer à la prévention du traitement de certains cancers. De manière beaucoup moins spécifique, certains antimitotiques comme la 5-aza-cytidine ou des substances comme les dérivés de l'acide rétinoîque pourraient aussi moduler l'expression des gènes et font l'objet d'essais thérapeutiques, en particulier dans les hémopathies malignes.

b) phénotypique : puiqu'il est démontré au moins expérimentalement qu'on peut faire différencier normalement jusqu'au stade terminal (c'est-à-dire jusqu'à la mort par différenciation) des cellules malignes. L'hormonothérapie des cancers du sein et de la prostate fait d'ailleurs figure de précurseur dans ce domaine. Ainsi, il apparait possible de contourner le niveau génique pour faire de la compensation, de la réparation à l'aide des molécules dont nous disposons, par exemple les interleukines et les facteurs de croissance.

Chez les souris, des succès ont été obtenus _in vivo_ dans le traitement de certaines tumeurs transplantées. Chez l'homme, l'injection de GM-CSF (granulocyte-macrophage colony-stimulating factor) une des interleukines qui joue un rôle important dans la prolifération et la différenciation des cellules souches myéloîdes, a permis d'obtenir des résultats prometteurs sur des patients atteints de syndrome myélodyslasique. Cette affection hématologique caractérisée par un défaut de maturation des précurseurs des lignées érythocytaires, granulocytaires de plaquettes accompagné le plus souvent d'un excès de cellules blastiques n'est pas véritablement une leucémie, bien qu'elle puisse le devenir mais son évolution est généralement mortelle en quelques mois ou années.

In vitro, il est possible d'obtenir la prolifération et la différenciation de cellules de leucémies aigues myéloîdes humaines qui conservent cependant les marqueurs caractéristiques du clone malin. Il est probable que des essais de traitement des leucémies humaines seront bientôt entrepris. L'acide rétinoîque, dont le récepteur présente des analogies importantes avec les récepteurs des hormones stéroîdiennes et thyroîdiennes illustre les relations étroites existant entre le système hormonal et les facteurs de croissance aussi bien au cours du développement embryonnaire, que dans l'organisme normal ou au cours de la cancérisation. Comme dans le cas de l'hormonothérapie, les traitements seront substitutifs et devront être poursuivis au long cours, ce qui implique une excellente tolérance des produits utilisés.

c) immunologique : car les interactions entre les systèmes de l'organisme commencent à être un peu plus connues, ainsi, le système endocrinien, le système nerveux central, le système immunitaire, l'hématopoîèse et même différents viscères (intestins, poumons ...) semblent reliés par des médiateurs comme les hormones, les neuropeptides, les lymphokines, et/ou interleukines ...
La découverte récente de la neuroleukine est venue renforcer la réalité des liaisons entre ces systêmes dans l'organisme.

Par exemple, le GM-CSF qui est capable d'augmenter la production des leucocytes pourrait être utilisé pour diminuer le risque d'infection en cas d'immunodéficience congénitale ou acquise. Il pourrait aussi améliorer les résultats de la greffe de moelle osseuse et diminuer les effets toxiques des drogues antimitotiques.

Les TNF α et β agiraient sur les tumeurs humaines (greffées chez la souris nude) par l'intermédiaire des cellules monocytaires-macrophagiques.

Le facteur nécrosant des tumeurs (TNFα et β) semble jouer un rôle de régulation de la prolifération des cellules fibroblastiques normales ; il serait couplé avec l'interféron β2, qui assurerait un contrôle négatif de son effet. Comme les interférons, les TNF ont des effets pléïotropiques et sur divers tissus comme par exemple :

a) l'augmentation des antigènes HLA classes I et II sur les cellules endothéliales et fibroblastiques.
b) une activité antivirale.
c) un effet sur la résorption osseuse.

De même, les interleukines 1 peuvent en plus de leur effet sur les lymphocytes T et B, induire un état de fièvre avec hypercatabolisme protidique, jouer un rôle dans l'inflammation et dans le contrôle de la production des glucocorticoïdes... Ainsi, comme le démontrent les premiers essais cliniques de traitement par l'interféron ou l'interleukine 2, la manipulation du système immunitaire par de fortes doses risque d'être limitée par des effets toxiques du fait du pléiotropisme de ces molécules. Ce qui pourrait constituer un écueil important à leur utilisation thérapeutique.

Malgré ces restrictions, il est probable que les recherches des années 90 seront portées par l'espoir de transformer la révolution biologique des années 80 en une révolution thérapeutique.

Symposium nausea, vomiting and chemotherapy

Nausées, vomissements et chimiothérapie

Neo-Adjuvant Chemotherapy. Ed. Cl. Jacquillat, M. Weil, D. Khayat. Colloque INSERM/John Libbey Eurotext Ltd. © 1988. Vol. 169, p.909.

Editorial

F.O. Oberling

In recent years, optimizing the use of drugs already available given at adequate doses individually, or in suitable combination, has led to improved control of emesis induced by highly emetogenic cytotoxic drugs.

However, the search for new agents with higher therapeutic indexes still remains the principal target in this field.

ALIZAPRIDE, a new benzamide derivative was one of them in these recent years.

The most emetogenic drug in use is CISPLATIN and none of the standard agent is satisfactory in controlling its vomiting.

Recent papers highlighted that the 5-hydrotryptamine receptor is the potential source for the nausea and vomiting induced by chemotherapy and/or radiotherapy. This is now a new way in research using 5-HT Receptor antagonists.

But, in high doses, METOCLOPRAMIDE interacts with 5-HT Receptors.

Neo-Adjuvant Chemotherapy. Ed. Cl. Jacquillat, M. Weil, D. Khayat. Colloque INSERM/John Libbey Eurotext Ltd. © 1988. Vol. 169, pp. 911-918.

Synthèse des travaux concernant l'alizapride dans les chimiothérapies

D. Cupissol et M. Caubel

Service d'Immunochimiothérapie, Centre Val-d'Aurelle, rue de la Croix Verte, 34094, Montpellier Cedex, France

Les nausées et les vomissements sont un facteur limitant quelques fois l'utilisation de la chimiothérapie chez le patient cancéreux. En effet, les troubles digestifs font partie des incidents secondaires liés aux traitements des cancers. Les médias retiennent souvent ce point, de telle sorte qu'il reste bien ancré dans les esprits du grand public.

L'introduction d'agents anti-émétisants dans la thérapeutique des cancers est un élément d'appoint absolument indispensable permettant à la fois de conforter le malade donc d'améliorer à terme le succès de la chimiothérapie. La tâche du thérapeute s'en trouve simplifiée.

Parmi les médicaments moyennement émétisants, il faut citer les nitrosourées, la cyclophosphamide et les antracyclines qui induisent des nausées de façon aléatoire chez les patients. Par contre, la Dacarbazine et l'Actinomycine sont des produits entrainant quasi systématiquement des nausées. Enfin, il faut citer tout spécialement comme champion toutes catégories le Cisplatine qui est l'un des produits les plus remarquables de la pharmacopée par cet aspect toxique.

Les mécanismes des vomissements passent par trois voies essentielles :

- par le cortex supérieur et le diencéphale, d'où l'importance des sensations olfactives et des phénomènes psychiques ;

- par le système nerveux para-sympathique ;

- par les chémorécepteurs : Trigger zone qui se situe dans la paroi postérieure du 4ème ventricule.

En fonction de ces mécanismes, quelles sont les possibilités d'améliorer ces nausées ?

- Les sédatifs ont été souvent utilisés mais se sont aussi révélés peu efficaces notamment pour les vomissements iatrogènes.

- Les dérivés du canabis induisent des effets secondaires, des phénomènes d'assuétude et d'accoutumance de telle sorte que la législation française n'a pas permis leur introduction sur notre territoire.

- Les corticoïdes sont des produits efficaces, mais leur mécanisme d'action est mal connu, on pense qu'ils agiraient par l'intermédiaire des prostaglandines. Toutefois ils présentent l'inconvénient de ne pas pouvoir être utilisés dans tous les cas, la cortisone étant souvent un facteur facilitant le développement des tumeurs.
- Les antihistaminiques sont un élément d'appoint, ils ont un impact essentiellement labyrinthique et qui se révèle efficace dans le mal des transports.
  Des progrès substantiels ont été réalisés avec les benzamides substitués.

Nous nous sommes attachés à l'étude d'un de ces composés connu sous le nom chimique d'Alizapride, (nom de spécialité "Plitican"). Ce benzamide est le N(Allyl-1-pyrrotidinyl-2) methyl) methoxy-2, azimide-4,5 benzamide-hydrochlorate. Ces principales caractéristiques pharmacologiques sont les suivantes:

- Il est peu toxique : DL 50, de 200 mg/kg en sous-cutané chez la souris, et de 370 mg/kg en sous-cutané chez le rat.

- La toxicité chronique montre qu'une dose de 100mg/kg/jour per os chez le rat, pendant 12 mois n'a pas entraîné de mortalité.

- Ce produit a deux demi-vies, la première à 0,125 $\pm$ 0,007 heures et la seconde à 2,51 $\pm$ 1,49 heures.

- En outre l'Alizapride exerce son action à plusieurs niveaux.

- Sur le système nerveux central, il se révèle un antagoniste très puissant à doses faibles vis-à-vis des poisons émétisants comme l'apomorphine. Il a le grand avantage de ne pas entraîner de manifestations dépressives centrales, il n'a pas de propriété anticonvulsivante, ni antianalgésique.

- sur le système para-sympathique il n'induit pas de phénomènes anticholinergiques.

- Sur le système sympathique, il entraîne une limitation des poussées hypertensives dues à l'adrénaline.

En conclusion, cette molécule n'a pas d'action sur le système neurovégétatif ce qui marque une différence fondamentale avec les phénothiazines. Sur la base de ces données pharmacologiques, les premières études de NICAISE ont montré en phase I, l'efficacité potentielle de ce produit à moindre dose (1). Effectivement, ce dernier était administré sous la forme de perfusions d'un quart d'heure toutes les deux heures. Les doses testées étaient de 1 mg/Kg à 5 mg/Kg. C'est uniquement pour cette dernière dose qu'il est apparu quelques hypotensions sévères. Mais une efficacité réelle était notée pour la dose de 4 mg/Kg.

D'autres essais de phase II ont montré qu'il était possible d'aller éventuellement au delà de la dose de 5 mg/ Kg. Les tests à 6 mg et 8 mg/kg ont montré des manifestations d'intolérance majeure chez 4 patients au cours des 4 cycles de chimiothérapie à la dose de 8 mg/kg, par contre à la dose de 6 mg/kg seulement six incidents ont été dénombrés chez 9 patients. Toutefois la dose de 4 mg était, là aussi, montrée comme la dose la mieux tolérée (2).

Les enseignements des phases I et II montraient donc une bonne tolérance globale du produit jusqu'à 5 mg/kg avec la possibilité compte-tenu du faible nombre d'incidents secondaires de pouvoir répéter les injections, d'autant que la demie-vie de ce médicament est relativement courte.

Il s'avérait donc nécessaire de multiplier les injections pour maintenir un taux sérique efficace et constant durant toute la période correspondant à la phase d'action des produits de chimiothérapie considérés. Si on prend le cas du Cisplatinum, ce produit a deux demi-vies, la deuxième demie-vie pouvant s'étaler jusqu'au delà de la troisième heure. Il nous parait donc nécessaire de couvrir toute la période d'administration du produit. Le but de l'administration de l'anti-émétique est de bloquer les centres nerveux, que ce soient les récepteurs ou les voies de communication afférentes ou efférentes. Il est donc nécessaire d'assurer : une couverture anti-émétique préventive, puis durant toute la période de perfusion de la chimiothérapie, et enfin il s'avère nécessaire de traiter après la perfusion dans la mesure où la pharmacologie du médicament indique des taux efficaces, au-delà de la perfusion dans les 24 à 48 heures suivant même l'arrêt de cette chimiothérapie. Des nausées et des vomissements se manifestent souvent dans cette période.

Sur la base de ces données, plusieurs protocoles ont donc été étudiés afin de couvrir toute la période des effets pharmacodynamiques liés au produits de chimiothérapie.

Compte-tenu de la diversité de la pharmacologie et de la pharmacodynamie des produits de chimiothérapie, il nous parait interessant de les distinguer en deux groupes :

- ceux qui sont donc moyennement émétisants

- ceux qui sont toujours émétisants comme le cisplatine.

De nombreuses études de phase III ont été menées afin de montrer l'efficacité de diverses associations d'Alizapride soit par rapport à des placébos, soit par rapport aux produits de référence habituellement utilisés tel que le Métodopramide ou les corticoïdes.

Pour J.J. VIALA et collaborateurs, il a été pratiqué une injection de 100 mg d'Alizapride ou de placébo I.V. avant chimiothérapie, puis une injection IM à la même dose quatre heures après. Le résultat était tel que les réponses positives étaient dénombrées chez les patients traités par Alizapride à 76% et 50% par placébo (3). La différence était importante mais n'avait pas de valeur significative compte-tenu du nombre de patients traités. De même pour l'essai qui évaluait l'intérêt d'une perfusion de 4 mg/kg trente minutes avant le Cisplatine puis une heure trente après le Cisplatine, puis trois heures, cinq et sept heures après le Cisplatine. Cette étude n'était réalisée que sur cinq patients qui ne montraient que quatre vomissements moyens sous Alizapride et sept vomissements moyens sous placébo. Ceci prouvait encore une efficacité réelle sans pour autant qu'il soit possible d'en tirer des conclusions statistiquement significatives.

Plus intéressantes sur le plan statistique en conclusion d'une autre étude randomisée, CLAVEL a montré une différence significative en faveur du Plitican par rapport à un placébo (4).

Les études de F. Oberlin montrent une efficacité réelle de l'Alizapride sur le métolopramide. Chez 57 malades étudiés en double aveugle, il était administré 100 mg d'alizapride pendant le traitement plus 100 mg IM quatre heures après versus 20 mg de métolopramide pendant le traitement et 20 mg quatre après. La différence est très hautement significative avec un p 0,05 en faveur de l'Alizapride (5).

Un consensus semble se détacher sur l'intérêt des effets anti-émétisants de l'alizapride dans les chimiothérapies ne comportant pas de cisplatinum. Nous nous sommes plus particulièrement intéressés à l'étude de l'alizapride dans les chimiothérapies associant du cisplatine.

Nous avons utilisé chez 50 patients vomisseurs de très fortes doses de produit de l'ordre de 600, 800 et 900 mg par jour alors que la dose habituelle était de 150 à 350 mg.

Le protocole d'administration était fractionné de sorte que les patients recevaient 200 mg au branchement de la perfusion de cisplatinum.
200 mg dans le flacon de cisplatinum, 100 mg en IV lente au débranchement de flacon de perfusion soit à la fin de perfusion et ils recevaient également 100 mg une heure ou deux heures après la fin de la perfusion par voie intra musculaire.

Cette méthode d'administration fractionnée a permis de montrer la bonne tolérance globale d'ensemble pour des fortes doses, avec des phénomènes de baisse de la vigilance. Ceci étant, il y avait un bénéfice en ce qui concerne les nausées et les vomissements (6).

Une étude analogue a été menée également par MENEGOLD et collaborateurs qui utilisaient l'alizapride avec le cisplatinum en ambulatoire. Ils ont mis en évidence l'action préventive du produit et insisté sur l'intérêt de traiter avant l'administration de platine (7).

Ceci rejoint le travail que nous avions réalisé puisque les patients recevaient 100 mg per os toutes les 6 heures avant le cisplatinum et 100 mg IV avec le cisplatinum.

Ces résultats ont montré un intérêt tout à fait significatif de l'amélioration des nausées et des vomissements et ont souligné l'importance fondamentale des traitements préventifs.

Il est donc possible d'utiliser le Plitican à très fortes doses avec une bonne tolérance. Il est donc nécessaire de fractionner la dose, particulièrement pour traiter préventivement les malades dans un espace de temps allant de 6 h à 1 h avant le début de la perfusion. Toutefois, le cisplatinum reste un produit difficile à administrer.

Des essais en double aveugle ont montré des résultats contradictoires. L'Alizapride comparée à la Dompéridone, n'a pas montré de modificationx significatives. Chaque patient recevait alternativement deux traitements : une injection 30 mn avant la chimiothérapie, puis 4 injections espacées de 2 heures (soit 4 mg/J d'Alizapride, soit 0,6 mg/J de Dompéridone).

La synthèse de ces études met en évidence une molécule ayant des potentialités anti-émétisantes formelles mais dont la maitrise reste encore à déterminer avec plus de précisions afin d'en dégager un meilleur effet pharmacodynamique.

L'introduction des études pharmacocinétiques et pharmacologiques plus systématiques doit faire appel aux méthodes d'ajustement de posologie des chimiothérapies. Des applications potentielles à l'Alizapride devraient permettre à terme une diminution encore plus systématique des nausées et des vomissements.

- REFERENCES -

1 - NICAISE C., ROZENWEIG M., ORTMANS M., FRISQUE C., BLEIBERG H.- Etude en phase I de l'Alizapride chez des patients cancéreux traités au cis-platine. Sem. Hôp. PARIS. 1983. 59. (31). 2161-2165

2 - JOSS R.A., GALEZZI R.L., BISCHOFF A.K., BRUNNER K.W.- Alizapride , a new substitued benzamide as an antiemetic during cancer chemotherapy. Eur. J. Clin. Pharmacology. 1985. 27-721

3 - VIALA J.J., GIRARD D., CORDIER J.F.- Etude en double insu d'un nouvel anti-émétique, l'Alizapride dans les nausées et vomissements de la chimiothérapie anticancéreuse. Sem. Hôp. 1982. 58 (6), 371-374

4 - POMMATAU E. Etude en double aveugle insu croisé alizapride placebo sur la prévention des nausées et des vomissements induits par la chimiothérapie antimitotique. Sem. Hôpi. 1982. 58. (6), 363-366

5 - OBERLING F.- Etude comparative en double aveugle. Alizapride-Métoclopramide. J. Med. Chir. Prat. 1984. 155. (5) 236-242

6 - CUPISSOL D., FAVIER F., FAVIER C., SERROU B.- Evaluation d'un nouvel antiémétique l'alizapride, en cancérologie. Sem. Hôp. 1982. 58. (22), 1370-1373

7 - MENEGOLD G., ABEL U., DROSS K., FRITZE D., HERMANN R.- The effect of Alizapride upon emesis induced by cytotoxic drugs clinical experience. Fourth NCI EORTC Symposium on new drugs in cancer therapy. Decembre 1983. BRUSSELS

Neo-Adjuvant Chemotherapy. Ed. Cl. Jacquillat, M. Weil, D. Khayat. Colloque INSERM/John Libbey Eurotext Ltd. © 1988. Vol. 169, pp. 919-923.

High-dose alizapride : clinical effectiveness and pharmacokinetic

E. Hiller*, K. Possinger* and G. Ehninger**

* *Medizinische Klinik III, University of Munich FRG.*
** *Medizinische Klinik, University of Tübingen, FRG.*

Inadequate antiemetic therapy during cancer chemotherapy may lead to a number of undesirable side effects, e.g. nausea and vomiting, non-compliance, dehydration and metabolic decompensation. Inadequate dosage of antiemetic drugs is probably a major cause for the large number of side effects. Since the original report by Gralla et al. (1) high-dose metoclopramide has been widely used for cisplatin - induced nausea and vomiting with better success than with conventional dosages. Alizapride is a newly substituted benzamide with similar central nervous properties to those of metoclopramide but without the gastro-kinetic properties of the latter drug. It has been claimed to possess a superior antiemetic efficacy and fewer side effects than metoclopramide (2, 5) but others reported a superiority of metoclopramide in cisplatin-induced emesis (3).

We studied the kinetics of alizapride in order to be able to define an optimal dose schedule. The purpose of the study was to evaluate

1) The safety and toxicity of the continuous high-dose infusion.
2) To evaluate a simple assay for alizapride.
3) To determine whether the hydration given to cisplatin therapy will lead to lower drug levels than in chemotherapy without hydration.
4) To establish a correlation between the serum level and antiemetic effect and the side effects of alizapride.

Patients and Methods

The clinical data of the patients are listed in table 1. Of the 18 patients who could be evaluated 8 received a combination chemotherapy including cisplatin, 10 were treated by combinations without cisplatin.

Following a loading dose of 200 mg alizapride a 24 hour continuous infusion with 15 mg/kg of alizapride was given. The processing of the serum samples and the HPTLC-chromatography system according to Dross are summarized in table 2.The detection limit of this method is 2 ng/ml, the day to day variation coefficient at a concentration of 150 ng/ml is 9%.

Results

Figure 1 depicts the course of the serum concentration in one patient who was given a loading dose of 5 mg/kg followed by a continuous infusion of 15 mg/kg over a 22 hour period. At the end of the loading dose a peak concentration of 4 µg/ml was achieved. During continuous infusion the serum concentrations of this patient were between 1 and 2 µg/ml.

Figure 2 depicts the serum concentrations of 18 patients under steady-state conditions. The average serum concentration amounted to 1.7 µg/ml with considerable intraindividual variation. Minimal serum levels amounted to 0.4 µg/ml and maximal values to 10 µg/ml. There was no difference in the group of cisplatin - treated patients with hydration as compared to the patients without cisplatin and thus without hydration.

Under antiemetic therapy with high-dose alizapride 9 out of 18 patients experienced no vomiting, 4 out of 18 no nausea.
Table 3 summarizes the degree of the objective efficacy. In this context the inhomogeniity of the diagnosis, the type of therapy and the number of pretreatments should be considered.

The subjective effects of high-dose alizapride therapy are summarized in table 4 and the observed side effects are listed in table 5.
Effects and side effects were correlated with the measured serum levels and evaluated in the 4-field-test.
The following conclusions could be derived:

Side effects:

1. Dryness of mouth (serum concentration 2-s-range)
2. Extensive vomiting (serum concentration 10 fold above median, intoxication?)
3. Diminished activity of the patient with high serum levels ($p=0.01$)
4. All other side effects showed no correlation.

Efficacy:

1. 4/4 cisplatin-treated patients with nausea grade 3 + 4 had serum levels $<$ median value.
2. 3/4 cisplatin-treated patients with nausea grade 1 + 2 had serum levels $>$ median value.

3. No correlation was found between extent of vomiting and serum level.

Discussion

Our data show that following an initial loading dose of 200 mg alizapride a continuous intravenous infusion with 15 mg/kg alizapride leads to a steady state level between 0.5 and 3.5 μg/ml (1.6±0.7 μg/ml). The hydration which is obligatory with cisplatin therapy did not lead to a decrease in serum concentration. The dosing regimen used circumvents unwanted high peak concentrations. The efficacy of the drug in this study was not very satisfactory ~~in this study~~ but this was not the purpose of the investigation, considering the heterogeneiity of patients, the number of pretreatments and differing Chemotherapy regimens.

Our clinical and pharmacological data suggest that in a future study the 24hour continuous infusion could be reduced to 12 hours to achieve higher serum levels and thus a more pronounced antiemetic effect.

Literature

1. Gralla, R.J., Intri, L., Pisko, L.M., Squillante, S.E., Kelsen, D.P., Braun, D.W., Bordin, L.A., Braun, T.J., Young, C.W.: Antiemetic efficacy of high dose metoclopramide: Randomized trials with placebo and prochlorperazine in patients with chemotherapy-induced nausea and vomiting. N. Engl. J. Med. (1981) 305, 905 - 909

2. Huys, J., Troch, M., Bourguignon, R.P., Smets, Ph.: High-dose alizapride versus high-dose domperidone: a double blind comperative study in the management of CIS-platinum-induced emesis. Curr. Med. Res. Opin.(1985) 9, 400 - 406

3. Joss, R.A., Galeazzi, R.L., Bischoff, A.K., Pirovino, M., Ryssel, H.J., Brunner, K.W.: The antiemetic activity of high-dose alizapride and high-dose metoclopramide in patients receiving cancer chemotherapy: A prospective, randomized, double-blind trial. Clin. pharmacol. Ther. (1986) 39, 619 - 624

4. Schütte, J., Niederle, N., Krischke, W., Giesche, U., Seeber, S.: Antiemetische Wirksamkeit von Alizapride bei Cisplatin-bedingtem Erbrechen.
Tumor-Diagnostik & Therapy (1983) 4, 146 - 149

5. Von Budach, V., Krüger, K.: Alizapride im Doppelblindversuch mit Metoclopramid bei Übelkeit und Erbrechen infolge einer Strahlentherapie. Fortschr. Med. (1983) 101, 1792 - 1794

Neo-Adjuvant Chemotherapy. Ed. Cl. Jacquillat, M. Weil, D. Khayat. Colloque INSERM/John Libbey Eurotext Ltd. © 1988. Vol. 169, pp. 925-928.

Pharmacokinetic study of alizapride in children receiving chemotherapy for solid tumors

E.R. Stettler*, G. Pons**, E. Rey, M.O. Richard**, J. Lemerle* and G. Olive**

* *Institut Gustave-Roussy, Service de Pédiatrie, 94805 Villejuif Cedex, France*
** *Département de Pharmacologie Clinique Périnatale et Pédiatrique, Hôpital Saint-Vincent-de-Paul, 75674 Paris Cedex, France*

Nausea, retching and vomiting represent the more distressing and feared side effects of chemotherapy and radiotherapy in children having a malignant solid tumor. In comparison, a real breakthrough for pain control has been achieved in the same clinical situations [1]. This breakthrough has been possible mainly for two reasons: 1) a fairly precise knowledge of the neurophysiological mechanisms involved; 2) the availability of a large choice of active drugs, allowing an individualized and flexible control of pain. Our understanding of the physiology of emesis is incomplete, and the available drugs are, in the best hands, active in 70% of the situations, allowing not more than a blunderbuss prevention of nausea and vomiting [2][3].

The chemotherapy of solid tumors in infants, children and adolescents include highly emetogenic agents such as cisplatinum, dacarbazine actinomycin D, mechlorethamine, cyclophosphamide, ifosfamide, doxorubicin, daunorubicin, cytarabine, procarbazine and high dose methotrexate. So the need for improved control of nausea and vomiting has become of important consideration in both pediatric oncology and supportive care.

Although not satisfactory in all respects [4], metoclopramide has become a reference molecule: a serious limitation of its use in children and young adults is the relative high incidence of acute dystonic reactions, such as trismus, torticollis, protrusion of the tongue, as well as hiccup and neurovegetative reactions. In this respect, alizapride, a congener molecule, shares only mildly and partially these side-effects. In order to optimalise the use of alizapride, a pharmacokinetic study of this antiemetic was decided, with the aim of giving an optimal protection without side effects.

A preliminary study done in our Division showed that a loading dose of 4 mg/kg, and a maintenance dose of 16 mg/kg/day of alizapride tend to show the best protective effect against nausea and vomiting. With these dosages, unpleasant side effects have rarely been encountered. The following study design has been chosen:

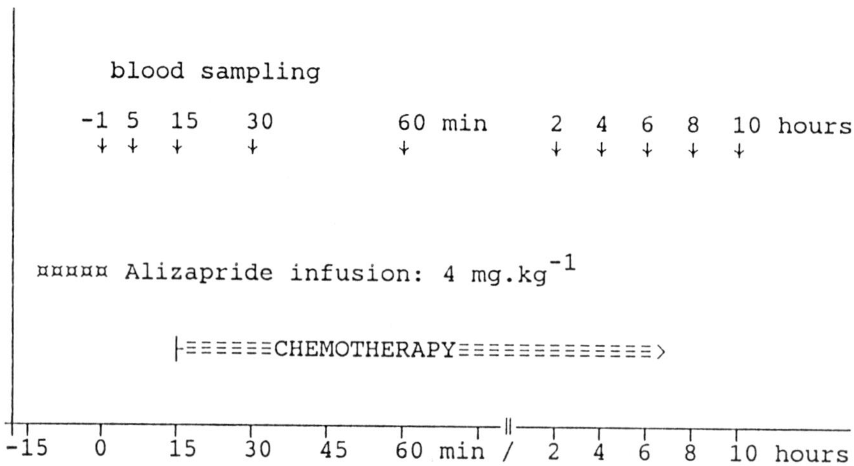

An alizapride infusion of 4 $mg.kg^{-1}$ body weight is given in a peripheral vein over 15 min, using an electric syringe. Fifteen minutes after the completion of the alizapride infusion, the anti-neoplasic chemotherapy is started, whatever its type. Blood sampling for alizapride is drawn from another veinous access as noted.

Blood samples are centrifugated immediately at 1500 RPM, and supernatant stored at - 30°C. In adolescents, urine has been collected in 2 hours fractions and stored in the same conditions. Analysis was done with HPLC and a spectrofluorometric detection. Calculations have been performed with the program TRIOMPHE. Three groups of patients have been selected:

- group A: 1 month to 2 years
- group B: 2 to 5 years
- group C: 10 to 15 years

The first group is still under investigation: we are presenting here partial results: patients of group B anc C.

Morphologic characteristics are as follows:
Group B: body weight: 15.0 ± 2.0 kg; body surface: 0.64 ± 0.07 m^2
Group C: body weight: 29.2 ± 3.7 kg; body surface: 1.10 ± 0.12 m^2
Mean age for group B is 3 years and 11 months, for group C 11 years and 10 months.

Summary of pharmacokinetic data

AUC [$\mu g.l^{-1}.h$]	5574 ± 1496	8100 ± 1410	P<0.05
Cl [$l.h^{-1}.kg^{-1}$]	0.770 ± 0.243	0.499 ± 0.105	P<0.05
Vd_β [$l.kg^{-1}$]	2.60 ± 1.30	1.60 ± 0.31	NS
$t_{\frac{1}{2}\beta}$[h]	2.27 ± 0.53	2.25 ± 0.37	NS
UE [%]		66 ± 12	

AUC: area under the plasma concentration - time curve; Cl: plasma clearance; Vd_β: volume of distribution; $t_{\frac{1}{2}\beta}$: elimination half life; UE: urinary elimination in % of the administered dose.

The peak plasma concentration, at the end of alizapride infusion, has reached a maximal individual value of 9 $mg.l^{-1}$ in group B and 13 $mg.l^{-1}$ in group C. The $t_{\frac{1}{2}\alpha}$, for both groups, is 6.5 min.

Plasma clearance is significantly higher in 2-5 yo infants, compared to older children and to values reported in adults ($Cl = 0.40 \pm 0.12\ l.h^{-1}.kg^{-1}$). The volume of distribution tends to be higher in group B than in group C, this last one showing values very close to adults ($Vd_{\beta} = 1.22 \pm 0.45\ l.kg^{-1}$). The elimination half life is similar in small children, adolescents and adults.

Conclusions

Targeting an optimal alizapride concentration among 2 - 5 years old children implies the following adjustments compared to adults or adolescents:

1) Loading dose can safely be increased by 25%, practically, 5 $mg.kg^{-1}$ is suggested.

2) Maintenance dose should be increased by 18% and reach 19 $mg.kg^{-1}.d^{-1}$, preferably as a continuous infusion.

References

[1] The Medical Clinics of North America, Volume 71, Number 2, March 1987. Cancer pain.

[2] Treatment of Cancer Chemotherapy-Induced Nausea and Vomiting. Edited by Don S. POSTER, John S. PENTA, and Salvador BRUNO, from NCI. Masson Publishing USA, Inc., 1981.

[3] Antiemetics and Cancer Chemotherapy. Edited by John LASZLO. Williams & Wilkins, USA, 1983.

[4] Eur J Clin Pharmacol (1987) 33: 161-165. TAYLOR W.B., SIMPSON J.M. and BATEMAN D.N. High-dose Metoclopramide by Infusion: a Double-Blind Study of Plasma Concentration-Effect Relationships in Patients Receiving Cancer Chemotherapy.

This work was supported by grant 774/86 of the FONDATION DE FRANCE, Comité Leucémies, and by DELAGRANGE LABORATORIES (France).

Neo-Adjuvant Chemotherapy. Ed. Cl. Jacquillat, M. Weil, D. Khayat. Colloque INSERM/John Libbey Eurotext Ltd. © 1988. Vol. 169, pp. 929-940.

Metoclopramide as an anti-emetic for cancer chemotherapy

Richard J. Gralla

Memorial Sloan-Kettering Cancer Center, New-York, NY, USA

Metoclopramide plays a major role in controlling the emesis induced by cancer chemotherapy. Studies to enhance the activity of metoclopramide and to examine its mechanism of action continue to be important. Recent trials have reported several findings that affect the understanding and application of this agent. These findings include the following: 1) high doses of metoclopramide are required for maximum efficacy against the emesis caused by the most difficult chemotherapeutic agents; 2) combinations of metoclopramide plus a corticosteroid are more effective than single agent antiemetic treatment; 3) metoclopramide is helpful in regimens preventing delayed emesis as well as in the treatment of acute chemotherapy induced emesis; and 4) in addition to blocking dopamine receptors, metoclopramide in high doses may exert its antiemetic effects through interactions with serotonin receptors. Studies with metoclopramide have established its utility as an antiemetic in patients receiving cancer chemotherapy and have helped to outline rational study designs for antiemetic trials.

It is certainly unusual for a pharmaceutical agent to be the subject of both clinical and laboratory investigation over two decades after its original introduction. Nonetheless, metoclopramide now plays a major role in controlling the emesis induced by cancer chemotherapy, and studies to enhance its activity and to examine its mechanism of action continue to be important.

Studies conducted in the 1960's demonstrated the potential utility of metoclopramide as an antiemetic and helped establish the agent as a useful addition to clinical practice (1,2). Although reports indicated that metoclopramide had efficacy in a variety of situations where emesis is a problem, it appeared to have limited usefulness as an antiemetic with chemotherapy (2,3). As newer chemotherapeutic drugs became available, and as the problem of emesis became even more pressing, the role of metoclopramide was reexamined. Studies in the 1980's found that different dosage schedules and markedly higher doses could result in greater efficacy, even against the emesis caused by cisplatin (4,5,6). With greater interest in antiemetic research, new emetic problems were identified, and additional uses for metoclopramide were found (7). To understand the utility of metoclopramide, it may be helpful to review the studies of the physiology of emesis and the mechanism of action of antiemetics.

BACKGROUND

The mechanism by which chemotherapy induces emesis is not completely understood, although the studies of Borison have been revealing (8). Studies support the hypothesis that reflex-induced emesis is caused by stimulation of receptors in the central nervous system or in the gastrointestinal tract. Receptor areas have been identified that affect the vomiting or emetic center in the lateral reticular formation of the medulla, which then coordinates the act of vomiting. An important area also located in the medulla is the chemoreceptor trigger zone (CTZ), in the area postrema. This receptor region is sensitive to chemical stimuli from both the blood and the cerebrospinal fluid. Chemotherapeutic agents or their metabolites may stimulate receptors in the CTZ, such as dopamine receptors. Impulses generated in the CTZ and transmitted to the vomiting center may then lead to the initiation of emesis. Neuroreceptors in the gastrointestinal tract, which has afferents to the vomiting center, may also play a role in chemotherapy-induced nausea and vomiting.

Metoclopramide exerts its activity in both the central nervous system and in the gastrointestinal tract (2). This agent may affect several different neuroreceptors, and its actions have been linked to dopamine, serotonin, and cholinergic receptors. The studies of Justin-Besancon indicated that the major antiemetic activity is likely exerted via dopamine receptors (1). Apomorphine, a substance which causes the rapid onset of emesis by stimulating these receptors, was administered parenterally to dogs who had been given various antiemetics. The most effective agent was metoclopramide (1). The CTZ has a variety of neurotransmitter receptors including dopamine receptors. It is widely acknowledged that metoclopramide affects the dopamine D2 receptors in the CTZ.

A gastrointestinal action was indicated by the antiemetic protection noted with metoclopramide when dogs were given oral doses of copper sulfate (1). This is supported by the known clinical gastrokinetic action of metoclopramide and by its effects on preparations of isolated gastric smooth muscle (2). Recent studies indicate that at higher doses, metoclopramide may exert its actions in the gut via serotonin (5-HT3) receptors as well as through dopamine receptors (9). Antiemetic agents that block neuroreceptors in the CTZ, the vomiting center, or in the gastrointestinal tract may be useful in preventing or controlling emesis. In addition to blocking the emesis induced by apomorphine and copper sulfate in dogs, metoclopramide was also effective in preclinical trials in reducing vomiting caused by the chemotherapeutic agent cisplatin (10).

CLINICAL TRIALS

Studies over the past few years have indicated that metoclopramide is the most effective antiemetic available for the emesis induced by chemotherapy. When metoclopramide was given in typical 10mg or 20mg oral doses, antiemetic contol with chemotherapy was variable, but generally not sufficient (3,11,12). When given in high intravenous doses; however, superior results occur (5,6).

A study was conducted which investigated gradually increasing doses of intravenous metoclopramide (4). Eleven dose levels were explored from 0.4 mg/kg to 3.0 mg/kg, with the agent given by rapid infusion or by continuous intravenous infusion. All levels were administered with safety, and encouraging antiemetic effects were reported (4). Random-assignment studies have shown metoclopramide to be superior, or at least equivalent, to all other antiemetic agents it has been compared with, against cisplatin-induced emesis (5,6,13,14,15,16). Several reports have indicated useful activity against the emesis associated with a number of other chemotherapeutic agents (17,18,19).

A pharmacologic trial demonstrated that efficacy was correlated with of high blood levels (>850 ng/ml) of metoclopramide in patients receiving cisplatin (20). Also important is insuring an adequate level of this antiemetic at the time of emetic vulnerability through the use of an appropriate dosing schedule. In preventing emesis induced by cisplatin or by cyclophosphamide plus doxorubicin, metoclopramide administration every two hours (beginning shortly before chemotherapy) appears to be the most effective schedule. With the late onset of emesis often seen with cyclophosphamide (typically at 9 to 18 hours after administration)(21), it is important to maintain effective blood levels of the metoclopramide at that time.

High oral doses of metoclopramide (using 50 mg and 100 mg tablets) can result in therapeutic blood levels and can be highly effective (22,23,24). A study comparing similar high doses and schedules of oral metoclopramide with the same agent given intravenously, in patients receiving cisplatin 60 mg/m2, reported similar results in both arms of the study. Emesis was completely controlled in half of the patients while two-thirds achieved a major response (two or fewer emetic episodes) (24).

The side-effects commonly associated with metoclopramide include mild sedation, dystonic reactions, akathisia (restlessness), and diarrhea (which may be an effect of specific chemotherapeutic agents, such as cisplatin) (5,25). In general, the side-effects are easy to control or prevent. Akathisia is easily prevented or treated with a benzodiazepine, and dystonic reactions can be dealt with similarly or with diphenhydramine. Acute dystonic reactions, such as trismus or torticollus, are age related. In a report reviewing nearly five hundred patient courses of high dose metoclopramide, dystonic reactions were unusual in patients above age 30 (1.8%), while 27% ($p<0.001$) of younger patients had this reversible reaction (26). When dopamine blocking antiemetics, such as metoclopramide, are given on several consecutive days, dystonic reactions are also more common (27). This can be of importance for younger patients in that several regimens for malignancies of this age group utilize chemotherapy on a daily schedule.

COMBINATIONS OF ANTIEMETIC AGENTS

Trials of single agents have indicated which are the most effective antiemetics, and which are most likely to be compatible with other active drugs. Effective combination regimens regimens should combine agents that have different mechanisms of activity and do not have overlapping toxicities. Additionally the drugs should be active as single agents, with the optimal doses, best routes of administration and proper schedules having been previously established.

Several recent studies have compared the activity of metoclopramide with the combination of metoclopramide plus a corticosteroid. In each of these studies, the combination of the two active antiemetics has been superior to the single agent (28,29,30,31). In addition to improved antiemetic efficacy with the steroid plus metoclopramide, the incidence of diarrhea was significantly reduced (28).

The preferred combination regimen for patients receiving high doses of cisplatin (120 mg/m2), at our institution has been as follows: metoclopramide 3 mg/kg IV at 30 minutes before cisplatin and at 90 minutes after the start of the cisplatin, plus dexamethasone 20 mg IV at 40 minutes before cisplatin, plus lorazepam 1.5 mg/m2 (or diphenhydramine 50 mg) IV at 35 minutes before chemotherapy. The cisplatin, following hydration and mannitol, is administered over 20 minutes. This same regimen, using high oral or intravenous doses of these antiemetics, is effective against the emesis induced by combinations of cyclophosphamide plus doxorubicin plus vincristine (32).

A recent study investigated the combination of metoclopramide plus dexamethasone plus either lorazepam or diphenhydramine, in a random-assignment design. The doses of the agents were as listed above, and all patients received cisplatin at 120 mg/m2. Both arms of the study had similar objective antiemetic efficacy, with over 60% of patients having complete control and nearly 90% having major control. The lorazepam containing regimen, however, was favored due to improved subjective results with reduced anxiety and akathisia (33).

Metoclopramide is effective in another problem in chemotherapy induced emesis. Delayed emesis is defined as nausea or vomiting beginning twenty-four hours or more after chemotherapy administration. This is a particular problem with major sources of emesis such as high-dose cisplatin. A recent natural history study observed that delayed emesis is less severe than that which occurs acutely, but still causes significant discomfort as well as difficulties with hydration and nutrition level. Although delayed emesis occurs less often in those patients who have complete emetic control on the day of chemotherapy, it still may occur in this group. The majority of patients treated with cisplatin at doses greater than 100 mg/m2 experience some degree of delayed emesis, with the onset being most frequent 48 to 72 hours after chemotherapy (7). A recent random-assignment trial demonstrated that oral metoclopramide plus dexamethasone, given for four days after high dose cisplatin, was significantly more effective than dexamethasone alone or than placebo (34). Over the four day study period, emesis was completely controlled in 61% of patients receiving the combination, as opposed to 40% given only the steroid and 18% receiving the placebo.

CONCLUSION

Metoclopramide continues to be an interesting and important agent in controlling chemotherapy induced emesis. Recent studies have indicated several findings that affect the understanding and application of this agent. First, in addition to blocking dopamine receptors, metoclopramide in high doses may exert its antiemetic effects through interactions with serotonin receptors. Second, high doses of metoclopramide are required for maximum efficacy against the emesis caused by the most difficult chemotherapeutic agents. Third, combinations of metoclopramide plus a corticosteroid are more effective than single agent antiemetic treatment. Fourth, metoclopramide is helpful in regimens preventing delayed emesis as well as in the treatment of acute chemotherapy induced emesis.

In addition to its utility as an antiemetic, studies with metoclopramide have helped to outline rational study designs and approaches for antiemetic trials. As newer agents become available, metoclopramide provides both the standard of activity by which new drugs should be judged, and an example of effective antiemetic agent development. While new drugs would be desirable to help address existing emetic problems, education in the most effective uses of metoclopramide could greatly improve antiemetic control today.

REFERENCES

1. Justin-Besancon L., Laville D.: Action antiemetique du metoclopramide vis-a-vis de l'apomorphine et de l'hydergine. C R Soc Biol(Paris) 158:723-7, 1964.

2. Pinder, RM, Brogden RN, Saywer PR, et al: Metoclopramide: a review of its pharmacological properties and clinical use. Drugs 12:81-131, 1976.

3. Moertel CG, Reitemeier RJ. Controlled clinical studies of orally administered antiemetic drugs. Gastroenterology 57:262-8, 1969.

4. Gralla RJ, Braun TJ, Squillante A, et al: Metoclopramide: Initial clinical studies of high dosage regimens in cisplatin-induced emesis. IN: Poster E (ed): The Treatment of Nausea and Vomiting Induced by Cancer Chemotherapy. New York, Masson Publishing, 1981, pp 167-176.

5. Gralla RJ, Itri LM, Pisko SE, et al: Antiemetic efficacy of high-dose metoclopramide: Randomized trials with placebo and prochlorperazine in patients with chemotherapy-induced nausea and vomiting. N Engl J Med 305:905-909, 1981.

6. Homesley HD, Gainey JM, Jobson VN, et al: Double-blind placebo-controlled study of metoclopramide in cisplatin-induced emesis. N Engl J Med 307:250-251, 1982.

7. Kris MG, Gralla RJ, Clark RA, et al: Incidence, course, and severity of delayed nausea and vomiting following the administration of high-dose cisplatin. J Clin Oncol 3:1379-1384, 1985.

8. Borison HL, Hawken MJ, Hubbard JI, Sirett NE. Unit activity from cat area postrema influenced by drugs. Brain Res. 92:153-6, 1975.

9. Miner WD, Sanger GJ: Inhibition of cisplatin-induced vomiting by selective 5-hydroxytryptamine M-receptor antagonism. Br. J. Pharmac. 88:497-99, 1986.

10. Gylys JA, Doran KM, Buyniski JP. Antagonism of cisplatin induced emesis in the dog. Res Commun Chem Pathol Pharmacol 23:61-8, 1979.

11. Kahn T, Elias EG, Mason GR. A single dose of metoclopramide in the control of vomiting from cis-dichlorodiammineplatinum(II) in man. Cancer Treat Rep 62:1106-7, 1978.

12. Arnold DJ, Ribiero V, Bulkin W. Metoclopramide (MCP) vs prochlorperazine (PCP) in the prevention of vomiting from diamminedichloroplatinum (DDP). Proc Am Assoc Cancer Res Am Soc Clin Oncol 21:344, 1980 (abstract)

13. Frustaci S, Tumolo S, Tirell U, et al: High dose metoclopramide versus dexamethasone in the prevention of cisplatin induced vomiting. Proc ASCO 2:87, 1983.

14. Aapro MS, Plezia PM, Alberts DS, et al: Double-blind crossover study of the antiemetic efficacy of high-dose dexamethasone vs. high-dose metoclopramide. Proc ASCO 2:93, 1983.

15. Grunberg SM, Gala KV, Lampenfeld M, et al: Composition of the antiemetic effect of high-dose intravenous metoclopramide and high-dose intravenous haloperidol in a randomized double-blind crossover study. J Clin ONcol 2:782-787, 1984.

16. Gralla RJ, Tyson LB, Borden LB, et al: Antiemetic therapy: A review of recent studies and a report of a random assignment trial comparing metoclopramide with delta-9-tetrahydrocannabinol. Cancer Treat Rep 68:163-172, 1984.

17. Strum SB, McDermed JE, Opfel RW, et al: Intravenous metoclopramide. An effective antiemetic in cancer chemotherapy. JAMA 247:2683-2686, 1982.

18. Tyson LB, Clark RA, Gralla RJ: High-dose metoclopramide: control of dacarbazine-induced emesis in a preliminary trial. Cancer Treat Rep 66:2108, 1982.

19. Bui NG, Marit G, Hoerni B: High-dose metoclopramide in cancer chemotherapy-induced nausea and vomiting. Cancer Treat. Reports 66:2107-8, 1982.

20. Meyer BR, Lewin M, Dreyer DE, et al: Optimizing metoclopramide control of cisplatin-induced emesis. Ann Intern Med 200:393-395, 1984.

21. Fetting JA, Grochow LB, Folstein MF, et al: The course of nausea and vomiting after high-dose cyclophosphamide. Cancer Treat Rep 66:1487-1993, 1982.

22. Garnick MB: Oral metoclopramide and cisplatin chemotherapy. Ann Intern Med 99:127, 1983.

23. Gralla RJ, Tyson LB, Clark RA, et al: An all oral combinatgion antiemetic regimen of patients receiving cytoxan + adriamycin + vinceistine (CAV). Proc ASCO 4:267, 1985.

24. Anthony LB, Krozely MG, Woodward NJ, et al: Antiemetic effect of oral versus intravenous metoclopramide in patients receiving cisplatin: A randomized double-blind trial. J Clin Oncol 4:94-103, 1986.

25. Von Hoff DD, Schilsky R, Reichert CM, et al: Toxic effects of cisdichlo-rodiammineplatinum (II) in man. Cancer Treat Rep 63:1527-1531, 1979.

26. Kris MG, Tyson LB, Gralla RJ et al: Extrapyramidal reactions with high-dose metoclopramide. N Engl J Med 309-433, 1983.

27. Allen JC, Gralla RJ, Reilly C, et al: Metoclopramide: Dose-related toxicity and preliminary antiemetic studies in children receiving cancer chemotherapy. J Clin Oncol 3:1136-1141, 1985.

28. Kris MG, Gralla RJ, Tyson LB, et al: Improved control of cisplatin-induced emesis with high-dose metoclopramide and with combinations of metoclopramide, dexamethasone, and diphenhydramine. Results of consecutive trials in 255 patients. Cancer 55:527-534, 1985.

29. Allan SG, Cornbleet MA, Warrington PS, et al: Dexamethasone and high dose metoclopramide: Efficacy in controlling cisplatin-induced nausea and vomiting. Br Med J 289:878-879, 1984.

30. Rosell R, Abad-Esteve A, Ribas-Mundo, Moreno I: Evaluation of a combination antiemetic regimen including IV high-dose metoclopramide, dexamethasone, and diphenhydramine in cisplatin-based chemotherapy regimens. Cancer Treatment Reports 69:909-10, 1985.

31. Roila F, Tonato M, Basurto C, et al: Antiemetic activity of high doses of metoclopramide (MTC) combined with methylprednisolone (P) vs. MTX alone in cisplatin treated cancer patients (PTS). A randomized double blind trial of the Italian Oncology Group for Clinical Research 9GOIRCO. Proc ASCO 5:263, 1986.

32. Tyson LB, Gralla RJ, Clark RA, Kris MG. Effective oral and intravenous antiemetic combinations using high-dose metoclopramide. Proc. 4th European Conference on Clinical Oncology, 1987; 280.

33. Kris MG, Gralla RJ, Clark RA, Tyson LB, Groshen S. Antiemetic control and prevention of side effects of anticancer therapy with lorazepan or diphenhydramine when used in combination with metoclopramide plus dexamethasone: A double-blind, randomized trial. Cancer 60:2816-2822, 1987.

34. Tyson LB, Kris MG, Gralla RJ, Clark RA. Double-blind, randomized trial for the control of delayed emesis: Comparison of placebo vs dexamethasone vs metoclopramide plus dexamethasone. Proc Am Soc Clinc Oncol 6:267, 1987.

Neo-Adjuvant Chemotherapy. Ed. Cl. Jacquillat, M. Weil, D. Khayat. Colloque INSERM/John Libbey Eurotext Ltd. © 1988. Vol. 169, pp. 941-944.

High dose metoclopramide continuous infusion versus intermittent infusion in cisplatinum-induced emesis

Pamela S. Warrington

Imperial Cancer Research Fund Medical Oncology Unit, Western General Hospital, Edinburgh, Scotland, UK.

High dose metoclopramide given as an intermittent infusion is an effective antiemetic against cisplatinum-induced emesis[1-5]. Various doses of metoclopramide have been used and in a previous study[5], there was a trend for better control at higher doses. The addition of dexamethasone has been shown to enhance the antiemetic effect of high dose metoclopramide[6] but there is still need for improvement as major control (two or fewer episodes of vomiting) was only achieved in 65% of patients.

Meyer et al[7] when using the intermittent infusion found that a minimum plasma level of metoclopramide of 0.85 µg/ml was required to achieve antiemetic control. It is well established[8] that intermittent infusions will give rise to peaks and troughs of drug and that the failure to control emesis could be the result of subtherapeutic concentrations of metoclopramide.

In our most recent study[9] we compared the antiemetic efficacy and incidence of side-effects of high dose metoclopramide given by intermittent infusion with that of metoclopramide given by continuous infusion, designed to produce plasma levels of metoclopramide greater than 0.85 µg/ml.

Thirty-three patients receiving cisplatinum combinations were randomised to receive a loading dose and continuous infusion of metoclopramide or an intermittent infusion of metoclopramide, and received the alternate antiemetic regimen with their second treatment. With both schedules, the patient received dexamethasone (20 mg) 30 minutes before the cisplatinum. The continuous regimen consisted of metoclopramide given as a loading dose of 3 mg/kg followed by a continuous infusion of 4 mg/kg given over 8 hours. The same total dose of metoclopramide, 7 mg/kg, was given with both regimens. In the intermittent regimen the total dose of metoclopramide was made up to 500 ml with 0.9% sodium chloride, and infused in 100 ml aliquots 15 minutes before the cisplatinum and then at 2 hourly intervals for a further 4 doses.

Blood samples for the measurement of plasma metoclopramide concentrations were taken at appropriate time points.

Nausea, retching, vomiting, diarrhoea and adverse reactions were recorded on a standard questionnaire which was completed in consultation with the patient and the medical and nursing staff 24 hours after the administration of cisplatinum.

All patients received both the intermittent and continuous infusion, and metoclopramide concentrations were measured in plasma from 13 patients receiving the continuous infusion and 14 patients receiving the intermittent infusion.

As indicated on the visual analogue scale, nausea was significantly reduced ($p<0.001$ Wilcoxon signed rank test) when patients received the continuous metoclopramide infusion compared with the intermittent infusion. There was no significant reduction in retching ($p<0.1$). Vomiting was significantly better controlled by the continuous infusion, major control (2 or fewer episodes) being achieved in 82% of patients compared with 55% of patients receiving the intermittent infusion. One patient experienced diarrhoea while receiving the continuous metoclopramide regimen compared with 8 patients receiving the intermittent infusion ($p<0.05$). Drowsiness was the most common side-effect experienced with both regimens. Eighteen patients preferred the continuous infusion compared with 5 who expressed a preference for the intermittent infusion ($p<0.05$); 10 patients expressed no preference.

The loading dose and continuous infusion of metoclopramide resulted in a mean plasma concentration of metoclopramide above 0.85 µg/ml throughout the 8-hour period whilst the intermittent infusion produced mean plasma concentration below this value during the first 4 hours, with accumulation of metoclopramide at 8 hours. There was marked inter-patient variation in plasma concentration of metoclopramide. In 2 patients in whom plasma concentrations of metoclopramide fell below 0.85 µg/ml during the continuous infusion regimen and antiemetic control was poor, nausea and vomiting were reduced by increasing the dose of the maintenance infusion during subsequent treatment.

The administration of high dose metoclopramide by continuous infusion allows for improved control of nausea and vomiting and a reduction in the number of patients experiencing diarrhoea. This regimen also allows for the optimisation of metoclopramide levels in individual patients to achieve antiemetic control.

The schedule of high dose metoclopramide and dexamethasone seems to be one of the most effective antiemetic combinations currently available for cisplatinum-induced emesis and has also proven useful with regimens containing Adriamycin with cyclophosphamide where 75% of patients have complete control of emesis[10].

References

1. Coates A, Abraham S, Kaye SB, et al. On the receiving end - patient perception of the side-effects of cancer chemotherapy. Eur J Cancer Clin Oncol 1983;19:203-8

2. Kris KMG, Gralla RA, Clark RA, et al. Incidence, course and severity of delayed nausea and vomiting following the administration of high dose cisplatinum. J Clin Oncol 1985;3:1379-84

3. Gralla RJ, Litri LM, Pisko SE, et al. Anti-emetic efficacy of high dose metoclopramide: randomised trial with placebo and prochlorperazine in patients with chemotherapy-induced nausea and vomiting. N Engl J Med 1981;305:905-9

4. Strum SB, McDermed JE, Opfell RW, Riech LP. Intravenous metoclopramide. An effective anti-emetic in cancer chemotherapy. JAMA 1982;247,2683-6

5. Allan SG, Cornbleet MA, Lockhart SP, Warrington PS, Leonard RCF, Smyth JF. Emesis due to cancer chemotherapy: results of a prospective, randomised, double-blind trial of varying doses of metoclopramide in the management of cisplatinum-induced vomiting. Eur J Cancer Clin Oncol 1984;20:1481-4

6. Allan SG, Cornbleet MA, Warrington PS, Leonard RCF, Smyth JF. Dexamethasone and high dose metoclopramide effective in controlling cisplatinum-induced vomiting. Br Med J 1984;289:878-9

7. Meyer RB, Lewin M, Drayer DE, et al. Optimizing metoclopramide control of cisplatinum-induced emesis. Ann Intern Med 1984;100:363-5

8. Taylor WB, Bateman DN. High dose metoclopramide - preliminary pharmacokinetic studies. Br J Clin Pharmacol 1983;16:341-2

9. Warrington PS, Allan SG, Cornbleet MA, Macpherson JS, Smyth JF, Leonard RCF. Optimising antiemesis in cancer chemotherapy: efficacy of continuous versus intermittent infusion of high dose metoclopramide in emesis induced by cisplatin. Br Med J 1986;293:1334-7

10 Allan SG, Cheyne AJ, Warrington PS, Cornbleet MA. Emesis and cancer chemotherapy. Eur J Cancer Clin Oncol 1988. In Press

Neo-Adjuvant Chemotherapy. Ed. Cl. Jacquillat, M. Weil, D. Khayat. Colloque INSERM/John Libbey Eurotext Ltd. © 1988. Vol. 169, pp. 945-953.

Individualizing metoclopramide dosage for the control of cisplatin-induced emesis : a pharmacokinetic approach

J.M. Brechot.[1], J.P. Dupeyron[2], F. Guyon[2], C. Delfour[2], C. Delattre[2], B. Lebeau[1] and J. Rochemaure[1]

[1] *Service de Pneumologie*
[2] *Laboratoire de Biochimie et Toxicologie, Hôtel-Dieu de Paris, 1, Place du Parvis Notre-Dame, 75181 Paris Cedex 04, France*

INTRODUCTION

High-dose metoclopramide (MCP), associated or not with other drugs, has been widely used for control of cisplatin-induced nausea and vomiting (1,2, 3). Plasma concentration of 0,85 mg/l seems to provide a good anti-emetic protection with minimal side effects (4, 5). Furthermore, constant intravenous infusions reduce plasma concentration variations of the drug (5, 6, 7). The wide interindividual variations in the drug's pharmaco-kinetic parameters have been shown (8,9) ; however the estimation of indi-vidual doses based on pharmacokinetic studies has not been previously used for this treatment. Therefore we conducted a prospective study aiming to enhance the benefit-risk ratio of MCP by using constant intravenous infusion ; in addition we determined for each patient the dosage necessary to obtain (loading dose) and maintain (maintenance dose) an efficient and stable plasma concentration. It clearly appears that it considerably dif-fers for one subject to another. A therapeutic approach has been proposed wich might be routinely used for metoclopramide as an antiemetic (10).

PATIENTS AND METHODS

A - Patients

We studied ten patients with advanced non-small cell lung cancer. Age of the subjects ranged from 38 to 69 years (mean 53,7). None of the patients had previous chemotherapy. All had normal renal function. Two had moderate liver abnormalities. All the subjects were included in a randomized clinical trial wich compared two different chemotherapies including both cisplatin at the same dose. Regimen A was a combination of adriamycin 45 mg/m2 IV day 1 (D1), vindesine 3 mg/m2 IV D1 and cisplatin 80 mg/m2 IV D1 ; regimen B associated VP 16 100 mg IV D1, cisplatin 80 mg/m2 IV D1, VP 16 100 mg IV D2, VP 16 200 mg/m2 per os D3 and D5. The cisplatin was infused in 250 ml of normal saline over 30 minutes. Intravenous prehydratation was obtained with 1000 ml normal saline and 1000 ml 5% dextrose over 5 hours. No other antiemetic, narcotic of sedative, neither corticosteroïds, were administed within 24 hours of cisplatin therapy. Prophylactic anti-diarrheic therapy or anticholinergic treatment with diphenhydramine were not used.

B - Pharmacokinetic study

Pharmacokinetic study was performed within the two days preceding chemotherapy. MCP (2 mg/kg) was intravenously infused with a constant flow rate during 15 minutes. Blood sampling (10 ml on lithium heparinate) was performed 1, 2.5 and 4 hours after the onset of infusion.

MCP concentration in plasma was obtained with a liquid-chromatographic assay, as previously described (11). After constant intravenous infusion of high-dose metoclopramide, two different phases are identified : the first one, during infusion, from 0 to 15 minutes, and the second one, following infusion and distribution, where decrease of plasma concentration is estimated as a mono-exponential elimination model.

Our three samples, performed at 1, 2.5 and 4 hours during this second phase, allow us to determine the elimination rate constant (K) and the plasma concentration at the end of infusion. The apparent volume of distribution (Vd) can be calculated, and then the total body clearance (CL) : $CL(\ell/kg/h) = K\ (h^{-1}) . Vd\ (\ell/kg)$. The loading dose (DL), necessary to obtain in 15 minutes a given plasma concentration Cx, is :

$DL\ (mg/kg) = Cx\ (mg/\ell)\ .\ Vd\ (\ell/kg)$. The maintenance dose (DM), necessary to hold a given plasma concentration Cx, is : $DM\ (mg/kg/h) = Cx\ (mg/\ell)\ .\ CL\ (\ell/kg/h)$.

In our study, the loading dose was calculated to obtain in 15 minutes a plasma concentration of 0,85 mg/l ; the maintenance dose was calculated to maintain this plasma concentration of 0,85 mg/l with a constant infusion during four hours ; cisplatin was administrered just after the MCP loading dose, simultanously with the first 30 mn of the maintenance dose.

RESULTS

A - Pharmacokinetic results

In this study we are able to determine for each subject the loading dose as well as the maintenance dose necessary to obtain and maintain a high and stable plasma concentration of metoclopramide.
Pharmacokinetic results are reported on Table I. A wide range of volume of distribution as well as total body clearance was observed. Thus the loading and maintenance doses necessary to obtain a 0,85 mg/l plasma concentration also considerably differed with a range of 1 to 4 and 1 to 10 fold respectively.
At the end of the intravenous MCP infusion, the mean plasma concentration obtained with the adjusted dosages was 0,84 mg/l and thus was very close to the 0,85 mg/l wich was sought after. These results validated our pharmacokinetic approach.
In addition, for 4 subjects, plasma metoclopramide concentration at the end of infusion was again tested 4 to 8 weeks after at the time of the next chemotherapy cycles ; there was only a very limited variation for a given patient. Therefore the total body clearance appeared stable in these subjects.

B - Clinical results

The antiemetic efficiency of this regimen was estimated by the patient, his family and the medical staff by means of a standardized check-list. Vomiting and nausea occuring during 24 hours following cisplatin infusion were taken into account as well as their exact timing. The criterion for antiemetic efficacy (ie. the number of forceful expulsions separated by free intervals) was the occurence of 2 antiemetic events during the first 24 hours following cisplatin. Antiemetic efficiency was tested only during the first cisplatin cycle. Side effects due to MCP treatment were always sought for : diarrhoea, drowsiness, akathisia, dystonia, rigidity.
The metoclopramide was efficient in 6 of the 10 subjects ; two patients had no vomiting. However 4 had an average of 5 emetic events despite a MCP plasma concentration above 0,85 mg/l (average 1 mg/l). Figure 1 shows the time of occurence of nausea and vomiting : all appeared from 1 to 7 hours after cisplatin infusion, although MCP plasma concentration was in the expected range. No significant side effects were reported ; indeed only two patients had mild diarrhoea and two had drowsiness.

DISCUSSION

High-dose metoclopramide is widely used as an antiemetic agent (1, 2, 3, 12-15). However its efficiency is not complete and adverse side effects may occur, mainly diarrhoea and extrapyramidal reactions (8, 16, 17). Our study indicates that determination of the volume of distribution and of the total body clearance prior to MCP treatment might have clinical implications. Indeed the pharmacokinetic analysis allowed to calculate the MCP doses for obtention for each patient of an optimal plasma concentration. Thus a mean MCP plasma concentration of 0,84 mg/l was obtained, wich was very close to that expected (ie : 0,85 mg/l) ; such a plasma concentration was consistent in previous studies with a good antiemetic effect (4, 5) and indeed this was the case for 6 of the 10 subjects treated.
However the MCP adjusted doses markedly differed from one patient to another ; the loading doses varied from 0,9 to 3,4 mg/kg and the maintenance doses from 0,6 to 0,65 mg/kg. The total doses per cycle varied from 1,17 to 6,10 mg/kg. With MCP treatment without individual adjusted dosage, even with continous infusion administration, substantial variations in the MCP plasma concentration have been observed (7).
In view of this, it should also be noted that our protocol, including adjusted dosage, might also permit to test higher MCP doses due to the absence of serious si effects. This appears to be important since 4 subjects still had more than 2 emetic episodes although the mean MCP plasma concentration averaged 1 mg/l. Altogether this approach would provide tools for a high-dose MCP therapy with adjusted doses to each patient. Its clinical efficiency as well as absence of side effects appear promising.

PHARMACOKINETIC RESULTS

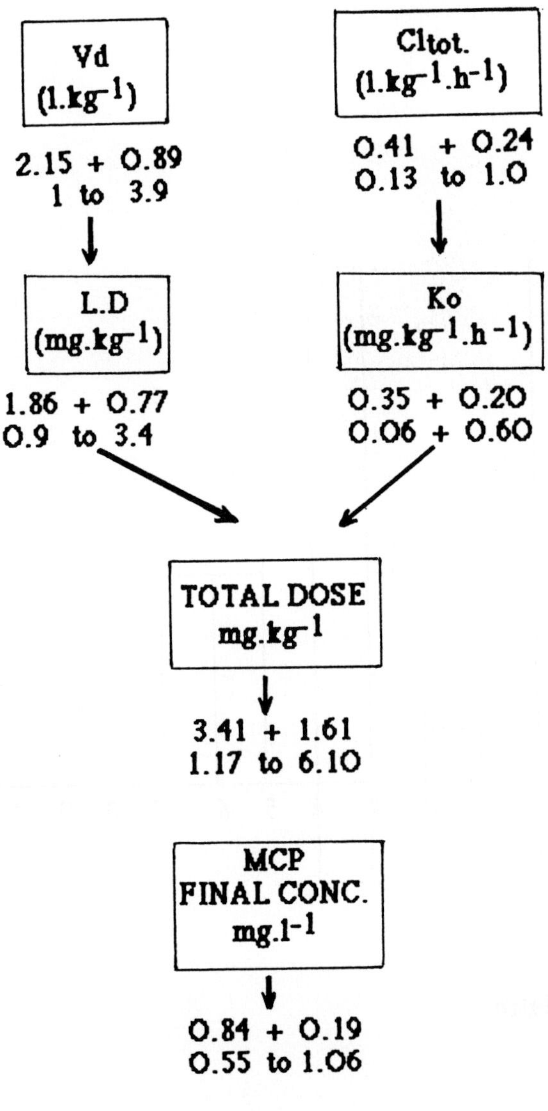

TABLE I

TIME OF OCCURRENCE OF NAUSEA AND VOMITING

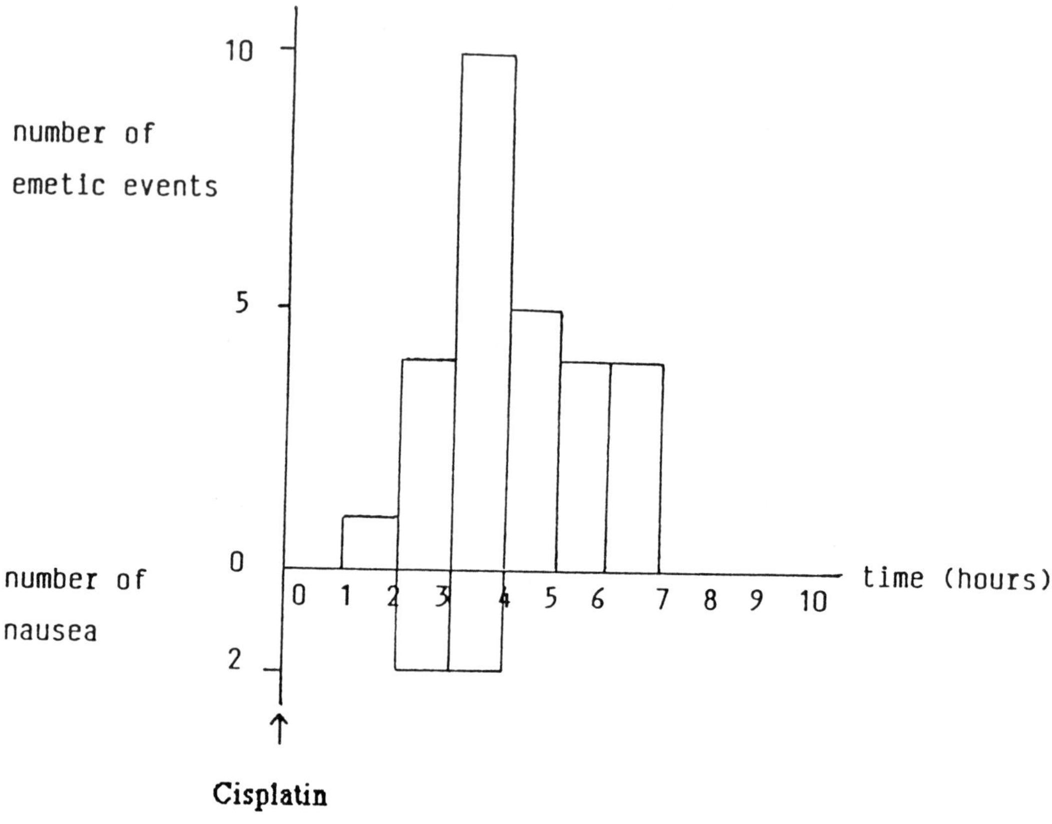

- **Figure 1** -

REFERENCES

1 - GRALLA RJ, ITRI LM, PISKO SE and al.
Antiemetic efficacy of high-dose metoclopramide : randomized trials with placebo and prochlorperazine in patients with chemotherapy-induced nausea and vomiting.
N. Engl. J. Med. 1981, 305 : 905-909.

2 - KRIS MG, GRALLA RJ, TYSON LB and al.
Improved control of cisplatin-induced emesis with high-dose metoclopramide and with combinations of metoclopramide, dexamethasone, and diphenhydramine : results of consecutive trials in 255 patients.
Cancer 1985, 55 : 527-534.

3 - RICHARDS PD, FLAUM MA, BATEMAN M, KARDINAL CG.
The antiemetic efficacy of secobarbital and chlorpromazine compared to metoclopramide, diphenhydramine, and dexamethasone : a randomized trial.
Cancer 1986, 58 : 959-962.

4 - MEYER BR, LEWIN M, DRAYER DE, PASMANTIER M, LONSKI L, REIDENBERG MM.
Optimizing metoclopramide control of cisplatin-induced emesis.
Ann. Intern. Méd. 1984, 100 : 393-395.

5 - KERR DJ, GRAHAM J, BLACKIE RG and al.
The relationship between steady state metoclopramide levels and control of emesis during treatment with cisplatinum.
Br. J. Clin. Pharmacol. 1985, 20 : 426-427.

6 - SALLER R, HELLENBRECHT Ph.D, BRIEMANN L and al.
Metoclopramide kinetics at high-dose infusion rates for prevention of cisplatin-induced emesis.
Clin. Pharmacol. Ther. 1985, 37 : 43-47.

7 - WARRINGTON PS, ALLAN SG, CORNBLEET MA, MACPHERSON JS, SMYTH JF, LEONARD RCF.
Optimizing antiemesis in cancer chemotherapy efficacy of continous versus intermittent infusion of high-dose metoclopramide in emesis induced by cisplatin.
Br. Med. J. 1986, 293 : 1334-1337.

8 - MC GOVERN EM, GREVEL J, BRYSON SM.
Pharmacokinetics of high-dose metoclopramide in cancer patients.
Clin. Pharmacokinet. 1986, 11 : 415-424.

9 - SALLER R, HELLENBRECHT D, HELLSTERN A, HESS H.
Improved benefit/risk ratio of higher-dose metoclopramide therapy during cisplatin-induced emesis.
Eur. J. Clin. Pharmacol. 1985, 29 : 311-312.

10 - BRECHOT JM, DUPEYRON JP, GUYON F et al.
Posologie individualisée du métoclopramide dans le contrôle des vomissements au cisplatine.
Premières journées de Pharmacocinétique clinique Oncologique. Paris 17-18 *Octobre* 1986.

11 - GUYON F, DELFOUR C, DELATTRE C, DUPEYRON JP.
Liquid-chromatographic assay of metoclopramide in human plasma.
Clin. Chem. 1987, 33 : 190-191.

12 - STRUM SB, MC DERMED JE, OPFELL RW, RIECH LP.
Intravenous metoclopramide : an effective antiemetic in cancer chemotherapy.
JAMA. 1982, 247 : 2683-2686.

13 - GRALLA RJ.
Metoclopramide : a review of antiemetic trials.
Drugs. 1983, 25 (suppl. 1) : 63-73.

14 - EYRE HJ, WARD JH.
Control of cancer chemotherapy-induced nausea and vomiting.
Cancer 1984. 54 : 2642-2648.

15 - TROPE C, DANNESKIOLD-SAMSOE P, HAUKSSON A.
High-dose metoclopramide in the treatment of cisplatinum induced emesis.
A dose-finding study.
Neoplasma 1985. 32 : 507-512.

16 - BATEMAN DN, RAWLINS MD, SIMPSON JM.
Extrapyramidal reactions with metoclopramide.
Br. Med. J. 1985, 291 : 930-932.

17 - BREITBART W.
Tardive dyskinesia associated with high-dose intravenous metoclopramide.
N. Engl. J. Med. 1986, 315 : 518.

Neo-Adjuvant Chemotherapy. Ed. Cl. Jacquillat, M. Weil, D. Khayat. Colloque INSERM/John Libbey Eurotext Ltd. © 1988. Vol. 169, pp. 955-962.

Proposition de schémas d'administration des anti-émétiques à partir de modèles pharmacocinétiques

H. Roche[1], P. Canal[1], M. Canal[2], C. Desanti[2] et A. Dufour[2]

[1] *Centre Claudius Regaud, 20-24 rue du Pont St-Pierre, 31052 Toulouse Cedex, France.*
[2] *Laboratoire Delagrange, 1 avenue Pierre Brossolette, 91380 Chilly-Mazarin Cedex, France*

Si l'efficacité des benzamides dans le traitement des vomissements provoqués par la chimiothérapie anticancéreuse n'est plus à prouver, l'utilisation optimale de ces agents est encore sujette à caution. Les administrations traditionnelles par injections bolus répétées sont responsables de grandes variations interindividuelles et d'écarts de concentrations plasmatiques préjudiciables probablement à l'efficacité thérapeutique tout en exposant à des accumulations potentiellement toxiques.

Il nous est apparu intéressant, de regrouper les informations pharmacocinétiques publiées tant pour le métoclopramide que l'alizapride, d'essayer d'établir un modèle mathématique qui servira de base à des propositions de schémas d'administration optimisés.

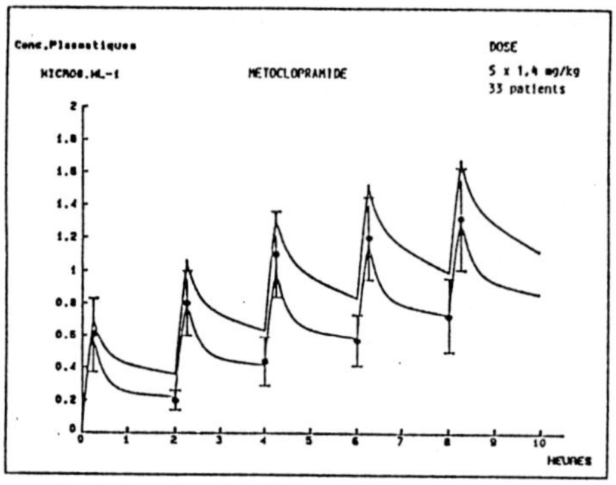

Modelisation des données moyennes (n = 33) après administration de 5 perfusions (15 minutes) de 1,4 mg/kg de metoclopramide (données observées par P.S. Warrington et Coll. 1986)

Fig. 1A

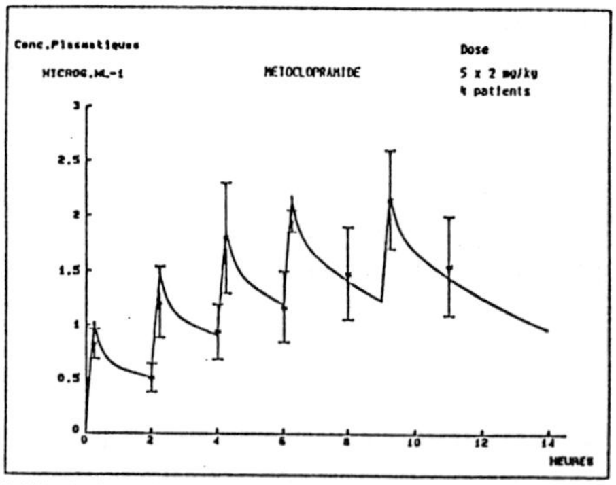

Modelisation des données moyennes (n = 4) après administration de 5 perfusions (15 minutes) de 2 mg/kg de métoclopramide (données observées par W.B. Taylor et D.N. Bateman 1983).

Fig. 1B

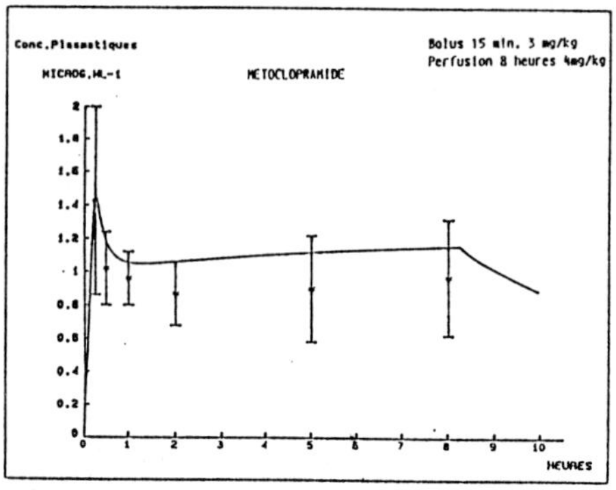

Modelisation des données moyennes (n = 33) après administration d'une dose de charge (15 min.) puis d'une dose d'entretien (8 heures) (données observées par P.S. Warrington et coll. 1986)

Fig. 2A

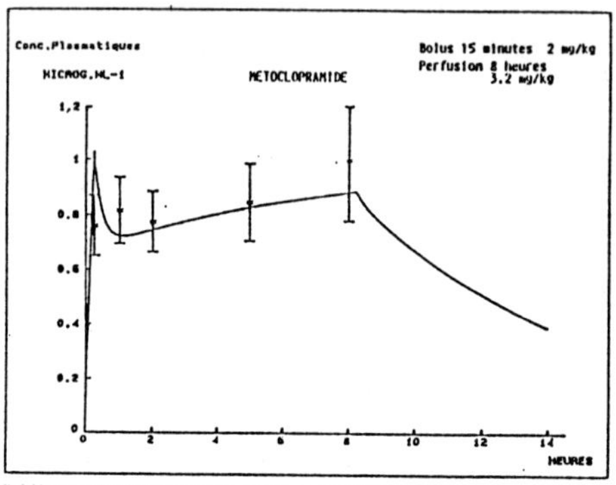

Modelisation des données moyennes (n = 6) après administration d'une dose de charge (15 minutes) puis d'une dose d'entretien (8 h) (données observées par W.B. Taylor et coll. 1984)

Fig. 2B

MODELES POSOLOGIQUES : BOLUS + PERFUSION

METOCLOPRAMIDE

AUTEURS	DOSE DE CHARGE BOLUS 15 minutes	DOSE D'ENTRETIEN PERFUSION DOSE	DOSE D'ENTRETIEN PERFUSION DUREE
W.B. TAYLOR (1984)	2 mg/kg	3.2 mg/kg	8 heures
P.S. WARRINGTON (1986)	3 mg/kg	4 mg/kg	8 heures
D.J. KERR (1985)	2 mg/kg	4.5 mg/kg	12 heures
J.M. BRECHOT (1986)	2 mg/kg	1.6 mg/kg	4 heures

Fig. 3A

MODELES POSOLOGIQUES : BOLUS + PERFUSION

METOCLOPRAMIDE

AUTEURS	CONCENTRATION PLASMATIQUE MOYENNE microg.ml-1 Au pic plasmatique 15 minutes	CONCENTRATION PLASMATIQUE MOYENNE microg.ml-1 En fin de perfusion
W.B. TAYLOR	0.76	1
P.S. WARRINGTON	1.43	0.97
D.J. KERR	-	0.82
J.M. BRECHOT	-	0.8

Fig. 3B

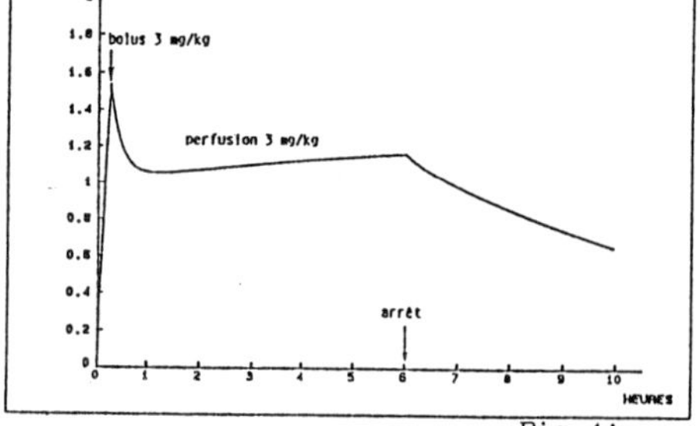

Fig. 4A

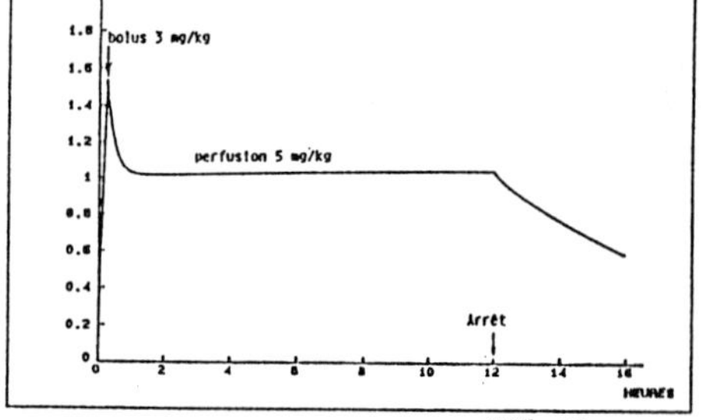

Fig. 4B

LE METOCLOPRAMIDE -

La variabilité intersujets après injections réitérées ou perfusions prolongées est grande, allant d'un facteur 4 (WARRINGTON) à 10 (MEYER) et même 12 (Mc DERMED). Nous avons, à partir de données publiées, établi un modèle pharmacocinétique moyen que nous avons comparé aux modèles de Warrington (fig. 1A) et Taylor (1B).

Après perfusions successives de 15 minutes toutes les 2 heures à la dose unitaire de 2 mg/kg, notre modèle semble plus proche des données expérimentales de Taylor que de celles de Warrington.

Le même modèle a été comparé aux données fournies par les auteurs précités après administration d'une dose de charge pendant 15 minutes suivie d'une dose d'entretien de 8 heures (fig. 2A et 2B). Ici également, le modèle moyen est plus proche des données de Taylor. Il est intéressant de noter que les "pics" et les "vallées" disparaissent comme prévu au profit d'un plateau de concentrations laissant espérer une meilleure efficacité thérapeutique et une moindre toxicité.

La validité de ce modèle s'affirme dès lors qu'il s'intègre dans les valeurs rapportées par d'autres auteurs (Kerr, Brechot) qui utilisaient des protocoles d'administration sensiblement différents (Fig. 3A, 3B).

Il est alors possible, grâce à des programmes informatiques de simulation, de rechercher des schémas posologiques précis. Le but est d'obtenir une concentration plasmatique de métoclopramide en plateau aux environs de 1 µg/ml. Cette valeur minimale proposée par Taylor et Brechot est proche de celle recommandée par Meyer et Warrington (0,85 µg/ml). Lors de perfusions réitérées elle n'est que rarement atteinte dans les vallées notamment pendant la période d'exposition maximale au risque émétisant du cisplatine. Lors de perfusions prolongées, les schémas posologiques proposés par les différents auteurs approchent de 20% cette concentration.

Les figures 4A et 4B montrent deux exemples de propositions posologiques permettant de répondre aux objectifs fixés sur des périodes de 6 à 12 heures. Le problème de l'adéquation aux variations pharmacocinétiques individuelles susceptibles de modifier cette planification a été abordé dans une autre communication par Brechot.

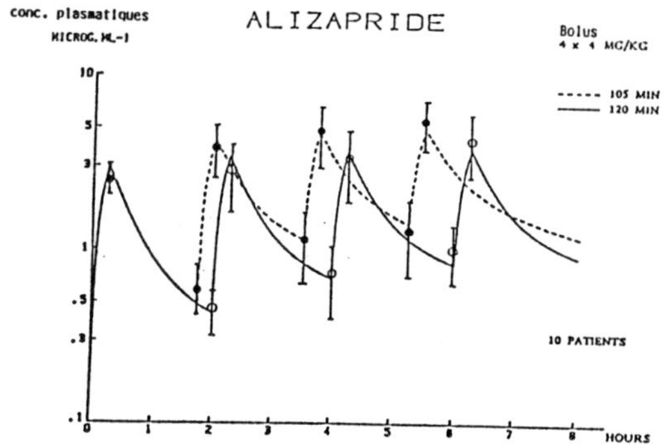

Modelisation des données plasmatiques (n = 10) après administration de 4 perfusions (15 minutes) de 4 mg/kg d'alizapride (données observées par P. Canal et coll. 1987)

Fig.5A

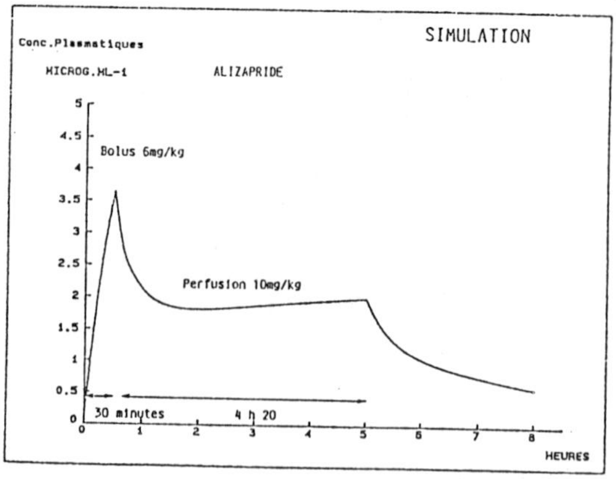

Fig.5B

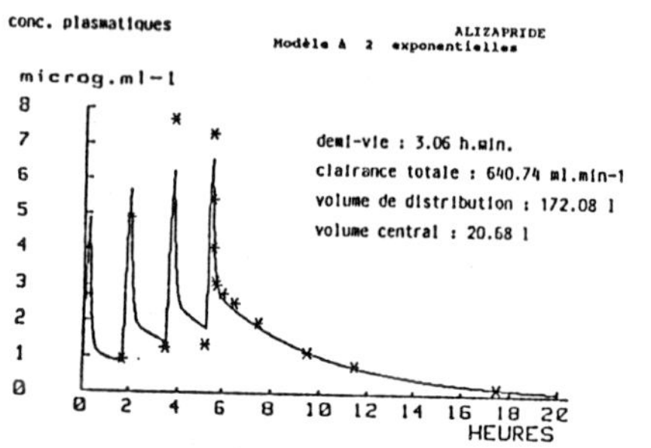

Alizapride : 4 doses de 4 mg/kg à 105 minutes d'intervalle
P. CANAL et coll. : Modélisation des données observées : patient n° 6

Fig.6A

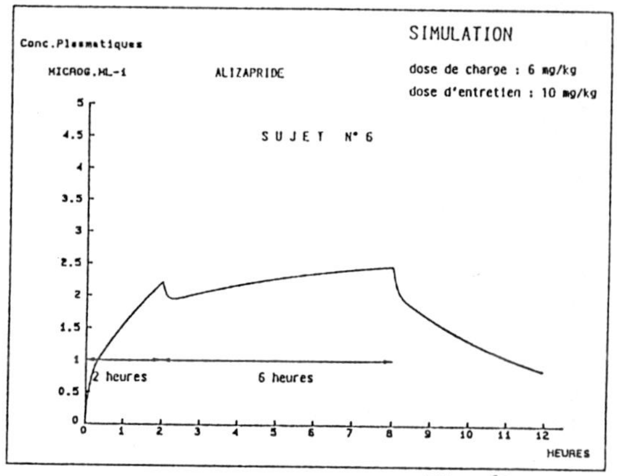

Fig.6B

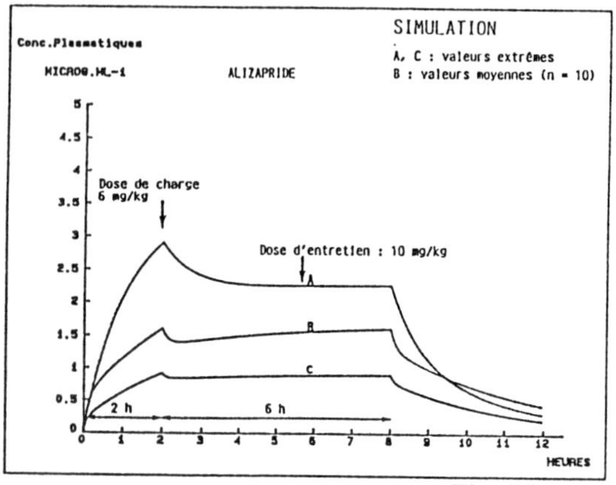

Fig.7A

ALIZAPRIDE

SIMULATION DES CONCENTRATIONS PLASMATIQUES MICROG.ML-1		
	PIC PLASMATIQUE	DOSE D'ENTRETIEN Conc. fin de perfusion
A	2.90	2.27
B	1.60	1.62
C	0.92	0.91

Fig.7B

L'ALIZAPRIDE -

Cette autre benzamide, d'utilisation plus récente, pose des problèmes très proches :

. quel est le schéma d'administration optimal : perfusions réitérées ou bolus suivi de perfusion lente ?

. existe-t-il de grandes variations individuelles et si oui, justifient-elles un ajustement individuel ?

Nous avons utilisé dans un premier temps les données d'un travail personnel (P. CANAL et coll.) s'intéresssant à la pharmacocinétique de l'alizapride chez 11 patients exposés au cisplatine. Deux schémas d'administration délivrant 4 mg/kg d'alizapride à 4 reprises toutes les 105 ou 120 minutes ont été utilisées.

Le raccourcissement de l'intervalle entre les injections était motivé par l'observation clinique de vomissements avant la 3ème injection lors du schéma toutes les 120 minutes et par la demi-vie plus courte de l'alizapride par rapport au métoclopramide (2,8 h versus 5 h). Nous avons observé des valeurs de pics plasmatiques se situant entre 3 et 4,8 µg/ml, des valeurs de vallées entre 0,43 et 1,4 µg/ml (fig. 5A).

Lors d'un autre travail personnel regroupant 77 patients recevant du cisplatine (non publié) nous avons noté une protection antiémétique beaucoup plus importante lorsque la concentration plasmatique à la 2ème heure après la fin de la perfusion du cisplatine était supérieure à 2 µg/ml. Il nous a donc semblé intéressant d'élaborer un modèle pharmacocinétique moyen, à partir de données obtenues par injections réitérées, et de rechercher le schéma posologique permettant d'obtenir une concentration stable de 2 µg/ml par injection bolus suivie de perfusion prolongée pour une même dose totale délivrée de 16 mg/kg (figure 5B)

Qu'en est-il des variations intersujets lorsque l'on utilise ce schéma thérapeutique ?

Nous avons étudié sur chacun des 10 patients pour lesquels nous disposions de données et en utilisant les paramètres pharmacocinétiques de chaque individu, les concentrations plasmatiques obtenues par perfusion de 6 mg/kg d'alizapride en 2 heures suivie d'une dose relai de 10 mg/kg étalée sur 6 heures (fig. 6A et B) : exemple du sujet n° 6. Ceci nous a permis de vérifier les importantes variations individuelles observées. Les conclusions qui ressortent des fig. 7A et 7B sont les suivantes :

. un même schéma thérapeutique, utilisé sur des sujets ayant des paramètres pharmacocinétiques différents, expose à des variations de concentrations plasmatiques importantes (sujets A et C).

. le modèle moyen (B) peut être éloigné des courbes individuelles extrêmes

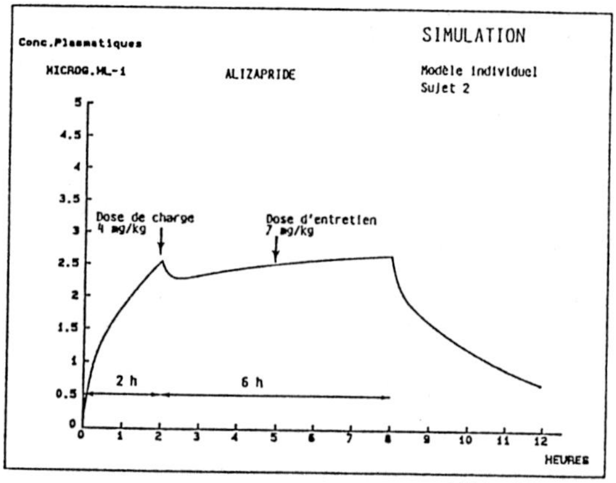

Fig.8B

SUJETS	Dose de charge en mg/kg perfusée en 2 h	Dose d'entretien en mg/kg perfusée en 6 h	Dose totale en mg/kg perfusée en 8 h
1	3	5	8
2	4	7	11
3	5	7	12
4	4	6	10
5	5	7	12

DOSES INDIVIDUELLES D'ALIZAPRIDE NECESSAIRES A L'OBTENTION D'UN PLATEAU PLASMATIQUE EGAL OU SUPERIEUR A 2 MICROG.ML-1 Fig.9A

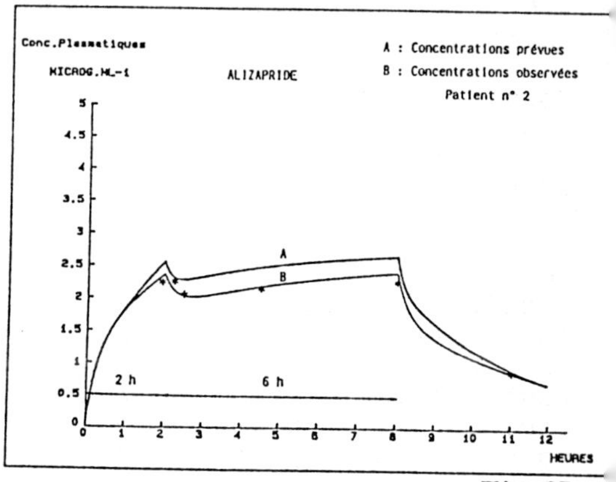

Fig.9B

ALIZAPRIDE CONCENTRATIONS PLASMATIQUES MICROG.ML-1						
	DOSE DE CHARGE		DOSE D'ENTRETIEN PERFUSION			
	PIC (2h)		VALLEE (2h30)		PLATEAU (8h)	
SUJETS	PREVUE	OBSERVEE	PREVUE	OBSERVEE	PREVUE	OBSERVEE
1	2.89	2.27	2.52	2.08	3.08	2.31
2	2.50	2.24	2.28	2.05	2.65	2.26
3	2.93	2.62	2.42	2.21	2.75	2.67
4	2.44	2.12	2.25	2.09	2.16	1.95
5	2.47	2.68	2.11	2.60	2.90	2.93
M	2.64	2.38	2.31	2.20	2.71	2.42
SD	0.24	0.25	0.16	0.23	0.34	0.38

CONCENTRATIONS PLASMATIQUES PREVUES A PARTIR DE LA DOSE-TEST, ET CONCENTRATIONS EXPERIMENTALES OBSERVEES LE JOUR DE LA CHIMIOTHERAPIE. Fig.10A

ALIZAPRIDE								
SUJETS N°	DEMI-VIE h		CLAIRANCE TOTALE ml/min-1		VOLUME DE DISTRUBUTION litre		VOLUME CENTRAL litre	
	Dose-test	Dose chimio.	Dose-test	Dose chimio.	Dose-test	Dose chimio.	Dose-test	Dose chimio.
1	3.00	4.96	365.5	366.8	95.9	157.9	12.7	27.9
2	2.45	3.08	457.4	488.6	96.9	130.1	20.5	25.4
3	3.13	3.83	449.5	451.4	122.2	149.7	17.0	26.7
4	3.18	5.90	262.8	222.8	72.2	113.8	19.0	20.9
5	5.55	2.73	344.4	451.4	165.6	106.8	19.4	21.5
M	3.46	4.10	375.9	396.2	110.5	131.6	17.7	24.5
SD	1.20	1.32	80.5	106.7	35.5	20.1	3.1	3.1

PARAMETRES PHARMACOCINETIQUES DE L'ALIZAPRIDE CALCULES APRES DOSE-TEST ET APRES CHIMIOTHERAPIE

Fig.10B

dans le cas présent, l'objectif souhaité d'une concentration de 2 µg/ml ne sera atteint ni pour le modèle moyen, ni pour la plupart des patients.

La conclusion évidente à cette étude expérimentale était la nécessité d'essayer de définir au préalable les caractéristiques de l'individu par une dose test.

Nous avons donc, chez 5 sujets n'ayant jamais reçu de cisplatine, perfusé en 15 minutes une dose test de 4 mg/kg d'alizapride 48 heures avant l'administration de la chimiothérapie, . Six prélèvements sanguins nous ont permis de déterminer les paramètres et le modèle pharmacocinétiques, puis de calculer, à l'aide d'un programme de simulation, les doses de charge et d'entretien nécessaires à l'obtention d'une concentration plasmatique en plateau de 2 µg/ml (figure 8)

La fig. 9A regroupe les résultats obtenus chez les 5 sujets : il est intéressant de noter que la dose totale calculée varie de 8 à 12 mg/kg.

Nous avons vérifié l'exactitude de nos prévisions en mesurant la concentration plasmatique lors de la chimiothérapie (grâce à des prélèvements sanguins en fin de perfusion de la dose de charge et au plateau de concentrations).

Les fig. 10 A et 10 B regroupent toutes les données concernant les 5 sujets. La concentration prévue n'a été atteinte qu'une seule fois chez un sujet présentant par ailleurs lors de la chimiothérapie une clairance totale plus élevée que lors de la dose-test, et un volume de distribution plus faible. Dans tous les autres cas, la valeur observée, si elle n'a pas atteint l'objectif souhaité, a toujours été supérieure à 2 µg/ml. Il est à retenir que dans la plupart des cas le volume de distribution lors de la chimiothérapie est de 20 à 60% plus grand que lors de la dose-test. Ce fait pourrait être expliqué par la nécessité d'une hyperhydradation avant toute administration de cisplatine. Néanmoins la différence entre la valeur observée et calculée est faible ce qui valide l'emploi d'une dose test pour établir un schéma posologique.

La méthodologie employée, c'est à dire le contrôle sanguin et l'utilisation de modèles élaborés, tant pour le métoclopramide que pour l'alizapride devrait maintenant nous permettre de répondre à la question fondamentale d'une relation concentration plasmatique - protection antiémétique.

BIBLIOGRAPHIE

. WARRINGTON P.S. et coll.
OPTIMISING ANTIEMESIS IN CANCER CHEMOTHERAPY : efficacy of continuous versus intermittent infusion in high dose metoclopramide in emesis induced by cisplatin.
Br. Med. J. 293 : 1334 , 1986

. MEYER B.R. et coll.
OPTIMIZING METOCLOPRAMIDE CONTROL OF CISPLATIN - INDUCED EMESIS
Ann. Int. Med. 100 : 393, 1984

. McDERMED J.E. et coll.
CLINICAL PHARMACOKINETICS OF HIGH DOSE METOCLOPRAMIDE IN CANCER PATIENTS RECEIVING CISPLATIN THERAPY
J. Clin. Oncol. : 3 :1400, 1985

. TAYLOR W.B. et coll.
PHARMACOKINETICS AND EFFICACY IN HIGH DOSE METOCLOPRAMIDE GIVEN BY CONTINUOUS INFUSION FOR THE CONTROL OF CYTOTOXIC DRUG - INDUCED VOMITING
Br. J. Clin. Pharm. 18 : 679, 1984

. KERR D.J.
THE RELATIONSHIP BETWEEN STEADY STATE METOCLOPRAMIDE LEVELS AND CONTROL OF EMESIS DURING TREATMENT WITH CIS-PLATINUM
Br. J. Clin. Pharmacol. 20 : 426, 1985

. CANAL P. et coll.
PHARMACOKINETICS OF HIGH-DOSE IV ALIZAPRIDE IN PREVENTION OF CISPLATIN-INDUCED EMESIS
Fundam. Clin. Pharmacol. 1 : 213, 1987

Symposium mitomycin C

Mitomycine C

Neo-Adjuvant Chemotherapy. Ed. Cl. Jacquillat, M. Weil, D. Khayat. Colloque INSERM/John Libbey Eurotext Ltd. © 1988. Vol. 169, pp. 965-970.

BCG (RIVM) immunoprophylaxis versus mitomycin chemoprophylaxis in patients with superficial bladder cancer

F.M.J. Debruyne[1] and A.P.M. Van der Meijden[1] (for the Dutch South-East Cooperative Urological Group) and C. Bollack[2] (for the EORTC GU-Group)

[1]*Department of Urology, University Hospital Nijmegen, The Netherlands*
[2]*Department of Urology, Hospices Civils de Strasbourg, France*

ABSTRACT

Intravesicale chemoprophylaxe wordt al langere tijd gebruikt ter voorkoming van recidieven van oppervlakkige blaascarcinomen. Van de gebruikte chemotherapeutica is het MMC het effectiefst gebleken. De laatste jaren neemt het gebruik van het BCG bij deze behandeling echter sterk toe, een superioriteit t.o.v. chemotherapie is echter in klinische trials niet volledig aangetoond c.q. bevestigd.

In deze voorliggende studie vergelijken we de effectiviteit van het MMC met die van het BCG RIVM. Het aantal patiënten in deze prospectief gerandomiseerde studie bedroeg 337. 213 Patiënten hadden een pTa, 114 een pT1 tumor en 10 een carcinoma in situ. Primaire carcinomen waren aanwezig bij 235 patiënten (=70%). Bijwerkingen waren vergelijkbaar in beide therapie-armen.

Dit geldt zowel voor de bacteriële als de chemische, drug-induced, cystitis. Ernstige toxiciteit trad bij geen enkele patiënt op. De recurrence rate na 1 jaar follow-up is voor beide therapie-armen gelijk (30% bij de met BCG RIVM behandelde patiënten vertoonden recidieven versus 25% bij de met MMC behandelde patiënten, dit verschil is niet statistisch significant. De resultaten laten een gelijkwaardig behandelingseffect zien van het MMC en het BCG RIVM, een mogelijke superioriteit van het BCG kan in deze studie niet aangetoond dan wel bevestigd worden.

KEYWORDS

Superficial bladder cancer, Mitomycin C, BCG RIVM, Prophylaxe.

INTRODUCTION

For more than two decades intravesical chemoprophylaxis has been used to prevent recurrence in superficial bladder cancer (pTa, pT1 and pTis). Different agents have proven to be effective (Soloway, 1980) in many studies conducted over the years, bur from more recent reports it could be concluded that MMC is the most effective agent for intravesical chemoprophylaxis of superficial bladder cancer (Bracken, 1980; Huland, 1984).

Morales et al. (1976) showed that bacillus Calmette-Guérin (BCG) intravesical immunotherapy was also effective in the prevention of recurrences and more recent reports have even claimed that BCG is superior to other forms of intravesical chemotherapy (Lamm, 1982). This suggestion, however, has not been fully evidenced by results of a sufficient number of prospective randomized clinial trials in which intravesical immunotherapy and chemoprophylaxis are compared.

Furthermore, several types of BCG vaccines -prepared from different BCG strains- have been used in different studies and it is not yet clear whether all strains are similarly effective.

In this study, a Dutch BCG strain produced at the Rijksinstituut voor Volksgezondheid en Milieuhygiene (RIVM) (National Institute of Public Health and Environmental Hygiene) was investigated in the prophylactic management of superficial bladder cancer after transurethral resection.

The BCG strain used for the RIVM vaccine was originally derived from a lot from the Pasteur institute in Paris. Immunostimulatory and antitumor activity has been observed both in experimental and spontaneous animal tumors.

MATERIAL AND METHODS

In January 1985 a clinical trial was initiated to compare BCG RIVM with MMC. The study was a joint effort of the EORTC Genitourinary (GU) Group (protocol No. 30845) and the Dutch South-East Urological Co-operative Group. Comparison with MMC was chosen since at that time MMC was assumed to be one of the most potent and least toxic drugs for intravesical chemotherapy (Huland, 1984).

The objective of the two-armed, prospectively controlled and randomized trial was to compare the prophylactic effect of intravesically administered BCG RIVM with that of MMC in patients with primary or recurrent superficial bladder tumors, including CIS. The parameters compared were recurrence rate (including evaluation of the number and size of recurrent tumors), duration of disease-free interval, rate of progression to a higher stage (T-category) of disease, incidence and severity of side effects.

Patients with resectable and histologically proven stage Ta and T1 papillary transitional cell carcinoma (TCC) of the bladder were eligible for the study. Patients were entered after complete transurethral resection and at random biopsies of the bladder mucosa of all visible lesions. Patients with primary carcinoma in situ (CIS) were also eligible.

Patients were randomly allocated to BCG RIVM or MMC intravesical instillation, which started between seven and fifteen days after complete transurethral resection of all papillary superficial tumors. Study regimens were as follows: BCG (1×10^9 bacilli in 50 ml saline) was given once a week for six consecutive weeks, and MMC (30 mg in 50 ml saline) was instilled once a week for one month (weeks one to four) and thereafter once a month for a total of six months. Control cystoscopies were performed at three-month intervals for three years. If recurrence was observed at 3 months in the BCG group, the tumor was again completely resected and additional intravesical BCG therapy was restarted for six weekly instillations. If recurrence was observed in the MMC group, the tumor was totally resected and the MMC treatment was continued monthly. If, however, at 3 months an increase in T category to T2 or higher was observed the patient went off-study. Patients were removed from the study at their first recurrence after completion of intravesical treatment; i.e. at six months or thereafter.

RESULTS

A total number of 337 patients were randomised in this study, which was closed October 1st, 1986.

Stratification for CIS, and Stages Ta and T1, as well as for G category, number of tumors, primary and recurrent tumors were similar in both treatment arms. Tables 1 and 2 compare the occurrence of bacterial and drug-induced, or chemical, cystitis by both patient and number of instillations. Drug-induced, or chemical, cystitis was observed after 57 from 934 instillations with BCG RIVM (6.1%) and after 92 from 1252 instillations with MMC (7.3%). In the same group bacterial cystitis occurred after 67 instillations with BCG RIVM (7.2%) and after 69 instillations with MMC (5.5%). 149 Patients were treated with BCG RIVM and 155 patients with MMC. No difference between the two treatment groups was observed. Severe systemic toxicity was absent in both treatment arms.

Table 1. Protocol 30845: no. of occurrences of chemical cystitis

	BCG	MMC	TOTAL
No. of patients	149	155	304
No. of instillations	934	1252	2186
No. of occurrences*	57 (6.1%)	92 (7.3%)	149 (6.7%)

* one patient may report several occurrences

Table 2. Protocol 30845: no. of occurrences of bacterial cystitis

	BCG	MMC	TOTAL
No. of patients	149	155	304
No. of instillations	934	1252	2186
No. of occurrences*	67 (7.2%)	69 (5.5%)	136 (6.2%)

* one patient may report several occurrences

Table 3 shows the recurrence rate for 308 patients for a follow-up period of twelve months. In the BCG-treated group (N=148), 44 (29.8%) patients had recurrent tumors, while in the mitomycin group (N=160) 40 (25%) patients had a recurrence. The recurrence rate for BCG-treated patients was 0.33. For MMC-treated patients, the rate was 0.29. This difference is not statistically significant (p=0.560).

Table 3. Protocol 30845: available follow-up until August, 1987

	BCG RIVM	MMC
Patients with follow-up	148	160
Mean follow-up (months)	11.63	11.78
Mean no. of cystoscopies	4	4
Total number of recurrences	47	45
Recurrence rate	0.33	0.29

DISCUSSION

Intravesical prophylaxis has become an important adjuvant treatment form after transurethral resection of superficial bladder tumors. After the initial use of different effective chemotherapeutic agents BCG immunotprophylaxis seems also to be of value.

It is not known how BCG really act and its use remains largerly empirical. The immunostimulating effect of intravesical BCG therapy is, however, clearly demonstrated by the local reaction in the bladder as well as by the conversion of the purified protein derivative (PPD) skin reaction, from negative to positive, which can be regarded as an expression of the systemic immunostimulating effect by BCG.

Different vaccines prepared from BCG have been used and most of the vaccines seem to have antitumor activity although it was also demonstrated that there was a relationship between treatment results and different lots of BCG. In fact, striking differences in the number of colony-forming units among BCG lots of the same preparation as well as among different preparations were revealed. Differences can range from 10^6 to 10^{12} colonies per ampule (Kelley, 1985). Furthermore, it is not only the number of bacilli present in the vaccin that is important but also the activity to multiply in vivo; i.e. the viability of the vaccine.

It is not known whether the culture method of BCG might influence its effectivity. In general, two different culture methods are used: the first (classic) way of preparing BCG is to grow it as a surface culture. This surface pellicle is subsequently homogenized in a ball mill such that together with viable bacilli, subcellular debris and dead bacilli also are harvested. In the second method, BCG is grown in a homogeneously stirred deep culture medium. Bacteriae are collected by centrifugation and resuspended. This culture method ensures a relatively high ratio of viable organisms and a small quantity of subcellular debris and dead microorganisms; BCG RIVM is prepared according to the second method. Other preparations (Tice, Connaught, Armand Frappier) are cultured as a surface pellicle.

It is possible that the difference in culture method is responsible for the significant difference in local side effects noted between BCG RIVM and other vaccines. In the present study, agent-induced cystitis was only seen in 16.7 per cent of the patients (comparable with the local toxicity of intravesical chemotherapy), whereas about 90 per cent of the patients complain of (transient) cystitis when the other strains are used (Lamm, 1986). On the other hand, the question arises whether the efficacy of the preparation may be related to its local toxicity: the adherence of the bacilli to the bladder wall is probably an important factor by which BCG excerts its effect. It is therefore possible that subcellular debris or cell products are necessary to achieve attachment of BCG to the bladder wall (Nickel, 1987). Ratliff et al. (1987) demonstrated that the protein fibronectin plays a role in the attachment of BCG.

The results pertaining to recurrence rate obtained so far in our study, although preliminary, do not indicate superiority of BCG RIVM over MMC. This is in contrast to other studies in which it has been demonstrated that BCG strains are superior to intravesical chemotherapy (Lamm, 1984; Netto, 1983). However, additional prospective studies are indispensable to prove the superiority of one agent over another and of one regimen over another. For example, it is not yet clear whether 6 weekly instillations are suboptimal, as suggested by Haaff et al. (1986). It has also yet to be determined whether maintenance therapy is necessary.

These questions can only be answered in further prospective, randomized clinical trials. As far as the BCG RIVM vaccine is concerned, the most urgent question to be answered is whether this preparation, with its minimal toxicity, is as effective as other strains of BCG. Such a randomized trial is now under study by the Dutch South-East Co-operative urological Group in which BCG RIVM is compared with BCG Tice and MMC.

This and other studies will certainly contribute to further elucidation of the exact value of active non specific immunotherapy with BCG in the treatment of superficial bladder cancer.

REFERENCES

Bracken, B.; Johnson, D.; Von Eschenbach, A.; Swanson, D.; De Furia, D.; Crook, S. (1980): Role of intravesical mitomycin in management of superficial bladder tumors. Urology 16, 11.

Haaff, E.O.; Dresner, S.M.; Ratliff, T.L.; Catalona, W.J. (1986): Two courses of intravesical bacillus Calmette-Guérin for transitional cell carcinoma of the bladder. J. Urol. 136, 820.

Huland, H.; Otto. U.; Droese, M.; Kloppel, G. (1984): Long-term mitomycin C instillation after transurethral resection of superficial bladder carcinoma: influence on recurrence progression and survival. J. Urol. 132, 27.

Kelley, D.R.; Ratliff, T.L.; Catalona, W.J.; Shapiro A.; Lage, J.M.; Bauer, W.C.; Haaff, E.O.; Dresner S.M. (1985): Intravesical bacillus Calmette-Guérin therapy for superficial bladder cancer: effect of bacillus Calmette-Guérin viability on treatment results. J. Urol. 134, 48.

Lamm, D.L.; Thor, D.E.; Stogdill, V.D.; Radwin, H.M. (1982): Bladder cancer immunotherapy. J. Urol. 128, 931.

Lamm, D.L.; Crawford, E.D.; Montie, J.E.; Scardino, P.T.; Grossman, H.B., Sullivan, J.W. (1985): BCG versus adriamycin in the treatment of transitional cell carcinoma in situ: a South-west Oncology Group Study. J. Urol. 133: 184A.

Lamm, D.L.; Stogdill, V.D.; Stogdill, B.J.; Crispen, R.G. (1986): Complications of bacillus Calmette-Guérin immunotherapy in 1278 patients with bladder cancer. J. Urol. 135, 272.

Morales, A.; Eidinger, D.; Bruce, A.W. (1976): Intracavitary bacillus Calmette-Guérin in the treatment of superficial bladder cancer. J. Urol. 116, 180.

Netto, M.R.; Lemos, G.C. (1983): A comparison of treatment methods for the prophylaxis of recurrent superficial bladder tumors. J. Urol. 129, 33.

Nickel, J.C.; Morales, A.; Heaton, J.P.W.; Costerton, J.W. (1985): Ultrastructural study of the interaction of B.C.G. with bladder mucosa after intravesical treatment of bladder cancer. J. Urol. 133, 268A.

Ratliff, T.L.; Palmer, J.O.; McGarr, J.A, Brown, E.J. (1987): Intravesical bacillus Calmette-Guérin therapy for murine bladder tumors: Initiation of the response by fibronectin-mediated attachment of B.C.G. Cancer Res. 47, 1762.

Soloway, M. (1980): Rationale for intensive intravesical chemotherapy for superficial bladder cancer. J. Urol. 123, 461.

ACKNOWLEDGEMENTS

The authors whish to thank all collaborating urologists, members of the EORTC-GU group, and their nursing staffs for their excellent contributions to this study; and thanks to Mrs. D. Litjens-de Heus for assistance in preparing and typing the manuscript.

Résumé

La chimioprophylaxie intravésicale est utilisée depuis longtemps dans la prévention de récidives des cancers de vessie superficiels. La MMC est restée la plus efficace des chimiothérapies utilisées. Ces dernières années, l'emploi du BCG dans cette indication a tendance à augmenter sans toutefois que sa supériorité par rapport à la chimiothérapie n'ait été détectée ou confirmée dans les essais cliniques.

Dans cette étude, nous avons comparé l'efficacité de la MMC et celle du BCG RIVM. Cette étude prospective randomisée a porté sur 337 patients, dont 213 avaient une tumeur pTa, 114 une tumeur pT1 et 10 un cancer in situ. Des cancers primitifs étaient en cause chez 235 malades (70 %). Les deux groupes thérapeutiques ont comporté des effets secondaires comparables.

Ceci concerne aussi bien la cystite bactérienne que la cystite chimique iatrogène. Aucun malade n'a révélé de toxicité aigüe. La fréquence des récidives après un an de suivi est la même dans les deux groupes thérapeutiques.

(30 % des patients traités par BCG RIVM contre 25 % chez ceux traités par MMC, la différence n'étant pas statistiquement significative). Les résultats ont fait apparaître une action thérapeutique de la MMC et du BCG RIVM de la même valeur et on n'a pas pu détecter ni confirmer de supériorité éventuelle du BCG au cours de cette étude.

Neo-Adjuvant Chemotherapy. Ed. Cl. Jacquillat, M. Weil, D. Khayat. Colloque INSERM/John Libbey Eurotext Ltd. © 1988. Vol. 169, pp. 971-974.

Intravesical mitomycin C for the treatment of superficial bladder cancer

Mark Stephen Soloway

Department of Urology, University of Tennessee, 956 Court, Box 10, Memphis, Tennessee 38163, USA

ABSTRACT

I have treated 80 patients with stages Ta, T1, or Tcis with intravesical Mitomycin C. After establishing the diagnosis by biopsy or partial transurethral resection, Mitomycin was instilled in a dose of 40 mg. in 40 ml. sterile water for a two-hour interval. The instillations were continued weekly for eight weeks. The first evaluation was at week 12.

The complete response rate for those with an initial Ta lesion was 37 per cent (15/41), for those with a T1 tumor it was 44 per cent (8/18), and for those with Tcis, 33 per cent (7/21).

Two thirds of the patients have been followed for at least three years or have had a cystectomy or have died of bladder cancer. Nineteen per cent of those with an initial Ta, 22 per cent of those with a T1, and 43 per cent of those with initial Tcis eventually had a cystectomy during the follow up interval. The likelihood of having a cystectomy or of dying from bladder cancer was much lower if they had a complete response at the first three-month evaluation.

Intravesical Mitomycin C for the treatment of residual superficial bladder cancer has an excellent chance of providing a complete response after an eight-week treatment period. Those who have a complete response are much more likely to retain their bladder than if they have persistent disease at the first three-month interval.

KEY WORDS

Mitomycin C, superficial bladder cancer

INTRODUCTION

Intravesical therapy may be used for either treatment of existing tumor or for the prevention of a subsequent tumor following removal of all tumor. In the first instance, tumor remains in the bladder prior to initiation of therapy and this can be documented by a positive cytology. Alternatively, a bladder diagram and/or endoscopic photography can document the extent and appearance of tumor.

It is preferable, when possible, to resect all tumor prior to instillations of an intravesical agent. In instances of multifocal carcinoma, however, this may not be possible.

I have now treated 80 patients with stages Ta, T1, or Tcis bladder cancer with intravesical Mitomycin C (MMC). There were 59 men and 21 women with ages ranging from 48 to 82 years (mean 65). All of the patients had multifocal tumor, almost all had a prior bladder tumor history, and in no case was all of the tumor resected prior to initiation to MMC. The mean follow up for the 80 patients is 40 months. Fifty-four (67.5 per cent) of the patients have been followed a minimum of three years and 27 (34 per cent) have been followed at least five years.

Seven to 14 days following the staging biopsy or partial transurethral resection, MMC was instilled in a dose of 40 mg. in 40 ml. sterile water fir a two-hour interval. Patients were asked to wash their hands and genitalia following the initial instillation and following the first several voidings. This has reduced the incidence of MMC associated rashes on the genitalia and hands. Forty-one of the 80 patients were placed on MMC as first line therapy. The remainder received at least one three-month course of intravesical Thiotepa. Almost all of these patients developed a recurrence on Thiotepa.

The initial evaluation for response was determined at 12 weeks - four weeks after the last of the eight weekly MMC instillations. A complete response required that there be no visible or histologic evidence of bladder cancer and that the bladder washing contain no tumor cells. Every patient with initial Tcis had selected site and random mucosal biopsies, and these must, of course, have no tumor to fulfill the criteria for a complete response. Initialy we did use a partial response category ; however, it was found that patients with a partial response, even if it was due only to a positive cytology without endoscopic evidence of tumor, performed similarly to the failure group and thus we have discontinued the partial response category.

Patients who had a complete response, and occasionally those with only a positive cytology, were continued on a monthly maintenance schedule of 40 mg./40 ml. MMC for 9-12 months. Endoscopic evaluation with bladder washing cytology was performed every three months for the first 12 months, and every three to six months subsequently.

RESULTS

The complete response rate for those with an initial Ta lesion was 37 per cent (15/41) and for those with a T1 tumor, 44 per cent (8/18). Thrity-three per cent (7/21) who had multifocal carcinoma in situ had a complete response. Ten additional patients with Tcis (48 per cent) had a positive cytology but no endoscopically visible abnormality and the biopsies obtained contained either normal mucosa or varying degrees of dysplasia.

The intent of an intensive course of intravesical therapy in this group of patients with multifocal disease is to eradicate tumor remaining in the bladder and prevent tumor progression as indicated by invasion into the muscle, cystectomy, or death from bladder cancer. Nine of 21 patients (43 per cent) with Tcis eventually had a cystectomy; however, only one of the seven who had a complete response at three months had a cystectomy. Only 14 per cent of the 21 patients with Tcis developed a tumor that invaded the muscle. One patient died of bladder cancer.

Nineteen per cent (8/41) of those whose tumor was limited to the mucosa (Ta) subsequently had a cystectomy. This was lower if they had a complete response, 13 per cent, than if they failed, 23 per cent. The incidence of a subsequent tumor with muscle invasion was twice as likely for the failures compared to the complete responders, 15 per cent versus seven per cent. The three deaths in the Ta category were all in those who had a recurrence following the initial treatment course of MMC.

Only 12 per cent (1/8) of those with an initial tumor with lamina propria invasion (T1) who had a complete response at three months eventually had a cystectomy. This contrasts with the 30 percent (3/10) cystectomy incidence for those who had residual tumor at 12 weeks.

Toxicity with intravesical MMC as been minimal. Three men had a penile rash and only one discontinued therapy as a result. Palmar erythema and/or dermatitis was observed in five patients. Bladder irritative symptoms were intermittent and mild.

DISCUSSION

Following the identification of a transitional cell carcinoma of the urinary bladder that is histologically confined to the urothelium (Ta or Tcis) or lamina propria (T1), a trial of an effective intravesical therapeutic agent is indicated. Drugs which have demonstrated activity include Thiotepa, Mitomycin C, Adriamycin, and BCG. MMC has been used for both the treatment and prophylaxis of superficial bladder tumors for several years. One of the advantages of MMC is its relatively high molecular weight, which accounts for its low level of absorption.

The majority of published studies dealing with MMC were designed to determine whether this agent was capable of eradicating existing superficial bladder tumors, i.e., treatment. The weekly dose was varied from 20 to 60 mg but most urologist have used 30 to 40 mg weekly for eight weeks. When the drug is used to prevent subsequent tumor following endoscopic resection, 20 mg. in 20 ml. sterile water delivered every other week has been a recent standard regimen.

Eighty patients who have residual superficial bladder cancer following biopsy or partial transurethral resection have now received MMC and two thirds have been followed at least five years. Thirty-eight per cent have had a complete response and importantly, only 13 per cent of these complete responders have subsequently had a cystectomy and only 10 per cent have subsequently developed a tumor which has invaded into the muscle. Only one of these patients (3 per cent) has died of bladder cancer. Thus, this initial 12-week evaluation has impressive prognostic import.

Neo-Adjuvant Chemotherapy. Ed. Cl. Jacquillat, M. Weil, D. Khayat. Colloque INSERM/John Libbey Eurotext Ltd. © 1988. Vol. 169, pp. 975-976.

Traitement prophylactique des cancers superficiels de la vessie : analyse de 130 cas de mitomycine C intravésicale

P. Léandri, G. Rossignol, J.R. Gautier, J. Caissel, C. Rudelle et L. Gabay

Département d'Urologie, Clinique Saint-Jean-Languedoc, 31077 Toulouse Cedex, France

RESUME

130 patients ont été traités de 1980 à 1986 par de la Mitomycine Intra-Vésicale (I.V.M.). Il s'agissait de patients présentant une tumeur urothéliale superficielle récidivante (44 cas, groupe A) ou la première atteinte d'une tumeur urothéliale surpeficielle (86 cas, groupe B).
L'I.V.M. à la dose de 40 mg par semaine pendant 20 semaines a été commencée 15 jours après une résection transuréthrale. La tolérance a été très bonne avec des effets toxiques mineurs dans huit cas. Dans 75 % des cas, il n'y a pas eu de récidives (7 récidives groupe A, 25 récidives groupe B).

MOTS CLEFS

Chimiothérapie locale, tumeurs superficielles de vessie

INTRODUCTION

130 patients ont été traités entre 1980 et 1986 par de l'Amétycine intra-vésicale (I.V.M.). Il s'agissait soit de patients présentant des tumeurs urothéliales superficielles récidivantes To ou T1 (groupe A), soit des patients présentant pour la première fois une tumeur urothéliale superficielle T1 ou un carcinome in situ (groupe B).

MATERIEL ET METHODE

Les patients reçoivent 40 mg d'Amétycine dans 40 ml d'eau, une fois par semaine pendant 20 semaines, 15 jours après avoir pratiqué une résection transuréthrale. Une cystoscopie et une cytologie sont effectuées 15 à 30 jours après la dernière I.V.M., puis tous les six mois pendant deux ans et tous les ans après la 2ème année sans récidive.
112 patients étaient de sexe masculin, 18 de sexe féminin. Les âges extrêmes étaient de 26 ans à 75 ans. 44 patients (groupe A) avaient des récidives multiples de To (28 cas) ou T1 (16 cas). La moyenne des récidives était de 2,3 et la moyenne des délais de récidives, 8 mois.
86 patients (groupe B) avaient soit une tumeur urothéliale de type T1 pour la 1ère fois (83 cas), soit un carcinome in situ (3 cas).

RESULTATS

La moyenne des contrôles a été de 33 mois après I.V.M.
Il n'y a pas eu de récidives chez 98 patients (75 % des cas).
Pour le groupe A, on a observé 7 récidives (To = 4, T1 = 3) avec un délai moyen de récidive de 14 Mois. Pour le groupe B, il y a eu 25 récidives (T1 = 23, C.I.S. = 2) avec un délai moyen d'apparition pour la première récidive de 11 mois.
Des effets toxiques mineurs ont été rencontrés chez huit patients = 3 dermatoses, 3 cystites chimiques, 2 cystites bactériennes. 3 patients n'ont pas terminé leur traitement.

DISCUSSION - CONCLUSIONS

L'Amétycine à visée prophylactique après résection de la tumeur a une efficacité certaine. Elle permet d'éviter les récidives dans plus de 60 % des cas de tumeurs superficielles et de diminuer significativement la fréquence des récidives (dans le groupe A, elle est passée de 8 mois à 14 mois). Ces résultats sont en accord avec ceux de Harrison, Devonec, MacFarlane.
La toxicité de ce produit est faible. Il n'y a pas de toxicité hématologique, les autres réactions sont minimes et régressent à l'arrêt du traitement. Elles n'obligent que rarement à cesser l'administration de la Mitomycine Intra Vésicale.

REFERENCES

MacFarlane, J.R. (1985) : Intravesical Mitomycin C Thérapy for superficial bladder cancer. Br. J. Uro. 57, 37-39

Devonec, M. (1983) : Intravesical instillation of Mitomycin C in the prophylactic treatment of recurring superficial transitionnal cell carcinoma of the bladder. Br. J. Uro. 55, 382-385

Harrison, G.S.M. (1983) : A phase II study of intravesical Mitomycin in the treatment of superficial bladder cancer. Br. J. Uro. 55

Mishina, T. (1986) : Absorption of anticancer drugs through bladder épithélium. Urology, volume XXVII, number 2, 148-157

Résumé

130 patients were treated between 1980 and 1986 using intravesical Mitomycin C (I.V.M.). 44 patients (Group A) had an elevated recurrence rate of stage To, T1 tumor ; 86 patients (group B) had first transitional cell carcinoma of the bladder. I.V.M. has been used as a prophylactic agent 15 days after transurétral resection. Patients received 40 mg weekly for 20 weeks. Cystoscopy and cytology evaluation were performed 15 days after the last I.V.M., and every 6 months. The average follow up was 33 months after I.V.M.. There were recurrences in 25 % cases (7 cases group A, 25 cases group B).
Minor toxic side effects occured in eight patients.

Neo-Adjuvant Chemotherapy. Ed. Cl. Jacquillat, M. Weil, D. Khayat. Colloque INSERM/John Libbey Eurotext Ltd. © 1988. Vol. 169, pp. 977-984.

The prophylactic use of mitomycin C bladder instillation for preventing the recurrence of superficial bladder tumours

T. Mishina*, M. Nakao** and S. Nakagawa**

Mishina Urological Office, Higashino-toin Sanjo-Sagaru, Nakagyo-ku, Kyoto 604, Japan.*
*Department of Urology, Kyoto Prefectural University of Medicine**, Kyoto 602, Japan*

ABSTRACT

A total of 238 patients with superficial bladder tumours who had undergone TUR-Bt or partial cystectomy between 1964 and 1983 were chosen for the study. The effect of preoperative bladder instillation(POI) of Mitomycin C (MMC) and periodic prophylactic bladder instillation (PPI) of a combination of MMC and 5-FU was evaluated in connection with the prevention of recurrence, progression and cancer death after surgery in 238 patients with superficial bladder tumours. Both POI and PPI significantly reduced the recurrence rate, the tumour progression and the cancer death rate in patients treated with POI or PPI or both, compared with patients treated with neither POI nor PPI. No carcinogenic action on the bladder epithelium was observed at all.

KEYWORDS

Prophylactic use of MMC for superficial bladder tumours, MMC, recurrence of bladder tumours, preoperative bladder instillation (POI), periodic prophylactic bladder instillation (PPI).

INTRODUCTION

Many urologists(Lutzeyer, 1982; Vakarakis, 1974) have observed that recurrent tumours were found in most patients with superficial bladder tumours who had been treated with transurethral resection. The incidence of recurrent tumour in the bladder after endoscopic treatment of the primary tumour has been between 40 per cent and 87 per cent, with the majority of reports giving an incidence of around 70 per cent (Heney, 1982). The risk of progression for superficial bladder tumours is 7-22 per cent (Lutzeyer, 1982; Henei, 1983). Progression may be defined as any change in the characteristics of a recurrent tumour that increases its threat to the patient and is principally a change in grade, depth of invasion or the development of metastases. Efforts to reduce the recurrence rate have so far been unsuccessful.

Subsequent tumour can be classified as follows: 1)tumours arising from carcinoma in situ or precancerous changes missed at surgery (Melicow,1952), 2)tumours implanted during surgery (Soloway,1980) and tumours arising from carcinoma in situ or precancerous changes which have developed in the bladder epithelium after surgery (Miller,1977).

Preoperative bladder instillation (POI) of Mitomycin C (MMC) was used to destroy carcinoma in situ or precancerous changes which might be missed by the naked eye (Mishina,1975 and 1982). In addition, periodic prophylactic bladder instillation (PPI) of a combination of MMC and 5-FU was carried out to destroy both tumour cells implanted during surgery and carcinoma in situ or precancerous changes developing after surgery. A combination of MMC and 5-FU was chosen from our clinical results in our comparative study of bladder instillation therapy for low stage bladder tumours using 8 anticancer drugs (Mishina, 1982). In this paper, the effect of both POI and PPI on the recurrence of bladder tumours will be evaluated.

MATERIALS AND METHODS

A total of 238 patients with superficial bladder tumours who underwent TUR-Bt or partial cystectomy in our clinic between January 1964 and December 1983 were chosen for the study. The cases consisted of 40 females and 198 males who ranged in age from 16 to 85, with an average age of 63.2 years. The 238 patients were divided into four groups. Group A (51 cases) was treated with POI and PPI, Group B (15 cases) with PPI but not POI, Group C (75 cases) with POI but not PPI and Group D (97 cases) with neither PPI nor POI. Group A consists of 51 cases among which 30 were treated with TUR-Bt and 21 with partial cystectomy. There are 15 cases in Group B. Six were treated with TUR-Bt and 9 with partial cystectomy. Group C consists of 75 cases, of which 42 were treated with TUR-Bt and 33 with partial cystectomy. Group D consists of 97 cases, of which 63 were treated with TUR-Bt and 34 with partial cystectomy "Table 1,2".

Table 1. 238 evaluated cases with superficial bladder tumours (1)

Group(No.pts)	Intravesical chemotherapy		Operation method	
	POI	PPI	TUR-Bt	Partial cystectomy
Group A (51)	+	+	30(59%)	21(41%)
Group B (15)	−	+	6(40%)	9(60%)
Group C (75)	+	−	42(56%)	33(44%)
Group D (97)	−	−	63(65%)	34(35%)
Total			141(59%)	97(41%)

Table 2. 238 evaluated cases with superficial bladder tumours (2)

Group(No.pts)	Stage		Grade				No. tumours	
	pTa	pT1	G0	G1	G2	G3	single	Multiple
Group A (51)	24(47%)	27(53%)	0(0%)	23(45%)	21(41%)	7(14%)	31(61%)	20(39%)
Group B (15)	6(40%)	9(60%)	0(0%)	7(47%)	5(33%)	3(20%)	8(53%)	7(47%)
Group C (75)	32(43%)	43(57%)	3(4%)	23(31%)	36(48%)	13(17%)	46(61%)	29(39%)
Group D (97)	43(44%)	54(56%)	4(4%)	67(69%)	19(20%)	7(7%)	66(68%)	31(32%)
Total	105(44%)	133(56%)	7(3%)	120(50%)	81(34%)	20(13%)	151(63%)	87(37%)

Histological malignancies are as follows: Group A consists of 23 cases (45 per cent) of G1, 21 cases (41 per cent) of G2, and 7 cases (14 per cent) of G3. Group B is made up of 7 cases (47 per cent) of G1, 5 cases (33 per cent) of G2 and 3 cases (20 per cent) of G3. Group C consists of 3 cases (4 per cent) of G0, 23 cases (31 per cent) of G1, 36 cases (48 per cent) of G2 and 13 cases (17 per cent) of G3. Group D is made up of 4 cases (4 per cent) of G0, 67 cases (69 per cent) of G1, 19 cases (20 per cent) of G2 and 7 cases (7 per cent) of G3. Histological stage is as follows: pTa in 24 cases (47 per cent) and pT1 in 27 cases (53 per cent), in Group A; pTa in 6 cases (40 per cent) and pT1 in 9 cases (60 per cent), in Group B; pTa in 32 cases (43 per cent) and pT1 in 43 cases (57 per cent), in Group C; pTa in 43 cases (44 per cent) and pT1 in 54 cases (56 per cent), in Group D. The numbers of tumours are as follows: Group A consists of 31 cases (61 per cent) with a single tumour and 20 cases (39 per cent) with multiple tumours. Group B is made up of 8 cases (53 per cent) with a single tumour and 7 cases (47 per cent) with multiple tumours. Group C consists of 46 cases (61 per cent) with a single tumour and 29 cases (39 per cent) with multiple tumours. Group D is made up of 66 cases (68 per cent) with a single tumour and 31 cases (32 per cent) with multiple tumours.

Patients who underwent POI of MMC for bladder tumour were requested to lie on the examination table after they had voided and 20mg of MMC in 20ml of sterilized distilled water was instilled into the bladder through a catheter. The drug was held in the bladder for as long as possible-on the average for about 3 hours. This procedure was performed daily or 3 times weekly for a total of 20 such procedures. PPI was performed twice a month, starting one month after surgery, using a combination of 20mg of MMC and 1000mg of 5-Fu, for 5 years. Cystoscopy, Papanicolaou's staining of urine, roentgenological examination of the chest and bone marrow and liver function tests were carried out every five months and DIP was performed once a year on all patients.

Recurrence-free rates and survival rates in each group were calculated by Kaplan-Meir's method.

RESULTS

The recurrence-free rates for the different Groups, one, three, five and seven years after surgery, is shown in "Fig.1" In Group A, treated with POI and PPI, recurrence-free rates 1,3,5 and 7 years after surgery were 98 per cent, 88 per cent 81 per cent and 81 per cent, respectively. In Group B treated with PPI but not POI, recurrence-free rates 1,3,5 and 7years after surgery were 93 per cent, 93 per cent, 93 per cent,and 93 per cent, respectively. In Group C, treated with POI but not PPI, recurrence-free rates 1,3,5 and 7 years after surgery were 88 per cent, 67 per cent, 62 per cent and 62 per cent, respectively. In Group D, treated with neither PPI nor POI, recurrence-free rates 1,3,5 and 7 years after surgery were 72 per cent, 50 per cent, 39 per cent and 34 per cent, respectively. Statistical significance was observed between Group A and Group C and or Group D, between Group B and Group C and or Group D and between Group C and Group D, respectively.

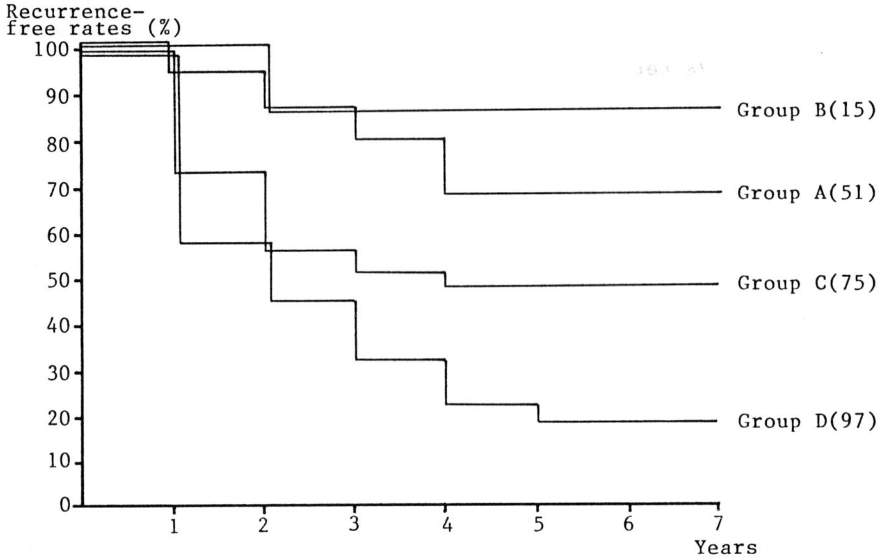

Feb.19.,1988. Mishina, et al.

Fig.1. Recurrence-free rates

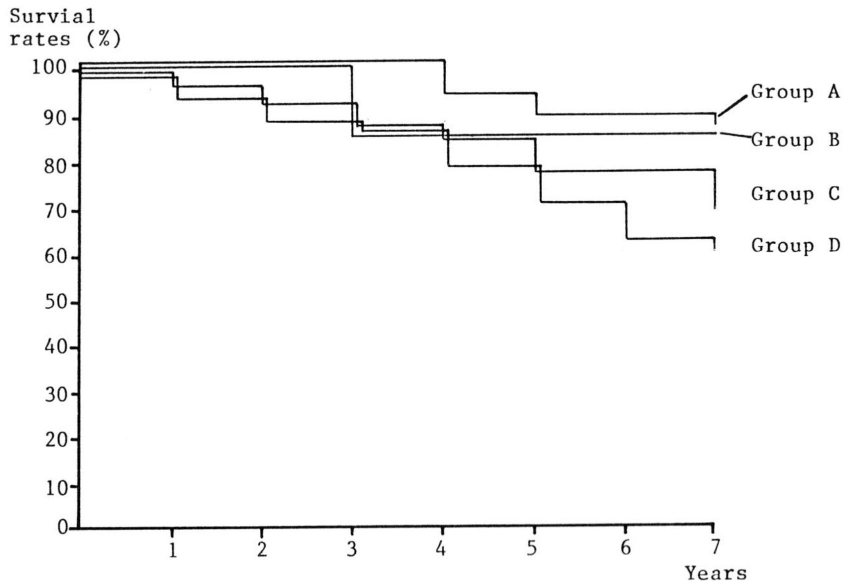

Feb.19.,1988. Mishina, et al.

Fig.2. Survival rates

The survival rate for the different groups, three, five and seven years after surgery, is shown in "Fig.2" In Group A, survivarl rates 3,5 and 7 years after surgery were 100 per cent, 90 per cent and 87 per cent, respectively. In Group B, survival rates 3,5 and 7 years after surgery were 86 per cent 86 per cent and 86 per cent, respectively. In Group C, survival rates 3, 5 and 7 years after surgery were 88 per cent, 78 per cent and 69 per cent, respectively. In Group D, survival rates 3, 5 and 7 years after surgery were 85 per cent, 71 per cent and 60 per cent, respectively. Stastistical significance was observed between Group A and Group C and or Group D, between Group B and Group C and or Group D, and between Group C and Group D, respectively.

The clinical results for all patients are described here. In Group A, 51 cases treated with POI and PPI, recurrence of bladder tumour was observed in 13 cases (26 per cent), progression in 4 cases (8 per cent) and cancer death in 2 cases (4 per cent). In Group B, 15 cases treated with PPI but not POI, recurrence was observed in 1 case (7 per cent), but neither progression nor cancer death was observed. In Group C, 75 cases treated with POI but not PPI, recurrence was observed in 27 cases (36 per cent), progression in 8 cases (11 per cent) and cancer death in 5 cases (7 per cent). In Group D, 97 cases treated with neither POI nor PPI, recurrence was observed in 56 cases (58 per cent), progression in 24 cases (25 per cent) and cancer death in 22 cases (23 per cent).

DISCUSSION

Subsequent tumours may develop from 1) carcinoma in situ or precancerous changes missed at surgery, 2) tumour cells implanted during surgery and 3) carcinoma in situ or precancerous changes which have developed in the bladder epithelium after surgery. In order to eradicate these factors, POI of MMC and PPI of a combination of MMC and 5-FU were carried out and evaluated.

1) The Significance of POI for The Prevention of The Recurrence of Bladder Tumours.
Melicow (1952) performed a histological study of the vesical urothelium intervening between gross neoplasms in the extirpated bladder. Epithelial hyperplasia, squamous metaplasia and carcinoma in situ were found in grossly normal regions of the bladders extirpated for cancer but not in the bladders extirpated for benign diseases. Soloway (1978) performed selected situ biopsies from apparently normal mucosa at the time of initial and subsequent endoscopy on 52 patients. Histological abnormalities were discovered in 33 per cent of the patients, with biopsies at initial endoscopy, while 77 per cent of 43 patients undergoing three-month selected situ biopsies had at least one abnormal biopsy during a one-year period. Subsequent follow-up of these patients revealed that 38 per cent of patients with epithelial hyperplasia, atypia or carcinoma in situ suffered from bladder cancer whereas only 16 per cent of those without such findings did. From these clinical studies, it is presumed that the recurrence of bladder tumours after surgery may arise from carcinoma in situ or precancerous changes which are missed at surgery.

In our series, the recurrence-free rate and the survival rate 7 years after surgery were 62 per cent and 69 per cent, respectively, in Group C treated with POI but not PPI. However, they were only 34 per cent and 60 per cent,respectively, in Group D, which didn't receive either POI or PPI treatment.
Statistical significance was observed in both the recurrence-free rate and the survival rate between these two groups. Tumour progression was observed in 8 cases (11 per cent) and cancer death in 5 cases (7 per cent) in Group C. In Group D, tumour progression was seen in 24 cases (25 per cent) and cancer death occured in 22 cases (23 per cent). These clinical results suggest that POI may destroy carcinoma in situ or precancerous changes and that it will reduce the recurrence and the progression of bladder tumours, resulting in improved prognosis for the patient.

2) <u>The Significance of PPI for The Prevention of The Recurrence of Bladder Tumours.</u>
Another contributing factor to the high recurrence rate might be the implantation of tumour cells on the urothelial surface traumatized during transurethral resection or fulguration. Burnand (1976) compared the recurrence rate between randomly selected patients who had received a single intravesical thiotepa instillation immediately after cystodiathermy and a control group of patients who had been treated by cystodiathermy alone. Recurrent tumours were recognized in significantly fewer patients in this thiotepa treated group. A single intravesical instillation seemed to inhibit the implantation of tumour cells on the urothelial surface during TUR-Bt. Veenema (1969) carried out a prophylactic program of thiotepa bladder instillation. They administered 30 to 60mg of thiotepa in 60ml of sterilized distilled water intravesically at intervals of one to two weeks for a total of four to eight instillations, starting seven to ten days after endoscopic or open surgery, followed by 30 to 60mg every four to eight weeks for at least one year. The 30 patients studied had a total of 45 recurrences and an average of seven tumours per recurrence before the beginning of the program. After the program, 15 patients had no recurrence at all for at least three years. The remaining 15 patients showed some recurrence but the frequency of recurrence and the number of recurrent tumours were definitely reduced.

Intravesical instillation of MMC for prophylaxis has been applied by several investigators (Oomaru, 1933; Kyushu Cooperative Urological Research Group, 1974; Mishina, 1979 and 1981; Huland, 1983). Niimura (1980) performed prophylactic instillation of 6mg of MMC dissolved in 20ml of saline solution twice a week or once a month for five years in 33 cases, starting one or two weeks after TUR-Bt or partial cystectomy. The one, three and five year recurrence rates were 18.2 per cent, 34.3 per cent and 34.3 per cent, respectively.

In our serise, the recurrence-free rate and the survival rate 7 years after surgery were 81 per cent and 87 per cent, respectively, for Group A treated with POI and PPI. The same rates for the same period of time were 62 per cent and 69 per cent, respectively, in Group C treated with POI but not PPI. Statistical significance was observed in both the recurrence-free rate and the survival rate between these two groups. Tumour progression and cancer death were observed in 4 cases (8 per cent) and in 2 cases (4 per cent), respectively, in Group A, while in Group C, 8 cases (11 per cent) of tumour progression and 5 cases (7 per cent) of cancer death were seen. In Group B, treated with PPI but not POI, the recurrence-free rate and the survival rate 7 years after surgery were 93 per cent and 86 per cent, respectively, while neither tumour progression nor cancer death was observed at all.

It is presumed from these results that PPI may destroy not only tumour cells implanted during surgery but also carcinoma in situ or precancerous changes which have developed in the bladder epithelium after sugery. Also, it appears to reduce the recurrence and the progression of bladder tumours, resulting in improved prognosis of patients with superficial bladder tumours.

3) <u>Side Effects of PPI</u>
Before accepting repeated long term use of intravesical chemotherapy, we must consider the possible long-term toxic effects. Hicks and Wakefield (1972) instilled a total of 6mg of N-methyl-N-nitrosourea into the bladder of 100 female Wister rats through a urethral catheter. All animals kept for more than 30 weeks developed a bladder tumour. From this experiment, we may conclude that some anticancer drugs might be carcinogenic when instilled into the bladder. Ohtani (1984) found that intravesical of ADR or MMC once a week for 12 weeks into rats pretreated for 4 weeks with BBN markedly enhanced development of bladder tumours.

In our study on random biopsies (Mishina, 1982), no carcinogenic action of MMC was seen in repeated, long term intravesical use. In other words, we have never experienced bladder carcinogenesis in intravesical use of MMC for repeated, long term use. As for the absorption of anticancer drugs and the local irritation caused by intravesical chemotherapy, MMC was found to be an ideal anticancer drug for topical use because it can not be absorbed through the bladder epithelium and it causes little local irritation (Mishina, 1986). No serious local or general side effects were observed in this study.

SUMMARY

The effect of preoperative bladder instillation (POI) and periodic prophylactic bladder instillation (PPI) of MMC was evaluated in connection with the prevention of recurrent bladder tumours after surgery. A total of 238 patients with pTa or pT1 tumours, including patients who underwent TUR-Bt and partial cystectomy between January 1964 and December 1983, were chosen for the study. They were divided into the following four groups: Group A (51 cases) was treated with POI and PPI, Group B (15 cases) with PPI but not POI, Group C (75 cases) with POI but not PPI and Group D (97 cases) with neither POI nor PPI. POI was performed daily or three times a week for a total of 20 applications of 20mg of MMC starting one or two months before surgery. PPI was performed twice a month, starting one month after surgery, with a combination of 20mg of MMC and 1000mg of 5-FU. The recurrence-free rate and the survival rate of these four groups were estimated by Kaplan-Meir's method. The seven-year recurrence-free rates in Groups A,B,C and D were 81 per cent, 93 per cent, 62 per cent and 34 per cent, respectively. The seven-year survival rates in Groups A,B,C and D were 87 per cent, 86 per cent, 69 per cent and 60 per cent, respectively. The number of cases in which cancer progression was observed in Groups A,B,C and D was 4 cases (8 per cent), 0 case (0 per cent), 8 cases (11 per cent) and 24 cases (25 per cent), respectively. The number of cancer death cases in Groups A,B,C and D was 2 cases (4 per cent), 0 case (0 per cent) 5 cases (7 per cent) and 22 cases (23 per cent), respectively. No carcinogenic action on the bladder epithelium was observed in the cases treated with POI or PPI.

It is presumed from our study that POI may destroy carcinoma in situ or precancerous changes and that PPI may destroy not only tumour cells implanted during surgery but also carcinoma in situ or precancerous changes which have developed in the bladder epithelium after surgery. Also, we have found that a combination of POI and PPI may markedly reduce the recurrence and the progression of bladder tumours, resulting in improved prognosis.

REFERENCES

Burnand,K.G.,Boyd,P.T.R., Mayo,M.E.,Shuttle Worth,K.E.D., Loyd-Davies,R.W.(1976): Single dose intravesical thio-tepa as an adjuvant to cystodiathermy in the treatment of transitional cell bladder carcinoma. Brit.J. Urol. 48, 55-59.

Heney. NM, Nocks BN, Daly JJ, Prout GR, Newall JB, Griffin PB, Perrone TL., Szyfelbein WA (1982): Ta and T1 bladder cancer; Location recurrence and progression. Br.J. Urol. 54, 152-157.

Henei NM, Ahmed S, Flanagan MJ, Frable W, Corder MP, Hafermann MD, Hawkins IR (1983): Superficial bladder cancer; progression and recurrence. J.Urol. 130, 1083-1086.

Hicks, RM, Wakefield JSTJ (1972): Rapid induction of bladder cancer in rats with N-methyl-N-nitrosourea. 1. Histology. Chem. Biol. Interactions. 5, 139-152.

Huland, H., Otto, U. (1983): Mitomycin Instillation to prevent recurrence of superficial bladder carcinoma, Results of a controlled, prospective study in 58 patients. Eur. Urol. 9, 84-86.

Kyushu Cooperative Urological Research Group (1974): Effects of intravesical instillation of mitomycin C on the recurrence rate of bladder tumours. Nishinihon J. Urol. 36, 535-539.

Luteyer, W., Rubben H, Dahm H (1982): Prognostic parameters in superficial bladder

cancer: an analysis of 315 cases. J. Urol. 127, 250-252.
Melicow, MM (1952): Histological study of vesical urothelium intervening between gross neoplasms in total cystectomy. J. Urol. 68, 261-279.
Miller, A. B.(1977): The etiology of bladder cancer from the epidemiological viewpoint. Cancer Res. 37, 2939-2942.
Mishina,T., Oda,K., Murata,S., Ooe,H., Mori,Y. and Takahashi,T. (1975): Mitomycin C bladder instillation therapy for bladder tumours. J. Urol. 114, 217-219.
Mishina,T. Miyakoda,K., Araki,H., Fujiwara,T., Kobayashi,T. and Maekawa,M. (1979): Bladder instillation therapy for bladder tumours. Jpn. J. Cancer Clin. 25, 845-855.
Mishina,T. Watanabe,H., Fujiwara,T., Kobayashi,T., Maegawa,M., Nakao,M., Nakagawa, S. (1982): Prophylactic use of mitomycin C bladder instillation for preventing the recurrence of bladder tumours. In Mitomycin C Current Impact on Cancer Therapy, M.Ogawa, M.Rozencweig, M.J.Staquet, pp 153-162, Amsterdam-Princeton-Geneva-London.; Excerpta Medica.
Mishina,T. Watanabe,H., Fujiwara,T., Kobayashi,T., Maegawa,M., Nakao,M., Nakagawa, S. (1982): Therapeutic use of mitomycin C bladder instillation: comparative study of bladder instillation therapy for low stage bladder tumours using eight anticancer drugs. In Mitomycin C Current Impact on Cancer Therapy, M.Ogawa, M.Rozencweig, M.J.Staquet, pp 163-175, Amsterdam-Princeton-Geneva-London.; Excerpta Medica.
Mishina,T. Watanabe,H., Kobayashi,T., Maegawa,M., Nakao,M., and Nakagawa,S. (1986): Absorption of anticancer drugs through bladder epithelium. Urol. 27, 148-157.
Niimura,K., Hayakawa,M., Fujioka,T., Okishio,N., Yamakoshi,T., Naide,Y. (1980): Clinical obserbation of intravesical instillation of mitomycin C for prophylaxis of the recurrence of bladder tumours. Jpn.J. Clin. Urol. 34, 749-753.
Ohtani,N., Fukushima,S., Okamura,T., Sakata,T., Ito,N., Koiso,K., Niijima.T. (1984): Effects of Intravesical instillation of antitumour chemotherapeutic agents on bladder carcinogenesis in rats treated with N-butyl-N-(4-hyroxybutyl) nitrosamine. Cancer 54, 1525-1529.
Oomaru,K., Hidaka,M. and Fujii,K. (1973): Effect of intravesical instillation of antitumour agent on prophylaxis for recurrence of bladder tumour. Nishinihon J. Urol. 35, 510-514.
Soloway,M.S., Murphy,W., Rav,MK, Cox,C. (1978): Serial multiple-site biopsies in patients with bladder cancer. J. Urol. 120, 57-59.
Soloway,M.S,Masters,S. (1980): Urothelial susceptibility to tumour cell implantation. Influence of cauterization. Cancer 46, 1158-1163.
Vakarakis MJ, Gaeta J, Moore RH, Murphy GP (1974) Superficial bladder tumour. Aspects of clinical progression. Urol. 4, 414-420.
Veenema,R.J., Dean,A.L.Jr., Uson,A.C., Roverts,M., Longo,F. (1969): Thiotepa bladder instillations: therapy and prophylaxis for superficial bladder tumours. J. Urol. 101, 711-715.

Résumé

238 malades ont subi une résection transurétrale ou cystectomie partielle pour tumeur superficielle de la vessie en 1964 et 1983 ont été chois choisis pour cette étude.

L'effet d'une instillation pré-opératoire de Mitomycine-C et l'instillation périodique d'une association de 5.Fu et de Mitomycine-C ont été évaluées avec pour critère la prévention des rechutes, la progression et la mort par cancer, après chirurgie de 238 malades atteints de cancer superficiel de la vessie. L'instillation pré-opératoire de la vessie ainsi que l'instillation prophylactique périodique ont réduit significativement le taux de récurrence, de progression des tumeurs, de décès par cancer chez les malades traités, par rapport aux malades qui n'ont reçu ni l'un ni l'autre. Nous n'avons observé chez aucun malade d'action carcinogénique sur la vessie.

Neo-Adjuvant Chemotherapy. Ed. Cl. Jacquillat, M. Weil, D. Khayat. Colloque INSERM/John Libbey Eurotext Ltd. © 1988. Vol. 169, pp. 985-989.

Résultat d'une étude de phase II associant méthotrexate, fluoro-uracile, doxorubicine et mitomycine C (M-FAM) dans les adénocarcinomes à point de départ inconnu

Th. Le Chevalier[1], C. Tremblay, D. Sevin[1], M. Spielmann[1], J. Treat[2] et J. Rouëssé[1]

[1]*Institut Gustave Roussy, Villejuif, France*
[2]*Lombardi cancer Center-Georgetown University Hospital, Washington DC, USA*

Le pronostic des malades porteurs d'adénocarcinome à point de départ inconnu est sombre, la survie médiane ne dépassant guère 4 mois (1). La combinaison de Fluorouracile, Doxorubicine et Mitomycine C (FAM) a permis d'obtenir chez de tels malades non pré-traités un taux de réponse de 30 % et une survie médiane de 10 mois (2). L'adjonction au FAM de Méthotrexate, basée sur son synergisme avec le Fluorouracile a donné des résultats encourageants (3,4) et nous avons testé cette combinaison chez les malades porteurs d'adénocarcinomes à point de départ inconnu.

MALADES ET METHODES

Dix sept malades, 7 hommes et 10 femmes, ont été inclus dans cette étude de Phase II entre Décembre 1984 et Janvier 1986. Leur âge moyen était de 47 ans (allant de 28 à 72 ans) et leur état initial, apprécié selon l'index de Karnofsky était de 100 % dans 9 cas, 90 % dans 2 cas, 80 % dans 5 cas et 60 % dans 1 cas.

Les localisations métastatiques étaient pulmonaires dans tous les cas, uniquement 5 fois, et associées à des métastases pleurales dans 4 cas, hépatiques dans 2 cas, osseuses dans 2 cas, surrénaliennes dans 1 cas. Enfin, 3 fois, il existait 3 sites métastatiques ou plus. La tumeur primitive n'était décelée ni à l'examen clinique, ni lors des examens complémentaires orientés par l'interrogatoire ou la symptomatologie clinique.

Tous les malades présentaient au moins une cible évaluable et aucun d'entre eux n'avait reçu un traitement de chimiothérapie auparavant.

L'examen clinique, la radiographie du thorax, et une échographie abdominale ne permettaient pas d'individualiser une tumeur primitive.

Le protocole de chimiothérapie administré est présenté ci-dessous :

METHOTREXATE	50 mg/m2	IV	Jour 1
FLUOROURACILE	600 mg/m2	IV	Jours 2, 8
DOXORUBICINE	30 mg/m2	IV	Jour 2
MITOMYCINE C	10 mg/m2	IV	Jour 2

- Le FAM est administré 18 heures après le Méthotrexate
- Une cure tous les 28 jours.
- La MITOMYCINE C n'est administrée qu'une cure sur deux.

RESULTATS

Les dix sept malades ont reçu en moyenne 7 cycles de chimiothérapie (allant de 2 à 16).

Une réponse objective a été constatée chez 5 malades (29 %) et 9 malades (53 %) ont présenté une stabilisation. La durée médiane de la réponse a été de 12 mois (allant de 2 à 14 mois) chez les malades répondeurs et de 6 mois (allant de 2 à 15 mois) chez les malades présentant une stabilisation. La survie médiane de l'ensemble de la population a été de 12 mois (allant de 3 à 19 mois). Cette survie médiane a été de 16 mois pour les 5 malades répondeurs (allant de 5 à 19 mois), et de 15 mois pour les malades présentant une stabilisation (allant de 3 à 19 mois).

Parmi les répondeurs, 3 présentaient des métastases pulmonaires seulement et 2 avaient par ailleurs des localisations osseuses.

Le traitement a été dans l'ensemble bien toléré et seul 1 malade a présenté une toxicité hématologique de grade IV OMS (5).

DISCUSSION

Le problème des cancers sans point de départ se pose fréquemment puisqu'il représente 3 à 15 % des malades vus dans les Centres spécialisés (1,6). Les Adénocarcinomes représentent environ la moitié de ces cas (6).

Le traitement de ces malades est dans l'ensemble décevant et l'impact de la chimiothérapie sur la survie parait marginal (6,8,9). Les résultats encourageants obtenus avec le FAM chez ces malades (2) et la potentialisation du Fluorouracile par le Méthotrexate (3,4,7) nous ont conduits à tester cette combinaison dans les Adénocarcinomes à point de départ inconnu.

Le taux de réponse constaté, la durée de la réponse et la survie de l'ensemble de nos malades ne sont pas supérieurs à ceux obtenus avec le FAM seul. Ils sont supérieurs à ceux classiquement rapportés en l'absence de chimiothérapie chez de tels malades (6) et la tolérance de ce protocole de chimiothérapie a été dans l'ensemble satisfaisante. Son efficacité a été par ailleurs au moins égale à celle rapportée dans d'autres études de la littérature (6,8,9).

En conclusion, l'adjonction de Méthotrexate au FAM n'a pas entraîné d'amélioration de la survie dans cette étude, reproduisant seulement les résultats obtenus avec cette combinaison.

REFERENCES

1) Nystrom JC, Weyner JM, Wolf RM. Bateman JR. Viola MV Identifying the primary site in metastatic cancer of unknown origin. JAMA 1979 241; 381-383

2) Goldberg RM, Smith FP, Ueno W, Ahlgren JD, Schein PS 5-Fluorouracil, Adriamycin and Mitomycin (FAM) in the treatement of adenocarcinoma of unknown primary. J. Clin. Oncol. 1986 4, 395 - 399

3) Benz C, and Cadman E : Modulation of 5 -Fluorouracil Metabolism and Cytotoxicity by Anti-metabolite Pretreatment in Human Colorectal Adenocarcinoma HCT -8. Cancer Res.1981-41 : 994-999,

4) Cadman E, Heimer R, and Davis L : Enhanced 5-Fluorouracil Nucleotide Formation After Methotrexate Administration : Explanation for Drug Synergism. Science 1979-205 : 1135-1137,

5) World Health Organisation. WHO Handbook for reporting the results of cancer treatment. Geneva, WHO Offset Publication 1979, N°48,

6) Moertel CG, Reitemeier RJ. Schutt AJ; Hahn QRG : Treatment of the patient with adenocarcinoma of unknown origin. Cancer 1972. 30. 1469-1479

7) Klein HO. Wickramanayake PD. Dieterle F. Mohr R. Oerkermann H. Gross R : High dose Methotrexate/5- Fluorouracil and Adriamycin for gastric cancer. Sem. Oncol. 1983. 10.2 - 29-31.

8) Nelson RB : Chemotherapy of metastatic adenocarcinoma of unknown origin. New Engl. J. Med. 1980, 303, 498.

9) Woods RL. Fox RM. Tattersall MHN. Levi JA. Brodie GN Metastatic adenocarcinomas of unknown primary site. A randomized study of two combination chemotherapy regimens. New Engl. J. Med. 1980, 303, 2, 87-89.

Résumé

The prognosis of patients (pts) with adenocarcinoma of unknown primary is poor, with studies of untreated pts showing a median survival of 3-4 months. The FAM chemotherapy regimen was reported to give 30 % response rate and 10 months median survival in previously untreated patients. Because Methotrexate has been shown to potentiate the activity of 5-FU both in vitro and in vivo, an attempt was made to exploit this synergy by incorporating Methotrexate into the FAM regimen.

Seventeen previously untreated pts (7 M, 10 F ; mean age 47, range 28-72 ; mean performance status 90 % ; range 60-100 %) with measurable adenocarcinoma of unknown primary (as defined by a negative clinical examination except for evidence of metastatic disease) were treated with 2-16 cycles (mean = 7) of Methotrexate 50 mg/m2 day 1, 29 ; 5-FU 600 mg/m2 day 2, 9, 30, 37 ; Doxorubicin 30 mg/m2 day 2, 30 ; Mitomycin 10 mg/m2 day 2 ; all drugs were recycled every 56 days. Five partial remissions (median duration 12 Months, range 2-14) were seen for an overall response rate of 29 %. Nine additional pts had stable disease for a median duration of 6 months (range 2-15).

Median survival for the entire group is 12 months (range 3-19). Toxicities included one grade IV leucopenia and thrombocytopenia but otherwise have been limited to grade I and II myelosuppression, nausea and vomiting, mucositis and alopecia. While accrual and follow-up on this study continue, preliminary results would suggest that the current regimen does not represent a significant improvement over the standard FAM regimen in this group of pts.

Summing-up lectures

Synthèses

Neo-Adjuvant Chemotherapy. Ed. Cl. Jacquillat, M. Weil, D. Khayat. Colloque INSERM/John Libbey Eurotext Ltd. Vol. 169, pp. 993-996.

The summing up lecture

Emil J. Freireich

The University of Texas System Cancer Center, Houston, Texas, 77030, USA

ABSTRACT

Neo-adjuvant chemotherapy is an important new strategy for the control of malignant disease. From a conceptual point of view it is an extremely attractive hypothesis. The notion that chemotherapy can treat micrometastatic disease at the earliest phase in the multimodality treatment of malignancy is in itself appealing. The in-vivo chemotherapy sensitivity assessment, that is, the determination of which chemotherapy is effective in controlling the detectable disease is additional important information for making the proper treatment decisions leading to the best outcome.

For several organ site tumors it is clear that neo-adjuvant therapy has an established role. For many others the data is too immature to be conclusive. Certainly it is a field like its precedent, that is adjuvant chemotherapy that will attract the attention of clinical scientists for many years to come. The organizers of this syposium are to be congratulated for what is undoubtedly a significant international meeting which will advance not only the knowledge of but the application of this important new strategy to cancer treatment.

KEY WORDS

Adjuvant, neo-adjuvant, organ preservation, survival, in vivo chemosensitivity, molecular genetics, biological therapy

Introduction

It is difficult to recall the time in the late 1940's, approximately four decades ago, when the concept that chemotherapy which had been so successful for the control of infectious diseases, malaria, etc., could conceivably be useful for the management of malignant disease. The notion that all of the biochemical and biological functions of tumor cells could also be identified in their counterpart normal cells led to a sense of deep frustration among clinical scientists. During that period only surgery was considered curative. The strategy of early detection and more radical excision was the prevailing clinical biological thought. In the early 1950's the first complete regressions in childhood leukemia and lymphoma raised the hope that chemotherapy might be effective. It was soon recognized by the early 1960's that achieving a complete hematological remission usually resulted in a change in the natural history of the advanced metastatic form of the disease and this knowledge greatly accelerated the interest in chemotherapy. It was not until the mid 1960's, less than 25 years ago that the hypothesis that systemic cancer could be cured with chemotherapy was advocated and it was soon recognized that a list of highly undifferentiated malignancies were associated with proven long term disease free survival. Today approximately 10-15% of patients with advanced metastatic systemic cancer can be cured with chemotherapy. Thus for the advanced metastatic phase of the disease, chemotherapy has become not only a significant therapy, but widely practiced.

Adjuvant Therapy

Once it was recognized that the systemic form of cancer could be cured with chemotherapy, and it was appreciated that most of the patients who achieved complete remission had recurrence of the disease, the biological conception of residual disease below the level of detection was formulated. A new discipline was introduced, adjuvant chemotherapy. Since therapy was proven effective against advanced disease, administration of such therapy to patients with minimal disease might convert patients from palliation to cure. For a large number of tumor diagnoses, adjuvant therapy has now been shown to be of proven value and is an established part of medical practice.

Neo-Adjuvant Chemotherapy

This Second International Congress has moved chemotherapy even further forward in the struggle to control cancer. At the first meeting, much of our intellectual and emotional energy was spent on the appropriateness of the term, neo-adjuvant. We recognized that like many of the terms we use in clinical work, this is also grammatically poor, non-descriptive, and almost certainly the worst possible name we could choose. Yet, I am afraid that I will have to admit that the term is here to stay, just as the term adjuvant is here to stay. It is a bold and important advance in clinical thinking to move chemotherapy to the front line as the primary treatment for patients with locally advanced malignancy. How far we have come in the short period of forty years from a discipline which was restricted to hopelessly ill, far advanced patients, with a treatment that was exclusively for palliation, to an international conference where we discuss chemotherapy as primary treatment for a number of prevalent malignancies. For malignancies which can be cured after failure of local treatment modalities, neo-adjuvant therapy was established early. In the case of acute leukemia where local treatment is rarely effective, neo-adjuvant and adjuvant treatment are well established principles of treatment, similarly for lymphoma and now for choriocarcinoma, testicular neoplasms, etc. But the move to the more frequent malignancies represents a dramatic change in our thinking about the management of disease.

Organ Preservation

During these three days of the Congress, we have heard papers which have dealt exhaustively with breast cancer, bladder cancer and other genitourinary malignancies, soft tissue sarcoma, squamous cancers of the head and neck, gynecological malignancies and even gastrointestinal tumors. The intellectual attractiveness of neo-adjuvant therapy is not only that it offers the potential for converting palliative treatments to curative treatments, but the dramatic evidence of preservation of organ function. The example of laryngeal cancer is striking here. For patients who have sensitivity to chemotherapy, local treatment can be administered to allow equally satisfactory control of the disease and preservation of organ function. There are similar findings in breast, and in the head and neck where local methods of treatment can be particularly disfiguring and disabling. Such preservation of function make cancer treatment not only more effective, but more humane. The preservation of organ function alone provides adequate justification for neo-adjuvant therapy as a science which is here to stay.

Survival

The potential for improving the cure rate and survival exists, but for most of the diagnoses, this remains to be clearly demonstrated. I suspect as with adjuvant therapy we will enter a period where a host of multi-institution, large, patient studies will be conducted to firmly establish the impact of neo-adjuvant therapy on survival. I predict that this will be demonstrated.

In Vivo Chemosensitivity

A major intellectual virtue of neo-adjuvant therapy is the in vivo chemotherapy assessment. There has been an enormous amount of professional time and money spent on developing the in vitro tests for predicting sensitivity to chemotherapeutic agents. All investigators hope that we will be able to have a test the equivalent of antimicrobial in vitro sensitivity for the selection of treatment before administration. Until that day however, neo-adjuvant therapy provides an important tool for the clinical scientist. For patients who respond completely to treatment, staging now includes surgical staging. For patients who have demonstrated in vivo chemosensitivity, the choice for adjuvant therapy is obvious. Of course, the important observations about selection of drug resistant clones will necessitate other strategies for adjuvant treatment such as non-cross-resistant multiple agent combination chemotherapy regimens to consolidate such remissions and hopefully convert them into curative treatments. It is already clear that the in vivo chemotherapy assessment is important for choice of adjuvant treatment.

Molecular Genetics

This clinical strategy is also important for the rapid utilization of the new knowledge of tumor biology. The powerful tool of molecular genetics has revealed the potential for having sophisticated molecular targets for treatment. For at least a few malignancies, the molecular targets are clear. In the case of chronic granulocytic leukemia, for instance, the breakpoint cluster region (BCR) has been cloned, the RNA transcript identified and even the protein product can be measured in vitro. This recombination resulting from a translocation between chromosomes 9 and 22 provides a unique molecular genetic structure that does not exist in normal cells. As emphasized in the opening paragraph, the notion that tumor specific biochemical targets can be found was unlikely forty years ago, today it has been established for many tumors that there are unique genes created by translocations, rearrangements and the insertion of viral macromolecules. Thus the hope for tumor specific targets are clearly available. Moreover it is likely that these unique genes result in gene products which are important in maintaining the biological characteristic of malignancy in the tumor cell. As a result the rearranged gene and the gene products are novel targets for the innovative clinical scientist. The important discovery that the polymerase chain reaction can be used to amplify rearranged genes that are unique to specific tumors represents an extremely promising approach to the problem of detecting minimal residual disease (1). Clearly such molecular genetic techniques should they be shown to be associated with the likelihood of recurrence of the original diagnosis will in themselves become important targets for further therapy.

Biological Therapy

Finally there is the important area of the biological response modifiers. The initial observations of the effect of BCG on disease free duration in a number of common malignancies demonstrated that host factors are important in regulating tumors. Subsequent demonstration that interferon produces substantial palliation and life prolongation in hairy cell leukemia demonstrated that biologicals will almost certainly play a role in the management of malignant disease. We are expectantly awaiting the outcome of clinical trials with interleukin-2 which can stimulate the growth of lymphoid cells in vivo and in vitro and the important description of the LAK cell therapy inducing remission in patients with melanoma and renal cell tumors again offers a bright new opportunity for neo-adjuvant, adjuvant, or the treatment of minimal residual disease.

RESUME

This conference marks an important transition for the discipline of chemotherapy. The science of chemotherapy has moved from a purely palliative treatment to the treatment of choice for newly diagnosed patients with malignancy. As our techniques for the diagnosis of cancer by needle aspiration and by serological testing advances, the importance of chemotherapy as primary treatment for malignancy will almost certainly continue to grow.

REFERENCE

Lee, M-S., Chang, K-S., Cabanillas, F., Freireich, E.J, Trujillo, J.M., and Stass, S.A. (1987): Detection of minimal residual cells carrying the t(14;18) by DNA sequence amplification. Science 237:175-178.

Neo-Adjuvant Chemotherapy. Ed. Cl. Jacquillat, M. Weil, D. Khayat. Colloque INSERM/John Libbey Eurotext Ltd. © 1988. Vol. 169, pp. 997-1001.

Induction chemotherapy. An overview

James F. Holland

Mount Sinai School of Medicine, New-York, NY, USA

Induction chemotherapy embraces the concepts implied in the phrase neo-adjuvant, and provides perspective of its relevance from other prior studies. Regression of the primary tumor, is a clear benefit thereby affecting the techniques of surgery and radiotherapy. Proof is still lacking of its difference from conventional adjuvant chemotherapy with respect to effect on micrometastasis. Organized comparative studies of induction therapy are needed to provide proof of its advantage, at which time the term primary therapy, as suggested by DeVita, will be appropriate. The primary therapist directly influences the patterns of medical care. In part this accounts for the taxonomic, strategic, political and economic importance of the topic.

Key words: Neoadjuvant, Induction chemotherapy, Primary chemotherapy, Chemotherapy.

Neoadjuvant is just as appropriate a term as it was when I was here at the First International Conference. At that time I thought that it was induction chemotherapy, and I still think it is induction chemotherapy, although I am appreciative of Dr. DeVita's term primary chemotherapy. What could induction chemotherapy do for cancer, and why the interest that sustains a conference with multicontinental input?

Induction chemotherapy could make tumors more operable by decreasing the viable cells in the tumor. But it could also make surgeons think the tumor more operable, which is a hazard in itself. It has been pointed out at this meeting that there are instances of failures at the primary site because the initial operative considerations for the tumor have not been respected. Induction chemotherapy could make the primary tumor more radiosensitive by a decrease in the population of tumor cells and by a decrease in the population density, thereby possibly avoiding surgery. But it might also compromise the delivery of a radiocurative dose because of the effects of drugs on the surrounding tissues.

Mutilating surgery might be avoided, with preservation of more nearly normal organ structure and function, because of induction chemotherapy and the substitution of less radical surgery or radiotherapeutic treatments for amputative or radical excisional surgery. Induction chemotherapy tests the candidate drug regimen, albeit in the most expensive way possible, using the human patient as the experimental animal (until we come upon more satisfactory techniques). Induction chemotherapy provides an early assessment of whether the drug regimen is active on the primary tumor and is likely to be active on micrometastases, an assay which is denied to adjuvant chemotherapy given after surgery. Induction chemotherapy also selects the patient that will have complete remission from the chemotherapy, and thus provides effective prognostication. The population that has complete responses contains those that are most effectively and successfully treated. In fact, chemotherapy really exists for and is justified by the patients who get complete remissions. In some diseases partial remissions are clinically meaningful, but they are often therapeutic incompletions.

Some potential pitfalls exist for induction chemotherapy. It might select a naturally resistant clone by killing sensitive clonal cells that themselves serve to impede proliferation of a more virulent subclone of tumor cell through some kind of paracrine effect of cell-cell interactions. Cells remaining in the primary tumor might then be less responsive to treatment. If successful treatment of the primary tumor is not achieved by surgery or radiotherapy, the outcome might be compromised. Induction chemotherapy might impair the potential effect of surgical amputation on the growth rate in micrometastases as described by Simpson-Herron. This has been demonstrated in experimental animals, but is not well established in man. Many of us believe that removal of the primary tumor changes some kind of humoral or cellular message to the micrometastases. Absence of the post excisional growth acceleration in micrometastases might diminish our chances of encountering a cell vulnerable to conventional adjuvant chemotherapy on kinetic grounds. Use of induction chemotherapy can decrease the tolerance for radiotherapy or for extensive surgery. The potential exists for inappropriate compromise radiation dose or for disastrous compromise of the extent of surgery. This could lead to a failure in the primary site because of induction chemotherapy; this could blemish an extremely promising area of research. Early backlash could cost us the opportunity to progress at a steady pace. There is some time loss if the first regimen of chemotherapy used in induction is unsuccessful, and even the possibility of the primary tumor becoming inoperable. It is often easier to give intensive chemotherapy post-operatively to patients who are well nourished and not suffering cachexia or the anatomical distortions of major primary tumors, particularly of the upper aerodigestive tract.

Most importantly, however, induction chemotherapy works. Induction chemotherapy started with vincristine and prednisone. The outlook for a child with acute lymphocytic leukemia is changed when normal function of the marrow is restored, thereby allowing major difference in drug tolerance and effectiveness of cytotoxic agents capable of cure. As was pointed out by Tubiana, chemotherapy prior to radiotherapy in certain instances of Hodgkin's disease significantly augments the impact of both treatments. Rosen made a masterful contribution in pioneering studies with induction chemotherapy for osteosarcoma that allows resection of the affected bone, preserving the limb. The technique has now been enhanced by my colleague at Mount Sinai, Michael Lewis, with his extendable and adjustable prosthesis. Even young children can have endoprostheses which "grow" with them every year, thereby avoiding amputation because of induction chemotherapy and reconstructive orthopedics.

The significant contribution of SOMPS has been to show that the breast can be salvaged as well as the cost of much disease later on, by use of induction chemotherapy and radiation treatment of breast cancer. How can one choose a regimen that is worthy of use in induction? It is not necessary to achieve a complete remission with chemotherapy alone in advanced tumors before adopting a treatment to be the induction chemotherapy to augment curing. The Food and Drug Administration in the United States has found in their papyri that it is necessary to demonstrate increased survival from use of a new cancer drug before it can be approved for marketing. As Dr. DeVita has stressed a number of times, and I completely agree with him, that is not a characteristic of chemotherapy that ought to be required. We made the unhappy experiment once, with Dr. Weil and Dr. Jacquillat, of treating children only with vincristine and prednisone because they were so effective an induction treatment. Even though there is no superior inducing regimen for children at presentation with advanced disease, the children relapsed very rapidly . I think a drug regimen should demonstrate effectiveness on about 40% of patients before being chosen for induction treatment. Forty percent was the level of activity we had seen for adriamycin in patients with advanced osteosarcoma. We were then able to demonstrate that adriamycin is a useful drug in adjuvant treatment of osteosarcoma. Jaffe and Frei saw a similar 40 percent for metastatic disease treated with methotrexate, and it proved efficacious as an adjuvant. Rosen combined these two regimens in adjuvant therapy and attained 70% cures of osteosarcoma in children.

I believe induction chemotherapy, followed by an additional treatment is feasible for most kinds of human cancer. I believe it will likely require a specific trial in each type and stage of cancer with demonstrated effectiveness before this will be accepted. Proponents of regional treatments, who are surgeons and radiotherapists, have had hundreds of years in the case of surgery and nearly 9 decades in radiotherapy, to establish their approach to the primary neoplasm. In properly staged patients, a study of chemotherapy versus no treatment, followed by surgery and/or radiotherapy will be required in at least several diseases to establish that induction chemotherapy is advantageous.

In acute leukemia of children, the people who changed the patterns of care of chemotherapy the most were mothers, not doctors. After reading about progress in the lay press, mothers demanded the most advanced treatment for their children. This often resulted in transfer to university pediatric centers and cancer research institutes. I expect that because of the proper role of the public media, induction chemotherapy will eventually become the primary therapy. As soon as the words "primary therapy" are used, an abundant number of surgeons and radiotherapists are affected by an all important pocketbook issue. The first cancer specialist who sees the patient is in reality the physician who determines the treatment. If we believe that first there should be a complex organization of chemotherapeutic and immunotherapeutic measures, and not of surgical or radiotherapeutic measures, a revolutionary change in the triage of patients will follow. Because of that we need unambiguous proof of the value of induction chemotherapy. In the United States a proof would doubtless shape testimony to the Congress, laying out in economic terms the savings that can be expected. Use of ambulatory induction chemotherapy is a cheap investment, if we thereby avoid metastatic disease with its huge cost in lives and lost potential, not to mention expenditures for patient care. An outcry of negative voices from other diminished medical specialties should be anticipated and should not be underestimated.

The effect of induction chemotherapy on micrometastases must be considered, since the foregoing has been limited almost entirely to the primary tumor. The superior impact of induction chemotherapy on micrometastases, as contrasted to conventional adjuvant treatment remains to be demonstrated. Studies remain to be conducted in which the chemotherapy is given before or after the local treatment. The great advantage, for example, of the Rosen technique in osteosarcoma or of the SOMPS technique in breast cancer is that the care of the primary tumor has been changed. It has not as yet been proved that they are better in their impact on the micrometastases than conventional adjuvant chemotherapy with the same regimens.

There are pitfalls along the way. Some cancer-bearing lymph nodes will, in all probability be sterilized by the chemotherapy that is used. There will doubtless be lawsuits and professional battles over the true staging of such down-staged patients and whether they were needlessly overtreated.

Although induction chemotherapy may be useful for node-negative patients, even more useful than for others, politically and strategically that is not the place to start. The strategy will be for trial in T3 and T4 tumors, usually with N_+ metastases although they are likely to provide the poorest results. Patients with T3 and T4 tumors, particularly those with head and neck cancer, are immuno-depressed, nutritionally impaired and have anatomical deformities that may constitute predilections to infection. Another pitfall is that some patients can be self-deluded into thinking their treatment has been so miraculous they need not go through with an agreed-upon operation. They will relapse rapidly. Surgeons will not excuse the oncologist involved in such an episode of failure for having let the patient escape. Medical therapies require patient compliance for a much longer time than does surgical therapy.

There are promises on the present horizon which are more dramatic than any we have so far experienced. One is a flower of one of the seminal studies that Freireich conducted in acute leukemia, demonstrating for the first time that a drug could have activity in patients already in complete remission. We have now demonstrated that a second combination of drugs has activity in the adjuvant treatment of breast cancer. Patients without clinically evident disease have a significantly longer disease-free interval and survival when treated with CMFVP followed by VATH compared to those treated throughout with CMFVP alone. We are also exploring, at the clinical level, combinations of interleukin-2 with chemo-therapy. In some diseases we have seen dramatic augmentation of effectiveness. The same phenomenon for interferon and chemotherapy has been seen in experimental systems. After the principle is established that chemoimmunotherapy is active as induction therapy, comparative studies will follow to determine if it is more active than chemotherapy alone.

The colony stimulating factors, the recombinant hematopoietins, will make therapy easier and safer. The oncologist will not be forgiven for a patient who dies of septicemia from chemotherapy-induced granulocytopenia prior to treatment of the primary disease. Even though the overall mortality of the treated group might be less death related to induction chemotherapy it will be unacceptable to everyone in our culture where surgery and radiotherapy are so well established as primary therapy.

Hryniuk has reported, from incisive analyses of the literature, that the intensity of drug dosing in chemotherapy regimens for breast cancer, and for ovarian cancer, is the most critical determinant of outcome. DeVita has extended this concept to the lymphomas. It is necessary to change our concepts, providing we exclude lethal toxicity, from treating at an acceptable drug level for the patient, to treating at an unacceptable drug level for the tumor. To accomplish this I believe there will be considerably greater modulation of chemotherapy: e.g. tetrahydrofolate cofactors on the activity of fluorouracil, interferons, and interleukin-2. Averbuch has reported an extraordinarily interesting molecule, an oxomorpholinyl dimer that modulates the toxicity of adriamycin.

It is incumbent upon us to recognize that there are types of chemotherapy and ways of administering it that will make it easier to give to patients. It appears sensible, and very probably better, to give chemotherapy to patients before they are involved in other kinds of local treatment. To get those points accepted, a somewhat different grand strategy is needed than is evident at this congress. It is disappointing to find at this meeting literally scores of approaches with tens of chemotherapeutic regimens, but little definitive data. Had the same resources and the same commitment been allied behind some of the original leaders and proponents of these concepts, we might have demonstrated, in tight designs with well-staged cancers in randomized controlled trials, evidence that would persuade surgeons and radiotherapists the world over that this is the proper approach. Many fewer studies, properly designed, and applied to hundreds of patients in many places will prove the worth of induction chemotherapy faster than the present array of uncontrolled tiny trials. Such a strategy will advance us down the road to where Jacquillat and Weil and Khayat have been taking us in this elegant neoadjuvant symposium. When we prove that induction chemotherapy or chemoimmunotherapy should be the first treatment, DeVita's statement should obtain that we call it primary therapy. But premature nomination as primary therapy challenges a powerful segment of today's medical establishment, with a predictable counter reaction. Everyone who has in his youth been something of a revolutionary, as Freireich and I can remember, realizes that revolutions don't always succeed. The old adage stipulates "If you can't lick 'em, jine 'em." Perhaps we should join them and help to guide them in the right direction.

Author Index
Index des auteurs

Colloques INSERM
ISSN 0768-3154

Other *Colloques* published as co-editions by John Libbey Eurotext and INSERM

133 Cardiovascular and Respiratory Physiology in the Fetus and Neonate. *Physiologie Cardiovasculaire et Respiratoire du Fœtus et du Nouveau-né.*
Scientific Committee : P. Karlberg, A. Minkowski, W. Oh and L. Stern;
Managing Editor : M. Monset-Couchard.
ISBN : John Libbey Eurotext 0 86196 125 0
INSERM 2 85598 340 1

134 Porphyrins and Porphyrias. *Porphyrines et Porphyries.*
Edited by Y. Nordmann.
ISBN : John Libbey Eurotext 0 86196 087 4
INSERM 2 85598 281 2

137 Neo-Adjuvant Chemotherapy. *Chimiothérapie Néo-Adjuvante.*
Edited by C. Jacquillat, M. Weil and D. Khayat.
ISBN : John Libbey Eurotext 0 86196 125 0
INSERM 2 85598 340 1

139 Hormones and Cell Regulation (10th European Symposium). *Hormones et Régulation Cellulaire (10e Symposium Européen).*
Edited by J. Nunez, J.E. Dumont and R. J.B. King.
ISBN : John Libbey Eurotext 0 86196 125 0X
INSERM 2 85598 340 1

147 Modern Trends in Aging Research. *Nouvelles Perspectives de la Recherche sur le Vieillissement.*
Edited by Y. Courtois, B. Faucheux, B. Forette, D.L. Knook and J.A. Tréton.
ISBN : John Libbey Eurotext 0 86196 125 0X
INSERM 2 85598 340 1

149 Binding Proteins of Steroid Hormones. *Protéines de liaison des Hormones Stéroïdes.*
Edited by M.G. Forest and M. Pugeat.
ISBN : John Libbey Eurotext 0 86196 125 0
INSERM 2 85598 340 1X

151 Control and Management of Parturition. *La Maîtrise de la Parturition.*
Edited by C. Sureau, P. Blot, D. Cabrol, F. Cavaillé and G. Germain.
ISBN : John Libbey Eurotext 0 86196 125 0
INSERM 2 85598 340 1

153 Hormones and Cell Regulation (11th European Symposium). *Hormones et Régulation Cellulaire (11e Symposium Européen).*
Edited by J. Nunez and J.E. Dumont
ISBN : John Libbey Eurotext 0 86196 104 8
INSERM 2 85598 324 X

158 Biochemistry and Physiopathology of Platelet Membrane. *Biochimie et Physiopathologie de la Membrane Plaquettaire.*
Edited by G. Marguerie and R.F.A.A. Zwaal.
ISBN : John Libbey Eurotext 0 86196 114 5
INSERM 2 85598 345 2

162 The Inhibitors of Hematopoiesis. *Les Inhibiteurs de l'Hématopoïèse.*
Edited by A. Najman, M. Guigon, N.-C. Gorin, and J.-Y. Mary
ISBN : John Libbey Eurotext 0 86196 125 0
INSERM 2 85598 340 1

164 Liver Cells and Drugs. *Cellules Hépatiques et Médicaments.*
Edited by A. Guillouzo
ISBN : John Libbey Eurotext 0 86196 128 5
INSERM 2 85598 341 X

165 Hormones and Cell Regulation (12th European Symposium). *Hormones et Régulation Cellulaire (12e Symposium Européen).*
Edited by J. Nunez, J.E. Dumont and E. Carafoli
ISBN : John Libbey Eurotext 0 86196 133 1
INSERM 2 85598 347 9

167 Sleep Disorders and Respiration. *Les Evénements Respiratoires du Sommeil.*
Edited by P. Lévi-Valensi and D. Duron
ISBN : John Libbey Eurotext 0 86196 127 7
INSERM 2 85598 344 4

171 Structure and Functions of the Cytoskeleton. *Structure et Fonctions du Cytosquelette.*
Edited by B.A.F. Rousset
ISBN : John Libbey Eurotext 0 86 196 149 8
INSERM 2 85598 351 7

172 The Langerhans Cell. *La Cellule de Langerhans.*
Edited by J. Thivolet and D. Schmitt
ISBN : John Libbey Eurotext 0 86 196 181 1
INSERM 2 85598 352 5

IMPRIMERIE LOUIS-JEAN
Publications scientifiques et littéraires
05002 GAP — Tél. : 92.51.35.23
Dépôt légal : 690 — Novembre 1988